SATALOFF'S COMPREHENSIVE TEXTBOOK OF OTOLARYNGOLOGY HEAD AND NECK SURGERY

Series Editor: **Robert T Sataloff** MD DMA FACS

OTOLOGY/NEUROTOLOGY/ SKULL BASE SURGERY

SATALOFF'S COMPREHENSIVE TEXTBOOK OF OTOLARYNGOLOGY HEAD AND NECK SURGERY

Series Editor: **Robert T Sataloff** MD DMA FACS

OTOLOGY/NEUROTOLOGY/ SKULL BASE SURGERY

Vol. 1

Volume Editor

Anil K Lalwani MD
Professor and Vice Chair for Research
Director, Division of Otology, Neurotology and Skull Base Surgery
Director, Columbia Cochlear Implant Program
Department of Otolaryngology—Head and Neck Surgery
Columbia University College of Physicians and Surgeons
New York, New York, USA

JAYPEE *The Health Sciences Publisher*
New Delhi | London | Philadelphia | Panama

Jaypee Brothers Medical Publishers (P) Ltd

Headquarters
Jaypee Brothers Medical Publishers (P) Ltd.
4838/24, Ansari Road, Daryaganj
New Delhi 110 002, India
Phone: +91-11-43574357
Fax: +91-11-43574314
E-mail: jaypee@jaypeebrothers.com

Overseas Offices
J.P. Medical Ltd.
83, Victoria Street, London
SW1H 0HW (UK)
Phone: +44-20 3170 8910
Fax: +44(0)20 3008 6180
E-mail: info@jpmedpub.com

Jaypee-Highlights Medical Publishers Inc.
City of Knowledge, Bld. 237, Clayton
Panama City, Panama
Phone: +1 507-301-0496
Fax: +1 507-301-0499
E-mail: cservice@jphmedical.com

Jaypee Medical Inc.
The Bourse
111 South Independence Mall East
Suite 835, Philadelphia, PA 19106, USA
Phone: +1 267-519-9789
E-mail: jpmed.us@gmail.com

Jaypee Brothers Medical Publishers (P) Ltd.
17/1-B, Babar Road, Block-B, Shaymali
Mohammadpur, Dhaka-1207
Bangladesh
Mobile: +08801912003485
E-mail: jaypeedhaka@gmail.com

Jaypee Brothers Medical Publishers (P) Ltd.
Bhotahity, Kathmandu, Nepal
Phone: +977-9741283608
E-mail: kathmandu@jaypeebrothers.com

Website: www.jaypeebrothers.com
Website: www.jaypeedigital.com

Inquiries for bulk sales may be solicited at: jaypee@jaypeebrothers.com

Sataloff's Comprehensive Textbook of Otolaryngology: Head and Neck Surgery: Otology/Neurotology/Skull Base Surgery (Vol. 1)

First Edition: **2016**

ISBN: 978-93-5152-455-7

Printed at Replika Press Pvt. Ltd.

Contributors

Robert A Adamson MD
Assistant Professor
School of Biomedical Engineering
Dalhousie University
Halifax, Nova Scotia, Canada

Sumit K Agrawal MD FRCSC
Associate Professor
Department of Otolaryngology—
Head and Neck Surgery
Western University
London, Ontario, Canada

Yuri Agrawal MD
Assistant Professor
Department of Otolaryngology—
Head and Neck Surgery
Johns Hopkins University
School of Medicine
Baltimore, Maryland, USA

Art Ambrosio MD
Head and Neck Surgeon at Marine Corps
Base Camp Lejeune
Jacksonville, North Carolina, USA

Simon I Angeli MD
Professor
Department of Otolaryngology
University of Miami
Miami, Florida, USA

Maris Appelbaum AuD
Clinical Preceptor
Department of Communication
Sciences and Disorders
Montclair State University
Montclair, New Jersey, USA

H Alexander Arts MD FACS
Professor of Otolaryngology
University of Michigan
Ann Arbor, Michigan, USA

Manohar Bance MB MSc FRCSC
Professor and Head
Division of Otolaryngology—
Head and Neck Surgery
Department of Surgery
Dalhousie University
Halifax, Nova Scotia, Canada

Gregory J Basura MD
Assistant Professor
Department of Otolaryngology—
Head and Neck Surgery
Kresge Hearing Research Institute
Ann Arbor, Michigan, USA

Carol Bauer MD
Professor/Chair
Department of Surgery
Division of Otolaryngology
Southern Illinois University
School of Medicine
Springfield, Illinois, USA

Joan M Besing PhD CCC-A
Professor
Department of Communication
Sciences and Disorders
Montclair State University
Montclair, New Jersey, USA

Jason A Beyea MD PhD FRCSC
Fellow
Department of Otolaryngology—
Head and Neck Surgery
The Ohio State University
Columbus, Ohio, USA

Dennis I Bojrab MD
CEO and Director of Research
Michigan Ear Institute
Director of Skull Base Surgery
Providence Hospital and
Medical Centers
Clinical Professor
Wayne State University
Farmington Hills, Michigan, USA

Derald E Brackmann MD
Clinical Professor of Otolaryngology—
Head and Neck Surgery and
Neurological Surgery
University of Southern California
School of Medicine
Associate
House Ear Clinic
Board of Directors
House Ear Institute
Los Angeles, California, USA

Kevin D Brown MD PhD
Associate Professor
Department of Otolaryngology—
Head and Neck Surgery
University of North Carolina at Chapel
Hill School of Medicine
Chapel Hill, North Carolina, USA

Roxanne Cano MD
University of Texas Medical School
Houston, Texas, USA

Divya Chari MD
Resident
University of California, San Francisco
San Francisco, California, USA

Daniel H Coelho MD FACS
G Douglas Hayden Associate Professor
Department of Otolaryngology—
Head and Neck Surgery
Virginia Commonwealth
School of Medicine
Richmond, Virginia, USA

C Eduardo Corrales MD
Brigham and Women's Instructor
Associate Surgeon
Department of Surgery
Harvard Medical School
Assistant Professor
Department of Otolaryngology
Massachusetts Eye and Ear Infirmary
Harvard Medical School
Boston, Massachusetts, USA

Maura K Cosetti MD
Assistant Professor
Departments of Otolaryngology—
Head and Neck Surgery and
Neurosurgery
Louisiana State University
Health Sciences Center—Shreveport
Shreveport, Louisiana, USA

Ryan A Crane MD
Resident Physician
Department of Otolaryngology—
Head and Neck Surgery
University of Cincinnati Medical Center
Cincinnati, Ohio, USA

Karen Jo Doyle MD PhD
Professor
Otology and Neurotology
University of California
Davis Health System
Department of Otolaryngology
Sacramento, California, USA

Robert W Eppsteiner MD
University of Massachusetts
Medical School
Worcester, Massachusetts, USA

Deema Fattal MD
Associate Professor
Director of Balance Disorders Clinic
Department of Neurology
University of Iowa
Iowa City, Iowa, USA

Alexander Filatov MD
Department of Radiology
Stony Brook University
Stony Brook, New York, USA

Richard A Goldman MD
Assistant Professor
Department of Otolaryngology—
Head and Neck Surgery
University of Kentucky
College of Medicine
Lexington, Kentucky, USA

Sachin Gupta MD
Neurotology Fellow
Department of Otolaryngology—
Head and Neck Surgery, University of
Texas—Southwestern Medical Center
Dallas, Texas, USA

Mari Hagiwara MD
Assistant Professor
Department of Radiology
New York University, School of Medicine
New York, New York, USA

Marlan R Hansen MD FACS
Professor
Departments of Otolaryngology—
Head and Neck Surgery and
Neurosurgery, University of Iowa
Iowa City, Iowa, USA

Mary J Hawkshaw BSN RN CORLN
Research Associate Professor
Department of Otolaryngology
Drexel College of Medicine
Philadelphia, Pennsylvania, USA

Selena E Heman-Ackah MD MBA
Director of Otology
Neurotology, and Audiology
Division of Otolaryngology
Beth Israel Deaconess Medical Center
Harvard Medical School
Boston, Massachusetts, USA

Michael E Hoffer MD
Otolaryngology
University of Miami Health System
Miami, Florida, USA

Brandon Isaacson MD FACS
Associate Professor
Department of Otolaryngology—
Head and Neck Surgery
University of Texas—
Southwestern Medical Center
Dallas, Texas, USA

Daniel Jethanamest MD
Assistant Professor
Department of Otolaryngology
New York University School of Medicine
New York, New York, USA

Steven K Juhn MD
Department of Otolaryngology—
Head and Neck Surgery
University of Minnesota
Minneapolis, Minnesota, USA

Robert W Jyung MD
Associate Professor
Department of Otolaryngology—
Head and Neck Surgery
Rutgers New Jersey Medical School
Newark, New Jersey, USA

Ruwan Kiringoda MD
Resident Physician
Otolaryngology—Head and Neck Surgery
University of California, San Francisco
San Francisco, California, USA

Ilkka Kivekäs MD PhD
Assistant Professor in Otolaryngology
Tampere University Hospital and
the University of Tampere
Tampere, Finland

Janet Koehnke PhD
Professor and Chair
Department of Communication
Sciences and Disorders
Montclair State University
Montclair, New Jersey, USA

Anil K Lalwani MD
Professor and Vice Chair for Research
Director
Division of Otology
Neurotology and Skull Base Surgery
Director
Columbia Cochlear Implant Program
Department of Otolaryngology—
Head and Neck Surgery
Columbia University College of
Physicians and Surgeons
New York, New York, USA

Lawrence R Lustig MD
Howard W Smith Professor and Chair
Department of Otolaryngology—
Head and Neck Surgery
Columbia University
Medical Center and New York
Presbyterian Hospital
New York, New York, USA

Dean M Mancuso AuD
Assistant Professor of Audiology
Department of Otolaryngology—
Head and Neck Surgery
Columbia University Medical Center
New York, New York, USA

Peter L Santa Maria MBBS PhD
Instructor
Department of Otolaryngology—
Head and Neck Surgery
Stanford University
Stanford, California, USA

Adam N Master MD
Resident Physician
Department of Otolaryngology—
Head and Neck Surgery
Louisiana State University
Health Science Center Shreveport
Shreveport, Louisiana, USA

Michael J McKenna MD
Director
Division of Otology and Neurotology
Massachusetts Eye and Ear
Boston, Massachusetts, USA

Sean O McMenomey MD
Professor of Otolaryngology and
Neurosurgery—Vice Chair
Department of Otolaryngology
New York University
Langone Medical Center
New York, New York, USA

Cliff A Megerian MD FACS
Julius W McCall
Professor and Chairman
Otolaryngology—Head and Neck Surgery
Case Western Reserve University
School of Medicine
Richard W and Patricia R
Pogue Endowed Chair
Director Ear, Nose and Throat Institute
University Hospitals Case Medical Center
Cleveland, Ohio, USA

Myles Melton
Medical Student
Weill Cornell Medical College
New York, New York, USA

Ted A Meyer MD PhD
Associate Professor
Department of Otolaryngology—
Head and Neck Surgery
Medical University of South Carolina
Charleston, South Carolina, USA

Alan G Micco MD FACS
Associate Professor
Department of Otolaryngology
Northwestern University
Feinberg School of Medicine
Chicago, Illinois, USA

Faith M Mogila ScD
Clinical Preceptor
Department of Communication
Sciences and Disorders
Montclair State University
Montclair, New Jersey, USA

Joseph J Montano EdD
Associate Professor of Audiology
Department of Otolaryngology
Weill Cornell Medical College
New York, New York, USA

Marc-Elie Nader MD
Assistant Professor
Department of Otolaryngology
University of Montreal
Montreal, Quebec, Canada

John K Niparko MD
Professor and Chair
Department of Otolaryngology—
Head and Neck Surgery
Keck School of Medicine of
University of Southern California
Los Angeles, California, USA

John S Oghalai MD
Associate Professor
Department of Otolaryngology—
Head and Neck Surgery
Stanford University
Stanford, California, USA

Steven R Otto
Chief Audiologist and Coordinator
Auditory Brainstem Implant
Program House Clinic
Los Angeles, California, USA

Lorne S Parnes MD FRCSC
Professor
Departments of Otolaryngology—
Head and Neck Surgery and
Clinical Neurological Sciences
Western University
London, Ontario, Canada

Dennis Poe MD PhD
Associate Professor in Otolaryngology
Boston Children's Hospital
Boston, Massachusetts, USA

Alicia M Quesnel MD
Instructor
Department of Otology and Laryngology
Harvard Medical School
Attending Surgeon
Department of Otolaryngology
Massachusetts Eye and Ear Infirmary
Boston, Massachusetts, USA

Habib Rizk MD
Neurotology Fellow
Otolaryngology Head and Neck Surgery
Medical University of South Carolina
Charleston, South Carolina, USA

Amy L Rutt DO
Assistant Professor
Department of Otolaryngology—
Head and Neck Surgery
Mayo Clinic
Rochester, Minnesota, USA

Robert T Sataloff MD
Professor and Chairman
Department of Otolaryngology—
Head and Neck Surgery
Senior Associate
Dean for Clinical
Academic Specialties
Drexel University College of Medicine
Philadelphia, Pennsylvania, USA

David A Schessel PhD MD
Associate Professor
Department of Surgery
Stony Brook University
Stony Brook, New York, USA

Marc S Schwartz MD
Neurological Surgery
House Ear Clinic
Los Angeles, California, USA

Samuel H Selesnick MD FACS
Professor and Vice-Chairman
Department of Otolaryngology—
Head and Neck Surgery
Weill Cornell Medical College
New York, New York, USA

Maroun T Semaan MD
Associate Professor
Ear Nose and Throat Institute
University Hospitals
Case Medical Center
Case Western Reserve University
Cleveland, Ohio, USA

J Caleb Simmons MD
Baylor College of Medicine
Houston, Texas, USA

Eric E Smouha MD
Associate Professor
Department of Otolaryngology—
Head and Neck Surgery
Icahn School of Medicine at
Mount Sinai
New York, New York, USA

Jaclyn B Spitzer PhD
Professor
Department of Otolaryngology—
Head and Neck Surgery
Columbia University
New York, New York, USA

Shawn M Stevens MD
Resident Surgeon
Department of Otolaryngology—
Head and Neck Surgery
Medical University of
South Carolina
Charleston, South Carolina, USA

Emily Z Stucken MD
Michigan Ear Institute
Farmington, Hills, Michigan, USA

Daniel Q Sun MD
Radiation Oncology Healthcare
Towson, Maryland, USA

Maja Svrakic MD
Bellevue Hospital—Otolaryngology
New York, New York, USA

Alex D Sweeney MD
Department of Otolaryngology—
Head and Neck Surgery
Vanderbilt University
Nashville, Tennessee, USA

Monica Tadros MD FACS
Assistant Professor of Otolaryngology—
Head and Neck Surgery
Director of Facial Plastic and
Reconstructive Surgery
Columbia University Medical Center
New York, New York, USA

Elizabeth H Toh MD FACS
Department of Otolaryngology—
Head and Neck Surgery
Lahey Hospital and Medical Center
Burlington, Massachusetts, USA

Andrea Vambutas MD FACS
Professor of Otolaryngology and
Molecular Medicine
Hofstra North Shore—
LIJ School of Medicine
New Hyde Park, New York, USA

Alejandro Vázquez MD
Resident
Department of Otolaryngology—
Head and Neck Surgery
Rutgers New Jersey Medical School
Newark, New Jersey, USA

Jeffrey T Vrabec MD
Professor of Otolaryngology—
Head and Neck Surgery
Baylor College of Medicine
Houston, Texas, USA

Cameron C Wick MD
Resident
Department of Otolaryngology—
Head and Neck Surgery
Case Western Reserve University
School of Medicine
Cleveland, Ohio, USA

Brent Wilkerson MD
Resident
Department of Otolaryngology
University of California
Davis Health System
Sacramento, California, USA

Eric P Wilkinson MD
Surgeon and Partner, House Clinic
Los Angeles, California, USA

Robert A Williamson MD
Assistant Professor of Otolaryngology—
Head and Neck Surgery
Baylor College of Medicine
Houston, Texas, USA

Justin D Wilson AuD
Mayo Clinic Health System
LaCrosse, Wisconsin, USA

Qiu Zhong MD
Resident
Department of Otolaryngology
Northwestern University
Feinberg School of Medicine
Chicago, Illinois, USA

Foreword

Sataloff's Comprehensive Textbook of Otolaryngology: Head and Neck Surgery is a component of the most extensive compilation of information in otolaryngology—head and neck surgery to date. The six volumes of the comprehensive textbook are part of a 12-volume, encyclopedic compendium that also includes a six-volume set of detailed, extensively illustrated atlases of otolaryngologic surgical techniques. The vision for the *Comprehensive Textbook* was realized with the invaluable, expert collaboration of eight world-class volume editors. Chapter authors include many of the most prominent otolaryngologists in the world, and coverage of each subspecialty is extensive, detailed and scholarly.

Anil K Lalwani, MD edited the volume on otology/neurotology/skull base surgery. Like all six of the volumes in the *Comprehensive Textbook*, the otology/neurotology/skull base surgery volume is designed not only as part of the multivolume book, but also to stand alone or in combination with the atlas of otological surgery. Dr Lalwani's volume covers anatomy and physiology of hearing and balance, temporal bone radiology, medical and surgical treatment of common and rare disorders of the ear and related structures, occupational hearing loss, aural rehabilitation, cochlear and brainstem implantation, disorders of the facial nerve, and other topics. Each chapter is not only replete with the latest scientific information, but also accessible and practical for clinicians.

The rhinology/allergy and immunology volume by Marvin P Fried and Abtin Tabaee is the most elegant and inclusive book on the topic to date. Drs Fried and Tabaee start with a history of rhinology beginning in ancient times. The chapters on evolution of the nose and sinuses, embryology, sinonasal anatomy and physiology, and rhinological assessment are exceptional. The volume includes discussions of virtually all sinonasal disorders and allergy, including not only traditional medical and surgical therapy but also complementary and integrative medicine. The information is state-of-the-art.

Anthony P Sclafani's volume on facial plastic and reconstructive surgery is unique in its thoroughness and practicality. The volume covers skin anatomy and physiology, principles of wound healing, physiology of grafts and flaps, lasers in facial plastic surgery, aesthetic analysis of the face and other basic topics. There are extensive discussions on essentially all problems and procedures in facial plastic and reconstructive surgery contributed by many of the most respected experts in the field. The volume includes not only cosmetic and reconstructive surgery, but also information on diagnosis and treatment of facial trauma.

The volume on laryngology edited by Dr Michael S Benninger incorporates the most current information on virtually every aspect of laryngology. The authors constitute a who's who of world experts in voice and swallowing. After extensive and practical discussions of science and genetics, the volume reviews diagnosis and treatment (traditional and complementary) of laryngological disorders. Chapters on laser physics and use, voice therapy, laryngeal dystonia, cough, vocal aging and many other topics provide invaluable "pearls" for clinicians. The volume also includes extensive discussion of surgery for airway disorders, office-based laryngeal surgery, laryngeal transplantation and other topics.

For the volume on head and neck surgery, Drs Patrick J Gullane and David P Goldstein have recruited an extraordinary group of contributors who have compiled the latest information on molecular biology of head and neck cancer, principles of radiation, immunobiology, medical oncology, common and rare head and neck malignancies, endocrine neoplasms, lymphoma, deep neck space infections and other maladies. The surgical discussions are thorough and richly illustrated, and they include definitive discussions of free flap surgery, facial transplantation and other subjects.

Dr Christopher J Hartnick's vision for the volume on pediatric otolaryngology was expansive, elegantly scholarly and invaluable clinically. The volume begins with information on embryology, anatomy, genetics, syndromes and other complex topics. Dr Hartnick's contributors include basic discussions of otolaryngologic examination in a pediatric patient, imaging, hearing screening and aural rehabilitation, and diagnosis and treatment of diseases of the ear, nose, larynx, oral cavity, neck and airway. Congenital, syndromic and acquired disorders are covered in detail, as are special, particularly vexing problems such as chronic cough in pediatric patients, breathing and obstructive sleep apnea in children, pediatric voice disorders, and many other subjects. This volume will be invaluable to any otolaryngologist who treats children.

All of us who have been involved with the creation of the six-volume *Sataloff's Comprehensive Textbook of Otolaryngology: Head and Neck Surgery* and its companion six-volume set of surgical atlases hope and believe that our colleagues will find this new offering to be not only the most extensive and convenient compilation of information in our field, but also the most clinically practical and up-to-date resource in otolaryngology. We are indebted to Mr Jitendar P Vij (Group Chairman) and Mr Ankit Vij (Group President) of M/s Jaypee Brothers Medical Publishers (P) Ltd., New Delhi, India, for their commitment to this project, and for their promise to keep this work available not only online but also in print. We are indebted also to the many otolaryngologists who have contributed to this work not only by editing volumes and writing chapters, but also by asking questions that inspired many of us to seek the answers found on these pages. We also thank especially the great academic otolaryngologists who trained us and inspired us to spend our nights, weekends and vacations writing chapters and books. We hope that our colleagues and their patients find this book useful.

Robert T Sataloff MD DMA FACS
Professor and Chairman
Department of Otolaryngology—Head and Neck Surgery
Senior Associate Dean for Clinical Academic Specialties
Drexel University College of Medicine
Philadelphia, Pennsylvania, USA

Preface

Though a subspecialty within otolaryngology—head and neck surgery, otology/neurotology/skull base surgery is as diverse as the field of medicine itself. And like medicine, it enthralls those who pursue it—whether as a generalist or a specialist. This textbook endeavors to capture the dynamic nature of otology/neurotology/skull base surgery in its pages while providing a broad foundation in its basic and clinical sciences. Written by experts, the chapters encompass the basics such as anatomy and physiology of hearing loss, vestibular dysfunction, facial nerve disorders, and skull base tumors. Radiology has its own chapter, and disease-specific imaging is reviewed in all relevant chapters. Building upon the basics, cutting-edge topics such as cochlear implantation, auditory brainstem implants, and implantable hearing aids are thoroughly covered in their own chapters. Ultimately, this textbook is distinguished by the expertise of its contributors—all leaders in otology/neurotology/skull base surgery. It is the reader who will benefit from absorbing their experience as articulated in this wonderful textbook.

Anil K Lalwani MD

Acknowledgments

The editor would like to thank Joseph Rusko, Marco Ulloa, Carol Rogers Field, Bridget Meyer, Thomas Gibbons and the rest of the Jaypee Brothers team. Without their perseverance and hard work, this volume would not have been possible. Special thanks are offered to the authors, who have shared their expertise and experience in order to improve the care of the otology/neurotology/skull base surgery patients.

I would also like to thank Mr Jitendar P Vij (Group Chairman), Mr Ankit Vij (Group President), Ms Chetna Malhotra Vohra (Associate Director), Mr Umar Rashid (Development Editor) and Production team of Jaypee Brothers Medical Publishers (P) Ltd., New Delhi, India.

Contents

Video Legend

Video 28.1: Transmastoid superior semicircular canal occlusion.

CHAPTER

1

Anatomy and Physiology of the Auditory System

Peter L Santa Maria, John S Oghalai

PINNA (AURICLE)

The pinna is composed of fibroelastic cartilage covered by skin. This cartilage is continuous with that of the external auditory canal (EAC). Anteriorly the cartilage is adherent to the skin, but posteriorly there is a loose areolar layer in between. The dimensions of characteristics of the pinna include (Fig. 1.1)[1,2] a height of 5-6 cm, width 55% of height, forms an angle that is 20° from the vertical plane, has an auricle that diverges from the occipital scalp at 21°–30°, forms an angle of < 90° at the conchal bowl to the mastoid and has a distance of 1–2 cm from the helical rim to the mastoid.

Clinical comment

- An end aural incision is placed between a fibrous band between the tragus and the crus helices where the cartilage is absent.

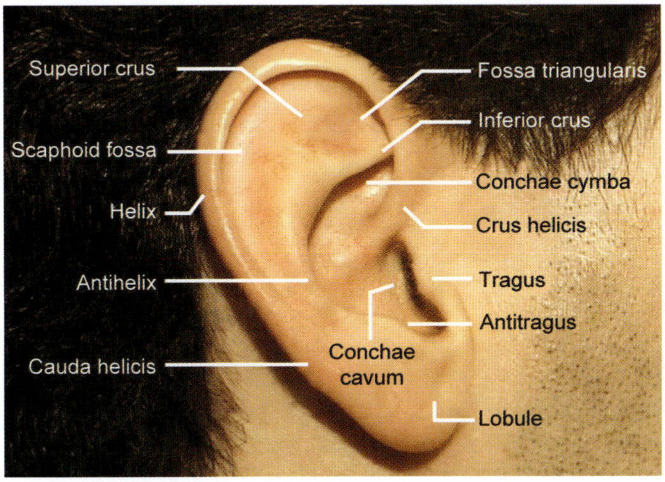

Fig. 1.1: The anatomical landmarks of the pinna.

There are two intrinsic and three extrinsic ligaments. There are six intrinsic and six extrinsic muscles. The major intrinsic ligaments attach from the crus helicis to the tragus and from the antihelix to the cauda helicis. The extrinsic ligaments are named anterior (from the tragus to the crus of helicis to the zygoma), superior (from the spine of the helix to the superior EAC), posterior medial (from the concha to the mastoid prominence). The muscles are divided into intrinsic (helix major, helix minor, tragus, antitragus, transverse, oblique) and extrinsic (auricularis posterior, auricularis superior, auricularis anterior).

The pinna and mastoid scalp area are supplied by branches of the external carotid artery (Fig. 1.2). Veins also accompany the named arteries. The postauricular artery[3] supplies the posterior surface of the pinna, except the lobule and the mastoid scalp. It has auricular, mastoid, transverse nuchal artery[4] branches. The occipital artery[5] supplies part of the mastoid scalp (via a lateral branch) and has a medial and a lateral branch. The superficial temporal artery[6] supplies the anterior pinna, the temporal scalp, and the superficial temporalis fascia. Its branches are[7] anterior (or superior), the temporal artery (via the main trunk or parietal branch), parietal, temporal, and middle temporal (Fig. 1.3).

The pinna is formed from the sixth gestational week from the six hillocks of His that originate from the first and second branchial arches (Fig. 1.1). It is completely formed by week 16. It reaches adult size by age five. Hillocks one to three are supplied by the auriculotemporal nerve and hillocks four to six are supplied by a branch from facial nerve, greater auricular and lesser occipital nerves (Figs. 1.4A and B).[8,9]

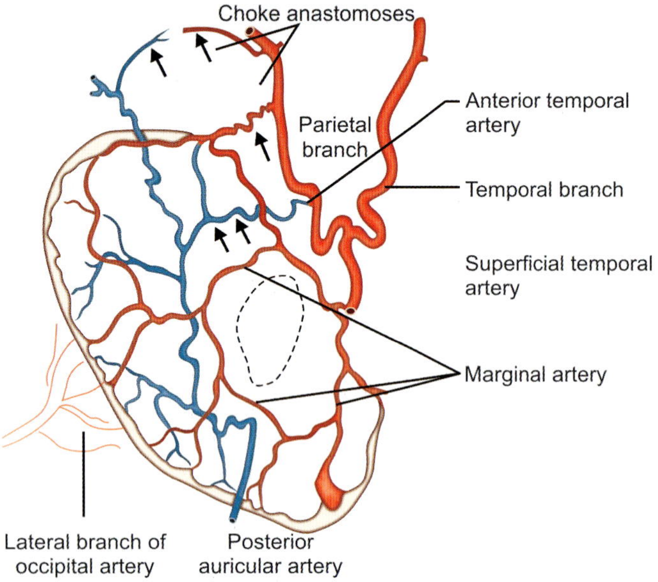

Fig. 1.2: The arterial supply of the pinna and mastoid region. *Source*: Adapted from Imanishi and Nakajima[3] and Alvernia et al.[5]

The external ear is important for sound localization.[10] The folds and crevices that create the shape of the pinna facilitate sound localization in vertical space. This design provides a 10 kHz dip with elevation of sound. In contrast, sound localization in horizontal space is provided by three mechanisms. The resonance gain of the near ear provides the gain of the ear closest to the sound. The head shadow effect attenuates frequencies <2 kHz so that there is a 5–15 dB interaural difference. There is an interaural time difference of 0.6 ms between sounds that is detected within the ascending brainstem nuclei.

EXTERNAL AUDITORY CANAL

The EAC is composed of cartilage in its lateral third (8 mm) and bone in its medial two thirds (16 mm). The cartilaginous EAC is deficient superiorly but there is a ligament between the helix and tragus. The EAC runs inferiorly and anteriorly in adults but more horizontally in neonates. The anterior wall of the EAC is longer than the posterior wall by 4 mm. It contains two sutures: the tympanosquamous (anteriorly) and the tympanomastoid (posteriorly) with the skin in the intervening area forming the "vascular strip". The EAC contains two constrictions, at the bony cartilaginous junction and at the isthmus. The isthmus is 5 mm lateral to the tympanic membrane (TM) produced from the anterior canal overhang. The tympanic ring is deficient superiorly at the tympanic incisura.[11]

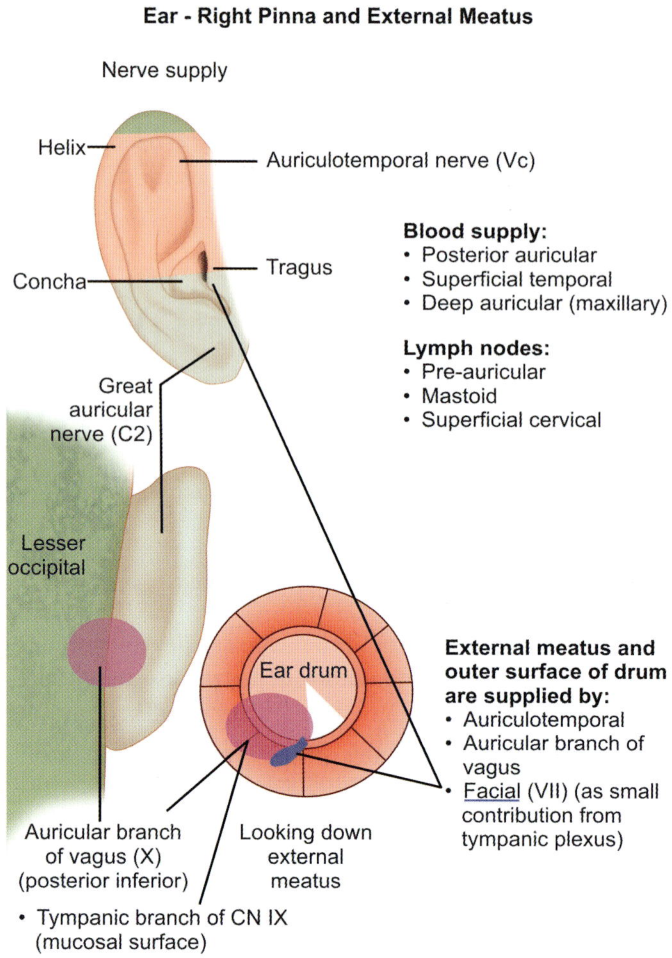

Fig. 1.3: The innervation of the pinna.

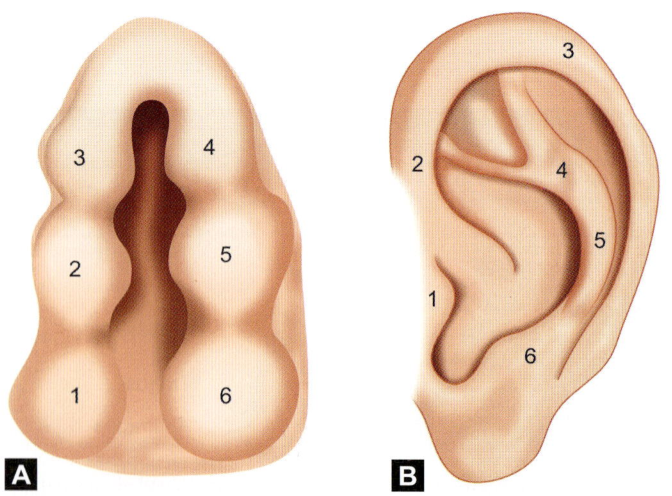

Figs. 1.4A and B: The embryology of the pinna. The six hillocks of His form as follows: one (tragus), two (helix crus), three (helix), four (antihelix), five (antitragus), and six (lobule, inferior helix).

Clinical comment

- The TM is visualized by pulling the pinna superiorly and posteriorly in adults or just posteriorly in children.

The EAC is largely supplied by the deep auricular artery, a branch from the internal maxillary artery that passes through the parotid, running posterior to temporomandibular joint (TMJ). The "vascular strip" is supplied by the anterior/superior auricular artery, a branch from the superficial temporal artery. The skin of the EAC is much thinner in the bony canal and lacks appendages (cerumen, sweat glands, and hair follicles). The cartilaginous EAC skin contains these appendages with cerumen glands being most prominent in the superior and inferior walls. The EAC is drained by the superficial temporal vein and postauricular vein.[11] The lymph drains mainly to parotid nodes and mastoid nodes.

The EAC is formed by ectoderm of the first pouch as it contacts the endoderm of first pouch with intervening mesoderm that forms the TM. The bony EAC is formed by four centers of ossification of the tympanic ring in the ninth week.

Clinical comment

- There are two routes of infection from the EAC in malignant otitis externa.[12] Fissures of Santorini run from anterior inferior in the cartilaginous canal to the parotid. The Foramen of Huschke is formed by anterior and posterior ossification centers that normally obliterate in adolescence. In 5% of people, this foramen persists in the anteroinferior canal and forms a connection to the TMJ.

TYMPANIC MEMBRANE

The TM is a trilaminar structure composed of an outer epidermal layer, middle connective tissue layer, and an inner mucosal layer. It forms an angle with the superior EAC of 140° and the inferior EAC of 55°. Its dimensions are 8 mm (horizontal) by 10 mm (vertical). It is composed of a pars tensa and a pars flaccida that has a thicker connective tissue layer. The epithelium of the TM migrates radially from the umbo at 1–2 mm per day.[13] Upon perforation, keratinocytes form from progenitor cells at the umbo and migrate across to close the perforation.[14,15] The middle connective tissue layer contains collagen fibers arranged in three patterns: radial, circular, and oblique (Fig. 1.5).

The lateral surface of the TM is supplied by the deep auricular artery. The medial surface is supplied by the anterior tympanic artery, stylomastoid artery (a branch from the postauricular artery) and also by branches of the middle meningeal artery.[16] The lateral surface of the TM is supplied by the auriculotemporal nerve from cranial nerve (CN) V, auricular branch of CN X (Arnold's nerve), and branches from CN VII, IX, X. The medial surface is supplied by CN VII and CN IX branches from the tympanic plexus.

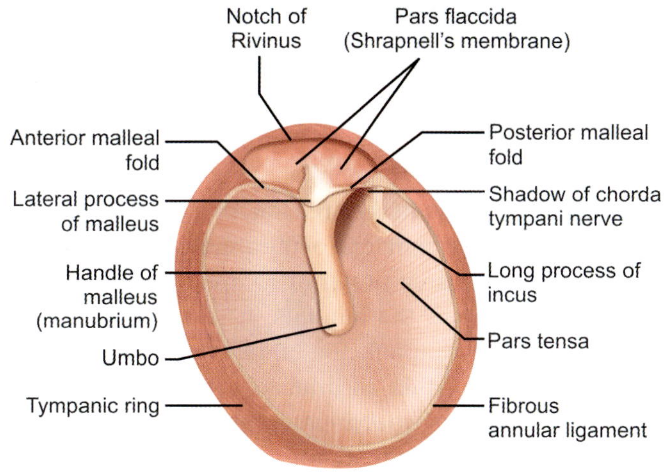

Fig. 1.5: The surface anatomy of the left tympanic membrane.

The TM is formed by ectoderm (epithelial layer) and endoderm (mucosal layer) with intervening mesoderm between these two layers (connective tissue layer) of the first branchial pouch.

Clinical comment

- A myringotomy should be placed away from the posterior-superior quadrant so as to avoid damage to the chorda tympani and incudostapedial joint. It should also be placed with awareness of a potential high riding jugular bulb in the posterior inferior quadrant or a dehiscent internal carotid artery in the anterior inferior quadrant.
- TM perforations can lead to a conductive hearing loss up to 30 dB. Small holes lead to more loss in the low frequencies, whereas large holes lead to a wider frequency hearing loss. The resulting hearing loss may be inversely proportional to the size of the mastoid.[17] The maximum conductive hearing loss is approximately 55 dB. Therefore, a patient presenting with a perforation and conductive hearing loss of >30 dB should alert the clinician to pathology beyond that of the perforation.

MIDDLE EAR

The middle ear is divided into areas above the level of the superior TM annulus (epitympanum), between the superior and inferior TM annulus (mesotympanum) and below the inferior TM annulus (hypotympanum). The protympanum refers to the area anterior to a vertical line level with the anterior margin of the annulus. The posterior tympanum is the area posterior to a vertical line at the posterior margin of the annulus. It includes the facial recess and sinus tympani. The middle ear contains three mucocilliary tracts that all drain toward the Eustachian tube. These are the hypotympanic (the largest tract), the epitympanic, and the promontorial tracts.

The walls of the middle ear contain some important landmarks. Its lateral wall is composed of the tympanic bone and TM. It has three holes. The posterior canaliculus for chorda[18] lies between the junction of posterior and lateral wall at the level of the malleus handle. The Petrotympanic (Glaserian) fissure[19] transmits the anterior malleolar ligament, the anterior tympanic artery, and the chorda tympani nerve (via the canal of Huguier). The roof of the middle ear is composed of the Petrous and Squamous bones. It has one hole, the petrosquamous suture[19] that transmits veins to the inferior petrosal sinus. The anterior wall has three holes. These communicate the superior and inferior caroticotympanic nerves (sympathetic branches from the carotid to the tympanic plexus) and the tympanic branches of the internal carotid artery. There are also two tunnels, the canal for the tensor tympani muscle and the Eustachian tube. On the medial wall is the oval window (fenestra vestibulae) and round window (fenestra cochleae). The oval window dimensions are 3.25 mm by 1.75 mm and contain the stapes footplate that has dimensions of 3 mm by 1.4 mm. The round window is closed by the secondary TM that communicates to the floor of the scala tympani of the cochlea. The round window membrane[20,21] has dimensions of 2.3 mm by 1.87 mm. It is composed of three layers: mucosal, fibrous, and an inner mesothelium. It is directed inferior and posterior. It sits within a niche[22] that is triangular in shape with anterior (1.5 mm), posterior superior (1.3 mm), and posterior inferior (1.6 mm) walls. Also on the middle wall is the facial nerve. The facial nerve runs in the middle ear from the first turn at the geniculate ganglion to the tympanic segment to the second genu and then to the mastoid (vertical) segment. The facial nerve may be dehiscent (defined as a nonpathological gap ≥0.4 mm) in the middle ear with an incidence 55% There is an incidence of more than one dehiscence in 22%. Dehiscences occur 90% at the tympanic segment (with 80% just above oval window and 25% also involving facial nerve prolapse) It may also occur next to tensor tendon, in the facial recess or in the anterior epitympanic recess. The remainder of the dehiscences (10%) occurs in the mastoid segment (Fig. 1.6).[23-27]

Clinical comment

- The surgeon should be wary of a soft tissue mass over the oval window, which may be a prolapsed facial nerve. A soft tissue mass on the promontory may be an anatomical variation of the facial nerve and must not be biopsied until this variation is ruled out. The facial nerve may be bifurcate or trifurcate. It may run anterior, posterior or through the stapes arch and then any variation of this before the stylomastoid foramen. It may also run anterior to the round window.

The posterior wall[28] of the middle ear contains the fossa incudis that itself contains the short process of the incus and a ligament connecting to the incus. The facial recess lies between the pyramidal process, facial nerve, and the TM. The sinus tympani[29] is bounded medially by the posterior semicircular canal and laterally by the pyramidal eminence and the facial nerve. It is bounded superiorly by the ponticulus (a ridge running from the pyramidal eminence to the oval window) and the lateral semicircular canal and inferiorly by the subiculum, styloid eminence, and the jugular wall (Fig. 1.7).

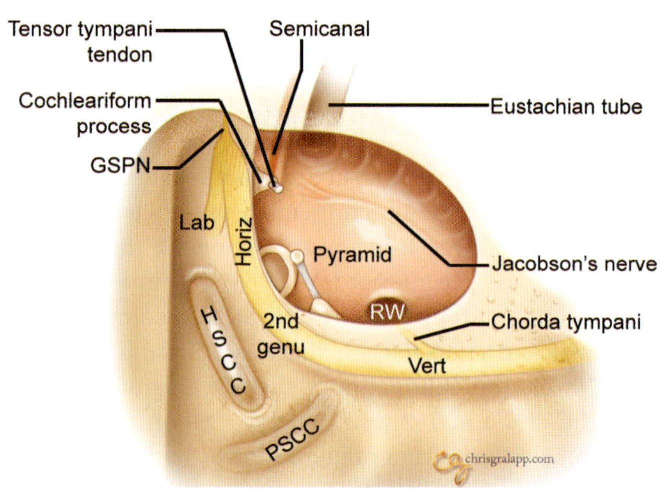

Fig. 1.6: The lateral wall of the middle ear and the path of the tympanic facial nerve. (RW, round window; HSCC, horizontal semicircular canal; PSCC, posterior semicircular canal; GSPN, greater superficial petrosal nerve). From C Gralapp and R Jackler, Stanford University, CA, USA.

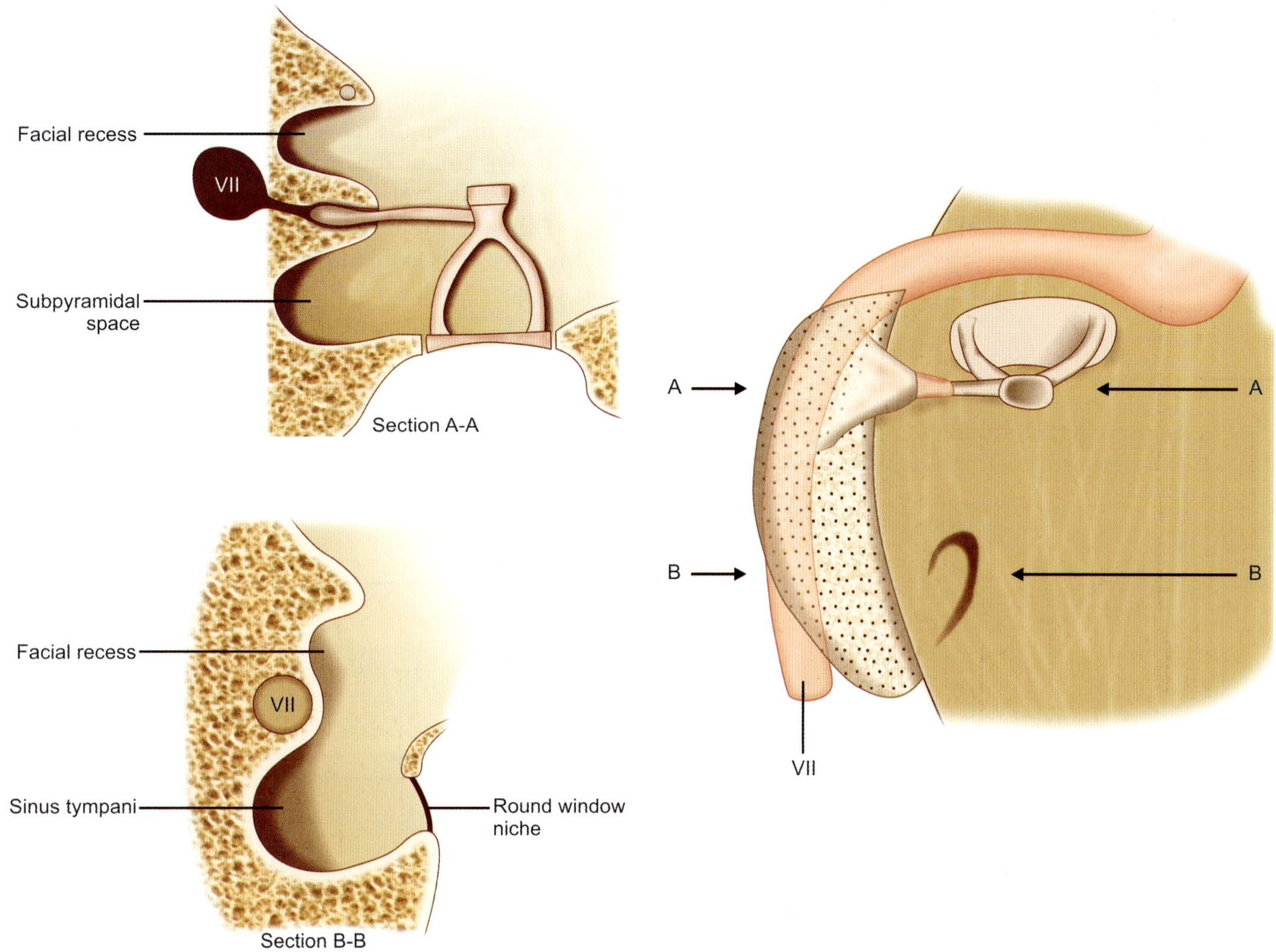

Fig. 1.7: The relations of the facial recess and sinus tympani.

Clinical comment

- The round window niche is a landmark for the singular nerve, which runs 1 mm deep (medial) and in line with parallel to the posterior attachment of the round window membrane.

The posterior wall of the mesotympanum also contains three eminences and three ridges (Fig. 1.8).

The epitympanum contains the head of the malleus, body of the incus, the malleolar and incudal ligaments and folds. The epitympanum communicates with the mastoid air cells via the mastoid antrum. The mastoid antrum is fully developed at birth with a volume of 1 mL. The supratubal recess (or anterior tympanic recess) is bounded by[30,31]: anteriorly, the petrosal tegmen, posteriorly by the cog (a ridge of bone extending down from the tegmen), superiorly by the middle cranial fossa tegmen, and laterally by the tympanic bone and chorda tympani nerve.

The malleus[32] consists of a head, neck, lateral and anterior process and manubrium. The lateral process attaches to the TM and the anterior process provides attachment for the anterior malleolar ligament to the petrotympanic fissure. The manubrium provides attachment of the malleus to the TM from the lateral process to the umbo. It has three ligaments. The anterior malleolar attaches the head to the anterior wall of epitympanum, the lateral malleolar attaches the neck to the notch of Rivinus, and the superior malleolar attaches the head to the roof of the epitympanum. The malleus also has three associated folds; an anterior malleolar fold attaching the lateral process to

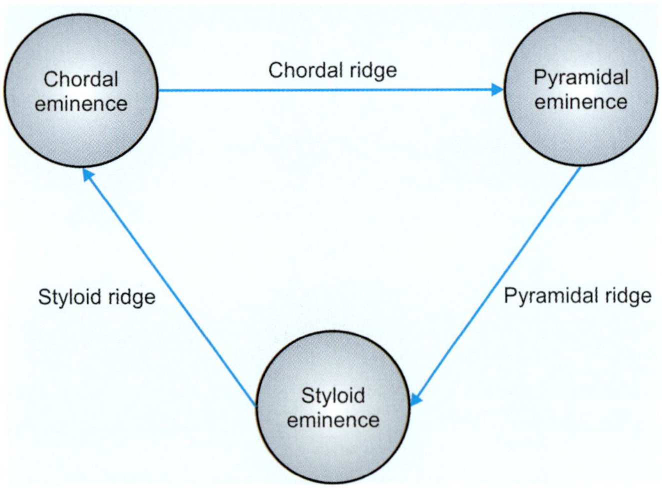

Fig. 1.8: A diagrammatic representation of the posterior wall of the mesotympanum.

the annulus, a posterior malleolar fold attaching the lateral process to the annulus, and a lateral malleolar fold attaching to the annulus (Figs. 1.9A to D).

The tensor tympani has an origin with its muscle fibers within the canal for the tensor tympani, turning to tendon that loops 90° around the cochleariform process[33] to insert onto the neck of malleus. It is innervated by the nerve to tensor tympani (a branch from CN V).

The incus[34] is composed of a body, short process, long process, and a lenticular process that articulates with stapes. The ligaments of the incus are the posterior incudal that attaches the short process to the incudal recess (in the area of the "incus buttress") posteriorly, a medial and lateral that attaches the body to the head of the malleus, and a superior incudal ligament which is variably present.

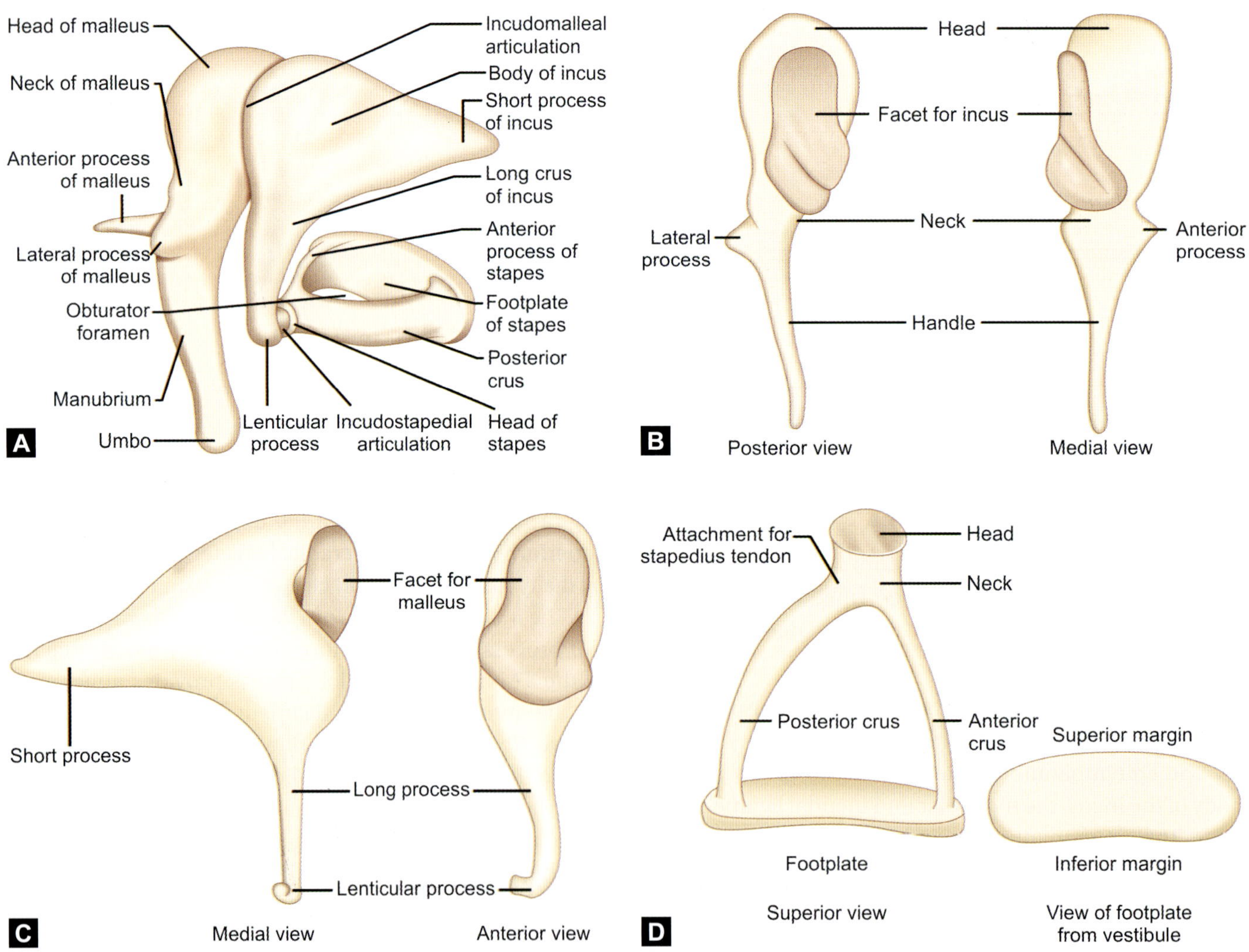

Figs. 1.9A to D: The left ossicular chain.

The stapes[35] parts are the head (capitulum) for articulation with the lenticular process of the incus and an anterior and posterior crus. The anterior crus is straighter, shorter, and thinner. The stapes footplate has dimensions of 1.75 mm by 3.25 mm. Its relations to the structures within the vestibule are important to consider and differ depending on the area of the footplate. The utricle is at 0.58 mm (posterior), 1.04 mm (middle) and 1.51 mm (anterior), compared to the saccule which is at 1.33 mm (middle) and 1.31 mm (anterior) (Fig. 1.10).[36]

The stapedius muscle[33] originates from the pyramidal process and inserts into the posterior crus of stapes just below its head. It is innervated by the nerve to stapedius (from CN VII). It has a number of hypothesized functions.[37,38] The stapedius protects from loud sounds by contracting at sounds louder than 80 dBHL with a latency of >10 ms. It is most efficient at 2 kHz. It provides rigidity and blood supply to the ossicular chain and reduces physiological noise from chewing and talking. The stapedial reflex[39] is the contraction of the stapedial muscle that occurs bilaterally to sound presented to one ear. The stapedial reflex is a measure of the integrity of the inner hair cells (IHCs). Contraction of the stapedial muscle occurs at approximately 70–100 (mean 85) dBHL above threshold. The ipsilateral reflex occurs at approximately 2–14 dB less than the contralateral ear. Stimulating both ears lowers the threshold by 3 dB. If a patient has hearing loss combined with the reflex threshold greater than the limits of the audiometer (approximately 120 dB), the reflex will be absent. It is also absent in 5–20% of normal people (Fig. 1.11).

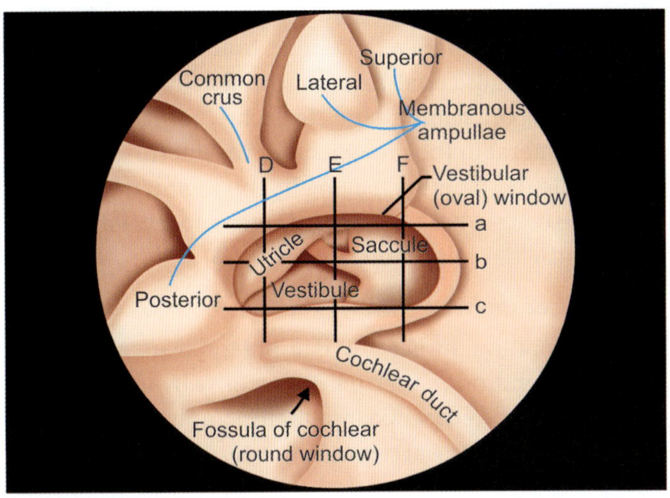

Fig. 1.10: The relationships of the stapes footplate to the utricle and the saccule.
Source: Adapted from Backous et al.[36]

The tympanic diaphragm is a series of mucosal folds that separate the epitympanum from the mesotympanum and the mastoid. Its components are the malleus head, body of incus, lateral incudal fold, medial incudal fold, anterior malleolar fold, lateral malleolar fold, and tensor tympani fold.[40] There are two narrow passages that breach the diaphragm, the anterior and posterior tympanic isthmuses. The anterior tympanic isthmus is medial to the body of the incus, passing between the stapes, long process incus, and the tensor tympani tendon. The posterior tympanic isthmus is between the pyramidal process, short process of incus and posterior incudal ligament, medial incudal fold, stapes and stapedial tendon (Fig. 1.12).

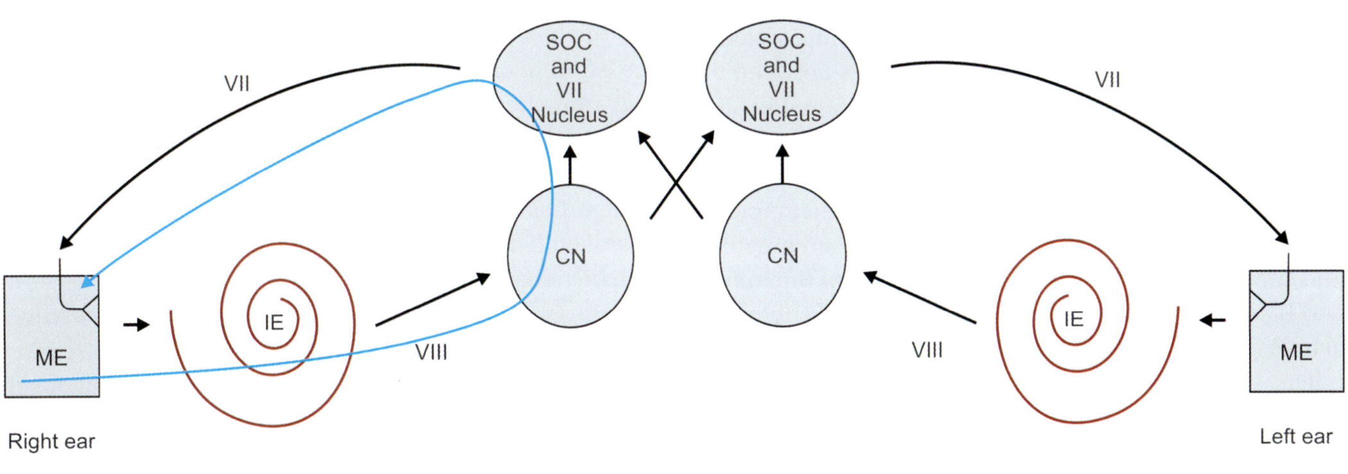

Figs. 1.11: The right ipsilateral stapedial (acoustic) reflex pathway.

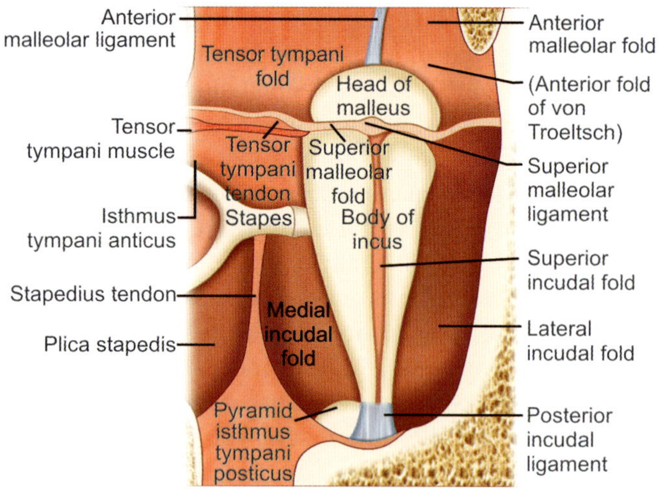

Fig. 1.12: The tympanic diaphragm and connections between the epitympanun and the mesotympanum. Areas of communication are highlighted.
Source: Adapted from Proctor.[40]

Clinical comment

- The tympanic diaphragm provides some resistance to the spread of cholesteatoma between the mesotympanum and epitympanum. The patency of the tympanic isthmus and aditus ad antrum are important for aeration of the mastoid.

In surgery for chronic otitis media, sometimes the head of the malleus and the body of the incus are removed with the attaching folds and ligaments to increase aeration between the middle ear and mastoid.

Beneath the floor of the attic and in the upper mesotympanum there are three compartments.[40] The inferior incudal space is from the inferior surface of the incus laterally to the posterior malleolar fold limited medially by the medial incudal fold and anteriorly by the interossicular fold. The posterior pouch of von Troeltsch is between the TM and the posterior malleolar fold. Its inferior edge often contains the chorda tympani. It opens inferiorly toward the posterior mesotympanum. The anterior pouch of von Troeltsch is between the TM and the anterior malleolar fold.

The chorda tympani[18,26] runs in the mesotympanum and supplies taste to the anterior two-thirds of the tongue and is secretomotor to the submandibular and sublingual glands. The taste cell bodies lie in the geniculate ganglion. It leaves the facial nerve, on average, 5 mm (a range of -1 to 11 mm) above the stylomastoid foramen and runs in the canaliculus of chorda tympani. It enters the middle ear via the ita chordae posterius (in the posterior lateral wall of the middle ear) with the posterior tympanic artery. It lies between the pyramidal eminence and the tympanic annulus. It runs through the middle ear lateral to the long process of the incus and the tendon of tensor tympani but medial to the neck of the malleus and posterior malleolar ligament. It exits the middle ear at the iter chordae anterius to run in the canal of Huguier. The chorda tympani may have a number of variations. In the middle ear it may pass lateral to the TM or may pass lateral to the malleus. In the mastoid it may arise distal to the stylomastoid foramen or may arise as high as the lateral semicircular canal.

The tympanic plexus[42] lies on the cochlea promontory. The incoming fibers include parasympathetics that come from Jacobson's nerve (CN IX) and Arnold's nerve (CN X) and sympathetic branches from the internal carotid artery Its outgoing fibers include the lesser superficial petrosal nerve that carry parasympathetic branches of CN IX. It leaves in a small canal beneath the tensor tympani. It is joined by parasympathetic branches of CN VII and emerges lateral to the greater superficial petrosal nerve in the middle fossa before leaving by the foramen ovale. The plexus also has a branch to the greater superficial petrosal nerve and TM mucosal branches.

Clinical comment

- A tympanic neurectomy is a potential treatment for Frey's syndrome after parotidectomy by interrupting the misdirected parasympathetic supply via the lesser superficial petrosal nerve.[43,44]

The hypotympanum lies beneath the floor of the bony EAC and contains hypotympanic air cells with the jugular bulb posterior inferiorly and the internal carotid artery anterior inferiorly. Either may be dehiscent in the hypotympanum.

The blood supply of the middle ear[45] is by branches of the external carotid, internal carotid, and basilar arteries. The branches of the external carotid artery branches include the anterior tympanic artery that runs from the internal maxillary artery through the petrotympanic fissure. It has a superior branch that supplies the anterior lateral epitympanum, a posterior branch that supplies the TM, incudostapedial joint and lateral tegmen, and an ossicular branch. The ossicular branch further divides into a mallear and incudal branch. The external carotid also gives the deep auricular artery via the maxillary internal maxillary artery through the inferior bony EAC. It has an anterior and posterior branch. The inferior tympanic artery runs from the ascending pharyngeal artery through the inferior tympanic canaliculus. The stylomastoid artery runs from the postauricular artery running up through the stylomastoid foramen. The stylomastoid artery also provides the posterior tympanic artery. There is a mastoid branch from the occipital artery. A tubal branch comes from the accessory meningeal artery. The superficial petrosal artery branches from the middle meningeal artery and runs with the greater superficial petrosal nerve. A superior tympanic artery branches from the middle meningeal artery through the superior tympanic canaliculus with the lesser superficial petrosal nerve. The internal carotid artery supplies blood to the middle ear via its caroticotympanic branches[2] that come direct from the internal carotid artery. The basilar artery supplies the middle ear via branches of the subarcuate artery, itself coming from the labyrinthine artery, or the anterior inferior cerebellar artery.

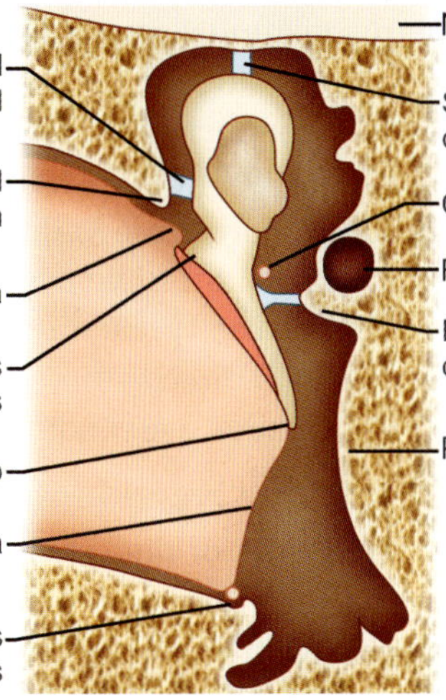

Fig. 1.13: A coronal view of the boundaries of Prussak's space.

Clinical comment

- A persistent stapedial artery is the persistence of the artery to the second brachial arch. It runs from the internal carotid artery over the promontory, through the stapes arch and enters the fallopian canal above the oval window. It then runs with the facial nerve upward to supply a region of dura. Its ligation may comprise cerebral function and therefore is a potential hazard during stapedectomy.[46]

The inferior tympanic artery is the usual blood supply to a glomus tympanicum tumor.[47]

The middle ear and Eustachian tube forms from the expansion of the first pouch. The epitympanum and antrum are developed by birth. The expansion of the first pouch leads to the development of four primary sacs.[40] The saccus medius forms the epitympanum and divides into three smaller spaces, the medial (to later form Prussak's space), the posterior, and the anterior. The saccus anticus forms the anterior pouch of von Troeltsch. The saccus superior forms the posterior pouch of von Troeltsch. The saccus posticus forms the posterior middle ear and hypotympanum (Fig. 1.13).

Clinical comment

- Knowledge of the folds and spaces in the middle ear helps with the understanding of the routes of spread of cholesteatoma.[48] The main routes of spread for cholesteatoma in decreasing order are via the posterior epitympanum, posterior mesotympanum, and anterior tympanum. From the posterior epitympanum, it can penetrate the superior incudal space (running lateral to the body of the incus), then to the antrum and then the mastoid. It may also go through the floor of Prussak's space to the posterior pouch of von Troeltsch (running between the TM and posterior malleolar fold) to the posterior mesotympanum then to the stapes, round window, sinus tympani, and facial recess. The posterior mesotympanum route forms as retraction forms a sac medial to the neck of the malleus and incus then to the sinus tympani and facial recess. The anterior epitympanum route forms by retraction anterior to the malleus head, then to the anterior pouch of von Troeltsch (between the TM and the anterior malleolar fold), then to the supratubal recess. This route often causes early facial nerve palsy.
- Acquired cholesteatoma is seen as squamous epithelium extending into Prussak's space. The boundaries of Prussak's space are the pars flaccida (laterally), the neck of the malleus (medially), the lateral process of the malleus (inferiorly), and the lateral malleolar fold (superiorly).[49]
- Meningitis may result from the spread of infection between the middle ear and the cerebrospinal fluid (CSF) via a number of anatomical and pathological routes. These potential connections are from the middle ear to the inner ear, from the middle ear directly to the CSF and from the inner ear to the CSF. The oval window connects the middle ear to the inner ear and is the most common route of spread. The middle ear may connect to the CSF via Hyrtl's fissure, a congenital cleft between the hypotympanum and the posterior

fossa, or the petrosquamous sinus (of Lushka) which is an occasional embryological remnant often open in infancy. It usually connects the middle ear and the transverse or sigmoid sinus (although it is highly variable). Retrograde spread from the middle ear can also occur via the internal auditory vein or the mastoid emissary vein. Infection can spread from the inner ear to the cerebrospinal fluid directly through the internal auditory canal (IAC) fundus, via modiolar end defects or via the cochlear aqueduct.

The resonant frequencies of the external and middle ears are determined by their design.[50] This results in a combined external ear gain of 15–20 dB over 2–7 kHz and 5 dB at 3 kHz in the middle ear. The resonance of the middle ear is includes the air space contained within the mastoid antrum. This effect is lost by blocking the antrum, as is sometimes performed in chronic ear surgery. The combined resonance of the external and middle ear is thought to produce the typical notch in the audiogram seen in sensory hearing loss associated with noise induced hearing loss. The gain provided via the various parts of the ear include[51] the concha with a 10 dB gain at 5 kHz and the EAC with a 10 dB gain at 2–5 kHz. In infants the EAC provides a 15 dB gain at 3 kHz (at approximately 8 kHz in infants) and reaches adult value after age two and a half. The middle ear[52] has a gain of 5 dB at 3 kHz and the TM has a gain at 800–1600 Hz.

Sound is transferred from the TM to the cochlear with a gain according to the transformer ratio theory.[53,54] It accounts for a total gain of approximately 25–30 dB. In normal subjects up to 25 dB variations in middle ear mechanics can occur. At 1 kHz, the ratio of gain from the TM to the cochlear is 82.5. This is a combination of three levers: the hydraulic, ossicular, and catenary. The hydraulic lever provides a gain of 17–20 times relates to the ratio of the area of the oval window to the TM. The ossicular lever has a gain of 1.3 represents the ratio of the long axis of the malleus to the long process of the incus. The catenary lever provides a gain of 2 due to the outward convexity of TM with its radial arrangement of collagen fibers.

The levers have greatest efficiency at 1 kHz. Frequencies >1 kHz lead to a reduction in the efficiency of the levers. Above 1 kHz, the hydraulic lever changes as vibrations are broken up into smaller vibratory patterns, while the ossicular lever provides more slippage in the axis of rotation of the ossicles. The TM has its greatest movement at its inferior edge at 2 kHz. Above 6 kHz vibrations are broken up into small zones. The annular ligament provides approximately 90% of the stiffness. No movement occurs at the malleoincudal joint at physiological sound pressures.

Clinical comment

- Sound is localized to the worse-hearing ear in a conductive hearing loss with the Weber test. One explanation of this in ossicular fixation is that increased ossicular chain stiffness leads to less shunting of pressure out of the cochlea, which increases bone vibration detection.[55]

INNER EAR

The cochlea is 5 mm in height. The cochlea duct is 34 mm and has two and three quarter turns around the helicotrema. The modiolus points laterally, anteriorly, and inferiorly. It has a similar orientation as the EAC.[56] The cochlea aqueduct transmits the periotic duct (perilymphatic duct) between the basal turn of the scala tympani to the media of the jugular fossa (Table 1.1 and Fig. 1.14).[21]

Clinical comment

- The cochlea aqueduct is a potential route of spread of meningitis. Its dissection during a translabyrinthine procedure releases cerebral spinal fluid pressure. During this procedure, it marks the inferior limit of dissection as further inferior dissection puts CN IX–XI at risk.[57]

Hair cells[62,63] do not possess true stereocilia, which require a nine plus two arrangement of microtubules and do not have kinocilia. They are like microvilli with an actin core. They increase in length along the cochlea duct. The first-order neurons of the cochlea nerve lie in the spiral ligament, compared to within the IAC for the vestibular nerve. The IHCs are arranged to form a single row of hair cells and are flask shaped. They have only afferent synapses. Their stereocilia do not attach into the tectorial membrane, they are deflected by fluid in between tectorial membrane and reticular lamina. Cilia deflection causes mechanically gated ion channels to open allowing potassium and calcium to enter the cell. This then causes voltage gated calcium channels to open, causing depolarization. Outer hair cells (OHCs)[64,65] are arranged in three rows and are cylinder shaped. They have both afferent and efferent synapses. They are unique to mammals. Their stereocilia attach into the bottom surface of the tectorial membrane. They are responsible for the sensitivity of hearing and provide the "cochlea amplifier". They do this by sensing the incoming sound wave, and then generating force in synchrony with

Table 1.1 Functions of the parts within the cochlea

Part	*Composition*	*Function*
Stria vascularis	Three epithelial layers (marginal, intermediate, basal), blood vessels, pericytes, melanocytes, endothelial cells	Produces endolymph Source of endocochlear potential Primary producer of energy for the cochlea
Spiral ligament	Mainly type I collagen Contains five types of aquaporins	Role in endocochlear potential Fluid homeostasis
Spiral prominence cells	Express pendrin and aquaporins	Ion + fluid regulation
Spiral limbus + Huschke's teeth cells		Ion + fluid regulation Tectorial membrane maintenance (glycosaminoglycans, tectorins) Potassium recycling from IHCs
Pillar cells Inner/outer		Maintain spatial relationships between hair cells
Dieter's cells (between the OHCs)		Mechanical support of organ of Corti
Hensen		Potassium recycling
Bottchers (Not in apical turn)		Secretory HCO_3 regulation
Claudius		Potassium recycling
Spaces of Nuel	Contain perilymph	
Basilar membrane	Inner/zona arcuata (under tunnel of Corti), thin Outer/zona pectinata Thick, striated Covered by vascular layer beneath Permits nearly unimpeded passage to organ of Corti (therefore fluid resembles perilymph)	Frequency tuning
Reissner's membrane		Possible area of fluid transport between scala
Tectorial membrane		Coupling of vibrations to OHC stereocilia

(IHCs, inner hair cells; OHCs, outer hair cells).

it to increase the vibration of the basilar membrane. This provides a gain of up to 60 dB. The plasma membrane of the OHC contains prestin, which is a motor protein that senses the voltage within the cell and generates force. This causes the length of the OHC to elongate and contract, a phenomenon called electromotility. By adding this additional energy to the cochlear traveling wave, viscous damping forces within the cochlea are overcome, leading to high-frequency hearing.

Clinical comment

- Otoacoustic emissions (OAEs) are a measure of OHC function. They are absent if hearing loss is >50 dBHL. There are various types of OAEs that can be measured, including spontaneous, transient evoked, stimulus frequency evoked, and distortion product evoked.[64,66] OAEs are the most common type of test used to screen for hearing loss in newborn babies.

Clinical comment

- OHCs are the most susceptible of the hair cells to ototoxicity. OHCs are also typically lost after loud noise exposure and with aging. Loss of OHCs leads to hearing loss and decreased word recognition ability. Recruitment is the perception of exaggerated sound and reduced dynamic range that also occurs when OHCs are lost.

The basilar membrane has a tonotopic organization. This is primarily because its stiffness decreases from base to apex, although its width (and hence its mass) also increases along the length of the cochlea. The traveling wave of the basilar membrane vibrates with maximum amplitude at a place along the cochlea that is dependent on the frequency of the sound presented. The corresponding hair cells stimulate the adjacent nerve fibers, which are organized according to the frequency at which they are

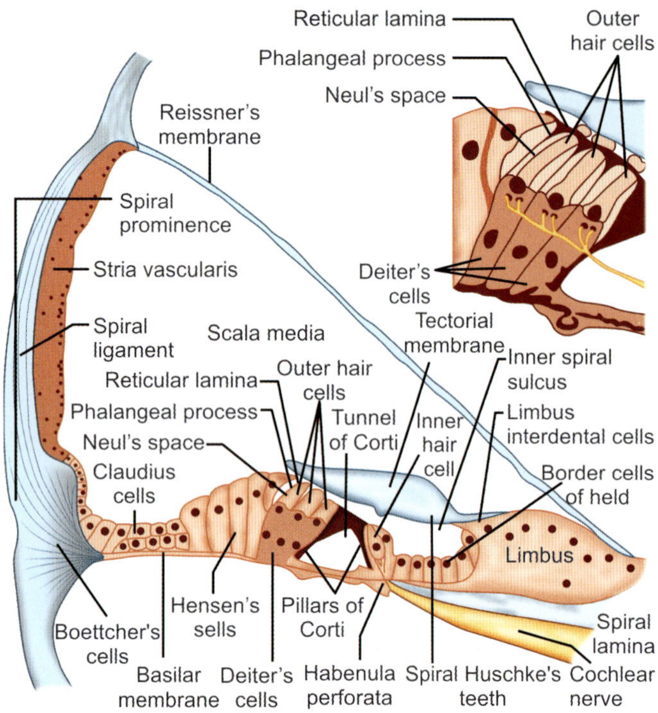

Fig. 1.14: A cross section of the cochlea.[58–61]

most sensitive. The lower frequencies travel further (to the apex). The basilar membrane response allows complex sounds to be broken up into narrow bands of frequencies.

The cochlea fluids[67,68] are predominantly composed of potassium (K^+) and sodium (Na^+). The difference in potassium concentrations between the compartments leads to an endocochlear potential of +80–100 mV. This is maintained by a Na^+/K^+ ATPase within the stria vascularis (Table 1.2).

Clinical comment

- β2 transferrin can be used to identify a cerebrospinal fluid or perilymphatic fluid leak.

The arterial supply[45,69,70] (Fig. 1.15) of the inner ear is via branches of the labyrinthine artery (a branch of the anterior inferior cerebellar artery, but sometimes comes from the basilar or superior cerebellar artery). It runs in the IAC before becoming the anterior vestibular artery. This will supply the utricle, superior semicircular canal, and lateral semicircular canal (the embryological pars superior)). From this, the common cochlear artery branches. This branches again into two further arteries, the main cochlear artery and the vestibulocochlear artery. The main cochlear artery supplies the apical three quarters of the cochlea and the modiolus. It gives the

Table 1.2: The fluid composition in the cochlea

Fluid	*Like*	*K^+*	*Na^+*	*Other*
Endolymph	Intracellular	High (144 mM)	Low (5 mM)	
Perilymph	Extracellular, CSF	Low (10 mM)	High (140 mM)	Contains β2 transferrin

(CSF, cerebrospinal fluid).

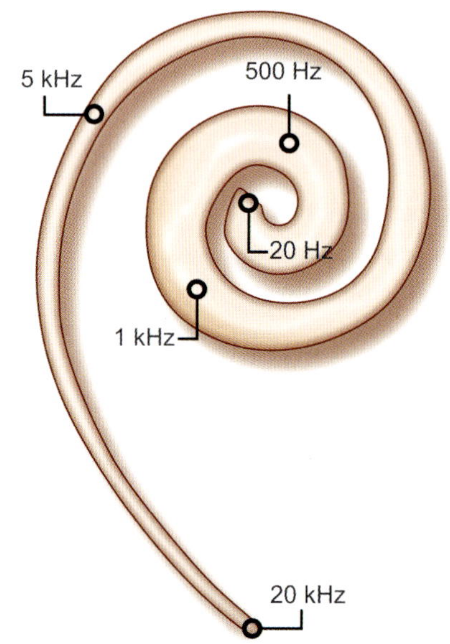

Fig. 1.15: The tonotopical arrangement of the cochlea.

external radiating arterioles, which gives four networks supplying the cochlea. The spiral ligament branches give branches to the scala vestibule and the scala tympani. The other networks are to the stria vascularis and the spiral prominence. The main cochlea artery also gives the internal radiating arterioles that provide the limbus vessels and marginal vessels. The vestibulocochlear artery gives the posterior vestibular artery that supplies the saccule and posterior semicircular canal (the embryological pars inferior). It also gives the cochlear ramus artery to supply the basal one quarter of the cochlea.

The venous drainage of the inner ear (Fig. 1.16) is similarly matched to the arterial supply. The anterior spiral vein, draining the spiral ligament and scala vestibule, and the posterior spiral vein, draining the scala media and scala tympani, both drain into the common modiolar vein. The anterior vestibular vein, draining the pars superior, the posterior vestibular vein, draining the pars inferior, and the vein of the round window all drain into the vestibulocochlear vein. The common modiolar vein joins the vestibulocochlear vein to form the inferior cochlear vein,

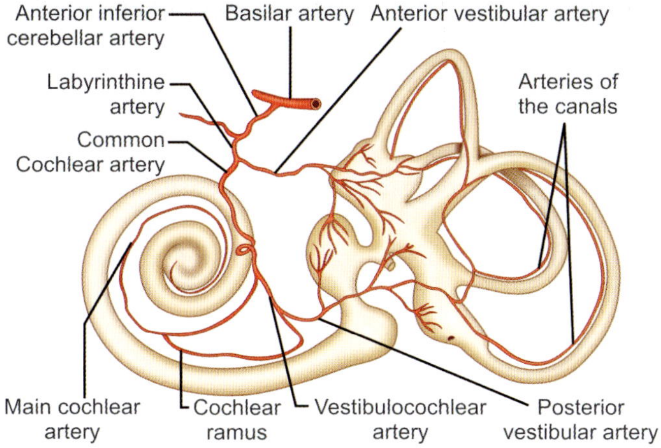

Fig. 1.16: The arterial supply of the cochlea.[72]

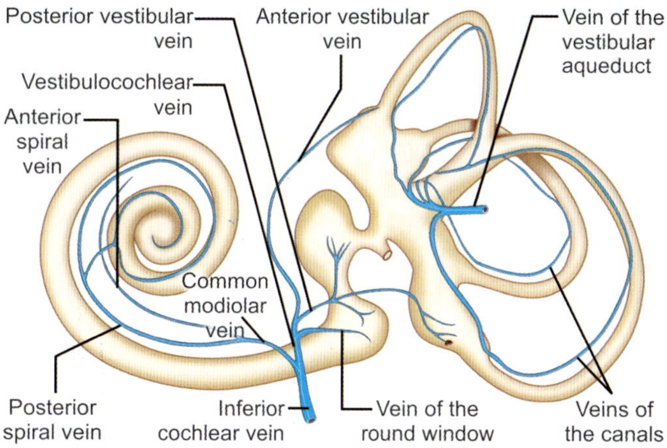

Fig. 1.17: The venous drainage of the cochlea.[72]

which then drains to the inferior petrosal vein via the canal of Cotugno. The membranous semicircular canals drain into the vein of the vestibular aqueduct that then joins the sigmoid sinus. Sometimes there is also an internal auditory vein that flows into the inferior petrosal sinus via the IAC (Fig. 1.17).

Cochlear neurons can be divided into type I or type II.[72] Afferent nerve fibers are unmyelinated and run from the organ of Corti, through the habenula perforata, to the spiral ganglion. Spiral ganglion neurons are bipolar and acquire the myelin in the modiolus. This can be compared to the vestibular neurons that are myelinated and gain their myelin sheath as they cross the basement membrane directly under the sensory epithelium. 95% of the afferent nerve fibers synapse with IHCs. These are called type I afferent neurons, and are the primary source of auditory input to the brain. Type II afferent neurons receive input from OHCs, and their purpose is unknown. Efferent fibers are the terminations of descending olivocochlear nerve fibers (Rasmussen's bundle). They come from the brainstem and synapse onto the OHCs. Their function is unknown at this time, but they may be important to understanding speech in noisy background environments. The sensory epithelium in the inner can be divided according to embryological origin into the pars superior (supplying the superior semicircular canal, lateral semicircular canal and utricle) and pars inferior (supplying the posterior semicircular canal and saccule) (Table 1.3).

The endolymphatic fluid[73] is produced predominantly by the stria vascularis but also by the planum semilunatum (around cristae), the dark vestibular cells and from the perilymph across the labyrinth membranes. Vasopressin plays a role in its formation. It moves by longitudinal flow

Table 1.3: A comparison of cochlear neurons

Type	*I*	*II*
Incidence	95%	5%
Hair cell supply	IHC	OHC
Number of neurons per row	1	3–5
Ratio of neuron to hair cell	10:1	1:10
Size	Large	Small
Myelination	Yes (acquire in the modiolus)	No

(IHCs, inner hair cells; OHCs, outer hair cells).

and radial exchange. Longitudinal flow is slow at 0.004–0.007 mm/min and flows from the stria vascularis to the scala media to the ductus reunions to the saccule and them to the endolymphatic sac. Radial exchange is rapid and occurs via an exchange and balance of chemicals.

INTERNAL AUDITORY CANAL

The IAC has a diameter of 4.5 mm with a <1 mm difference between sides. If a CT scan demonstrates that there is a >2 mm difference in an individual between sides, it is suggestive of a pathological condition (such as a vestibular schwannoma). Its length along the posterior wall measures 8 mm with <2 mm between sides. It runs at an angle of 80°–90° (in 60%) or 90°–100° (in 40%) to the sagittal plane.[74] Anatomical variations include an absence of the bony partition on its lateral end associated with a stapes gusher. It may be too narrow (<3 mm). If this occurs with normal facial nerve function it typically means there is coexisting cochlea nerve aplasia. It may have a vertical orientation, associated with hearing loss. The IAC may also be too wide (>10 mm) and associated with a stapes gusher. The IAC contains the facial nerve, cochlear nerve, superior vestibular nerve, inferior vestibular nerve, internal auditory artery (labyrinthine artery), the singular nerve (branches from the inferior vestibular nerve at the fundus and passes through its own foramen to supply the posterior semicircular canal), the intracanalicular cistern and meninges.[75] The relations of the contents of the IAC are important.[76] At the brainstem the cochlear nerve is below all, with the facial nerve anterior and the vestibular nerve posterior. At the porus,[77] the facial nerve is above all, the vestibular nerve is posterior inferior and the cochlear nerve is anterior superior. The relationship at the fundus is shown in Figure 1.18. The nerves rotate 90° within the canal and the cerebellopontine angle so that the facial nerve is superior to the vestibulocochlear nerves and is separated at the brainstem by the anterior inferior cerebellar artery.[76]

Clinical comment

- At the brainstem the vestibular nerve appears grey compared to the cochlear nerve, which is white. The vestibular nerve is closest to CN V. This helps with its identification during vestibular nerve section.

There are at least two acousticofacial anastomoses within the IAC between the nervus intermedius and the superior vestibular nerve (Figs. 1.19 and 1.20).[78]

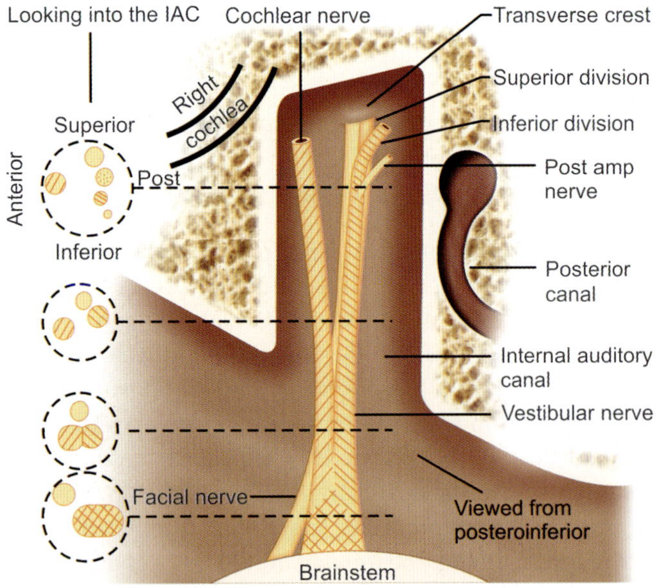

Fig. 1.18: The relationships of the nerves within the internal auditory canal.
Source: Adapted from Rhoton and Tedeschi.[77]

Embryologically, the vestibular system develops before the cochlea.[79] The inner ear develops from the otic placode that forms on each side of the neural groove between the second and third branchial arches. The otic placode then forms the otic pit and then the otic vesicle. This then develops into two compartments. The medial compartment will form the endolymphatic sac. The lateral compartment will form the utriculosaccular chamber, which, after undergoing a series of complex folds, forms two chambers: the utricular and the saccular chamber. The utricular chamber forms the utricle and semicircular canals. The superior forms first, then the posterior with the lateral canal forming last. As the lateral semicircular canal develops the slowest, it is the most commonly maldeveloped canal. The saccular chamber forms the saccule and

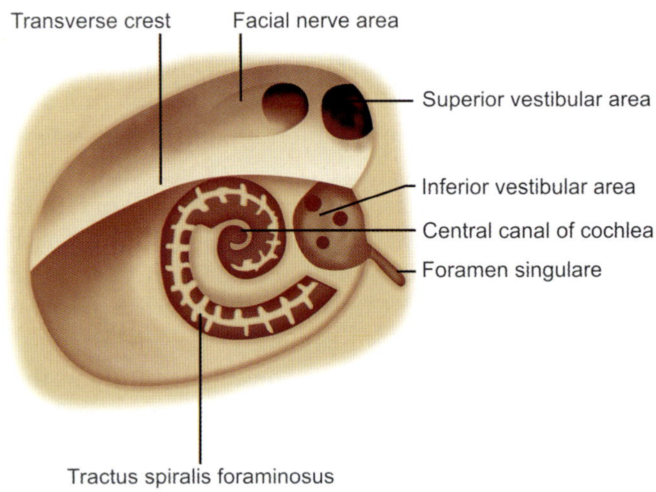

Fig. 1.19: The fundus of the right internal auditory canal.

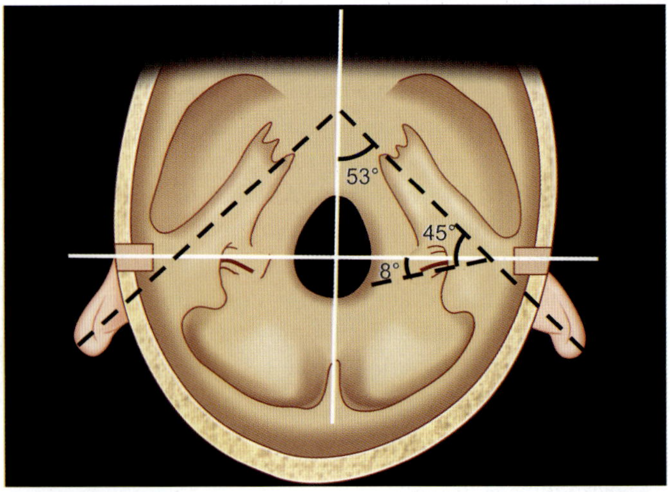

Fig. 1.20: The angle of the internal auditory canal and petrous ridge.

cochlear. This explains the connection between them called the ductus reunions. The cochlea develops by intrachondral bone within endochondral bone and therefore heals by fibrous healing. At gestational week 20 the cochlea reaches adult length. At week 25 the organ of Corti is fully developed. The bony labyrinth develops as mesoderm and surrounds the membranous labyrinth. Ossification then occurs from 14 ossification centers from week 15. The vestibular aqueduct develops from a diverticulum in the otocyst in week 4 (Table 1.4 and Fig. 1.21).

Clinical comment

- As the cochlea heals by fibrous healing following temporal bone fracture, cochlea implantation can involve a difficult insertion if left long after the injury.

Inner ear malformations[81–83] can be classified as membranous/osseous or membranous. Membranous malformations account for 80% of congenital deafness. Membranous/osseous malformations can be further classified as total aplasia (Michel's) or partial. Cochlear deformities can be complete aplasia, hypoplasia, common cavity (the most common), or Mondini's malformations. Mondini's malformation is described as a cochlea with only one and a half turns, a large vestibule, normal labyrinth, and enlarged vestibular aqueduct (EVAS). It is the most common malformation and is associated with other syndromes including Pendred's, branchial-oto-renal, Waardenburg's, Wildervancks (cervico-oculo-acoustic syndrome), Klippel Feil (fusion of cervical vertebrae), and Treacher Collins. Lateral semicircular canal dysplasia is the most common labyrinthine abnormality as it is the last canal to develop. The most common radiological abnormality is EVAS. The cochlear aqueduct is thought to be abnormal when >1 mm. It is usually patent, but neither transmits pressure or allows free spinal fluid to flow. Membranous abnormalities can either be incomplete or complete. Scheibe is an incomplete type, cochleosaccular dysplasia (of the pars inferior) with a malformed membranous canal. The organ of Corti is partially or totally missing with a normal bony canal. Alexander is also an incomplete type and is partial (localized to the basal turn) aplasia of cochlea duct occurring with high-frequency sensory hearing loss. Bing Siebemann malformations involve complete membranous dysplasia and are associated with Jervell and Lange-Nielsen syndrome and Usher's syndrome (Table 1.5 and Fig. 1.22).

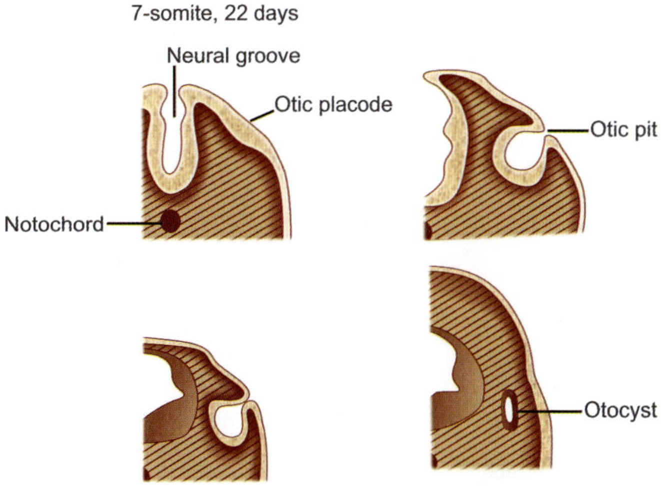

Fig. 1.21: The embryological development of the otocyst.

Table 1.4: The embryological development of the inner ear[83]

Primordium	*Week complete*
Otic placode	3
Otic pit	4
Otic vesicle (otocyst)	5
Ventral pouch of otocyst	
Cochlea duct	8
Saccule	11
Dorsal pouch of otocyst	
Endolymphatic duct	11
Utricle and semicircular ducts	11
Semicircular canals	19–22
Labyrinthine ossification	23
Total development	26

Table 1.5: Classification of inner ear malformations[84,85]

Arrested development	*Features*
3rd week (early)	Michel's deformity (complete labyrinthine aplasia, i.e. no inner ear)
3rd week (late)	Cochlea aplasia (absent cochlea, deformed vestibule)
4th week	Common cavity (same chamber)
5th week	Cochlear agenesis (incomplete partition type I, labyrinth is cystic but separate) Normal vestibular aqueduct
6th week	Cochlear hypoplasia (≤1 turn of cochlea, hypoplastic labyrinth)
7th week	Incomplete partition (Mondini's) 1½ turns (cystic appearance of cochlea apex only)
8th week	Normal

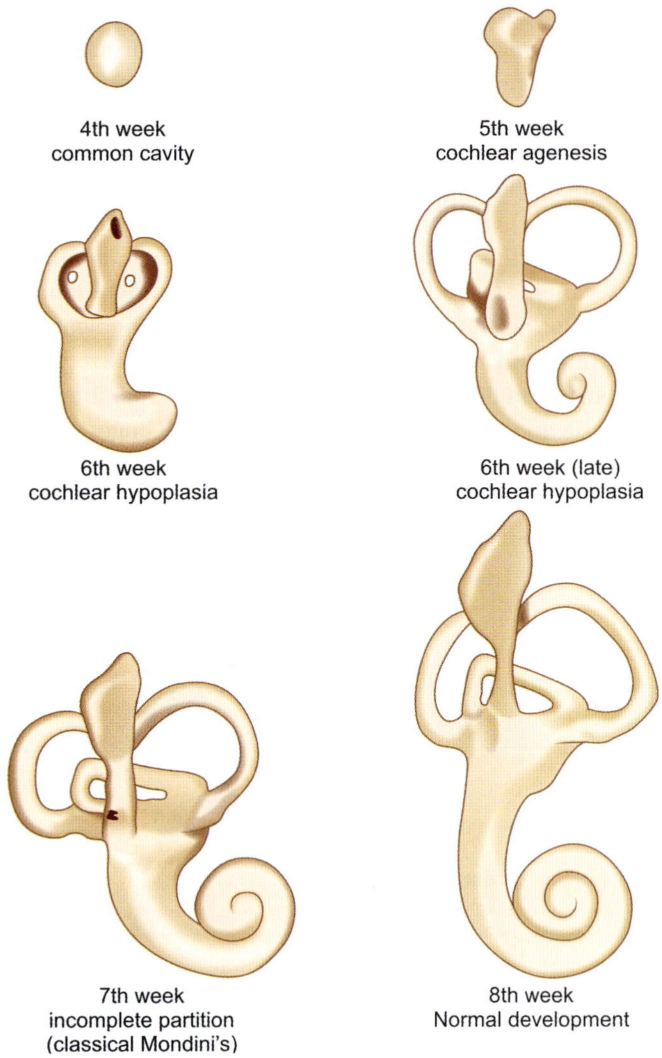

Fig. 1.22: A classification of inner ear malformations.
Source: Redrawn from Jackler et al.[84]

AUDITORY CORTEX

The auditory cortex is in the lateral (Sylvian) fissure.[84] It is arranged with low frequencies superior and high frequencies inferior. The auditory cortex exhibits plasticity in that it has the ability to modify or reorganize. Although this plasticity occurs throughout life, it occurs to a greater extent at younger ages. Modification of the tonotopic organization of the auditory cortex occurs after hearing loss and with rehabilitation of hearing (Fig. 1.23).

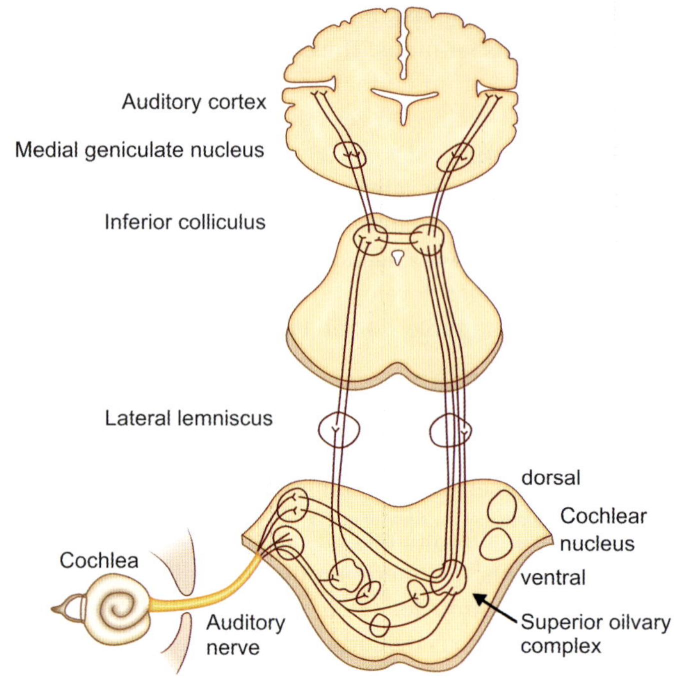

Fig. 1.23: The central auditory pathway.
Source: Redrawn from Nieuwenhuys.[87]

Clinical comment

- The auditory brainstem response is a test of the auditory pathway[85,86] Electrodes are placed at the mastoid and record the response to broadband clicks (centered on 3 kHz) or frequency specific tone bursts played by ear phones. It is absent when the pure tone average is >65 dB or age greater than approximately 65. Typically, five to seven peaks occur within 10 ms. The waves correspond to the following areas of the auditory pathway: Wave I—distal eighth nerve, corresponds with the action potential in electrocochleography, Wave II—proximal VIII/cochlear nuclei (dorsal + ventral), Wave III—superior olivary nucleus, Wave IV—lateral lemniscus, Wave V—contralateral inferior colliculus, Wave VI—Medial geniculate nucleus, Wave VII—Auditory cortex.

Note: Most fibers cross midline at superior olivary nucleus, while some continue uncrossed to inferior colliculus.[88-90]

REFERENCES

1. Petersson RS, Friedman O. Current trends in otoplasty. Curr Opin Otolaryngol Head Neck Surg. 2008;16(4):352-8.
2. Adamson PA, Litner JA. Otoplasty technique. Otolaryngol Clin North Am. 2007;40(2):305-18.
3. Imanishi N, Nakajima H, Aiso S. Arterial anatomy of the ear. Okajimas Folia Anat Jpn. 1997;73(6):313-23.
4. McKinnon BJ, Wall MP, Karakla DW. The vascular anatomy and angiosome of the posterior auricular artery. A cadaver study. Arch Facial Plast Surg. 1999;1(2):101-4.
5. Alvernia JE, Fraser K, Lanzino G. The occipital artery: a microanatomical study. Neurosurgery. 2006;58(1 suppl): ONS114-22; discussion ONS-22.
6. Houseman ND, Taylor GI, Pan WR. The angiosomes of the head and neck: anatomic study and clinical applications. Plast Reconstr Surg. 2000;105(7):2287-313.

7. Song R, Song Y, Qi K, et al. The superior auricular artery and retroauricular arterial island flaps. Plast Reconstr Surg. 1996;98(4):657-67; discussion 68-70.
8. Wright CG. Development of the human external ear. J Am Acad Audiol. 1997;8(6):379-82.
9. Klockars T, Rautio J. Embryology and epidemiology of microtia. Facial Plast Surg. 2009;25(3):145-8. Epub 2009/10/08.
10. Whitfield IC. Mechanisms of sound localization. Nature. 1971;233(5315):95-7. Epub 1971/09/10.
*11. Kelly KE, Mohs DC. The external auditory canal. Anatomy and physiology. Otolaryngol Clin North Am. 1996;29(5):725-39.
12. Chandler JR. Malignant external otitis and osteomyelitis of the base of the skull. Am J Otol. 1989;10(2):108-10.
13. Alberti PW. Epithelial migration on the tympanic membrane. J Laryngol Otol. 1964;78:808-30.
14. Santa Maria PL, Redmond SL, McInnes RL, et al. Tympanic membrane wound healing in rats assessed by transcriptome profiling. Laryngoscope. 2011;121(10):2199-213. doi: 10.1002/lary.22150.
15. Santa Maria PL, Redmond SL, Atlas MD, et al. Histology of the healing tympanic membrane following perforation in rats. Laryngoscope. 2010;120(10):2061-70.
16. Applebaum EL, Deutsch EC. Fluorescein angiography of the tympanic membrane. Laryngoscope. 1985;95(9 Pt 1):1054-8.
17. Mehta RP, Rosowski JJ, Voss SE, et al. Determinants of hearing loss in perforations of the tympanic membrane. Otol Neurotol. 2006;27(2):136-43.
18. Gray O. The chorda tympani. J Laryngol Otol. 1953;67(3):128-38.
19. Proctor B, Nielsen E, Proctor C. Petrosquamosal suture and lamina. Otolaryngol Head Neck Surg. 1981;89(3 Pt 1):482-95..
20. Bellucci RJ, Fisher EG, Rhodin J. Ultrastructure of the round window membrane. Laryngoscope. 1972;82(6):1021-6.
21. Su WY, Marion MS, Hinojosa R, et al. Anatomical measurements of the cochlear aqueduct, round window membrane, round window niche, and facial recess. Laryngoscope. 1982;92(5):483-6.
22. Stewart TJ, Belal A. Surgical anatomy and pathology of the round window. Clin Otolaryngol Allied Sci. 1981;6(1):45-62.
23. Monkhouse WS. The anatomy of the facial nerve. Ear Nose Throat J. 1990;69(10):677-83, 86-7.
24. Proctor B, Nager GT. The facial canal: normal anatomy, variations and anomalies. I. Normal anatomy of the facial canal. Ann Otol Rhinol Laryngol Suppl. 1982;97:33-44.
25. Sando I, English GM, Hemenway WG. Congenital anomalies of the facial nerve and stapes: a human temporal bone report. Laryngoscope. 1968;78(3):316-23.
26. Nager GT, Proctor B. The facial canal: normal anatomy, variations and anomalies. II. Anatomical variations and anomalies involving the facial canal. Ann Otol Rhinol Laryngol Suppl. 1982;97:45-61.
*27. Proctor B. The anatomy of the facial nerve. Otolaryngol Clin North Am. 1991;24(3):479-504.
28. Proctor B. Surgical anatomy of the posterior tympanum. Ann Otol Rhinol Laryngol. 1969;78(5):1026-40.
29. Donaldson JA, Anson BJ, Warpeha RL, et al. The surgical anatomy of the sinus tympani. Arch Otolaryngol. 1970;91(3):219-27.
30. Petrus LV, Lo WW. The anterior epitympanic recess: CT anatomy and pathology. AJNR Am J Neuroradiol. 1997;18(6):1109-14.
31. Gluth MB, Cohen MA, Friedland PL, et al. Surgical anatomy of the anterior supralabyrinthine air cell tract. J Laryngol Otol. 2011;125(10):1009-13. Epub 2011/06/15.
32. Richany SF, Anson BJ, Bast TH. The development and adult structure of the malleus, incus and stapes. Q Bull Northwest Univ Med Sch. 1954;28(1):17-45.
33. Anson BJ, Donaldson JA, Warpeha RL, et al. The surgical anatomy of the ossicular muscles and the facial nerve. Laryngoscope. 1967;77(8):1269-94.
34. Todd NW, Creighton FX Jr. Malleus and incus: correlates of size. Ann Otol Rhinol Laryngol. 2013;122(1):60-5.
35. Anson BJ, Bast TH. Anatomical structure of the stapes and the relation of the stapedial footplate to vital parts of the otic labyrinth. Ann Otol Rhinol Laryngol. 1958;67(2):389-99.
36. Backous DD, Minor LB, Aboujaoude ES, et al. Relationship of the utriculus and sacculus to the stapes footplate: anatomic implications for sound-and/or pressure-induced otolith activation. Ann Otol Rhinol Laryngol. 1999;108(6):548-53.
37. Margolis RH, Levine SC. Acoustic reflex measures in audiologic evaluation. Otolaryngol Clin North Am. 1991;24(2):329-47.
38. Borg E, Counter SA. The middle-ear muscles. Sci Am. 1989;261(2):74-80.
39. Hall CM. Stapedial reflex decay in retrocochlear and cochlear lesions. Review of procedures and methods for conducting SRD tests. Ann Otol Rhinol Laryngol. 1977;86(2 pt. 1):219-22.
*40. Proctor B. The development of the middle ear spaces and their surgical significance. J Laryngol Otol. 1964;78:631-48.
41. McMinn RMH, Last RJ. Last's anatomy: regional and applied, 9th edn. Edinburgh: Elsevier Health Sciences; 1994. 705p.
42. Tekdemir I, Aslan A, Tuccar E, et al. An anatomical study of the tympanic branch of the glossopharyngeal nerve (nerve of Jacobson). Ann Anat. 1998;180(4):349-52.
43. Daud AS, Pahor AL. Tympanic neurectomy in the management of parotid sialectasis. J Laryngol Otol. 1995;109(12):1155-8.
44. Thomas RL. Tympanic neurectomy and chorda tympani section. Aust N Z J Surg. 1980;50(4):352-5. Epub 1980/08/01.
45. Janfaza P, Nadol JB Jr, Galla RJ, et al. Surgical anatomy of the head and neck. Cambridge, MA: Harvard University Press; 2011. 932 p.
46. Pahor AL, Hussain SS. Persistent stapedial artery. J Laryngol Otol. 1992;106(3):254-7. Epub 1992/03/01.
47. Hesselink JR, Davis KR, Taveras JM. Selective arteriography of glomus tympanicum and jugulare tumors: techniques, normal and pathologic arterial anatomy. AJNR Am J Neuroradiol. 1981;2(4):289-97.
*48. Jackler RK. The surgical anatomy of cholesteatoma. Otolaryngol Clin North Am. 1989;22(5):883-96.

*References with asterisks refer to critical sources.

49. Palva T, Northrop C, Ramsay H. Aeration and drainage pathways of Prussak's space. Int J Pediatr Otorhinolaryngol. 2001;57(1):55-65. Epub 2001/02/13.
50. Huttenbrink KB. The mechanics of the middle-ear at static air pressures: the role of the ossicular joints, the function of the middle-ear muscles and the behaviour of stapedial prostheses. Acta Otolaryngol Suppl. 1988;451:1-35.
51. Caiazzo AJ, Tonndorf J. Ear canal resonance and temporary threshold shift. Otolaryngology. 1978;86(5):ORL-820.
52. Garcia-Gonzalez A, Gonzalez-Herrera A. Effect of the middle ear cavity on the response of the human auditory system. J Acoust Soc Am. 2013;133(5):3544.
53. Koike T, Wada H, Kobayashi T. Modeling of the human middle ear using the finite-element method. J Acoust Soc Am. 2002;111(3):1306-17.
54. Gan RZ, Reeves BP, Wang X. Modeling of sound transmission from ear canal to cochlea. Ann Biomed Eng. 2007;35(12):2180-95.
55. Sichel JY, Freeman S, Sohmer H. Lateralization during the Weber test: animal experiments. Laryngoscope. 2002;112(3):542-6.
56. Toth M, Alpar A, Bodon G, et al. Surgical anatomy of the cochlea for cochlear implantation. Ann Anat. 2006;188(4):363-70.
57. Gopen Q, Rosowski JJ, Merchant SN. Anatomy of the normal human cochlear aqueduct with functional implications. Hear Res. 1997;107(1-2):9-22.
58. Kimura RS. The ultrastructure of the organ of Corti. Int Rev Cytol. 1975;42:173-222.
59. Lim DJ. Cochlear anatomy related to cochlear micromechanics: A review. J Acoust Soc Am. 1980;67(5):1686-95.
*60. Lim DJ. Functional structure of the organ of Corti: a review. Hear Res. 1986;22:117-46.
61. Harada Y, Tagashira N, Takunida M, et al. Three-dimensional ultrastructure of cochlea: a review. Adv Otorhinolaryngol. 1990;45:49-68.
62. Roberts WM, Howard J, Hudspeth AJ. Hair cells: transduction, tuning, and transmission in the inner ear. Ann Rev Cell Biol. 1988;4:63-92.
63. Meyer AC, Moser T. Structure and function of cochlear afferent innervation. Curr Opin Otolaryngol Head Neck Surg. 2010;18(5):441-6.
64. Brownell WE. Outer hair cell electromotility and otoacoustic emissions. Ear Hear. 1990;11(2):82-92.
65. Dallos P. The role of outer hair cells in cochlear function. Prog Clin Biol Res. 1985;176:207-30.
66. Shulman A, Goldstein B, Strashun AM. Final common pathway for tinnitus: theoretical and clinical implications of neuroanatomical substrates. Int Tinnitus J. 2009;15(1):5-50. Epub 2009/10/22.
67. Zorowka PG. Otoacoustic emissions: a new method to diagnose hearing impairment in children. Eur J Pediatr. 1993;152(8):626-34.
68. Guinan JJ, Jr, Salt A, Cheatham MA. Progress in cochlear physiology after Bekesy. Hear Res. 2012;293(1-2):12-20.
69. Schratzenstaller B, Janssen T, Alexiou C, et al. Confirmation of G. von Bekesy's theory of paradoxical wave propagation along the cochlear partition by means of bone-conducted auditory brainstem responses. ORL J Otorhinolaryngol Relat Spec. 2000;62(1):1-8.
70. Anniko M, Wroblewski R. Ionic environment of cochlear hair cells. Hear Res. 1986;22:279-93.
71. Waltner JG, Raymond S. On the chemical composition of the human perilymph and endolymph. Laryngoscope. 1950;60(9):912-8.
72. Anson BJ, Winch TR, Warpeha RL, et al. The blood supply of the otic capsule of the human ear, with special reference to that of the cochlea. Ann Otol Rhinol Laryngol. 1966;75(4):921-44.
73. Anson BJ, Warpeha RL, Rensink MJ. The gross and macroscopic anatomy of the labyrinths. Ann Otol Rhinol Laryngol. 1968;77(4):583-607.
74. Mazzoni A. The vascular anatomy of the vestibular labyrinth in man. Acta Otolaryngol Suppl. 1990;472:1-83.
75. Spoendlin H. Anatomy of cochlear innervation. Am J Otolaryngol. 1985;6(6):453-67.
76. Wangemann P. K+ cycling and the endocochlear potential. Hear Res. 2002;165(1-2):1-9. Epub 2002/05/29.
77. Rhoton AL, Jr, Tedeschi H. Microsurgical anatomy of acoustic neuroma. Otolaryngol Clin North Am. 1992;25(2):257-94.
78. Mazzoni A, Hansen CC. Surgical anatomy of the arteries of the internal auditory canal. Arch Otolaryngol. 1970;91(2):128-35.
79. Silverstein H, Norrell H, Haberkamp T, et al. The unrecognized rotation of the vestibular and cochlear nerves from the labyrinth to the brain stem: its implications to surgery of the eighth cranial nerve. Otolaryngol Head Neck Surg. 1986;95(5):543-9.
80. Mazzoni A. Internal auditory canal arterial relations at the porus acusticus. Ann Otol Rhinol Laryngol. 1969;78(4):797-814.
81. Unel S, Yilmaz M, Albayram S, et al. Anastomoses of the vestibular, cochlear, and facial nerves. J Craniofac Surg. 2012;23(5):1358-61.
82. Pujol R, Lavigne-Rebillard M, Uziel A. Development of the human cochlea. Acta Otolaryngol Suppl. 1991;482:7-12; discussion 3.
83. Freeman S, Geal-Dor M, Sohmer H. Development of inner ear (cochlear and vestibular) function in the fetus-neonate. J Basic Clin Physiol Pharmacol. 1999;10(3):173-89.
*84. Jackler RK, Luxford WM, House WF. Congenital malformations of the inner ear: a classification based on embryogenesis. Laryngoscope. 1987;97(3 Pt 2 Suppl 40):2-14.
85. Suehiro S, Sando I. Congenital anomalies of the inner ear: introducing a new classification of labyrinthine anomalies. Ann Otol Rhinol Laryngol Suppl. 1979;88(4 Pt 3 Suppl 59):1-24.
86. Sennaroglu L, Saatci I. A new classification for cochleovestibular malformations. Laryngoscope. 2002;112(12):2230-41.
87. Nieuwenhuys R. Anatomy of the auditory pathways, with emphasis on the brain stem. Adv Otorhinolaryngol. 1984;34:25-38.
88. Borg E. Physiological mechanisms in auditory brainstem-evoked response. Scand Audiol Suppl. 1981;13:11-22.
89. Miller CA, Brown CJ, Abbas PJ, et al. The clinical application of potentials evoked from the peripheral auditory system. Hear Res. 2008;242(1-2):184-97.
90. Luxon LM. The anatomy and pathology of the central auditory pathways. Br J Audiol. 1981;15(1):31-40.

*References with asterisks refer to critical sources.

CHAPTER 2

Evaluation of Auditory Function

Janet Koehnke, Faith M Mogila, Maris Appelbaum, Joan Besing

This chapter is designed to provide an overview of the profession of audiology. It begins with a brief history of audiology followed by a description of the scope of practice of audiologists and some facts and figures on the incidence of hearing loss. The remainder of the chapter describes the diagnostic test procedures conducted by audiologists. These include subjective measures such as pure tone air conduction and bone conduction thresholds, speech recognition thresholds, and speech intelligibility tests as well as objective measures such as middle ear immittance, evoked otoacoustic emissions (OAEs), auditory brainstem tests, and vestibular tests. Each procedure is described briefly along with examples of typical test results and a discussion of the interpretation of results. The chapter concludes with some ideas about the future of audiologic assessment.

BRIEF HISTORY

The profession of audiology emerged in the late 1940s as many soldiers from World War II returned home suffering from prolonged exposure to the sounds of artillery, grenades, sirens, aircraft, and the like. The term itself was coined by three different individuals at about the same time in the mid-1940s, an otolaryngologist, Norton Canfield, a speech pathologist, Raymond Carhart, and an auditory scientist, Hallowell Davis.[1] Shortly thereafter, specialized institutions were developed to serve the needs of military personnel returning from active duty who were experiencing difficulty hearing and understanding speech and hearing essential sounds such as alarms, honking horns, and other important auditory information.

Since then the field of audiology has developed and grown into a flourishing profession, serving the needs of individuals across the lifespan who experience hearing and/or vestibular problems. Dr. James Jerger, one of Carhart's first audiology students, was one of the pioneers of the profession; he developed many of the early test methods and procedures, including the Carhart-Jerger method for the measurement of pure-tone thresholds.[2] This procedure is followed to this day and is the foundation of audiometric threshold testing that is the basis for all differential diagnosis in audiology. Dr. Jerger has also written a book entitled *Audiology in the USA*, which details the history and development of the profession.[1]

Audiology is the study of hearing and balance function and disorders; audiologists evaluate auditory and vestibular function and provide rehabilitation for individuals across the lifespan identified with pathologies of these systems. It is also important to note that audiologists strive to inform and educate people about ways to prevent hearing loss as well as cope with the challenges presented by their hearing loss.

The professional activities of audiologists are clearly defined by the two largest organizations representing them, the American-Speech-Language-Hearing Association (ASHA), and the American Academy of Audiology (AAA). In addition, all 50 states license or certify audiologists and have established guidelines for practicing in those states. According to the ASHA Scope of Practice for audiologists, "The practice of audiology includes both the prevention of and assessment of auditory, vestibular, and related impairments as well as the habilitation/rehabilitation and maintenance of persons with these impairments.

The overall goal of the provision of audiology services should be to optimize and enhance the ability of an individual to hear, as well as to communicate in his/her everyday or natural environment".[3] Similarly, the AAA Scope of Practice states, "Audiologists identify, assess, diagnose, and treat individuals with impairment of either peripheral or central auditory and/or vestibular function, and strive to prevent such impairments".[4] Both of these documents also stipulate that practicing audiologists must, at all times, adhere to the Code of Ethics of the respective organization.

SCOPE OF PRACTICE

The scope of practice for the profession has grown dramatically over the past 30–40 years. It was not until 1977 that audiologists began dispensing hearing aids and other assistive devices. As technology has advanced, hearing aids have evolved from body worn analog devices to completely in-the-ear and small behind the ear digital devices. Along with the progress in hearing aid technology came the development of the cochlear implant and the bone anchored hearing aid in the 1960s. Cochlear implants have evolved from single channel devices that were first available commercially in 1972, to multiple channel systems that were introduced in 1984 and provide remarkably accurate auditory input to individuals with profound hearing loss.[5] All of these advances in remediation have resulted in the expansion of the profession of audiology and the need for skilled audiologists.

Although the middle latency response (MLR) and the late auditory evoked potentials (AEPs) were first discovered in the late 1950s, the introduction of clinical electrophysiologic tests including auditory brainstem testing and evoked OAEs testing did not commence until the late 1970s. Together, these diagnostic procedures have contributed to the growth of the profession of audiology. More recently, audiologists have become involved in the evaluation and treatment of vestibular pathologies and in intraoperative monitoring of brainstem and cortical responses during surgical procedures. Clearly, audiology is a rapidly growing and developing profession. Currently, there are >12,000 audiologists in the United States.[6] According to the US Bureau of Labor Statistics this number is expected to grow to about 17,000 by the year 2020.[7] This is a rate of 37%, which is much more rapid than most professions.

Audiologists work as independent practitioners in a variety of settings including private practice, schools, hospitals, community clinics, otolaryngology offices, industry, university clinics, and the military. They may also be involved in the education of audiology students as well as medical residents and interns and other health professionals. Audiologists serve a diverse population across the lifespan including individuals of all races, genders, religions, national origins, and sexual orientations.

DEMOGRAPHICS OF HEARING LOSS

Along with the expanding breadth of the profession, there is an increased need for audiologists and audiologic services. This is, of course, due to the growing numbers of individuals with hearing loss. According to the National Institute on Deafness and Other Communicative Disorders (NIDCD) of the NIH, 17% (36 million) of American adults report some degree of hearing loss. More specifically, the NIDCD reports that "18 percent of American adults 45–64 years old, 30 percent of adults 65–74 years old, and 47 percent of adults 75 years old or older have a hearing loss".[8] World Health Organization statistics indicate that, worldwide, 360 million people (including 328 million adults and 32 million children) experience "disabling" hearing loss. They define disabling as "hearing loss >40 dB in the better hearing ear in adults and a hearing loss >30 dB in the better hearing ear in children".[9]

In the newborn population, the incidence of hearing loss continues to be reported as two or three individuals per 1000 births in the United States.[8] As a result of the 1993 NIH Consensus Conference on Newborn Screenings, programs to evaluate every newborn have been established in all 50 states. This has led to earlier identification of hearing loss and auditory pathologies, which, in turn, results in appropriate intervention at an earlier age. Despite earlier detection of hearing loss in newborns, according to Niskar et al.[10], about 12.5% of children and adolescents in the United States aged 6–19 years (approximately 5.2 million) experience permanent hearing loss due to exposure to loud sounds. These numbers have likely increased in the past decade due to the use of personal listening systems and the popularity of clubbing and concert-going among teenagers and young adults. According to the NIDCD, approximately 15% of Americans age 20–69 have high-frequency hearing loss due to exposure to loud sounds or noise in some aspect of their daily lives.[8] Other important statistics regarding hearing loss and auditory pathologies can be obtained from the NIDCD, the Centers for Disease Control, the World Health Organization, and the Hearing Health Foundation to name just a few sources.

In our work as audiologists, it is imperative that we collaborate with other professionals to ensure that we provide the best possible care for our patients. Clearly, it is necessary for us to refer to and consult frequently with otolaryngologists. By working together closely and conferring with each other, we can effectively monitor the auditory status of our patients. Individuals receiving implantable devices and those experiencing pathologies such as Meniere's Disease, acoustic neuroma, or cholesteatoma represent just a few of the many individuals for whom collaborative care between audiologists and otolaryngologists is so essential.

Of course, there are many other health professionals with whom audiologists work on a regular basis. When diagnosing an infant with hearing loss it is imperative to consult with social workers, psychologists, and speech-language pathologists as well as physicians. For children with hearing loss, audiologists confer with teachers and other support personnel in the schools. Adults with gradual or sudden onset hearing loss may need not only hearing aids or other assistive devices, but also help obtaining accommodations in the workplace. In such instances, audiologists are likely to interact with vocational counselors and possibly other individuals in state and local agencies to assist their patients. For geriatric patients, audiologists consult with home healthcare workers, personnel at senior centers and assisted living facilities, and others to achieve optimal auditory input in the environment where these individuals spend their time. Clearly, the overall goal is to work cooperatively to meet the needs of our patients.

CLINICAL AUDIOLOGIC PROCEDURES

A complete audiologic evaluation typically includes assessment, using insert or circumaural earphones, of pure-tone air and bone conduction thresholds as well as spondee thresholds and word recognition testing. In addition to these tests, an immittance battery and OAEs should always be included. The results of these procedures should provide comprehensive evidence for differential diagnosis. These findings also provide direction for habilitation/rehabilitation of the patient.

As with most clinical protocols, changes and adjustments in technique may be required to address any special needs or concerns of the patients. However, these adaptations should not sacrifice the fundamentals on which the following tests are designed and implemented.

Air and Bone Conduction

Audiometric assessment is an integral component in otologic evaluation of a patient who is suspected of having an auditory and/or vestibular pathology. Testing should be completed by a state licensed audiologist in a quiet room

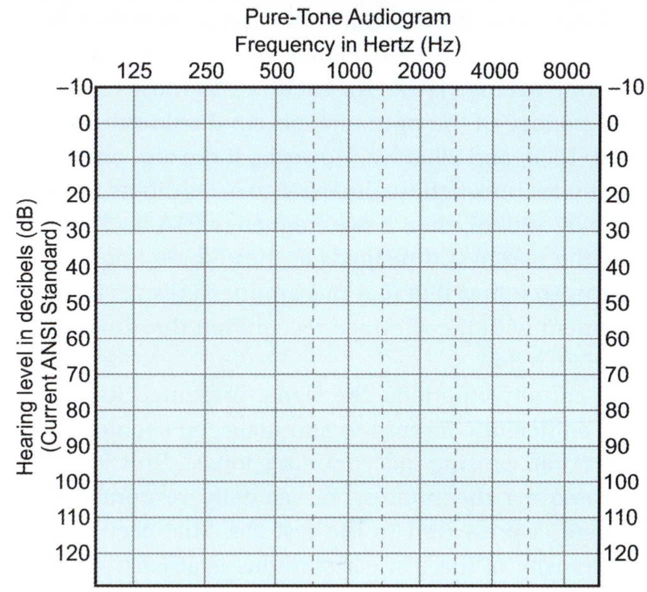

Fig. 2.1: Typical audiogram form used to record audiometric air and bone conduction thresholds.

with minimal ambient noise. Test results may be recorded on a table or displayed on an audiogram such as the one shown in Figure 2.1.

Prior to audiometric testing, a case history and otoscopy should be performed. Any obstruction in the outer ear could potentially affect pure tone responses. The tympanic membrane should be visible bilaterally during otoscopy. Obtaining a case history can provide information to assist the audiologist in determining the order in which the tests are conducted.

Optimally, air conduction, as well as bone conduction testing, is completed in a double-walled sound-treated booth with the patient wearing insert or circumaural earphones. All equipment utilized for testing should be calibrated annually. Air conduction stimuli pass through the outer, middle and ultimately, the inner ear on the way to the auditory cortex. Bone conduction stimuli are delivered directly to the cochlea through a bone oscillator placed on the mastoid bone. Pure tone signals are used to establish thresholds at specific frequencies. For air conduction, the octave frequencies from 250 to 8000 Hz are tested. In addition, if there is a 20 dB or greater difference between the thresholds at these adjacent frequencies, the interoctaves, 1500, 3000, and/or 6000 Hz, should be tested. Bone conduction thresholds are obtained in response to signals at the octave frequencies from 250 to 4000 Hz. Threshold testing should follow a standardized method such as those outlined by the American National Standards Institute,[11] the American Speech-Language-Hearing Association,[12] or the Carhart-Jerger procedure.[2]

Once air conduction and bone conduction thresholds are obtained, it is standard clinical practice to calculate the pure tone average (PTA) for each ear. In most cases, this is the average of the pure tone air conduction thresholds at 500, 1000, and 2000 Hz. However, if the air conduction threshold at one of these three frequencies differs from the others by >20 dB, then a two frequency PTA is calculated using the two best thresholds at these three frequencies. It has been found that that this approach results in better agreement with the spondee recognition threshold (SRT) described below.

In certain situations, the signal presented to the test ear is sufficiently intense to stimulate the cochlea of the nontest ear, causing inaccurate responses. This is known as crossover; the nontest ear actually responds when the tone is presented to the test ear. This occurs when the intensity of the test ear stimulus is at least 40 dB or greater (circumaural earphone) or 55 dB or greater (insert earphone) than the bone conduction threshold in the nontest ear. The term interaural attenuation is used to describe the amount of sound absorbed by the head before the sound presented to the test ear is intense enough to stimulate the opposite cochlea. The specific value varies as a function of frequency as well as the transducer used for testing. The values cited above are conservative estimates used clinically to ensure that crossover is not occurring during testing. To be certain the nontest ear is not being stimulated resulting in inaccurate responses, masking procedures must be employed. Thus, if the presentation level of the pure-tone in the test ear exceeds the bone conduction threshold in the nontest ear by these values (40 and 55 dB for circumaural and insert earphones, respectively), masking is presented to the nontest ear via air conduction using an insert or circumaural earphone.

For bone conduction testing, the interaural attenuation is 10 dB. This means that if the bone conduction stimulus level and the air conduction threshold differ by >10 dB in the ear being tested or in the nontest ear, masking is necessary at that frequency. The reason for this value is because when a stimulus is presented via bone conduction, all of the bones in the skull are stimulated, not just the ones in the cochlea closest to the bone oscillator. The interaural attenuation is thus minimal resulting in the use of the 10 dB value for determining the need for masking. Use of appropriate masking techniques is essential to obtain accurate threshold measurements.

Example audiograms are provided in Figures 2.2 to 2.5 to illustrate typical results obtained for bilateral and/or unilateral losses as well as conductive (Fig. 2.4), sensorineural (Fig. 2.2), mixed type hearing loss (Fig. 2.5), and a functional hearing loss (also referred to as malingering, Fig. 2.3). Each case includes results for pure tone air and bone conduction tests as well as many of the other tests described below such as OAEs, tympanometry, word recognition, etc.

Speech Testing

The SRT is used as a reliability check for the pure tone findings. The PTA described above should be within ±6 dB of the spondee threshold.[13] The SRT is measured by presenting two syllable words, called spondee words, with equal stress on each syllable. The words can be presented using either recorded speech or monitored live voice. Standardized testing procedures must be employed. The outcome of this measure is a threshold for speech and should be in good agreement with the average of the pure-tone thresholds at 500, 1000, and 2000 Hz (PTA). There may be times when traditional SRT testing cannot be employed. Examples of this might be with non-native speakers of English, infants, or difficult to test patients. In cases such as these, a speech detection threshold (SDT) or a speech awareness threshold (SAT) would be obtained. The preferred term according to ASHA[14] is SDT because it is an accurate description of the task of exhibiting a behavioral change to spondee words or cold running speech. The SDT is often lower than the expected SRT because it requires the patient only to detect rather than recognize and correctly repeat speech stimuli.

The other speech test typically administered is used to obtain the word recognition score (WRS), using monosyllabic words. This suprathreshold test should be administered 30–40 dB above the SRT.[15] The goal of word recognition testing is to determine the best score a patient can attain. In some cases, this test may need to be administered at more than one intensity to find the level of maximum performance. This level is known as PB max (phonetically balanced) and is the highest speech recognition score that is determined using a PI function (performance intensity).

According to Gelfand,[16] speech recognition measures are used in every phase of audiology such as (1) to describe how hearing loss affects speech understanding, (2) in the differential diagnosis of auditory disorders, and (3) for determining the need for amplification and other forms of audiologic rehabilitation. Word recognition measures can also be used as part of a monitoring protocol, when needed. In patients with a sensorineural hearing loss, it is expected that the WRS will decrease as the severity of the loss increases. When dealing with a conductive loss, however, WRSs often approach the "excellent" range due to the normal bone conduction scores, when the words

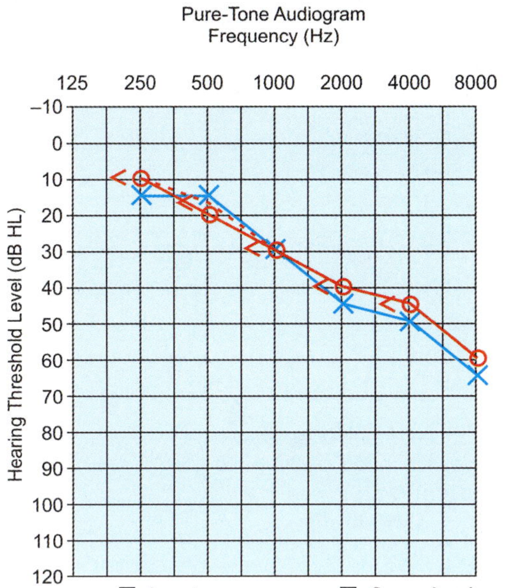

☑ Inserts ☐ Supra-Aural

	PTA	SRT/SAT	WRS	
Right (AD)	30	30	76%	60 dB HL
Masked				
Left (AS)	50	50	80%	80 dB HL
Masked				50 dB HL

	MCL	UCL	WRS	
Right (AD)				
Masked				
Left (AS)				
Masked				

TEOAE	Right Ear	Left Ear
	Fail	Fail

Key:

Right		Left
o	Air	x
<	Bone	>
Δ	Masked Air	☐
[	Masked Bone	]
↓	No Response	↓
R	Aided soundfield	L
	Soundfield ~ or s	

RE		LE
1.2 cc	V_{ea}	1.4 cc
0 daPa	Pk Press	–30
9 mmho	Pk St Comp	1 mmho
80	Tymp Width	90 daPa
A	Type	A

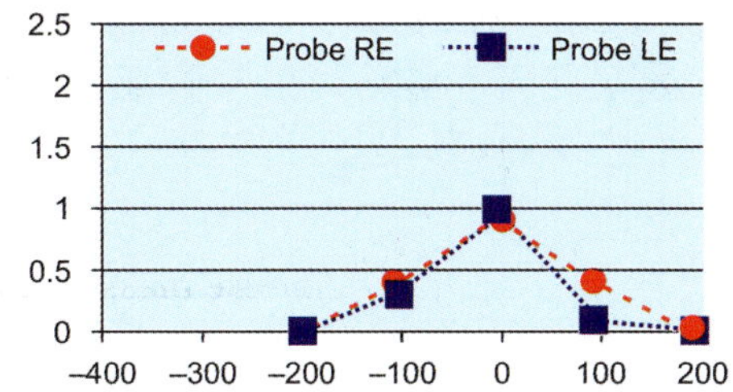

Otoscopy: RE: Clear
LE: Clear

Stimulus–500 Hz

Probe	RE	LE	Decay
RE	85	95	NEG
LE	90	90	NEG

Stimulus–1000 Hz

Probe	RE	LE	Decay
RE	95	95	NEG
LE	95	95	NEG

Stimulus–2000 Hz

Probe	RE	LE	Decay
RE	95	100	DNT
LE	95	95	DNT

Fig. 2.2: Results for a 75-year-old patient. The pure tone results indicate a bilateral, symmetrical sensorineural hearing loss. Hearing thresholds are normal through 500 Hz, sloping to a mild sensorineural loss at 1000 and 2000 Hz, with a moderately severe loss at 8000 Hz. Good agreement between the PTA and SRT is noted. Immittance results indicate normal middle ear function. The patient has good word recognition scores bilaterally. TEOAE results indicate refer bilaterally. Audiologic recommendations for this patient would include hearing aids and perhaps other assistive devices. (PTA, pure-tone average; SRT, spondee recognition threshold; TEOAE. transient evoked otoacoustic emissions).

are presented at 30–40 dB above the SRT. In contrast, individuals with cochlear pathology usually have WRSs between 60% and 90% when measured at the same relative level. Scores for this group vary widely depending upon the degree and configuration of hearing loss. For patients with retrocochlear pathologies, an often observed result is WRS much poorer than expected based on the degree of hearing loss. For example, a patient with a PTA of 30 dBHL may obtain a WRS of 54% when tested at 30 or 40 dB above the PTA.

In addition to the traditional word lists used to obtain speech scores, there are other tests that can accomplish the same goal. When testing a child or a patient who is unable to verbally respond, tests such as the Word Intelligibility by Picture Identification—WIPI,[17] Northwestern University Children's Perception of Speech—NU-CHIPS,[18] or Pediatric Speech Intelligibility Test—PSI may be utilized.[19] These tests require the patient to point to a picture in a closed set that corresponds to the word they heard the audiologist speak. Tests also exist to assess how well a patient can hear in noise. In these tests, a target stimulus (word or sentence) is presented in the presence of background noise. Examples of these tests are the BKB-SIN, the Quick-SIN and the Revised Speech Perception in Noise Test.[20]

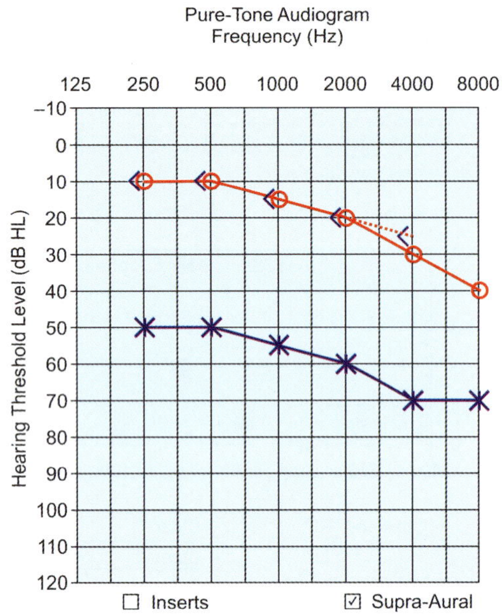

	PTA	SRT/SAT	WRS	
Right (AD)	15	10	100%	45 dB HL
Masked				
Left (AS)	55	10	100%	45 dB HL
Masked				35 dB HL

	MCL	UCL	WRS	
Right (AD)				
Masked				
Left (AS)				
Masked				

TEOAE	Right Ear	Left Ear
	Pass	Pass

Key:

Right		Left
o	Air	x
<	Bone	>
Δ	Masked Air	□
[	Masked Bone	]
↓	No Response	↓
R	Aided soundfield	L
	Soundfield ~ or s	

RE		LE
1.3 cc	V_{ea}	1.4 cc
0 daPa	Pk Press	0 daPa
1.9 mmho	Pk St Comp	1 mmho
80 daPa	Tymp Width	90 daPa
A	Type	A

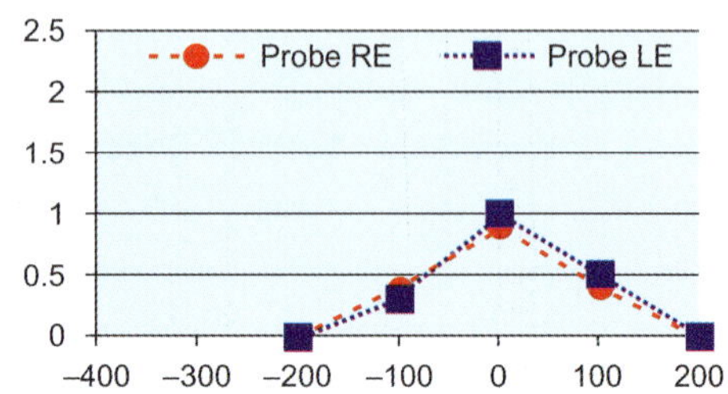

Otoscopy: RE: ____
LE: ____

Stimulus–500 Hz

Probe	RE	LE	Decay
RE	80	90	
LE	90	85	NEG

Stimulus–1000 Hz

Probe	RE	LE	Decay
RE	85	90	
LE	90	85	NEG

Stimulus–2000 Hz

Probe	RE	LE	Decay
RE	80	90	
LE	90	90	DNT

Fig. 2.3: These are results for a 15-year-old male who reported a sudden hearing loss in his left ear following an automobile accident. Test results were inconsistent. Right ear thresholds indicate normal hearing from 250 to 2000 Hz with a mild high frequency loss. Left ear results indicate a moderate hearing loss from 250 to 1000 Hz, sloping to moderately-severe from 2000 to 8000 Hz. Left ear thresholds reveal a shadow curve because interaural attenuation has been exceeded; therefore, crossover cannot be ruled out. The poor PTA–SRT agreement, normal tympanogram and acoustic reflexes, as well as "pass" OAE results for the left ear suggest that this patient is malingering. Recommendations for this patient would include a complete audiologic re-evaluation in 3–6 months. (PTA, pure-tone average; SRT, spondee recognition threshold; OAE, otoacoustic emission).

Immittance

An integral part of a complete audiologic evaluation is the inclusion of the immittance test battery. Immittance protocols are used to evaluate middle ear status and the function of the ipsilateral and contralateral reflex patterns.

Otoscopy should be performed prior to immittance to rule out any complications or pre-existing conditions that may contraindicate the use of this battery. Some examples of conditions that may preclude the use of tympanometry include a draining ear or cerumen that occludes the ear canal. The series of tests administered includes tympanometry, determination of the ipsilateral and contralateral reflex thresholds, and observation of reflex decay (if any).

In order for the tests to be performed, a pneumatic seal between the probe assembly and the patient's outer ear must be obtained. Failure to obtain a seal prevents completion of the test.

Tympanometry is the first portion of the immittance battery. Once the seal is obtained, a probe tone is presented

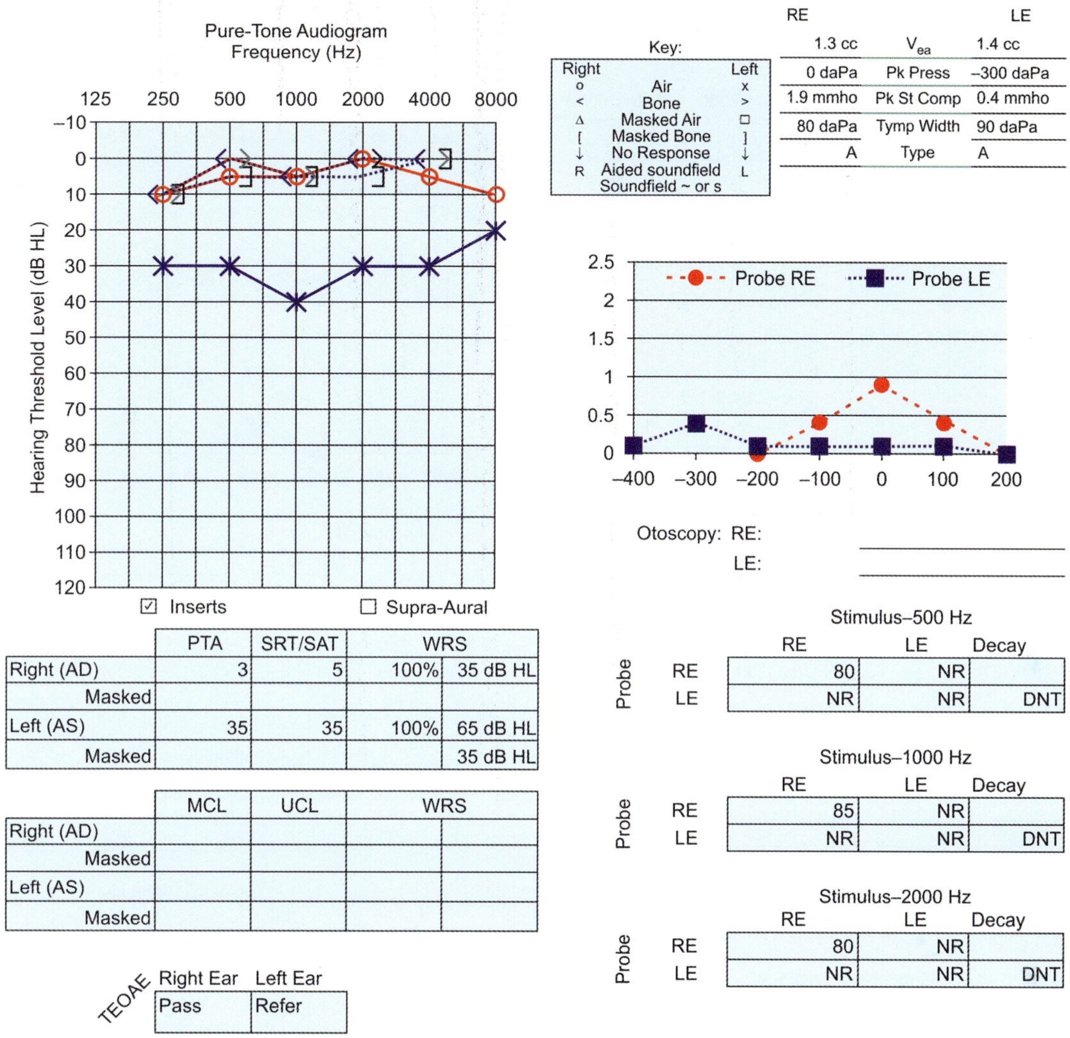

Fig. 2.4: Audiometric results for a 6-years-old with a history of chronic, recurrent otitis media. Pure tone thresholds in the right ear are within normal limits by air and bone conduction. Left ear thresholds indicate a mild flat conductive loss from 250 to 4000 Hz, gently rising to normal hearing at 8000 Hz. Note the excellent word recognition scores in the left ear, which are expected with a purely conductive loss. The air-bone gaps present from 250 to 4000 Hz in the left ear are also indicative of a conductive component. Tympanometry reveals negative pressure and reduced compliance in that ear. This patient "referred" on OAE results left ear, and "passed" right ear. Recommendations for this patient would include referral to an otolaryngologist. (OAE, otoacoustic emission).

to the patient's outer ear and the pressure in the canal is varied to determine the point of maximum compliance of the middle ear system. The probe tone used for individuals over 6 months of age is 226 Hz, while a 1000 Hz probe tone is used for patients who are newborn to 6 months old. More information regarding the use of tympanometry in the pediatric population can be found in several pediatric audiology textbooks.[21]

Tympanograms are interpreted on several parameters: (1) ear canal volume, (2) equivalent peak pressure, and (3) static admittance. In more recent years, tympanometric width has been added to the parameters that are used in the assessment of middle ear function. Table 2.1 summarizes the normative data for these tympanometric parameters described by ASHA.[22]

Interpretation of tympanometric width (or gradient) was introduced in 1968 by Brooks. It is a measure of the sharpness of the peak of the tympanogram. The gradient can be measured by bisecting the distance from the peak to the positive end of the tympanogram. Tympanometric width is reported in dekapascals (daPa). According to ASHA,[22] the normal range is 60–150 daPa for children

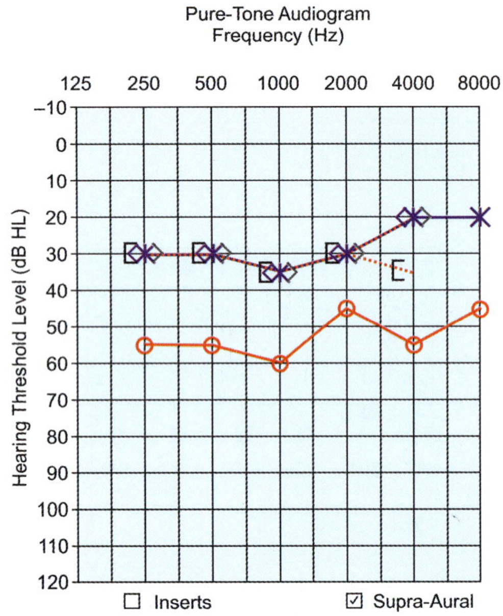

Right	Key:	Left
o	Air	x
<	Bone	>
Δ	Masked Air	□
[	Masked Bone	]
↓	No Response	↓
R	Aided soundfield	L
	Soundfield ~ or s	

RE		LE
1.3 cc	V_{ea}	1.4 cc
0 daPa	Pk Press	NA
1.3 mmho	Pk St Comp	1 mmho
NA	Tymp Width	80 daPa
A	Type	A

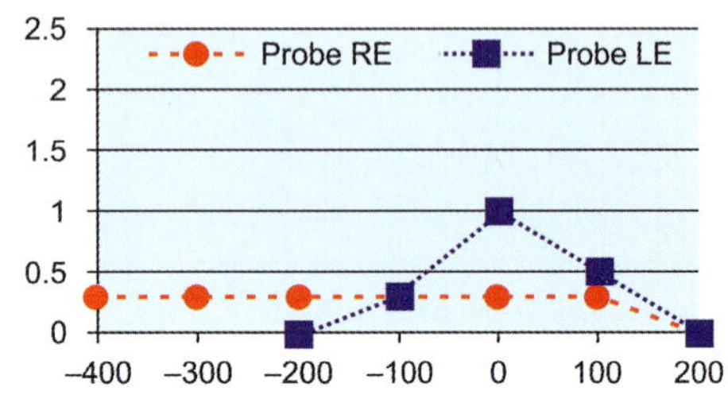

Otoscopy: RE: ______

LE: ______

	PTA	SRT/SAT	WRS	
Right (AD)	55	55	80%	85 dB HL
Masked				65 dB HL
Left (AS)	13.3	15	88%	55 dB HL
Masked				

	MCL	UCL	WRS	
Right (AD)				
Masked				
Left (AS)				
Masked				

TEOAE	Right Ear	Left Ear
	Pass	Pass

Stimulus–500 Hz

Probe	RE	LE	Decay
RE	NR	NR	
LE	NR	95	NEG

Stimulus–1000 Hz

Probe	RE	LE	Decay
RE	NR	NR	
LE	NR	90	NEG

Stimulus–2000 Hz

Probe	RE	LE	Decay
RE	NR	NR	
LE	NR	95	DNT

Fig. 2.5: These results are for a 55-year-old patient with a history of a mild sensorineural hearing loss. He came to the clinic complaining of stuffiness and pressure in the right ear. Left ear thresholds reveal a mild sensorineural loss from 250 to 2000 Hz, rising to normal hearing at 4000 Hz. Right ear thresholds reveal a moderate mixed loss at 250 and 500 Hz, sloping to a moderate loss at and above 1000 Hz. The air-bone gaps present from 250 to 4000 Hz, and the bone conduction thresholds >25 dBHL indicate a conductive component in that ear. Tympanometry reveals a flat configuration in the right ear, and a normal result in the left ear. TEOAE responses were "refer", bilaterally. Recommendations for this patient should include referral to an otolaryngologist, and annual audiologic evaluations.

and 50–100 daPa for adults. Abnormal tympanometric width should be considered an indication of middle ear dysfunction.[23]

In 1970, Jerger introduced a classification system for tympanograms using a 226 Hz probe tone that is still in use today. Based on this system, tympanograms are characterized as either type A, A_d, A_s, C, or B.[24]

During tympanometry, the external ear canal pressure is changed from atmospheric pressure (0 daPa) to 200 daPa above the ambient pressure and down to 200–600 daPa below the ambient pressure. As would be expected, maximum compliance will be obtained when the pressure on each side of the tympanic membrane is the same. So, in order to evaluate middle ear status in a clinical population, the pressure in the outer ear is adjusted to find the point of maximum compliance. In some cases, there is no point of maximum compliance (Jerger type B). This is commonly seen in patients whose ears have middle ear effusion or have patent ventilating tubes in the tympanic membrane.

In cases where the pressure in the external canal has to be a negative value to achieve maximum compliance, the tympanic membrane has been shown to be retracted into the middle ear space (Jerger type C).

Table 2.1: Normative data for use in interpretation of tympanograms*

Type	*Ear canal volume (ECV) in cc*	*Tympanometric peak pressure (daPa)†*	*Admittance (mmho)*
A	0.6–1.5 (adults) 0.4–1.0 (children)	+100 to −100 daPa	0.3–1.4 mmho (adults) 0.2–0.9 mmho (children)
A_d	0.6–1.5 (adults) 0.4–1.0 (children)	+100 to −100 daPa	>1.4 mmho
A_s	0.6–1.5 (adults) 0.4–1.0 (children)	+100 to −100 daPa	<0.3 mmho (adults) <0.2 mmho (children)
C	0.6–1.5 (adults) 0.4–1.0 (children)	>−100 daPa	0.3–1.4 mmho (adults) 0.2–0.9 mmho (children)
B	Varies based on pathology: PE tubes, perforations, etc. = larger ECV	No peak recorded	Essentially flat

*Values in this table are taken from ASHA.[22]

†It should be noted that there is no clear cutoff in terms of peak pressure which definitely indicates the presence of middle ear effusion. The norms listed above should be considered in conjunction with case history, otoscopy, and audiometric findings.

For patients who have normal middle ear pressure (i.e. the point of maximum compliance is at ambient pressure) (Jerger type A), there can be changes in mobility of the middle ear system. The mobility may be reduced (Jerger type A_s) or greater than normal (Jerger type A_d). These tympanogram types may be seen in patients with stapes fixation or ossicular discontinuity, respectively.

It should be noted that these Jerger classifications that were established in the 1970s are still in use but are not adequate to completely describe middle ear function. Further, the use of these classifications is limited to findings obtained with a 226 Hz probe tone in adults. Because the typical middle ear system is stiffness dominated, the use of this probe frequency does not allow an analysis of the effects of changes in mass on the middle ear system.

In order to further assess the effects of changes in middle ear stiffness and the possible effects of changes in mass components on the middle ear, multifrequency, multicomponent tympanometric protocols have been developed. The details of this type of tympanometry are beyond the scope of this chapter but interested readers should consult Wiley and Fowler.[25]

An area of middle ear assessment that is beginning to be used clinically is wideband reflectance. This is a procedure that does not require a pneumatic seal or adjustment of pressure in the outer ear canal to evaluate the middle ear system. In the future, wideband reflectance may prove to be a more flexible tool than tympanometry. This technique relies on measurement of amount of energy that is transferred through the middle ear system and so gives information about the input impedance of the middle ear. Using this technique, we get an estimate of the magnitude of reflectance as a function of frequency. The reflectance is a ratio of the reflected sound to the input sound. A low reflectance value indicates that most of the sound power in the incident wave is delivered to the middle ear system. In contrast, a high reflectance value indicates that most of the sound power is reflected back into the ear canal. For more information regarding this tool, *see* Keefe and Feeney.[26]

Figures 2.6 to 2.10 provide examples of the most commonly observed tympanograms elicited in response to a 226 Hz probe tone.

Acoustic Reflexes

Measurements of acoustic reflexes are useful in the evaluation of middle ear function, auditory nerve function, brainstem function, and facial nerve function. It is important to note that the acoustic reflex threshold is an indirect measure of the integrity of the reflex pathway. In order to measure an acoustic reflex, the stapedius muscle must contract. Contraction of the muscle creates a change in middle ear compliance that can be observed. The acoustic reflex is a bilateral event. Observation of a compliance change in the same ear as the reflex activating stimulus (RAS) is referred to as an ipsilateral reflex. In contrast, an observation of a change in compliance in the ear opposite the RAS is referred to as a contralateral reflex. The lowest stimulus level that produces a change in acoustic admittance is the acoustic reflex threshold. Studies document normal thresholds of 70–100 dB SPL for tonal stimuli ranging from 500 to 2000 Hz. Reflex thresholds that are >100 dB SPL are considered elevated. Elevated or absent acoustic

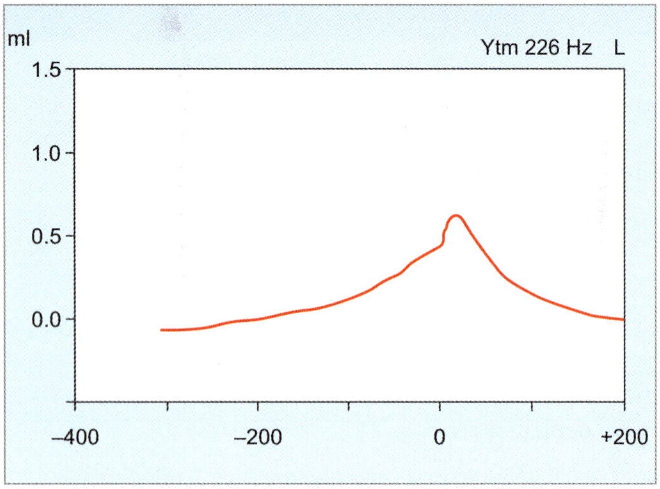

← 600/200daPa/s daPa

Earcanal Volume: 1.1

Tymp 1: daPa ml
Typm 2: 15 0.6
Tymp 3:
Gradient: 100 daPa

Fig. 2.6: Example of a normal, type A tympanogram. This is typically seen in individuals with normal hearing or sensorineural hearing loss. Note the peak at 0 daPa.

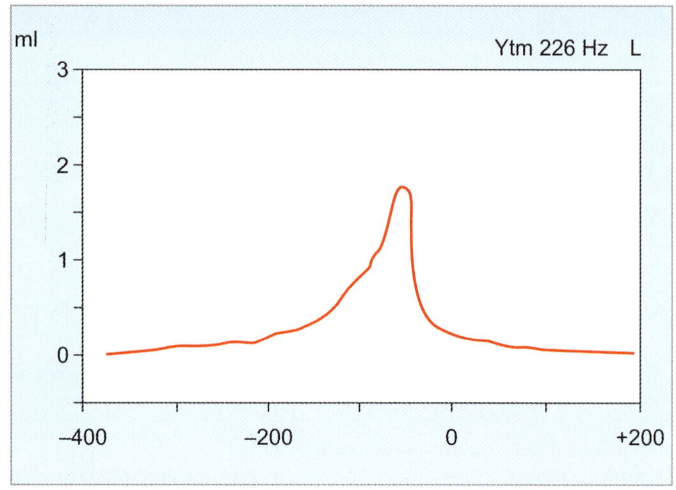

← 600/200daPa/s daPa

Earcanal Volume: 1.4

Typm 1: daPa ml
Typm 2: –50 1.8
Typm 3:
Gradient: 45 daPa

Fig. 2.7: Example of a hypermobile tympanic membrane, a type A_d tympanogram. This is typically seen in individuals with an ossicular discontinuity or a flaccid tympanic membrane. Note the peak at 0 daPa.

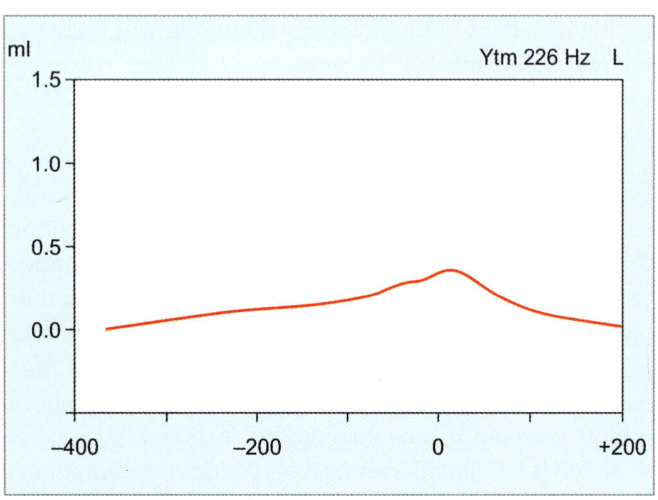

← 600/200daPa/s daPa

Earcanal Volume: 0.8

Tymp 1: daPa ml
Tymp 2: 10 0.4
Tymp 3:
Gradient:

Fig. 2.8: Example of a hypomobile tympanic membrane, a type A_s tympanogram. This is typically seen in individuals with an otosclerosis. Note the peak at 0 daPa.

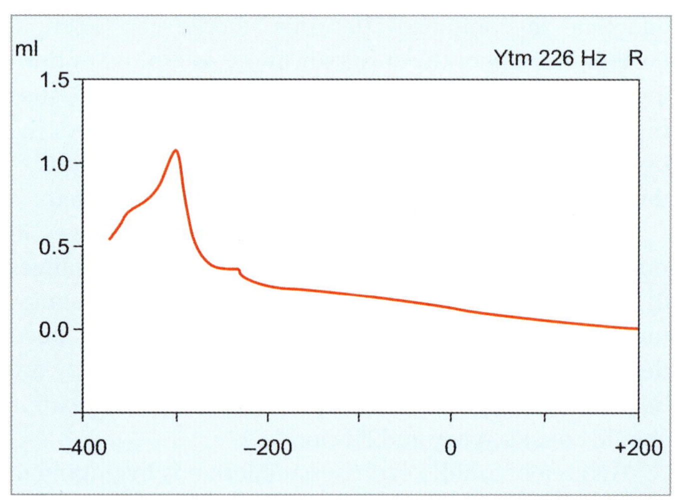

← 600/200daPa/s daPa

EARCANAL VOLUME: 0.9

Tymp 1: daPa ml
Tymp 2: –295 1.1
Tymp 3:
Gradient: 85 daPa

Fig. 2.9: Example of a middle ear with negative peak pressure, a type C tympanogram. This is typically seen in individuals with a retracted tympanic membrane. Note the peak at –300 daPa.

reflex thresholds in an individual with normal hearing or a sensorineural hearing loss may be indicative of a retrocochlear lesion and require further investigation. Acoustic reflex thresholds <70 dB SPL are consistent with cochlear hearing loss. If a patient exhibits a type B tympanogram, and/or has significant other middle ear pathology, acoustic reflexes will most likely be absent. Figures 2.11A and B provide examples of acoustic reflex thresholds measured at 500 and 1000 Hz.

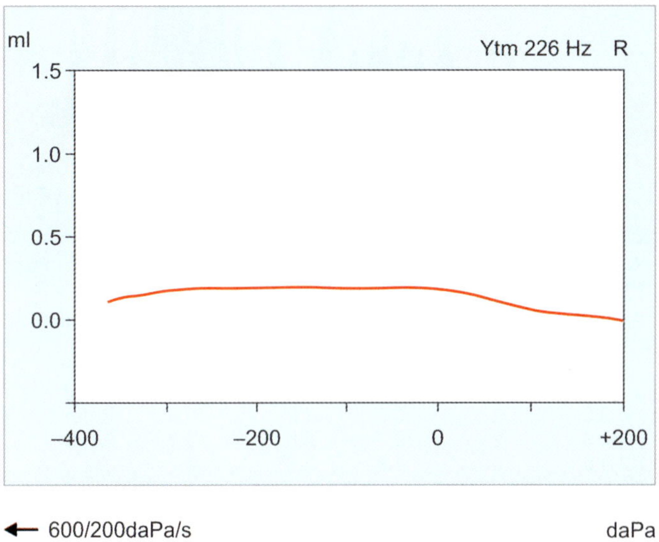

Earcanal Volume: 0.6

	daPa	ml
Tymp 1:		
Tymp 2:	–155	0.2
Tymp 3:		
Gradient:		daPa

Fig. 2.10: Example of a tympanic membrane with little or no mobility, a type B tympanogram. This is typically seen in individuals with a fluid filled middle ear or impacted cerumen. Note the absence of a peak in the tympanogram.

A decrease in the strength of the stapedius contraction during continuous stimulation is referred to as acoustic reflex decay.[27] Acoustic reflex decay is usually tested contralaterally at 500 and 1000 Hz. Reflex decay testing involves the presentation of a tone at 10 dB above the contralateral acoustic reflex threshold. The tone is presented for 10 seconds. If, during that time, the response decreases by 50% or more, decay is considered to be positive. Abnormal, or positive, reflex decay is often a sign of possible retrocochlear pathology. This finding should be considered together with the rest of the test battery and analyzed in conjunction with other results.

Otoacoustic Emissions

Robust OAEs are indicative of healthy outer hair cell function. These emissions are typically observed in response to an evoking stimulus. Clinically, OAEs are used to measure small changes in hearing status that may not be detectable by traditional audiometry. This is an excellent tool for monitoring cochlear status in patients with noise-induced hearing loss or exposed to any ototoxic medications or radiation. OAE testing is objective and does not require a behavioral response from a patient. Thus, it is also used to rule out functional hearing loss. The test is noninvasive, easy to administer, and provides rapid results; therefore, OAEs are often used as part of a newborn hearing screening process.

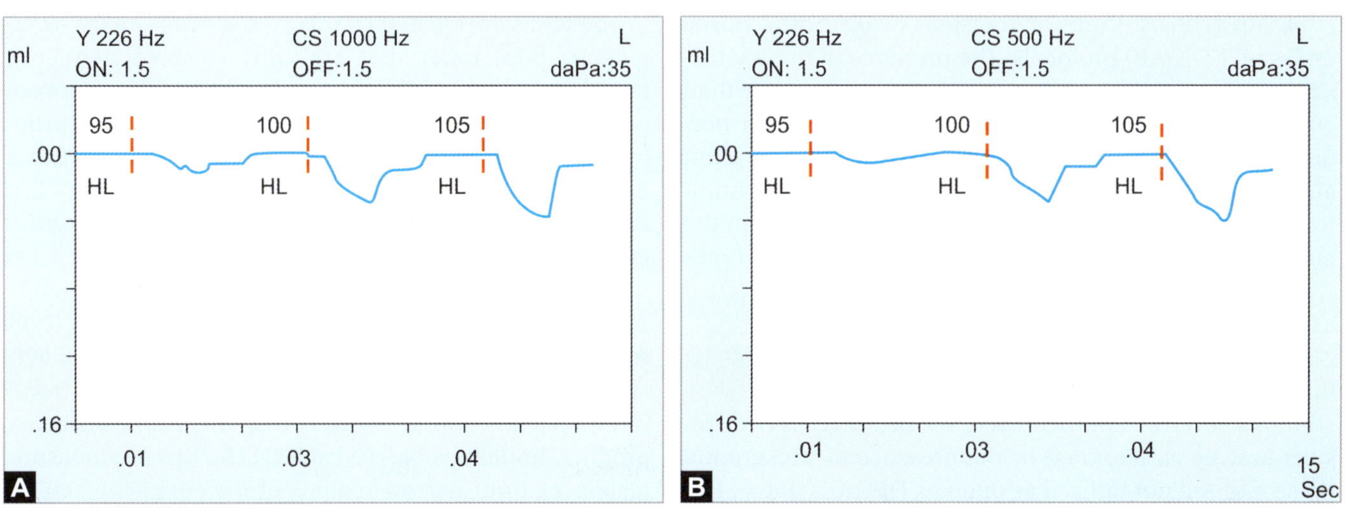

Figs. 2.11A and B: Contralateral acoustic reflex thresholds measured at 500 and 1000 Hz in the patient's left ear. According to these results the reflex threshold at both 500 and 1000 Hz is at 100 dBHL.

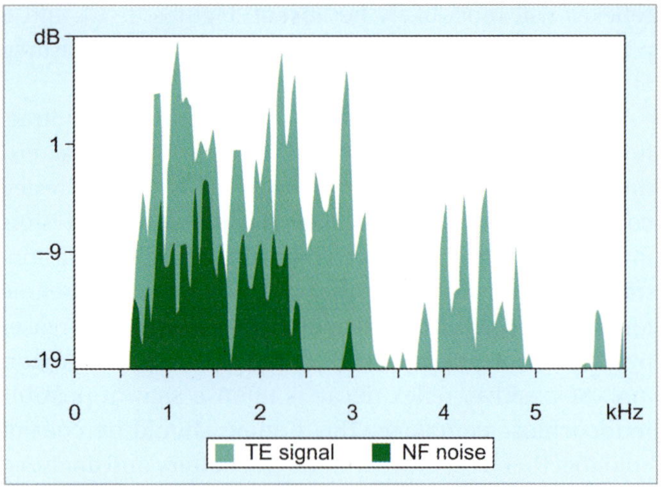

Left: 23-Apr-13: Stab: 99% : TE test: 13D23T01. TE

Frq(kHz)	Repor(%)	TE(dB)	NF(dB)	TE-NF(dB)	Result
1.0	94	15.1	0.7	14.4	–
1.5	73	12.2	4.1	8.1	–
2.0	91	15.5	1.5	14.0	–
3.0	99	11.4	–6.3	17.7	–
4.0	96	5.0	–11.0	16.0	–
1.2-3.4	83	18.2	6.3	11.9	–

Fig. 2.12: Transient emissions recorded from 1000 to 4000 Hz. Note that the reproducibility percentage is higher than 70% at all frequencies and the TE-NF (transient emission-noise floor) ratio is of sufficient amount (10 dB for adults, 15–20 dB for children, at all frequencies.[30] This TEOAE test would be considered a "pass" overall.

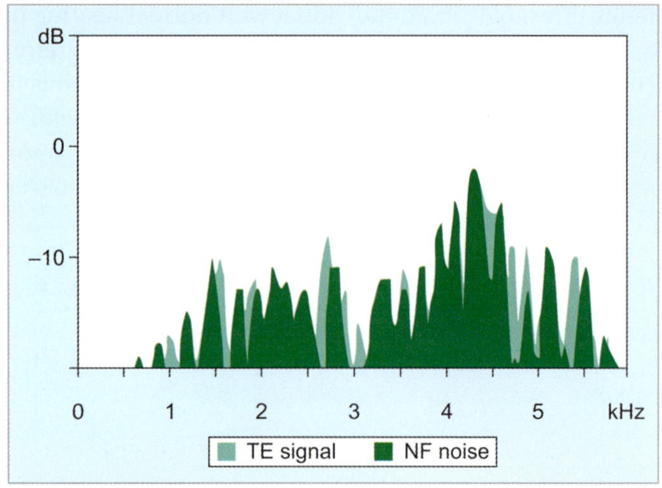

Right: 03-May-13: Stab: 100% : TE screen: 70% at 3/4 freq. for Pass: 13E03T00. TE

Frq(kHz)	Repor(%)	TE(dB)	NF(dB)	TE-NF(dB)	Result
1.0	0	–9.0	–7.7	–1.3	–
1.5	0	–4.8	–4.5	–0.3	Refer
2.0	0	–4.1	–1.5	–2.6	Refer
3.0	2	–0.8	–1.2	0.4	Refer
4.0	2	6.7	6.6	0.1	Refer
1.2-3.5	0	1.9	2.6	–0.7	–

Fig. 2.13: Transient emissions tested from 1000 to 4000 Hz. Note the reproducibility percentage is between 0% and 2% at all frequencies and that the TE-NF ratio is poor at all frequencies. This TEOAE test would be considered an overall "refer".

Testing is done by placing a probe assembly in the external auditory meatus to both present a stimulus and record a response. The indirect evaluation of the cochlea obtained by using OAE protocols helps to separate the effects of changes in cochlear and neural function. Common clinical practice utilizes distortion product otoacoustic emission (DPOAE) and/or transient evoked otoacoustic emission (TEOAE) protocols. The presence of these emissions indicates that hearing sensitivity is no poorer than 30 dBHL. Interpreting OAE results is an important portion of an audiometric evaluation, especially for ruling out auditory neuropathy and functional hearing loss. Auditory neuropathy is a result of the lack of synchrony in the auditory nerve. It should be noted that there will be times when an emission may be present, but cannot be recorded as a result of middle or outer ear pathology.

TEOAEs are recorded in the range of 250–4000 Hz for children[28] and from 500 to 6000 Hz for adults[29] at a stimulus level of approximately 80 dB SPL. TEOAE results may be confounded by the presence of background noise and are not utilized as often as DPOAEs due to this phenomenon. These emissions are recorded between stimulus presentations; therefore, TEOAEs evaluate the outer hair cell status in a resting state. Figures 2.12 and 2.13 provide examples of TEOAE measures. Test results shown in Figure 2.12 reveal a robust response indicating normal outer hair cell functioning. In contrast, results shown in Figure 2.13 suggest abnormal outer hair cell function.

DPOAEs are elicited by presenting two primary simultaneous pure tones that are fairly close in frequency; the emission is usually observed at one of the distortion products that is created. The most prominent distortion product is the cubic distortion product that occurs at $2F_1 - F_2$. Examples of DPOAEs are shown in Figures 2.14 and 2.15. In a clinical setting, the primary tones used to elicit the OAEs are typically in a frequency ratio of 1.1 to 1.3; and the levels may be equal or may be separated by 10 dB. For example, the first row of frequencies and levels shown in Figure 2.14 below are F_1 = 4922 Hz and F_2 = 6000 Hz (F_1:F_2 ratio = 1.2) and the levels are separated by 9.9 dB (L_1 = 63.8 dB and L_2 = 54.9 dB). The cubic distortion product should be observed at 3884 Hz. This test measures responses from narrow regions of the cochlea when the outer hair cells are active. DPOAEs are most reliable when recorded in the frequency range from 750 to 16,000 Hz.

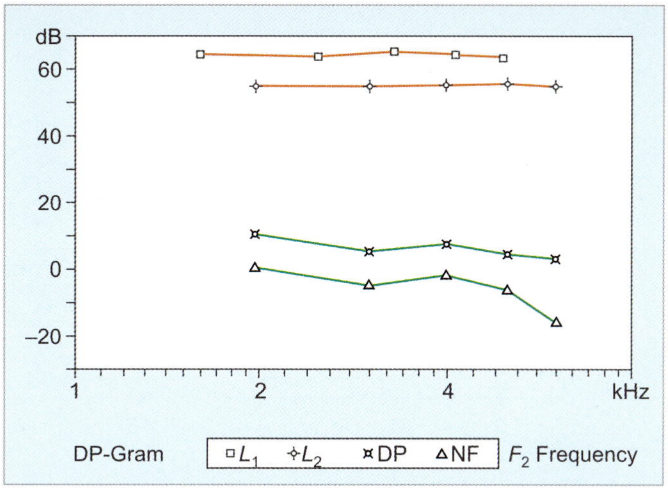

Left: 10-Nov-11: Pass: 2-6 kHz Screen, 3/5 for Pass: 11K10D01.OAE

L_1(dB)	L_2(dB)	F_1(Hz)	F_2(Hz)	GM(Hz)	DP(dB)	NF(dB)	DP-NF(dB)	Result
63.8	54.9	4922	6000	5434	4.9	−16.2	19.1	Pass
64.9	55.6	4125	5016	4549	4.4	−6.4	10.8	Pass
65.7	55.4	3281	3984	3616	7.5	−1.6	9.1	Pass
64.3	55.2	2484	3000	2730	5.1	−4.8	9.9	Pass
64.8	55.1	1594	1969	1771	10.4	0.6	9.8	Pass

Fig. 2.14: Distortion product emissions recorded from 2000 to 6000 Hz. Note the L_1 and L_2 values are 65 and 55 dB, respectively. The output shown above also reports the geometric mean (GM) of F_1 and F_2, which is a value in between the F_1 and F_2. Note the DP-NF ratio is well above 6 dB at all frequencies and the DP itself is above –6 dB. This patient would be considered to have "passed" the test.

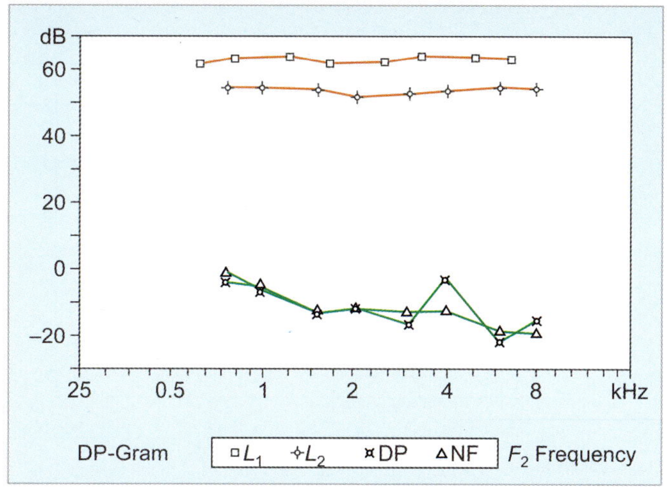

Left: 26-Apr-13: 750-8000 HzTest: 13D26D01.OAE

L_1(dB)	L_2(dB)	F_1(Hz)	F_2(Hz)	GM(Hz)	DP(dB)	NF(dB)	DP-NF(dB)
64.1	55.0	6516	7969	7206	−15.0	−18.9	3.9
64.6	55.5	4922	6000	5434	−21.6	−18.2	−3.4
64.7	54.4	3281	3984	3616	−2.2	−12.1	9.9
63.2	53.3	2484	3000	2730	−16.4	−12.3	−4.1
62.7	52.6	1641	2016	1818	−11.5	−11.4	−0.1
64.6	54.5	1219	1500	1352	−14.1	−12.5	−1.6
63.9	55.2	797	984	886	−5.1	−6.4	1.3
62.4	55.0	609	750	676	−3.9	−1.0	−2.9

Fig. 2.15: Distortion product emissions tested from 750 to 8000 Hz. Note the L_1 and L_2 values are 65 and 55 dBHL, respectively. Note the DP-NF ratio is below 6 dB at all except for one frequency and that the DP itself is not above 6 dB at all frequencies. This patient would be considered a "refer" response.

A determination of a "pass" versus "refer" depends on the protocol employed by each clinical setting and/or recording instrument. For TEOAEs many audiologists will accept a reproducibility rate of anywhere from 50% to 70% for an emission to be considered present, in addition to the ratio of emission over noise floor. The program employed for recording TEOAEs generates a wave reproducibility value that is expressed as a percentage. The closer this reproducibility value is to the preset determining value, the stronger the emission. For DPOAEs, they must be measured at least 6 dB above the noise floor and the DP itself must not be <-6 dB.

Auditory Brainstem Responses

Physiologic testing of the auditory portion of the brainstem is referred to by many different acronyms. These include BSER (brainstem evoked response), AEP (auditory evoked potential), BAER (brainstem auditory evoked response), ABAER (automated brainstem auditory evoked response), or the most commonly used acronym, ABR (auditory brainstem response). Although there is considerable variability among individuals, it is generally expected that the ABR will be seen in the first eight milliseconds following the auditory stimulus.

An ABR records the electrical response to an auditory stimulus in the brainstem using electrodes. This is accomplished using equipment to present the stimuli and amplifiers and signal averaging equipment to amplify and record the response. A normal ABR response is characterized by five distinct peaks in the waveform. These peaks are marked using Roman numerals and are thought to be generated from the lower portion of the brainstem. Traditionally, waves I, III, and V offer the most clinical utility. Evoked potential protocols that are used to record responses from higher up the brainstem and cortex are also available, and are referred to as middle latency response (MLR) and late auditory evoked potentials (cortical ERPs); these are not typically used in the clinical setting.

Evoked potential testing may be used as part of a neuro-otologic evaluation or in threshold estimation for difficult to test patients. Often times, newborn hearing screening programs use an automated ABR protocol called ABAER. Typically, click stimuli are used for evaluation of

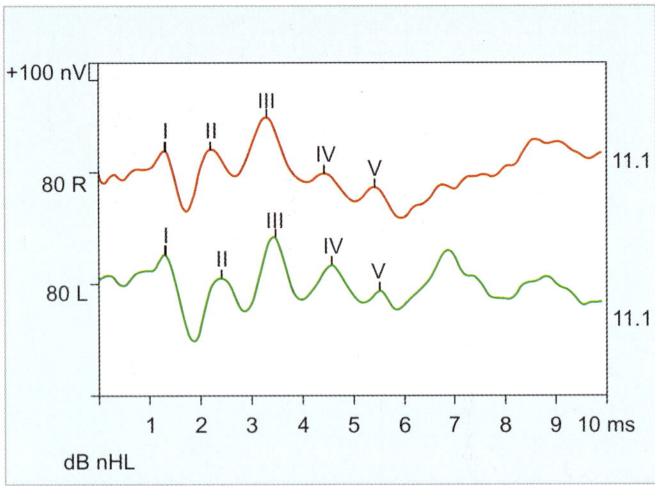

Fig. 2.16: Neurologic ABR for a 26-year-old male known to have normal audiometric thresholds. Testing completed using click stimuli with two channel electrode array with low forehead as ground. The intensity level was 80 dB, which is suprathreshold to obtain accurate recording with a rate of 11.1 clicks per second. Note that waves I–V are marked for the right ear (80R) and the left ear (80L). This is a normal neurologic ABR based on the absolute latencies, interpeak latencies, and interaural latencies.

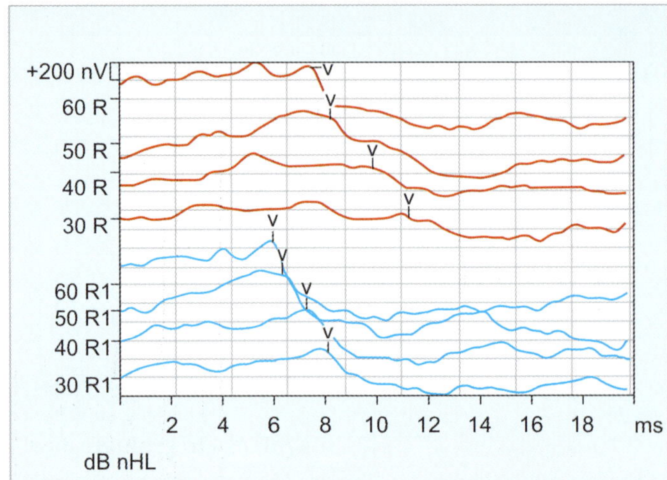

Fig. 2.17: Results for a 23-year-old female known to have normal audiometric thresholds bilaterally. ABR obtained using tone burst stimuli (top 4 waves) and using CE-Chirp (Interacoustics EP25) stimuli (bottom 4 waves) with 1 channel electrode array using nontest ear as ground. Note that threshold search for both stimuli begins at 60 dBHL and continues in 10 dB decrements to 30 dBHL to determine threshold. Presence of wave V is marked, indicating hearing is present at that frequency and intensity. Note that as recording intensity decreases and approaches the threshold of the patient, the latency of wave V increases and the amplitude of wave V decreases.

neurologic integrity as shown in Figure 2.16. In contrast, toneburst stimuli from 500 to 4000 Hz are used for threshold evaluation. An example of toneburst responses is provided in Figure 2.17. If a conductive loss is suspected, bone conduction ABR threshold testing is available.

The evaluation of individual ABR tracings includes assessment of the morphology of the waveform as well as the peak latencies, the interpeak latencies and interaural intervals. Otoneurologic evaluation using ABR is done at suprathreshold levels and is designed to evaluate the integrity of the auditory nerve and/or cochlear status. For threshold evaluation, in difficult to test populations, the presence of wave V is used to estimate thresholds. The ABR response is influenced by the degree of hearing impairment of the subject. For example, if a patient has a moderate sensorineural hearing loss, their wave V will disappear at a higher intensity tone burst level when compared to a subject with normal hearing or a mild hearing loss. In order for hearing impairment to be estimated, the ABR recordings done in nHL need to be converted to an eHL (equivalent). The eHL value varies with the type of ABR system and the normative data obtained by each clinical site. In addition, depending on which equipment is being used, the evoked response may be affected by degree of patient arousal.

Electrocochleography

Electrocochleography (ECochG) is a physiologic examination of the relationship between the summating potential (SP) and the action potential (AP) of the eighth nerve. Clinically, it is useful for diagnosis and monitoring of patients with suspected Meniere's disease. The ECochG is most likely to be clinically significant when the patient is exhibiting active symptoms of Meniere's disease. A common ECochG analysis approach is calculation of SP and AP amplitude (in microvolts) from a common baseline, and then computation of an SP/AP amplitude ratio.[31] Normative data indicate a mean SP/AP amplitude ratio to be 0.26 μV using a tympanic membrane electrode site,[32] 0.24 μV using an ear canal electrode site[33] and 0.16 μV using a transtympanic electrode site.[34] The SP/AP ratio can be recorded using a transtympanic electrode or a far-field array. The far-field recording technique is used more commonly as it is less invasive; however, it should be noted that due to the distance between the electrode and the generation site of interest, responses may be difficult to interpret. Far-field recordings typically place an electrode against the skin of the ear canal or the surface of the tympanic membrane.

Video Nystagmography

Video nystagmography (VNG) is used by audiologists to assess the peripheral and central vestibular systems. As with all assessments, a case history is a crucial part of assessing a dizzy patient. Testing is conducted using infrared goggles connected to a computer system to record eye movement and to deliver visual stimuli. In addition, a caloric irrigator is necessary for the peripheral system to be evaluated. There are three main components of a VNG test battery: ocular motor, positional/positioning, and caloric testing. Results are analyzed based on presence and degree of nystagmus, if any, and subjective dizziness experienced by the patient. The VNG is an integral test to evaluate dizziness because it relies on objectively recording eye movements. The test results can provide information about inner ear function that may be missed by imaging and electrophysiologic testing. During all portions of the VNG, horizontal and vertical eye movements are measured.

The ocular motor portion of the test battery includes assessing saccadic, pursuit, and optokinetic movements of the eye as well as the ability to gaze-hold in different directions. The presence of nystagmus may indicate a possible ocular disorder, peripheral vestibular disorder or a central vestibular issue that may be contributing to the patient's complaint of dizziness. Positional testing allows the audiologist to evaluate the posterior, anterior and horizontal semicircular canals by having the patient manipulate their head and body into various positions. The positional portion of the evaluation is analyzed for the presence and degree of nystagmus within the different positions, with and without fixation. The presence of nystagmus, as well as any consistent pattern, can provide the audiologist with information about how the central or peripheral vestibular system is functioning.

Caloric testing is the final portion of a complete VNG test battery. Prior to beginning testing, an otoscopic examination should be completed to be sure that the tympanic membrane is intact and there is no obstruction in the ear canal. An irrigator with air or water is used to present the stimulus to the ear canal. By changing the temperature of the stimulus in the external auditory canal, the endolymph within the semicircular canals is affected. Once the endolymph begins to move, the vestibulo-ocular reflex is elicited producing nystagmus. Typical caloric procedures employ the bithermal and bilateral method. This requires that cool air (or cool water) and warm air (or warm water) be presented to each ear in separate trials. It is important to remember that test protocols may vary by clinic and audiologist.

Further information on vestibular anatomy and physiology and assessment can be found in additional chapters of this text.

THE FUTURE OF AUDIOLOGY

Audiology at its heart is a problem-solving profession. As members of the hearing healthcare team we are faced with the need to properly assess the communication challenges that our patients face and to determine intervention strategies that will maximize their ability to function in society.

There are many techniques that can be used to assess sensory functions related to hearing and balance and evaluate impairments of the ear and related functions. There are also intervention strategies (described elsewhere in this text) to facilitate the removal of barriers to participation. In particular, the use of products for communication (e.g. hearing aids and other assistive devices) may mitigate, at least in part, the effects of the changes in sensory function and auditory impairment that may limit participation in meaningful life activities.[35]

Audiology, like other disciplines, never seems to stand still. Assessments of hearing, balance and communication function are all essential elements of audiologic practice. The rapid increases in available technology have rendered many of the behavioral tests used prior to the 1980s (e.g. Short Increment Sensitivity Index and Alternate Binaural Loudness Balance) as antiquated and of little use. In their place, electrophysiologic tests of (1) the middle ear system (multi-frequency acoustic immittance test battery, wideband power reflectance), (2) the outer hair cells of the inner ear (OAE), (3) the inner ear and the lower brainstem (acoustic reflexes, OAE, masking level difference, and ABR), and (4) the rest of the auditory pathway [MLRs, event-related potentials (ERPs)]. MLRs and ERPs are a sophisticated evaluation of the brain's response to acoustic signals and multimodal signals (visual and auditory interactions) in ecologically valid conditions. To date, MLR and ERP assessments of an individual's brain response have been limited to research laboratories. Given the equipment required for these measurements this is unlikely to change in the near future. Nonetheless, there is a consistent pressure to assess our patients where they live.

Thus, we are challenged to examine each patient's sensory function, ear and vestibular impairment, and restrictions on communication in realistic environments and with tasks that are representative of the demands made on them. Adequate assessment and intervention requires the special expertise of audiologists, but must be done in a way in which the patient is at the center of the team; expertise from a number of professionals (e.g. otolaryngologists, optometrists, social workers, and speech-language pathologists) is brought to bear in order to reduce the effects of the changes in sensory function and impairment on the individual's communication and day-to-day activities.

Exciting changes are in the future regarding assessment and intervention of auditory function. Through the use of simulations, patients can be tested in situations that are more representative of their everyday life than those situations found in the typical audiometric test booth (i.e. listening to pure tones and monosyllabic words in quiet). For example, virtual tests have been developed to evaluate localization ability and speech understanding in realistic environments containing both reverberation and background noise.[36,37]

There have also been a multitude of assessment tools in which the tasks are made more demanding by the introduction of noise so that the perceptual system is taxed in a way that more closely approximates everyday listening experiences. These tools are making their way into the clinical arena and will improve the ability of audiologists to assess function and impairment. In order to provide more appropriate intervention we need to do more ecologically valid assessment of communication function. In the future, we will likely find ourselves assessing not only the sensitivity and function of the auditory and vestibular systems but also doing multimodal assessments and examining the brain's response to experiences that are closely related to everyday experiences.

Another area of growth that has significant effects on our patients is the impact of the ever-increasing knowledge of genetics that is being held by clinicians of all perspectives. For example, understanding the role of the inheritance of the *POU4F3* gene in progressive hearing loss in humans changes the way that intervention is planned. This knowledge also increases the need to address possible limitations in participation by all members of the family—those affected and those unaffected by the mutation. Knowledge about the impact of mutations in the *GJB2* gene can influence decisions made by a clinician or a team of clinicians with regard to the use of a cochlear implant over conventional amplification. An understanding of the role of mitochondrial 12S rRNA mutations in nonsyndromic hearing loss and aminoglycoside sensitivity will allow prediction of individuals who are at risk for ototoxicity and will improve the outcomes of individuals who may undergo such therapy.

As our profession changes with advances in technology to facilitate assessment and intervention, we will remain rooted in one of the most important clinical tasks—listening to our patients as they describe their symptoms and the barriers that they face that limit their participation and activity in their everyday lives. There is an exciting future ahead for audiologists, particularly with the move toward interprofessional care of our patients.

REFERENCES

1. Jerger J. Audiology in the USA. San Diego: Plural Publishing; 2009.
2. Carhart R, Jerger J. Preferred methods for clinical determination of pure-tone thresholds. J Speech Hear Disord. 1959;24:330-45.
3. ASHA. Scope of Practice in Audiology, 2004.
4. AAA. Scope of Practice 2004.
5. Niparko J. Cochlear implants: principles and practices. Philadelphia, PA: Lippincott Williams & Wilkins; 2009.
6. ASHA. Highlights and Trends: Member and Affiliate Counts, Year-End 2012. 2012.
7. US Department of Labor. Occupational Outlook Handbook 2010.
8. NIDCD. http://www.nidcd.nih.gov/health/statistics/Pages/quick.aspx. 2010 [cited 2013 July 1].
9. World Health Organization. http://www.who.int/mediacentre/factsheets/fs300/en/. 2013 [cited 2013 July 1].
10. Niskar A, Kieszak S, Holmes A, et al. Estimated prevalence of noise induced hearing threshold shifts among children 6 to 19 years of age: The third national health and nutritional examination survey 1988-1994, United States. Pediatrics. 2001;108:40-3.
11. American National Standards Institute. Methods of manual pure-tone threshold audiometry. ANSI 53.21-1978 (R1997). New York: ANSI; 1997.
12. ASHA. Guidelines for manual pure-tone threshold audiometry [Guidelines] 2005.
13. Chaiklin JB, Ventry IM. Spondee threshold measurement: A comparison of 2- and 5-dB steps. J Speech Hear Disord. 1964;29:47-59.
14. ASHA. Guidelines for determining threshold level for speech. 1988;(suppl 30):85-9.
15. Maroonroge S, Diefendorf A. Comparing normal hearing and hearing-impaired subjects' performance on the Northwestern Auditory Test Number 6, California Consonant Test and Pascoe's High-Frequency Word Test. Ear Hear. 1984;5:356-60.
16. Gelfand S. Essentials of audiology, 3rd edn. New York: Thieme Publishing; 2009.
17. Ross M, Lerman J. Word intelligibility by picture identification-WIPI. Auditec, St. Louis, Mo.; 1972.
18. Elliot L, Katz D. Northwestern University Children's Perception of Speech (NU Chips). Auditec, St. Louis, Mo.; 1980.

19. Jerger J, Jerger S. Pediatric Speech Intelligibility Test-PSI. Auditec, St. Louis, Mo.; 1984.
20. Bilger RC, Nuetzel JM, Rabinowitz WM, et al. Standardization of a test of speech perception in noise. J Speech Hear Disord. 1984;23:330-45.
21. Gravel J, Seewald R, Tharpe A. Comprehensive handbook of pediatric audiology. San Diego: Plural Publishing; 2010.
22. ASHA. Committee on Audiometric Evaluation. Guidelines for Audiometric Symbols. 1990;(suppl 32):25-30.
23. Margolis R, Hunter L. Tympanometry: basic principles and clinical applications. In: Rintelmann WF, Musiek F (eds), Contemporary perspectives on hearing assessment. Boston: Allyn & Bacon; 1999. pp. 89-130.
24. Jerger J. Clinical experience with impedance audiometry. Arch Otolaryngol. 1970;92:311-24.
25. Wiley TL, Fowler CG. Acoustic immittance measures in clinical audiology: a primer. San Diego: Singular; 1997.
26. Keefe DH, Feeney MP. Principles of acoustic immittance and acoustic transfer functions. In: Katz J, Medwetsky L, Burkard R, Hood L (eds), Handbook of clinical audiology, 6th edn. Baltimore, MD: Lippincott Williams & Wilkins; 2009. pp. 125-56.
27. Wilson R, Steckler J, Jones H, et al. Adaptation of the acoustic reflex. J Acoust Soc Am. 1978;64:782-91.
28. Glattke TJ, Pafitis IA, Cummiskey C, et al. Identification of hearing loss in children using measures of transient otoacoustic emission reproducibility. Am J Audiol. 1995;4:71-86.
29. Robinette M. Clinical observations with transient evoked otoacoustic emissions with adults. Semin Hear. 1992;13: 23-36.
30. Prieve B, Fitzgerald T, Schulte L. Basic characteristics of click-evoked otoacoustic emissions in infants and children. J Acoust Soc Am. 1997; 102:2860-70.
31. Hall JWI. Handbook of auditory evoked responses. Needham Heights, MA: Allyn and Bacon; 1992.
32. Margolis R, Rieks D, Fournier M, et al. Tympanic electrocochleography for diagnosis of Meniere's Disease. Arch Otolaryngol Head Neck Surg. 1995;121:44-55.
33. Koyuncu M, Mason SM, Shinkwin C. Effect of hearing loss in electrocochleographic investigation of endolymphatic hydrops using tone-pip and click stimuli. J Laryngol Otol. 1994;108:125-30.
34. Densert B, Arlinger S, Herglis L. Reproducibility of the electric response components in clinical electrocochleography. Laryngoscope. 1994;33:254-63.
35. World Health Organization. International classification of functioning, disability and health. Geneva, Switzerland: WHO. Available at: http://www.who.int/classifications/icf/en/.
36. Besing J, Koehnke J. A test of virtual auditory localization. Ear Hear. 1995;16(2):220-29.
37. Koehnke J, Besing J. A procedure for testing speech intelligibility in a virtual listening environment. Ear Hear. 1996; 17(3):211-17.

CHAPTER 3

Middle Ear Mechanics in Normal Hearing, in Diseased Ears, and in Hearing Reconstruction

Manohar Bance, Robert A Adamson

INTRODUCTION

Ear surgeons acknowledge that it is very difficult to achieve consistently good hearing results from middle ear surgery. There are a host of factors at play, only some of which are due to the mechanical properties of any replacement prostheses or reconstructions, and many of which are difficult to control. Stability of the reconstruction is a key challenge, and scarring and ventilation in turn heavily affect this. Both of these factors also affect the ability of the eardrum to vibrate, and this is key to any hearing reconstruction. We will see below that a functioning eardrum is the "engine" of the transformer action that allows middle ear pressure gain, and that no impedance matching can happen without a vibrating eardrum. In the end, all the biological factors have an effect on hearing by their mechanical impact on vibrations of the middle ear structures.

Achieving a vibrating eardrum is the start of the process; the vibrations have to be transmitted to the inner ear without loss, and many factors affect this, including stability of the connector, compliances or losses in the connector or its interfaces with its connecting surfaces, or scarring of the connector. For most reconstructions, the final point for acoustic entry to the inner ear is the footplate, and this has to be mobile, as does the round window (RW) to allow the incompressible cochlear fluids to move. Biological processes such as scarring, biocompatibility, inflammation, and ventilation dominate many of these factors.

With all these factors at work, it is not surprising, then, that successful hearing reconstruction is a challenge with an enormous range of hearing outcomes.[1]

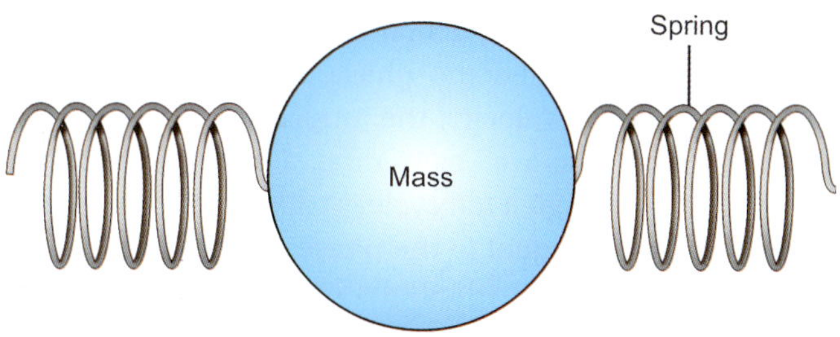

Fig. 3.1: A simple mass–spring system. The mass is set in motion and then exchanges kinetic energy in its inertia with the potential energy stored in the springs.

In this chapter, we focus on temporal bone studies, in which the various factors affecting outcomes can be more easily separated and examined, which is not possible in clinical studies. Prosthesis in this context will refer to any connector between two vibrating structures in the middle ear, whether allograft or homograft.

A few acronyms that will be used in this chapter include TM for tympanic membrane, OW for oval window, RW for round window, and EAC for external ear canal.

Basic Concepts in Vibration

The middle ear can be regarded as a series of masses and springs arranged in a complex network.

Figure 3.1 shows a simple mass–spring system. Such a system vibrates because once displaced from its resting position by a force, the restoring force of the stretched spring, which has "stored" the energy, moves the mass toward the initial position, but the inertia of the mass also "stores" energy, and this carries it past the starting point toward the other side, until the cycle starts again. In each cycle, energy is converted from kinetic energy associated with the motion of the mass to elastic energy associated with compression of the springs, and then back again. If displaced from its equilibrium position and allowed to vibrate freely, the mass will move in such a way that its location as a function of time will be sinusoidal. This sinusoidal motion has an amplitude determined by the size of the initial displacement, a frequency determined by the relative size of the mass and the spring constants, and a phase if measured relative to another sinusoid. We call the time to complete one full cycle the period, which is the inverse of the frequency.

The above description assumes point-like masses and springs that can instantaneously deliver forces from one side to another. In real materials, both mass and stiffness are distributed in three dimensions and mechanical vibrations have finite propagation velocities. In such systems vibrations of a particular frequency travel with a particular speed called the phase velocity. As a result of the finite phase velocity, the amplitude of a vibration changes in space as well as in time, and the length over which it goes through a full cycle is called the wavelength. The wavelength is equal to the phase velocity/frequency, so that low-frequency vibrations have long wavelengths and high-frequency vibrations short wavelengths (at least in structures in which the vibration propagation phase velocity does not change with frequency).

In vibration, we have to think not only about the resistance to movement from friction, but a more general concept called impedance that encapsulates other processes by which motions can give rise to forces opposing that motion. Both inertia of masses and the compression of springs give rise to impedances. In general, impedance will vary with frequency, often in a complex way. Any system containing springs and masses such as the one shown in Figure 3.1 will vibrate at different amplitudes at different frequencies when a sinusoidal equal amplitude driving force is applied to it. The impedance is defined as the ratio of the force applied to a system to the velocity at which it moves. Since we are usually interested in the response as a function of frequency, it is convenient to make impedance a complex number which, at each frequency has a real and imaginary part or, equivalently, a magnitude and a response velocity phase relative to the driving force phase. It turns out that the real part of the impedance describes dissipative processes that resist motion like friction, while the imaginary component describes reactive processes like springs and inertia that store energy in such a way as to create a counterforce opposing the motion.

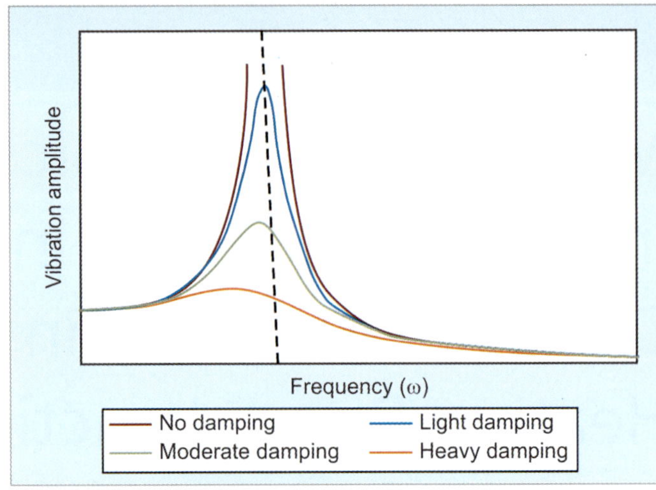

Fig. 3.2: Vibration amplitude by driving vibration frequency. In a simple mass–spring resonator such as Figure 3.1, there will be a simple resonance peak frequency as shown above. Damping from friction will lower this peak, broaden its response, and lower the peak response frequency.

For a given combination of spring stiffness and masses, a system will exhibit its maximal response amplitude at a particular frequency called the resonance frequency. Figure 3.2 shows the displacement of a simple series-connected mass–spring system subjected to a frequency-independent driving force. The peak in the displacement response of the system is the resonance frequency. Simple systems consisting of single mass–spring combination will have a single resonance. More complex systems consisting of multiple masses and springs can exhibit many resonance peaks. When driven at the resonance frequency the amplitude of the displacement will grow until frictional losses or nonlinearities become sufficient to limit further increases. As a result, the stronger the frictional damping, the lower the peak displacement on resonance.

In general, the stiffer the springs and the lighter the mass, the higher the resonance frequency is. Conversely, the more compliant the springs, and the larger the mass, the lower the resonant frequency is. Since mass inertia is low at low frequencies and high at high frequencies, the system response is usually determined by the stiffnesses at low frequencies by the masses at the higher frequencies. This is shown in Figure 3.3. At resonance, neither mass nor stiffness dominates, and the impedances to motion of the stiffness and the mass cancel, leading to a large increase in the response. The resonance frequency of a simple mass–spring system can be calculated from the equation in Figure 3.3.

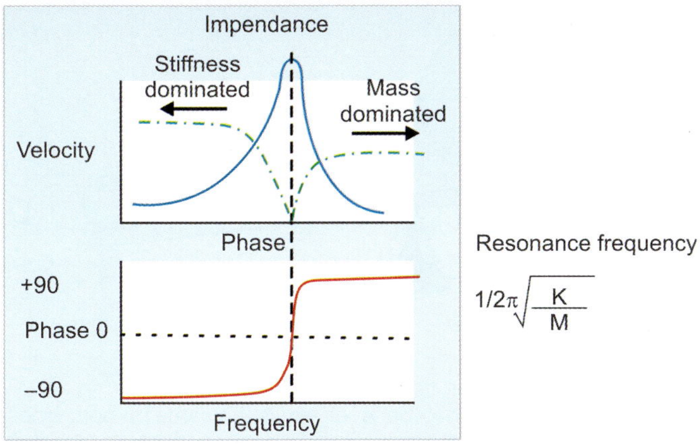

Fig. 3.3: The solid line represents vibration velocity of a driven system with a simple resonance, and the dot-dash gray line the impedance, plotted by frequency. Also shown in the lower plot is the phase of the driving force to the velocity of the driven body.

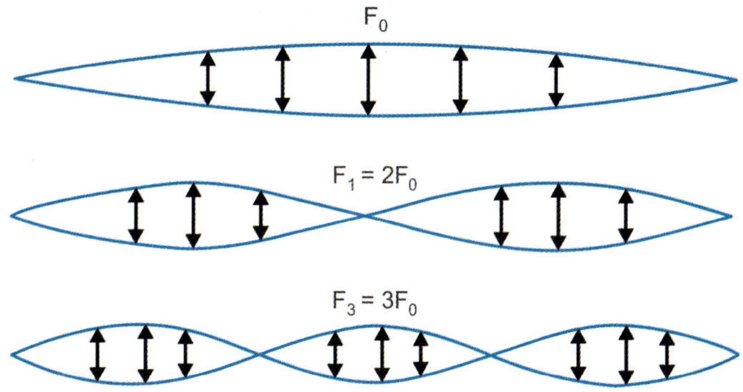

Fig. 3.4: Modes of vibration of a vibration string. At increasingly higher frequencies, the string takes on different modal patterns of vibration, with nodes and antinodes of vibration.

Another important concept in vibration is that of impedance phase that describes how the system response is delayed or advanced in time relative to the driving force. Phase is expressed in degrees, or fractions of a period. At low frequencies, the main impedance arises due to stiffness. Springs generate a force proportional to the amount of displacement they experience that opposes further changes in displacement. Since velocity is the time derivative of displacement it is advance by 90° in phase relative to the displacement (always assuming that all motions and forces are sinusoidal) and is larger than the displacement by a factor $2\pi f$, where f is frequency. Since impedance phase is based on the velocity relative to the driving force, it follows that the impedance phase of a spring dominated system is -90° and that the impedance of a spring decreases linearly with frequency. This is why stiffnesses are most important at low frequencies.

The impedance of a mass is determined by its inertia. When a mass is accelerated it generates a force $F = ma$ opposing the acceleration. Velocity lags acceleration by 90°, so in a mass dominated system, force leads velocity and the phase of the impedance is +90°. Since the ratio of the acceleration to the velocity is $2\pi f$, the impedance of a mass increases linearly with frequency which is why inertia is more important at high frequencies.

For a mass-spring system at resonance, the size of the impedance of the spring and the mass are equal, but since they are 180° out of phase with each other they cancel out, leaving only the impedance due to friction and other dissipative losses (Fig. 3.3). This explains why the amplitude of the motion can grow so much on resonance. In experimental systems, measurements of phase can be very useful in determining whether a system is mass or stiffness dominated, or at one of multiple resonances.

Mechanical systems that are extended in space also exhibit "modes" of vibration. Simply put, this means that at low frequencies, the entire unit might move as a rigid body if it is stiff enough, i.e. all parts move in phase and of equal amplitude. Compliant structures such as drum-skins or strings may move more at the center than at the edges, but all parts move in the same direction at low frequencies, i.e. all parts move in phase. At higher frequencies when the propagation delays involved in traversing the structure become comparable to the period of the wave, the different parts of the structure will start moving out of phase with each other, resulting in multimodal vibration patterns. This is shown for a vibrating string in Figure 3.4.

Structures tend to have multiple normal modes of vibration which are determined by the geometry of the structure and the speed of sound through it. One can think of each normal mode frequency as being set by the time it takes a wave to propagate along a path through the structure that reflects back to point of excitation. When this round trip time is a whole number of periods, the wave amplitude will add constructively on each pass through the structure and a resonance is formed. The amplitude of the wave will vary with location in the structure and is characterized by fixed minima and maxima called nodes and antinodes—again, the waves on a string in Figure 3.4 are a good example of this. Since the mode number is determined by the number of periods contained in the round-trip time through the structure, every additional period added adds an extra node. For the waves on a string the first mode has zero nodes, the second one node, the third two nodes etc. A string has a single, frequency-independent speed

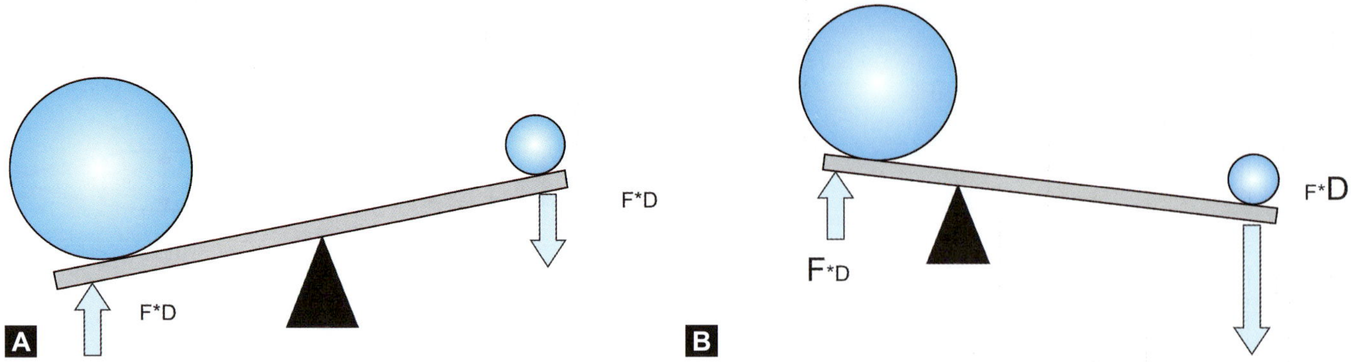

Figs. 3.5A and B: On the left (A), a simple lever is shown with the fulcrum in the middle so that the lever arm is the same on both sides. The mass on the right exerts a force *F*, which cannot lift the larger mass on the left. The width of the arrow represents the force exerted, and the length of the arrow the distance *D* it would travel. In (B), on the right, the fulcrum is moved, so that distance travelled is further for the smaller mass, but the force is proportionally magnified at the other end of the fulcrum, allowing it to move the larger mass load, but through a smaller distance.

of sound and so the round trip condition is met when the string length is a whole number of half wavelengths. The resonant frequencies are, therefore, $f = c/2L$, $f = c/L$, $f = 3c/L$, etc., where L is the length of the string. The ear canal has normal modes that occur roughly at odd multiples of $c/4L$, where c is the speed of sound and L is the length of the ear canal. Normal modes also characterize the vibration of the eardrum, of sound pressure in the pinna and, at the highest audible frequencies, the internal vibration of the middle ear.

Basic Concepts in Mechanics of Hearing

Hearing can only occur if the basilar membrane is forced to vibrate, and in the human ear for acoustic hearing, this means that a pressure difference has to be established between the oval window (OW) and the RW. Two windows are needed because the fluid in the cochlea is essentially incompressible, and so a "relief" valve is needed in the RW in order for the basilar membrane to move away from the scala vestibuli and toward the scala tympani. There are not known to be other significant compliances, or relief windows, in the normal human cochlea. Hence, the driving force on the basilar membrane is proportional to the pressure difference between the oval and RWs. It is important, then, that the RW be shielded from the pressure driving the OW, in any surgical restoration of the middle ear. The basic problem that the middle ear has to solve is that acoustic pressure in air cannot efficiently drive the cochlear fluids to vibrate. This is primarily achieved by creating a large ratio between the area of the tympanic membrane and that of the stapes footplate to increase

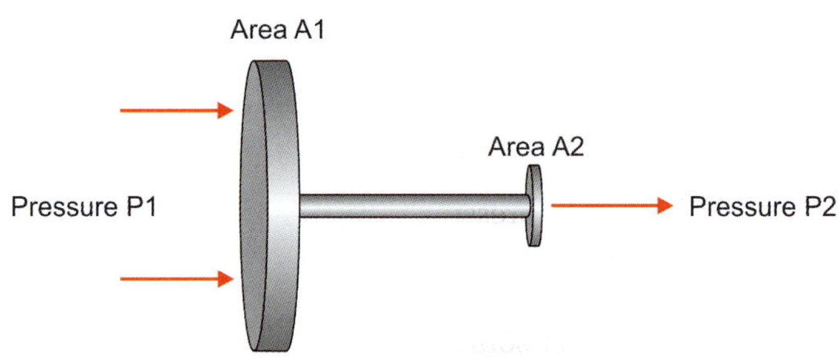

Volume velocity A1 × Pressure A1 = Volume velocity A2 × Pressure A2 Pressure P2 = P1*A1/A2

Fig. 3.6: This shows the pressure transformation from collecting pressure over a large surface area, and focusing it on a smaller surface area. This is similar to the hydraulic lever in the middle ear.

pressure at the OW. Since pressure is force divided by the area, the force delivered to the ossicles increases in proportion to the area of the TM. This effect is depicted in the diagram in Figures 3.5A and B.

The other means that pressure at the footplate is increased is through the pivoting action of the ossicles about the incudomalleolar joint. The middle ear can be thought of as a lever and just as a lever can use a small force to lift a large weight, if the fulcrum is placed appropriately (Fig. 3.6), the middle ear can use a large displacement of the TM driving the malleus and incus to create a larger force (with a smaller displacement) at the stapes footplate.

Both the effect of the TM to footplate area ratio and the middle ear lever act to generate a pressure "gain" at the footplate relative to the TM. It is important to understand

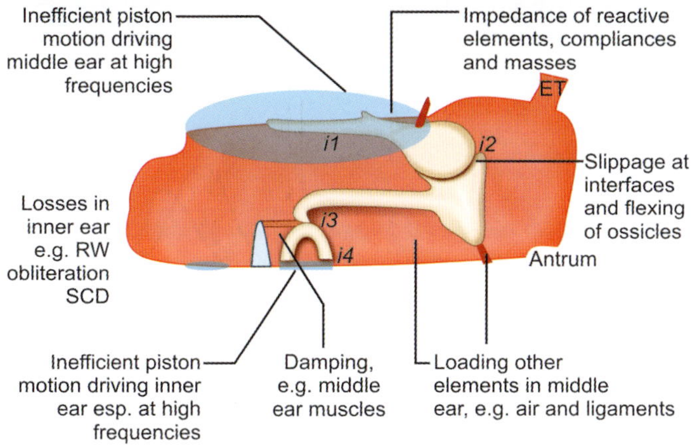

Fig. 3.7: Vibration losses in the normal middle ear. The interfaces (*i1* to *i4*) are labeled, *i1* is the TM to manubrium interface, *i2*, the incudomalleolar joint, *i3* the incudostapedial joint and *i4* the stapes to vestibule interface. Ligaments are shown in red, and the two windows, oval and round window, are shown. (TM, tympanic membrane).

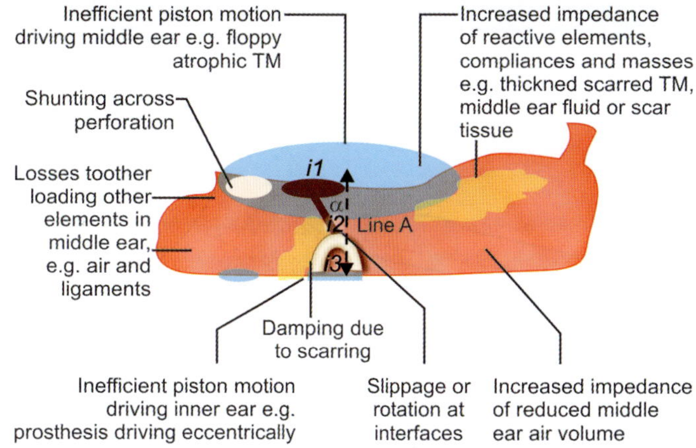

Fig. 3.8: Vibration losses in the diseased or reconstructed ear, similar to Figure 3.7. The Line A represents a line perpendicular to the footplate. The angle α represents the angle between this perpendicular line and a prosthetic connecting the TM to the remaining ossicles. (TM, tympanic membrane).

that the gain of the middle ear does not represent a gain in power, just a conversion of the power collected by the TM from a high-area, low pressure form to a high-pressure low area form, which can more efficiently drive impedance load of the inner ear fluids and the basilar membrane.

There are several sources of loss of vibrations in the middle ear. Some of these are shown schematically for the normal middle ear (Fig. 3.7) and the diseased and reconstructed middle ear (Fig. 3.8), and these will be referred to later in the chapter.

In the following sections, we will review the basic concepts as they apply to normal hearing, and then as they apply to diseased and reconstructed ears.

External Ear Canal

Any physical object in space will change the characteristics of sound propagating past it. There will be slight increase in pressure on the incident side (baffle), and a decrease in pressure on the opposite side (shadow), but the exact nature of the changes depend on the frequencies involved, and the size and shape of the object. Complex objects like the pinna and ear canal can create a variety of resonances that can cause a strong frequency-dependence of the sound pressure at the eardrum, even for a sound source emitting the same pressure at all frequencies. Because this frequency-dependence changes depending on the direction of the sound incident on the pinna, it can be used to help localize the sound source. The pinna is particularly important in localization of elevation.

The various effects of the head, concha, body, and EAC contribute to a sizeable increase in the sound pressure at the eardrum as compared to what it would be at the same point in space in the absence of the head. The head, pinna, ear canal, and TM resonances increase the pressure at the eardrum by up to 22 dB, and while peaking at about 2100 Hz, continues to provide a gain of over 10 dB from 1500 to 6000 Hz.[2] In this frequency range, these external ear effects actually contribute more to the pressure gain than the middle ear.

Teranishi and Shaw[2] performed many of the measurements that underpin our understanding of these effects. Their estimates for the pressure gain due to the baffle created by the head, the concha, the pinna flange, and the ear canal are summarized in Figure 3.9.

The gain of the ear canal can be largely understood as being due to its behavior as a quarter wave resonator with a typical resonance frequency at 2.5 kHz. Canal wall down mastoidectomy changes this resonance, but not drastically. Jang et al.[4] and Evans[5] studied the effects of canal wall down versus canal wall up mastoidectomies on external canal resonance (Fig. 3.10), and found it changed the normal resonance of around 2900 Hz (in the Evans study) by about 300–400 Hz.

The Middle Ear

There are several concepts that are important to understand when examining the function of the normal middle ear, and of the reconstructed middle ear, and despite this

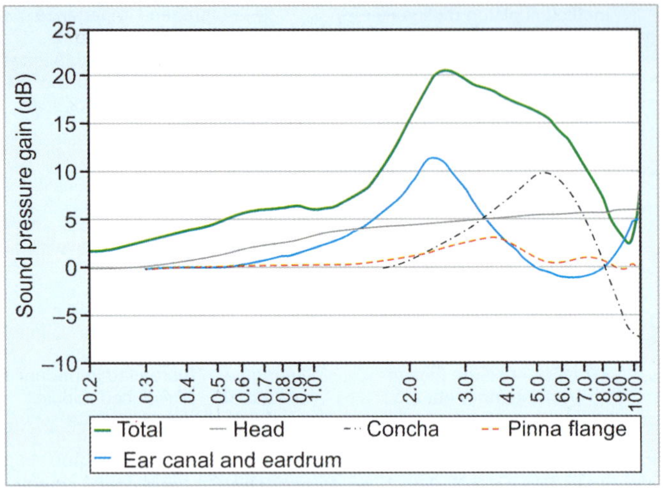

Fig. 3.9: The pressure at the TM for a sound source at 45° in the horizontal azimuth source. (TM, tympanic membrane).
Source: Modified from Shaw.[3]

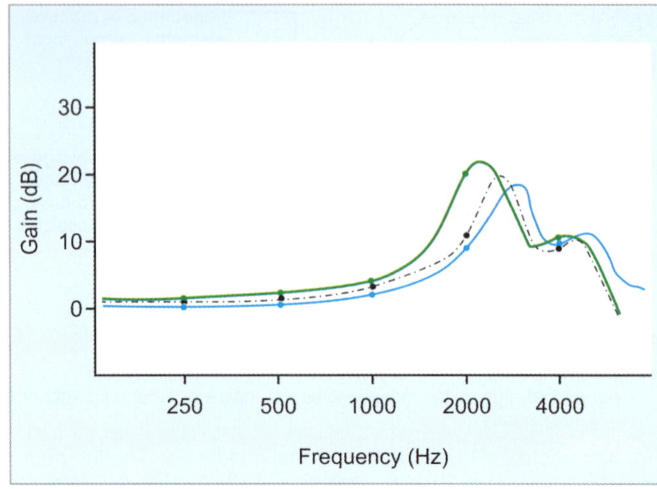

Fig. 3.10: The pressure gain at the eardrum for normal patients (blue line), open mastoid patients (green line), and obliterated or filled mastoid patients (dotted grey line).
Source: Modified from Jang et al.[5]

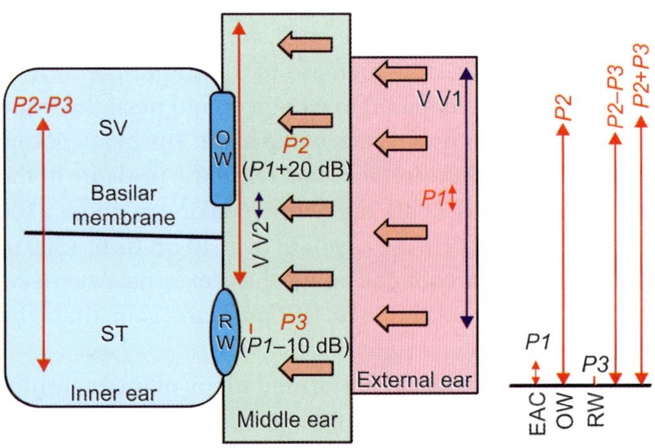

Fig. 3.11: The pressure transformations from the external ear to the vestibule, through the middle ear. The length of the lines for pressure (in red) and volume velocity (blue) are shown to scale in relative values. *P1* is the pressure in the external ear canal (EAC), *P2* is the pressure at the oval window (OW), *P3* is the pressure at the round window (RW), SV is the scala tympani, and ST is the scala tympani. VV represents volume velocity. Also shown on the right are the pressures relative to each other on a scale.

artificial separation, they are all intimately related. Some of these concepts are outlined below, and used to structure a discussion of the normal and diseased middle ear.

THE MIDDLE EAR IS A PRESSURE GAIN TRANSFORMER

Acoustic energy applied to a body can be transmitted, reflected, or dissipated into other kinds of energy. How much of each happens depends on how well the force is matched to the impedance load it is trying to drive. Since energy cannot be created or destroyed, in levers, power (energy/time) is conserved, but other quantities are traded off. In the classic simple lever (*see* Fig. 3.6), force is traded for distance travelled. The middle ear is essentially a lever for increasing the pressure at the stapes footplate, because the pressure in air is not sufficient to drive the inner ear fluid load directly. Without the middle ear, most of the incident acoustic power would reflect off the inner ear, and little would be transmitted. The middle ear does not have any energy source to amplify the acoustic power, so the power of the stapes driving the cochlear fluids is the same as the power of the TM driving the umbo less any losses incurred in the middle ear. The lever in the middle ear classically consists of three different levers working together. Figure 3.11 shows some of the pressure transformations in the middle ear.

The first and most important lever in the middle ear is the hydraulic lever (*see* Fig. 3.5). This lever works as a result of the difference in surface area of the TM and the stapes footplate. The acoustic power at the eardrum is the volume velocity of the air at the eardrum (average linear velocity × the surface area) multiplied by the average pressure over the eardrum. If the stapes were directly connected to the TM, the displacement of the two would be the same, but the differences in area between them would cause the volume displaced by the TM and stapes to differ. As Figure 3.11 shows, at the footplate, the volume velocity is lower because the surface area is lower, and since the power is conserved the pressure the footplate exerts on the OW is greater than the pressure exerted by the sound field on the TM. The ratio of the eardrum surface area to stapes footplate area is about 20. This difference creates a 26 dB increase in pressure from the TM to the stapes.

In addition to the hydraulic lever action, there is a contribution to middle ear gain from the ossicular lever, which results from the difference in lengths of the incus and malleus. The ratio of the lengths of the incus and malleus is about 1.3,[6] which translates to a further 2 dB increase in sound pressure at the stapes footplate.

A third lever, the catenary lever, which results from the curved shape of the eardrum, may also exist. It is postulated that this mechanism translates large movements in the curved regions of the eardrum between the fixed annular rim and the manubrium to smaller displacement but higher force movements at the manubrium.[7] This mechanism is dependent on the special curved geometry of the TM. It is consistent with measured movements at the center of the TM being larger than those on the umbo and manubrium.[8,9] Whether this mechanism actually exists is somewhat controversial, but it may add up to 6 dB if it does exist.[10] Even ignoring the catenary lever effect, there should be a 28 dB pressure gain in the ideal middle ear if all these levers worked completely. Since these lever models do not include any masses or springs they can be taken to describe a system that is massless and rigid in the sense that none of the elements of the TM and middle ear have any compliance to them. In this case, there should also not be any frequency dependence to the middle ear gain.

The actual measured pressure gain from the ear canal to the inner ear, as measured in the vestibule, is shown in Figure 3.12.[11,12]

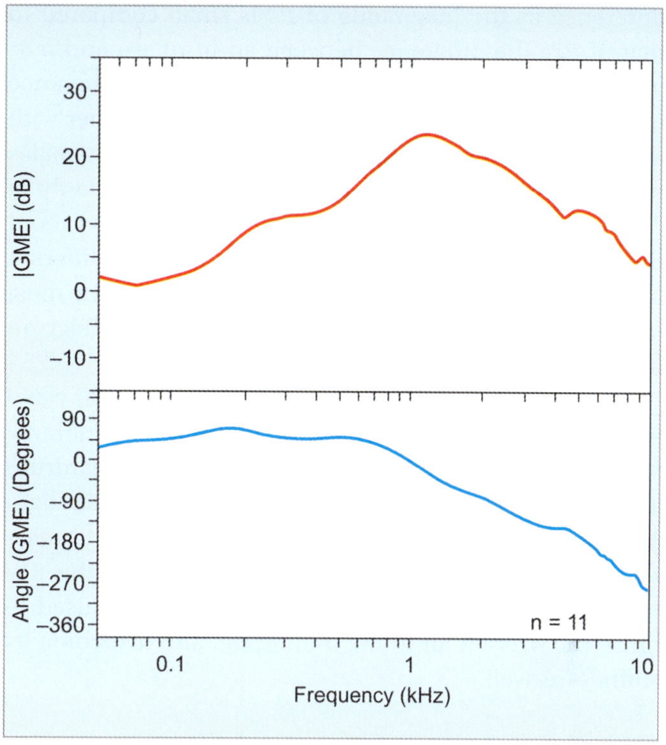

Fig. 3.12: Pressure measured in the vestibule using a hydrophone, compared to the pressure in the external ear canal (EAC), gain in dB (GME, gain middle ear). Also shown is the phase angle of the pressure transfer function.
Source: Modified from Aibara et al.[11]

The pressure gain reaches a maximum gain of only 24 dB at a frequency of around 1 KHz and the gain exhibits a strong frequency dependence. This demonstrates that the middle ear acts best as a lever between 1 and 3 kHz, with decreasing gain above and below this range. The reasons for the frequency dependence are manifold, but as we will discuss below, not all the energy is used to drive the inner ear, some is lost to elements in the middle ear, and some is dissipated.

Figure 3.11 shows the pressure transformations in the normal ear. The lengths of the arrows are to scale in sound pressure levels, i.e. in SPL not in HL sound pressure terms. The arrow in the ear canal represents an arbitrary EAC pressure. The pressure at the OW is then increased by 20 dB or 10 times. The pressure at the RW is decreased by 10 dB, i.e., about a third of the EAC pressure. In absolute terms, the drop in pressure at the RW from the ear canal pressure is relatively unimportant compared to the much larger pressure gain at the OW. For instance, if the EAC pressure was 1 unit, the OW pressure would be 10 units, and the RW pressure about 0.32 units. The driving pressure to the inner ear is the difference between the OW and RW pressures, and it can be seen that whether the RW is dropped to 0.32 units or stays completely at 1 unit has little effect on the total difference in the OW to RW pressure, which is dominated by the much larger gain at the OW. Indeed, in normal ears, we have shown that shielding the RW makes little difference to the stapes vibrations.[13] This kind of normal pressure coupling has been termed "ossicular coupling".[14] It can also be seen from Figure 3.11 that whether the RW pressure is in phase with the OW (which it mostly is because of the long wavelengths of audiologically relevant sounds compared to the distance between the RW and OW), in which case the inner ear driving pressure is *P2–P3*, or whether it is out of phase, in which case the driving pressure is *P2* + *P3*, makes little difference as the magnitude of *P3* is small compared to that of *P2*. The difference between an in-phase and out-phase RW pressure makes to the total pressure difference is about 0.5 dB. This small difference taken together with the fact that over the audiologically-relevant frequencies the driving pressure at the RW and OW will be nearly in phase in any realistic scenario means that concerns about the "phase cancellation" effects of perforations at different locations, i.e. over the RW, are entirely specious. The most important factor by far about a perforation's effect on hearing is its size, not its location.[15]

In the normal ear, the acoustic energy in the ear canal is not all directed toward moving the basilar membrane. Some is used to overcome the stiffness of the eardrum and ligaments in the middle ear such as the annular ligament, move the ossicular mass and inner ear fluid masses, damping in the inner ear and stiffness of the RW membrane and basilar membrane. Some is also used to move the mass of air in the middle ear, and overcome its stiffness as well.

APPLICATIONS TO HEARING RECONSTRUCTION

One of the key concepts that emerges from the actions of the middle ear as a lever is that without a functioning TM, little lever action occurs, and it is impossible to get normal levels of hearing. There are several other areas in which this impedance matching function is relevant.

Piston Diameter

A confusing aspect of middle ear function for many students in this area is that it is often referred to only in terms of pressure gain. Using this metric alone, then a very small pin-like connection to the stapes footplate, or very small diameter stapedotomy piston ought to give the best pressure gain, and best hearing results. In actual fact, the hearing is more linked to the volume velocity generated in the inner ear. A very small prosthesis stem placed on the footplate might result in a high pressure, but the pressure is averaged over the whole stapes footplate. For stapedotomy pistons, a smaller piston diameter results in less volume displacement, despite the high pressure, so that total volume velocity is smaller with smaller pistons. Estimates of the ideal piston diameter suggest that the ideal area would in fact be an area similar to the normal stapes footplate.[16]

Ossicular versus Acoustic Coupling

This is a fundamental concept in hearing reconstruction, proposed by Peake et al.[14] As described above, the middle ear produces a pressure differential between the oval and RWs, primarily by increasing the pressure at the OW by about 20 dB compared to the EAC, a much smaller effect is decreasing the pressure at the RW by about 10 dB (*see* Fig. 3.11). This normal situation has been termed ossicular coupling.[14]

APPLICATION OF ACOUSTIC AND OSSICULAR COUPLING TO HEARING RECONSTRUCTION

Figures 3.13A and B show two different ways in which hearing can be reconstructed.

In damaged ears without the normal pressure gain at the OW, there is still a small pressure difference between the OW and the RW, because there is some RW shielding in the normal ear. This pressure difference is about 1/100 of the pressure in the EAC, or about -40 dB relative to EAC pressure. Hence, the inner ear driving pressure is now 1/100 of the EAC pressure, whereas it normally is 10 × the EAC pressure. This difference between the normal driving pressure and the pressure with no middle ear function is 1000 times or 60 dB. Hence, with loss of the middle ear, we might expect a hearing loss of 60 dB, provided the stapes footplate mobility doesn't change. This form of hearing by the pressure difference between the OW and RW has been termed "acoustic coupling."[14]

Clearly, in the acoustic coupling scenario, it would be much better if we could get the entire EAC pressure to drive the inner ear, instead of just 100th of it, which is the normal pressure differential between the OW and RW. One way to do this is to shield the RW, so that the pressure here is as close to zero as possible. This is the classic Wullstein type IV tympanoplasty.[17] Wullstein's tympanoplasty classification is given in Table 3.1. The mechanics of this procedure have been investigated in detail by Rosowski and Merchant.[18,19] In this reconstruction (Fig. 3.13B), essentially the OW is left exposed as much as possible to EAC pressure by using a thin split thickness skin graft, and a thick cartilage shield shields the RW from the EAC pressure. It is important that the RW area is connected somehow to the Eustachian tube to ventilate this area, otherwise if fluid or scar tissue forms in this area, the RW membrane cannot move, and so neither can the stapes footplate as the inner ear fluid is

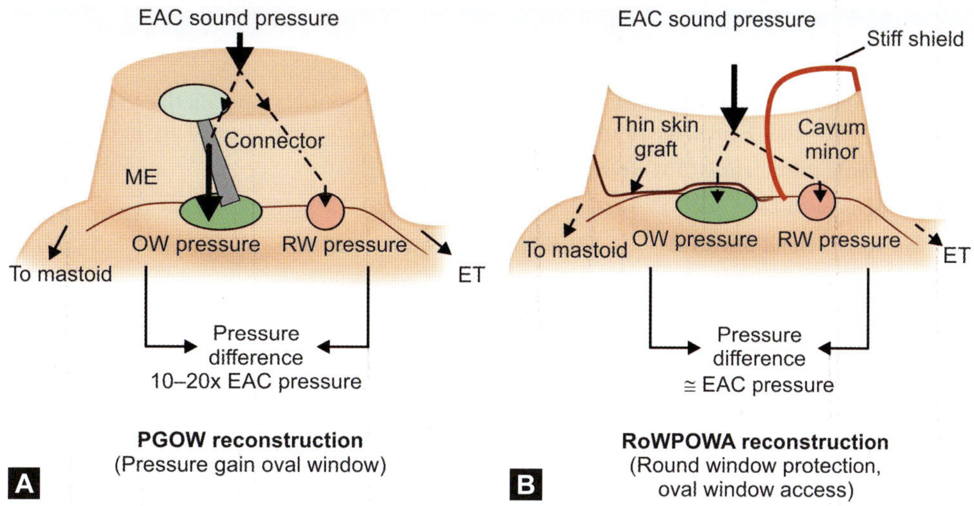

Figs. 3.13A and B: This shows two different ways that hearing can be reconstructed. In the first type, on the left, a pressure gain is attempted to the round window by reconstructing the hydraulic lever, by connecting the TM to the remaining ossicles. This is termed PGOW, pressure gain at the oval window. The right side shows a typical Wullstein type IV reconstruction. In this case, there is no attempt to reconstruct the hydraulic lever, but rather to allow unimpeded access to the OW (oval window) and to shield the RW (round window) as much as possible (RoWPOWA). (TM, tympanic membrane).

Table 3.1: Wullstein classification of tympanoplasty

Type I	Myringoplasty only
Type II	Tympanic membrane (TM) to remaining incus
Type III	TM to stapes head
Type IV	TM to stapes footplate
Type Va	Lateral canal fenestration
Type Vb	TM to vestibule with removal of stapes footplate and fat graft

essentially incompressible. This shielded cavity containing the RW and connected to the ET forms a small cave, a "cavum minor." Theoretically, if all the EAC pressure is applied to the OW, then the loss from normal hearing is only the 20 dB gain of the normal middle ear acoustic transformer, and so air-bone closure to within 20 dB should be possible.[18,19]

Just as in the normal ear, the hearing reconstruction surgeries can be classified into the following types (Figs. 3.13A and B):

Type I: Pressure gain at the OW (PGOW): This attempts to restore the hydraulic lever ratio from the eardrum to the footplate, by attaching the volume velocity of the eardrum to any remaining ossicles. This is analogous to ossicular coupling in the normal ear. The "engine" of this kind of reconstruction has to be a vibrating eardrum. This can be by connecting the eardrum directly to any remaining ossicles (such as a Wullstein type III tympanoplasty) or through allograft or autograft connectors, such as artificial prostheses or sculpted ossicles.

Type II: RW protection with OW access (RoWPOWA): This is an attempt to optimize acoustic coupling. Basically, the entire EAC pressure is delivered to the OW (hence unimpeded OW access without scarring is important), and the RW is protected as much as possible, so that the pressure differential from OW to RW is the entire EAC pressure. As described above, this needs the formation of a cavum minor and ventilation around the RW. These kind of reconstructions are the Wullstein type IV (eardrum to stapes footplate) or type V (eardrum to vestibule with footplate removed and fat graft in OW) tympanoplasties. Important to note is that these type of tympanoplasties do not require a vibrating eardrum, as there is no attempt to recreate the hydraulic lever. Without this pressure gain, however, they are limited at the very best to about a 20-25 dB air-bone closure,[20,21] which is the maximum pressure differential that can be achieved between the OW and RW without the hydraulic lever action.

In practice, achieving a good result from RoWPOWA reconstruction can be difficult. Scarring over the OW will severely attenuate the EAC pressure experienced by the footplate, so only very thin split thickness skin and not fascia (which scars to a thicker state) is used, the annular ligament has to be mobile, the round window has to be mobile, and the cavum minor has to be ventilated and well

Table 3.2: Classification of middle ear hearing reconstruction techniques

A. Pressure gain at OW (PGOW) reconstruction

In general, the lateral and medial and mid-prosthesis interface/stabilizers should be specified, e.g. medial ± footplate shoe, lateral ± cartilage overlay, mid-shaft ± cartilage or other stabilizer. The most commonly used are in bold face.

(I) Direct connection tympanic membrane (TM) to residual ossicles

(a) Direct connection incus onto TM	(D-IOT- Wullstein type II)
(b) Direct connection stapes head onto TM	**(D-SHOT-Wullstein type III)**

(II) Connectors between TM and residual ossicles

Connecting	*Acronym*	*Current terminology or examples*
Stapes head onto TM	**SHOT**	**PORP**
Stapes head onto malleus	**SHOM**	**PORP**
Stapes head onto incus	SHOI	e.g. Cement, Applebaum
Stapes head onto both TM and malleus	**SHOTM**	**PORP**
Stapes head to artificial or	SHOAM	PORP to relocated malleus
Stapes FP onto TM	**FOT**	**TORP**
Stapes FP onto malleus	**FOM**	**TORP**
Stapes FP onto incus	FOI	e.g. stapes piston on mobile FP
Stapes footplate onto both TM and malleus	**FOTM**	**TORP**
Stapes footplate onto relocated or artificial malleus	**FOAM**	**TORP to relocated malleus**
Vestibule to TM	VOT	TORP with stapedotomy
Vestibule to malleus	**VOM**	**Malleostapediopexy**
Vestibule to incus	**VOI**	**Standard stapedotomy**
Vestibule to both TM and malleus	VOB	
Vestibule to artificial or relocated malleus	VOAM	Rarely used
Incus to TM	IOM	Rarely used
Incus to malleus	IOT	e.g. cementing IM joint, rarely used

B. OW access with RW protection (RoWPOWA) hearing reconstruction

RoWPOWA-FP: Stapes footplate access (Wullstein type IV)

RoWPOWA-V: Inner ear access with removal of stapes footplate (Wullstein type Vb)

RoWPOWA-HC: Inner ear access with lateral canal fenestration (Wullstein type Va)

shielded from EAC pressure. All of these can be difficult to achieve, but perhaps not as difficult as achieving a thin, vibrating eardrum with middle ear ventilation connected without scar tissue to the remaining ossicles in a severely diseased ear, as required for a PGOW type reconstruction. Lateral canal fenestration is similar in concept to the RoWPOWA.

Table 3.2 shows a more comprehensive and inclusive classification scheme for middle ear reconstruction, developed by one of the authors (Bance) to aid in more precise descriptions of middle ear surgery.

DIFFERENCE BETWEEN HIGH- AND LOW-FREQUENCY RESPONSE OF THE MIDDLE EAR

Like most mechanical structures with compliant components, the middle ear responds differently at high and

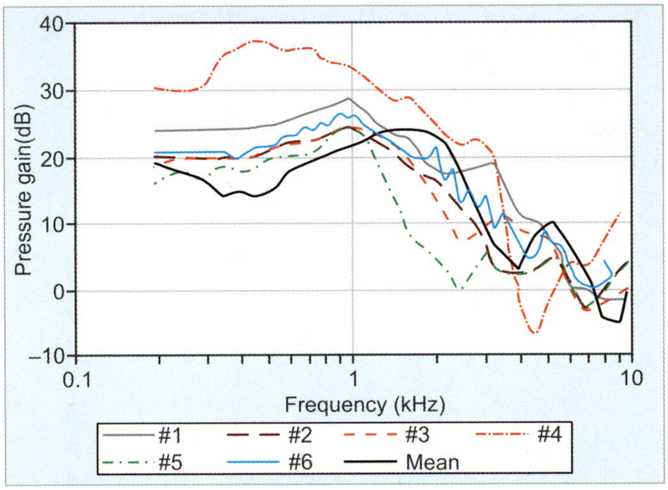

Fig. 3.14: The sound pressure gain in the middle ear estimated by the SPL needed to achieve equivalent displacements of the stapes footplate with and without the middle ear intact. Results are from six temporal bones, and the gray line is the mean. *Source*: Modified from Kurokawa and Goode.[28]

low frequencies. At higher frequencies above 2kHz, like the string in Figure 3.4, there are multimodal vibrations in the eardrum, and parts of the eardrum start moving out of phase exhibiting modal patterns.[8,22] At lower frequencies, the ossicles and eardrum all move in phase (although at different amplitudes), much closer to the idealized hydraulic lever model. At higher frequencies, the coupling of the eardrum to the umbo is less efficient, because of these complex vibration modes.

At these higher frequencies, the ossicles can also start to flex and bend, as well as exhibiting slippage at the interossicular joints.[23,24] The axis of rotation of the ossicles also moves at higher frequencies, from the axis at lower frequencies that passes through the posterior incudal ligament-anterior malleolar ligament axis,[23,25,26] and rotations become more complicated. In addition, the stapes footplate develops a more rocking motion rather than the more piston-like motion at lower frequencies.[27] This is not as efficient at inner ear fluid displacement, as part of the footplate is displacing outward while another part is displacing inward, so that there is reduced net volume displacement. However, there is evidence that these modes can still cause some inner ear stimulation.[27]

All these factors taken together mean that the middle ear is not nearly as efficient as an acoustic transformer at high frequencies as it is at lower frequencies.

This is illustrated by the findings of Kurokawa and Goode.[28] In the idealized case, the ratio of the areas of the eardrum and footplate is about 20 × (29) or 26 dB, so if the middle ear acted as an ideal hydraulic lever, we might expect a gain of 26 dB in pressure at the footplate from the EAC. Kurokawa and Goode attempted to measure the pressure gain of the middle ear by measuring the stapes footplate vibrations with and without the middle ear present. The increase in pressure required to achieve equivalent stapes footplate motion without the middle ear is a measure of the pressure gain of the cochlea. The results are shown in Figure 3.14. The gain calculated for the middle ear is close to the "ideal" hydraulic lever gain of 26 dB for frequencies below 1 kHz, but rapidly falls above this frequency, as the middle ear becomes less efficient as a pressure/volume velocity transformer.

The difference between Figures 3.12 and 3.14 is that some part of the energy transduced by the middle ear does not actually drive the inner ear fluids, but rather is used to overcome the stiffness of the annular ligament, and the stapes itself. So, the pressure experienced by the inner ear is actually that of Figure 3.12.

CLINICAL RELEVANCE OF HIGH- AND LOW-FREQUENCY MIDDLE EAR FUNCTION

It is clear from the measured data that the gain of the middle ear at high frequencies is poor. This means that no middle ear reconstruction is likely to improve the high frequencies past 4 kHz, since the middle ear contributes little gain at these frequencies. However, the high frequencies can be preferentially attenuated more than the low frequencies, for instance by an earplug or similar obstruction in the ear canal. Another point worth noting is that the vibration amplitudes are smaller for high frequencies. This means that small series compliances can "soak up" high frequencies better than higher low frequencies. This may arise, for instance, if there is subluxation of the incudomalleolar joint, or a tenuous connection of the incudostapedial joint. In general, however, most middle ear pathologies preferentially affect the lower frequencies.

While the eardrum has complicated modal patterns of motion at the higher frequencies and it may not be well coupled to the umbo at these higher frequencies, placing cartilage or covering dimeric segments of the TM seems to change the TM vibration patterns substantially in the areas where the cartilage is placed, but has little effect on overall modal patterns of vibration, umbo or stapes vibration amplitudes.[8,29-31] What's more important is to restore the baffle effect of the TM, i.e. to be able to create a pressure differential across it in the case of a perforation, and the material used may not matter too much.[32]

However, the modal patterns of vibration do have an application in that if only a small part of the eardrum is sampled by a prosthesis (e.g. a very small diameter prosthesis head, or stapes classic type III reconstruction), this point may only sample an node in the TM, or have a complicated frequency response because the vibrations of the point of contact may vary dramatically with frequency. On the other hand, large prothesis head sizes are difficult to handle and place, and may increase the stiffness of the TM by tenting it up. Bance et al.[33] compared stapes head to TM prosthesis head sizes of 4 × 4 mm, 4 × 3 m, and 3 × 2.3 mm in temporal bones, and found no differences in performance. Zahnert et al.[34] looked at 1 mm, 3 mm, and 4 mm head diameter prostheses, and found the 1 mm prosthesis head size to be worse than the other two, possibly because of the effects of sampling of a small area of a TM. Indeed, the effect that Mehta et al.[35,36] noted of improvement of type III tympanoplasty function improvement when a cartilage sheet is placed on the head of the stapes may be for the same reasons.

STIFFNESS AND MASS EFFECTS IN THE MIDDLE EAR

There are many compliances and mass elements in the middle ear that affect its frequency response. Among the most important are the stiffness of the TM, the masses of the ossicles, and the stiffness of the various ligaments in the middle ear.

As noted above, the TM is the main factor in the hydraulic lever action of the middle ear.[37] As the first line of transformation of acoustic energy to vibrations in the middle ear, its frequency response shapes the frequency response of the whole middle ear. The frequency response of the umbo in response to EAC sound pressure is shown in Figure 3.15 from Ravicz et al.[38]

In the lower frequency range (i.e. below 1 kHz), the eardrum and its associated ligaments dominate the frequency response, which is primarily stiffness dominated, as seen by the approximately 0.2 period phase lag in the phase plot. Since in a stiffness-dominated system pressure is proportional to displacement, a pressure–velocity plot of a stiffness dominated system should exhibit a 0.25 cycle phase shift. The fact that the measured phase is somewhat less indicates that there is also a frictional component to the response. Between 2 and 8 kHz, there is a combination

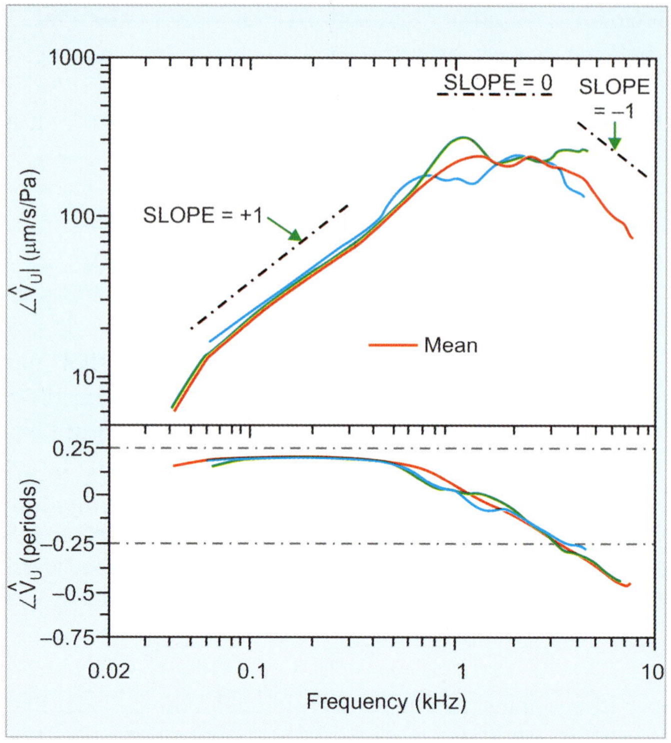

Fig. 3.15: Umbo velocity relative to sound pressure in the ear canal in 9 fresh temporal bones.
Source: Modified from Ravicz et al.[38]

of resistive (damping from the inner ear and middle-ear losses) and mass effects, with a phase angle between sound pressure and umbo response of between 0 and –0.2 periods. At higher frequencies above 4 kHz, the increasing phase lag also points to some kind of delay, such as travelling waves on the TM.

APPLICATIONS TO HEARING RECONSTRUCTION

From Figure 3.3, and the introduction, we can surmise that in general, changes in the stiffness of the eardrum and middle ear or annular ligaments will primarily affect the low frequencies (i.e. the stiffness dominated zone), whereas changes in the TM or ossicular mass are more likely to affect the higher frequency transmission through the middle ear.[39]

Changes in the TM Stiffness and Mass

The TM is clinically reconstructed with a wide variety of materials, including fascia, perichondrium, and cartilage of varying thicknesses. These have very different stiffnesses, and it might be expected that cartilage would have a worse low-frequency responses than fascia, and thicker cartilage worse than thinned cartilage.[40] However, clinical studies seem to show similar air–bone gap closures for both, with lower reperforation rates for cartilage.[41,42] It is difficult to extrapolate from clinical studies the underlying mechanisms for this apparent contradiction, as there are so many confounding factors to consider. It is possible that there is better coupling of the cartilage to the ossicles or prosthesis,[35] so that cartilage is more efficient at transmitting the pressure over its whole surface area to the ossicle or prosthesis connection. Other factors that may affect the air–bone gap are that fascia may more often have small breakdowns or perforations, more often form retraction pockets, and be better at creating a larger pressure difference across by having fewer thinned areas that act as acoustic shunts to the middle ear. Because it is stiffer, cartilage may also not break up into multimodal vibrations at frequencies above 2 kHz, hence resulting in a more efficient high-frequency hydraulic lever mechanism. However, when the whole TM is replaced, without any compliant hinge areas at the edges or within the cartilage shield itself, then it might be expected to result in worse low-frequency hearing results.

According to our simple mass and stiffness models, adding mass to the TM might be expected to reduce high-frequency responses above 2 kHz. In fact, experimental work does not seem to suggest this kind of response. For instance, Nishihara et al.[43] reported only narrowband drops in umbo velocity, increasing with mass size when loading masses between 3 and 20 mg on the TM. Overall effects were small, and even less marked for the stapes than for the umbo.

Changing the Prosthesis Tension

Another factor that will change stiffness in the middle ear transmission path is the tension that a prosthesis is placed under. This can increase the stiffness both at the TM, and at the stapes annular ligament ends, and both of which contribute to middle ear stiffness in the low-frequency stiffness dominated zone.[44] In clinical practice, it can be hard to control this tension, as the tympanomeatal flap or TM reconstruction is simply laid over the prosthesis, but scarring and ventilation of the middle ear will affect the final tension. Sometimes, in reconstruction to a more fixed object such as the malleus, more careful control of tension can be achieved. Tension can, however, be controlled in cadaveric temporal bone models. For instance, Morris et al.[45] found that increased tension on a stapes head onto TM

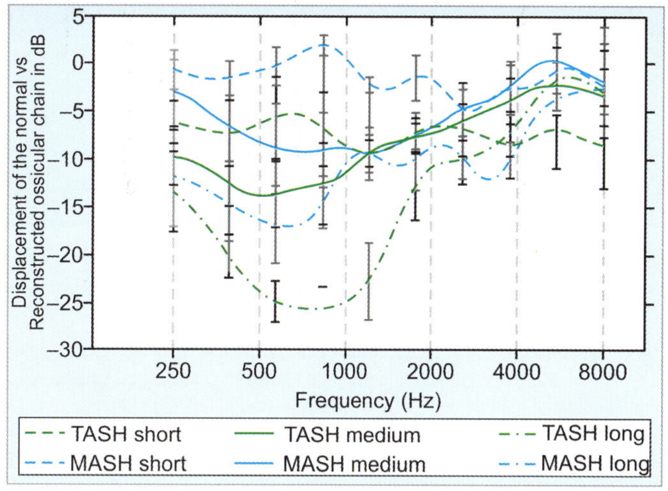

Fig. 3.16: Effect of tension in prosthetic reconstruction to the malleus and TM. Y-axis is stapes displacement with respect to intact ear with normal ossicles. The stapes displacement is shown for three different tensions of prosthesis from stapes head to malleus, and from stapes head to TM. The legend are: long = tight, medium = medium, short = loose, from stapes head to malleus (MASH- now called SHOM in this chapter) or stapes head to tympanic membrane (now called SHOT in this chapter). Modified from Bance et al.[48] of each of the reconstructions.(TM, tympanic membrane).

(SHOT) type reconstruction, achieved by varying the length, resulted in worsening of the low-frequency responses below 1 kHz especially. This has been confirmed by other authors.[46,47] This study was repeated by the same group[48] with reconstructions to the malleus, with similar findings, lower tension resulted in better low-frequency responses. This is shown in Figure 3.16. Clinically, surgeons have to balance the need for stability of the prosthesis with the need for low tension in its placement.

Stiffness of the prosthesis itself is unlikely to be a major determinant of middle ear responses, provided it is stiff enough to not flex or bend significantly at audio frequencies and pressures, and almost all kinds of commonly used prostheses are "rigid" enough. If they are relatively stiff, they will not contribute much to the overall middle ear input stiffness, as that will be more determined by the more compliant terminations at the TM and the footplate. Cartilage, unless thick in cross-sectional area, may flex, at least in FEM models.[49]

Changes in Prosthesis or Ossicular Mass

While simple models of the ear suggest that adding mass might decrease higher frequency responses,[39] more sophisticated circuit,[16] finite element[50] and physical[51] models

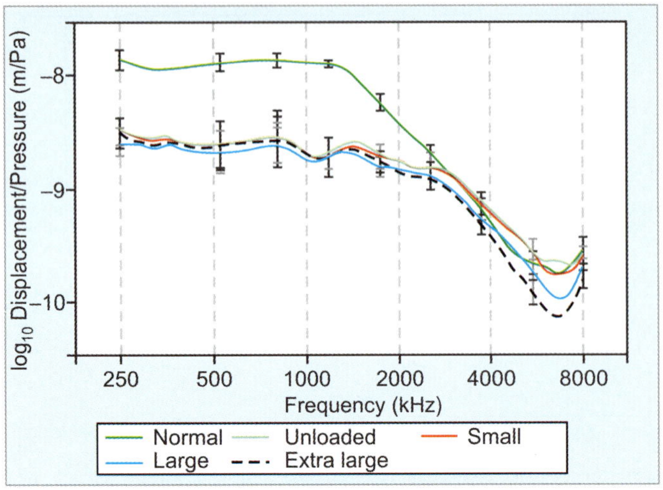

Fig. 3.17: Effects of mass loading the stem of a SHOT prosthesis on stapes displacements. Mean ±SE are shown for eight temporal bones. Normal = intact ear. Weights were loaded on the stem, with the initial unloaded prosthesis mass of 25 mg, small = 27 mg, large = 37 mg, and extra large = 55 mg.
Source: Modified from Bance et al.[52]

suggest that changes in ossicular mass would have only a minor effect on the middle ear responses. Experimental data from Nishihara and Goode[43] on two temporal bones obtained by adding 3–5 mg to the head of the malleus or stapes, and the incus long process found little impact overall, apart from some an increase in the size of the minima and maxima in narrow frequency regions. Stapes displacement was even less impacted. Bance et al.[52] added masses to a SHOT prosthesis (Fig. 3.17). There was only a mild drop with adding masses up to 55 mg to the prosthesis, and only at higher frequencies past 3 kHz.

Clinically, lighter prostheses may be more stable to sudden head impulse accelerations such as head trauma, but can be difficult to place if too light, as they adhere easily to blood clots, are moved by suction and can easily fall over during placement unless given a low center of gravity.

Fluid and Middle Ear Ventilation

The larger the volume of air, the lower its stiffness, i.e. the lower the pressure needed to compress it. The normal middle ear has a highly variable degree of pneumatization, from 2 to 20 mL, with a mean of about 6 mL,[24] with only 1–2 mL of this in the actual middle ear cleft behind the TM. Even with only 2 mL of air, this volume of air is so compressible that it does not play a part in the input impedance of the middle ear, the other elements such as the eardrum are much stiffer and dominate this impedance. Even mastoid obliteration has little effect on this. The volume of air in the middle ear has to fall to <10% of normal values (i.e. 0.2 cc or less) to have a significant effect on the impedance of the middle ear,[38] but this can easily happen in diseased ears.

Another aspect in which the compressibility of the middle ear can affect hearing is in the presence of a tympanic membrane perforation. Many studies show that the size of the perforation primarily determines the ensuing hearing loss, regardless of location[29,32,53] (because of the loss of the trans-TM eardrum pressure difference, and not because the hydraulic lever ratio changes significantly), but the volume of the middle ear determines the amount of drop of pressure across the TM. This means for equivalent size perforations, smaller middle ear spaces will have a larger hearing loss than larger spaces.[54]

Fluid has two effects in the middle ear. By displacing air, it reduces the middle ear air volume and hence increases its stiffness, which results in a low-frequency hearing loss.[38] Viscosity of the fluid had little effect. As it touches the TM, the fluid mass loads the TM and results in a higher frequency hearing loss as well.[38] As the authors point out, clinically, there may be additional low frequency losses from the negative pressure that often accompanies middle ear fluid.

INTERFACES BETWEEN VIBRATING STRUCTURES

At every interface between two mechanical structures, there is a potential for loss of power transmission. It can be lost in slippage at the interface, dissipated in friction, reflected, or converted to a directional vector that does not perform useful work for hearing, or reflected back. There are numerous interfaces in the middle ear. These include the air to TM interface, the TM to ossicular interface, the joints between the ossicles, and the footplate to inner ear interface. All of these have the potential to lose mechanical power. In addition, even "solid" structures such as the ossicles can flex and bend at higher frequencies, preventing efficient power transmission. At these same higher frequencies, the footplate may lose its efficient piston-like motion in the OW, and take on a rocking motion.[27]

To some extent, as mentioned earlier, the separation of the middle ear function into the distinct headings used in this chapter is somewhat artificial, in that the various factors are intimately related and interactive. For instance, coupling interfaces become more of a problem at high frequencies than at low frequencies, and so this is also related to the differences in the function of the ear at low and high frequencies. The coupling interface or air with the TM is dominated by the mass and stiffness characteristics of the TM for instance, as it often is at the interface between two mediums with very different mechanical impedance to vibrations. In this section, we will focus more on transferring power from two structures with relatively similar impedances, e.g. between ossicles, or between prostheses and the TM or other ossicles, rather than from air to a solid structure.

The interfaces in the normal ear are labeled in Figure 3.7 as *i1*: eardrum to malleus, *i2*: incudo-malleolar joint, *i3*: incudostapedial joint, and *i4*: stapes-vestibule incorporating the annular ligament. For the eardrum to malleus interface, was mentioned earlier, the eardrum appears to take on complicated multimodal vibration patterns in the higher frequencies. This means that rather than being an idealized hydraulic lever, the coupling between the eardrum and the manubrium becomes increasingly inefficient at higher frequencies, and by about 6 kHz, the eardrum is quite decoupled from the manubrium.[55] There is some controversy as to the role of the radial fibers in the eardrum, with some authors suggesting they contribute to this high-frequency coupling.[56] From Figure 3.12, however, it can be seen that the gain of the middle ear is negligible at these higher frequencies. The incudomalleolar joint (i2) also shows increased slippage at higher frequencies,[24] particularly in the important rotational axis through the short process of the incus and head of the malleus. In fact, Willi et al.[24] ascribe much of the steep loss in the transfer function of the middle ear between 1 and 3 kHz (12–15 dB/octave loss) to loss at this interface. The role of this joint is unknown, but it may protect against static pressure changes.[57] The incudostapedial joint also changes its behavior to become more complex at higher frequencies. It has been suggested that this joint may be converting the rotational movements of the incus tip to the largely piston-like movements of the stapes.[58] There is a fairly large degree of flexibility at this joint, but fixing this joint does not seem to change the middle ear transmission very much.[59] It is difficult to functionally immobilize the joints, but Offergeld et al.[60] tried to fixate the incudomalleolar joint and the incudostapedial joint, and found a modest drop in the low frequencies, and a slight increase in the high-frequency response. Interestingly, the low-frequency loss was much worse at negative middle ear pressures. The interface with the middle ear (*i4*) has already been commented on, in that a piston-like movement is most efficient for generating inner ear pressure, but this may change to more rocking movements at higher frequencies.[27]

Application to Reconstruction

The interfaces in the reconstructed ear are shown in Figure 3.8. These are *i1*, the interface between the umbo and the prosthesis, and *i2*, the interface from the prosthesis to the remaining ossicles, this could be to the head of the stapes, or to the footplate. The footplate interface to the inner ear is unchanged, although the annular ligament might well be stiffer than normal from processes such as tympanosclerosis, scarring, and otosclerosis. This will significantly increase the stiffness at this i3 interface, which might affect the low frequencies more than the high frequencies.

Because of these interfaces, there can be problems with slippage, as there are in the normal ossicular chain. These interfaces in reconstruction are less constrained than the normal ossicular joints, as there are no capsules around the joints, and so rotation at these interfaces also becomes an issue. Ideally, it would be best to achieve in-line piston like transmission from the eardrum to the stapes footplate, as that creates the most volume of displacement of inner ear fluids, but there is also a rotational moment around *i1* and *i2*, which could result in rotation of the prosthesis instead if its translation. The force in line with the perpendicular axis of the footplate, Line A in Figure 3.8 (i.e. that causing piston-like movements) is $\text{Cos}^2\alpha$, where α is the angle of the prosthesis from this axis (α in Figure 3.8). So even at 45° tilt, only about half (–6 dB) of the force at the TM is directed along Line A. Because of this, a prosthesis directed toward the TM (such as a SHOT or FOT in Table 3.2) will have a better force vector than one directed to the malleus (SHOM or FOM). This is particularly true if the malleus is very anterior. Vlaming and Feenstra[47] showed increasing tilting and less volume displacement by the stapes footplate as a SHOM type prosthesis was tilted more anteriorly. However, there may be other reasons to go to the malleus, such as increased stability, better averaging from the whole TM to the malleus instead of sampling just one part of the TM, and the possible catenary lever pressure gain at the malleus.[7]

At the *i2* interface, many modern prostheses of the SHOM or SHOT type have deep cups to encase the stapes head, which constrain rotational movement slippage (but still result in some tilting of the footplate if the prosthesis is angled). This is difficult to do with prosthesis that connects to the stapes footplate instead of to its head.

The TM–Prostheis Interface (i1)

There are numerous variables at this interface that could be manipulated in hearing reconstruction. Examples of some clinically relevant variables are whether the prosthesis connects to the TM or to the malleus, the presence of cartilage covering the head of the prosthesis at this interface and the size of prothesis head.

Prothesis to malleus (FOM or SHOM) versus to prosthesis to TM (FOT or SHOT) reconstruction: Clinically, whether one is better than the other is difficult to determine. There are some reports suggesting superior results in reconstructions to the malleus,[2,61,62] but there are many confounding factors in clinical reconstruction that may affect results. While there may be an increase in pressure at the malleus if the catenary lever concept is correct, there is also an increase in angulation of the prosthesis as it is positioned more anteriorly to fit under the malleus.

There are few temporal bones studies to draw upon. An older study[63] using less sensitive measuring apparatus in only one bone found better high-frequency responses in a SHOM compared to a SHOT reconstruction. Bance et al.[48] compared SHOM to SHOT reconstructions at differing levels of tension. Tension was a much larger effect than the TM termination point, but the SHOM seemed to perform better than the SHOT (Fig. 3.16). This could be, however, because greater tension can be achieved in the SHOT reconstruction. Also the SHOM reconstruction angulates the prosthesis more than a SHOT type reconstruction, and with a very anterior or medialized malleus, this may dominate the mechanics.

In an interesting study in which the prosthesis angulation was not changed, Shimizu and Goode[64] performed a SHOM interposition, and then took out the malleus and replaced the prosthesis to the same position on the TM and found little difference in the results. It is possible that a prosthesis becomes a new "fixed point" for a catenary lever action, even if the malleus is not present, although this point is unproven.

Another point to consider is where on the malleus the prosthesis should be connected. The umbo vibrates about 10 dB more than the short process, but only below 1 kHz,[65] above that vibration amplitudes are similar. Goode and Nishihara[66] also tried connecting rods from the stapes head to the short process, mid-manubrium and umbo, but only in two bones. While the short process was worse than the other two sites below 1kHz, above this, the stapes vibrations were similar. On the other hand, Zahnert et al.[34] report worse results at the umbo for high frequencies, and similar results for short process, manubrium and umbo at low frequencies. It is difficult to connect to the umbo clinically as this requires significant angulation and is difficult to stabilize.

Cartilage overlay over prosthesis: Clinically, cartilage is often used to cover prostheses to prevent extrusion. This will also have a mechanical effect on vibration transmission.

In a study by Morris et al.,[67] looking at the effects of different size cartilages over the prosthesis, glass (a rigid material) or a softer spongy material in this interface,[67] it was found that none of these changed vibration transmission very much, except for the spongy material causing some drop at the very highest frequencies. Large pieces of cartilage, however, dropped the low-frequency vibrations measured on the stapes footplate, probably by increasing the tension at the TM by tenting it. In unpublished observations by Bance et al., we have also tested different thicknesses of cartilage covering the prosthesis, without noting any difference in stapes responses. Clinically, larger pieces of cartilage are often used to prevent retractions, and to stabilize the TM.

The effect of prosthesis head size has been discussed in the section on high- and low-frequency responses.

i2 Interface (Prosthesis to Remaining Ossicles)

Surgeons often have a choice to either reconstruct to the stapes head (SHOT or SHOM) or to the stapes footplate (FOM or FOT) if the supra structure is still present.

While the stapes head allows better stabilization, and constraint of rotation, sometimes it can be very angulated, and a better vector of reconstruction can be achieved on the footplate. Clinical data on this question are confused and contradictory.

In temporal bone studies, Alian et al.[68] compared a SHOT to a FOT reconstruction, i.e. from TM to stapes head or to footplate. In this case, there is little change in the angulation of the prosthesis, as it terminated on the same point on the TM. Little difference was found in stapes vibrations in the two conditions. Murugusu et al.[69] performed a similar study comparing FOM to SHOM type prosthesis, i.e. footplate to malleus versus stapes head to malleus. These authors found an advantage of about 6.2 dB in going to the footplate compared to the stapes head, but it must be remembered that the SHOM is much more angulated than the FOM reconstruction, and their prosthesis did not have a deep cup, so may have had significant rotational slippage on the head of the stapes.

If considering a FOM or FOT type reconstruction to the footplate, it is not clear where on the footplate is the best place to locate the prosthesis. Placing it off-center may cause significant tilting movements. Vlaming and

Feenstra[47] examined reconstructions to the footplate center to one in the anterior half of the footplate, and calculated the displacement volume of the footplate, finding little difference. Others have found a frequency-specific effect. Indeed, the normal footplate exhibits much more tilting and rocking motions in the higher frequencies.[70] For instance Asai et al. formed cement rods in-situ from various parts of the footplate to the malleus, and clearly found the center of the footplate to be the best site of contact at higher frequencies particularly. The anterior footplate was second best, and was better than the posterior footplate by 10–15 dB at the higher frequencies. Cottle and Khanna (1966) reported similar findings in the cat.[71]

Again, the geometry of the ear may determine the most stable prosthesis placement, and this may dominate the clinical decision.

DAMPING

Damping refers to processes that tend to take energy out of the system. Damping can arise from frictional losses or through the transmission of energy to other systems. All physical systems have some damping; otherwise, if they ever began to oscillate they would continue to do so forever. The effects of damping are shown in Figure 3.2. In the middle ear, damping can be active (e.g. from the actions of the middle ear muscles, the stapedius and tensor tympani) or passive, from friction in the middle ear. The action of the middle ear muscles is primarily to damp the low frequencies.[72]

CLINICAL RELEVANCE OF DAMPING

In the reconstructed or diseased ear, damping from scar tissue or prosthesis or ossicular restriction is very important cause of hearing loss, and failure of reconstruction. As shown in Figure 3.8, scar tissue commonly surrounds an allograft prosthesis. In the diseased ear, damping can occur because of tympanosclerotic fixation of the ossicles, otosclerotic fixation of the stapes, or soft tissue scarring around the ossicles or around the eardrum itself. This scar tissue also adds a mass load, and causes loss of compliance. It is difficult to examine scarring in cadaveric temporal bones as the mechanical properties of scar tissue are hard to simulate. We[73] have tried to simulate scarring in the temporal bone using cynoacrylates and slow setting cements around prostheses, and noted losses of 15–25 dB, larger than the effect size of almost any other modification of the prosthesis, aside from disconnecting it. Clearly scarring has the potential to have a huge effect on hearing reconstruction results.

The actions of the middle ear muscles have only a small impact during most sound stimulation,[74,75] and cutting the stapedius tendon had little effect on the actions of a middle ear prosthesis to the stapes head in a temporal bone model.[52]

CONCLUSION

We have examined many of the factors that are relevant to normal middle ear function, and to diseased ears. The normal middle ear is primarily a volume velocity/pressure transformer that increases pressure at the OW. The main factor in this pressure gain is the hydraulic lever, dependent on the area ratio difference between the TM and OW, of about 20 to 1. It is most effective between 1 and 3 kHz, with roll-offs in the pressure gain above and below this. At high frequencies over 2 kHz, the middle ear exhibits more complex multimodal vibration patterns, and the TM becomes increasingly decoupled from the umbo. At high frequencies, the EAC may provide more of a pressure gain than the middle ear.

We have also considered factors most important to successful hearing reconstruction. While we have focused on the controllable factors in middle ear reconstruction, many of the factors dominating hearing results are not under the surgeon's control, such as ventilation and scarring. These have deep biological underlying mechanisms that are poorly understood in the ear, or indeed in any other part of the body.

To summarize important lessons in reconstruction, the TM is the key to the hydraulic lever, and hence to pressure gain at the OW. The TM can only function if it is not thickened from scarring, or damped from fixation, and if there is middle ear ventilation. Having achieved this, connections without slippage or rotational losses are required to the stapes footplate. This again requires that these connectors are not damped by scar tissue or ankylosis to surrounding structures, and are securely stabilized to both the TM and to their medial connection. This has to allow for changes in the position of the TM with healing, as it can lateralize or medialize with healing. The footplate itself has to be mobile, which can be a limiting factor in itself. An alternative is to avoid the hydraulic lever reconstructions (PGOW) and aim for RW protection (RoWPOWA). This is also not easy, as it requires good access to the OW without scarring, a mobile footplate, and ventilation and shielding of the RW.

It is no surprise then, that hearing reconstruction surgery is unpredictable in its outcomes, and often delivers less than ideal results.

REFERENCES

1. Merchant SN, Ravicz ME, Voss SE, et al. Toynbee Memorial Lecture 1997. Middle ear mechanics in normal, diseased and reconstructed ears. J Laryngol Otol. 1998;112(8):715-31.
2. Shaw EA, Teranishi R. Sound pressure generated in an external-ear replica and real human ears by a nearby point source. J Acoust Soc Am. 1968;44(1):240-49.
3. Shaw EAG. The external ear. In: Kiedel WD, Neff WD (eds), Handbook of sensory physiology. Berlin: Springer-Verlag; 1974. pp. 455-90.
4. Jang CH. Changes in external ear resonance after mastoidectomy: open cavity mastoid versus obliterated mastoid cavity. Clin Otolaryngol Allied Sci. 2002;27(6):509-11.
5. Evans RA, Day GA, Browning GG. Open-cavity mastoid surgery: its effect on the acoustics of the external ear canal. Clin Otolaryngol Allied Sci. 1989;14(4):317-21.
6. Kirikae I. The structure and function of the middle ear. Tokyo: University of Tokyo Press; 1960.
7. Helmholtz H. The mechanism of the ossicles of the ear and membrana tympani. Pfluger Archiv fur Physiologie. 1868;1.
8. Cheng JT, Hamade M, Merchant SN, et al. Wave motion on the surface of the human tympanic membrane: holographic measurement and modeling analysis. J Acoust Soc Am. 2013;133(2):918-37.
9. Tonndorf J, Khanna SM. The role of the tympanic membrane in middle ear transmission. Ann Otol Rhinol Laryngol. 1970;79(4):743-53.
10. Tonndorf J, Khanna SM. Tympanic-membrane vibrations in human cadaver ears studied by time-averaged holography. J Acoust Soc Am. 1972;52(4):1221-33.
11. Aibara R, Welsh JT, Puria S, et al. Human middle-ear sound transfer function and cochlear input impedance. Hear Res. 2001;152(1-2):100-9.
12. Nakajima HH, Dong W, Olson ES, et al. Differential intracochlear sound pressure measurements in normal human temporal bones. JARO. 2009;10(1):23-36.
13. Alian WA, Majdalawieh OF, Van Wijhe RG, et al. Effect of Silastic sheeting over the round window niche on sound transmission in the intact human middle ear. J Otolaryngol Head Neck Surg [Le Journal d'oto-rhino-laryngologie et de chirurgie cervico-faciale]. 2012;41(1):1-7.
14. Peake WT, Rosowski JJ, Lynch TJ, 3rd. Middle-ear transmission: acoustic versus ossicular coupling in cat and human. Hear Res. 1992;57(2):245-68.
15. Voss SE, Rosowski JJ, Merchant SN, et al. Non-ossicular signal transmission in human middle ears: experimental assessment of the "acoustic route" with perforated tympanic membranes. J Acoust Soc Am. 2007;122(4):2135-53.
16. Rosowski JJ, Merchant SN. Mechanical and acoustic analysis of middle ear reconstruction. Am J Otol. 1995;16(4):486-97.
17. Wullstein HL. The surgical restoration of hearing in chronic otitis media and its audiological basis. Ann Otol Rhinol Laryngol. 1958;67(4):952-63.
18. Merchant SN, Ravicz ME, Rosowski JJ. Mechanics of type IV tympanoplasty: experimental findings and surgical implications. Ann Otol Rhinol Laryngol. 1997;106(1):49-60.
19. Merchant SN, Rosowski JJ, Ravicz ME. Middle ear mechanics of type IV and type V tympanoplasty: II. Clinical analysis and surgical implications. Am J Otol. 1995;16(5):565-75.
20. Lempert J. Endaural fenestration of external semicircular canal for restoration of hearing in cases of otosclerosis. Arch Otolaryngol. 1940;31:711-79.
21. Montandon P, Chatelain C. Restoration of hearing with type V tympanoplasty. ORL; journal for oto-rhino-laryngology and its related specialties. 1991;53(6):342-5.
22. Rosowski J, Cheng J, Merchant S, et al. New data on the motion of the normal and reconstructed tympanic membrane. Otol Neurotol. 2011;32(9):1559-67.
23. Decraemer W, Khanna S. Measurement, visualization and quantitative analysis of complete three-dimensional kinematical data sets of human and cat middle ear. In: Gyo K, Wada H, Hato N, Koike T (eds), Middle ear mechanics in research and otology. Singapore: World Scientific; 2004. pp. 3-10.
24. Willi U, Ferrazzini M, Huber A. The incudo-malleolar joint and sound transmission loss. Hear Res. 2002;174:32-44.
25. Wever E, Lawrence M. Physiological acoustics. Princeton: Princeton University Press; 1954.
26. Dahmann H. Zur Physiologie des Hörens; experimentelle Untersuchungen über die Mechanik der Gehörknöchelchenkette, sowie über deren Verhalten auf Ton und Luftdruck. Zeits f Hals- Nasen- Ohrenheilk. 1929;24:462-97.
27. Eiber A, Huber A, Lauxmann M, et al. Contribution of complex stapes motion to cochlea activation. Hear Res. 2012; 284:82-92.
28. Kurokawa H, Goode RL. Sound pressure gain produced by the human middle ear. Otolaryngol Head Neck Surg. 1995; 113(4):349-55.
29. Voss SE, Rosowski JJ, Merchant SN, et al. Middle-ear function with tympanic-membrane perforations. I. Measurements and mechanisms. J Acoust Soc Am. 2001;110(3 Pt 1): 1432-44.
30. Morris DP, Bance M, Van Wijhe RG. Vibration characteristics and function of atelectatic segments in the tympanic membrane in fresh human cadaveric temporal bones. Clin Otolaryngol Allied Sci. 2004;29(2):133-7.
31. Aarnisalo AA, Cheng JT, Ravicz ME, et al. Middle ear mechanics of cartilage tympanoplasty evaluated by laser holography and vibrometry. Otol Neurotol. 2009;30(8): 1209-14.
32. Voss SE, Rosowski JJ, Merchant SN, et al. Middle-ear function with tympanic-membrane perforations. II. A simple model. J Acoust Soc Am. 2001;110(3 Pt 1):1445-52.
33. Bance M, Campos A, Wong L, et al. How does prosthesis head size affect vibration transmission in ossiculoplasty? Otolaryngol Head Neck Surg. 2007;137(1):70-3.
34. Zahnert TBM, Huttenbrink K-B (eds.) Calculations and experiments on the influence of prosthesis coupling to the middle ear transfer function. Middle ear mechanics in research and otology: Proceedings of the Third Symposium, Matsuyame, Ehime, Japan 9-12 July 2003; World Scientific Publishing Co.

35. Mehta RP, Ravicz ME, Rosowski JJ, et al. Middle-ear mechanics of type III tympanoplasty (stapes columella): I. Experimental studies. Otol Neurotol. 2003;24(2):176-85.
36. Merchant SN, McKenna MJ, Mehta RP, et al. Middle ear mechanics of Type III tympanoplasty (stapes columella): II. Clinical studies. Otol Neurotol. 2003;24(2):186-94.
37. Rosowski JJ. Outer and middle ear. In: Popper A, Fay R (eds), Springer handbook of auditory research: comparative hearing: mammals. The Springer Series in Auditory Research. IV. New York: Springer-Verlag; 1994. pp. 172-247.
38. Ravicz ME, Rosowski JJ, Merchant SN. Mechanisms of hearing loss resulting from middle-ear fluid. Hear Res. 2004; 195(1-2):103-30.
39. Relkin EM. Introduction to the analysis of middle-ear function. In: Jahn AF, Santos-Sacchi J (eds), Physiology of the ear. New York: Raven Press; 1988.
40. Murbe D, Zahnert T, Bornitz M, et al. Acoustic properties of different cartilage reconstruction techniques of the tympanic membrane. Laryngoscope. 2002;112(10):1769-76.
41. Kim JY, Oh JH, Lee HH. Fascia versus cartilage graft in type I tympanoplasty: audiological outcome. J Craniofac Surg. 2012;23(6):e605-8.
42. Caye-Thomasen P, Andersen J, Uzun C, et al. Ten-year results of cartilage palisades versus fascia in eardrum reconstruction after surgery for sinus or tensa retraction cholesteatoma in children. Laryngoscope. 2009;119(5):944-52.
43. Nishihara S, Aritomo H, Goode RL. Effect of changes in mass on middle ear function. Otolaryngol Head Neck Surg. 1993;109(5):899-910.
44. Rabinowitz WM. Measurement of the acoustic input immittance of the human ear. J Acoust Soc Am. 1981;70(4): 1025-35.
45. Morris DP, Bance M, van Wijhe RG, et al. Optimum tension for partial ossicular replacement prosthesis reconstruction in the human middle ear. Laryngoscope. 2004;114(2): 305-8.
46. Yamada H, Goode RL. A self-adjusting ossicular prosthesis containing polyurethane sponge. Otol Neurotol. 2010; 31(9):1404-8.
47. Vlaming MS, Feenstra L. Studies on the mechanics of the reconstructed human middle ear. Clini Otolaryngol Allied Sci. 1986;11(6):411-22.
48. Bance M, Morris DP, Vanwijhe RG, Kiefte M, Funnell WR. Comparison of the mechanical performance of ossiculoplasty using a prosthetic malleus-to-stapes head with a tympanic membrane-to-stapes head assembly in a human cadaveric middle ear model. Otol Neurotol. 2004;25(6): 903-9.
49. Koike TWH, Toshimitsu K. Analysis of the finite element method of transfer function of reconstructed middle ear and their postoperative changes. In: Rowsowski JJ, Merchant SN (eds), The Function and Mechanics of Normal, Diseased and Reconstructed Middle Ears. The Hague, Netherlands: Kugler Publications; 2000. pp. 309-20.
50. Gan RZ, Dai C, Wang X, et al. A totally implantable hearing system—design and function characterization in 3D computational model and temporal bones. Hear Res. 2010;263 (1-2):138-44.
51. Mojallal H, Stieve M, Krueger I, et al. A biomechanical ear model to evaluate middle-ear reconstruction. Int J Audiol. 2009;48(12):876-84.
52. Bance M, Morris DP, Van Wijhe R. Effects of ossicular prosthesis mass and section of the stapes tendon on middle ear transmission. J Otolaryngol. 2007;36(2):113-19.
53. Lerut B, Pfammatter A, Moons J, et al. Functional correlations of tympanic membrane perforation size. Otol Neurotol. 2012;33(3):379-86.
54. Voss SE, Rosowski JJ, Merchant SN, Peake WT. How do tympanic-membrane perforations affect human middle-ear sound transmission? Acta Otolaryngol. 2001;121(2):169-73.
55. Tonndorf J, Khanna SM. The tympanic membrane as a part of the middle ear transformer. Acta Otolaryngol. 1971; 71(2):177-80.
56. O'Connor KN, Tam M, Blevins NH, et al. Tympanic membrane collagen fibers: a key to high-frequency sound conduction. Laryngoscope. 2008;118(3):483-90.
57. Huttenbrink KB. Die Mechanik der Gehorknochelchen bei statischen Drucken. I.: Normales Mittelohr. Z. Laryngol Rhinol Otol. 1988;67:45-52.
58. Funnell WR, Heng Siah T, McKee MD, et al. On the coupling between the incus and the stapes in the cat. JARO. 2005;6(1):9-18.
59. Alian W, Majdalawieh O, Kiefte M, et al. The effect of increased stiffness of the incudostapedial joint on the transmission of air-conducted sound by the human middle ear. Otol Neurotol. 2013;34(8):1503-9.
60. Offergeld CFE HtK-B, Zahnert T, et al. Experimental investigations of ossicular joint ankylosis. In: JJ Rosowski, Merchant SN (eds), The function and mechanics of normal, diseased and reconstructed middle ears. Hague, the Netherlands: Kugler Publications; 2000. pp. 177-186.
61. Goldenberg RA. Ossiculoplasty with composite prostheses. PORP and TORP. Otolaryngol Clin N Am. 1994;27(4): 727-45.
62. De Vos C, Gersdorff M, Gerard JM. Prognostic factors in ossiculoplasty. Otol Neurotol. 2007;28(1):61-7.
63. Elpern BS, Elbrond O. Restoration of ossicular continuity with methyl methacrylate. Arch Otolaryngol. 1966;84(3): 320-24.
64. Shimizu Y, Goode RL. Effect of absence of malleus on ossiculoplasty in human temporal bones. Otolaryngol Head Neck Surg. 2008;139(2):301-6.
65. Goode RL, Killion M, Nakamura K, et al. New knowledge about the function of the human middle ear: development of an improved analog model. Am J Otol. 1994;15(2): 145-54.
66. Nishihara S, Goode RL. Experimental study of the acoustic properties of incus replacement prostheses in a human temporal bone model. Am J Otol. 1994;15(4):485-94.

67. Morris DP, Bance M, Van Wijhe RG. How do cartilage and other material overlay over a prosthesis affect its vibration transmission properties in ossiculoplasty? Otolaryngol Head Neck Surg. 2004;131(4):423-8.
68. Alian WA, Majdalawieh OF, Van Wijhe RG, et al. Prosthetic reconstruction from the tympanic membrane to the stapes head or to the stapes footplate? A laser Doppler study. J Otolaryngol Head Neck Surg [Le Journal d'oto-rhino-laryngologie et de chirurgie cervico-faciale]. 2012;41(2):84-93.
69. Murugasu E, Puria S, Roberson JB, Jr. Malleus-to-footplate versus malleus-to-stapes-head ossicular reconstruction prostheses: temporal bone pressure gain measurements and clinical audiological data. Otol Neurotol. 2005;26(4): 572-82.
70. Asai M, Huber AM, Goode RL. Analysis of the best site on the stapes footplate for ossicular chain reconstruction. Acta Otolaryngol. 1999;119(3):356-61.
71. Cottle RD, Tonndorf J. Mechanical aspects of stapedial substitution: an experimental study. Arch Otolaryngol. 1966;83 (6):547-53.
72. Bance M, Makki FM, Garland P, et al. Effects of tensor tympani muscle contraction on the middle ear and markers of a contracted muscle. Laryngoscope. 2013;123(4): 1021-7.
73. Morris DP, Wong L, van Wijhe RG, et al. Effect of adhesion on the acoustic functioning of partial ossicular replacement prostheses in the cadaveric human ear. J Otolaryngol. 2006; 35(1):22-5.
74. Voss SE, Rosowski JJ, Merchant SN, et al. Acoustic responses of the human middle ear. Hear Res. 2000;150(1-2):43-69.
75. Rosowski JJ, Ravicz ME, Songer JE. Structures that contribute to middle-ear admittance in chinchilla. J Comp Physiol. 2006;192(12):1287-311.

CHAPTER

4

Anatomy and Physiology of the Vestibular System

Daniel Q Sun, Yuri Agrawal

The vestibular system senses movement of the head and the orientation of the head with respect to gravity. The vestibular system accomplishes these tasks through the five sensory end organs: the three semicircular canals (SCCs) that sense head rotations and the two otolith organs that sense linear translations and tilts of the head. The information collected by the vestibular system is then transmitted centrally and used by the brain to perform a number of tasks. Most of the best-characterized functions subserved by the vestibular system relate to balance and postural stability. However, emerging research is also demonstrating a role for vestibular information in regulating the autonomic nervous system, spatial navigation and memory, and even cognitive function and affective states. Vestibular information is used to drive homeostatic reflexes, e.g. the vestibulo-ocular reflex (VOR) that stabilizes gaze and the vestibulospinal reflex (VSR) that stabilizes posture. Vestibular inputs also feed into cortical and cerebellar networks that are involved in higher order functions such as motor planning and adaptation. This section on vestibular anatomy and physiology will review gross and cellular anatomy of the peripheral vestibular sensory system, and basic principles of its physiology, including mechanoelectric transduction, vestibular afferent organization, and the physiology of the best-characterized vestibular reflex: the VOR.

GROSS ANATOMY

The vestibular labyrinth is a complex three-dimensional structure located within the otic capsule in the petrous temporal bone and contiguous with the auditory regions of the inner ear. The physiology of the vestibular system arises directly from its anatomical structure, and an in-depth understanding of its system behavior and characteristics requires first a detailed understanding of the gross and cellular anatomy of the vestibular labyrinth.

Bony and Membranous Labyrinth

The vestibular labyrinth (Fig. 4.1) consists of a series of fluid-filled bony canals and chambers located within the otic capsule, referred to as the bony labyrinth. Suspended within the bony labyrinth is a series of similarly shaped fluid-filled tubes and sacs termed the membranous labyrinth. The fluid filling the space between bony and membranous labyrinth is termed perilymph, which resembles

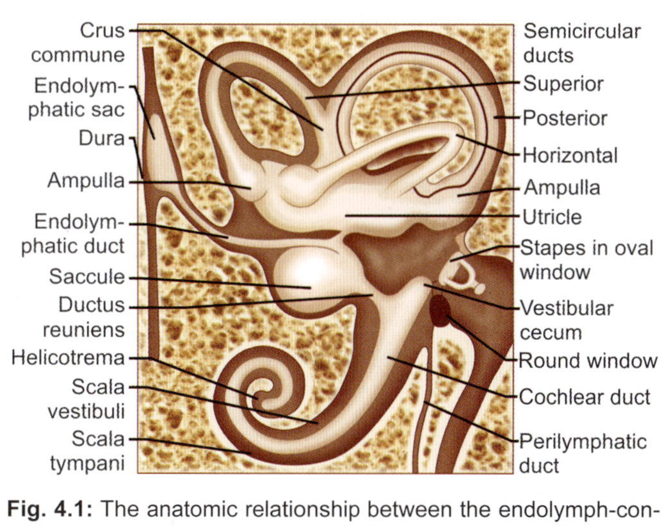

Fig. 4.1: The anatomic relationship between the endolymph-containing membranous and perilymph-containing bony labyrinths, showing the three semicircular canals as well as the utricle and saccule located within the vestibule, contiguous with the cochlea.

cerebral spinal fluid in composition with a high concentration of sodium relative to potassium. The lumen of the membranous labyrinth is also filled by fluid, termed endolymph, which contains a high concentration of potassium relative to sodium. The perilymphatic space of the vestibular system is contiguous with the scala vestibuli of the cochlea via the vestibule, from where the basal turn of the cochlea arises. The endolymph in the vestibular labyrinth communicates with the endolymph-containing scala media (cochlear duct) of the cochlea via the ductus reuniens. These connections between the vestibular labyrinth and the cochlea allow not only for equilibration of molecules but also the transmission of both physical (e.g. pressure waves in sound conduction) and chemical (e.g. diffusion of ototoxic drugs) perturbations of clinical relevance. The perilymph communicates with CSF via the perilymphatic duct (cochlear aquaduct), while the endolymph circulates to the endolymphatic sac located in the posterior cranial fossa via the endolymphatic duct.

The membranous labyrinth on each side includes three SCCs and two otolith organs, which together make up the five end organs of the vestibular system. These end organs, together with their identical but mirror image pairs on the other side, provide vestibular sensory input to the central nervous system (CNS) by detecting head motion and position relative to gravitation.

Semicircular Canals

Each vestibular labyrinth is composed of three SCCs arranged approximately orthogonal to each other (Figs. 4.2A and B). The horizontal (lateral) SCC lies approximately 30° from Earth horizontal when the head is upright, with the anterior limb tilted more superiorly compared to the posterior limb, while the superior and posterior SCCs are aligned 45° anterior and posterior, respectively, to the interaural line and 90° to the plane of the horizontal SCC. When the SCCs in the contralateral vestibular labyrinth are taken into account, three planes are created by the orientation of the SCCs. The horizontal canal plane lies parallel to the two horizontal SCCs and is pitched 30° from Earth horizontal. The right anterior left posterior (RALP) canal plane is formed by the right superior (anterior) and left posterior SCCs and is orthogonal to the horizontal canal plane while angled at 45° from the midsagittal plane. Similarly, the left anterior right posterior (LARP) canal plane is formed by the left superior and right posterior SCCs, and lies 45° off the midsagittal plane in the opposite direction as LARP. The planes in which these three canals lie are therefore mutually orthogonal and approximate an XYZ Cartesian coordinate system.

One end of each SCC is dilated at its connection to the vestibule. Termed the ampulla, it is the site of the sensory

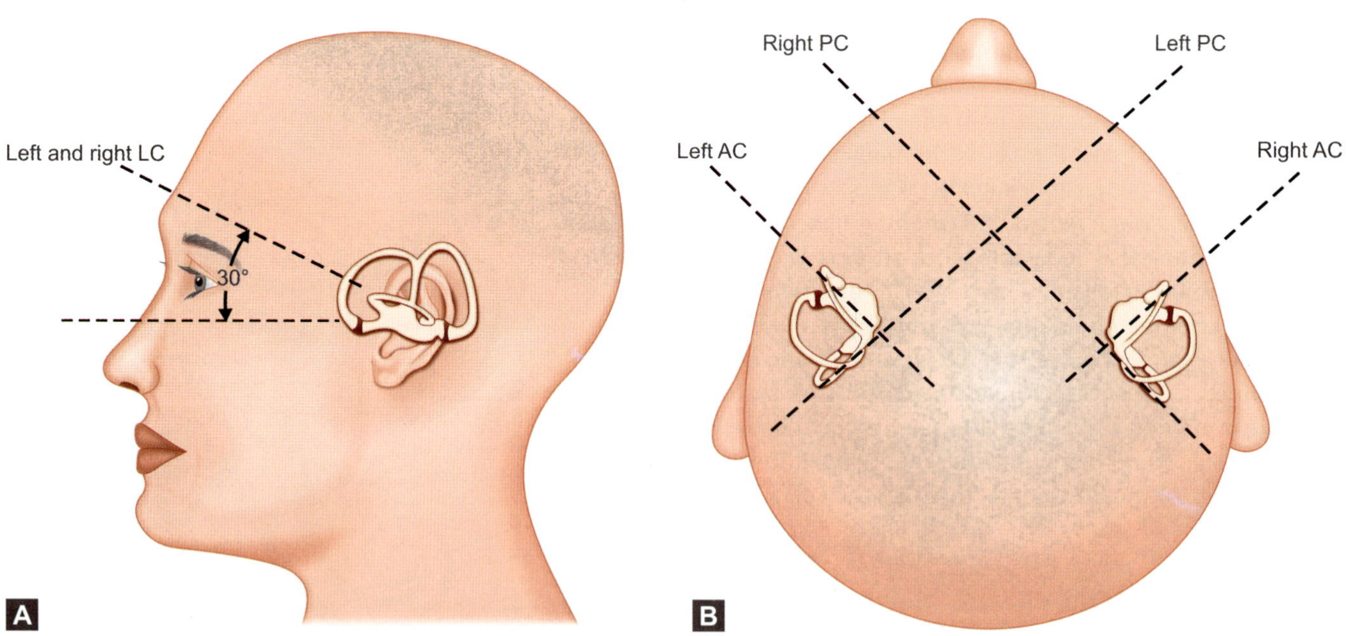

Figs. 4.2A and B: Orientation of the semicircular canals (SCCs) in head. The lateral SCCs (A) are pitched upward 30° from Earth horizontal and form the horizontal canal plane. The anterior and posterior SCCs (B) are oriented 45° from the midsagittal plane and 90° from each other. The right anterior and left posterior canals form the RALP plane and the left anterior and right posterior canals form the LARP plane. [LC: Lateral (horizontal) SCC; AC: Anterior (superior) SCC; PC: Posterior SCC].

neuroepithelium and innervation for that SCC. Each ampulla consists of a saddle-shaped neuroepithelial membrane termed the crista ampullaris that contains vestibular hair cells (HCs) (Fig. 4.3). Akin to HCs in the cochlea, vestibular HCs also project stereocilia from their surface. In each crista, these stereocilia project into a gelatinous matrix comprised of mucopolysaccharides and keratin,[1] termed the cupula, which extends across the cross-section of the ampulla. The cupula is deflected by the movement of endolymph in that SCC, which in turn causes deflection of the associated stereocilia, leading to mechanotransduction in vestibular HCs. In the horizontal SCCs, flow of endolymph toward the ampulla (centripetal) activates vestibular HCs while in the superior and posterior SCCs, flow of endolymph away from the ampulla (centrifugal) activates vestibular HCs. As a consequence of the toroidal shape of each SCC and the arrangement of the cupula across the cross-section of the ampulla, each SCC is maximally sensitive to rotational movement in the plane of that canal.

If a rotational movement of the head is thought of as a three-dimensional angular acceleration vector with a direction and magnitude, the SCCs faithfully represent the direction of this vector via the geometric alignment of its canals and the magnitude via the differential modulation of the firing rate of vestibular HCs from each side. Since an SCC is only activated by rotational movement in the plane of that canal, any head rotation is resolved into its respective components in the horizontal, LARP, and RALP canal planes. The magnitude of angular acceleration is encoded by the firing rate of vestibular HCs. Unlike cochlear HCs, vestibular HCs have a nonzero baseline firing rate (~100 pps in humans).[2] Any head motion (e.g. turning head to left) results in activation or increased firing rate of one canal (e.g. left horizontal) and inhibition or decreased firing rate of the complementary canal (e.g. right horizontal) in that plane. Therefore, direction of the head rotation is encoded in the specific activation pattern of the SCCs, while the magnitude of acceleration is encoded by the firing rate in the affected canals.

Otolith Organs

The vestibule contains two otolith organs, utricle and saccule, which sense linear acceleration. Each organ's neuroepithelium, termed macula, is a planar structure that also contains directionally polarized vestibular HCs (Figs. 4.4A and B). Stereocilia of macular HCs project into an overlying gelatinous matrix, which contains small crystals of calcium carbonate termed otoconia. The planar shape of each macula along with its overlying otoconial membrane renders it sensitive to shear forces as a result of linear acceleration. The maculae of the utricle and saccule are oriented orthogonal to each other. The utricular macula is approximately coplanar with Earth horizontal with the head upright, and the saccular macula is oriented vertically, 90° to the utricular macula. Therefore, this anatomic arrangement also provides a basis for encoding of linear forces along three mutually orthogonal axes (interaural, nasal-occipital, and rostral-caudal).

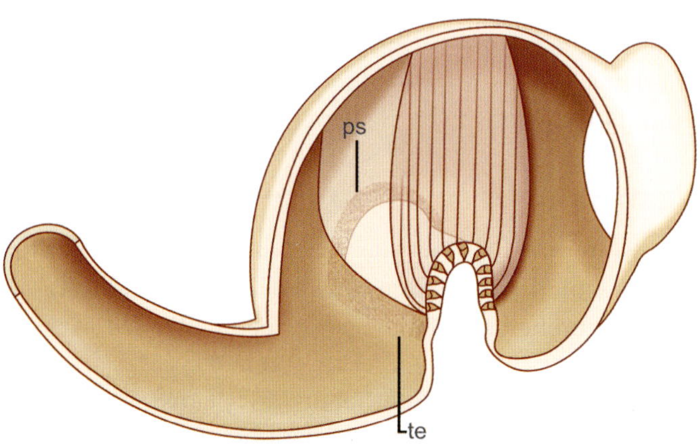

Fig. 4.3: Schematic representation of crista ampullaris in a semicircular canal (SCC). The neuroepithelium is saddle shaped and located within the ampulla. The cupula extends from the crista to the roof of the ampulla, allowing it to detect inertia movement of endolymph contained in the SCC and ampulla. The crista is innervated from below by ampullary nerve fibers and surrounded by a transitional epithelium (TE) and planum semilunatum (PS).

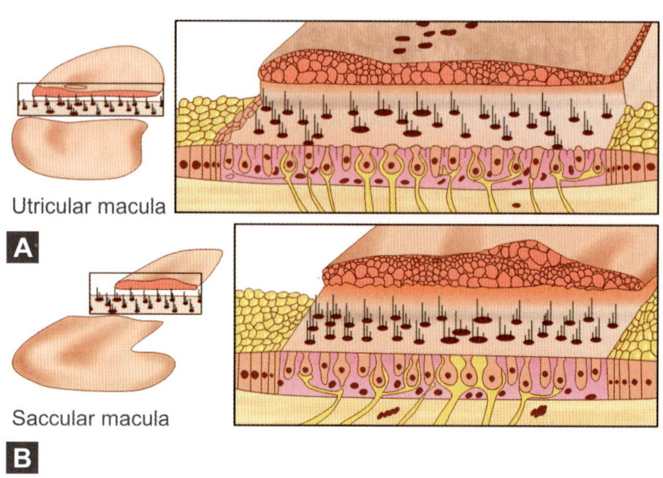

Figs. 4.4A and B: Schematic representation of utricular (A) and saccular (B) maculae. The neuroepithelium is mostly flat with an overlying otoconial membrane. In contrast to the semicircular canals, the hair cells in the maculae are not all polarized in the same direction.

These linear forces include not only gravity but also others such as forward motion and bobbing head movements during walking. The otolith organs detect forces both dynamic, such as translation, and static, such as tilt, to generate appropriate compensatory eye movements and/or musculoskeletal activation. The response characteristics of the otolith organs are also more complex than in the SCCs, as HCs in each macula are not all polarized anisotropically, i.e. their stereocilia are not all tuned to the same direction. In fact, a static head tilt will lead to activation and inhibition of HCs from different sectors within each macula. How this information is encoded in the peripheral end organs and integrated in the CNS remains an area of active research.

Vestibular Neuroanatomy

Each vestibular neuroepithelium is innervated by a terminal branch of the vestibular portion of cranial nerve VIII. Afferent neuronal bodies are located in Scarpa's ganglion, which is hour-glass shaped and divided into superior and inferior halves, corresponding to superior and inferior divisions of the vestibular nerve. The superior and horizontal SCC cristae, utricular macula, and a small portion of anterior saccular macula are innervated by the superior division, whereas the posterior SCC crista and posterior saccular macula are innervated by the inferior division. The terminal ampullary branch innervating the posterior SCC is also termed the singular nerve. Centrally, afferent projections enter the brainstem at the ventrolateral aspect of pontomedullary junction, then course between the inferior cerebellar peduncle and the descending tract of the trigeminal nerve to synapse in the ipsilateral vestibular nuclei, which is divided into medial, lateral, superior, and inferior divisions.[3] Afferent fibers also project to the cerebellum and other brainstem nuclei. In contrast to the organizational pattern of sensory systems such as vision, hearing, and touch, the receptive fields of the peripheral vestibular end organs are not mapped topographically to the vestibular nuclei. Indeed, a single vestibular nucleus neuron may receive convergent afferent input from more than one ipsilateral neuroepithelium. Neurons in the vestibular nuclei also receive downstream input from other sensory processes, such as optokinetic and neck proprioceptive information.

From the vestibular nuclei, neurons send projections to the motor neurons in the abducens, trochlear, and oculomotor nuclei (Figs. 4.5A and B). Each individual vestibular nucleus neuron may project to multiple extraocular motor neuron pools, both ipsi- and contralateral, to generate conjugate eye movements.[3] Ipsilateral projections tend to be inhibitory, using neurotransmitters glycine and GABA, whereas contralateral pathways tend to be excitatory, using glutamine.[4] These pathways form the neuroanatomical basis for the angular vestibulo-ocular reflex (aVOR) that is first encoded in the SCCs. Many eye movements, including the aVOR, require conversion of angular head velocity signal encoded in the SCCs into head position signal to generate accurate extraocular muscle movements. The neural integrator is a collection of neurons that performs this mathematical function. The nucleus prepositus hypoglossi (NPH), which lies just medial to the medial vestibular nucleus, and the interstitial nucleus of Cajal (INC), which lies adjacent to the oculomotor nucleus, are neural integrators for the horizontal and vertical aVORs, respectively.[5]

Central pathways also exist for the vestibulo-ocular and VSRs subserved by the otolith organs. Similar to aVOR, projections exist from the vestibular nucleus to the ipsi- and contralateral oculomotor nuclei for the linear VOR (lVOR) and ocular counter-roll (OCR). The pathways for vestibulocervical and VSRs lie in the lateral and medial vestibulospinal, and the lateral and medial reticulospinal tracts that originate in the vestibular nucleus to terminate on motor, and other neurons in the spinal cord.[6] These pathways link the reflex control of the cervical and trunk musculature to the vestibular system.

The peripheral vestibular end organs are also innervated by an efferent system originating adjacent to the abducens nucleus. These efferent fibers also travel along cranial nerve VIII to terminate along the base of type II vestibular HCs (*see* next section). The physiologic significance of the efferent system is not well understood, but likely serves to modulate HC sensitivity via hyper- or depolarization.[7]

Vestibular Vascular Anatomy

The primary blood supply is through the labyrinthine artery, which most commonly arises from the anterior inferior cerebellar (45%), superior cerebellar (24%), basilar (16%), or posterior inferior cerebellar (5%) arteries.[8] It travels through the internal auditory canal and divides into the anterior vestibular and common cochlear arteries, the latter of which further divides into the spiral modiolar and vestibulocochlear arteries. The vestibular branch of the vestibulocochlear artery supplies the posterior SCC ampulla and most of the saccule, while the anterior vestibular artery supplies the horizontal and superior SCC ampullae, utricle, and part of the saccule.

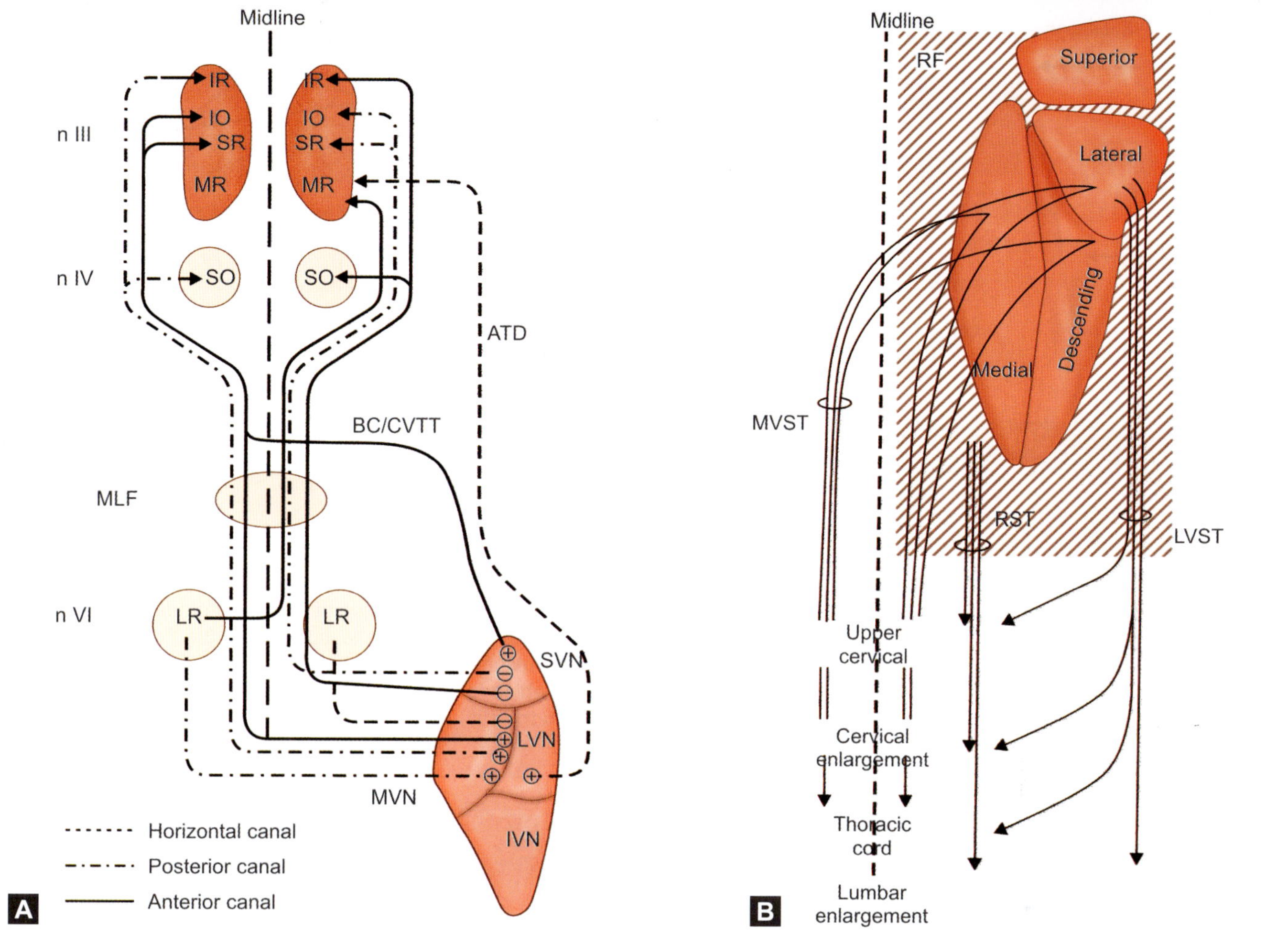

Figs. 4.5A and B: Connectivity diagram of vestibular nucleus projections to oculomotor (A) and vestibulocervical and -spinal (B) pathways in the central nervous system.

VESTIBULAR END ORGANS

Hair Cells

Vestibular HCs are specialized sensory epithelial cells that transduce mechanical signals into electrochemical impulses, and share many cellular and morphological features with auditory HCs in the cochlea. Stereocilia are macrovilli of varying height that project from the apical surface of a vestibular HC into the endolymphatic space. There are 20–100 stereocilia per HC.[9] Each stereocilium has a rigid actin core, and stereocilia bundles are arranged in a staircase configuration such that the shortest stereocilium is at one end and the tallest, termed the kinocilium, at the other. In contrast to stereocilia, the kinocilium has a microtubular support structure. Tip links[10] are proteins that span from the tip of one stereocilium to the side of the adjacent, taller stereocilium (Fig. 4.6). They are physically connected to the mechanoelectrical transduction (MET) channels expressed at the tip of each stereocilium and therefore couple the opening of an MET channel to physical deflection of its neighboring stereocilium, which serves as the molecular basis for MET in vestibular HCs[11] (*see* next section).

For each HC, deflection of stereocilia toward or away from the kinocilium results in an increase (excitation) or decrease (inhibition) in afferent discharge, respectively. As a consequence of the anisotropic configuration of stereocilia by height toward the kinocilium, each vestibular HC has a polarization vector along which it is most sensitive to stereocilia deflection and which forms a cosine relationship with the vector of rotational or translational force (Fig. 4.7). Therefore, force vectors that are parallel to the height gradient of the stereocilia and act toward the kinocilium of an HC cause maximum excitation while

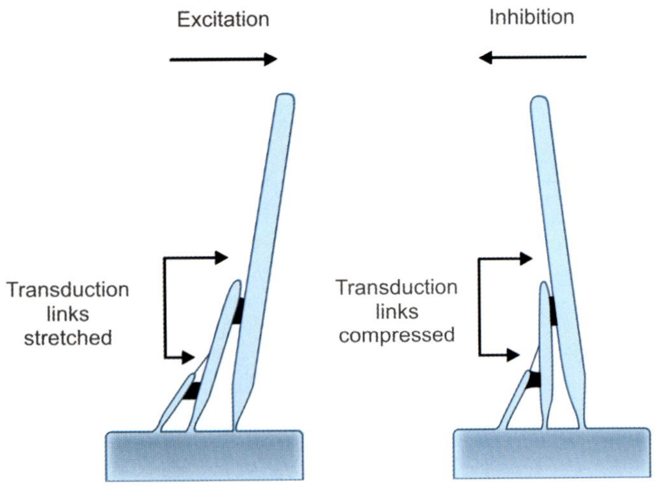

Fig. 4.6: Schematic representation of the relationship between hair cell stereocilia and tip links (dark lines) leading to mechanoelectrotransduction. Deflection of the stereocilia may stretch or compress the tip links, leading to excitation or inhibition, respectively.

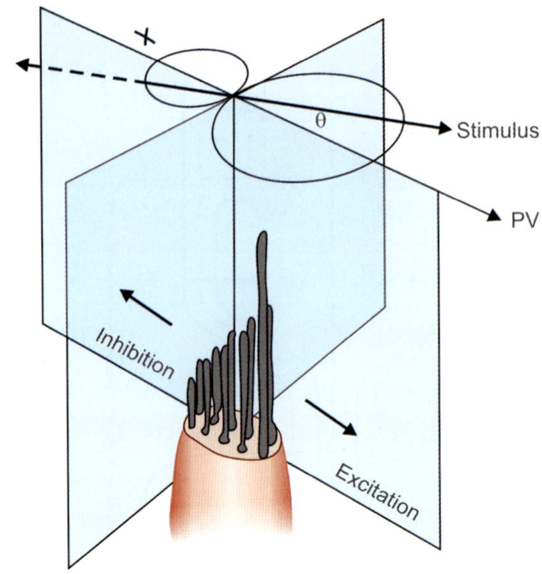

Fig. 4.7: Schematic representation of the directional sensitivity of a hair cell due to the orientation of the height gradient of its stereociliary bundle. Stereocilia deflection toward the kinocilium causes maximal excitation and form the hair cell (HC's) polarization vector (PV), which forms a cosine relationship with its angle (θ) with respect to the stimulus vector.

those that are perpendicular to the height gradient of the stereocilia cause minimal kinocilium deflection and are not sensed by the HC.

Vestibular HCs are innervated by afferent nerve terminals on their basolateral surface (Fig. 4.8). On HC activation, glutamate is released from synaptic ribbons located along the basolateral aspect of each HC and leads to action potential generation in the afferent nerve. Vestibular HCs exist in two types characterized by differences in morphology and afferent innervation.[12] Type I HCs are flask shaped with a rounded base and each is innervated by a calyx afferent nerve terminal in the shape of a chalice that almost completely surrounds the HC body. Type II HCs are cylindrically shaped and innervated by bouton nerve terminals of both afferents and efferents.[13] Although regional variations exist within a neuroepithelium, type II HCs synapse with multiple afferent boutons while each type I HC may synapse with only 1 calyx.

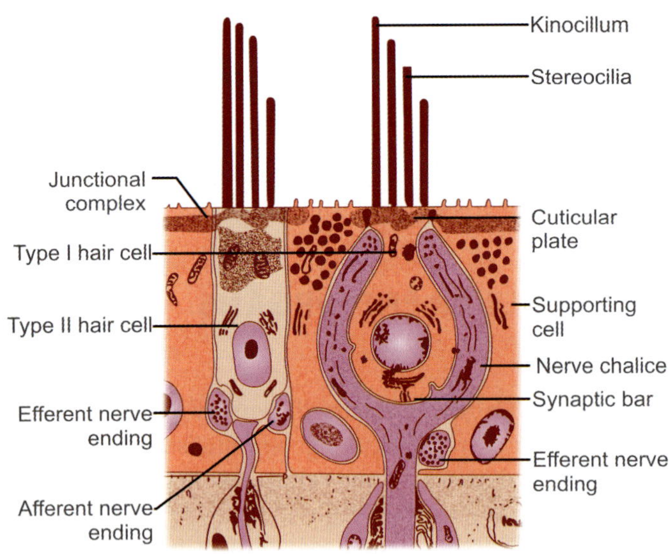

Fig. 4.8: Hair cell (HC) ultrastructure showing the difference between type I (right) and II (left) HCs. The flask-shaped type I HC is innervated by a calyx ending from a single vestibular nerve afferent, whereas the type II HC is cylindrical and innervated by multiple bouton endings.

Crista Ampullaris

All vestibular neuroepithelia share a common cellular architecture. A single layer of support cells lie directly above the basement membrane. They play important roles in maintaining the overlying cupula or otoconial membrane, and the homeostatic microenvironment around HCs and afferent nerve terminals, including removal of neurotransmitters. Type I and II HC nuclei are located above those of the support cells and they form tight junctions along their apical, endolymphatic surface. Immediately surrounding the neuroepithelium is a region known as the transitional zone, which contains cells similar to support cells, but not HCs. Dark cells, which play an important role in ion transport to maintain the potassium-rich endolymph, surround the transitional zone and melanocytes are found in the connective tissue stroma below.[14]

The crista forms a saddle shape and can be divided into central, intermediate, and peripheral zones with anatomical and functional distinctions. The total HC surface density in human cristae has been found to be approximately 60–80/0.01 mm^2.[15] The central zone includes the apex of the crista and in humans, ratio of type I to II HCs is approximately 1.6–2.4[15] and consequently, most calycal afferent terminals are also found here. The peripheral zone includes the slopes of the crista and contains a more even ratio of type I to II HCs. As such, bouton terminals that innervate type II HCs are more prevalent here. The intermediate zone lies between the central and peripheral zones. The functional implications of the morphological variations in afferent nerve terminals will be covered in the next section. Stereocilia of HCs in the crista of an SCC are all polarized in the same direction (Fig. 4.9A). That is, the height gradient of stereociliary bundles are all oriented in the plane of that canal, toward the direction of maximum sensitivity. This anisotropic arrangement of stereocilia within the HC population of an SCC thereby allows detection of the component of rotational force coplanar with that SCC.

Macula

The cellular architecture of the otolithic macula is similar to that of the crista, except that it is mostly flat and kidney shaped rather than saddle shaped. Instead of a central zone, a narrow ribbon-shaped band, termed the striola, runs across its length. The striola is characterized by decreased HC density and a predominance of type I HCs.[16] In contrast to the cristae, macular HCs are not all polarized in the same direction. In the saccular macula, HCs on either side of the striola are polarized away from it and in the utricular macula, HCs are polarized toward the striola (Figs. 4.9B and C). Therefore, otolithic neuroepithelia do not have a single direction of sensitivity and any force vector produces sector-specific excitation and inhibition within each neuroepithelium.

MECHANOELECTRIC TRANSDUCTION

MET is the process by which endolymph displacement associated with head movement is sensed by the vestibular HCs and converted into a modulation of the firing rate of the primary vestibular afferents. MET involves six steps: (1) endolymph acceleration (rotation or translation), (2) hair bundle deflection, (3) opening of MET channels, (4) HC depolarization, (5) increase in basolateral transmitter release, and (6) increase in rate of action potentials in the primary vestibular afferent neuron (Figs. 4.10A and B).

When the head either rotates or translates, the membranous labyrinth that is attached to the bony labyrinth moves with the head. However, inertial forces resist endolymph movement and lead to a relative movement of endolymph in the opposite direction to the head movement. The relative movement of the endolymph results

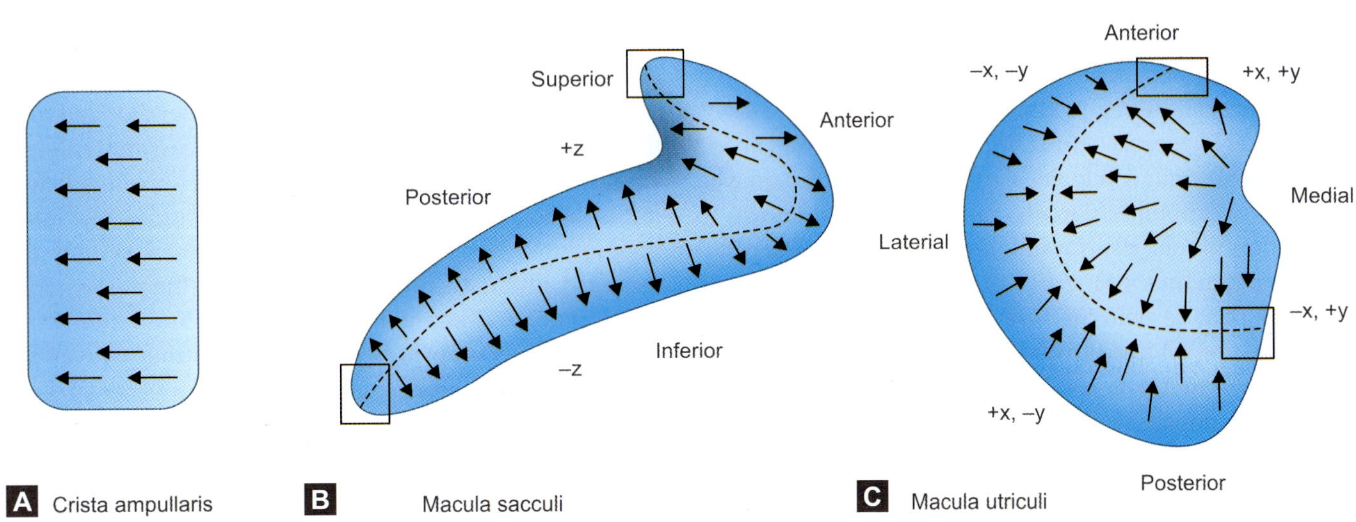

Figs. 4.9A to C: Schematic representation of hair cell (HC) polarization in vestibular end organs. In the crista ampullaris (A), all HCs are polarized in the same direction. The saccular (B) and utricular (C) maculae contain a striolar region (dashed line) that runs along its length. Hair cells are polarized away from the striola in the saccule and toward the striola in the utricle.

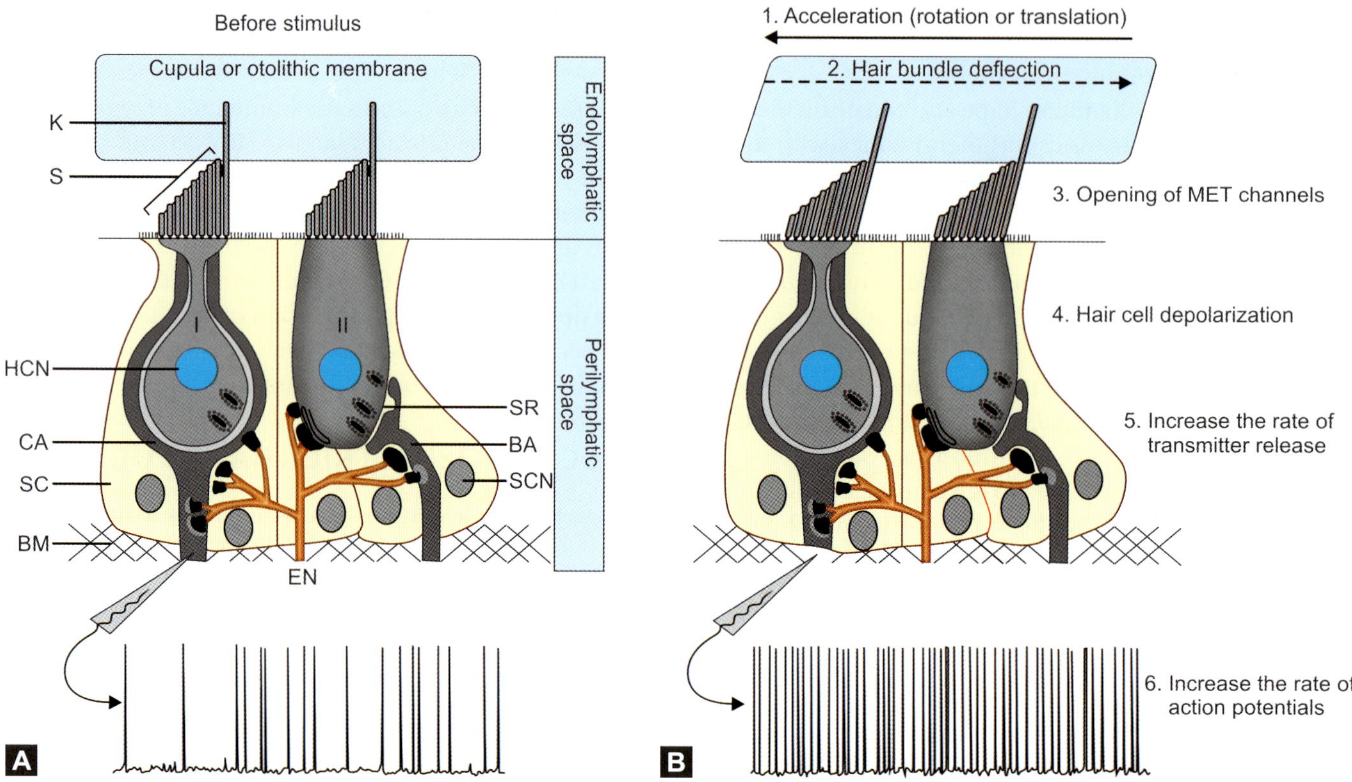

Figs. 4.10A and B: Hair cell (HC) mechanoelectric transduction. (A) HCs continuously release neurotransmitter from synaptic ribbons (SR) on their basolateral surface to depolarize afferent nerve terminals, leading to a baseline firing rate in the vestibular nerve. (B) This baseline firing rate is modulated by hair bundle deflection as a result of inertial forces in the endolymph generated by head movement. (BA, bouton afferent; BM, basement membrane; CA, calyx afferent; EN, efferent neuron; HCN, hair cell nucleus; I, type I hair cell; II, type II hair cell; K, kinocilia; S, stereocilia; SC, supporting cell).

in deflection of the cupula (or otolithic membrane in the otoliths), and a shear force is applied to the underlying HCs bundles that insert into the cupula. Endolymph and cupular dynamics have been modelled using the torsion-pendulum model, whereby cupular deflection is a function of head acceleration and endolymph viscosity. Moreover, this model suggests that the cupula integrates this acceleration input into a velocity signal, which is then relayed centrally. Vestibular afferents, for instance, are known to fire action potentials as a function of head angular velocity. The dynamic properties of the otolithic membrane have not been as well-characterized as the cupula. Models variously predict that the otolithic membrane responds to linear acceleration or jerk, the derivative of acceleration.

As mentioned in the previous section, depending on whether the shear force is in the direction toward the kinocilium or away from the kinocilium, the tip links between HC projections mechanically increase or decrease the probability of MET channel opening respectively.[11] In the SCCs, the HC stereocilia and kinocilia are all arrayed in the same direction such that all cells are similarly excited by the same direction of endolymph flow. In contrast, in the otoliths, the HCs are organized along multiple polarization vectors and respond differentially to various directions of head translation or tilt.[17] Increased opening of the MET channels leads to a potassium ion influx into the HC from the endolymph and HC depolarization. Depolarization of the HC in turn results in opening of voltage-gated calcium channels on the basolateral end of the HC, and calcium influx into the HC. The calcium ions stimulate vesicle release into the synaptic cleft of the neurotransmitter glutamate. Glutamate binds to receptors on the postsynaptic membrane, and stimulates an increase in afferent firing rate and generation of action potentials that convey the head movement information centrally.

It is important to note that a background level of glutamate release at the basolateral end of the HC occurs, leading to a resting level of afferent discharge. Thus if the HC is hyperpolarized rather than depolarized (through head movements that deflect the HC bundles away from the kinocilium), calcium conductance decreases and the background level of glutamate release decreases. The ability of the afferent neuron to be modulated both in the excitatory and inhibitory direction give the vestibular afferent system the important property of bidirectional sensitivity, which explains why loss of unilateral labyrinthine function can be compensated for to a certain extent by an intact contralateral labyrinth.

VESTIBULAR AFFERENT ORGANIZATION

Primary vestibular nerve afferents can be classified based on morphological characteristics into calyceal, bouton and dimorphic.[18,19] Calyceal afferents have a calyx nerve ending that exclusively contacts and envelops the type I HC. Bouton afferents have small rounded terminals that exclusively contact type II HCs. Dimorphic afferents have nerve endings that are both calyceal and bouton-like, and thus make connections with both type I and type II HCs (Figs. 4.11A to D).[20] Dimorphic afferents constitute the majority of afferents, followed by the bouton then calyceal afferents. Given that type I HCs are located in the central region of the SCC cristae (or in the striolar region of the otolithic maculae), calyceal afferents terminate largely in the central region. Type II HCs are located at the periphery of the cristae; as such bouton afferents largely terminate in the periphery. Dimorphic afferents terminate in both central and peripheral regions of the cristae, given that they contain both calyceal and bouton-type nerve endings.

Calyceal afferent nerve fibers can also be distinguished from bouton afferents based on their resting discharge rate. Calyceal fibers are irregularly discharging at baseline, whereas bouton fibers are regularly discharging. Again, dimorphic fibers span a spectrum from irregular to regular resting discharge rates (Figs. 4.12A and B).[2] Differences in potassium ion channel conductance following afferent neuron hyperpolarization are thought to underlie differences in afferent discharge regularity (Fig. 4.13).[21] The afferent nerve generates an action potential through inward sodium currents, and following the action potential an outwardly directed potassium current hyperpolarizes the afferent. The hyperpolarized potential then decays to ready the neuron for the next action potential. In regular afferents, nerve potential increases in a deterministic fashion to threshold levels, and an action potential is triggered at regular intervals. However, in irregular afferents, nerve potential is increased only to just below threshold, such that stochastic neurotransmitter release from the basolateral end of the HCs causes action potential firing at random intervals.

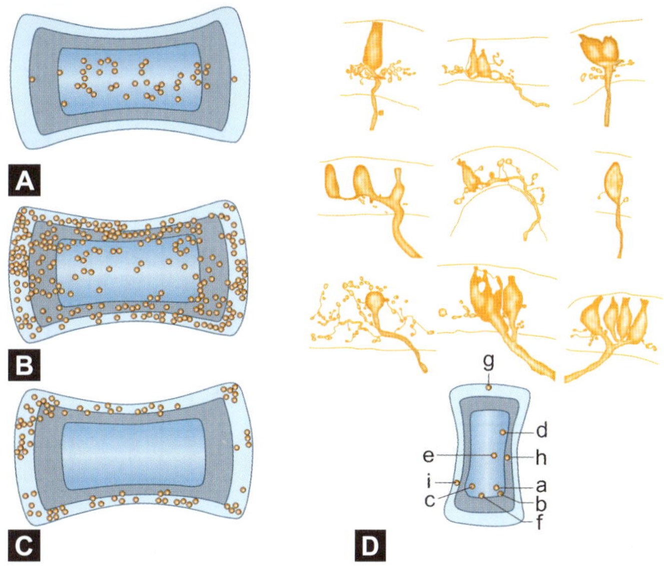

Figs. 4.11A to D: Variations in morphology of afferent terminals, which can be classified into calyceal, bouton, or dimorphic. Calyceal terminals innervate type I HCs and are mostly found in the central zone of the crista (A) whereas dimorphic (B) and bouton (C) terminals are mostly concentrated in the intermediate and peripheral zones. (D) Reconstruction of dimorphic units in chinchilla.

A large body of work suggests that the differences in afferent discharge regularity are associated with functional differences between the afferent classes. Irregular afferents are most responsive to changes in stimulus velocity. These changes occur at stimulus onset and offset; thus irregular afferents have also been termed "phasic" afferents.[22] Irregular afferents are typically activated by fast (high-frequency), transient head movements and are more sensitive to galvanic stimulation, which directly stimulates the vestibular afferents (bypassing the MET mechanism).[23] Additionally, irregular afferents have been suggested to be involved in context-specific adaptation of vestibular responses, e.g. with vergence or with the use of magnifying or minifying spectacles.[24,25] In contrast, regular afferents are thought to encode stimulus magnitude, and are thus also referred to as "tonic" afferents.[22] Regular afferents are most responsive to slow (low frequency), sustained head movements, and are less sensitive to galvanic stimulation.

A population of 400–600 efferent neurons also innervates the peripheral vestibular end organs. These fibers originate in the brainstem adjacent to the vestibular nuclei, and synapse onto the basolateral surface of type II HCs or on the calyceal endings of primary vestibular afferents synapsing with type I HCs. The efferent neurons are excitatory to the vestibular afferents, particularly the irregular

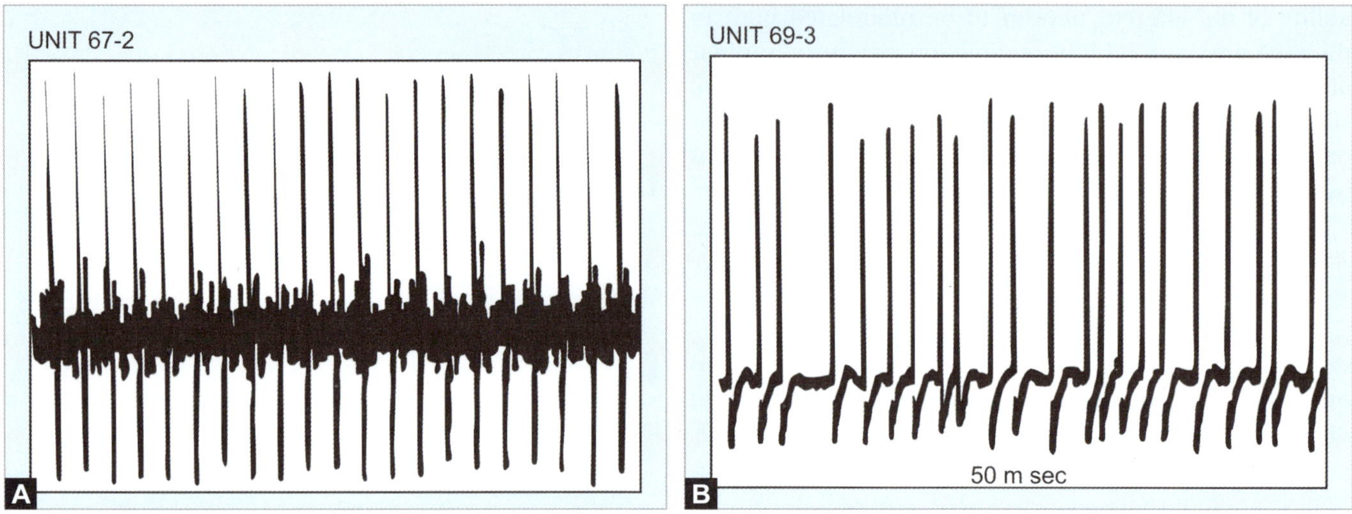

Figs. 4.12A and B: Action potentials recorded during rest from the vestibular nerve of a squirrel monkey showing two types of neurons. Unit 67-2 and Unit 69-3 demonstrate a regular and irregular resting discharge rate, respectively.

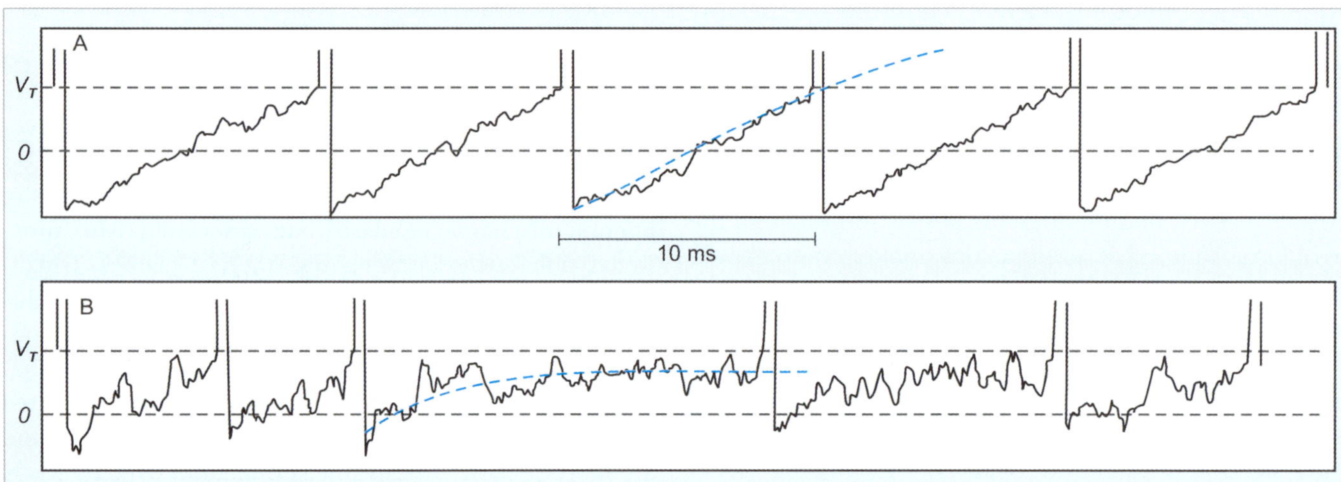

Fig. 4.13: Mathematical modeling of differences in afferent discharge regularity. Time- but not voltage-dependent potassium conductance leads to afterhyperpolarization in afferent terminals. This stochastic model demonstrates that two factors, the post spike voltage trajectory (dotted line in B) and synaptic noise, are relevant in determining discharge regularity. Horizontal dashed lines are the resting potential (*0*) and critical firing level (V_T).

afferents. Their function is not fully understood: they have been postulated to increase the baseline firing rate of the primary vestibular afferents, or balance the firing rates of afferents on the right and left sides.[26]

VESTIBULO-OCULAR REFLEX

The VOR is an important reflex driven by vestibular sensory signaling that maintains a stable visual image on the retina. Through a three neuron arc, information about head movement is transduced by the vestibular HC receptor into an electrical signal in the primary vestibular afferent neuron. The primary afferent synapses onto a neuron in the vestibular nucleus in the brainstem, which in turn synapses with a neuron in one of the oculomotor nuclei (III, IV, or VI). The oculomotor neuron then innervates an extraocular muscle, which drives an eye movement that compensates for the head movement in order to keep the eye's position in space fixed. Several other visually driven reflexes also serve to minimize retinal slip and stabilize gaze (i.e. eye-in-space). These include the smooth pursuit system, which tracks a target moving across the field of view, and the optokinetic system, which follows the movement of the visual field. However, these systems involve cortical processing, which imposes a latency of at least 100 milliseconds.[27] As such, these systems break down at retinal slip velocities greater than 50°/second and frequencies greater than 1 Hz. Many natural head movements reach much higher velocities and frequencies (e.g. 90°/second velocity during walking, and 15–20 Hz during running).[28] The VOR, which has a latency on the order of 7 milliseconds, can uniquely stabilize gaze in the high-velocity, high-frequency range.[29]

Head movements along the plane of a SCC drive compensatory eye movements that are equal and opposite along the plane of that SCC. In other words, eye movements occur in a canal-fixed (or head-fixed) frame of reference rather than in an eye-fixed frame of reference. This principle is referred to as Ewald's First Law, based on the German physiologist who stimulated the SCCs of pigeons and observed the resultant eye movements occurring in the canal plane.[30] The SCCs are organized into three sets of coplanar pairs that are roughly orthogonal to each other: the right and left horizontal canals, the left anterior and right posterior canals (LARP pair), and the right anterior and left posterior canals (RALP pair) (Fig. 4.2).[31] The extraocular muscles are roughly aligned along similar planes as the SCCs. The medial and lateral recti align with the horizontal SCCs, the anterior SCCs are aligned with the ipsilateral superior and inferior recti and the contralateral obliques, and the posterior SCCs are aligned with the ipsilateral obliques and the contralateral superior and inferior recti. The roughly parallel orientation of the SCCs and eye movements may be advantageous in that fewer neural computations are required to generate the VOR.[32] This may explain the extremely fast latency of this reflex. It should be noted that most natural head movements do not occur along a single canal plane. A series of experiments in cats by Cohen et al demonstrated that the perceived head rotation represents a vector sum of all the component rotations along individual canal planes.[33]

An additional property of the VOR is that it functions as a "push-pull" system. Rotation of the head along the plane of a canal produces an excitatory stimulus to the canal ipsilateral to the direction of head rotation, and an inhibitory stimulus to its coplanar paired canal. The excitatory stimulus leads to contraction of the eye muscles that generate a compensatory eye movement in the opposite direction as the head movement. Meanwhile, the inhibitory stimulus leads to a relaxation of the eye muscles that generate an anticompensatory eye movement in the same direction as the head movement. For example, leftward horizontal rotation of the head leads to excitation of the left horizontal SCC and inhibition of the right horizontal canal. Excitation of the left horizontal canal then leads to contraction of the left medial and right lateral recti in order to drive the eyes rightward (Fig. 4.14). Additionally, leftward head rotation leads to inhibition of the right horizontal SCC. This leads to relaxation of the left lateral and right medial recti (Fig. 4.15).

Although each labyrinth is capable of encoding both excitatory and inhibitory stimulation, labyrinthine responses to excitation are greater than to inhibition. Ewald made this observation when stimulating the SCCs of pigeons, and this excitation-inhibition asymmetry has been codified as Ewald's Second Law. There are several reasons why the labyrinth responds asymmetrically to excitatory vs inhibitory stimuli. First, vestibular HCs generate larger receptor potentials for stereociliary deflection in the excitatory (toward the kinocilium) vs inhibitory (away from the kinocilium) direction. Additionally, as discussed previously, vestibular primary afferents have a nonzero baseline firing rate (of 50–100 spikes/second), giving them bidirectional sensitivity.[18] Thus, one canal in a coplanar pair can sense movements in either direction (i.e. in both the excitatory and inhibitory directions) along the canal plane. However, if the excitatory stimulus is large enough, vestibular afferents enter the inhibitory cutoff range, because baseline firing rate can only go as low as zero whereas it can increase to 300–400 spikes/second. In the inhibitory cutoff range, only the afferent response to excitation is encoded.

This excitation-inhibition asymmetry is the basis for the clinical head impulse test, where the head is rotated along the plane of a SCC with high velocity (150–200°/sec), high acceleration (3000–4000°/sec^2), small amplitude (10–20°) and in an unpredictable direction.[34,35] These head impulses exceed the inhibitory cutoff of the SCCs, such that the function of a single canal can be tested in isolation without the contribution of its coplanar paired canal. For example, in a patient with right unilateral vestibular loss (e.g. post right labyrinthectomy), a slow head rotation to the right would not be sensed by the right horizontal canal but would be sensed by the left horizontal canal. The contralesional functional canal would experience an inhibitory stimulus, and would drive an eye movement response that mirrors the response that would have been given by the right horizontal canal. However, if a right head impulse is delivered to this patient, the left horizontal canal could only mount a small compensatory eye movement response before it is driven into inhibitory cutoff, leading to an insufficient eye movement response that can be observed by the examiner as a refixation saccade (Figs. 4.16A to D).[36]

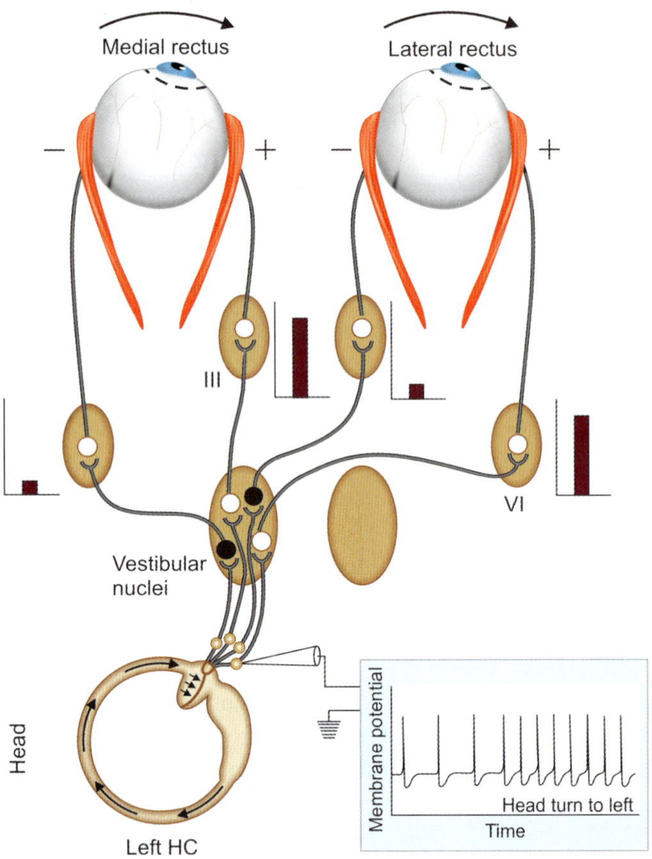

Fig. 4.14: The vestibular ocular reflex (VOR) generates compensatory eye movements via a push-pull system. Seen from above, a leftward head turn produces relative endolymph movement that is clockwise in the left horizontal semicircular canal (HC). The resultant cupular deflection leads to increased firing in the left HC afferent (inset). These action potentials travel to the ipsilateral vestibular nucleus, which then sends excitatory signals to the ipsilateral oculomotor (III) and contralateral abducens (VI) nuclei, and inhibitory signals to ipsilateral abducens and contralateral oculomotor nuclei. The end result is contraction and relaxation of the lateral and medial recti, respectively, in the right eye, and vice versa in the left eye, to generate a compensatory eye movement to the right. Bar graphs indicate firing rate in the respective motor nuclei.

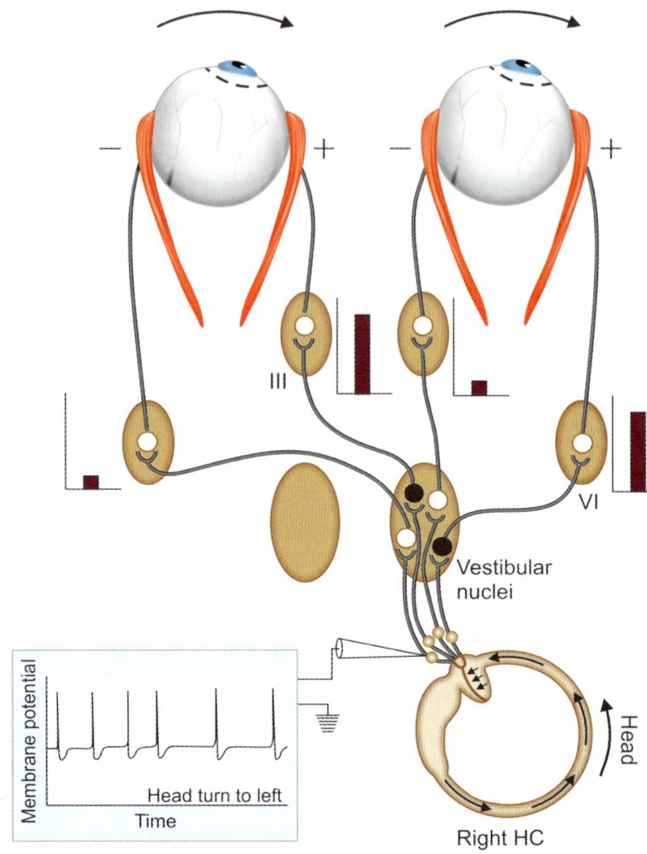

Fig. 4.15: A leftward head turn also leads to inhibition of the right horizontal canal (HC), and compensatory eye movements that are concordant with excitation of the contralateral canal. A leftward head turn produces relative endolymph movement that is clockwise in the right HC. The resultant cupular deflection leads to decreased firing in the right HC afferent (inset). These action potentials travel to the ipsilateral vestibular nucleus, which then sends inhibitory signals to the ipsilateral oculomotor (III) and contralateral abducens (VI) nuclei, and excitatory signals to ipsilateral abducens and contralateral oculomotor nuclei. The end result is contraction and relaxation of the lateral and medial recti, respectively, in the right eye, and vice versa in the left eye, to generate a compensatory eye movement to the right and which is identical as the eye movement generated by excitation of the left HC. Bar graphs indicate firing rate in the respective motor nuclei.

At rest, in the absence of head movement, both vestibular labyrinths fire at their baseline rate and provide fairly symmetric inputs to the brain. This leads to stability of the eyes-in-space. During a head movement, vestibular afferents fire asymmetrically conveying the magnitude and direction of the head movement, and compensatory eye movements are triggered by the VOR. However, asymmetries between vestibular afferent firing rates can arise for reasons other than a head movement. These reasons may be either physiologic or pathologic, and give rise to the symptom of vertigo and the sign of nystagmus (rapid to-and-fro movement of the eyes). The nystagmus pattern observed can be interpreted in the context of the physiologic principles of the VOR. For example, during caloric irrigation, the ear irrigated with warm water experiences an excitatory stimulation of the ipsilateral horizontal canal. The brain interprets this increase in firing (relative to the contralateral side) as an ipsilateral head rotation, and the VOR drives a compensatory eye movement response in the contralateral direction. Under sustained caloric stimulation the eye can only be rotated so far in the orbit, and the brainstem generates a quick resetting eye movement to recenter the eye. The eye movement driven

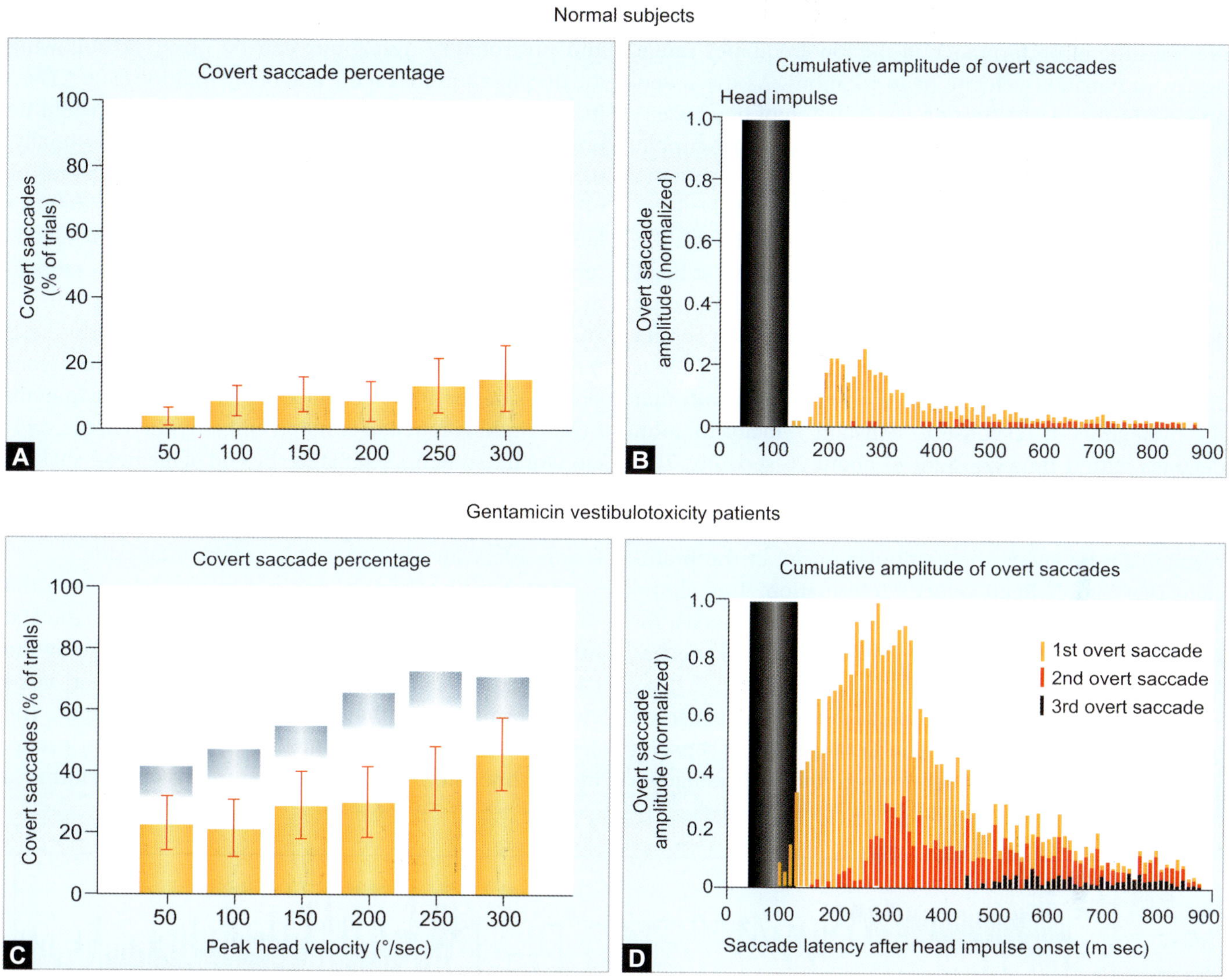

Figs. 4.16A to D: Covert and overt saccades in normal subjects and patients with gentamicin vestibulotoxicity after head impulse test (HIT). Patients with gentamicin-induced vestibulotoxicity (C and D) show a greater number of both covert and overt saccades than normal subjects after HIT (A and B).

by the VOR is called the slow-phase of nystagmus, and the quick resetting eye movement is termed the fast-phase. Nystagmus is typically described with respect to its fast phase, which is more clinically apparent. Thus, for a warm caloric irrigation, there is a contralateral slow phase eye movement and an ipsilateral fast phase eye movement, hence the mnemonic "COWS" (cold opposite, warm same, which relates to the fast phase of the caloric nystagmus).

An example of a pathologic asymmetric eye movement is posterior-canal benign paroxysmal positional vertigo (BPPV). Free-floating otoconia disperse from the utricular macula and typically settle in the posterior canal. When the head is moved into the provocative Dix-Hallpike position, the otoconial debris migrate to the most dependent position in the canal and excite the posterior canal HCs and afferents. The brain perceives a head movement along the plane of that canal backwards, and a downward and torsional compensatory slow phase eye movement is generated by the VOR. Fast phase eye movements occur in the upbeating direction, which is the classic nystagmus pattern observed clinically with BPPV. Depending on the direction the eye is looking, a geotropic torsional nystagmus can also be seen. This occurs because the eye movement is occurring within a canal-fixed frame of reference and the pupil is just a surface feature on the globe moving within this reference frame.

A further important property of the VOR relates to the boosting of performance in the low-frequency range (e.g. with constant velocity head rotation). As discussed previously, cupular deflection is a function of head acceleration. During a constant head rotation, the cupula deflects initially as head velocity changes from zero to its steady-state velocity (i.e. during the step of head acceleration). A nystagmus eye movement is generated, with the slow phase beating contralateral to the direction of head rotation. However, as the head reaches its steady state velocity, head acceleration becomes zero and the cupula returns to its normal position with a time constant of about 13 seconds.[37] However, it has been observed clinically that the nystagmus in response to constant velocity rotation declines with a time constant of about 20 seconds. This enhanced maintenance of the vestibular eye movement response has been attributed to velocity storage, a neural mechanism involving the vestibular nuclei in the brainstem that "store" head velocity information. This allows for compensatory eye movement responses to persist for longer than would be expected based on cupular mechanics alone.

The phenomenon of velocity storage can be observed clinically during rotational testing. During a step of constant velocity rotation in one direction, prerotatory nystagmus can be observed following the initial step of acceleration, and postrotatory nystagmus can be observed following the deceleration step at the end of the rotation (Fig. 4.17).[38] In both cases, the nystagmus lasts longer than would be predicted based on cupular mechanics. Additionally, in patients with labyrinthine dysfunction (unilateral or bilateral), time constants are reduced on the side(s) of labyrinthine dysfunction, given that peripheral vestibular input is required for maintenance of the velocity storage mechanism. Another clinical example involving velocity storage is the head-shake nystagmus test.[39] In this test, the patient's head is rotated in the horizontal plane from side-to-side for 10–20 seconds at 1–2 Hz. Any asymmetry in labyrinthine function is stored and amplified in the velocity storage system, such that at the end of the head-shaking maneuver, the brain perceives an ongoing head rotation to the intact side, and generates a slow phase toward the lesion side, with a fast phase toward the intact side.

Another important phenomenon associated with the VOR is neural integration. As discussed previously, the first integration of the head acceleration signal occurs by the cupula and endolymph system, which relay head velocity information to the primary vestibular afferent. The second integration of the head movement signal occurs in the brainstem neural integrator, which performs a

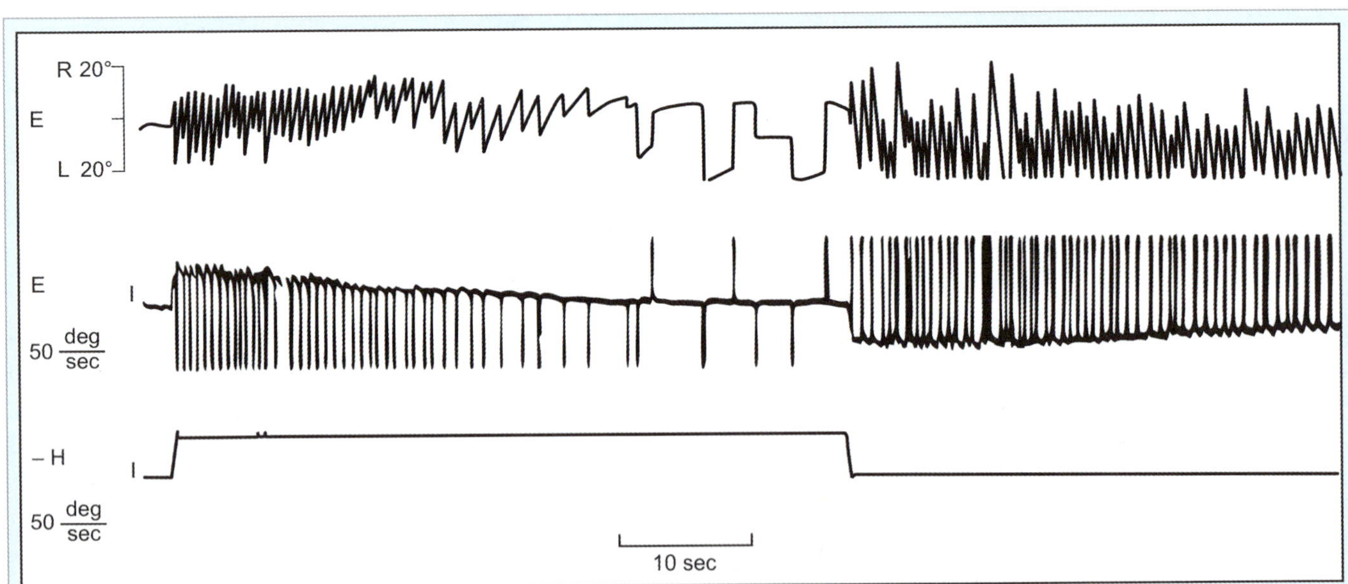

Fig. 4.17: Velocity storage in a monkey, which was rotated about an Earth-vertical axis in total darkness at 50° per second constant velocity. Shown in tracings top to bottom are horizontal eye position, eye velocity, and chair velocity, respectively, as a function of time. During the velocity step, the initial nystagmus decays slower than would be predicted based on the cupula's time constant. After the rotation stops, an oppositely directed nystagmus appears that also decays slower than expected, which is evidence of velocity storage in the brainstem.

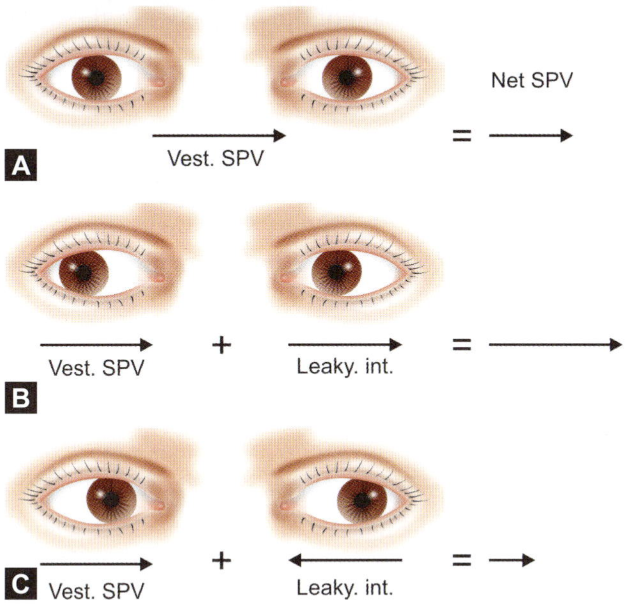

Figs. 4.18A to C: Illustration of Alexander's law in a case of left acute vestibular hypofunction. The net slow phase velocity (SPV) is a vector sum of the SPVs due to the peripheral vestibular system (vest.) and the leaky neurointegrator (Int.). In neutral gaze (A), only the vest SPV is manifest. In eccentric gaze away from the side of the lesion (aka toward the fast phase), vest SPV and leaky int SPV are summative, leading to a larger net SPV (B). In eccentric gaze toward the lesioned side (C), the leaky int SPV is in the opposite direction as the vest SPV and the net SPV decreases, and sometimes becomes clinically nondetectable (i.e. nystagmus disappears).

velocity-to-position integration.[40] The neural integrator sends the command to the extraocular muscles to maintain eye position at a given orientation in space (e.g. in eccentric gaze). In the absence of the neural integrator, the elastic forces of the globe and the antagonistic pairs of extraocular muscles would passively bring the eye back to neutral position. A clinical example that illustrates the function of the neural integrator is Alexander's law, which relates to the nystagmus pattern observed with unilateral labyrinthine dysfunction (Figs. 4.18A to C).[41] In the acute setting of unilateral labyrinthine dysfunction, the neural integrator is also impaired and becomes "leaky". Alexander's Law states that the nystagmus has the greatest magnitude when the eye is looking in the direction of the fast phase of the eye movement, because the slow phase eye movement and the drift of the eye back to center associated with a leaky neural integrator are additive and increase the amplitude of the slow phase velocity. As a corollary, nystagmus is attenuated when the eye is looking in the direction of the slow phase of the eye movement.

OTOLITH PHYSIOLOGY

Otolith physiology has not been as well characterized as SCC physiology. An otolith-mediated reflex that is gaining widespread recognition is the sacculocollic reflex. This reflex forms the basis of the sound-evoked cervical vestibular-evoked myogenic potential (cVEMP) clinical test.[42] The saccule was a hearing organ earlier in evolution and maintains some vestigial acoustic sensitivity. High amplitude sounds delivered to the ear stimulate a vestibular afferent response, which persists in the setting of sensorineural hearing loss and is abolished with vestibulopathy. Selective inner ear lesion studies have shown that the saccule is likely the organ of origin of the cVEMP. Abnormalities of the cVEMP can be observed with vestibular pathology.[43] In Menière's disease (also known pathologically as cochleosaccular hydrops), an initially elevated cVEMP can be observed followed by an attenuated or absent cVEMP. This may correspond with the irritative then impaired states characteristic of Menière's disease. Given that the saccular afferents travel centrally via the inferior vestibular nerve, the cVEMP has also been used to localize lesions in the case of vestibular neuritis or vestibular schwannomas. Vestibular neuritis typically involves the superior vestibular nerve; therefore, the cVEMP may be normal despite an abnormal caloric or head impulse test.[44,45] Loss of the cVEMP response in the setting of an acoustic neuroma may suggest an inferior vestibular nerve origin for the tumor. However, due to compressive effects of the tumor this may not always be the case.

As mentioned previously, the utricle is a horizontally oriented otolith organ that responds to head tilts or linear translations. Utricular HCs are polarized with respect to the striola, the central inversion line running through the utricle. Although this reversal in polarization gives the utricle bidirectional sensitivity, the zone medial to the striola is larger than the lateral zone thus the utricle appears to be most sensitive to ipsilateral head tilts and contralateral linear head translations.[46] A fundamental question that vestibular physiologists have grappled with over the years is how the brain resolves the ambiguity between tilt and translation signals coming from the utricle.[47] Both an ipsilateral head tilt and contralateral head translation produce the same force on the otoconial mass and increase in afferent response. However, the eye movement response would be different for a head tilt (torsional rotation of the eyes in the direction opposite the head tilt) compared to linear translation (horizontal movement of

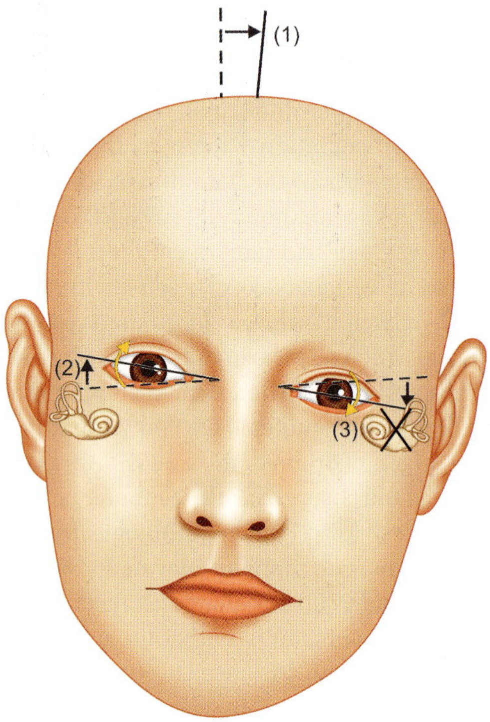

Fig. 4.19: Illustration of the ocular counter roll in a case of left acute utricular hypofunction, resulting in head tilt to the left (1), elevation of the right eye and depression of the left eye (2), and roll of the superior pole of each eye to the patient's left (3).

the eyes in the direction opposite the translation). Several theories have been advanced, including the difference in frequency content between tilt vs. translation. The brain may be able to distinguish low-frequency tilts from high-frequency translations. Alternatively, the brain may use canal signals to distinguish tilt from translation. Head tilts activate the canals whereas linear translations do not.

The ocular tilt reaction is a classic triad of findings associated with acute unilateral loss of utricular function (Fig. 4.19).[48] The brain perceives the unilateral loss of function as a head tilt directed to the intact side, and therefore makes adjustments to eye and head position to compensate for the head tilt. The ocular tilt reaction includes (1) a head tilt to the lesioned side (to compensate for the perceived head tilt to the intact side), (2) a vertical skew deviation with the intact side eye up and the lesioned side eye down, and (3) a torsional rotation of the eyes with the superior poles rotated toward the lesioned side. The skew deviation can be observed clinically with the alternate cover test, where each eye is covered sequentially and vertical eye movements can be observed bringing the eye back to center gaze once it is uncovered. Torsion of the eyes can be viewed clinically using fundoscopy, and observing the orientation of the line between the macula and optic nerve that should be approximately horizontal. Additionally, the subjective visual vertical (SVV) or subjective visual horizontal (SVH) tests can be used, where the patient is asked to orient a line vertically or horizontally. Patients with unilateral utricular dysfunction will typically orient the line toward the lesion side due to the torsional rotation of their eyes.[49,50] The brain compensates fairly well for unilateral utricular dysfunction therefore these symptoms may only be observable in the acute phase of the lesion. However, a persistent deviation of the SVV or SVH can persist for long term.

REFERENCES

1. Dohlman GF. The attachment of the cupulae, otolith and tectorial membranes to the sensory cell areas. Acta Otolaryngol. 1971;71:89-105.
2. Goldberg JM, Fernandez C. Physiology of peripheral neurons innervating semicircular canals of the squirrel monkey. I. Resting discharge and response to constant angular accelerations. J Neurophysiol. 1971;34:635-60.
3. Highstein SM, Holstein GR. The anatomy of the vestibular nuclei. Prog Brain Res. 2006;151:157-203.
4. de Waele C, Muhlethaler M, Vidal PP. Neurochemistry of the central vestibular pathways. Brain Res Brain Res Rev. 1995;20:24-46.
5. Scudder CA, Kaneko CS, Fuchs AF. The brainstem burst generator for saccadic eye movements: a modern synthesis. Exp Brain Res. 2002;142:439-62.
6. Shinoda Y, Sugiuchi Y, Izawa Y, et al. Long descending motor tract axons and their control of neck and axial muscles. Prog Brain Res. 2006;151:527-63.
7. Meredith GE. Comparative view of the central organization of afferent and efferent circuitry for the inner ear. Acta Biol Hung. 1988;39:229-49.
8. Wende S, Nakayama N, Schwerdtfeger P. The internal auditory artery: (embryology, anatomy, angiography, pathology). J Neurol. 1975;210:21-31.
9. Holt JC, Newlands SD. Vestibular function and anatomy. In: Johnson JT, Rosen CA (eds), *Bailey's Head and Neck Surgery—Otolaryngology*. Philadelphia, PA: Lippincott Williams & Wilkins; 2014. p. 2291.
10. Gillespie PG, Muller U. Mechanotransduction by hair cells: models, molecules, and mechanisms. Cell. 2009;139:33-44.
11. Pickles JO, Corey DP. Mechanoelectrical transduction by hair cells. Trends Neurosci. 1992;15:254-9.
12. Wersall J, Hawkins JE, Jr. The vestibular sensory epithelia in the cat labyrinth and their reactions in chronic streptomycin intoxication. Acta Otolaryngol. 1962;54:1-23.
13. Fernandez C, Lysakowski A, Goldberg JM. Hair-cell counts and afferent innervation patterns in the cristae ampullares of the squirrel monkey with a comparison to the chinchilla. J Neurophysiol. 1995;73:1253-69.

14. Boettger T, Hubner CA, Maier H, et al. Deafness and renal tubular acidosis in mice lacking the K-Cl co-transporter Kcc4. Nature. 2002;416:874-8.
15. Lopez I, Ishiyama G, Tang Y, et al. Regional estimates of hair cells and supporting cells in the human crista ampullaris. J Neurosci Res. 2005;82:421-31.
16. Desai SS, Zeh C, Lysakowski A. Comparative morphology of rodent vestibular periphery. I. Saccular and utricular maculae. J Neurophysiol. 2005;93:251-66.
17. Jaeger R, Takagi A, Haslwanter T. Modeling the relation between head orientations and otolith responses in humans. Hear Res. 2002;173:29-42.
18. Goldberg JM. Afferent diversity and the organization of central vestibular pathways. Exp Brain Res. 2000;130: 277-97.
19. Eatock RA, Songer JE. Vestibular hair cells and afferents: two channels for head motion signals. Annu Rev Neurosci. 2011;34:501-34.
20. Fernández C, Baird R, Goldberg J. The vestibular nerve of the chinchilla. I. Peripheral innervation patterns in the horizontal and superior semicircular canals. J Neurophysiol. 1988;60:167-81.
21. Smith CE, Goldberg JM. A stochastic after hyperpolarization model of repetitive activity in vestibular afferents. Biol Cybern. 1986;54:41-51.
22. Goldberg JM, Lysakowski A, Fernandez C. Structure and function of vestibular nerve fibers in the chinchilla and squirrel monkey. Ann N Y Acad Sci. 1992;656:92-107.
23. Hullar TE, Minor LB. High-frequency dynamics of regularly discharging canal afferents provide a linear signal for angular vestibuloocular reflexes. J Neurophysiol. 1999;82: 2000-5.
24. Lasker DM, Ramat S, Carey JP, et al. Vergence-mediated modulation of the human horizontal angular VOR provides evidence of pathway-specific changes in VOR dynamics. Ann NY Acad Sci. 2002;956:324-37.
25. Clendaniel RA, Lasker DM, Minor LB. Horizontal vestibuloocular reflex evoked by high-acceleration rotations in the squirrel monkey. IV. Responses after spectacle-induced adaptation. J Neurophysiol. 2001;86:1594-611.
26. Cullen KE, Minor LB. Semicircular canal afferents similarly encode active and passive head-on-body rotations: implications for the role of vestibular efference. J Neurosci. 2002; 22:1-7.
27. Meyer CH, Lasker AG, Robinson DA. The upper limit of human smooth pursuit velocity. Vision Res. 1985;25: 561-3.
28. Grossman G, Leigh R, Abel L, et al. Frequency and velocity of rotational head perturbations during locomotion. Exp Brain Res. 1988;70:470-6.
29. Tabak S, Collewijn H, Boumans LJ, et al. Gain and delay of human vestibulo-ocular reflexes to oscillation and steps of the head by a reactive torque helmet. I. Normal subjects. Acta Otolaryngol. 1997;117:785-95.
30. Ewald JR. Physiologische Untersuchungen ueber das Endorgan des Nervus octavus v.... J [ul.] Richard Ewald, Prof.... ad Univ. Strassburg: JF Bergmann; 1892.
31. Della Santina CC, Potyagaylo V, Migliaccio AA. et al. Orientation of human semicircular canals measured by three-dimensional multiplanar CT reconstruction. J Assoc Res Otolaryngol. 2005;6:191-206.
32. Robinson D. The use of matrices in analyzing the three-dimensional behavior of the vestibulo-ocular reflex. Biol Cybern. 1982;46:53-66.
33. Cohen B, Suzuki J, Bender M. Eye movements from semicircular canal nerve stimulation in the cat. Ann Otol Rhinol Laryngol. 1964;73:153-69.
34. Aw ST, Haslwanter T, Halmagyi GM, et al. Three-dimensional vector analysis of the human vestibuloocular reflex in response to high-acceleration head rotations. I. Responses in normal subjects. J Neurophysiol. 1996;76:4009-20.
35. Halmagyi GM, Curthoys IS. A clinical sign of canal paresis. Arch Neurol. 1988;45:737-9.
36. Weber KP, Aw ST, Todd MJ, et al. Head impulse test in unilateral vestibular loss: vestibulo-ocular reflex and catch-up saccades. Neurology. 2008;70:454-63.
37. Rabbitt RD, Damiano ER, Grant JW. Biomechanics of the semicircular canals and otolith organs. The vestibular system. New York: Springer; 2004. pp. 153-201.
38. Cannon S, Robinson D. Loss of the neural integrator of the oculomotor system from brain stem lesions in monkey. J Neurophysiol. 1987;57:1383-409.
39. Hain T, Fetter M, Zee D. Head-shaking nystagmus in patients with unilateral peripheral vestibular lesions. Am J Otolaryngol. 1987;8:36-47.
40. Cannon SC, Robinson DA, Shamma S. A proposed neural network for the integrator of the oculomotor system. Biol Cybern. 1983;49:127-36.
41. Robinson DA, Zee DS, Hain TC, et al. Alexander's law: Its behavior and origin in the human vestibulo-ocular reflex. Ann Neurol. 1984;16:714-22.
42. Colebatch J, Halmagyi G, Skuse N. Myogenic potentials generated by a click-evoked vestibulocollic reflex. J Neurol Neurosurg Psychiatry. 1994;57:190-7.
43. Welgampola MS, Colebatch JG. Characteristics and clinical applications of vestibular-evoked myogenic potentials. Neurology. 2005;64:1682-8.
44. Fetter M, Dichgans J. Vestibular neuritis spares the inferior division of the vestibular nerve. Brain. 1996;119 (Pt 3): 755-63.
45. Goebel JA, O'Mara W, Gianoli G. Anatomic considerations in vestibular neuritis. Otol Neurotol. 2001;22:512-8.
46. Fernandez C, Goldberg J. Physiology of peripheral neurons. J Neurophysiol. 1976;39:996-1008.
47. Angelaki DE, McHenry MQ, Dickman JD, et al. Computation of inertial motion: neural strategies to resolve ambiguous otolith information. J Neurosci. 1999;19:316-27.
48. Halmagyi GM, Gresty MA, Gibson WP. Ocular tilt reaction with peripheral vestibular lesion. Ann Neurol. 1979;6:80-3.
49. Böhmer A, Rickenmann J. The subjective visual vertical as a clinical parameter of vestibular function in peripheral vestibular diseases. J Vestib Res. 1995;5(1):35-45.
50. Curthoys I, Dai M, Halmagyi G. Human ocular torsional position before and after unilateral vestibular neurectomy. Exp Brain Res. 1991;85:218-25.

CHAPTER

5

Evaluation of Vestibular Disorders

Justin D Wilson, Art Ambrosio, Roxanne Cano, Michael E Hoffer

INTRODUCTION

Balance disorders are among the most common etiologies for individuals seeking medical care. Some estimates have postulated that as many as 50% of individuals will suffer a balance disorder at some point during their lifetime. These disorders may be mild but in many cases can have a significant impact on quality of life. Moreover, if the balance disorder becomes more severe, individuals can suffer other health implications as a result of immobility or falls. In the past, evaluating balance function was a difficult task, but recent advances combined with a basic understanding of balance physiology have dramatically improved our diagnostic capability. Fundamental to treating balance patients is understanding the available methods for evaluating balance function.

EVALUATION OF VESTIBULAR FUNCTION

Information regarding vestibular function is a valuable tool in evaluating the "dizzy" patient. Evaluating vestibular function can be used in making a diagnosis, providing prognostic information to patients, evaluating return to work status, and planning rehabilitation.

The evaluation of vestibular function begins with an accurate history. In fact, in many cases, history alone will allow the clinician to significantly narrow the differential diagnosis. In addition to a complete medical, surgical, family, medication, and social history, there are many acceptable history formats as well as several key questions that help elucidate the dizziness history as follows:

1. Can you describe your dizziness? Attempt to try to classify the dizziness as unsteadiness, vertigo, lightheadedness, visual flow, or motor—which of note is not true dizziness but rarely such individuals get referred to an otolaryngologist because they appear significantly imbalanced/uncoordinated, warranting a neurology consult.
2. Is the dizziness constant or intermittent? If intermittent, please describe the frequency and length of attacks.
3. How severe are your symptoms? To what extent do they interfere with your day-to-day life, job or activities of daily living?
4. What is the natural history of the dizziness from primary onset to present, including anything that may have caused the dizziness (head trauma, URI, etc.)?
5. What associated symptoms are there, including headaches, hearing loss, nausea/vomiting, etc.?
6. What exacerbating/alleviating factors are there, if any?
7. Have you received any treatment to date?

In addition to a complete head and neck physical exam, we add the following elements to the examination:

1. *Examination of ocular smooth pursuit*: The examiner has the individual follow his finger through the cardinal directions of gaze and examines how the eyes track the finger. The eyes should move smoothly. Jerking motions or corrective saccades are abnormal. It is important here that the examiner's finger be at least 12 inches from the eyes.

2. *Examination of nystagmus in all positions of the eye*: The examiner has the patient look in all six cardinal direction of gaze and examines for the presence of nystagmus. It is important here that the examiner not take the patient to the extremes in each position as a certain amount of end-point nystagmus can be normal.
3. *Head thrust examination*: The examiner has the individual stare at an object in the midpoint (e.g. the examiner's nose). The head is then moved quickly a short direction to either side. One corrective saccade is normal. Any more than one corrective saccade is defined as abnormal. This head thrust can be performed in the direction of any canal/pair of canals. It is important here that the examiner performs the head motion rather than the patient moving their own head as a certain amount of physiologic guarding can change the value of the test if self-motion is allowed.
4. *Romberg and Tandem Romberg*: This test is done in a variety of different manners. We choose to have individuals stand with feet together, arms out palms up and the eyes closed (Romberg). We look for body sway. Tandem Romberg is done in the same manner except that the feet are positioned heal to toe. It is important that this test be done with both the right foot in front of the left and the left foot in front of the right as orthopedic abnormalities can create an abnormal tandem Romberg with one foot forward and not the other, whereas vestibular abnormalities usually are abnormal in both right and left foot forward conditions.
5. *Fukuda step test*: The individual is instructed to hug themselves and then march in place with eyes closed. There are a variety of different criteria for judging abnormalities, but generally a turn of more than 90° over 30 seconds is abnormal in our laboratory.
6. *Gait, tandem gait, and museum gait (walking while turning hear side to side and up and down)*: We instruct the patient to walk down the hall normally, walk down the hall heal to toe, walk down the hall while turning the head slowly rightward and leftward, and walk down the hall while moving the head up and down. For the side to side and up and down motion (museum gait) it is important that the examiner call out the cadence and that head motion is full (e.g. all the way over the shoulders on side to side and all the way flexed and extended on up and down).
7. *Cerebellar tests*: A variety of different tests can be utilized as preferred by the examiner. We like rapid alternating motion of finger to nose, in which the patient brings their own finger from their own nose to the examiner's nose. This action is repeated several times and at increasing speed.
8. *Dix-Hallpike (and log roll maneuver, if indicated) is performed if positional vertigo is described*: The Dix-Hallpike maneuver is performed by starting with the patient in a sitting (legs out) position and then lying them back while turning the head to one side. If nystagmus is present to either side, the test is abnormal. There are a variety of different positional vertigo tests to examine other canals and other types of benign positional vertigo. The description of these tests is covered elsewhere in this text.

After completion of the history and physical, the clinician must decide what vestibular function tests need to be ordered. The remainder of this chapter will focus on the types of vestibular function tests with an added emphasis of what information these tests provide. This is important because as with most tests in medicine, the clinician must only order tests that provide valuable and necessary information. Further, audiograms are also integral ancillary studies, which are typically obtained in all balance disorder patients; however, these are reviewed elsewhere in the text. In addition, we will not discuss some very specialized tests that are available in only a few laboratories around the country. A list of the common tests is included in Table 5.1. A corresponding list of the characteristics of the most common balance disorders is shown in Table 5.2.

For the purposes of this review, we will divide the tests into three basic categories: evaluation of vestibulo-ocular-reflexes (VORs) and isolated functionality of the inner ears, examination of posture and gait, and lastly, tests involving audiometric measures.

VOR TESTS

Videonystagmography

Assessing the VOR is important in a patient with dizziness, and videonystagmography (VNG) is the test of choice to assess and determine if the vestibular organ is responsible for the abnormal eye movements seen on examination. Over the last 10–15 years, video eye recording has replaced electric eye recording, and electronystagmography (ENG) has been replaced with VNG due to ease of use, quick test results, and minimal patient preparation. Like its

Table 5.1: Common tests

Test	*Description*	*Elements tested*
Videonystagmography	Four separate tests with video goggles	Vestibulo-ocular-reflex (VOR) and central
Rotational chair	Seated in a chair in a darkened booth	VOR over many frequencies and otolith
Head impulse test	Short, fast, passive head motion	VOR (can examine all canals)
Posturography	Standing on platform	Passive posture
Functional gait index	Performing gait tasks	Active gait
Vestibular-evoked myogenic potential	Sound initiated measurement of muscle reaction	Otoliths
Electrocochleography	Auditory test	Hydrops

Table 5.2: Characteristics of the most common balance disorders

	History	*Physical examination*	*Tests*
Benign positional vertigo (BPV, BPPV)	Positional vertigo that last seconds to minutes	Dix-Hallpike or other positional test	Dix-Hallpike or other positional test with recording of eye movement
Meniere's disease	Episodic vertigo lasting minutes to hours associated with pressure and ringing in the involved ear(s) and hearing loss in the involved ear(s)	No unique characteristic finding. Can be normal between attacks	*Audiogram*: Low frequency hearing loss *ECoG*: Expanded SP/AP ratio *VNG*: Reduced vestibular response *VEMP*: Reduced amplitude *MRI*: abnormal
Vestibular neuronitis	Acute severe vertigo for day(s) followed by gradually improving unsteadiness	Abnormalities in any test of the vestibulo-ocular-reflex	VNG: Reduced or absent vestibular response Rotational chair: VOR abnormalities Audiogram: Mild or no hearing loss. If hearing loss is more severe think labyrinthitis or other abnormality
Vestibular migraines	Episodic dizziness with headaches as a dominant component. Usually episodes vary in quality and length	No unique findings	No unique findings
Superior canal dehiscence	Dizziness with load noises, pressure into ear, or external pressure changes	Abnormal fistula test	*VEMP*: Involved ear has the presence of a VEMP at a lower sound presentation level than normal *Audigram*: Low frequency conductive hearing loss
Post-traumatic dizziness	Can have a variety of complaints but most significant are unsteadiness (with or without true vertigo), headache, hearing complaints, cognitive disability/memory issues, and sleep disorders	No unique findings	Rotational chair "footprint" in development

(ECoG, electrocochleography; VNG, videonystagmography; VEMP, vestibular-evoked myogenic potential; VOR, vestibulo-ocular-reflex).

predecessor, VNG is not a single test but is actually a four-part test. In a VNG, the following items are measured:

1. *Ocular mobility/smooth pursuit*: The ability of the eyes to follow objects that move smoothly or jump from place to place
2. *Optokinetic nystagmus*: The ability of the eyes to track a target in continuous motion (like a rotating drum)
3. *Positional nystagmus*: The ability of the eyes to remain still with various head and eye positions
4. *Caloric tests*: The amount of eye motion initiated with warm and cold water/air placed in the external auditory canal.

Whereas the ocular mobility and optokinetic tests evaluate eye or central vestibular pathology, positional and caloric tests evaluate peripheral vestibular pathologies. The most objective outcomes of VNG are calculated from the caloric tests. While there are a number of potential parameters, the two most commonly used are unilateral weakness (reduced vestibular response) and directional preponderance. These parameters are calculated by Jongkees' equation.[1]

For reduced vestibular response (unilateral weakness or RVR), the sum of the responses obtained from each ear (cold and warm) are subtracted and then divided by the total responses, then multiplied by 100%, e.g. $\{(a - b/a + b) \times 100\%\}$, which gives a percent RVR. A significant positive or negative number indicates that one ear is stronger than the other. Often the absolute value is used and the weak side is simply stated (e.g. 30% right-sided weakness). The exact amount of difference that is significant varies from laboratory to laboratory but is normally approximately 30%.

For directional preponderance (DP), the sum of the responses that drive nystagmus one direction (right beating (RW + LC) – left beating (LW + RC) are divided by the total response (RW + RC + LW + LC), then multiplied by 100% to arrive at a DP%. A significant positive or negative number indicates a directional preponderance. Often, the absolute value is used and the side stated (e.g. 35% left-sided DP). The significant amount of DP generally lies within the 35% range and can differ from laboratory to laboratory. RVR indicates if one ear is weaker than the other and as such might point to peripheral pathology in the weaker ear. The significance of DP has been debated, but some believe this involves neurons higher upstream in the balance system.[2]

There are a number of variants on the caloric portion of the VNG, most adopted for efficiency. One common variant is to simultaneously irrigate the ears with the same temperature of air or water. While this will help distinguish which ear is stronger (if there is a big difference), this technique has been shown to be less accurate than doing each of the four irrigations separately.[3] Another variation of the caloric test is to irrigate an ear with ice to see if the ear has any response. A total unilateral vestibular loss will result in no response. On the other hand, a normal ear might result in a vigorous and unpleasant (sometimes for both the patient and the technician) vestibular response.

Rotational Chair Testing

Another aspect to testing VORs is the rotational chair test, which has become more advanced in its abilities since the first use in the early 1900s. Although becoming increasingly more common, rotational chair testing is still most often utilized in specialized vestibular laboratories. As such, many of the chair tests go beyond the scope of this chapter. Moreover, there is a great deal of variability in the capabilities of different chairs based on manufacturer, age of chair, and custom features designed by different laboratories.

Among the more common tests are sinusoidal chair motion and step velocity testing. In addition, most chairs have the ability to perform at least the first two components of a VNG (smooth pursuit and optokinetic). Both sinusoidal testing and step velocity testing are peripheral vestibular tests, but unlike caloric testing both of these tests function over a range of frequencies, providing more information about the balance system than caloric tests. In sinusoidal testing, individuals are rotated back and forth in both directions at a fixed velocity but over a variety of different frequencies. Since this involves changes in acceleration, nystagmus is seen as the ears are alternately stimulated. The slow phase of nystagmus is calculated by averaging several runs at each different frequency. Relevant parameters are gain (peak eye velocity divided by peak head velocity), phase (time of initiation of eye movement vs. head movement), and symmetry [comparison of clockwise (right ear) to counter-clockwise (left ear)] chair motion. Each of these parameters can be tested for each direction and at each frequency. In an ideal situation, eye movement is equal but opposite of the head movement and occurs at the same time and speed. That would produce a gain of 1.0 and no phase lag or lead. In reality, gain values above 0.7 or 0.8 are usually normal, and there is often a very short phase lag or lead. Some individuals believe that symmetry (the comparison of CW to CCW responses at the same frequency) can be used to determine the side of the lesion, but this is still unclear because there are other inputs on eye motion with head rotation.[4,5]

In step velocity testing, the patient is rotated in a constant direction and periodically accelerated in that direction. At the conclusion of acceleration the chair is maintained at a constant speed (or abruptly stopped). Either stimulus leads the patient to feel as if they are moving in the opposite direction, and there is a natural nystagmus that decays (disappears since the body is no longer accelerating and is at constant velocity whether it be moving or at rest). The time it takes for this nystagmus to decay to a certain percentage of its maximum is termed the time constant. Time constants can be a sensitive measure of peripheral vestibular function.[6]

Head Impulse Test

In the head impulse test, the examiner moves the patient's head a short distance at a high rate of speed while requesting that the patient remain focused on an object in the center of the field. The test was popularized for clinical use by Halmagyi and Curthoys in 1988 and is often referred to as the Halmagyi head thrust test.[7] It is critical that the head thrust be passive (e.g. done by the examiner and not imitated by the patient) and given at random intervals.

In the clinical setting, we utilize this test as part of our physical examination and perform the test to both sides at a variety of different speeds. We consider the test abnormal if the patient requires more than one catch-up saccade for any thrust.

More recently, there has been a considerable improvement in eye tracking and recording technology. As such, the tests can now be recorded and analyzed electronically, allowing more parameters to be recorded. The video recording of the head thrust was initially reported several years ago, but is beginning to gain popularity as we write this chapter.[8,9] Video recording of the head thrust test gives a better assessment of the VORs than simply by the examiner alone.

POSTURE AND GAIT TEST

Posturography

The most common posture test done in most vestibular laboratories is computerized dynamic posturography.[10] In this test both the surround and the force platform can be sway referenced, allowing the clinician to isolate different parts of the balance system. Dynamic posturography devices perform a variety of tests, but the most common are the sensory organization test (SOT) and the motor control test (MCT).

In condition 1, neither the eyes nor the feet are sway referenced, and quiet posture is observed. In condition 2, the eyes are closed or blindfolded, and posture is observed. This means the patient must rely on proprioception and balance alone. In condition 3, the surround is sway referenced, fooling the eyes into believing that the patient is perpendicular to the ground even if the patient moves forward. In this condition, proprioception and the vestibular organs must be able to maintain balance in order to overcome any erroneous eye symptoms. In condition 4, the floor, but not the surround, is sway referenced, so the eyes and ears must work together to maintain balance. Conditions 5 and 6 are the most challenging balance conditions. In condition 5, the ground is sway referenced (moving with the patient) and the eyes are closed/blindfolded, so the patient only has inner ear function to rely on to maintain balance. In condition 6, both the surround and the ground are sway referenced, so the inner ears need to maintain balance and overcome erroneous eye and/or proprioceptive information. Up to three tries are allowed in each condition and a computer generated (SOT) score is obtained. The SOT score is important, but in order to determine the performance of the patient, each condition must be analyzed to decipher which part of the system is working and, if applicable, not working.

In the MCT, an unexpected forward and backward perturbation occurs and the ability of the intake system to compensate quickly is analyzed. While this test looks at the whole balance system, knowing the status of the eyes and proprioceptive system may allow inference to be made about the inner ears. Posturography has been validated over years of use and is an excellent way to evaluate postural balance function.

Functional Gait Tests

Posturography measures passive upright balance. Active motion is a second component of upright balance. There are a number of emerging technologies to measure active balance quantitatively, but these are not yet in widespread use. Most often, active balance function is measured in the physical therapy laboratory. Therapists utilize two common active motion tests, the dynamic gait index and the functional gait index. In both cases, the therapist asks the patient to perform a series of gait tasks, grading each task on a 0-3 scale (with zero being could not perform and 3 being performed well). Detailed discussion of these tests goes beyond the scope of this chapter, but these tests are reliable and internally consistent.[11]

AUDIOMETRIC-BASED TESTS

Vestibular-Evoked Myogenic Potentials

Vestibular-evoked myogenic potentials (VEMPs) testing is a balance test traditionally conducted in the audiology laboratory. These tests are used to measure otolith function via the medial vestibulospinal tract.[12] In VEMP testing, traditionally a stimulus (tone burst, forehead tap, or auditory clicks) is presented to the patient and short latency responses are recorded at the sternocleidomastoid (cVEMP) or the eyes (oVEMP). This test was initially popular for screening/diagnosing for superior canal dehiscence, where the cVEMP response occurred at lower intensities (60–70 dB) than normal (80–90 dB). Over time it has been realized that VEMP testing provides an excellent chance to assess otolithic function.[13] It is generally assumed that oVEMPs measure primarily utricular responses and cVEMPs primarily saccular responses. As stimuli and recording sites have increased, investigators have begun to examine the utility of these tests for diagnosing other vestibular disorders, particularly Meniere's disease.[14] It is likely that over time with the variety of stimulus patterns and output parameters, more utility will be discovered for VEMPs. Figure 5.1 shows the pathway of the cervical VEMP and Figure 5.2 represents the pathway for the ocular VEMP. Figures 5.3 and 5.4 show normal and abnormal cervical and ocular VEMP tracing, respectively. In each case, the normal tracing for each side is on the top and the abnormal on the bottom.

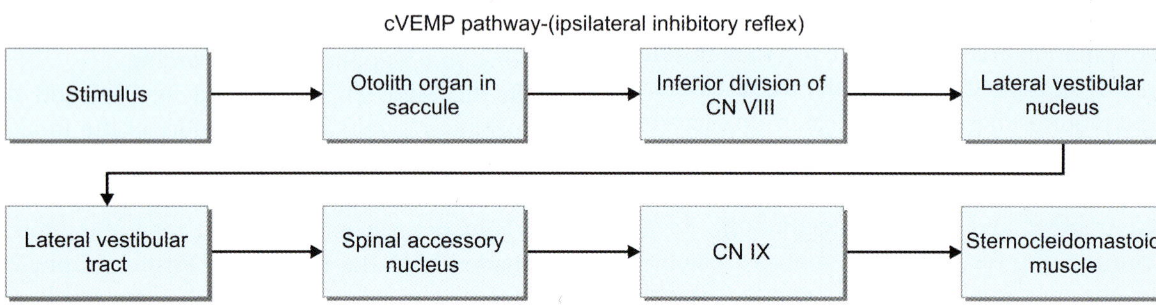

Fig. 5.1: Pathway for cervical vestibular-evoked myogenic potential (cVEMP).

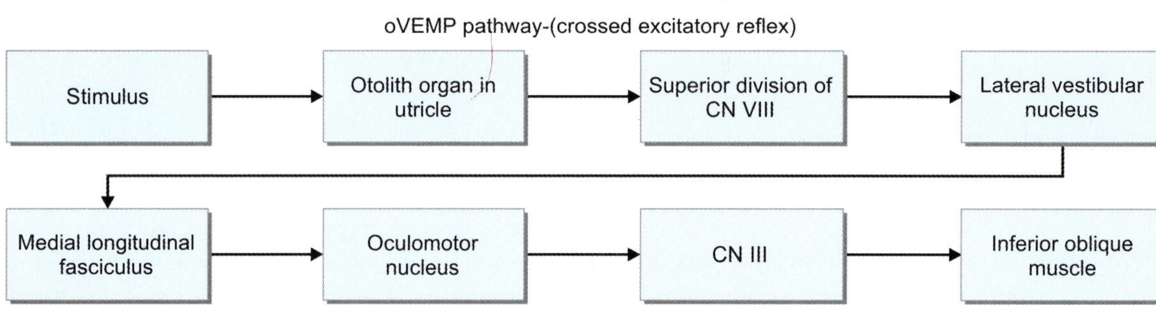

Fig. 5.2: Pathway for ocular vestibular myogenic potential (oVEMP).

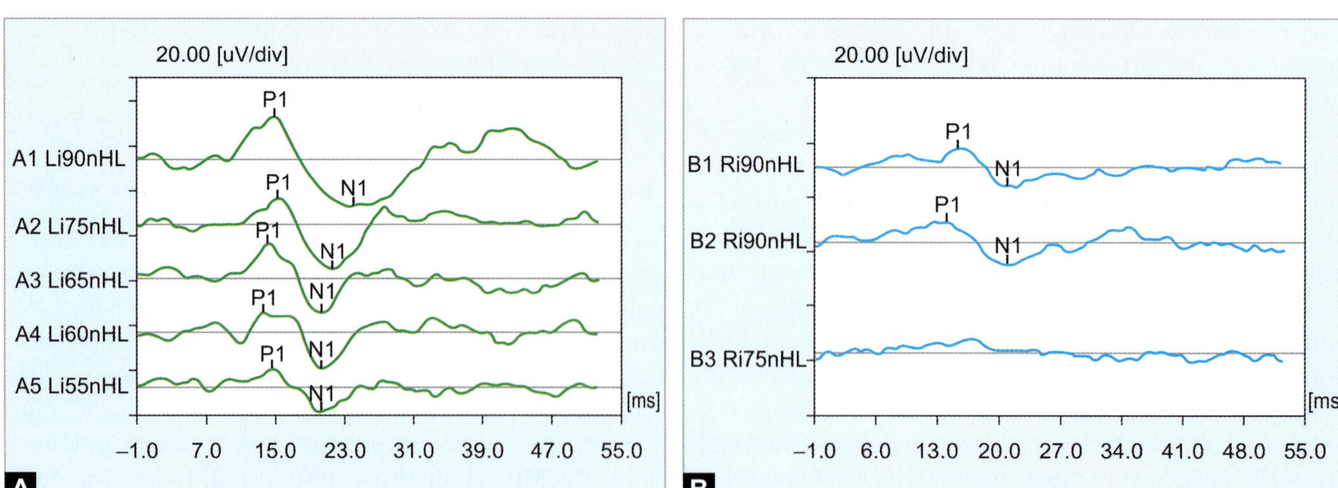

Figs. 5.3A and B: oVEMP with tracing identified at lower than normal intensity on the left. oVEMP, ocular vestibular myogenic potential.

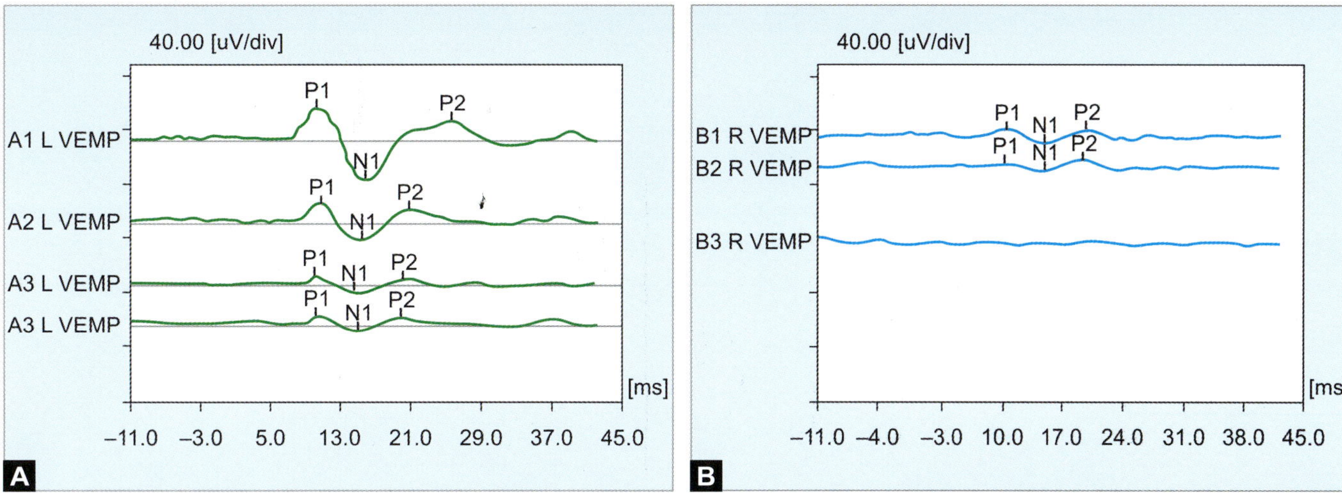

Figs. 5.4A and B: oVEMP with tracing identified at lower than normal intensity on the left. oVEMP, ocular vestibular myogenic potential.

Electrocochleography

Electrocochleography (ECoG) is an auditory test mentioned here for completeness. It is covered in more detail elsewhere in this text. Two parameters of the ECoG are relevant in assessing the vestibular system. The summating potential is a very early potential followed by the action potential. If there is an increase in the summating potential to action potential ratio (usually over 0.4 but laboratory dependent), this may be indicative of endolymphatic hydrops. The specificity and sensitivity of ECoG in the diagnosis of Meniere's disease remains controversial.[15] Nonetheless, ECoG continues to have a prominent role in the work-up of Meniere's disease, as it remains one of the best available tests in helping to make this diagnosis.

REFERENCES

1. Furman JM, Cass SP. Laboratory Testing 1: Electronystagmography and rotational testing. In: Baloh RW, Halmagyi M (eds), Disorders of the vestibular system. New York: Oxford University Press, 1996, p. 201.
2. Halmagyi GM, Cremer PD, Anderson J, Murofushi T, Curthoys IS. Isolated directional preponderance of caloric nystagmus: I. Clinical significance. Am J Otol. 2000;21(4):559-67.
3. Furman JM, Wall C, 3rd, Kamerer DB. Alternate and simultaneous binaural bithermal caloric testing: a comparison. Ann Otol Rhinol Laryngol. 1988;97(4 Pt 1):359-64.
4. Peterka RJ, Benolken MS. Relation between perception of vertical axis rotation and vestibulo-ocular reflex symmetry. J Vestib Res. 1992;2(1):59-69.
5. Hanson JM, Goebel JA. Comparison of manual whole-body and passive and active head-on-body rotational testing with conventional rotary chair testing. J Vestib Res. 1998;8(3):273-82.
6. Bertolini G, Ramat S, Bockisch CJ, et al. Is vestibular self-motion perception controlled by the velocity storage? Insights from patients with chronic degeneration of the vestibulo-cerebellum. PLoS One. 2012;7(6):e36763.
7. Halmagyi GM, Curthoys IS. A clinical sign of canal paresis. Arch Neurol. 1988;45:737-9.
8. Weber KP, MacDougall HG, Halmagyi GM, et al. Impulsive testing of semicircular-canal function using video-oculography. Ann N Y Acad Sci. 2009;1164:486-91.
9. Macdougall HG, McGarvie LA, Halmagyi GM, et al. Application of the video head impulse test to detect vertical semicircular canal dysfunction. Otol Neurotol. 2013;34(6):974-9.
10. Black FO. What can posturography tell us about vestibular function? Ann N Y Acad Sci. 2001;942:446-64.
11. Wrigley DM, Machete GF, Kuharsky DK, et al. Reliability, internal consistency, and validity of data obtained with the functional gait assessment. Phys Ther. 2004;84(10):906-18.
12. Colebatch JG, Halmagyi GM. Vestibular evoked potentials in human neck muscles before and after unilateral vestibular deafferentation. Neurology. 1992;42(8):1635-6.
13. Rauch SD. Vestibular evoked myogenic potentials. Curr Opin Otolaryngol Head Neck Surg. 2006;14(5):299-304.
14. Manzari L, Tedesco AR, Burgess AM, et al. Ocular and cervical vestibular-evoked myogenic potentials to bone conducted vibration in Ménière's disease during quiescence vs. during acute attacks. Clin Neurophysiol. 2010;121(7):1092-101.
15. Fukuoka H, Takumi Y, Tsukada K, et al. Comparison of the diagnostic value of 3 T MRI after intratympanic injection of GBCA, electrocochleography, and the glycerol test in patients with Meniere's disease. Acta Otolaryngol. 2012;132(2):141-5.

CHAPTER

6

Anatomy and Physiology of the Eustachian Tube

Ilkka Kivekäs, Dennis Poe

INTRODUCTION

The conduit connecting the nasopharynx and middle ear was named after the anatomist, Bartholomeus Eustachius, who published a detailed anatomical and physiological description of it in 1562.[1] The function of the Eustachian tube, with its secretory, ciliary and dilatory components, is critical for aeration and drainage of the middle ear, and for the optimal conduction of sound through the tympanic cavity. Treatments for Eustachian tube disorders have not met with satisfactorily long-term success in the past, but novel technologies and better understanding of the anatomy, physiology and pathophysiology have led to improved diagnostic capabilities as well as strategies and advances in surgical intervention that will be discussed in this chapter.

Anatomy and Physiology

The Eustachian tube, also called the auditory tube or pharyngotympanic tube, measures approximately 31–38 mm in length in adults but only 21 mm in an infant. It is a dynamic link between the nasopharynx and the middle ear.[2–3] The Eustachian tube is comprised of two portions, a proximal osseous portion representing about one third of the total length that is contained within the petrosal portion of the temporal bone, and the remaining distal two-thirds is the cartilaginous portion. The proximal and distal parts of the Eustachian tube are defined according to the mucociliary clearance flow within the lumen. It flows from the proximal orifice in the middle ear cavity, to the distal end in the nasopharynx.[4]

The bony portion is funnel shaped and lined with cuboidal respiratory epithelium and it is always patent under normal condition.[5] The segment where the cartilaginous and bony portions connect has been termed the junctional portion. The lumen becomes its narrowest within the proximal cartilaginous portion, a few millimeters from the bony-cartilaginous junction.[6]

The cartilaginous portion gradually flares out as it extends and opens into the nasopharynx and it is lined with pseudostratified columnar respiratory epithelium that is taller and more densely ciliated than in the bony portion. It is composed of a single segment of cartilage, approximately 20–24 mm in length in adults and is anchored superiorly to the basisphenoid bone and distally to medial pterygoid plate. It contains abundant secreting goblet cells, especially in the inferior aspect of the cross-sectional area.[2–3,7] The lumen of the cartilaginous portion, particularly the proximal portion, is closed at rest and opens through active muscular action against the curved cartilaginous skeleton that has a spring-like memory action to reclose the lumen after dilation.

Peritubal Muscles and their Function

There are four peritubal muscles regulating Eustachian tube function: the tensor veli palatini (TVP), the levator veli palatini (LVP), the tensor tympani, and the salpingopharyngeus. The most important muscle for the opening action of the Eustachian tube is the TVP, which is innervated by the mandibular part of the trigeminal nerve.[8] The TVP muscle originates from the basisphenoid bone and the anterior–lateral lip of cartilaginous auditory tube and it is composed of two muscle fiber bundles. They course anteriorly and inferiorly, converging in a tendon that runs under, or sometimes inserts into, the hamulus of the medial pterygoid before inserting into palatine aponeurosis in the soft palate. The dilator tubae portion of the TVP originates directly along the anterolateral membranous wall of the Eustachian tube and is important for actively distracting the wall from the lumen in the process of tubal dilation. The bulk of the relaxed TVP muscle contributes to the closure of the tube as well.[7]

The main action of the LVP is elevating and supporting the soft palate, as well as the torus tubarius (posterior cushion) throughout Eustachian tube dilation. The LVP originates from the petrous portion of the temporal bone. It runs along the floor of the Eustachian tube, and finally inserts into the soft palate. It is innervated by the vagus nerve.[9] The tensor tympani muscle arises from the cartilaginous portion of the Eustachian tube and attaches in the middle ear cavity to the neck of the malleus. It is innervated by the mandibular branch of the trigeminal nerve.

The salpingopharyngeus muscle depresses the floor of the Eustachian tube's lumen in an action that appears to facilitate dilation, and prevents backward displacement of the LVP muscle. It originates from the medial and inferior borders of the cartilaginous Eustachian tube and inserts into the lateral pharynx wall. It is innervated by the pharyngeal plexus.

General Physiological Aspects

Intermittent tubal dilation through swallowing or yawning is the main mechanism for equilibration of middle ear pressure to the ambient atmosphere.[10] Gases within the middle ear and mastoid air cells exchange continuously with the gases dissolved in the mucosa and its venous blood supply. As the partial pressure of gases in the mucosa and blood are lower than those in the incoming air, there is a continual net absorption of gases with a resulting progressively lowering pressure within the middle ear between ventilations of air from the Eustachian tube. If the Eustachian tube stays persistently closed, middle ear pressure can decrease by as much as 150 daPa in just a few hours.[11]

At rest, there is a bulge of soft tissue from the anterolateral wall that approximates the posteromedial wall to close the tubal lumen. During dilation, muscular contractions of the TVP, LVP and salpingopharyngeus muscles initiate rotational movements of the cartilaginous framework, thereby creating tension with effacement and even a concavity of the anterolateral wall leading to active dilation of the lumen and a brief opening of the Eustachian tube. Surfactants are produced within the tubal mucosa and likely decrease the surface tension of the lumen thus reducing the work required to dilate the tube.[12]

Fluid and secretions in the middle ear are cleared by mucociliary activity,[13] combined with the muscular pumping action.[14] Reflux of nasopharyngeal secretions as well as breathing sounds and vocalizations into the middle ear are prevented by the airtight closed position of the cartilaginous portion of the Eustachian tube and by the remaining gas volume in the middle ear and mastoid bone.[1]

Eustachian Tube Dilation and Closure

The cartilaginous portion of the pharyngotympanic tube is closed in the resting state. The closure occurs over a variable length, about a 10–15 mm stretch, extending from within a few millimeters distal from the junction portion down to near the nasopharyngeal orifice. This dynamic portion of the cartilaginous Eustachian tube that intermittently dilates actively and closes serves as a functional valve and is termed "the valve". Tubal dilation occurs in two distinct phases (Figs. 6.1A and B). Tubal dilation is initiated through contraction of the LVP muscle that causes palatal elevation along with medial rotation of the torus tubarius and the posteromedial wall of the cartilaginous Eustachian tube. The LVP contraction is maintained throughout the tubal dilation. It serves as a scaffold against which the TVP subsequently contracts. The second phase of tubal dilation involves the contraction of the TVP, which dilates the functional valve of the Eustachian tube, thereby exerting a lateral traction force on the anterolateral membranous wall. Full contraction of the TVP results in maximal opening of the valve and creates a rounded Eustachian tube lumen. Due to the pyramidal shape of the cartilaginous Eustachian tube, dilation propagates from the nasopharyngeal orifice toward the proximal end of the Eustachian tube.

In a recent study, the dynamic opening of the Eustachian tube was investigated with cine CT.[15] Sequential "peristaltic-like" movement of an air bolus was observed passing through the Eustachian tube in normal subjects, but not in subjects with Eustachian tube dysfunction. These results are preliminary, but sequential opening of the Eustachian tube with progressive travel of air boluses may be an important newly recognized mechanism that contributes to middle ear ventilation, rather than a requirement for opening of the entire tube.

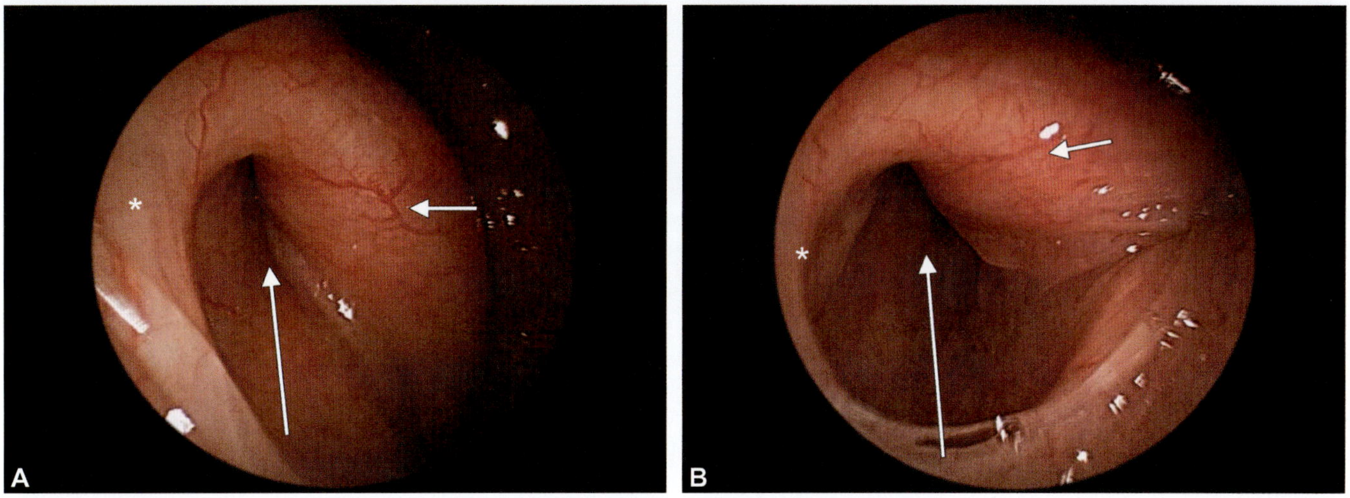

Figs. 6.1A and B: Normal left Eustachian tube depicting the torus tubarius (short arrow), lumen (long arrow), and anterolateral wall (asterisk). A 30° rigid endoscope in the ipsilateral nasal cavity was used to capture the images. (A) Closed resting position. (B) Open dilated position.

The closing of the Eustachian tube proceeds in the opposite direction, from the isthmus to the nasopharynx and the functional valve creates an air- and watertight seal. Under normal conditions, the Eustachian tube dilates approximately 1.4 times per minute throughout waking hours, with openings lasting approximately 400 milliseconds when swallowing and possibly exceeding several seconds in yawing. Dilatory activity is substantially decreased during sleep.[16–17]

Middle Ear Gas Exchange

Nitrogen, which is the dominant component of air within the middle ear air, diffuses very slowly into the venous system. Other air gases, such as carbon dioxide and oxygen, diffuse much more rapidly into the mucosa and blood, and the partial pressure of water vapor being always saturated remains stable. The slower diffusion rate of the residual nitrogen creates a greater percentage of nitrogen within the middle ear space compared to surrounding ambient air. If Eustachian tube dilation occurs insufficiently widely or frequently to adequately aerate the middle ear, the pressure within the middle ear will remain negative. As nitrogen slowly dissolves into the blood over hours and days, there will be a continual tendency for progressively negative pressure within the middle ear until such time as ventilation or filling of the space with fluid (middle ear effusion) occurs. The gradient of the partial pressure of nitrogen relative to that of the blood is believed to play an important role in the regulation of pressure within the middle ear. The Eustachian tube actively dilates by voluntary and involuntary actions such as yawning and swallowing, and by autonomic reflex stimulation due to alterations in gas composition and pressure in the middle ear that are detected by baroreceptors and chemoreceptors.[18–19]

Clearance of the Middle Ear

The most active mucociliary clearance in the middle ear has been observed to be within the anterior half to two-thirds of the tympanic cavity, increasing toward the Eustachian tube lumen. The mucociliary mechanisms serve to move secretions, fluids, and debris toward the nasopharyngeal orifice. The process is aided by the pyramidal shape of the Eustachian tube, which closes progressively from proximally to distally creating a "muscular pumping" effect with an expelling force from the relaxing cartilage and peritubal muscles.[1,14] However, in the case of extremely viscous secretions, mucociliary clearance can be hindered. Surfactants have been found in the Eustachian tube and may serve to help decrease surface tension within the lumen, effectively aiding mucociliary clearance, tubal dilation, and exchange of gases across the mucosal barrier.[20–21]

Protection of the Middle Ear

The air- and watertight functional valve of the Eustachian tube protects the middle ear against the reflux of sounds and material from the nasopharynx.[1] During the periods of intermittent tubal patency, the existing air pressure within the middle ear and mastoid cavity provides a gas cushion that further inhibits the reflux of material from reaching the middle ear.[16]

PATHOGENESIS OF EUSTACHIAN TUBE DYSFUNCTION

Endoscopic evaluation of the Eustachian tube has revealed that most patients with Eustachian tube dysfunction have identifiable pathology within the cartilaginous portion.[5,22] Insufficient dilation of the Eustachian tube (dilatory dysfunction) is the most common type of tubal dysfunction and the patulous Eustachian tube; the failure of proper closure of the tubal valve is significantly less common.

Dilatory dysfunction is commonly due to functional obstruction or insufficient dilation rather than true blockage of the lumen. The most common finding in dilatory dysfunction is mucosal inflammation within the cartilaginous portion of the Eustachian tube. The inflammation appears to involve the lymphoid tissues in the torus tubarius and tubal orifice, seen as cobblestoning of the mucosa. There is also edema, erythema, and increased mucus secretion at the orifice and extending into the lumen with the inflammation being most pronounced in the gland containing mucosa of the torus tubarius and posteromedial wall. The mucosa deeper within the lumen, i.e. closer to the isthmus, is typically less affected. In a study of dilatory obstructive dysfunction, mucosal edema near the orifice was found in 83% of the subjects and 74% had reduced anterolateral wall movement of the Eustachian tube, most likely due to the thickness of the inflamed mucosa.[23] It is common that the adenoid is also inflamed and hypertrophied. In a study of adults, inflammation correlated significantly with the presence of allergies and gastroesophageal reflux, raising suspicions that these factors may be important contributors to dilatory dysfunction.[22-23] Mucosal inflammation due to infection can result from diseases in the respiratory tract including those affecting the sinuses, nasal cavity, nasopharynx and the remainder of the upper and lower airway. Rare primary disorders of the mucosa or submucosa such as Wegener's disease, Samter's triad, and granulomatous diseases may also affect the nose and ears as well as the Eustachian tube. Most children are affected by frequent upper respiratory infections that are increased with day care, reflux disease in younger children and exposure to tobacco smoke or wood-burning stoves.[24] Smoke impairs both the mucociliary function and causes mucosal inflammation. Increased viscosity of secretions and primary ciliary disorders are other possible causes for compromised mucociliary clearance function. Hormone level changes, in particular progesterone, that are increased during pregnancy or oral contraceptive intake may induce mucosal hypertrophy.

Adenoid hypertrophy commonly causes a functional obstruction without physically blocking the tubal orifice by encroaching on the torus tubarius and compromising the dilatory process. The contraction of the pharyngeal constrictors during swallowing can press the enlarged adenoid into the torus tubarius thereby preventing its medial rotation or even causing an anterior thrusting of the torus that further blocks the tubal orifice instead of dilating it open (Figs. 6.2A and B).[23,25] Anatomical obstruction of the Eustachian tube from benign or malignant neoplasms is much less common. Other possible benign processes include large Thornwaldt cysts, mucus retention cysts, teratomas and dermoids, and synechia after surgeries. Malignant tumors may include most typically nasopharyngeal carcinoma followed by lymphoma, mucosal melanoma, and chondrosarcoma.[26]

Dynamic causes of Eustachian tube dilatory dysfunction occur less frequently and may be due to hypoactive, hyperactive, or uncoordinated contraction of TVP or LVP muscles. Muscular dysfunction and weakness of the TVP muscle is the most common dynamic cause of impairment in anterolateral wall dilatory movement. Decreased or disorganized TVP contractions may reduce the lateral excursion of the anterolateral wall in the second phase of dilation. Extreme contractions have been observed in both TVP and LVP muscles leading to a bulky mass effect, thereby paradoxically impairing the valve dilation at the moment it should be opening (Figs. 6.3A and B). Uncoordinated contractions may result in inadequate dilation should the LVP relax prematurely prior to the contraction of the TVP. This provides additional evidence that the LVP serves an important scaffold function against which the weak action of the TVP is dependent for adequate dilation function.

The pediatric Eustachian tube shows critical anatomical differences compared to adults that may play a significant role in the pathogenesis of otitis media. Compared to adults, the Eustachian tube of children is of considerably shorter length, has a narrower lumen, is more compliant, more horizontally oriented, and contains more luminal mucosal folds.[7] These anatomical differences may expose children to a decreased mucociliary clearance and increased reflux from the nasopharynx of pathogens, nasogastric contents, allergic or other inflammatory mediators.

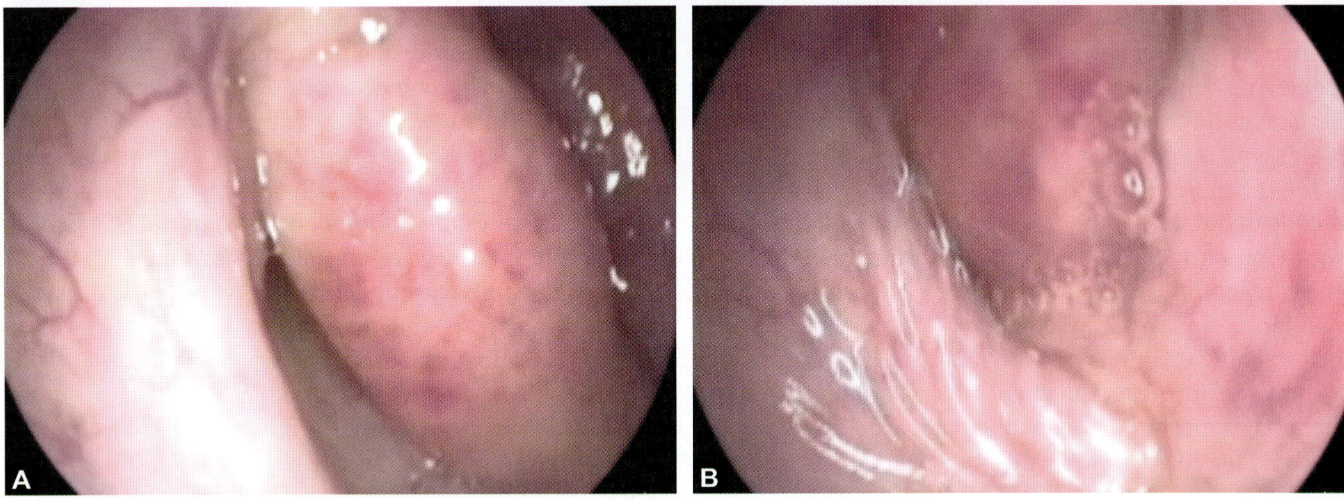

Figs. 6.2A and B: Right Eustachian tube and inflamed adenoid in the upper-right corner. The adenoid reaches and contacts the inflamed torus tubarius and prevents sufficient dilation. Additional, otitis media with effusion is seen. (A) Closed resting position. (B) Swallow with attempt to dilate the Eustachian tube. The swollen torus tubarius is compressed against the adenoid thus forcing the torus anteriorly and preventing opening of the lumen.

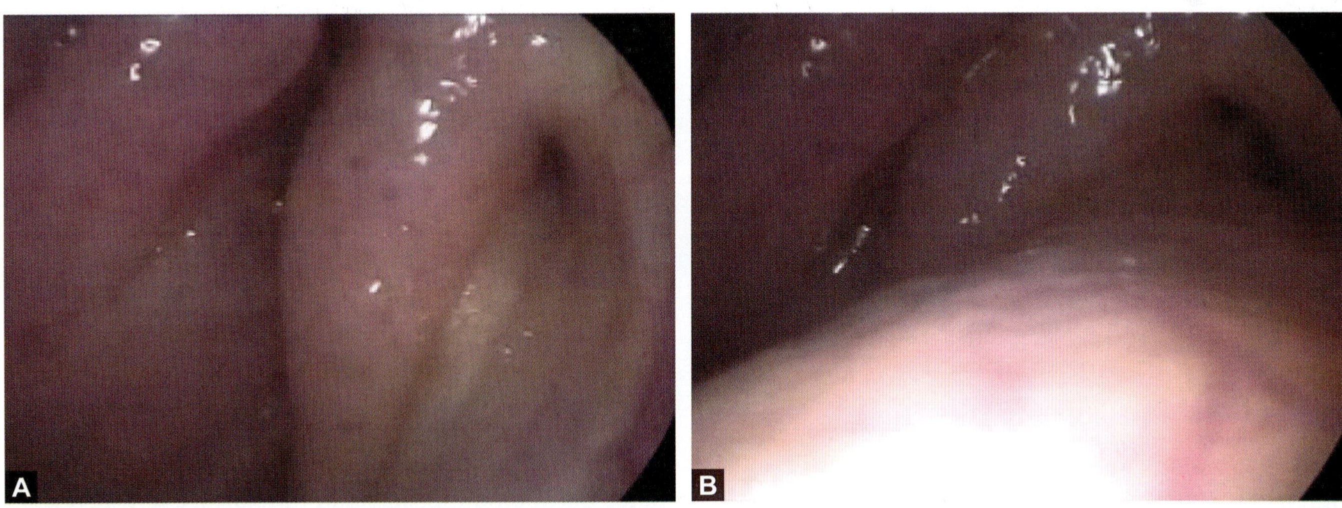

Figs. 6.3A and B: Left Eustachian tube demonstrating dysfunction of the LVP muscle. The muscle contracts abnormal high during swallows thus blocking the lumen during the dilatory effort. Otitis media with effusion is seen. (A) Resting closed position. (B) Swallow with high elevation of the soft palate; LVP muscle blocks the tubal lumen.

CLINICAL FINDINGS: SYMPTOMS AND SIGNS

Typical clinical findings in Eustachian tube dysfunction include negative middle ear pressure and tympanic membrane atelectasis, adhesive otitis media, pressure equalization problems with elevators, mountain driving, diving or flying, chronic otitis media with effusion, and conductive hearing loss. It may play a role in recurrent otitis media and it leads to complications of otitis media such as retraction pocket formation, cholesteatoma, and persistent tympanic membrane perforation.

EVALUATION OF THE EUSTACHIAN TUBE: LABORATORY, OTOLOGIC, AND NEUROTOLOGIC TESTING

History and Physical Examination

A comprehensive history and physical examination are the most important means for evaluation of Eustachian tube dysfunction. In patients with dilatory Eustachian tube dysfunction, mucosal inflammation of the cartilaginous portion of the Eustachian tube is the most common pathological finding. The Eustachian tube is an extension of the nasal cavity and as such, it may be affected by any diseases that may impact the nose or sinuses. Patients should therefore be questioned about inflammatory disorders such as allergies, chronic rhinosinusitis, reflux disease, vasomotor rhinitis, and in refractory cases, other less common causes such as granulomatous disease or Samter's triad should be considered. In children, it is important to additionally inquire about recurrent or persistent otitis media, respiratory infections, smoke or wood stove exposure, daycare attendance, and immune deficiency.[24] Mucociliary clearance is known to be negatively affected by tobacco use or smoke exposure. Eustachian tube disorders may have a familial genesis. Refractory pediatric cases should be evaluated for ciliary motility disorders such as Kartageners syndrome.

Patients with dilatory dysfunction typically complain of aural fullness, and varying degrees of conductive hearing loss, and there may be symptoms associated with otitis media such as otalgia, otorrhea, and fever. Patients with chronic aural fullness but without tympanic membrane retractions, effusion, or abnormalities and no difficulties with changes in altitude are unlikely to have Eustachian tube dilatory dysfunction, especially if tympanostomy tubes have not been of benefit. In these cases, other possible causes should be investigated including minor's third window syndrome (including superior semicircular canal dehiscence), temporomandibular joint disease, patulous Eustachian tube, and endolymphatic hydrops.

Endoscopic Examination of the Eustachian Tube

A flexible or Hopkins rod endoscope is used to evaluate the Eustachian tube. A systematic examination assessing the nasal mucosa, nasopharynx, pharynx, larynx, hypopharynx, and subglottic space for signs of inflammation or underlying allergy, granulomatous disease, laryngopharyngeal reflux, or other pathology should be performed prior to evaluating the Eustachian tube in detail.[27]

When examining the Eustachian tube with a flexible endoscope, the best view into the depths of the tubal lumen may be obtained by either advancing the instrument through the ipsilateral nostril or via the contralateral nostril, passing it behind the vomer, and positioning it close to the nasopharyngeal orifice of the auditory tube. To optimally inspect the tubal valve during swallowing and yawning, the endoscope should be directed along the longitudinal axis of the lumen, which courses approximately 45° laterally and 45° superiorly from the floor of the nasal cavity. Fiberoptic endoscopy is a convenient and well tolerated means for viewing all of the upper respiratory tract as well as the Eustachian tubes. However, the best resolution can be achieved with a rigid endoscope, 3 or 4 mm scopes with a 30° or 45° viewing angle are ideal. As the instrument is introduced into the nasal cavity, the scope is usually initially directed laterally to watch the turbinates. Then it can be rotated if needed to bring the Eustachian tube orifice into view when entering the nasopharynx.[28] When the healthy and intact lumen is closed, the tissues of the anterolateral wall create a convex bulge and create an S-shaped appearance from the opposed mucosal walls.

The orifice can be readily identified just posterior to the inferior turbinate by the prominence of the torus tubarius, also known as the posterior cushion. This structure contains the mobile medial cartilaginous lamina. The lateral cartilaginous lamina is immobile, considerably smaller and anchored to the medial pterygoid plate by a broad attachment. The cross-section of the cartilaginous skeleton in its entirety resembles an inverted "J" hook. It is important to differentiate between the tubal orifice and the fossa of Rosenmüller, also called the pharyngeal recess, just posterior to the torus tubarius. At the apex of the fossa courses the internal carotid artery (ICA) and in some cases it may be located just under the mucosa.[29] Within the midportion of the cartilaginous Eustachian tube, the mucosal surfaces of the anterolateral and posteromedial walls meet in apposition to close the lumen in resting position. This important, approximately 15-mm long section is termed the "functional valve" and is comprised of the mucosa, submucosa, Ostmann's fat pad, lateral cartilaginous lamina, and the relaxed bulk of TVP muscle. The distance between Eustachian tube and ICA is lowest at the osseous portion of the Eustachian tube and the distance between the Eustachian tube orifice and ICA is on average 23 mm, but it may be 10 mm or less if there is an aberrant ICA.[29]

The most common findings in Eustachian tube dilatory dysfunction are mucosal inflammation in the torus tubarius with edema, hypertrophy, excessive mucus secretion, hyperemia, and a cobblestone appearance from lymphoid hyperplasia (Fig. 6.4).[30]

Assessment with slow-motion endoscopy aids to differentiate between obstructive and dynamic causes of Eustachian tube dilatory dysfunction. To evaluate the principal peritubal muscle function, the patient is initially asked to say the letter "K" repeatedly. This causes isolated contraction of the LVP muscle and medial rotation of the posterior cushion without tubal dilation. Normal tubal dilation is then evaluated during repeated swallows, and lastly, the patient is asked to forcefully yawn to produce a maximal

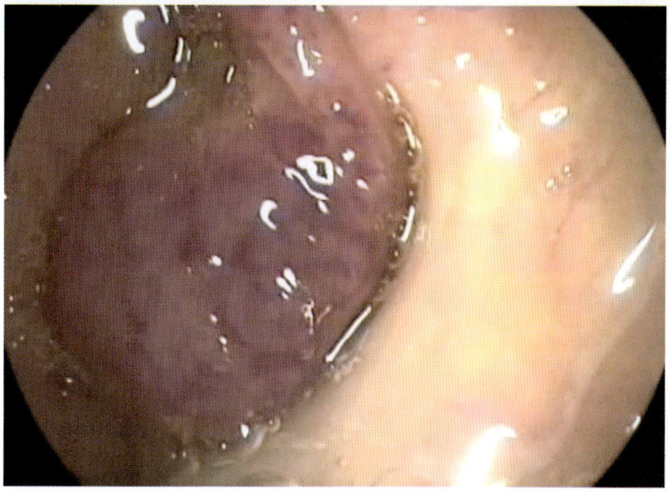

Fig. 6.4: Left Eustachian tube with significantly inflamed torus tubarius and lymphoid hyperplasia. Clinically the patient shows otitis media with effusion.

voluntary dilatory effort. Afterward video endoscopy can be reviewed in slow motion for a better view, allowing for a detailed assessment of the tubal dilatory phases, with the orifice seen changing from its resting S-shaped convexity into a rounded opening.

EVALUATION: RADIOLOGIC IMAGING

Imaging may be important during the diagnostic evaluation of dilatory dysfunction, particularly when there is a suspicion for nasal and sinus diseases or middle ear disease. Imaging, usually with contrast, is necessary to rule out nasopharyngeal neoplasms in adults with unilateral middle ear effusion. For patients being considered for surgical management of their Eustachian tube disorders, preoperative high resolution, noncontrasted CT imaging including the temporal bone and nasopharynx may be appropriate to assure that there is no dehiscence of the ICA within the skull base or any suggestion of aberrant course that may bring it into proximity with the cartilaginous Eustachian tube.[29]

TREATMENT OF EUSTACHIAN TUBE DYSFUNCTION

Medical Treatment for Eustachian Tube Dilatory Dysfunction

Mucosal disease is the most common cause of Eustachian tube dilatory dysfunction. Identifying the underlying etiology of the disease and treating it as thoroughly as possible is advised. Allergies may be the most common cause of dilatory dysfunction, especially in the case of children who fail to outgrow otitis media by age six and an allergy evaluation is often indicated.[31] Allergen avoidance, oral antihistamines, nasal topical steroid drops (available in Europe, but not in United States) or steroid sprays (less effective than drops), saline irrigations, nasal antihistamine, mast cell stabilizer sprays, leukotriene inhibitors, combination therapy, and immunotherapy may all be considered. A recent randomized, placebo-controlled, double blinded study in which nasal corticosteroid spray was given for Eustachian tube dilatory dysfunction without specified etiologies found that corticosteroid nasal spray provided no benefit in Eustachian tube dysfunction.[30] A total of 91 patients with otitis media with effusion, negative middle ear pressure, or both were treated with nasal corticosteroid spay or placebo for 6 weeks. There were no significant differences in tympanometry findings or symptoms scores between active treatment group and placebo group.

Recurrent nasal or sinus infections should be treated as indicated. Granulomatous diseases usually require immunosuppressant therapy and rheumatology should be consulted, but some topical treatments may be indicated. Laryngopharyngeal reflux should be treated with behavioral and dietary modifications as well as thoroughly with antireflux medications as indicated. True anatomical obstruction requires contrast enhanced imaging and a biopsy to determine the etiology.

Surgical Treatment for Eustachian Tube Dilatory Dysfunction

Persistence of dilatory dysfunction despite maximal efforts to control various underlying etiologies may imply that the tubal mucosa has become irreversibly injured or perhaps involved with bacterial biofilms. An anatomical compromise or defect of the Eustachian tube may be present in patients with familial predisposition for tubal dysfunction, cleft lip or palates, syndromic and other craniofacial anomalies.

Inserting tympanostomy tubes into the tympanic membrane may temporarily alleviate the negative pressure within the middle ear and relieve tympanic membrane retraction, effusion, and atelectasis. Adenoidectomy can provide significant relief to patients with otitis media and demonstrated chronic adenoid hypertrophy, especially if the hypertrophied adenoid tissue is in close contact with the torus tubarius.[32-33] Endoscopic-assisted adenoidectomy permits more complete removal of the tissue encroaching on the torus and it also allows for some gentle monopolar debulking of the hyperplastic tissue of the torus if considered necessary.

Eustachian Tuboplasty

In last decade, Eustachian tuboplasty has received increased attention as a safe and possibly effective surgical option for patients with dilatory dysfunction. Eustachian tuboplasty can be accomplished by removing presumably irreversibly inflamed soft tissue and, when necessary, cartilage bulges that may limit the lumen as they protrude from the posteromedial wall. Laser and microdebrider techniques have been used with reasonably good results (Figs. 6.5 and 6.6). More recently, balloon dilation of the cartilaginous Eustachian tube has been assessed for feasibility, safety, and the early clinical results have been promising. The authors employ a sinuplasty balloon system (Acclarent Corp, Palo Alto, CA, USA) that is not FDA approved for Eustachian tube dilation. It is most commonly being done under general anesthesia, although it can be done under local anesthesia with sedation, but it is not easy to obtain adequate local anesthesia in this area. A curved guiding catheter with a tip angle of 70° is inserted through the ipsilateral nostril, passing it along the floor of the nasal cavity avoiding any mucosal trauma. It is important to recognize that the Eustachian tube initially curves slightly medially before coursing laterally toward the ear. The lumen should be opened gently by retracting medially on the torus tubarius with the guiding catheter allowing for a view deep into the lumen before beginning the insertion. Failure to rotate the torus medially before inserting the catheter could result in mucosal laceration with bleeding or a false passage into the submucosal tissues. The balloon catheter is passed superiorly into the lumen atraumatically, advanced gently and slowly until meeting resistance as the catheter engages the bony-cartilaginous isthmus. The catheter should never be forcefully inserted. There is a yellow marker on the catheter that is 31 mm

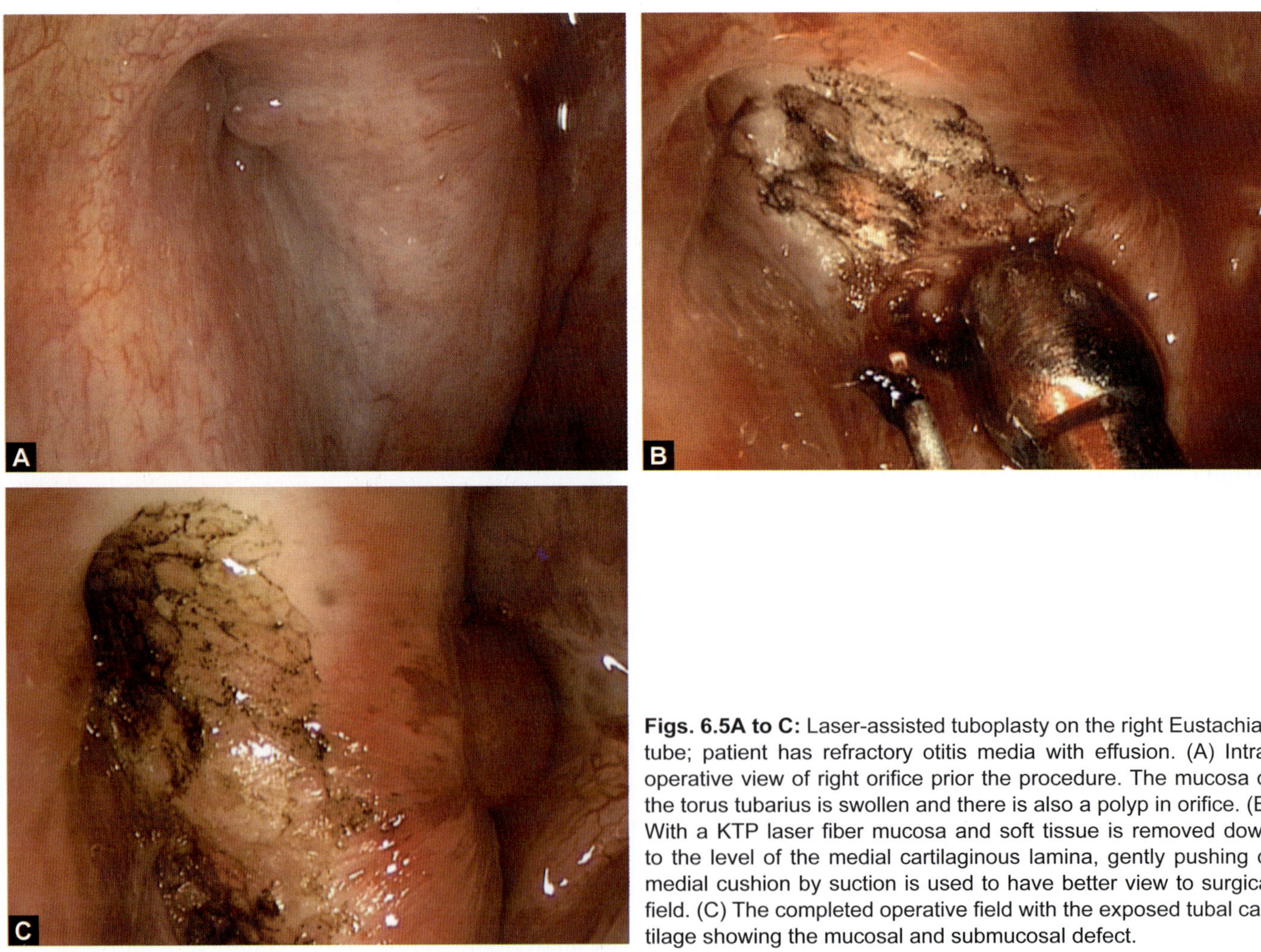

Figs. 6.5A to C: Laser-assisted tuboplasty on the right Eustachian tube; patient has refractory otitis media with effusion. (A) Intraoperative view of right orifice prior the procedure. The mucosa of the torus tubarius is swollen and there is also a polyp in orifice. (B) With a KTP laser fiber mucosa and soft tissue is removed down to the level of the medial cartilaginous lamina, gently pushing of medial cushion by suction is used to have better view to surgical field. (C) The completed operative field with the exposed tubal cartilage showing the mucosal and submucosal defect.

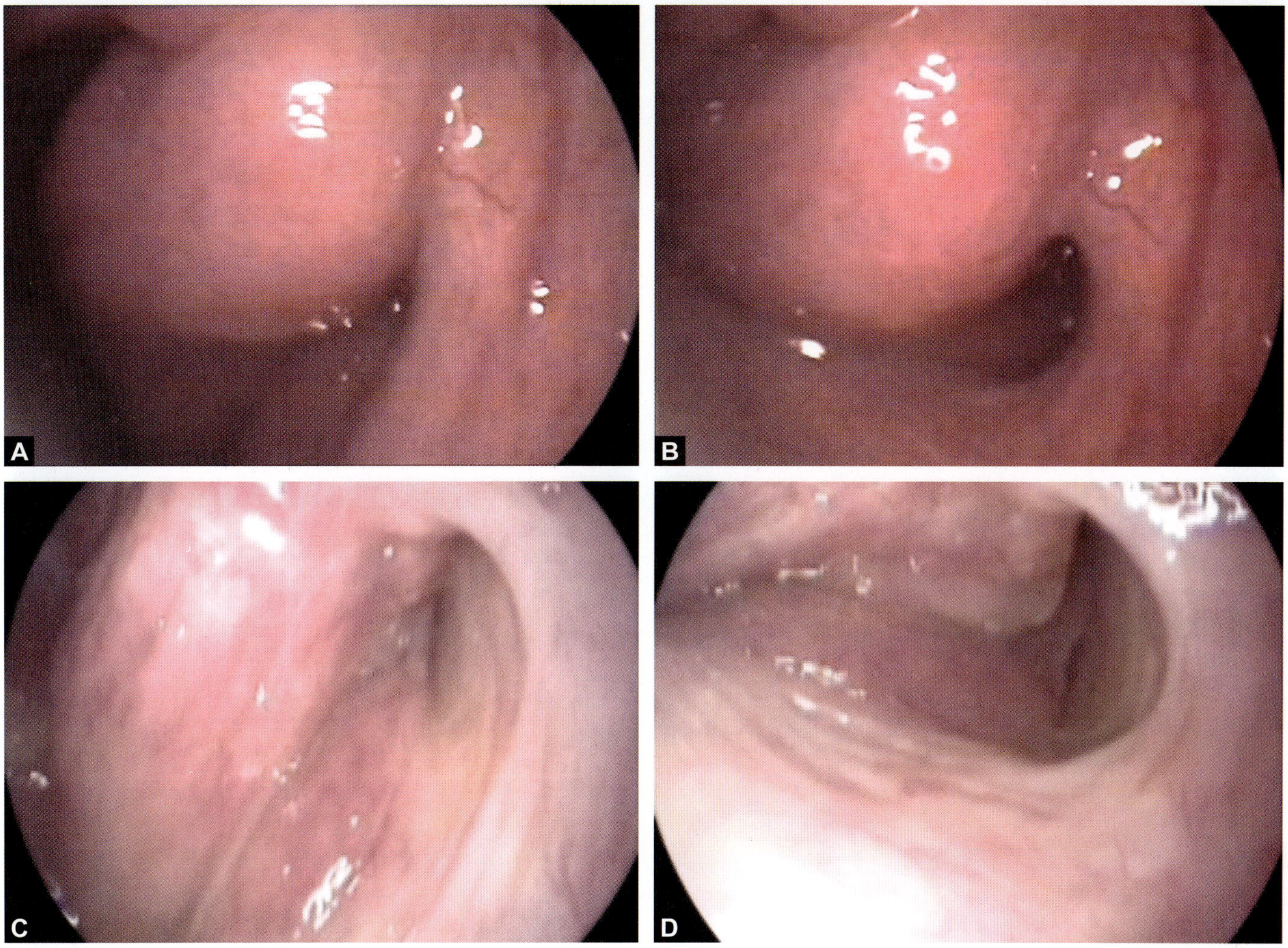

Figs. 6.6A to D: Pre- and postoperative photos of left Eustachian tube orifice laser Eustachian tuboplasty. The patient has refractory otitis media with effusion and underlying severe allergic disease. (A) Preoperative, resting position, where the posterior cushion is bulbous and edematous. (B) Preoperative, dilated position. The lumen is revealed only minimally. (C) Postoperative, resting position. The torus shows a scaphoid defect on the luminal surface and the mucosal inflammation is markedly reduced. (D) Postoperative, dilated position. The lumen is now open widely.

from the distal tip and it should be positioned outside of the orifice, this assures the balloon catheter is inserted at the proper depth into the tubal lumen. The balloon is inflated to 12 atm and it often drifts down to 10 atm during the 2 minutes of inflation, after which the balloon is deflated and removed (Figs. 6.7A to D). The procedure may be done bilaterally. Adverse events, such as minor tears in the mucosal lumen have been observed. Neither osseous or significant cartilaginous fracture nor trauma to the internal carotid has been reported.[34]

PROGNOSIS

Preliminary result from balloon dilation Eustachian tuboplasty has been assessed for feasibility, safety, and clinical application. In a pilot study on 11 patients with chronic otitis media with effusion of over 5 years duration, postoperatively 11/11 (100%) were able to perform a Valsalva maneuver, whereas they had previously been unable to do so, but this declined to 7/11 (64%) at the end of the follow-up period from 6–14 months. Resolution of middle ear effusion occurred in all of the 5/11 (45.4%) who had an intact tympanic membranes (no perforation or tube);[35] Ockermann et al. have reported comparable results in which 12/12 cases were able to perform a Valsalva maneuver 8 weeks postoperatively; and Schöder et al. have reported that 13/15 (87%) were able to perform a Valsalva maneuver in 1 year follow-up visit.[36–37] These authors employed a 10-point Eustachian tube score that included subjective measurement of Eustachian tube function in swallowing,

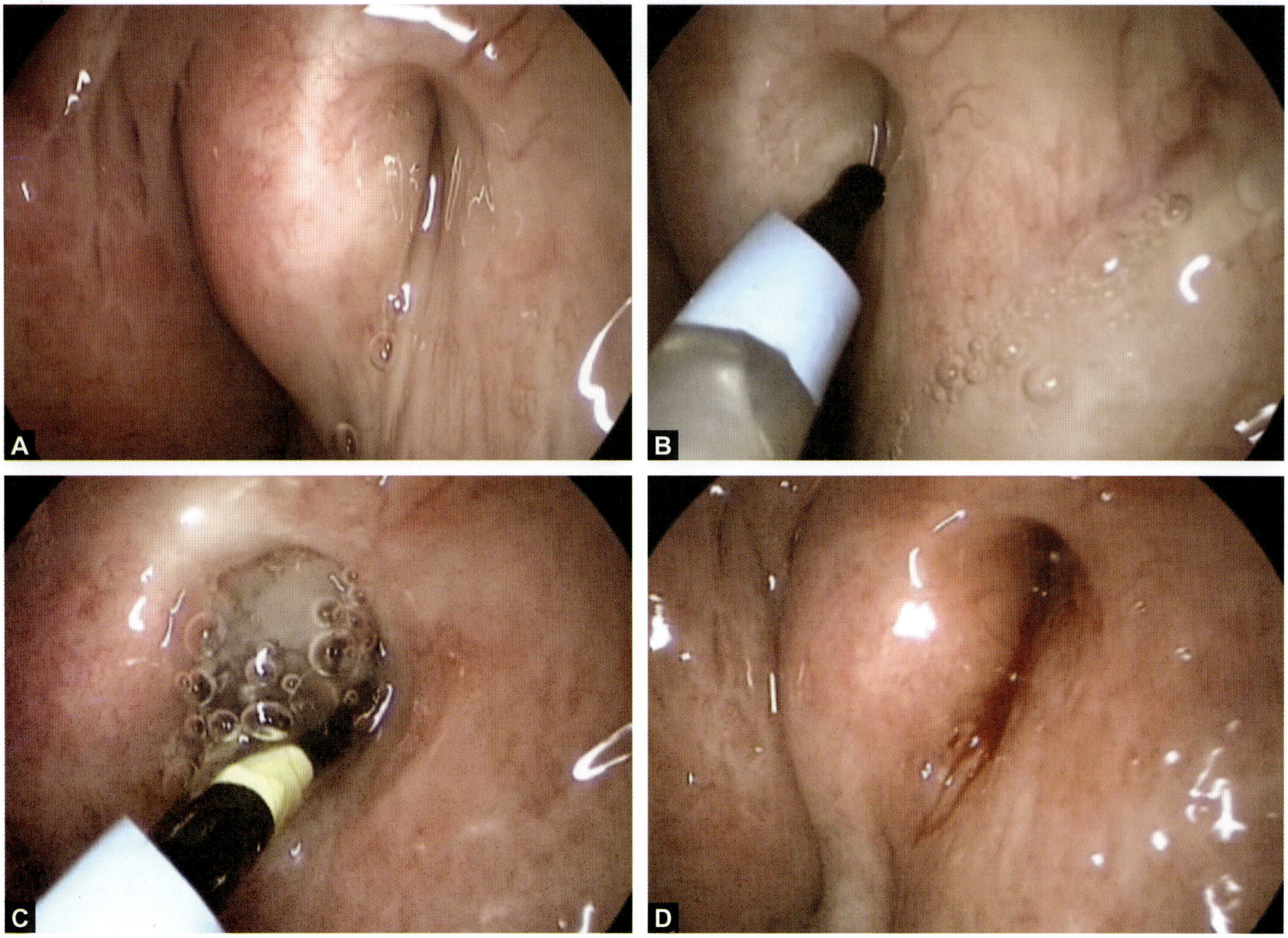

Figs. 6.7A to D: Balloon dilation of the left Eustachian tube. The patient shows chronic otitis media with effusion. (A) Preoperative resting position of the Eustachian tube with edema and inflammation of the torus tubarius. (B) A guide catheter is inserted into the tubal lumen. (C) The balloon catheter, 7 x 16 mm has been inserted fully and inflated to 12 atm for 2 minutes. (D) The balloon catheter has been removed. A widened lumen and minimal mucosal lacerations are appreciated.

Valsalva maneuver, and tubomanometry results. The scores improved from preoperative value 1.1 to postoperative value 7.5.[36] McCoul et al. has shown the improvement in tympanometry results in 34/35 (97%) cases in 6 weeks follow-up and improvement from B or C to A in 25/28 (89%) cases.[38]

The laser-assisted tuboplasty is mostly now reserved for the unusual circumstances in which there is a very limited amount of mucosal disease and circumferential dilation may risk a patulous tube or in the event of a prominent bulge of cartilage from the torus tubarius into the lumen that might interfere with the balloon dilation. The laser can be combined with the balloon techniques as well. Longer term experience with the laser has shown that positive Valsalva maneuver results have varied from 67% to 72%.[39-41] Long-term follow-up results are still lacking for Eustachian tuboplasty, and also, more controlled studies are needed to evaluate the meaning of surgical treatment in different kind of pathological conditions of Eustachian tube dysfunction.

PATULOUS EUSTACHIAN TUBE DYSFUNCTION

Overview, Etiology, and Pathophysiology

Patulous Eustachian tube dysfunction refers to persistent patency of the tubal lumen with disturbing symptoms. Air and sound can pass unrestricted between the nasopharynx and the middle ear space. Patients with this disorder complain of a disturbing amplified perception of their own voice and nasal breathing sounds (autophony), with sensation of aural fullness, and in few cases otalgia.

Although benign, patulous dysfunction, and the resulting autophony cause a range of symptom severity from asymptomatic to severe psychological impairment. Symptoms are often intermittent and can last from seconds to hours, but in extreme cases they may persist continuously throughout the day. Symptoms may be worsened with decongestants or nasal steroids, and improved with upper respiratory tract infections. Etiologically, symptoms may occur after a dramatic and substantial weight loss such as during postpregnancy, cachectic diseases, dietary weight loss, or bariatric surgery. An average of one-third of cases of patulous Eustachian tube have a history of substantial weight loss, one-third have an associated systemic rheumatologic disorder such as arthritis or Raynauds disease, and the remaining third are idiopathic. Oral contraceptives may contribute to the disorder. It is commonly seen that exercise initiates or exacerbates symptoms. Symptoms tend to abate in the supine or head dependent positions. Loss of tubal tissue volume especially within the valve is the likely etiology for many patients. A longitudinal concavity in the anterolateral wall in the resting position of the auditory tube resulting in inadequate closing of the tubal lumen that can be recognized in endoscopic evaluation (Fig. 6.8).[42] The anterolateral wall normally contains a convex bulge into the lumen in the resting position that contributes to the valve function. This bulge is usually diminished or absent in these patients. A majority of cases have anatomically an underdeveloped lateral cartilaginous lamina constituting a potential risk for patulous Eustachian tube. Patients with a thin build may have smaller Ostmann's fat pad and if combined with a lack of cartilage in the bulge of the valve may lead to patulous Eustachian tube. CT scans may reveal smaller Ostmann's fat pad and glandular tissues in patulous patients compared to normal control subjects.[43]

The symptoms of patulous Eustachian tube can be similar with other conditions, making the differential diagnosis more difficult. Examination should be done while patients are experiencing active autophony symptoms. Otoscopy or micro-otoscopy in the sitting position will usually reveal the pathognomic sign of a patulous tube with medial and lateral movements of the tympanic membrane during nasal breathing while the opposite nostril is held shut. A few minutes of vigorous physical activity prior to otoscopy can trigger symptoms if they are not initially present.

Impedance tympanometry is the most sensitive and objective test to aid in the diagnosis of patulous Eustachian tube dysfunction. Tympanometry shows ventilatory fluctuations in the compliance of the tympanic membrane, while a 15-second run is performed with the instrument set for reflex decay testing. Irregular moderately deep breathing (similar to breathing for auscultation of the lungs) through the ipsilateral nostril with the opposite nostril occluded should show sawtooth-like perturbations of the baseline tympanogram tracing. The breathing is performed irregularly to not confuse the tracing with the regular sawtooth waveforms that may occur from intracranial pulsations.

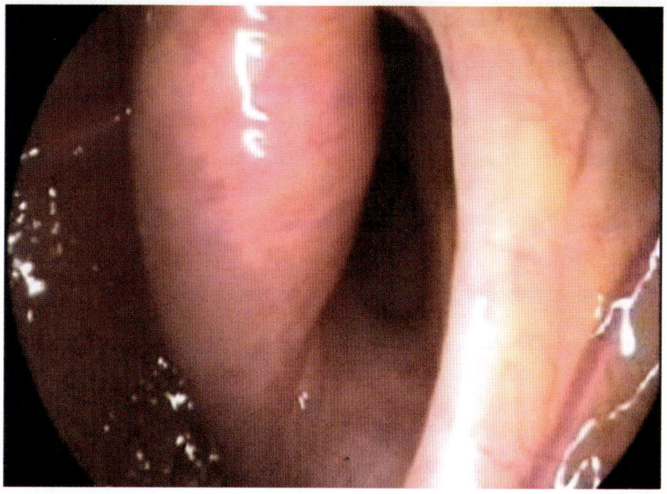

Fig. 6.8: Left patulous Eustachian tube. It shows a marked scaphoid lateral wall. No visible lateral cartilaginous lamina or evidence of a significant Ostmann's fat pad.

If clinical findings are lacking and the tympanogram is negative despite the patient having active autophony, other pathologies should be considered, such as Minor's third labyrinthine window syndrome (semicircular canal dehiscence syndrome). Vestibular evoked myogenic potential (VEMP) and electrocochleography testing can help in differentiating patulous dysfunction from Minor's third window syndrome. Although less common, endolymphatic hydrops can sometimes cause recruitment with hyperacusis and autophony. Patients with Minor's syndrome usually lack prominent autophony of their nasal breathing sounds, in contrast to the loud bone-conducted autophony of their voice. These patients show an abnormally low reflex threshold on VEMP. If the patient has tympanostomy tubes still in place, ventilatory excursions can still be observed as a following method: a drop of clear topical otologic medication is placed on top of the tympanostomy tube and movements of the fluid meniscus forming on top of the tube can be observed.

Sonotubometry research with recent improvements in detecting tubal patency status has demonstrated a correlation between the severity of autophony and measured tubal patency.[44]

Medical Treatment for Patulous Eustachian Tube Dysfunction

The goals for patulous Eustachian tube treatment are the restoration of the healthy humidified mucosa and competence of the tubal valve. Patients should be treated in a stepwise fashion. The first step is to reassure the patients that although the condition may be extremely disturbing, it is entirely physiologically benign. The next steps are the discontinuation of possible exacerbating medications such as decongestants, topical nasal corticosteroid, and oral contraceptives. Patients are encouraged to increase their fluid intake, particularly during exercise and adding nasal saline drops or irrigations to improve hydration of the mucosa.

Although roughly one-third of patulous patients have a history of significant weight loss, weight gain is generally not advised unless medically indicated. The following medications have been used off-label and with variable results. The concept behind these medications is to stimulate a closure of the Eustachian tube. Among them, saturated solution of potassium iodide, 8–10 drops diluted in orange juice, taken three times daily, enhances the viscosity of the mucus. Application of irritants such as boric and salicylic acid powder, silver nitrate, nitric acid, and phenol cause tissue inflammation and increased mucus production. Hydrochloric acid based drops are available without prescription, but have had variable success in long-term control rates. The off-label use of Premarin (25 mg in 30 mL normal saline topical nasal drops, three drops three times daily for a 6 week trial) or depo-estradiol estrogens (same schedule using 5 mg in 30 mL normal saline) may provide some relief by causing localized mucosal hypertrophy and increased mucus secretion, thus temporarily closing the open Eustachian tube.

Drops are most effectively applied in the supine position with the nose pointed straight upward, then turning the head 45° to the ipsilateral side as the drops pass through the nasal cavity. A tickle or sensation of irritation should radiate toward the affected ear when the drops come in contact with the tubal orifice.

Surgical Treatment of Patulous Eustachian Tube Dysfunction

When medical treatments lead to insufficient relief and symptoms are sufficiently disturbing, surgical options may be considered. Myringotomy with tympanostomy tube placement is commonly tried as an initial procedure, but this procedure is most effective for aural fullness and tympanic membrane excursions.[45] However, it is usually not very effective for treating autophony. To alleviate autophony, reconstruction of the valve of the Eustachian tube lumen may be considered and an attempt is made to restore the competency of the tubal valve without compromising dilatory function.

In an effort to treat the patulous symptoms while preserving tubal function, a shim can be inserted into the lumen as the most commonly performed and initial procedure. A shim made from catheter can be introduced into the nasopharyngeal orifice, wedging it into position within the isthmus. Being long and thin, the shim can be positioned into the length of the longitudinal concave defect of the valve to effectively restore the competency of the valve, yet avoiding the development of middle ear effusions or a need for tympanostomy tubes in most cases. A shim is made from an intravenous catheter filled with bone wax can be employed in this off-label application. A 14 gauge (2.1 mm diameter) intravenous catheter will appropriately fit most adult patients. A CT scan is necessary for all patients preoperatively to confirm that there is bony coverage of the ICA. Dehiscence of the artery into the tubal lumen is a contraindication for catheter insertion.

The catheter insertion is performed under general anesthesia. Bone wax is heated until molten and then aspirated through the intravenous catheter using a syringe and then the wax quickly cools and solidifies. Then the catheter is cut to 36–38 mm length for most females and 38–40 mm for most males. It is inserted under endoscopic guidance using a specific insertion tool that consists of a hollow tube that is passed through the oral cavity and an internal piston that pushes the catheter forward and outward toward the distal end. The insertion tool is also utilized to push the torus slightly medially. This maneuver reveals the curvature of the Eustachian tube. Directly viewing this anatomy through the endoscope is essential prior to introducing the catheter to avoid any unnecessary mucosal tears. The catheter should pass easily and atraumatically at all times and the insertion should be bloodless. The catheter will begin to meet some resistance at the isthmus region and is allowed to straighten itself out. It can then be enhanced with some firmer pressure to wedge it into position within the isthmus. Proper catheter placement is achieved when the catheter end is protruding from the nasopharyngeal orifice at a level just inside the anterior cushion (Figs. 6.9A to D). A smaller 16 gauge catheter may be used if the 14 gauge is too large to pass smoothly. A bigger 12 gauge catheter is rarely used. In most cases, the catheters stay in place nicely and are not felt by the patients at all.

19. Bluestone CD. Introduction. In: Bluestone MB (ed.), Eustachian tube: structure, function, role in otitis media. Hamilton, Ont.; Lewiston, NY: BC Decker; 2005. pp. 1-9.
20. McGuire JF. Surfactant in the middle ear and Eustachian tube: a review. Int J Pediatr Otorhinolaryngol. 2002;66:1-15.
21. Grace A, Kwok P, Hawke M. Surfactant in middle ear effusions. Otolaryngol Head Neck Surg. 1987;96:336-40.
22. Edelstein DR, Magnan J, Parisier SC, et al. Microfiberoptic evaluation of the middle ear cavity. Am J Otol. 1994;15: 50-55.
23. Poe DS, Abou-Halawa A, Abdel-Razek O. Analysis of the dysfunctional Eustachian tube by video endoscopy. Otol Neurotol. 2001;22:590-95.
24. Bluestone CD. Epidemiology. In: Bluestone MB (ed.), Eustachian tube: structure, function, role in otitis media. Hamilton, Ont.; Lewiston, NY: BC Decker; 2005. pp. 11-24.
25. Kindermann CA, Roithmann R, Lubianca Neto JF. Obstruction of the Eustachian tube orifice and pressure changes in the middle ear: are they correlated? Ann Otol Rhinol Laryngol. 2008;117:425-9.
26. Muzzi E, Cama E, Boscolo-Rizzo P, et al. Primary tumors and tumor-like lesions of the Eustachian tube: a systematic review of an emerging entity. Eur Arch Otorhinolaryngol. 2012;269(7):1723-32.
27. Poe DS, Gopen Q. Eustachian tube dysfunction. In: Snow JB, Wackym PA, Ballenger JJ (eds), Ballenger's otorhinolaryngology: head and neck surgery. Lewiston, NY: BC Decker; 2009. pp. 201-8.
28. Poe DS, Pyykko I, Valtonen H, et al. Analysis of Eustachian tube function by video endoscopy. Am J Otol. 2000;21: 602-7.
29. Bergin M, Bird P, Cowan I, et al. Exploring the critical distance and position relationships between the Eustachian tube and the internal carotid artery. Otol Neurotol. 2010; 31(9):1511-5.
30. Takahashi H, Honjo I, Fujita A. Endoscopic findings at the pharyngeal orifice of the Eustachian tube in otitis media with effusion. Eur Arch Otorhinolaryngol. 1996;253:42-4.
31. Hurst DS. Association of otitis media with effusion and allergy as demonstrated by intradermal skin testing and eosinophil cationic protein levels in both middle ear effusions and mucosal biopsies. Laryngoscope. 1996;106:1128-37.
32. Gates GA. Adenoidectomy for otitis media with effusion. Ann Otol Rhinol Laryngol Suppl. 1994;163:54-8.
33. Nguyen LH, Manoukian JJ, Yoskovitch A, et al. Adenoidectomy: selection criteria for surgical cases of otitis media. Laryngoscope. 2004;114:863-6.
34. Poe DS, Hanna BM. Balloon dilation of the cartilaginous portion of the Eustachian tube: initial safety and feasibility analysis in a cadaver model. Am J Otolaryngol. 2011;32: 115-23.
35. Poe DS, Silvola J, Pyykko I. Balloon Dilation of the Cartilaginous Eustachian Tube. Otolaryngol Head Neck Surg. 2011;144:563–569.
36. Ockermann T, Reineke U, Upile T, et al. Balloon dilatation Eustachian tuboplasty: a clinical study. Laryngoscope. 2010;120(7):1411-6.
37. Schröder S, Reineke U, Lehmann M, et al. Chronic obstructive Eustachian tube dysfunction in adults: long-term results of balloon Eustachian tuboplasty. HNO. 2013;61(2):142-51.
38. McCoul ED, Anand VK. Eustachian tube balloon dilation surgery. Int Forum Allergy Rhinol. 2012;2(3):191-8.
39. Kujawski OB, Poe DS. Laser Eustachian tuboplasty. Otol Neurotol. 2004;25(1):1-8.
40. Poe DS, Grimmer JF, Metson R. Laser Eustachian tuboplasty: two-year results. Laryngoscope. 2007;117(2):231-7.
41. Jumah MD, Jumah M, Pazen D, et al. Laser Eustachian tuboplasty: efficiency evaluation in the pressure chamber. Otol Neurotol. 2012;33(3):406-12.
42. Poe DS. Diagnosis and management of the patulous Eustachian tube. Otol Neurotol. 2007;28:668-77.
43. Kikuchi T, Oshima T, Ogura M, et al. Three-dimensional computed tomography imaging in the sitting position for the diagnosis of patulous Eustachian tube. Otol Neurotol. 2007;28:199-203.
44. Hori Y, Kawase T, Oshima T, et al. Objective assessment of autophony in patients with patulous Eustachian tube. Eur Arch Otorhinolaryngol. 2007;264:1387-91.
45. Dyer RK Jr, McElveen JT Jr. The patulous Eustachian tube: management options. Otolaryngol Head Neck Surg. 1991; 105:832-5.
46. Wolraich D, Zur KB. Use of calcium hydroxylapatite for management of recalcitrant otorrhea due to a patulous Eustachian tube. Int J Pediatr Otorhinolaryngol. 2010;74 (12):1455-7.
47. Doherty JK, Slattery WH, 3rd. Autologous fat grafting for the refractory patulous Eustachian tube. Otolaryngol Head Neck Surg. 2003;128:88-91.

CHAPTER

7

Radiology of the Temporal Bone

Alexander Filatov, Mari Hagiwara

INTRODUCTION

Imaging is essential in the diagnostic evaluation, presurgical planning, and post-treatment monitoring of temporal bone pathologies. In this chapter, the imaging techniques utilized in the evaluation of temporal bone pathologies and the indications and advantages/disadvantages of each imaging modality will be reviewed. Classic imaging findings of the more common pathologies of the temporal bone will also be described, with pathologies classified based on location and/or structure of involvement: the outer ear, middle ear, inner ear, petrous apex, and the facial nerve. Imaging of temporal bone trauma will be discussed at the end of the chapter.

IMAGING TECHNIQUES

Plain Radiography

Plain radiography of the temporal bone is a seldom-utilized imaging technique in modern practice due to the complex anatomy of the region and widespread availability, high resolution and multiplanar capability of computed tomography (CT).[1] However, standard radiographical views of the temporal bone remain in use in other parts of the world and include the Law, Schuller, Mayer, Owen, Chausse III, transorbital, Stenvers, submentovertical, and Towne projections.

Conventional radiography still remains useful in the assessment of correct intracochlear electrode array positioning status postcochlear implantation. Stenvers, or oblique posteroanterior view, obtained with the patient facing the film with the head slightly flexed and tilted 15° and rotated 35° away from the side being imaged with 12° cranial angulation of the incident X-ray beam, allows the long axis of the petrous pyramid to become parallel to the plane of the film, and thus permits examination of the entire pyramid.[2] On intra- or postoperative evaluation of a cochlear implant, it is important to observe the smooth curve of the array within the basal turn of the cochlea, with the electrodes regularly spaced (Fig. 7.1). Counting the number of electrodes relative to the cochlear promontory

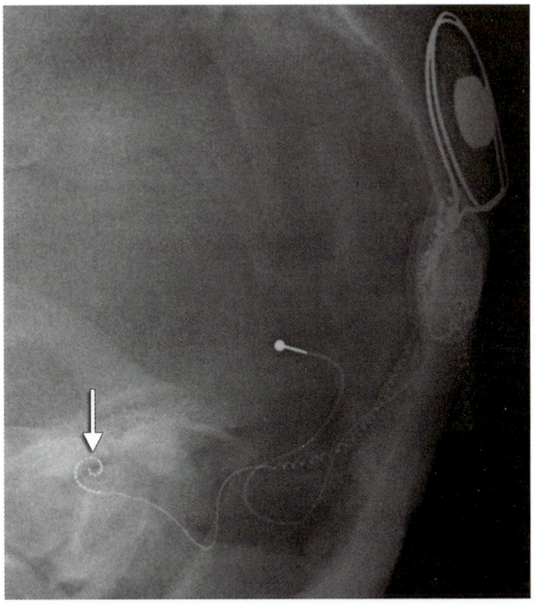

Fig. 7.1: Radiograph of cochlear implant. Normal Stenvers radiograph status post multichannel intracochlear electrode placement showing a normal curvature (arrow) of the electrode array within the cochlea and an intact wire leading from the array to the receiver-stimulator.

may be utilized to assess depth of insertion. Full insertion is reported when all 22 active electrodes are determined to be intracochlear in location.[3]

Computed Tomography

In many cases, noncontrast high-resolution CT is the initial imaging study of choice when evaluating the temporal bone. Compared with MR, CT is much more accessible, particularly in the acute setting, less expensive and has a significantly shorter acquisition time, making images less susceptible to motion artifact. High-resolution CT is also the imaging modality of choice for evaluating bony detail as well as air-containing spaces and therefore best depicts the complex anatomy of the temporal bone. Bony fractures, osseous erosion, osseous masses, and calcifications are best demonstrated with CT. Similarly, abnormalities involving the dense bone of the otic capsule as in the case of otospongiosis are also best evaluated with CT. CT also best delineates replacement of the air-containing middle ear cavity and mastoid air cells with fluid, blood, inflammatory cells and tumor, and therefore is used in the evaluation of inflammatory and neoplastic processes involving the temporal bones. Because of its superior depiction of anatomic detail, CT is also essential for presurgical planning, particularly for localization of the facial nerve canal.

Most CT scans of the temporal bones are performed without intravenous contrast administration. Enhancement with iodinated contrast may be difficult to appreciate on CT due to high density of the adjacent bony structures. Intravenous contrast may be indicated in the setting of acute inflammatory processes such as mastoiditis in order to evaluate for extratemporal pathology such as a subperiosteal abscess. Intravenous contrast may also be administered in order to evaluate the extratemporal soft tissue extent of a neoplasm, though contrast may still not be necessary if a concurrent contrast-enhanced MR is also acquired. Contrast may also be ordered in the setting of tinnitus and evaluation of vascular variant anatomy and pathology, though a dedicated CT angiogram (CTA) or CT venogram (CTV) may better depict arterial and venous abnormalities, respectively. A contrast-enhanced CTA is timed for maximum opacification of the intracranial arterial system with minimal venous contamination using bolus-triggering technique, while a delay of approximately three minutes following injection of intravenous contrast results in a CTV with a fully opacified venous system. It must be noted that intravenous contrast is contraindicated in patients with prior severe allergic reaction to contrast media (in the absence of steroid premedication), those with history of multiple myeloma, and patients with impaired renal function (creatinine value >1.5–2 mg/dL, depending on the institution) who are not on dialysis.

Characterization of soft tissue and intracranial and cranial nerve pathology, however, is limited with CT compared to magnetic resonance imaging (MRI). Another disadvantage of CT is the radiation exposure to the patient, which is of particular concern in the pediatric population.

Traditionally, a CT study of the temporal bone was acquired in axial and coronal planes. Modern high-resolution multidetector spiral CT systems are capable of producing nearly isotropic voxels for multiplanar reconstruction in any desired plane. Multiple thin sections (0.6–1.5 mm) are acquired using a high-resolution (512 × 512) matrix. Axial sections are acquired in a plane 30° superior to the anthropologic base line intersecting the inferior orbital rim and external auditory canal (EAC). Coronal images are obtained directly at an angle of 120° from the anthropologic baseline or reconstructed at 90° to the axial plane. Sagittal, oblique (particularly at 45° between the sagittal and coronal planes to approximate Stenvers view), Pöschl short axis [parallel to the superior semicircular canal (SSCC)], curved and three-dimensional surface-rendered projections may be reconstructed in postprocessing for problem-solving purposes. In particular, the Pöschl and Stenvers views best depict the arcuate eminence overlying the SSCC and should therefore be included in examinations where SSCC dehiscence is clinically suspected.

Magnetic Resonance Imaging

MRI demonstrates excellent soft tissue contrast and resolution and has become the primary imaging modality for evaluation of nonosseous temporal bone structures, including fluid spaces (cerebrospinal fluid, membranous labyrinth), nerves, muscle, cartilage, and fat. Unlike on CT, enhancement of masses involving the temporal bone is easily appreciated following gadolinium administration. Perineural tumor spread and vascular and intracranial extension of a mass or infectious process are shown with a better advantage with MRI rather than CT. However, the architecture of the normal bone and air spaces is not well defined as compared with CT; cortical bone and air are seen as signal voids on MR and therefore localization of pathology, particularly in the middle ear cavity, can be difficult. While CT is superior to MR for the evaluation of cortical bony erosion, MRI is superior for evaluating bone marrow invasion, particularly in the skull base and petrous apex.

MRI is often obtained as a complementary imaging modality to CT. MR can help differentiate pathologic lesions seen on CT based on the lesion's enhancement or signal characteristics. For instance, in the evaluation of a tympanic cavity soft tissue mass seen on CT, MRI can help differentiate a glomus typanicum from a cholesteatoma based on its appearance on postcontrast and diffusion-weighted sequences. Similarly, in the evaluation of an expansile petrous apex mass seen on CT, MRI can help differentiate a cholesterol granuloma from an aneurysm or a Meckel's cave meningocele based on the signal characteristics of the lesion. MRI is also often used as a complementary imaging tool to CT to evaluate the intracranial or soft tissue extent of an inflammatory or neoplastic process involving the temporal bones.

MRI may be the initial imaging modality of choice in the setting of sensorineural hearing loss. Vestibular schwannomas in the internal auditory canal (IAC) or cerebellopontine angle (CPA) are best depicted on a contrast-enhanced MR. MR is used to evaluate the cranial nerves and therefore is indicated to evaluate for cochlear nerve hypoplasia and aplasia as well as Bell's palsy. MRI with a routine brain survey may also be performed to exclude potential central pathologies unrelated to the temporal bone.[1]

Intravenous contrast is typically administered in the MRI evaluation of the temporal bones, particularly in the setting of inflammatory and neoplastic processes. However, contrast is not required in the evaluation of recurrent cholesteatoma, for which diffusion-weighted imaging (DWI) is the diagnostic sequence. Intravenous contrast is also not indicated in the evaluation of cochlear nerve aplasia/hypoplasia and congenital inner ear anomalies. Intravenous contrast is contraindicated in patients with renal insufficiency on dialysis or with GFR <30 mL/min/1.73 m^2 due to the risk of nephrogenic systemic fibrosis, or rarely, in those patients with severe allergy to gadolinium.

Various MR sequences are used in the routine evaluation of temporal bone pathology. High-resolution fluid-weighted sequences, including high-resolution T2-weighted fast spin echo (FSE), three-dimensional constructive interference in steady state (3D CISS), or FIESTA (fast imaging employing steady state acquisition) sequences, are obtained without contrast administration and allow evaluation of small fluid-containing structures including the membranous labyrinth and the delineation of the cisternal portions of cranial nerves. This sequence is therefore essential in the evaluation of cochlear nerve hypoplasia/aplasia, IAC/CPA pathology, and inner ear pathology.

Precontrast T1-weighted MRIs are necessary for the evaluation of fat-containing lesions such as lipomas and postsurgical fat-packing material, as well as hemorrhage, which appear intrinsically bright in signal. Fat saturation techniques are utilized to confirm the presence of fat-containing lipomas or fat-packing material. In addition, precontrast T1-weighted images best delineate bone marrow invasion with replacement of normal bright fatty marrow by abnormal soft tissue.

Postcontrast T1-weighted images are obtained following the intravenous administration of gadolinium. Gadolinium increases the signal of enhancing lesions due to neoplastic, inflammatory, and infectious conditions on T1-weighted images. Postcontrast images are typically obtained with fat-suppression in order to increase the conspicuity of bright enhancing lesions from fatty marrow in the surrounding temporal bone. Fat-suppression also helps differentiate abnormal enhancing soft tissue from fat-packing material in postsurgical examinations.

DWI is based on the Brownian motion of water molecules in tissue and assesses for restriction of such motion in certain disease processes by addition of a diffusion-sensitizing gradient. In the temporal bone, DWI is useful in the evaluation of cholesteatomas, particularly in the postoperative setting where cholesteatoma can be difficult to differentiate from granulation/inflammatory tissue on clinical examination and CT. Due to the densely packed keratin, cholesteatomas restrict the diffusion of water and demonstrate bright signal on DWI. Susceptibility artifacts are particularly troublesome in the temporal bone region due to the interface between brain tissue, air, and bone. To circumvent this issue, non-echoplanar-based diffusion-weighted sequences have been developed. Turbo spin echo (TSE) or FSE-based diffusion-weighted sequences are less affected by susceptibility and demonstrate higher spatial resolution capable of producing thinner slices (down to 2 mm).[4] These innovative sequences have proven instrumental in detection of recurrent cholesteatomas and are able to pick up lesions <5 mm in size.[5]

MR angiography (MRA) and MR venography (MRV) are useful in evaluation of arterial and venous anatomy, respectively, and are typically performed without contrast using phase contrast or time of flight (TOF) imaging techniques. MRV may also be performed following the administration of gadolinium. MRA is indicated in the evaluation of suspected vascular aneurysm, stenosis, occlusion, malformation, or dissection. MRV is frequently used to assess for dural venous sinus thrombosis or search for developmental venous anomalies. The noncontrast TOF technique is susceptible to signal loss due to flow-related artifacts seen in slow or turbulent flow and susceptibility artifacts at bone and air interfaces. Because the resolution of MRA/MRV is not as high as that of the analogous CT studies, CTA/CTV or direct angiography may be used to confirm or further evaluate a finding seen on MR.

NORMAL IMAGING ANATOMY

General Concepts

The petrous portion of the temporal bone may be anatomically divided into the outer ear, middle ear, inner ear, and petrous apex. The external ear (auricle) and the EAC form the outer ear. The lateral part of the EAC is fibrocartilaginous and is continuous with the auricle at the external auditory meatus while the medial part is osseous. The tympanic membrane, made up of the larger pars tensa and smaller pars flaccida portions, separates the outer ear from the middle ear. The middle ear cavity, also known as the tympanic cavity, contains the ossicles: the malleus, incus, and stapes. Posteriorly, the middle ear cavity communicates with the mastoid antrum and mastoid air cells via the additus ad antrum and anteriorly, with the nasopharynx via the Eustachian tube. The medial wall of the tympanic cavity serves as the division between the middle and inner ear, which consists of the bony labyrinth containing the cochlea, semicircular canals, and vestibule, and the membranous labyrinth composed of the semicircular ducts, cochlear duct, utricle, and saccule.[6]

CT: Axial Plane

Normal anatomical landmarks visualized on axial images through the temporal bone, proceeding from superior to inferior, include the SSCC oriented perpendicular to the long axis of the temporal bone in the most cephalad slice, with mastoid air cells visualized laterally (Fig. 7.2A). Proceeding inferiorly, the inner ear structures come into view including the vestibule and lateral semicircular canal (LSCC) oriented nearly parallel to the vestibular aqueduct (VA) (Fig. 7.2B). The VA approximates the posterior semicircular canal in size and should not exceed 1.5 mm in diameter. Further inferiorly, the epitympanum containing the head of malleus and body of the incus in an "ice cream cone" configuration is seen (Figs. 7.2C and D). Medially, the labyrinthine segment of the facial nerve canal emerging from the IAC courses anteriorly, forming a hairpin turn known as the anterior genu before heading posterolaterally as the tympanic segment.[7]

The slices further inferiorly demonstrate the "snail-like" cochlea located anterolateral to the IAC (Figs. 7.2D to G) within the dense otic capsule. At the more superior level of the cochlea, the tympanic segment of the facial nerve is seen coursing posterolaterally along the medial aspect of the middle ear cavity (Fig. 7.2D). The cuts below show the manubrium of the malleus and long process of the incus (Fig. 7.2F). The lenticular process of the incus connects to the stapes with its footplate at the oval window. The round window niche can be seen as an air-filled spaced posterior to the basal turn of the cochlea (Fig. 7.2F). Further caudad, the cochlear aqueduct is visualized medially; the vertically oriented mastoid segment of the facial nerve and mastoid air cells are seen posteriorly and laterally (Fig.7.2G).[8]

CT: Coronal Plane

Coronal images aid in understanding the complex three-dimensional relationships between the intricate temporal bone structures. The vertical orientation of the middle ear cavity lends to visualization of its components - the epitympanum, mesotympanum, and hypotympanum. Normal anatomical landmarks visualized on coronal images through the temporal bone, proceeding from anterior to posterior, begin with the helicotrema of the cochlea, located inferior to the "snake eye" appearance of the facial nerve canal formed by the labyrinthine (medial) and tympanic (lateral) segments (Fig. 7.3A). More posteriorly, the pointed scutum can be identified at the medial superior margin of the EAC and Prussak's space can be seen lateral to the neck of the malleus and inferomedial to the scutum (Fig. 7.3B). The epitympanum, or the attic, is located above the level of the scutum and contains the head of the malleus and body and short process of the incus.

Further posteriorly, the mesotympanum is seen containing the long and lenticular processes of the incus and stapes inserting upon the oval window (Fig. 7.3C). The hypotympanum is located inferior to the level of the EAC

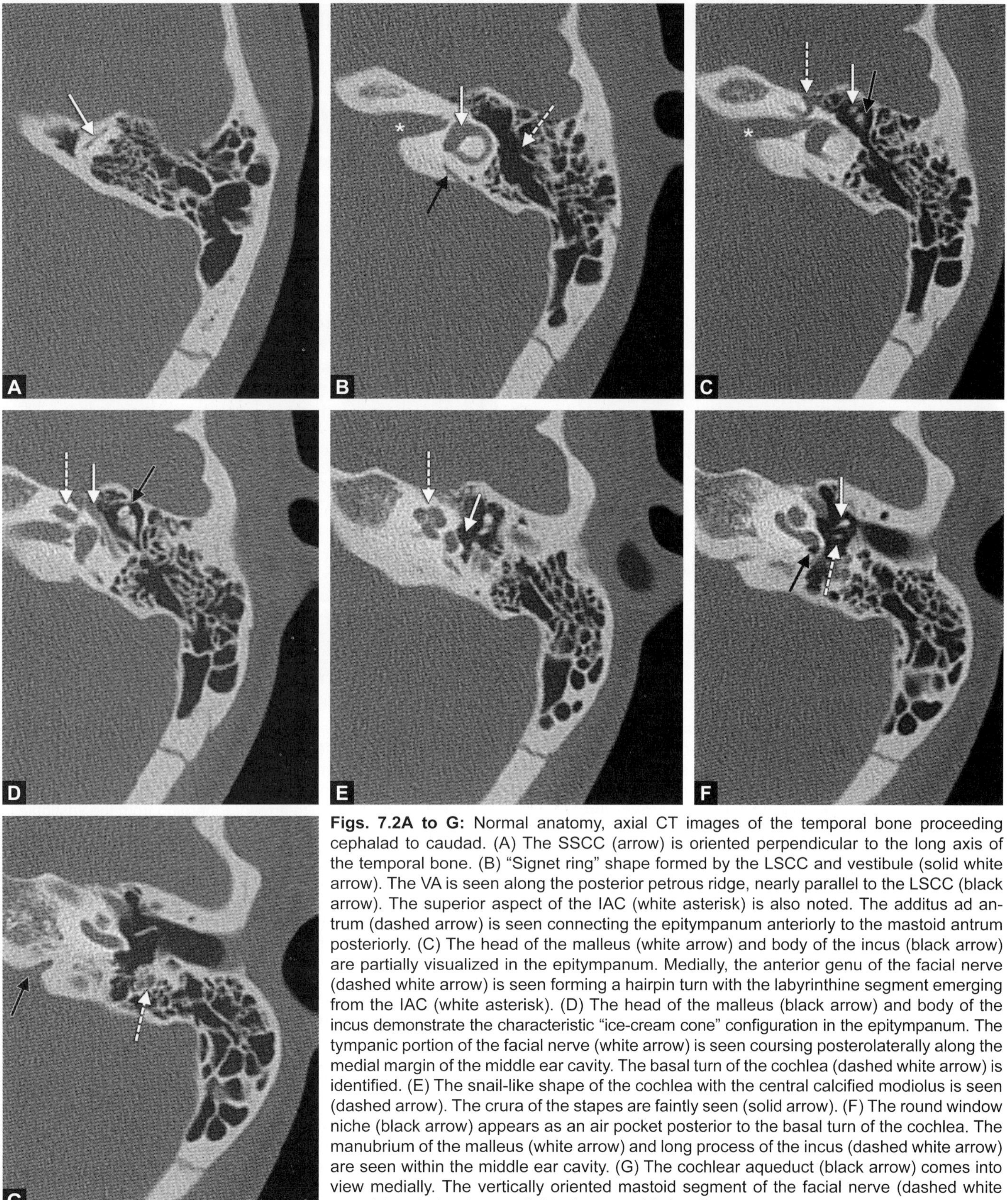

Figs. 7.2A to G: Normal anatomy, axial CT images of the temporal bone proceeding cephalad to caudad. (A) The SSCC (arrow) is oriented perpendicular to the long axis of the temporal bone. (B) "Signet ring" shape formed by the LSCC and vestibule (solid white arrow). The VA is seen along the posterior petrous ridge, nearly parallel to the LSCC (black arrow). The superior aspect of the IAC (white asterisk) is also noted. The additus ad antrum (dashed arrow) is seen connecting the epitympanum anteriorly to the mastoid antrum posteriorly. (C) The head of the malleus (white arrow) and body of the incus (black arrow) are partially visualized in the epitympanum. Medially, the anterior genu of the facial nerve (dashed white arrow) is seen forming a hairpin turn with the labyrinthine segment emerging from the IAC (white asterisk). (D) The head of the malleus (black arrow) and body of the incus demonstrate the characteristic "ice-cream cone" configuration in the epitympanum. The tympanic portion of the facial nerve (white arrow) is seen coursing posterolaterally along the medial margin of the middle ear cavity. The basal turn of the cochlea (dashed white arrow) is identified. (E) The snail-like shape of the cochlea with the central calcified modiolus is seen (dashed arrow). The crura of the stapes are faintly seen (solid arrow). (F) The round window niche (black arrow) appears as an air pocket posterior to the basal turn of the cochlea. The manubrium of the malleus (white arrow) and long process of the incus (dashed white arrow) are seen within the middle ear cavity. (G) The cochlear aqueduct (black arrow) comes into view medially. The vertically oriented mastoid segment of the facial nerve (dashed white arrow) is noted anteromedial to the mastoid air cells.

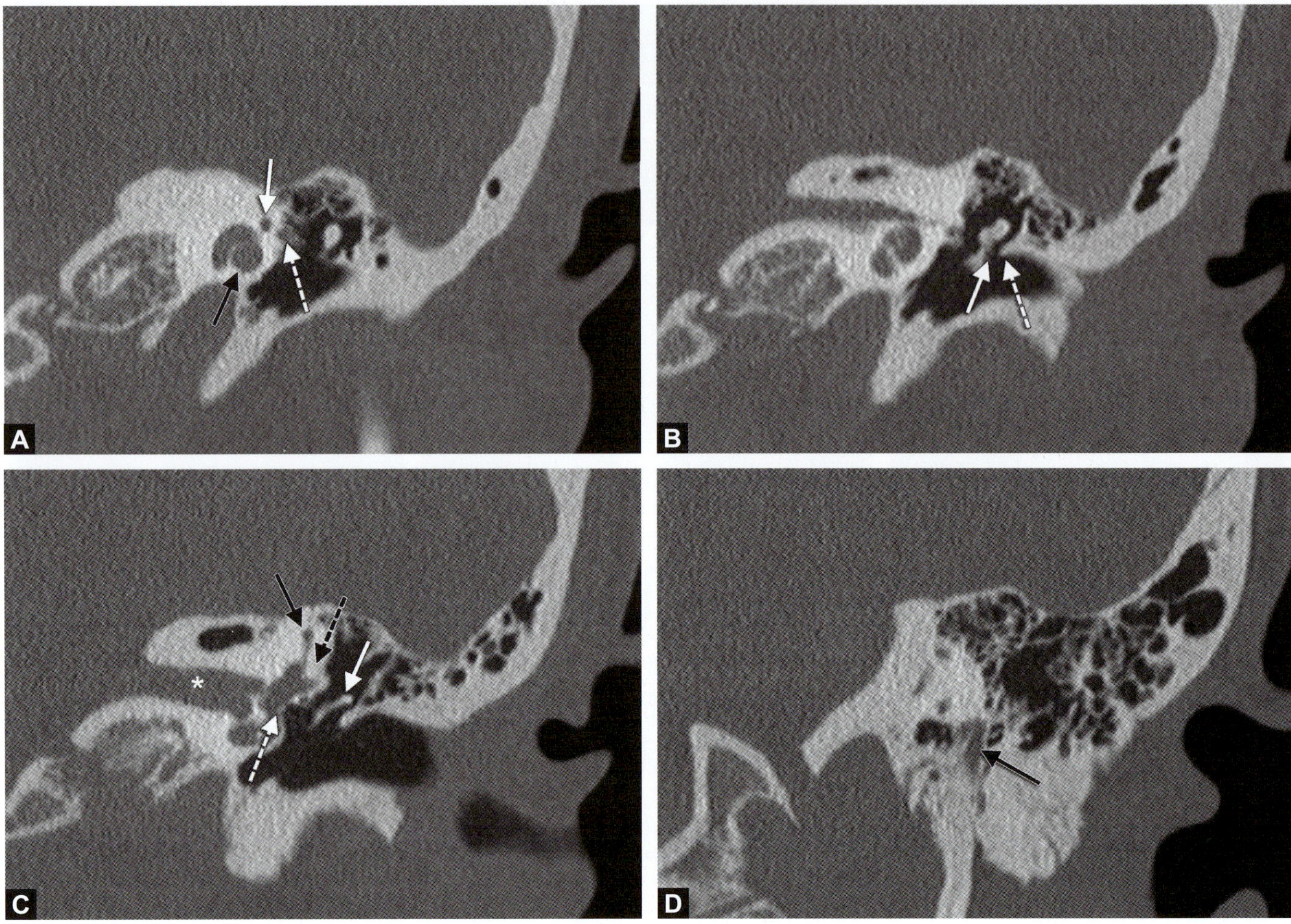

Figs. 7.3A to D: Normal anatomy, coronal CT images of the temporal bone proceeding anterior to posterior. (A) Helicotrema of the cochlear apex (black arrow) is located inferomedial to the "snake-eye" configuration of the facial nerve canal, with the labyrinthine segment (white arrow) medial to the tympanic segment (dashed white arrow). The head of the malleus is seen within the epitympanum. (B) Prussak's space (white arrow) is seen lateral to the neck of the malleus and inferomedial to the scutum (dashed white arrow). (C) The incus (white arrow) inferiorly joins the stapes, which attaches at the oval window (dashed white arrow). Emerging from the vestibule in a Y-configuration are the SSCC medially (black arrow) and the LSCC laterally (dashed black arrow). The posterior IAC (white asterisk) is seen medially. (D) The vertically oriented mastoid segment of the facial nerve (black arrow) is noted.

floor. The horizontally oriented IAC can be seen medially. The canals extending superiorly from the vestibule in a Y-configuration are the SSCC and LSCC. At the level of the oval window, the tympanic segment of the facial nerve canal can be seen coursing inferior to the LSCC. Further posteriorly, the vertical course of the mastoid segment of the facial nerve canal (Fig. 7.3D) can be seen, extending towards the stylomastoid foramen.

MRI

The described CT anatomy of the temporal bone is directly applicable to that seen on MR. However, it must be remembered that normal osseous structures and air-containing spaces appear as areas of signal void. Normal fluid-containing structures such as the membranous labyrinth and IAC appear bright on fluid-weighted images. The facial and vestibulocochlear nerves within the IAC appear as hypointense linear structures (Fig. 7.4).

PATHOLOGY OF THE OUTER EAR

Congenital Anomalies

EAC Stenosis and Atresia

Stenosis and atresia of the EAC represent a continuum of congenital pathology associated with auricular deformity.

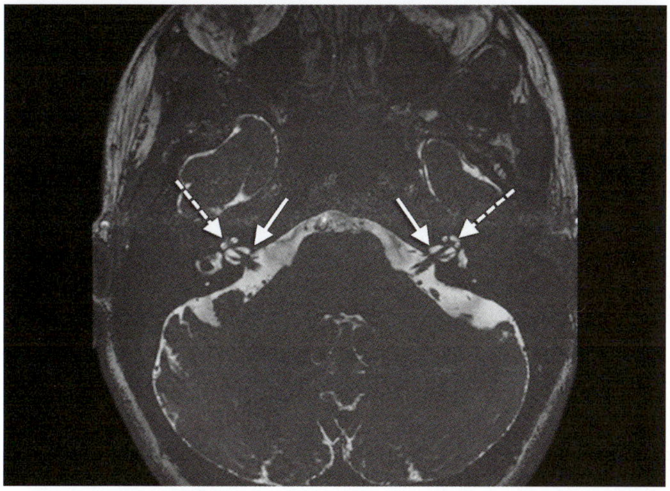

Fig. 7.4: CISS image. Normal axial CISS MRI demonstrates the normal hypointense linear branches of the vestibulocochlear nerves within the internal auditory canals (solid arrows) bilaterally. The fluid-filled cochleae (dashed arrows) and vestibules are also seen bilaterally.

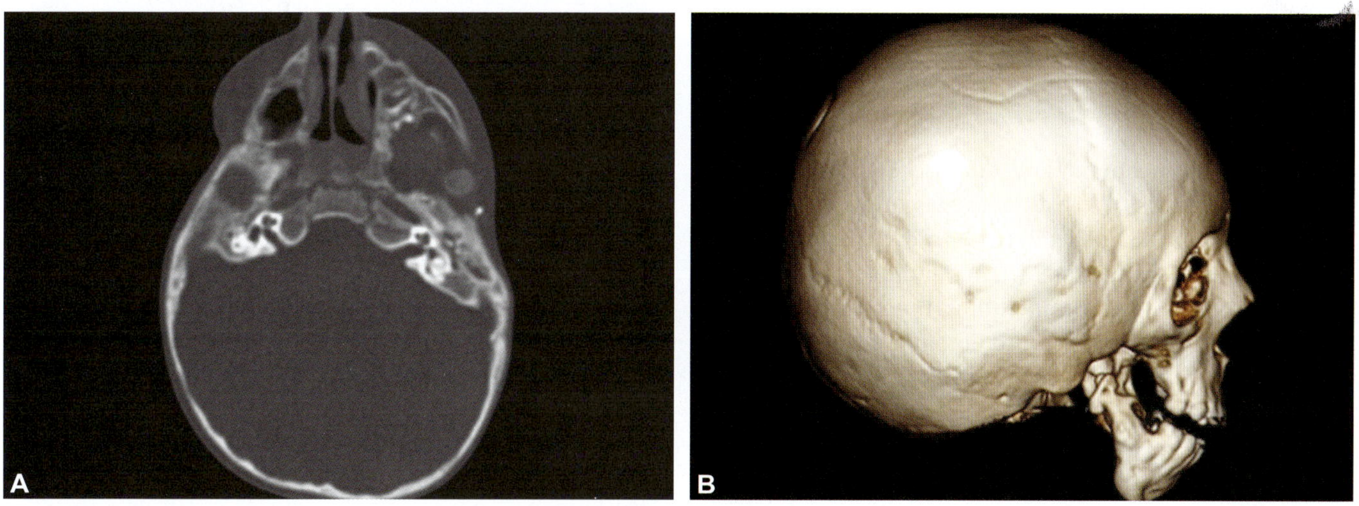

Figs. 7.5A and B: Bilateral EAC atresia, Goldenhar syndrome. (A) Axial CT image in a patient with Goldenhar syndrome demonstrates bilateral EAC atresia associated with marked middle ear cavity hypoplasia. (B) Craniofacial 3D reconstruction demonstrates absence of the EAC meatus, as well as dysplasia of the mandible and maxilla.

Some cases are syndromic as part of Crouzon, Goldenhar or Pierre Robin syndromes and are more likely to be bilateral. Given the altered complex anatomy in patients with EAC atresia, CT is the imaging modality of choice, particularly for presurgical planning and localization of the facial nerve canal which is often aberrant in its course. Key findings on CT include osseous or membranous stenosis or atresia of the EAC with hypoplasia of the mastoid air cells and a diminutive middle ear cavity (Figs. 7.5A and B). Ossicular malformations, particularly affecting the malleus and incus, with fusion to the lateral middle ear cavity wall are common. The inner ear and IAC are typically normal. As mentioned above, an aberrant anterior course of the mastoid segment of the facial nerve is frequently noted.[9]

Infection

Necrotizing External Otitis

Necrotizing external otitis (NEO) is a potentially life-threatening condition usually occurring in elderly diabetics and is most commonly secondary to *Pseudomonas aeruginosa* infection. Contrast-enhanced CT is the initial imaging modality of choice, given its accessibility and rapid acquisition in these acutely ill patients, as well as its superior delineation of bony erosion. On CT, NEO appears as swelling of the EAC soft tissues with or without osseous erosion on bone windows (Fig. 7.6). Both contrast-enhanced CT and MRI can demonstrate associated extratemporal soft tissue inflammatory changes, with heterogeneous

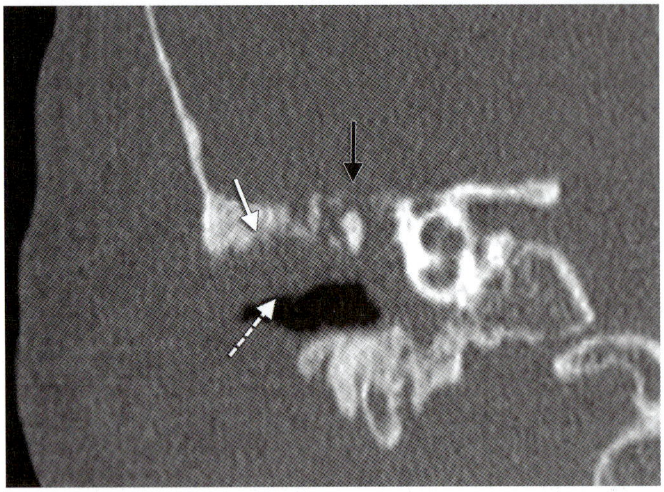

Fig. 7.6: Necrotizing external otitis. Noncontrast coronal CT image of the right temporal bone demonstrates marked soft tissue swelling overlying the EAC with soft tissue within the EAC (dashed arrow) and middle ear cavity. There is erosion of the EAC (solid white arrow) and tegmen tympani (black arrow).

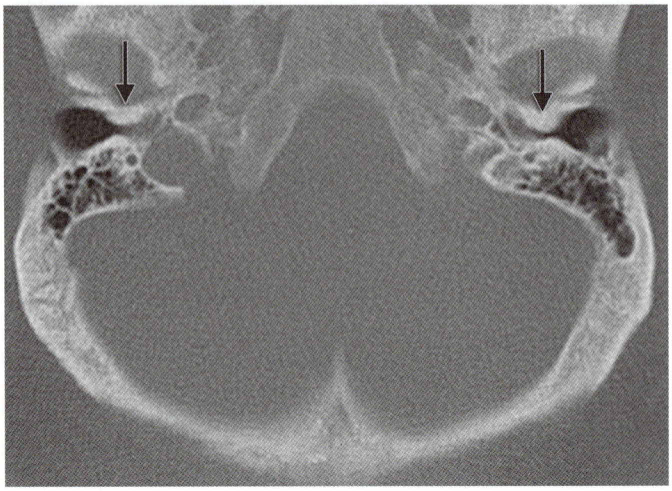

Fig. 7.7: Exostoses. Noncontrast axial CT image demonstrates broad-based osseous excrescences (black arrows) narrowing the medial EACs bilaterally.

ill-defined enhancement and edema of the soft tissues compatible with cellulitis; abscess formation manifests as rim-enhancing fluid collections within the adjacent soft tissues. Contrast-enhanced MRI better depicts intracranial extension of the infection including meningitis· subdural empyema, epidural abscess and parenchymal abscess.[10]

Inflammatory Lesions

Acquired Cholesteatoma

Cholesteatoma essentially reflects skin in an abnormal location, pathologically classified as exfoliated keratin debris within a sac of stratified squamous epithelium. On noncontrast CT, acquired cholesteatoma of the outer ear appears as a focal soft tissue mass eroding the EAC wall and classically contains intramural osseous fragments. Cholesteatomas demonstrate restricted diffusion manifested as bright signal on DWI. Contrast-enhanced MRI can also help differentiate cholesteatoma from neoplasm, demonstrating lack of enhancement of the cholesteatoma with or without peripherally enhancing granulation tissue.[9]

Keratosis Obturans

A rare, frequently bilateral condition in which desquamated keratin abnormally accumulates within the EAC, keratosis obturans manifests on CT as homogeneous soft tissue density filling the EAC without evidence of aggressive osseous changes or middle ear involvement. CT is the initial imaging modality of choice. If performed, an MRI shows the lesion to be of homogeneously low signal intensity on T1-weighted images and isointensity on T2-weighted images, with no enhancement on postcontrast T1-weighted images.[9] Minimal peripheral enhancement may be present due surrounding granulation/inflammatory tissue.

Osseous Lesions

Exostoses

Also known as surfer's ear, exostoses occur as a result of frequent cold water exposure and appear as broad-based overgrowth of the osseous EAC with lack of aggressive features. Well-defined bony protuberances circumferentially line and narrow the osseous EAC, typically involving the medial EAC bilaterally (Fig. 7.7). Exostoses are best demonstrated on noncontrast CT without the need for MRI. If performed, MRI shows the lesion follows signal intensity of bone without enhancement.[10] There may be abnormal soft tissue medial to the exostoses reflecting impacted cerumen or cholesteatoma.

Osteoma

The rare osteoma of the EAC presents as a focal, well-circumscribed pedunculated osseous overgrowth without associated soft tissue abnormality, best depicted on CT. Unlike exostoses, osteomas are typically unilateral and solitary (Fig. 7.8).

Neoplasm

Malignant tumors of the EAC are rare and typically occur in the elderly population, with squamous cell and basal cell carcinomas the most common types. Secondary involvement of the EAC by an extra-auricular squamous cell carcinoma (SCC) is more common than a primary lesion. Both CT and MR are typically obtained to evaluate EAC malignancies, with CT better demonstrating bony erosion and extension into the middle ear and mastoid air cells. On CT, SCC appears as an aggressive soft tissue mass with variable degrees of osseous destruction. On MRI, the mass is hypo- to isointense on T1-weighted images and hyperintense on T2-weighted images, with heterogeneous or homogeneous enhancement on postcontrast images (Figs. 7.9A and B). Assessment of SCC on MRI should include evaluation for intracranial extension, perineural tumor spread along the facial nerve, and invasion of the parotid gland.[10] Both CT and MR well demonstrate enlarged or necrotic metastatic lymph nodes, with drainage most commonly to the intraparotid lymph nodes.

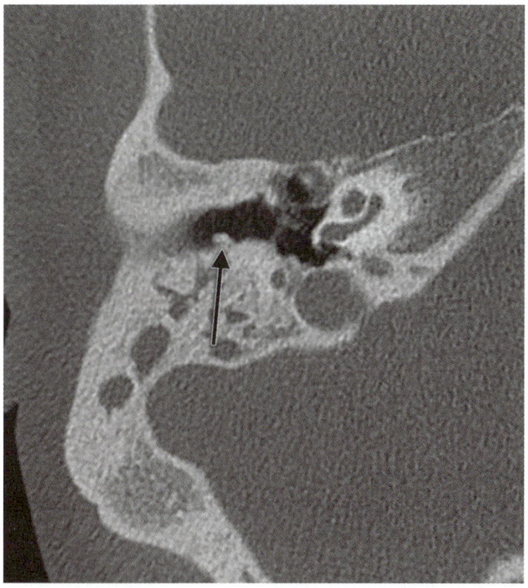

Fig. 7.8: EAC osteoma. Noncontrast axial CT image of the right temporal bone shows a solitary osseous protuberance along the posterior wall of the right EAC.

PATHOLOGY OF THE MIDDLE EAR

Vascular Anomalies

Aberrant Internal Carotid Artery

Maldevelopment of the cervical internal carotid artery (ICA) resulting in a congenitally aberrant ICA is important to identify in the presurgical CT evaluation of pulsatile tinnitus. Misdiagnosis of this apparent hypotympanic lesion and subsequent biopsy or middle ear surgery may lead to disastrous consequences. With the more common

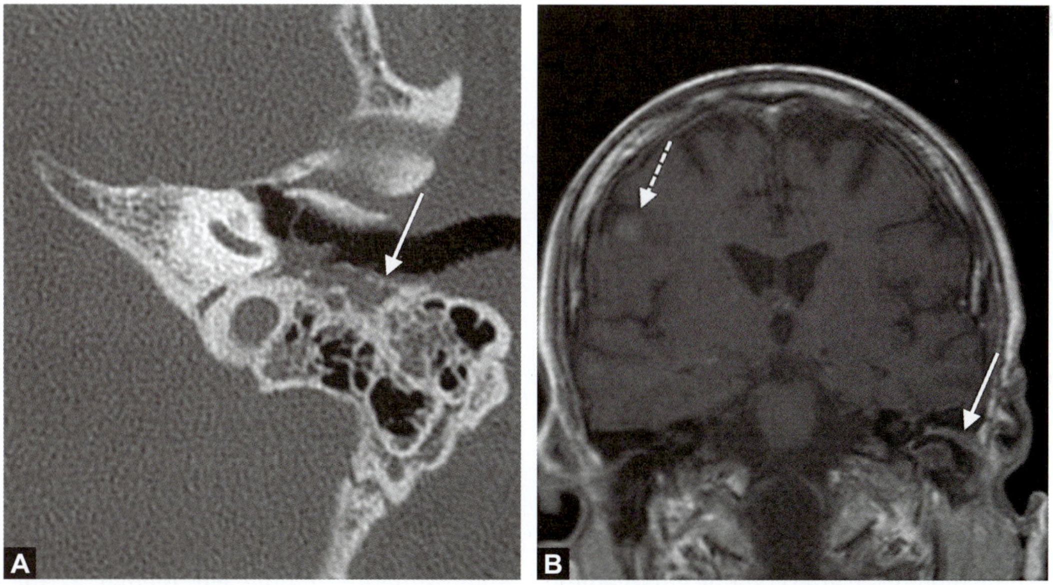

Figs. 7.9A and B: Squamous cell carcinoma of the EAC. (A) Axial noncontrast CT image of the left temporal bone demonstrates a markedly abnormal left external auditory canal with irregular thickened soft tissue and extensive bony erosion circumferentially (arrow). (B) Coronal contrast-enhanced T1-weighted MRI shows asymmetric enhancing soft tissue lining the left EAC (solid arrow). Also note an enhancing lesion within the brain parenchyma (dashed arrow) reflecting a metastatic focus.

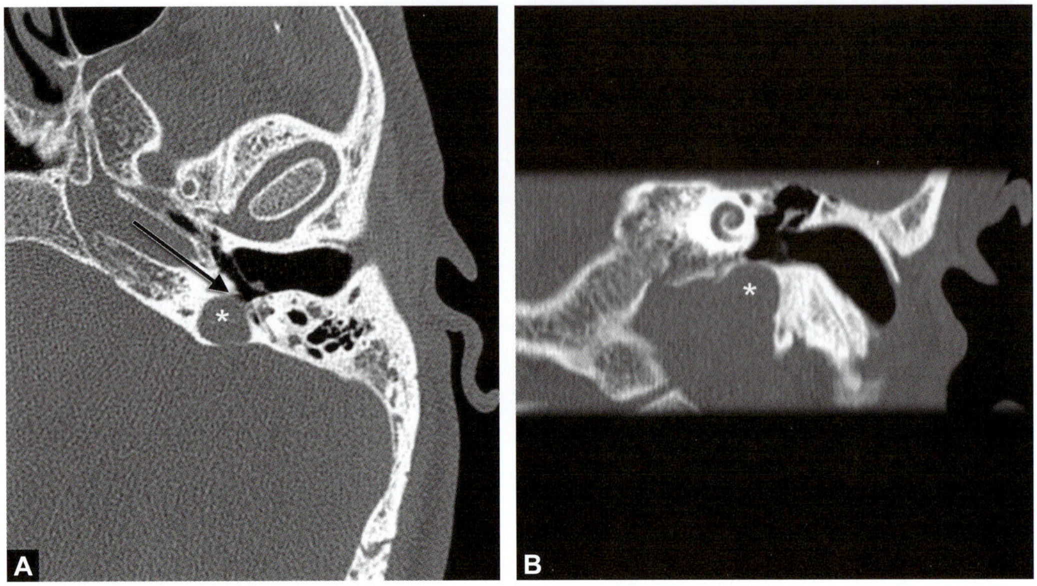

Figs. 7.10A and B: Dehiscent jugular bulb. Axial (A) and coronal (B) noncontrast CT images of the left temporal bone show protrusion of the jugular bulb (asterisk) into the middle ear cavity with dehiscence of the overlying bone (arrow).

variant, an aberrant intratympanic ICA is seen as a tubular enhancing lesion with a reduced diameter compared to a normal ICA, entering through an enlarged inferior tympanic canaliculus and traversing the inferior middle ear cavity from posterior to anterior along the cochlear promontory; anteriorly, the aberrant ICA joins the horizontal carotid canal through a dehiscent carotid plate.[11] An aberrant ICA can typically be demonstrated on a routine contrast-enhanced CT, though may be better depicted with a dedicated CTA. MRA is frequently only helpful in the frontal projection where the sharp turn of the aberrant ICA appears as a "7" or "reverse 7," depending on the affected side.[9]

Persistent Stapedial Artery

Frequently associated with aberrant ICA, persistence of the stapedial artery is found in 0.48% of the population and represents a normally transient anastomosis between the ICA and branches of the external carotid artery. The vessel arises from the vertical part of the petrous ICA, traverses the obturator foramen of the stapes and terminates within the extradural middle cranial fossa as the middle meningeal artery. CT clues to the diagnosis include an absent foramen spinosum on the affected side that usually contains the middle meningeal artery, subtle enlargement of the anterior tympanic segment of the facial nerve canal, and a curvilinear structure crossing the medial wall of the middle ear cavity over the cochlear promontory.[9]

High-Riding and Dehiscent Jugular Bulb

The jugular bulb is the dilated superior part of the jugular vein at the junction where it joins the sigmoid sinus. Extension into the middle ear above the level of IAC floor defines it as high-riding. A dehiscent jugular bulb lacks a complete osseous covering and protrudes into the middle ear (Figs. 7.10A and B). CT with contrast administration is the diagnostic imaging modality of choice. The abnormality may also be defined using MR venogram, though MR will not show any associated bony dehiscence. Another variant is a jugular diverticulum, which is a protrusion of the jugular bulb superior and medial to the jugular fossa.[12]

Congenital Lesions

Congenital Cholesteatoma

Representing a minority (5%) of temporal bone cholesteatomas, congenital cholesteatoma presents in children or young adults with unilateral conductive hearing loss and may originate in any part of the temporal bone, most commonly the middle ear. Unlike acquired cholesteatomas, the tympanic membrane is intact. On noncontrast CT, congenital cholesteatoma classically appears as a well-circumscribed soft tissue mass located in the anterosuperior middle ear medial to the ossicles and adjacent to the Eustachian tube. In advanced disease, erosive changes of the wall, ossicular dehiscence involving the long process of the incus and stapes, and labyrinthine

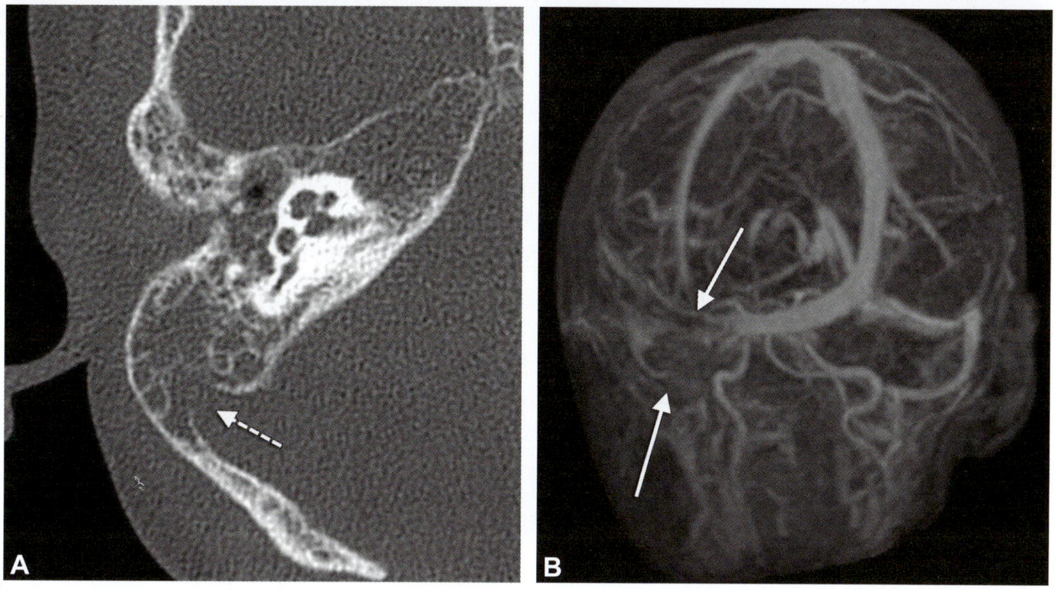

Figs. 7.11A and B: Coalescent otomastoiditis with dural venous thrombosis. Noncontrast CT of the temporal bone (A) shows opacification and destruction of the mastoid air cells with erosion of the cortical plate overlying the right sigmoid sinus (dashed white arrow). Contrast-enhanced MRV (B) demonstrates thrombosis of the sigmoid sinus and jugular vein (solid arrows).

extension may be present. MR can help differentiate congenital cholesteatoma from a glomus tympanicum, which is often found in a similar location. Congenital cholesteatoma demonstrates lack of central enhancement and diffusion restriction, whereas glomus tympanicum demonstrates avid enhancement and lack of diffusion abnormality.

Infection

Otitis Media

Acutely, otitis media with effusion may present on imaging as fluid and debris within the normally pneumatized middle ear, mastoid, and petrous bone. While fluid–fluid levels may be observed, there is no erosion of the mastoid air cells or ossicles. If fluid behind the tympanic membrane does not resolve in 3 months, otitis media is clinically considered to be chronic. Chronic otitis media may result in multiple complications, including postinflammatory ossicular erosion and tympanosclerosis.[10] A noncontrast CT is sufficient to evaluate patients with otitis media, though contrast may be administered if there is clinical concern for extratemporal extension of the infectious process.

Coalescent Otomastoiditis

Coalescent otomastoiditis is a feared complication of acute otitis media in which osseous erosive changes are present. Contrast-enhanced CT is the initial imaging modality of choice given its accessibility and rapid acquisition in these acutely ill patients, as well as its superior delineation of bony erosion. The most specific CT finding is erosion of the sigmoid plate (Figs. 7.11A and B), while the most common finding is destruction of the mastoid septae. Both postcontrast CT and MRI can demonstrate associated soft tissue inflammatory changes, including cellulitis which appears as diffuse enhancement and edema of the soft tissues, as well as abscess formation, which appears as a rim-enhancing fluid collection. A Bezold abscess occurs when osseous erosion and abscess formation occurs medial to the sternocleidomastoid muscle at the insertion of the posterior belly of the digastric muscle and extends into the infratemporal fossa.[13] Contrast-enhanced MRI better depicts intracranial extension of the infection, including meningitis, subdural empyema, epidural abscess, and parenchymal abscess.[9] Dural sinus thrombosis can be diagnosed on both contrast-enhanced CT and MR, seen as a filling defect within the enhancing venous sinus.

Inflammatory Lesions

Acquired Cholesteatoma

Acquired cholesteatoma is the most common type of cholesteatoma, making up 98% of these lesions. Pars flaccida cholesteatomas comprise 80% of the acquired cholesteatomas and arise within Prussak's space; Prussak's space is limited laterally by the pars flaccida portion of the tympanic membrane, inferiorly and medially by the lateral process and neck of the malleus, and superiorly and anteriorly by the lateral malleolar ligament.

In contrast to the pars flaccida cholesteatoma, the less common pars tensa cholesteatoma arises in the posterior and inferior middle ear cavity medial to the ossicles, displacing them laterally, and commonly results in ossicular erosion. The posterior recesses including the sinus tympani and facial recess may be involved.[10]

High-resolution noncontrast temporal bone CT is the examination of choice, with multiplanar contrast-enhanced MR reserved for assessment of complications and recurrence. The classic CT finding of a pars flaccida cholesteatoma is that of a soft tissue mass in Prussak's space with medial deviation of the ossicles and blunting of the scutum or erosion of the lateral attic wall (Fig. 7.12). Extension into the mastoid antrum and ossicular erosion may be seen. Serious complications include intracranial extension through an eroded tegmen tympani and labyrinthine fistula, most commonly involving the LSCC.[9]

On MRI, cholesteatomas appear isointense to cerebrospinal fluid on T1- and T2-weighted images, with enhancement only seen in the granulation tissue in the periphery of the nonenhancing soft tissue mass. As stated previously, cholesteatomas restrict the diffusion of water and therefore demonstrate bright signal on DWI; DWI is therefore useful for diagnostic purposes and in particular to detect recurrence in postoperative cases.[5]

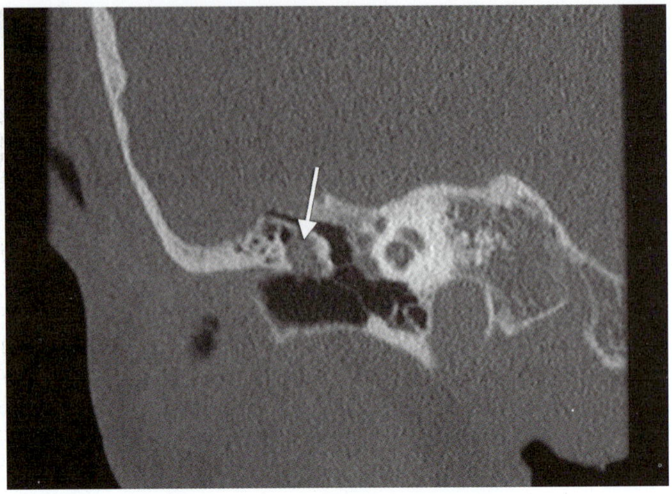

Fig. 7.12: Pars flaccida cholesteatoma. Coronal CT image of the right temporal bone shows a soft tissue mass (arrow) in Prussak's space resulting in scutal blunting as well as erosion and medial deviation of the ossicles.

Osseous Lesions

Ossicular Fixation-Fusion

Fibrous or osseous fixation of the ossicular chain is most commonly postinflammatory in nature. CT, the examination of choice, demonstrates an intact ossicular chain with nondependent soft tissue adjacent to the ossicles, oval window and/or Prussak's space in fibrous fusion. In fibro-osseous fusion or tympanosclerosis, calcification is seen in the middle ear cavity or along the suspensory ossicular tendons or ligaments, tympanic membrane or oval window. The ossicles typically become abnormally laterally located within the middle ear cavity.[10]

Neoplasm

Glomus Tympanicum

A glomus tympanicum tumor is a paraganglioma originating from the cochlear promontory. Both CT and MR are typically used as complementary imaging tools to evaluate this tumor. On CT, glomus tympanicum appears as a focal soft tissue mass without osseous erosion. Depending on the size, these lesions may be present in the hypotympanum or fill the entire middle ear cavity. MRI shows enhancement of the mass following gadolinium administration (Figs. 7.13A and B). The typical "salt-and-pepper" appearance characteristic of most paragangliomas is often not seen with glomus tympanicum given its small size, though this appearance can occasionally be seen with larger lesions; the salt and pepper appearance with mixed hyperintense and hypointense foci on precontrast T1-weighted images represent hemorrhagic foci and flow voids, respectively. Angiography is not necessary for diagnosis but would demonstrate a prominent ascending pharyngeal artery and its inferior tympanic branch feeding the mass via the inferior tympanic canaliculus.[9]

PATHOLOGIES OF THE INNER EAR

Congenital Anomalies

Vestibulocochlear Dysplasia

There is a broad spectrum of vestibulocochlear dysplasia, from complete aplasia of the entire labyrinth to underpartitioning of the cochlea. Either CT or MR can be used to evaluate such dysplasias. MRI is often preferred to avoid radiation exposure, as these dysplasias often manifest in the pediatric population; in addition, MRI can simultaneously assess whether there is hypoplasia/aplasia

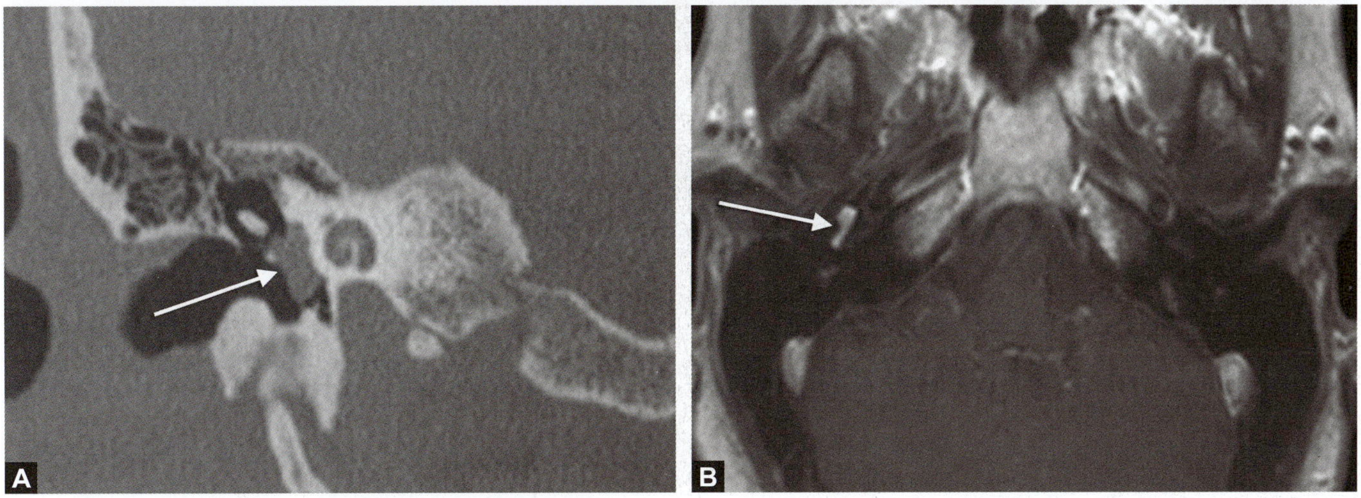

Figs. 7.13A and B: Glomus tympanicum. (A) Coronal CT image of the right temporal bone demonstrates a soft tissue mass within the middle ear cavity along the cochlear promontory. (B) Postcontrast T1-weighted MRI demonstrates avid enhancement of the mass.

of the cochlear nerve, an important factor for cochlear implantation. CT is more sensitive for subtle findings such as underpartitioning of the cochlea, and is more useful for presurgical planning, in particular to evaluate for a possible aberrant course of the facial nerve canal.

Also known as the Michel anomaly or deformity, complete aplasia of the labyrinth is diagnosed when absence of the entire inner ear including the cochlea, vestibule, and semicircular canals is seen. In the severe form of disease, ossicular abnormalities, hypoplasia or lack of the IAC and vestibulocochlear nerve, and absence of the petrous apex may be noted. The facial nerve is typically well developed but takes an abnormal course; the facial nerve canal may be prominent. High-resolution fluid-weighted MR demonstrates absence of normal fluid signal in the expected location of the membranous labyrinth.[14] A significant differential consideration is labyrinthitis ossificans, diagnosed on CT when dense bone is seen obliterating the membranous labyrinth. The lateral wall of the otic capsule tends to be convex in labyrinthitis ossificans and flat in labyrinthine aplasia.

Along the same spectrum but less severe than Michel anomaly, the absent cochlea is associated with variably affected vestibule, semicircular canals and/or IAC, which may be normal, hypoplastic, or cystic. Thin-section CT shows the labyrinthine, anterior genu, and anterior tympanic portions of the facial nerve occupy the expected location of the cochlea. On high-resolution fluid-weighted MR, dark signal of dense bone replaces the normally fluid-filled cochlea. With cochlear underpartitioning dysplasia, the cochlea has less than the expected 2½ to 2¾ turns.[15] Mondini deformity refers to an underpartitioning of the cochlea with 1½ turns as well as enlargement of the VAs.

Large VA Syndrome

The VA is normally narrow, measuring <1.5–2 mm in diameter or less than the diameter of the posterior semicircular canal. When abnormally enlarged, it is funnel-shaped and most dilated at its posterior aspect (Fig. 7.14). An enlarged VA is the most common imaging finding in pediatric patients with sensorineural hearing loss. While CT is the most sensitive imaging modality that can demonstrate this significant cause of sensorineural hearing loss, MRI may also be utilized.[15]

Infectious/Inflammatory Lesions

Labyrinthitis

Many etiologies of labyrinthitis exist, including post-traumatic and postoperative causes. Infectious labyrinthitis may be bacterial or viral. The bacterial form is an unusual complication of acute middle ear infection via a breach of the round window, or may occur due to a labyrinthine fistula resulting from a cholesteatoma or hematogenous spread via the cochlear vessels. Perinatal exposure to rubella or cytomegalovirus has been shown to affect the labyrinth. Herpes zoster, measles and mumps are the causative pathogens of labyrinthitis in the adult population. The imaging modality of choice is gadolinium-enhanced MRI which shows abnormal contrast enhancement of the labyrinth.

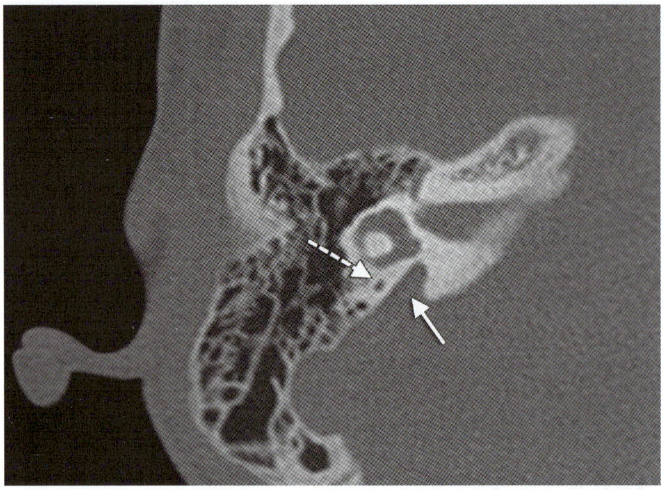

Fig. 7.14: Large vestibular aqueduct syndrome. Noncontrast axial CT image of the right temporal bone shows enlargement of the vestibular aqueduct (solid arrow), greater than the diameter of the posterior semicircular canal (dashed arrow), here seen in cross section. Note the normal size of the vestibular aqueduct in Figure 17.2B.

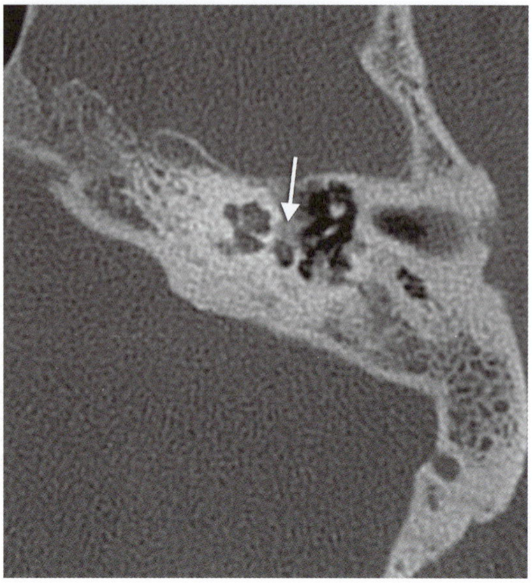

Fig. 7.15: Fenestral otospongiosis. Noncontrast axial CT image of the temporal bone demonstrates lucency (arrow) of the otic capsule in the region of the fissula ante fenestrum.

Herpes zoster oticus, or Ramsay Hunt syndrome, is a vesicular eruption on the auricle and EAC secondary to reactivation of the virus within the geniculate ganglion of the facial nerve with resultant pain and possible hearing loss, facial paralysis and vertigo. MRI findings include abnormal enhancement of the facial and vestibulocochlear nerves, membranous labyrinth, and pontine facial nerve nucleus.

Labyrinthitis Ossificans

Ossification of the membranous labyrinth occurs as a reparative response to an infectious, inflammatory, or surgical event, most commonly seen after meningitis. CT shows osseous deposition within the membranous labyrinth with obliteration seen in severe disease. The diagnosis may be more challenging in its early stages when fibro-osseous material gives the labyrinth a subtle hazy appearance on CT. High-resolution fluid-weighted MR imaging show these findings more easily as abnormal low-intensity foci within the normally bright labyrinth, making high-resolution fluid-sensitive MR the examination of choice for diagnosis of early labyrinthitis ossificans.

SSCC Dehiscence

Patients with SSCC dehiscence present with conductive hearing loss and Tulio's phenomenon, occurring when loud sounds result in vestibular symptoms such as vertigo, nausea, or nystagmus. The diagnosis is best made thin-section CT images through the temporal bone showing dehiscence of the arcuate eminence, or bony covering, of the SSCC. This is best demonstrated on Pöschl and Stenvers reconstructions oriented parallel and perpendicular, respectively, to the SSCC. High-resolution fluid-weighted MRIs in the coronal, Pöschl, or Stenvers plane may be used to suggest thinning or absence of bone in this location, although it is significantly more challenging.[9]

Otospongiosis

Otospongiosis, also known as otosclerosis, is a lytic disorder of the endochondral layer of the osseous labyrinth causing progressive conductive hearing loss and tinnitus. It is often bilateral (in 85% of cases). Otospongiosis can be categorized as fenestral or retrofenestral (cochlear), with fenestral otospongiosis involving the fissula ante fenestrum located just anterior to the oval window. Retrofenestral otospongiosis involves more extensive areas of the otic capsule, including around the cochlea, and most commonly occurs in the presence of the fenestral otosclerosis. Otospongiosis is best evaluated on CT, which reveals lucency replacing the normal dense bone of the otic capsule. In fenestral otospongiosis, there are subtle lytic foci at the fissula ante fenestrum (Fig. 7.15), whereas more extensive lucencies are seen involving the otic capsule in retrofenestral otospongiosis. Intravenous contrast is not required to diagnose otospongiosis. If performed,

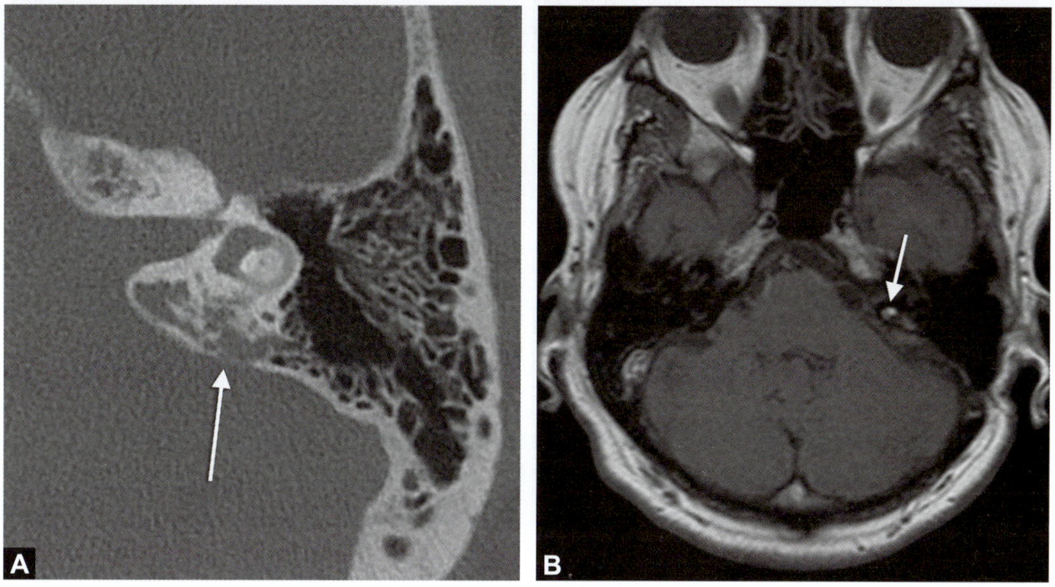

Figs. 7.16A and B: Endolymphatic sac tumor. (A) Noncontrast axial CT image of the left temporal bone shows an extensive permeative lytic lesion of the posterior aspect of the petrous pyramid and otic capsule (arrow) centered in the region of the vestibular aqueduct. (B) Noncontrast T1-weighted MRI shows intrinsic T1 hyperintense signal (arrow) within the lesion indicative of hemorrhage.

gadolinium-enhanced MRI may show multiple enhancing foci in the otic capsule,[9] though localization is often difficult.

Neoplasm

Endolymphatic Sac Tumor

The papillary cystadenomatous tumor of the endolymphatic sac occurs in a characteristic retrolabyrinthine location of the posterior petrous temporal bone, centered at the endolymphatic sac and VA. Both CT and contrast-enhanced MR play complementary roles in the evaluation of these tumors. On CT, endolymphatic sac tumors appear as an osteolytic soft tissue mass containing central osseous spiculations. A thin rim of calcification may be observed at the posterior aspect of the lesion. MRI classically shows intratumoral T1-hyperintense signal foci indicative of hemorrhage and T1-hypointense flow voids (Figs. 7.16A and B). Administration of gadolinium results in heterogeneous enhancement. CPA cistern, middle ear, and jugular foramen extension may be seen when the tumor is large. An association with Van Hippel-Lindau syndrome has been described.[16]

Schwannoma

Schwannoma of the inner ear occurs directly within the membranous labyrinth. It is typically not discernible on CT, and is best defined on MRI as a filling defect within the normally bright fluid-filled labyrinth on high-resolution fluid-weighted imaging and demonstrating enhancement on postcontrast images (Figs. 7.17A and B). Schwannomas in the IAC and CPA are also best depicted on contrast-enhanced MRI.

PATHOLOGY OF THE PETROUS APEX

Infection

Apical Petrositis

Apical petrositis is an uncommon complication of infectious otomastoiditis that occurs when the infection spreads medially into the petrous apex. Initially CT images show opacification of the petrous apex cells with purulent material in conjunction with findings of otomastoiditis but eventually, the cortical and cancellous osseous trabeculae undergo destruction and extension into adjacent bone marrow occurs, resulting in osteomyelitis. Advanced infection can result in erosion of the carotid canal and vasospasm or arteritis of the ICA, venous extension resulting in dural sinus thrombosis and meningitis, encephalitis, cranial neuritis, and intracranial abscess. Gadolinium-enhanced MRI is more sensitive in assessing for early apical petrositis since 30–50% bony demineralization is necessary before diagnosis may be confidently made on CT. MR is also more suited for visualization of intracranial complications and evaluation of the soft tissues.[17]

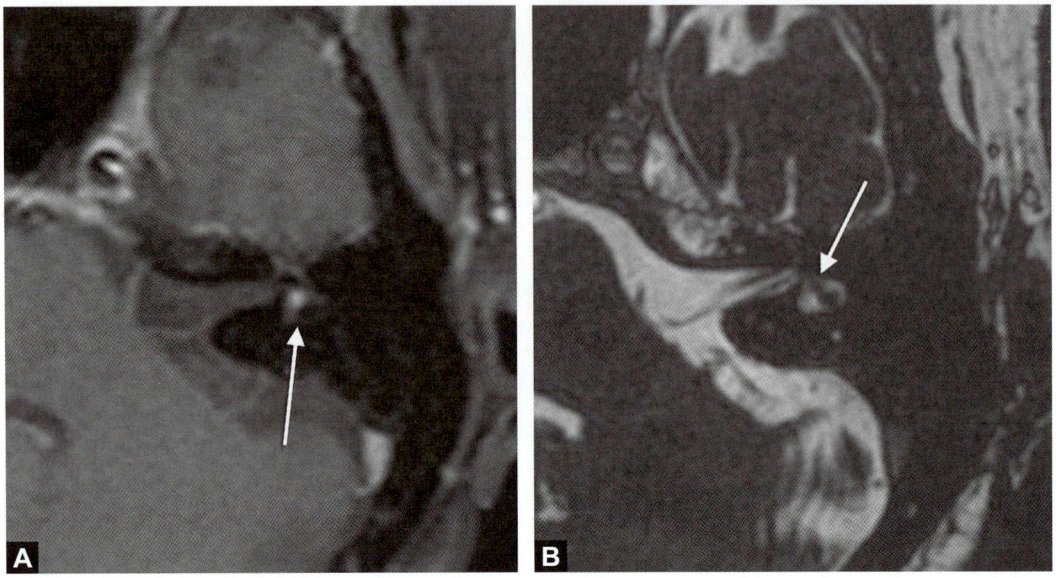

Figs. 7.17A and B: Intra-labyrinthine schwannoma. (A) Axial contrast-enhanced T1-weighted MRI of the left temporal bone shows a small enhancing nodule within the anterior vestibule (arrow). (B) The lesion is seen as a filling defect within the normally bright vestibule on the CISS image (arrow).

Inflammatory Lesions

Cholesterol Granuloma

A cholesterol granuloma represents granulation tissue occurring as a result of recurrent hemorrhage. The most common lesion originating in the petrous apex, cholesterol granulomas may be large at diagnosis, causing smooth osseous remodeling and expansion without frank destruction. The imaging modality of choice is MRI, which shows the lesion to be T1- and T2-hyperintense without enhancement (Fig. 7.18).[18] The T1 hyperintensity is due to the paramagnetic properties of methemoglobin, a hemoglobin breakdown product. Hemosiderin deposition may render the periphery of the lesion hypointense on both sequences.[9] The MR appearance is often diagnostic for cholesterol granuloma, though occasionally a CTA or MRA may need to be performed to exclude aneurysm if the lesion cannot be separated from the petrous ICA on conventional MRI.

Petrous Apex Cephalocele

Petrous apex cephaloceles occur due to abnormal herniation of arachnoid or dura matter into the petrous apex; bilateral lesions may be associated with an empty sella, Usher syndrome, and neurofibromatosis type 1. CT demonstrates a smoothly remodeled lytic lesion within the petrous apex, and when large enough can demonstrate central fluid attenuation and communication with Meckel's cave.[18] Fluid-weighted MRI best demonstrates the central fluid signal and communication with Meckel's cave, even with smaller lesions.[19]

Neoplasms

Chondrosarcomas most commonly arise off midline from the petroclival syndrondroses and are indistinguishable from chondromas, their benign counterpart, on imaging. These tumors are best evaluated with both CT and MRI. On CT, these tumors may show lytic destruction centered at the petroclival fissure, and may show the classic chondroid matrix with central "rings and arcs" calcifications. MRI shows a characteristic T2-hyperintense lesion reflecting the high-fluid content of cartilage, with central signal voids in the presence of calcifications. Enhancement is variable, sometimes in a "honeycomb" pattern typical of the lesion.[20]

The petrous apex is also the most common site of metastases in the temporal bone, most commonly from breast carcinoma; plasmacytoma, lymphoma, and nasopharyngeal carcinoma may also involve the petrous apex.[18]

PATHOLOGIES OF THE FACIAL NERVE

CT best depicts the normal caliber and course of the facial nerve canal within the temporal bone. However, abnormal enhancement of the nerve typically cannot be appreciated on CT due to its small size and the high density

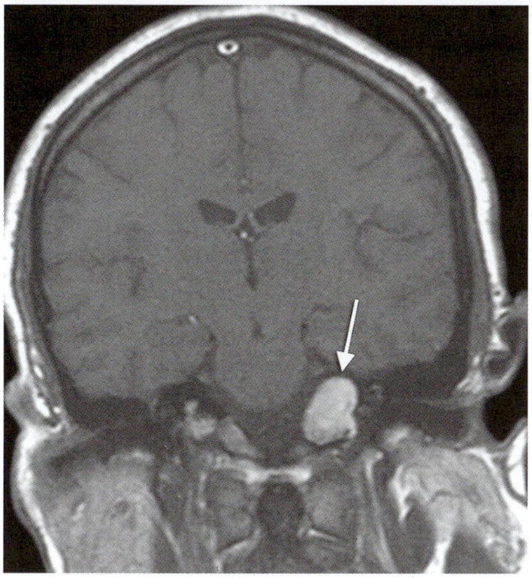

Fig. 7.18: Cholesterol granuloma. Coronal precontrast T1-weighted MRI shows a lobulated T1-hyperintense lesion within the petrous apex (arrow).

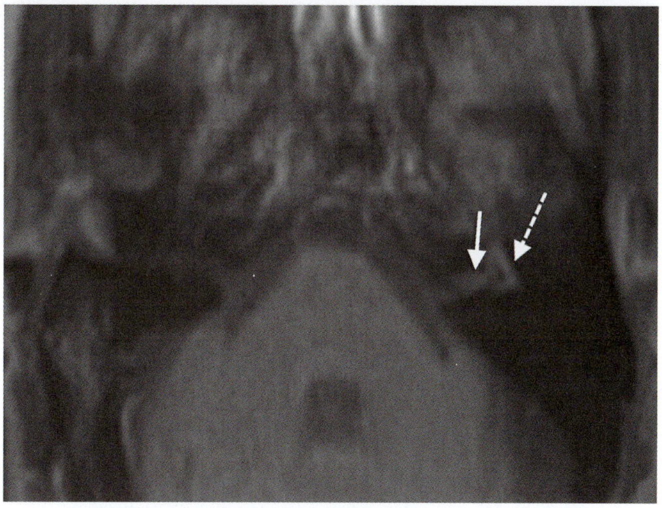

Fig. 7.19: Bell's palsy. Axial fat-saturated, contrast-enhanced T1-weighted MR image shows abnormal, linear asymmetrical enhancement of the left labyrinthine (solid arrow), anterior genu and proximal tympanic (dashed arrow) segments of the facial nerve, compatible with Bell's palsy.

of the adjacent bony structures. MRI best depicts the cisternal and intracanalicular portions of the facial nerve, particularly on high-resolution fluid-weighted images. Abnormal enhancement of the facial nerve, including where it courses through the temporal bone, is also best evaluated on MRI.

Normal enhancement of the facial nerve on T1-weighted postcontrast MRIs is symmetric and smooth, and normally seen along the geniculate, tympanic, and mastoid segments of the facial nerve where there is a normal surrounding venous plexus. For these normally enhancing segments of the facial nerve, asymmetry with increased caliber or intensity of enhancement is considered abnormal. Any enhancement along the cisternal, intracanalicular, labyrinthine, and extracranial segments is considered abnormal.

Infection

Bell's Palsy

Bell's palsy signifies facial paralysis occurring due to viral infection. MRI with contrast is the imaging modality of choice and should be reserved for atypical clinical presentations. Postcontrast images reveal asymmetric linear, uniform, and contiguous enhancement of the facial nerve, most commonly involving its fundal and labyrinthine segments (Fig. 7.19). Mild enlargement of the nerve may be observed.[21] Abnormal enhancement may persist beyond clinical improvement or even complete recovery.[9]

Lyme Disease

Neurologic manifestations of borreliosis occur with stage 2 (1–4 months after infection) and stage 3 (up to several years later) of the infection. Although nonspecific white matter lesions constitute the vast majority of MRI findings, abnormal cranial nerve enhancement may be seen, frequently involving the seventh and eighth cranial nerves.[22]

Hemangioma

Facial nerve hemangiomas present early with facial nerve paralysis and occur most commonly in the region of the geniculate fossa, arising from capillaries around the facial nerve. Several types have been described—capillary, cavernous, and ossifying hemangiomas, with the ossifying type producing spicules of lamellar bone. On CT, an ossifying hemangioma appears as a small, irregular soft tissue lesion with a "honeycomb" matrix.[23] MR demonstrates an avidly enhancing mass that cannot be distinguished from a facial nerve schwannoma.

Neoplasm

Schwannoma

Schwannomas of the facial nerve are tubular soft tissue masses that smoothly enlarge the facial nerve canal and homogeneously enhance on MRI following gadolinium

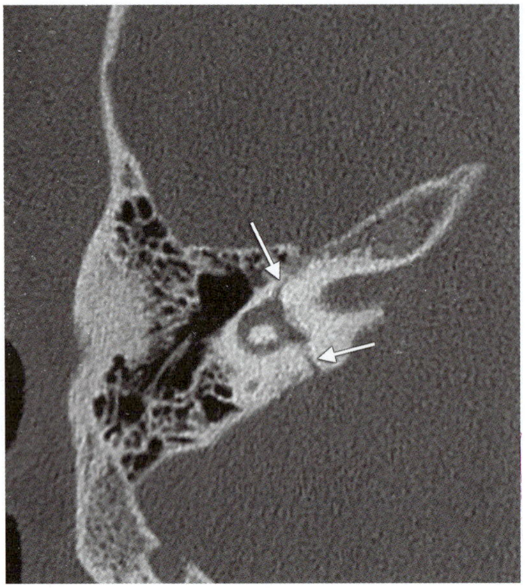

Fig. 7.20: Transverse temporal bone fracture. Noncontrast axial CT image of the temporal bone shows a transverse linear lucency (solid arrows) traversing the vestibule.

administration.[24] Differentiation of a facial nerve schwannoma in the IAC from an acoustic schwannoma may be difficult unless extension into the labyrinthine segment is present.

Perineural Tumor Spread

In the setting of parotid or periauricular skin malignancy, retrograde perineural spread of the tumor may occur, best evaluated with contrast-enhanced MRI. Fat-saturated postcontrast MRIs through the temporal bone demonstrate abnormal asymmetric enhancement of the facial nerve, which can be nodular or smooth; nodular enhancement favors perineural tumor spread over infectious/inflammatory etiologies.[9] Skip lesions may be present. CT may also demonstrate perineural tumor spread, though with decreased sensitivity compared with MR. On CT, perineural tumor spread may manifest as a soft tissue mass widening the stylomastoid foramen and facial nerve canal on the affected side with obliteration of the surrounding fat and possible mastoid invasion.

TRAUMA

CT is the imaging modality of choice in the evaluation of temporal bone trauma, given its easy accessibility, rapid acquisition, and superior bony detail.

Fractures

Although most fractures through the temporal bone do not conform to a strict pattern due to obliquity or complexity, classically they are described as longitudinal or transverse, depending on their orientation to the axis of the petrous temporal bone. Longitudinal fractures comprise the vast majority of fractures (85%) and result from blunt impact to the temporoparietal region. Longitudinal fractures are typically extralabyrinthine and result in conductive hearing loss due to tympanic membrane perforation, hemotympanum, or ossicular interruption. In the anterior subtype, the glenoid fossa is involved; it is spared in the posterior subtype. Transverse fractures result from frontal or occipital trauma and may be divided into the medial subtype where the fracture plane proceeds through the fundus of the IAC commonly resulting in complete sensorineural hearing loss, and the lateral subtype with extension through the labyrinth (Fig. 7.20), leading to a perilymphatic fistula. Thin-section CT readily shows the orientation of the fracture plane, opacification of mastoid air cells, and involvement of the ossicles and inner ear structures including presence of pneumolabyrinth.[25]

Ossicular Dislocation

Presence of ossicular chain discontinuity on CT images of the temporal bone, especially in the setting of a longitudinal fracture, should lead one to suspect ossicular dislocation. Incudo-stapedial disruption, best seen on axial images, shows abnormal widening at the incudo-stapedial joint. Disruption of the malleo-incudal joint is present when the head of the malleus is abnormally separated from the short process of incus on axial images; Y-shaped configuration of the laterally dislocated incus may be seen on coronal images. The stapes may become dislocated into the vestibule, leading to perilymph extravasation into the middle ear and perilymphatic fistula.[26]

REFERENCES

1. Som PM, Curtin HD. Head and neck imaging, 5th ed. St. Louis, MO: Mosby; 2011.
2. Gleeson M, Browning GG, Burton MJ, et al. Scott-Brown's otorhinolaryngology: head and neck surgery, 7th edn. London: Hodder Arnold; 2008.
3. Shpizner BA, Holliday RA, Roland JT, et al. Postoperative imaging of the multichannel cochlear implant. AJNR Am J Neuroradiol. 1995;16:1517-24.

4. De Foer B, Vercruysse J-P, Spaepen M, et al. Diffusion-weighted magnetic resonance imaging of the temporal bone. Neuroradiol. 2010;52(9):785-807.
5. Schwartz KM, Lane JI, Bolster Jr BD, et al. The utility of diffusion-weighted imaging for cholesteatoma evaluation. AJNR Am J Neuroradiol. 2011;32:430-36.
6. Hiatt JL, Gartner LP. Textbook of Head and Neck Anatomy, 4th ed. Philadelphia, PA: Lippincott Williams & Wilkins; 2009.
7. Fatterpekar GM, Doshi AH, Dugar M, et al. Role of 3D CT in the evaluation of the temporal bone. Radiographics. 2006;26:S117-32.
8. Fatterpekar GM, Doshi A, Delman BN. 3D CT of the temporal bone: anatomy and pathology. Terarecon Clin Case Stud. 2005;4:187-208.
9. Harnsberger HR, Glastonbury CM, Michel MA, et al. Diagnostic imaging: head and neck, 2nd edn. Manitoba, Canada: Amirsys; 2010.
10. Trojanowska A, Drop A, Trojanowski P, et al. External and middle ear diseases: radiological diagnosis based on clinical signs and symptoms. Insights Imaging. 2012;3:33-48.
11. Dimmick SJ, Faulder KC. Normal variants of the cerebral circulation at multidetector CT angiography. Radiographics. 2009;29:1027-43.
12. Weissman JL, Hirsch BE. Imaging of tinnitus: a review. Radiology. 2000;216:342-9.
13. Castillo M, Albernaz VS, Mukherji SK, et al. Imaging of Bezold's abscess. AJR Am J Radiol. 1998;171:1491-5.
14. Marsot-Dupuch K, Dominguez-Brito A, Ghasli K, et al. CT and MR findings of michel anomaly: inner ear aplasia. AJNR Am J Neuroradiol. 1999;20:281-4.
15. Urman SM, Talbot JM. Otic capsule dysplasia: clinical and CT findings. Radiographics. 1990;10:823-38.
16. Mukherji SK, Albernaz VS, Lo WW, et al. Papillary endolymphatic sac tumors: CT, MR imaging, and angiographic findings in 20 patients. Radiology. 1997;202(3):801-8.
17. Chapman PT, Shah R, Curé JK, et al. Petrous apex lesions: pictorial review. AJNR Am J Neuroradiol. 2011;196: WS26-37.
18. Razek AA, Huang BY. Lesions of the petrous apex: classification and findings at CT and MR imaging. Radiographics. 2012;32:151-73.
19. Moore KR, Fischbein NJ, Harnsberger HR, et al. Petrous apex cephaloceles. AJNR Am J Neuroradiol. 2001;22:1867-71.
20. Murphey MD, Walker EA, Wilson AJ, et al. Imaging of primary chondrosarcoma: radiologic-pathologic correlation. Radiographics. 2003;23:1245-78.
21. Saremi F, Helmy M, Farzin S, et al. MRI of cranial nerve enhancement. AJR Am J Radiol. 2005;185: 1487-97.
22. Agarwal R, Sze G. Neuro-Lyme disease: MR imaging findings. Radiology. 2009;253:167-73.
23. Gupta S, Mends F, Hagiwara M, et al. Imaging the facial nerve: a contemporary review. Radiol Res Pract. 2013. Article ID 248039.
24. Wiggins III RH, Harnsberger HR, Salzman KL, et al. The many faces of facial nerve schwannoma. AJNR Am J Neuroradiol. 2006;27:694-9.
25. Swartz JD. Temporal bone trauma. Semin Ultrasound CT MR. 2001;22:219-28.
26. Meriot P, Veillon F, Garcia JF, et al. CT appearances of ossicular injury. Radiographics. 1997;17:1445-54.

CHAPTER

8

Diseases of the External Ear

Myles Melton, Kevin D Brown, Samuel H Selesnick

INTRODUCTION

Anatomy

Morphology

The pinnae of the external ear are cartilaginous frames that aid in focusing and localizing sound. Each pinna is anchored to the cranium by skin, cartilage, the auricular muscles, and extrinsic ligaments. The anatomy of the pinna is illustrated in Figure 8.1.

The external auditory canal (EAC) is typically 24 mm in length with a volume of 1–2 mL. The lateral third of the canal is made of fibrocartilage, whereas the medial two-thirds are osseous. During early childhood, the canal is straight, but takes on an "S" shape by the age of 9. The EAC has an important relationship with the mastoid segment of the facial nerve, which lies posterior to the EAC as it descends toward the stylomastoid foramen. The temporomandibular joint is anterior to the EAC, and disease processes affecting this joint may lead to otalgia.[1]

Skin

The EAC is lined by stratified squamous epithelium that is continuous with the skin of the pinna and the epithelial covering of the tympanic membrane. The subcutaneous layer of the cartilaginous portion of the canal contains hair follicles, sebaceous glands, and ceruminous glands, and is up to 1 mm thick. The skin of the osseous canal does not have subcutaneous elements and is only 0.2 mm thick (Fig. 8.2). The epithelium of the EAC migrates laterally, allowing the canal to remain unobstructed by debris.

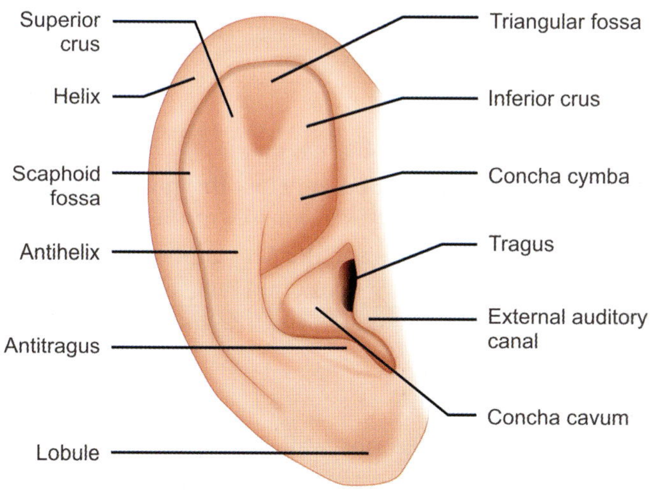

Fig. 8.1: Anatomy of the pinna.

The rate of epithelial migration is 0.07 mm per day and is thought to occur at the basal cell layer.

The ceruminous glands are modified apocrine sweat glands surrounded by myoepithelial cells; they are organized into apopilosebaceous units (Fig. 8.3). Cerumen prevents canal maceration, has antibacterial properties, and has a normally acidic pH, all of which contribute to an antibacterial effect of cerumen.

Innervation

The pinna is innervated laterally, inferiorly, and posteriorly by the great auricular nerve (cervical plexus). Arnold's nerve (a branch of the vagus nerve) innervates the inferior bony canal, the posterosuperior cartilaginous

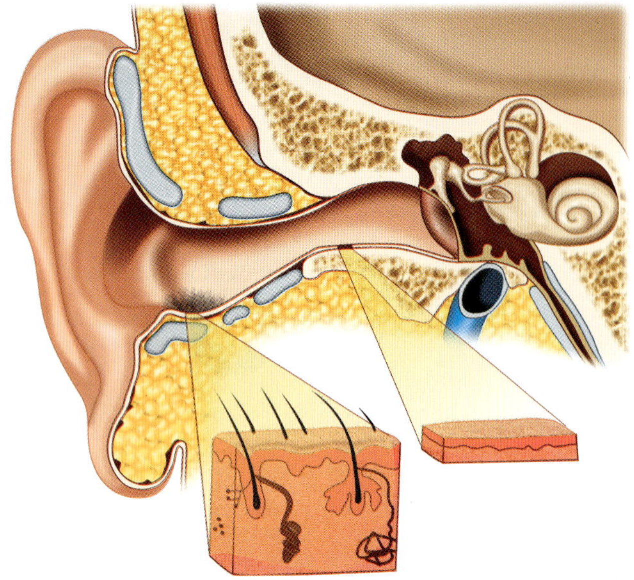

Fig. 8.2: Coronal section of the ear canal. The skin of the cartilaginous and osseous canals is magnified.

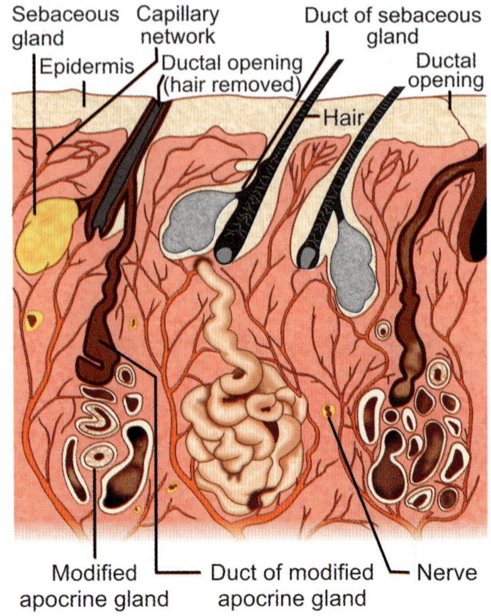

Fig. 8.3: Skin of the cartilaginous portion of the external auditory canal depicting apopilosebaceous units.

canal, and corresponding segments of the tympanic membrane and the cymba concha. The posterosuperior bony EAC is innervated by branches of the facial nerve. The auriculotemporal branch of V3 supplies the anterior portion of the pinna. The glossopharyngeal nerve contribution to the external ear is not well delineated.

Lymphatic Drainage

The anterior and superior wall of the EAC and tragus are drained by the preauricular lymph nodes. The infra-auricular lymph nodes drain the helix and the inferior wall of the EAC, whereas the concha and antihelix are drained by the mastoid nodes.

Vascular Supply

The posterior auricular artery and the superficial temporal artery arise from the external carotid artery and supply the auricle and lateral EAC. The deep auricular branch of the maxillary artery supplies the more medial aspects of the canal and the external surface of the tympanic membrane. The posterior auricular and superficial temporal veins drain the external ear.

Physiology

The external ear aids in the efficient transmission of sound to the tympanic membrane by serving as a functional resonator and, in particular, boosts transmission in the speech frequencies.

The hairs in the lateral canal, as well as the depth and tortuosity of the EAC, protect the tympanic membrane and structures of the middle ear.

Embryology

The mammalian ear is divided into external, middle, and inner ear components, which differ in their embryologic origin (Fig. 8.4). The external ear consists of the pinna, the EAC, and the tympanic membrane, and is embryologically derived from the first and second branchial arches, and includes both ectodermal and mesodermal components. The mesenchymal tissue of the arches is composed of paraxial mesoderm and neural crest cells. The pinna is formed by the gradual change in shape and fusion of components of the six auricular hillocks, which are derived from the first and second branchial arches (Figs. 8.5A to C). Formation of the external auditory meatus results from an ingrowth of a solid epithelial plate of ectodermal cells, the meatal plug, which eventually resorbs with only the lining of the canal remaining. The canal is lined by epithelial cells of ectodermal origin. The tympanic membrane begins to develop during the 28th week of gestation and arises from the most medial aspect of the meatal plug, which eventually becomes the external layer of the tympanic membrane.

CONGENITAL ANOMALIES OF THE EXTERNAL EAR

Introduction

Congenital anomalies of the external ear include a spectrum of malformations of the pinna as well as varying degrees of atresia and stenosis of the EAC. The causes of these disorders may be genetic or secondary to environmental exposures. These disorders include variants of microtia, lop ear, cup ear, Stahl's ear, cryptotia, and prominent ear.

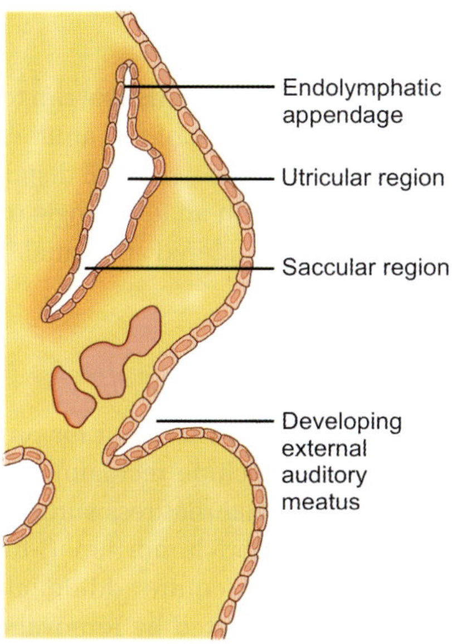

Fig. 8.4: Development of the ear at 29 days' gestation.

Patient evaluation requires a thorough head and neck examination to exclude additional congenital anomalies. The list of associated syndromes is extensive and includes Goldenhar (hemifacial microsomia), branchio-otorenal, Treacher Collins, and Robinow syndromes.

Pathogenesis

Multiple genes may have redundant roles in outer ear formation, which can account for phenotypically similar malformations. The sequence of such dysregulation is only beginning to be understood with the help of murine knock-out and knock-in models. The auricular hillocks that give rise to the pinna arise during the 6th week of embryogenesis, whereas the inner two thirds of the EAC are not formed until the 26th week. Untoward events throughout this period could give rise to structural anomalies of the external ear.

Microtia

Clinical Findings

Patients typically present at birth with obvious auricular malformations. Several classification systems are used to further subcategorize this entity, which are detailed below.[2,3]

Grade I: The ear exhibits mild deformity, typically with a slightly dysmorphic helix and antihelix. This group includes low-set ears, lop ears, cupped ears, and mildly constricted ears. All major structures of the external ear

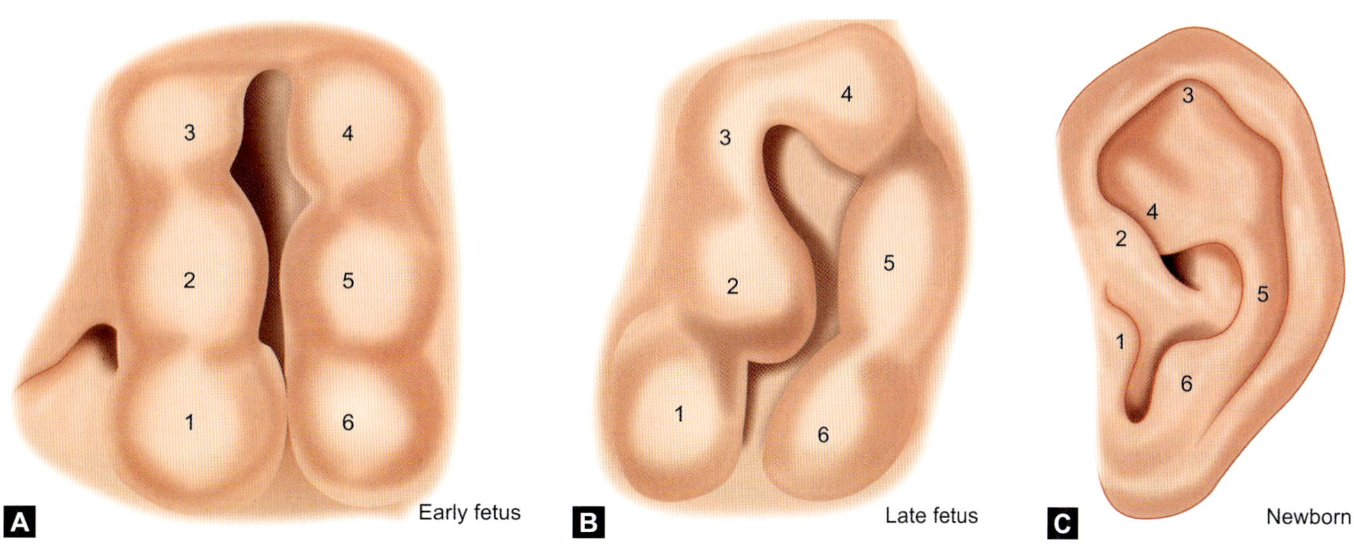

Figs. 8.5A to C: Differentiation of the six auricular hillocks.

are present to some degree. The lop ear is characterized by inferiorly angled positioning of the auricular cartilage and poor development of the antihelical fold, whereas the cup ear protrudes with a deep conchal bowl.

Grade II: All pinna structures are present, but tissue deficiency and significant deformity exist.

Grade III: Also known as classic microtia or peanut ear, type III microtia has few or no recognizable landmarks of the auricle. The ear lobule is usually present and anteriorly positioned. This subgroup includes anotia, which is complete absence of the external ear.

Treatment

Classically, microtia has been treated by a multistage auricular reconstruction.[4] Patients undergo observation until the age of 5 to allow for growth of rib cartilage, which is harvested for reconstruction, and the development of the contralateral ear. This approach offers the benefit of reconstruction with autogenous material, which ultimately requires little or no maintenance. However, it is difficult to achieve a perfect cosmetic result. Typically, reconstruction occurs in following four stages.

Stage I: cartilage implantation: Rib graft is typically harvested from the chondrosis of ribs 6, 7, and 8. The goals of this stage include symmetry in the position of the reconstructed cartilaginous ear framework with the normal ear. Postoperatively, the patient must be assessed for pneumothorax, which may arise with rib harvest.

Stage II: lobule transfer: This procedure should be performed 2–3 months after Stage I reconstruction and aligns the lobule with the reconstructed cartilage framework.

Stage III: postauricular skin grafting: A postauricular sulcus is created to allow the ear to project away from the mastoid. This step should be performed 3 months after stage II reconstruction. Skin for the creation of the sulcus may be harvested from the groin, lower abdomen, buttocks, contralateral postauricular sulcus, or back.

Stage IV: tragal reconstruction and soft tissue debulking: This should be performed several months after Stage III reconstruction.

Other treatment options: Another option for reconstruction includes the placement of a prosthesis. This can be either glued on or anchored to bone. If the patient selects a bone-anchored prosthesis rather than auricular reconstruction, he or she must be aware that daily maintenance is required and that the anchor may compromise the vascularity of the surgical site, complicating future reconstructive surgery if the patient becomes dissatisfied with the prosthesis. A prosthesis does offer the advantage of a minor surgical procedure and allows for auricular replacement at an earlier age than surgical reconstruction. Complications of all types of auricular reconstructions include infection, hematoma formation, skin-flap necrosis, scar contracture, and poor contouring.

Protruding Ears

Clinical Findings

An increase in distance from the helical rim to the mastoid is thought to be due to a lack of the antihelical fold and prominence of the conchal bowl. Ideal distance has been described as 15–20 mm with an ideal angle of 30°. Greater than 45° angulation is considered abnormal.[5] This entity is most frequently bilateral.

Treatment

Otoplasty is the mainstay of treatment for protruding ears. Often used techniques include recreating the antihelical fold utilizing 3–4 horizontal mattress sutures through the cartilage and anterior perichondrium (Mustarde technique).[6] Stiff cartilage may require additional contouring.[7] Conchal excess may be treated by removal of soft tissue and skin from the postauricular sulcus followed by concha to mastoid sutures at the fossa triangularis, cavum concha, and cymba concha.

Complications

Excessive overcorrection of the middle third of the ear should be avoided to prevent development of the "telephone ear" deformity.[8] Hematoma is the most common complication following otoplasty occurring in approximately 3% of cases. Lack of patient satisfaction, although not a true complication, is not an uncommon occurrence as loss of correction up to 40% has been reported.

Atresia and Stenosis of the EAC

Clinical Findings

Congenital anomalies of the EAC range from mild stenosis to complete atresia. These are often seen in association

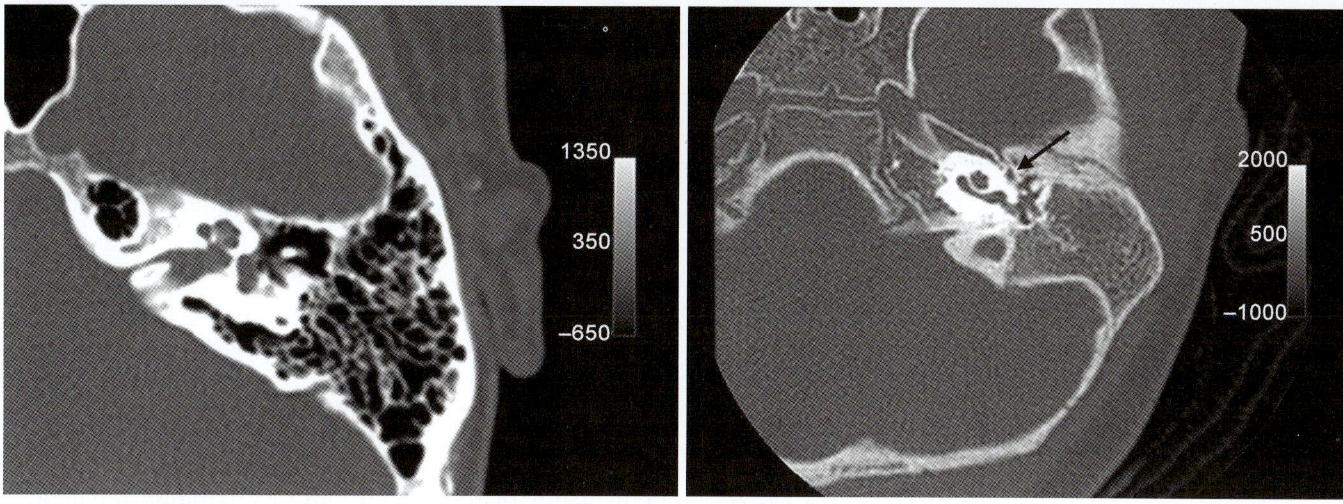

Fig. 8.6: High-resolution coronal CT scans demonstrating an excellent candidate for atresiaplasty in the left panel and a poor candidate in the right panel. Note abnormal position of facial nerve on promontory of cochlea (arrow) in poor candidate and limited aeration of mastoid and middle ear.

with malformations of the pinna and the structures of the middle ear. A canal cholesteatoma can develop in the face of severe EAC stenosis, and may also occur with epithelial rests left behind the atresia plate.

Evaluation

Audiologic evaluation via behavioral or electrophysiologic measures should be performed to confirm normal hearing in the contralateral ear in unilateral disease, and to assess for ipsilateral sensorineural hearing loss. The typical pattern of hearing loss in affected ears is a conductive hearing loss of 50–70 dB. Axial and coronal computed tomography (CT) scans are essential in the evaluation of patients with canal atresia or stenosis. CT scanning assesses for ossicular, facial nerve, and otic capsule abnormalities as well as for the degree of temporal bone pneumatization (Fig. 8.6).[9] In addition, CT scanning can be used to identify a cholesteatoma that would necessitate earlier surgical intervention.

Treatment

In congenital bilateral atresia, it is necessary to apply a bone-conduction hearing aid as early as possible, ideally as soon as the third or fourth week of life. This is not necessary in unilateral cases as long as the contralateral ear exhibits normal auditory function, although benefits of binaural acoustic stimulation are lost. Ultimately, meatoplasty can be used to treat mild stenosis of the EAC, and atresiaplasty is used to restore hearing in fully atretic cases.[9] Atresiaplasty is technically difficult, and long-term reductions in the air–bone gap to 30 dB or less are experienced in about 50% of primary cases.[10,11] Clinical outcomes are improved by careful patient selection using the Jahrsdoerfer criteria.[12]

First Branchial Cleft Anomalies

Pathogenesis

First branchial cleft anomalies occur as a result of anomalous fusion of the first and second branchial arches, with incomplete obliteration of the first branchial cleft.

Clinical Findings

Patients may present with a cyst or tract along the anterior border of the sternocleidomastoid muscle near the angle of the mandible. A membranous band between the medial aspect of the floor of the ear canal and the tympanic membrane at the manubrium of the malleus is also highly associated with first branchial cleft anomalies. The patient may have a history of recurrent infection and drainage from the ear or neck.

The Work classification system has been used to describe first branchial cleft cysts.[13] A Work type 1 anomaly duplicates the membranous EAC only. It is lined with squamous epithelium and opens to the external skin. It is located superficial to the facial nerve. A Work type 2 anomaly duplicates both the membranous and cartilaginous EAC. It has a variable relationship with the facial nerve. In addition, it has become evident through the analysis of certain cases that some first branchial cleft anomalies do not neatly fit the Work classification system due to the presence of elements of both Work type 1 and Work type 2 characteristics within a single case.[14]

Treatment

The treatment for first branchial cleft anomalies is complete excision. Incomplete excision predisposes the patient to recurrence and reinfection. The tract may be intimately involved with the facial nerve, which is at risk during excision. This necessitates early identification of the facial nerve as it exits the stylomastoid foramen and tracing distally through the lesion. A superficial parotidectomy type approach may be required for complete excision.[15]

EXTERNAL EAR TRAUMA

Introduction

The external ear is subject to a wide variety of injuries. All trauma patients require appropriate stabilization and triage of associated injuries based on their severity. Adherence to basic surgical principles and wound care prevents complications and improves the likelihood of a successful outcome.

Auricular Hematoma

Pathogenesis

Auricular hematoma refers to the accumulation of blood in the subperichondrial space, usually secondary to blunt trauma. Cartilage lacks its own blood supply and instead relies on the vascularity of the perichondrium via diffusion. Shearing forces secondary to blunt trauma to the pinna lead to an accumulation of blood in the subperichondrial space. This creates a barrier for diffusion between the cartilage and the perichondrial vascularity, leading to necrosis of the cartilage and predisposing it to infection and further injury.[16]

Clinical Findings

A patient with an auricular hematoma usually presents with an edematous, fluctuant, and ecchymotic pinna, with loss of the normal cartilaginous landmarks. Failure to evacuate the hematoma may lead to infection and/or cartilage necrosis and permanent disfigurement known as "cauliflower ear."

Treatment

The evacuation of hematomas can be performed using a skin incision parallel with the natural auricular skin folds. The irrigation of evacuated hematomas with topical antibiotics reduces the likelihood of infection. Splinting after drainage prevents the reaccumulation of hematomas, and options include cotton bolsters, plaster molds, silicon putty, and water-resistant thermoplastic splints. Through-and-through whip-type absorbable mattress sutures without a bolster have also been described.[17]

Auricular Lacerations

Sharp or severe blunt trauma may lead to laceration or avulsion of the auricle. The expeditious repair and prevention of infection are essential. Auricular lacerations should be cleansed and débrided prior to repair. Simple lacerations can be closed primarily, whereas extensive injuries with tissue loss may require undermining, flap reconstruction, or tissue grafts. In the case of a near-total ear avulsion still attached at the helical root, the ear can be successfully reattached as the supply of the upper auricular-helical artery seems to be sufficient for the entire ear. Leech therapy may be required to support venous outflow until neovascularization occurs. Repairs should be covered with pressure dressings to prevent edema and hematoma formation, and cartilage-penetrating antibiotics such as quinolones should be prescribed. Excellent cosmetic results can be achieved, even with extensive lacerations.[18]

Auricular Frostbite

Pathogenesis

Freezing temperatures lead to both direct cellular injury as well as vascular compromise. Prolonged exposure to cold temperatures can lead to vasoconstriction, cold-mediated dehydration, endothelial injury, thrombosis, and ischemia of auricular tissue. In the early stage, this process may be reversible, but over time, it leads to tissue necrosis.

Clinical Findings

Temperatures below 10°C may lead to hypesthesia, and the person is frequently unaware of impending frostbite. The ear is initially pale and then cyanotic. Ultimately, as the ear thaws, pain, erythema, and subcutaneous bullae secondary to extravasated extracellular fluid or blood may develop.

Treatment

The initial treatment for auricular frostbite consists of rapid rewarming of the ear to 40–42°C. Nonhemorrhagic blisters may be débrided, and patients should be given pain medicine and antibiotics. Aloe vera has antithromboxane properties and, together with ibuprofen, may aid in re-establishing circulation. More aggressive débridement should be delayed for several weeks until demarcation is complete.[19]

Auricular Burns

General Considerations

Thermal injury can be classified by the degree of the burn. Superficial burns involve the superficial layer of the epidermis. Partial-thickness burns extend into, but not through, the dermis. Full-thickness burns extend through the full thickness of the dermis. Subdermal burns extend into the subcutaneous tissue, including fat, muscle, tendon, cartilage, and bone.

Clinical Findings

Superficial auricular burns present with erythema secondary to dermal capillary dilation and vessel congestion. These burns are red and moderately painful. Patients with partial-thickness burns usually present with blisters that blanch on direct pressure and are very painful. Deep partial-thickness burns are associated with less pain, and there may be an eschar. Full-thickness and subdermal burns are painless because dermal nerve endings have been destroyed. The wound surface is of varying color, but may be gray or black and charred.

Treatment

Superficial burns do not scar and may be treated with moisturizing creams. The blisters of partial-thickness burns should be débrided, and antibiotic ointment applied. When not deep, these burns heal without scarring as well. Full-thickness, subdermal, and deep partial-thickness burns of the auricle heal with scarring and contracture and may be complicated by suppurative chondritis. These burns should be treated with both topical (usually silver based) and systemic cartilage penetrating antibiotics. Early débridement and closure with skin grafts should be considered. Secondary reconstruction is usually performed at approximately 1 year after injury.[20]

INFECTIOUS DISEASES OF THE EXTERNAL EAR

Otitis Externa

General Considerations

Otitis externa is an inflammatory and infectious process of the EAC. *Pseudomonas aeruginosa* and *Staphylococcus aureus* are the most commonly isolated organisms. Other commonly isolated organisms include *Proteus species*, *Staphylococcus epidermidis*, diphtheroids, and *Escherichia coli*.[21] Fungal otitis externa is discussed in the next section. Otitis externa is the most common otolaryngologic problem experienced by underwater divers.[22]

Pathogenesis

In the preinflammatory stage, the ear is exposed to predisposing factors, including heat, humidity, maceration, the absence of cerumen, and an alkaline PH. Loss of acidity has been shown to be proportionate to degree of infection. This can cause edema of the stratum corneum and occlusion of the apopilosebaceous units. In the inflammatory stage, bacterial overgrowth ensues, with progressive edema and intensified pain. Incomplete resolution or persistent inflammation for >3 months refers to the chronic inflammatory stage.

Clinical Findings

Symptoms of otitis externa may vary, depending on the stage and extent of disease. The clinical diagnosis is suggested by the presence of otalgia, otorrhea, aural fullness, pruritus, tenderness to palpation, and varying degrees of occlusion of the EAC. The patient may also present with hearing loss that results from occlusion of the EAC by edema and debris. Signs of otitis externa include pain on distraction of the pinna, EAC erythema, edema, otorrhea, crusting, and, in more advanced disease, lymphadenopathy of the periauricular and anterior cervical lymph nodes. Skin changes of cellulitis may be present as well. In the chronic stage, the skin of the EAC may be thickened.[23] A culture may be helpful for infections that are refractory to treatment.

Treatment

Treatment for otitis externa involves meticulous atraumatic debridement of the EAC with the aid of a microscope.

Analgesia can be achieved with nonsteroidal anti-inflammatory drugs (NSAIDs), opioids, or topical steroid preparations. After cleansing is complete, steroid, antibiotic, or acidifying otic preparations should be used. A recent Cochrane review did not reveal any meaningful differences regarding clinical cure rates among these otic preparations except that acetic acid may not be as effective as antibiotic, steroid, or antibiotic plus steroid drops at 2–3 weeks.[24] If the degree of stenosis of the canal is severe, a wick must be placed in an effort to stent open the EAC and permit delivery of drops to the medial portion of the canal.

Available antiseptic preparations include acetic and boric acids, ichthammol, phenol, aluminum acetate, gentian violet, thymol, thimerosal (e.g. Merthiolate), cresylate, and alcohol. Available antibiotic preparations include ofloxacin, ciprofloxacin, colistin, polymyxin B, neomycin, chloramphenicol, gentamicin, and tobramycin. Polymyxin B and neomycin preparations are often used in combination for the treatment of *S. aureus* and *P. aeruginosa* infections. Ofloxacin and ciprofloxacin are single-agent antibiotics with an excellent spectrum of coverage for pathogens encountered in otitis externa. Preparations with steroids help to reduce edema and otalgia. Systemic antibiotics are indicated for infections that spread beyond the EAC. For chronic otitis externa, a canalplasty may be indicated for thickened skin that has caused canal obstruction. Patients must be instructed to avoid EAC manipulation and water exposure if they have a history of recurrent otitis externa.

Otomycosis

General Considerations

Otomycosis is an inflammatory process of the external ear canal due to infection with fungi and is responsible for >9% of the diagnoses of otitis externa.[25] In 80% of cases, the etiologic agent is *Aspergillus*, whereas *Candida* is the next most frequently isolated fungus. Other more rare fungal pathogens include *Phycomycetes*, *Rhizopus*, *Actinomyces*, and *Penicillium*.

Pathogenesis

Otomycosis has similar predisposing factors to bacterial otitis externa. Patients with diabetes mellitus or an immunocompromised state are particularly susceptible to otomycosis. Patients with a mastoid bowl after a canal wall down procedure are predisposed to development of otomycosis as well.

Clinical Findings

Patients with otomycosis most frequently present with pruritus, aural fullness, and otorrhea, and may also complain of otalgia and hearing loss. The hearing loss associated with otomycosis usually results from the accumulation of mycotic debris.

Otoscopy often reveals mycelia, establishing the diagnosis. The EAC may be erythematous and fungal debris may appear white, gray, or black. Patients have typically been tried on topical antibacterial agents with no significant response. The diagnosis can be confirmed by identifying fungal elements on a KOH preparation or by a positive fungal culture.

Treatment

The treatment of otomycosis includes cleansing and debriding the EAC, acidifying the canal, and administering antifungal agents. Nonspecific antifungal agents include thimerosal (e.g. Merthiolate) and gentian violet. Commonly used specific antifungals include clotrimazole, Nystatin (otic drops or powder), and ketoconazole. Topical ketoconazole, cresylate otic drops, and aluminum acetate otic drops were all relatively effective with >80% resolution rate on initial application.[25] CSF powder (chloramphenicol, sulfamethoximazole, and fungizone) is also an excellent option.

Necrotizing Otitis Externa

General Considerations

Skull base osteomyelitis, also known as malignant otitis externa or necrotizing otitis externa (NOE), is a bacterial infection of the EAC and skull base. This disease process is most frequently seen in elderly diabetics and immunocompromised patients. It most commonly begins as an external otitis that progresses to involve the temporal bone, and may progress to fatal meningitis, sepsis, and death if unrecognized or untreated.

Pathogenesis

Skull base osteomyelitis commonly begins as an external otitis that progresses to cellulitis, chondritis, osteitis, and, ultimately, osteomyelitis. Unlike otitis media, which spreads through the pneumatized portion of the temporal bone, NOE disseminates through the haversian canals and vascularized spaces of the skull base. As this progresses

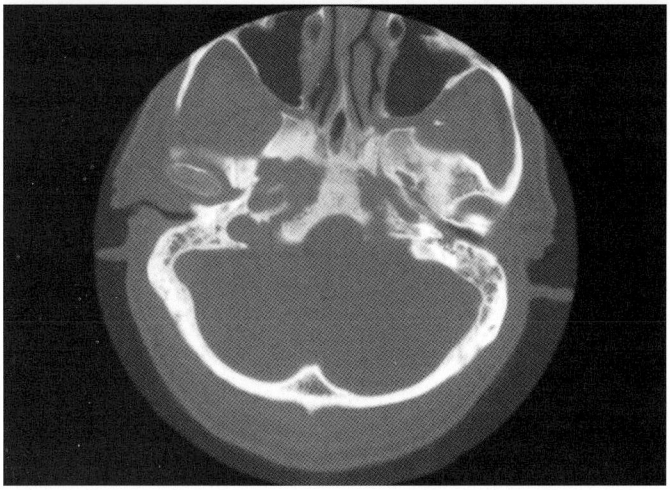

Fig. 8.7: Axial high-resolution CT scan demonstrating skull base osteomyelitis with evidence of petroclival bone erosion.

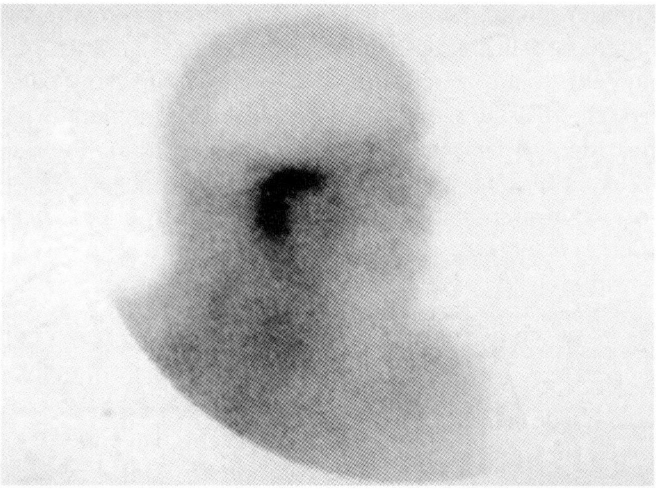

Fig. 8.8: Sagittal image of a bone scan in a patient with skull base osteomyelitis revealing focal enhancement of the skull base.

along the base of the skull, the facial nerve (stylomastoid foramen); hypoglossal nerve (hypoglossal canal); the abducens and trigeminal nerves (petrous apex); and the glossopharyngeal, vagus, and spinal accessory nerves (jugular foramen) may be involved. Cranial neuropathy has classically been considered to portend a poor prognosis, although recent data have not supported a difference in mortality.

The most frequently isolated causative organism is *P. aeruginosa*, which may exhibit high levels of antibiotic resistance. *Aspergillus* may also be an etiologic organism and is thought to originate from the middle ear or mastoid. Elderly diabetics are thought to be particularly susceptible because of the microangiopathic changes that blunt an already attenuated immune response. The cerumen of diabetic patients has also been described to be more acidic in nature, further contributing to their susceptibility.

Clinical Findings

Symptoms and signs: Patients may present with intense otalgia, otorrhea, aural fullness, pruritus, and hearing loss. As the disease advances to involve the temporal bone, granulation tissue is seen on the floor of the EAC at the osteocartilaginous junction. Bony sequestra can also be found in the EAC. Edema, periaural lymphadenopathy, and trismus may be present. Cranial neuropathies occur in more advanced presentations of disease, and the facial nerve is the most frequently affected cranial nerve. Further progression may lead to sigmoid sinus thrombosis, meningitis, sepsis, and death.

Diagnostic tests: Inflammatory markers such as ESR and CRP may be elevated. Cultures and sensitivity should be obtained to aid in selecting appropriate antibiotics.

CT and MRI are useful in the initial evaluation to determine the extent of disease (Fig. 8.7). Retrocondylar fat infiltration is the earliest indication of spread of disease beyond the ear canal and is best identified on MRI.[26] A technetium scan is the most sensitive test for diagnosing bony involvement but is not specific. Asymmetric uptake may be seen in severe cases of otitis externa. Gallium scans are used to track the resolution of the infection, since bone scans often remain positive long after the infection has resolved (Fig. 8.8).

Differential Diagnosis

Carcinomas of the EAC, chronic granulomatous disease, Paget disease, fibrous dysplasia, and nasopharyngeal carcinomas must be considered in the differential diagnosis. As carcinoma of the EAC mimics many features of NOE, a biopsy is requisite to rule out carcinoma.

Treatment

Long-term parenteral antibiotics are the treatment of choice. Aminoglycosides (e.g. tobramycin) and antipseudomonal β-lactam antibiotics, including piperacillin, ticarcillin, or ceftazidime, may be used. Some physicians recommend the use of outpatient fluoroquinolones such as ciprofloxacin or ofloxacin; however, this is appropriate only for patients with early presentations who can be followed up closely. Control of hyperglycemia and immunosuppression is necessary to maximize treatment. Surgical debridement may be necessary to remove necrotic tissue. Circumferential petrosectomy has been described as a method for surgical debridement with hearing and facial nerve function preservation. The use of hyperbaric oxygen has been described in cases refractory to antibiotics, with variable results. In an effort to prevent skull base osteomyelitis, all diabetic and immunocompromised patients must be followed up closely and treated aggressively if they present with symptoms suggestive of external otitis.[27]

DERMATOLOGIC DISEASES OF THE EXTERNAL EAR

Atopic Dermatitis

General Considerations

Atopic dermatitis is a chronic skin disease of immune-mediated origin. It may remit spontaneously or endure as a chronic condition. Lesions presenting on the ear may be pruritic and erythematous. Patients often have a personal or family history of atopy and allergy.

Atopic dermatitis often manifests in infancy on extensor surfaces and the face. Children may present with skin lesions on flexural areas and on the hands.

Pathogenesis

Though not completely understood, the clinical presentation of atopic dermatitis is thought to be secondary to immune dysfunction. Atopic skin lesions have been shown to have higher levels of Th2 T-lymphocytes, which produce inflammatory mediators such as interleukin 4, 5, and 10.

Clinical Findings

The diagnosis of atopic dermatitis is a clinical one. There is variability in skin lesions ranging from erythematous patches to weeping plaques. Lesions presenting on the ear are often pruritic and erythematous. Lesions typically persist for > 1 month. Secondary infections with *S. aureus*, herpes simplex virus, vaccinia, and malassezia may occur.[28]

Atopic dermatitis is characterized by the absence of specific laboratory and histologic markers. Elevated IgE and eosinophilia may be present yet are not specific for the diagnosis.

Differential Diagnosis

The differential diagnosis includes seborrheic dermatitis and psoriatic dermatitis.

Treatment

Topical corticosteroids are the mainstay of treatment. Antihistamines and lubricants may be used for the treatment of accompanying pruritus. Moisturizers and mild soaps are preferred to minimize exposure to potential allergens found in many cosmetic products. Food elimination and desensitization are not recommended. Though often self-limited, the disease may recur spontaneously and can become chronic. Bacterial superinfection may require topical and systemic antibiotics.[29]

Psoriasis

General Considerations

Psoriasis is a chronic inflammatory disorder of the skin. Eighteen percent of patients with psoriasis have some involvement of the ear, which may be secondary to extension from the scalp.[30] Plaques may present on the concha and meatus of the EAC and are variably pruritic.

The incidence of psoriasis in the United States ranges from 2% to 5%. Males and females are equally affected, with the onset of disease typically occurring in adolescence.

Pathogenesis

The cause of psoriasis is unknown, yet there is a strong genetic component. Attacks of psoriasis may be triggered by certain drugs such as NSAIDs, beta blockers, lithium carbonate, and antimalarial agents, as well as by infection, trauma, and stress.

Clinical Findings

Psoriasis is characterized by erythematous papules that coalesce to form round or oval salmon-pink plaques with silvery white scales found on the elbows, knees, scalp, and buttocks. These lesions bleed in pinpoint areas when scratched (Auspitz sign). Opacification or "oil spots" of the nails, as well as pitting and subungual hyperkeratosis, are also suggestive of this disease. Psoriatic lesions may present over areas of trauma, an entity known as Koebner phenomenon. Psoriatic arthritis occurs in 5–10% of all psoriatic patients.

Treatment

Patients should avoid excessive drying of the skin. For the ears and face, treatment includes low-dose topical nonfluorinated corticosteroids such as alclometasone, mometasone, desonide, clocortolone, hydrocortisone valerate, and butyrate creams and topical calcipotriene. Warm-water soaks, 1–5% coal tar treatment, and topical anthralin C may also be helpful. Oral psoralens and UVA phototherapy for patients with widespread disease may be necessary. Antihistamines are used to treat the associated pruritus. Methotrexate may be required for severe cases and for psoriatic arthritis. The response to treatment is variable, and the condition may become chronic.

Contact Dermatitis

General Considerations

Contact dermatitis can be an acute or chronic inflammatory disorder of the skin caused by contact with an allergen or irritant. This process may occur anywhere along the pinna or the EAC. Eruption may occur secondary to instrumentation, foreign objects - including jewelry, ear plugs, and hearing aids - and other objects used to scratch pruritic lesions. In addition, cosmetics and hair products are frequent culprits.

Pathogenesis

Allergic contact dermatitis is a type IV hypersensitivity reaction, and cutaneous manifestations are often delayed by 1–3 days. This is in contrast to irritant-mediated contact dermatitis, which usually manifests earlier.

Clinical Findings

Allergic contact dermatitis is characterized by an indurated, erythematous, pruritic, and poorly demarcated process. This is in contrast to irritant dermatitis, which often presents with well-defined areas of exposure.

Skin testing to identify contact allergens may be of use.

Treatment

The avoidance of exposure to irritants and allergens and high-dose topical glucocorticoids are the mainstays of therapy.

NEOPLASMS OF THE EXTERNAL EAR AND EAR CANAL

Basal Cell Carcinoma of the Auricle

General Considerations

Basal cell carcinomas are the most common malignant neoplasm of the auricle, representing 45% of auricular carcinomas.

Pathogenesis

Chronic long-term sun exposure is the predominant cause of basal cell carcinoma. Specifically, UVB radiation has been identified as a major carcinogen. The incidence of cancer increases with age. Other risk factors include fair skin, outdoor occupations, and a history of skin carcinoma.

Clinical Findings

Patients may initially present with a skin lesion that is nodular, ulcerated, and/or bleeding. Basal cell carcinomas of the auricle typically occur on the posterior surface of the pinna and in the preauricular area. The diagnosis of any suspicious lesion should be confirmed with biopsy. CT scans and MRI may be used to evaluate advanced disease with tumor extension to the adjacent temporal bone and soft tissue structures of the head and neck. The overall rate of metastasis is 0.003–0.1%.[31]

Staging

Basal cell carcinomas of the EAC can be staged using the American Joint Committee on Cancer (AJCC) general staging system for nonmelanoma cancer of the skin, which is a TNM (tumor, node, metastases) staging system. This staging system is limited by the fact that it does not account for histologic subtypes or the anatomic variability of the skin of the external ear compared with other skin sites.

Differential Diagnosis

Given the variability of subtypes, the differential diagnosis includes benign nevi, amelanotic melanomas, cutaneous squamous cell carcinomas, eczema, and scleroderma.

Treatment

Nonsurgical measures:

1. Topical 5-fluorouracil
2. Radiation therapy indicated for poor surgical candidates or unresectable lesions

Surgical measures:

1. *Curettage with electrodissection*: Operator dependent and typically used to excise nodular lesions and desiccate the base
2. *Cryosurgery*: Indicated for small basal cell carcinomas (< 1 cm) with well-defined borders

3. *Local excision*: Ninety-five percent of basal cell carcinomas <2 cm in size can be successfully treated with local excision with a surgical margin of at least 4 mm. Auricular reconstruction may be required for large defects
4. *Mohs surgical technique*: Refers to complete micrographic excision of the tumor using intraoperative histopathology to assess for positive margins. This technique is particularly useful for recurrent basal cell carcinomas, those larger than 2 cm, or those with an aggressive histology. Five-year cure rates using Mohs technique should approach 97.1%[32]

Cutaneous Squamous Cell Carcinoma

General Considerations

Squamous cell carcinomas account for 20% of all cutaneous malignant neoplasms and commonly occur in elderly males.[33]

Pathogenesis

Risk factors for squamous cell carcinoma include immunosuppression, advanced age, a nonhealing ulcer, and exposure to chemicals such as arsenic, soot, coal, tar, paraffin, and petroleum oil. The most important risk factor is exposure to UV radiation.

Clinical Findings

The appearance of these tumors is variable and includes plaques, nodules, and ulcerations. They may be friable and prone to bleeding. Auricular lesions frequently occur on the helix or preauricular region, but may occur on any sun-exposed areas.

CT scanning and MRI may be used to evaluate advanced disease with tumor metastasis to the adjacent temporal bone and soft tissue structures of the head and neck. The proper diagnosis should be made with biopsy. The overall risk of metastasis for cutaneous squamous cell carcinoma of the external ear is approximately 6–18%.

Staging

The AJCC system may be utilized for carcinoma of the external ear. AJCC staging systems for nonmelanoma cancer of the ear canal may also be utilized, but the University of Pittsburgh system[34] (Table 8.1) is more frequently utilized for staging squamous cell carcinoma of the temporal bone, as the AJCC does not account for histologic subtypes or the anatomic variability of the external ear skin compared with other skin sites.

Table 8.1: University of Pittsburgh staging system for squamous cell carcinoma

T1	Tumor limited to EAC without bony erosion or soft tissue extension
T2	Tumor with limited EAC bony erosion (not full thickness) or limited (<0.5 cm) soft tissue involvement
T3	Tumor eroding the osseous EAC (full thickness) with limited (<0.5 cm) soft tissue involvement, or tumor involving middle ear and/or mastoid, or patients presenting with facial paralysis
T4	Tumor eroding the cochlea, petrous apex, medial wall of the middle ear, carotid canal, jugular foramen, dura, or with extensive soft tissue involvement

Differential Diagnosis

The differential diagnosis includes basal cell carcinoma, actinic keratosis, seborrheic keratosis, keratoacanthomas, scars, psoriatic lesions, melanomas, and sarcomas.

Treatment

Nonsurgical measures: Radiation therapy may be indicated for unresectable lesions or those that may lead to significant cosmetic disfigurement with surgery.

Surgical measures:
1. *Local excision*: Ninety-five percent of squamous cell carcinomas <2 cm limited to the external ear can be successfully treated with local excision with a surgical margin of at least 6 mm. Auricular reconstruction may be required for large defects. T1 lesions of the EAC may be treated with sleeve excision with careful attention to deep margins. T2 lesions or greater necessitate lateral temporal bone resection. Subtotal temporal bone resection involves the piecemeal removal of structures medial to the tympanic membrane and may be necessary for T3 and T4 lesions. Facial nerve involvement may necessitate its resection and grafting with a nerve graft remote to the site of the tumor (i.e. sural nerve)
2. *Mohs surgical technique*: This technique is particularly useful for recurrent lesions, those >2 cm, or those with an aggressive histology

3. *Neck dissection and parotidectomy*: In all cases of palpable disease in the parotid and neck, and in the case of T3 and T4 squamous cell carcinomas, parotidectomy, neck dissection and adjuvant radiation should be strongly considered

Prevention

As with basal cell carcinoma, minimizing sun exposure between 10:00 am and 3:00 pm, wearing protective clothing, using UVB-protective sunscreens, and avoiding the sun are paramount for risk reduction.

Prognosis

In addition to the patient's age and overall immune status, the prognosis for squamous cell carcinoma is dependent on the histologic subtype, size, and location of the tumor. A better prognosis is associated with a well-differentiated histology. The 5-year cure rate for squamous cell carcinomas of the external ear range from 75% to 92%.

Squamous cell carcinoma of the EAC carries a much more dire prognosis with recent studies suggesting 5-year survival of T1 tumors of 83% and T4 tumors of 25%. Completeness of resection is highly correlated with recurrence. Facial nerve involvement and nodal disease are poor prognostic findings.

Melanoma of the External Ear

General Considerations

The incidence of melanoma in the United States is 11.1 cases per 100,000 individuals. Auricular melanoma accounts for < 1% of all melanomas.[35] Melanomas of the ear have a 10-year survival rate of 70%.

Clinical Findings

Most melanomas involving the ear present on the helix. Though initially painless, these lesions may change in size, ulcerate, and bleed. A thorough head and neck examination requires attention to enlarged lymph nodes that may occur with regional spread of disease.

The diagnosis of melanoma is dependent on the histologic evaluation of a biopsy. At a minimum, metastatic evaluation should include a chest X-ray to rule out lung metastases and liver function tests to rule out liver metastases. CT scanning and MRI have added sensitivity in detecting metastatic disease. Radio-nuclide bone scans can be used to diagnose bony metastases.

Staging

Melanomas may be staged using the staging system of the AJCC. This system incorporates the depth of invasion, measured in millimeters. Deeper lesions and lesions with ulceration are associated with higher stages and higher mortality rates.

Differential Diagnosis

The differential diagnosis is diverse and includes benign lesions as well as basal cell and squamous cell carcinomas.

Treatment

Nonsurgical measures: Adjunctive radiation therapy may have a role in palliation.

Surgical measures: The extent of excision, including surgical margins, is dependent on the histologic type and stage of disease. Management of the regional lymphatics is controversial and may include elective regional lymph node dissection and parotidectomy. Recently, sentinel lymph node biopsy has become a well-accepted approach in the management of the N0 neck for lesions > 1 mm deep.

Prevention

The avoidance of and protection from sun exposure are important in preventing disease, as is early detection. Early detection is also extremely important in improving prognosis.

Glandular Tumors of the EAC

Classification

Glandular tumors of the EAC are rare and include four types: (1) adenoid cystic carcinomas; (2) ceruminous adenomas; (3) ceruminous adenocarcinomas; and (4) pleomorphic adenomas.

Adenoid cystic carcinoma: These are capsular tumors most often found in salivary gland tissue. They have a predilection for perineural, perivascular, and fatty infiltration. Patients with perineural invasion often present with otalgia. Histologically, these tumors may show cribriform, tubular, or solid patterns of cellular arrangement. Lymph node metastases are rare, but late distant metastasis in particular to the lung are not an uncommon feature of these tumors.

Ceruminous adenoma: Ceruminous adenoma consists of benign painless masses that may grow undetected for

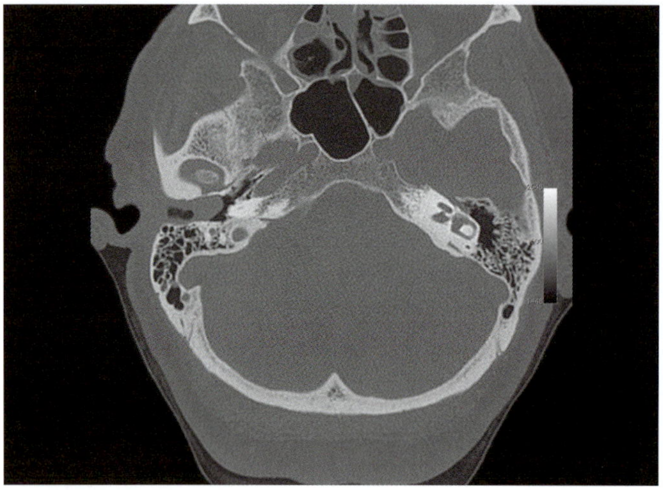

Fig. 8.9: Clinical T2 carcinoma of the right ear canal. Patient was ultimately demonstrated to have limited extension into the temporomanidbular joint at the time of surgery.

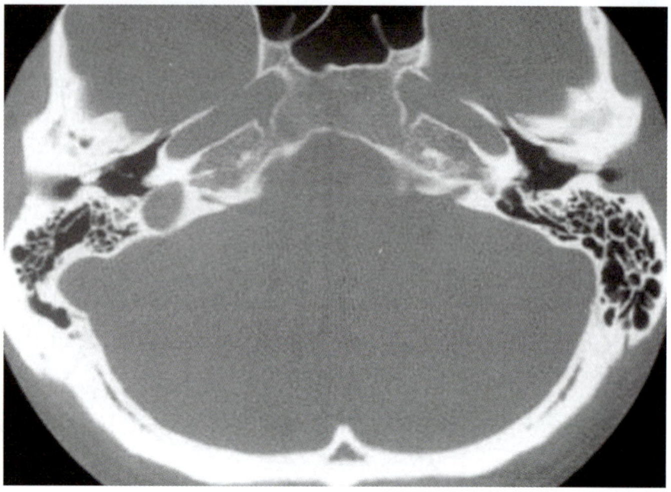

Fig. 8.10: High-resolution axial CT scan revealing right anterior and posterior external auditory canal exostoses.

prolonged periods of time. Patients may present with a conductive hearing loss or otitis externa. They are histologically characterized by double-layered cuboidal or columnar cells, and the epithelium may show apical "snouts" of apocrine secretion.

Ceruminous adenocarcinoma: These tumors share histologic features with ceruminous adenomas, but they have higher rates of mitoses and cellular atypia. Invasion into adjacent structures may be present, and lymph node metastases are rare.

Pleomorphic adenoma: These tumors vary histologically but are characterized by epithelial and mesenchymal elements. These benign tumors do not display features of invasion.

Clinical Findings

Patients with glandular tumors of the EAC may present with otorrhea, aural fullness, otalgia, and conductive hearing loss. Sensorineural hearing loss signifies tumor extension into the inner ear. CT imaging is helpful in determining the amount of bony erosion and the size of the tumor. Generous tissue samples are important for histologic diagnosis.

Treatment

Benign glandular tumors are treated with wide local excision. Malignant tumors are treated with a variant of temporal bone resection, and consideration should also be given to adjuvant radiation. In the case of adenoid cystic carcinoma parotidectomy should be considered as it has been associated with increased survival.[36]

Osteomas and Exostoses of the EAC

General Considerations

Osteomas are benign osseous neoplasms. Exostoses are firm, bony, broad-based lesions composed of lamellar bone (Fig. 8.9). Exostoses are formed by reactive bone formation and have been associated with cold water exposure. Both osteomas and exostoses arise from the bony portion of the EAC (Fig. 8.10).

Clinical Findings

Osteomas are usually pedunculated and often have a vascular core (Fig. 8.11). Exostoses commonly present as multiple lesions. Although most osteomas and exostoses are asymptomatic, occlusion of the EAC with an enlarged lesion may lead to cerumen impaction, recurrent external otitis, and a conductive hearing loss on audiogram.

Treatment

Most exostoses and osteomas require no intervention. If surgery is necessary, a transcanal or postauricular approach can be used, depending on the size of the lesions. The preservation of skin flaps speeds healing.

When used long term, ear plugs have been shown to be protective against exostoses in patients with frequent cold water exposure.

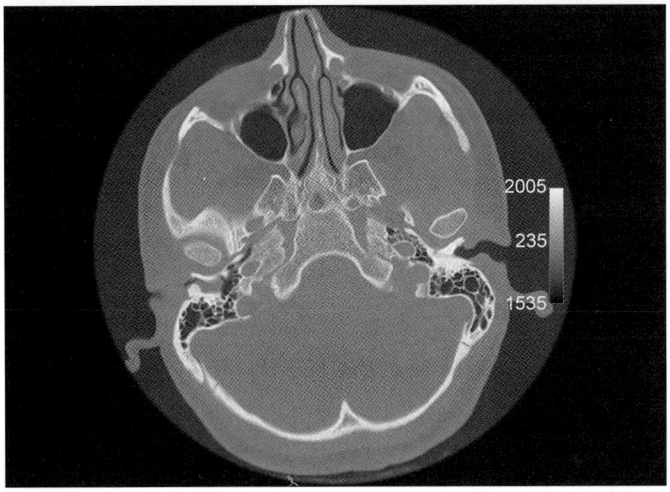

Fig. 8.11: High-resolution coronal CT scan demonstrating an inferiorly based osteoma of the right external auditory canal.

REFERENCES

*1. Prowse SJ, Kelly G, Agada F. Temporomandibular joint herniation and the foramen of Huschke: an unusual external auditory canal mass. J Laryngol Otol. 2011;125(12):1279–81.
2. Bartel-Friedrich S, Wulke C. Classification and diagnosis of ear malformations. GMS Curr Top Otorhinolaryngol Head Neck Surg. 2007;6:Doc05.
3. Weerda H. Classification of congenital deformities of the auricle. Facial Plast Surg. 1988;5(5):385-8.
4. Sivayoham E, Woolford TJ. Current opinion on auricular reconstruction. Curr Opin Otolaryngol Head Neck Surg. 2012;20(4):287-90.
5. Blitzer A, Guida R, Levenson MJ. Office-based surgery in otolaryngology. New York: Thieme; 1998. xix, 478pp.
6. Mustarde JC. The correction of prominent ears using simple mattress sutures. Br J Plast Surg. 1963;16:170-78.
7. Nazarian R, Eshraghi AA. Otoplasty for the protruded ear. Semin Plast Surg. 2011;25(4):288-94.
8. Adamson PA, Litner JA. Otoplasty technique. Facial Plast Surg Clin North Am. 2006;14(2):79-87, v.
9. Brackmann DE, Shelton C, Arriaga MA. Otologic surgery, 3rd edn. Philadelphia, PA: Saunders/Elsevier; 2010. 1 online resource (xxi, 831pp.).
10. De la Cruz A, Teufert KB. Congenital aural atresia surgery: long-term results. Otolaryngol Head Neck Surg. 2003;129(1):121-7.
11. Teufert KB, De la Cruz A. Advances in congenital aural atresia surgery: effects on outcome. Otolaryngol Head Neck Surg. 2004;131(3):263-70.
12. Kountakis SE, Helidonis E, Jahrsdoerfer RA. Microtia grade as an indicator of middle ear development in aural atresia. Arch Otolaryngol Head Neck Surg. 1995;121(8):885-6.
13. Work WP. Newer concepts of first branchial cleft defects. Laryngoscope. 1972;82(9):1581-93.
14. Ebelhar AJ, Potts K. An unusual otoscopic finding associated with a type II first branchial cleft anomaly. J Laryngol Otol. 2012;126(3):316-8.
15. Goff CJ, Allred C, Glade RS. Current management of congenital branchial cleft cysts, sinuses, and fistulae. Curr Opin Otolaryngol Head Neck Surg. 2012;20(6):533-9.
16. Greywoode JD, Pribitkin EA, Krein H. Management of auricular hematoma and the cauliflower ear. Facial Plast Surg. 2010;26(6):451-5.
17. Mudry A, Pirsig W. Auricular hematoma and cauliflower deformation of the ear: from art to medicine. Otol Neurotol. 2009;30(1):116-20.
*18. Pham TV, Early SV, Park SS. Surgery of the auricle. Facial plastic surgery: FPS. 2003;19(1):53-74.
*19. Petrone P, Kuncir EJ, Asensio JA. Surgical management and strategies in the treatment of hypothermia and cold injury. Emer Med Clin N Am. 2003;21(4):1165-78.
*20. DeSanti L. Pathophysiology and current management of burn injury. Adv Skin Wound Care. 2005;18(6):323-32; quiz 32-4.
21. Roland PS, Stroman DW. Microbiology of acute otitis externa. Laryngoscope. 2002;112(7 Pt 1):1166-77.
22. Azizi MH. Ear disorders in scuba divers. Int J Occup Environ Med. 2011;2(1):20-26.
23. Kesser BW. Assessment and management of chronic otitis externa. Curr Opin Otolaryngol Head Neck Surg. 2011; 19(5):341-7.
24. Kaushik V, Malik T, Saeed SR. Interventions for acute otitis externa. Cochrane Database Syst Rev. 2010(1):CD004740.
25. Ho T, Vrabec JT, Yoo D. Otomycosis: clinical features and treatment implications. Otolaryngol Head Neck Surg. 2006; 135(5):787-91.
26. Lee JE, Song JJ, Oh SH, et al. Prognostic value of extension patterns on follow-up magnetic resonance imaging in patients with necrotizing otitis externa. Arch Otolaryngol Head Neck Surg. 2011;137(7):688-93.
*27. Rubin Grandis J, Branstetter BFt, Yu VL. The changing face of malignant (necrotising) external otitis: clinical, radiological, and anatomic correlations. Lancet Infect Dis. 2004;4(1):34-9.
28. Bieber T. Atopic dermatitis. N Engl J Med. 2008;358(14): 1483-94.
29. Correale CE, Walker C, Murphy L. Atopic dermatitis: a review of diagnosis and treatment. Am Fam Physician. 1999;60(4):1191-8, 209-10.
30. Farber EM. Ear psoriasis. Cutis. 1992;50(2):105-7.
31. Witmanowski H, Lewandowicz E, Sobieszek D. Facial skin cancers: general information and an overview of treatment methods. Postep Derm Alergol. 2012;XXIX(4):240-55.
32. Mohs F, Larson P, Iriondo M. Micrographic surgery for the microscopically controlled excision of carcinoma of the external ear. J Am Acad Dermatol. 1988;19(4):729-37.
33. Alam M, Ratner D. Cutaneous squamous-cell carcinoma. N Engl J Med. 2001;344(13):975-83.
34. Moody SA, Hirsch BE, Myers EN. Squamous cell carcinoma of the external auditory canal: an evaluation of a staging system. Am J Otol. 2000;21(4):582-8.
35. Cole MD, Jakowatz J, Evans GR. Evaluation of nodal patterns for melanoma of the ear. Plast Reconstr Surg. 2003;112(1):50-56.
*36. Devaney KO, Boschman CR, Willard SC. Tumours of the external ear and temporal bone. Lancet Oncol. 2005;6(6): 411-20.

*References with asterisks refer to critical sources.

CHAPTER

9

Malignant Tumors of the Temporal Bone

Amy L Rutt, Mary J Hawkshaw, Robert T Sataloff

INTRODUCTION

Temporal bone malignant neoplasms remain particularly challenging problems for otolaryngologists. Traditionally, surgical excision of the temporal bone has been subtotal. Consequently, it has been hampered by transgression of tumors and incomplete excision. The emergence of skull base surgery as a distinct discipline that incorporates neurotological, neurosurgical, and head and neck surgical skills has opened new frontiers in surgery of anatomically complex areas of the skull base. In an effort to improve upon treatment results, a new approach to temporal bone resection was devised and performed first in the anatomy laboratory, then in humans. As mentioned previously, the first report published of total en bloc resection of the temporal bone and carotid artery was in 1984.[1] Two additional cases were performed by the author (RTS) in 1984, and others have been operated upon at our center since that time. This experience and additional cadaver dissection have resulted in modifications of the technique and recognition of additional pitfalls.

Accurate assessment and treatment planning for temporal bone malignancies are dependent on computed tomography (CT) scanning of the bone erosion, and MR imaging of soft tissue involvement. Biopsy and clinical staging based on involvement of the ear, surrounding structures, and lymph nodes are required, of course. However, preoperative assessment often underestimates tumor extent. Though Leonetti et al.[2] found fairly good correlation between CT scanning, magnetic resonance imaging (MRI), and intraoperative findings, they emphasized critical exceptions in their series of 26 patients. Three patients had infratemporal fossa extensions without radiographic evidence, only 8 of 16 patients with posterior extension into the mastoid were identified, and superior extension was underestimated in nine patients. Surgically proven otic capsule involvement was not seen radiographically in four patients, and carotid canal extension was found in six patients who were believed to be clear in this area on MR imaging. These patients did poorly because their disease was more advanced. The only radiographic overestimation occurred in the otic capsule in which only one of three patients had actual invasion. Other studies also have reported difficulty estimating tumor extent with radiographs.[3,4]

All treatment of temporal bone cancer is based on whether the carcinoma has extended beyond the external auditory canal. In the development of surgery for temporal bone carcinoma, larger operations have evolved as surgical techniques for dura repair, carotid bypass, and reconstruction have developed. The three operations utilized include (1) piecemeal removal, (2) various modifications of subtotal total temporal bone resection (STBR), and (3) total temporal bone resection (TTBR).[5,6]

PATHOGENESIS

Temporal bone malignancy is rare, with squamous cell carcinoma the most common cancer of the external auditory canal, middle ear, and mastoid. Carcinoma of the temporal bone accounts for <0.2% of all tumors of the head and neck. Approximately 200 new cases of temporal bone cancer are diagnosed each year across the United States. That number includes cancers arising from skin of the pinna that spread to the temporal bone; primary tumors of the external auditory canal, middle ear, mastoid, or petrous apex; and metastatic lesions to the temporal bone.[7] There is no gender predominance, and most cases occur in the fifth and sixth decades of life. Definitive information about the treatment and prognosis of squamous cell carcinoma of the temporal bone is not easy to obtain due to a multitude of factors: the rarity of its malignancy, the lack of an accepted staging system prior to 1990, and the wide variety of individualized treatments. Also, many authors include tumors of various histologies in their reports of treatment outcomes, which further complicate intepretation.[8]

Human papillomavirus has been implicated in squamous cell carcinomas of the middle ear[9] as well. Lim et al.[10] reported a series of temporal bone cancers in seven patients who had undergone radiotherapy for nasopharyngeal carcinoma and with poor outcomes.

Chondrosarcomas account for 0.1% of all head and neck tumors and almost 6% of all skull base lesions.[11] There are a few different theories proposed as to how chondrosarcomas develop in the temporal bone. The bones of the skull base mature predominantly by endochondral ossification, while the bones of the skull vault develop primarily by intramembranous ossification.[12] The areas of the petro-occipital, spheno-occipital, and spheno-petrosal synchondroses, as well as a large part of the petrous portion of the temporal bone, are sites in the mature skull that underwent endochondral development.[13]

Osteosarcoma is a highly aggressive malignant tumor that usually presents in the metaphysis of long bones. The majority of cases occur between the ages of 10 and 30 years with the median age of 28. There are about 7400 new cases and 4200 deaths from osteosarcoma occurring annually in the United States. Approximately 10% of cases occur in the head and neck, and this accounts for about 900 new cases per year.[14,15] In a review of world literature, Sataloff et al.[16] found 19 reported cases of osteosarcoma involving the temporal bone, with the largest series reporting three cases. An additional three have been reported since then for a total of 22 cases,[16-21] since 1910. Almost every bone of the skull has been involved as a primary site; however, the mandible was clearly the most common primary location in the head and neck.[14,19-21]

Glomus jugulare tumors are rare, but when they occur, they may be extensive (Fig. 9.1). Usually they are histologically benign paragangliomas, but they can be aggressive and locally malignant in their behavior. Occasionally, they are malignant histologically and can metastasize.[22-36]

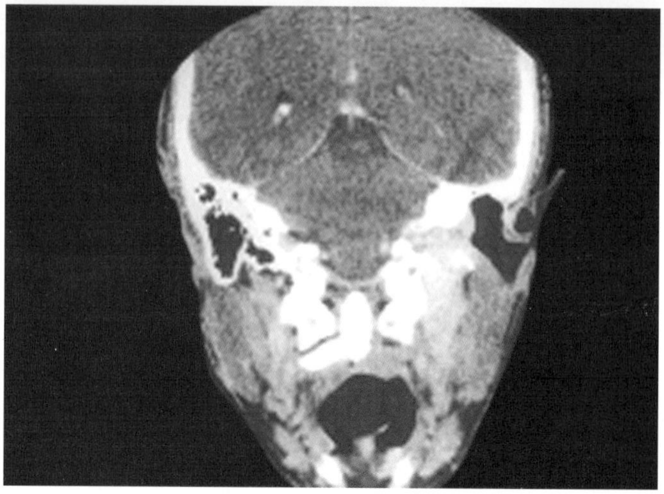

Fig. 9.1: Computed tomography (CT) scan shows a large recurrent glomus jugulare tumor in a 54-year-old man who had undergone incomplete, partial resection elsewhere followed by radiation. He presented with spontaneous hemorrhage through his mastoid cavity and is the only patient who has undergone total temporal bone resection for histologically benign disease.

CLINICAL FINDINGS: SYMPTOMS AND SIGNS

Defining specific etiologic factors for cancers in this area is very difficult. However, fair-skinned Caucasians are more prone to nonmelanomatous skin cancers throughout the body, especially areas exposed to ultraviolet radiation including the region of the ear. A genetic predisposition to skin cancer also may exist. Chronic otitis media and cholesteatoma are common in patients with temporal bone cancers and have been implicated as etiologic factors.[37,38]

Most of the time, it is the prolonged symptomatology nonresponsive to treatment that prompts further investigation; thus, the diagnosis often is delayed from 1 month to 5 years.[7,39,40] Hearing loss is present in many cases. The red flags should be history of persistent aural discharge associated with change in quality and/or quantity, development or increase in otalgia, cranial nerve VII paralysis, aural or mastoid polyp, and vertigo.

If complete resolution of symptoms does not occur after 2-to-3 weeks of vigorous medical therapy, it might be advisable to offer biopsy for temporal bone malignancy. Multiple authors have cautioned against reliance on a single biopsy results. They recommended strongly obtaining multiple deep biopsies including a cuff of normal tissue, even if general anesthesia or CT guidance is required. Inadequate biopsy may show only extensive inflammation and lead to delayed or missed diagnosis.[41,42-45]

Squamous cell carcinoma of the temporal bone remains a complex, challenging, and incompletely understood disease. However, it is not hopeless. Through aggressive treatment, even rare patients with advanced disease can be cured. Nevertheless, considerably more experience is needed before optimal treatment of all stages can be established with confidence.[8]

Primary sarcomas of the temporal bone are even more rare than primary carcinomas, but some are aggressive and lethal, such as osteogenic sarcoma. The literature contains scattered small series, case reports, and literature reviews of temporal bone sarcomas; however, most have too few cases to determine scientifically a superior treatment approach. Nevertheless, most reports provide an opinion or theory on how to handle these rare and aggressive tumors.[8] Nonrhabdomyosarcomas usually are treated with wide and/or radical surgical resection with varying protocols utilizing pre- and postoperative radiation and chemotherapy. Proton beam radiation has been used increasingly to treat chondrosarcomas and osteosarcomas of the temporal bone and skull base, with encouraging results. Further research and wider application may confirm this as a good radiation modality for all skull base sarcomas.[8]

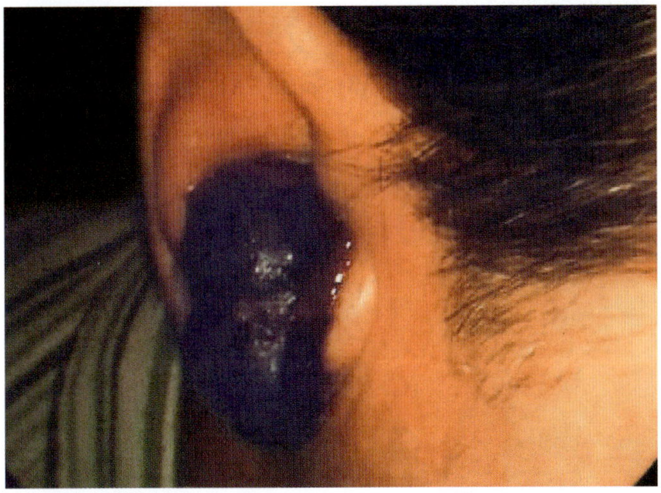

Fig. 9.2: A 52-year-old man with a nasopharyngeal chondrosarcoma protruding from the external auditory canal. Otoscopic examination revealed occlusion of the ear canal by the neoplasm.

Several clinical presentations have been reported for chondrosarcomas of the skull base. The symptoms correlate with the anatomic site of destruction or compression. Initial complaints may include hearing loss, pulsatile tinnitus, vertigo/unsteadiness, aural fullness, and headache (Figs. 9.2 to 9.5). Multiple cranial neuropathies are common and present as diplopia, facial pain, paresthesias, hemifacial spasm, facial paresis, dysphagia, hoarseness, shoulder weakness, and hemi-tongue weakness and atrophy.

In most studies of head and neck osteosarcoma, the most common presentation is pain and swelling over the area of the bone containing the lesion[15] (Fig. 9.6). In their review of 19 patients with osteosarcoma of the temporal bone, Sataloff et al.[16] reported that the most common presenting symptoms and signs were a mass in the temporal fossa, mastoid, or external ear canal in 84% (16/19), facial paralysis in 47% (9/19), conductive hearing loss

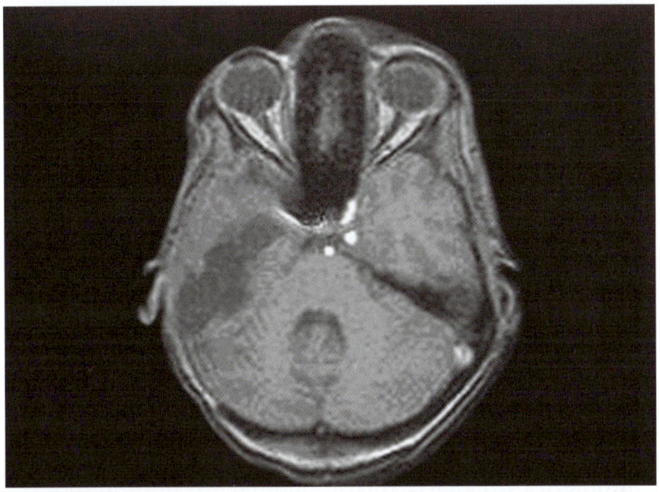

Fig. 9.3: Magnetic resonance imaging (MRI) of the brain and internal auditory canals revealing a right skull base chondrosarcoma measuring at least 5 cm with a small area of extra-axial extension into the right posterior fossa over the cerebellar hemisphere.

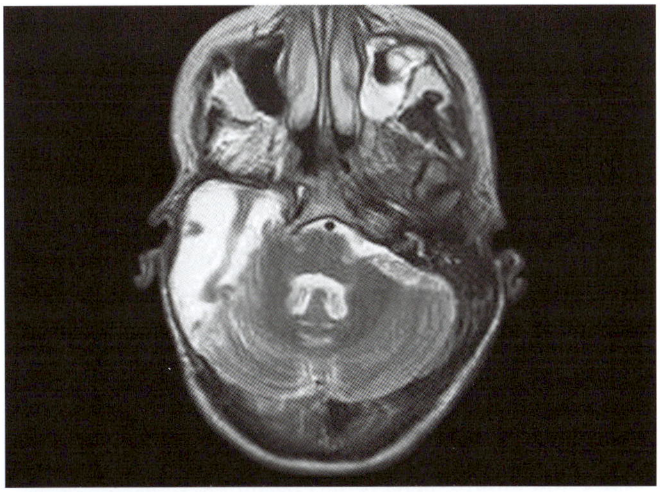

Fig. 9.4: Computed tomography (CT) of the brain and internal auditory canals revealing a right skull base chondrosarcoma measuring at least 5 cm with a small area of extra-axial extension into the right posterior fossa over the cerebellar hemisphere.

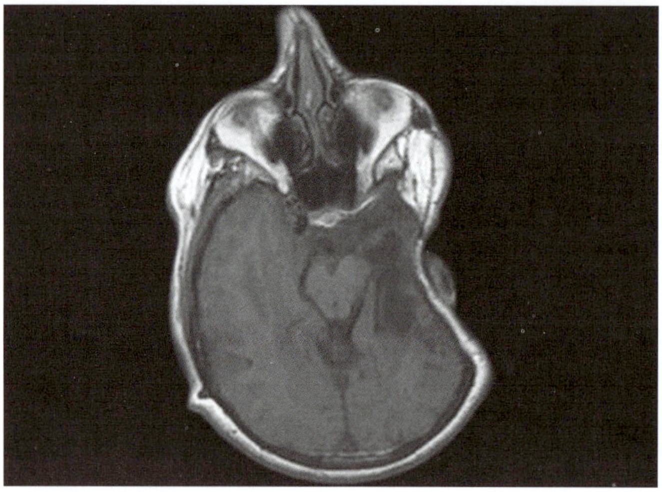

Fig. 9.5: Magnetic resonance imaging (MRI) showing a portion of resection of a patient with a grade 2 chondrosarcoma. Gross total tumor resection was accomplished.

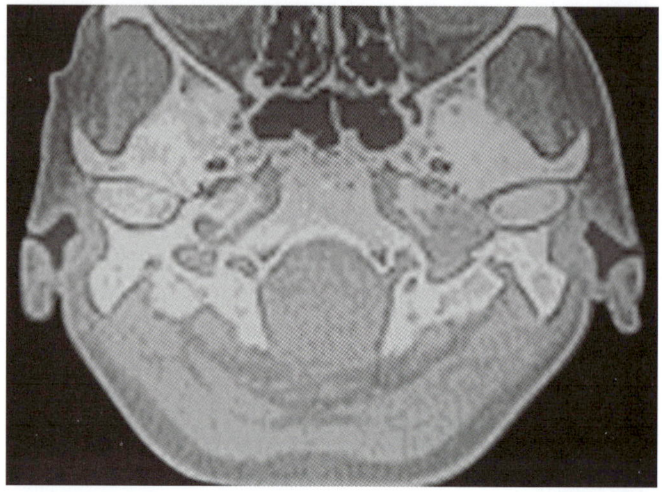

Fig. 9.6: Computed tomography (CT) scan shows malignant destruction of the left temporal bone in a 37-year-old woman with osteosarcoma.

in 37% (7/19), otalgia in 32% (6/19), bloody or purulent otorrhea in 16% (3/19), and other cranial nerve deficits in 16% (3/19). As with other skull base and temporal bone malignancies, symptoms caused by cranial nerve deficits are determined by the site of tumor involvement. Hearing loss and tinnitus are frequently the only symptoms of typical glomus tumors. This peculiar neoplasm arises from cells around the jugular bulb and expands to involve the neighboring structures[46] (Fig. 9.7).

In doing so, the neoplasm most frequently extends to the floor of the middle ear, causing conductive hearing loss and pulsatile tinnitus. As the disease progresses, it may appear as chronic otitis media and may even extend through the eardrum and appear to be granulation tissue in the ear canal. Biopsy of this apparent granulation tissue may cause profuse bleeding because of the marked vascularity of the tumor. As the disease extends, it may destroy portions of the temporal bone and jugular bulb and can extend intracranially.[8]

EVALUATION

The assessment of tumor invasion into soft tissue along fascial planes, perineural spread, and CNS infiltration is accomplished best with MRI.[47,48] MRI with contrast is now the study of choice for evaluation of the skull base, especially the common sites of invasion: the petroclinoid fissure and foramen lacerum (Fig. 9.8).

Despite the great sensitivity of radiological studies, intra-operative evaluation is of undisputed importance, and limitations of radiography have been recognized.[8]

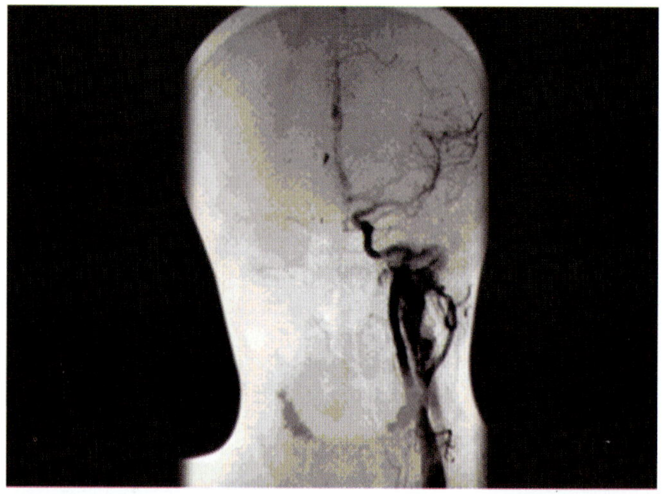

Fig. 9.7: Angiogram of the same 54-year-old man from Figure 9.1 with a large recurrent glomus tumor with intracranial extension.

A comprehensive neurotologic workup is indicated when temporal bone lesions are suspected. The workup includes pure tone and speech audiometry, CT of the temporal bones and brain, MRI/MRA, as well as any other tests that are indicated clinically[13,49] (Figs. 9.9 and 9.10).

Radiological evaluation is now the mainstay of glomus tumor diagnosis. CT of the temporal bone is used to assess bone erosion, and MRI, MR angiography, traditional arteriography, and retrograde jugular venography are used to define the extent of the neoplasm. Four vessel arteriograms are now being recommended by some otologists because of the high incidence of associated tumors. Up to 10% of patients with glomus tumors of the ear have associated contralateral glomus tumors, glomus vagale, carotid

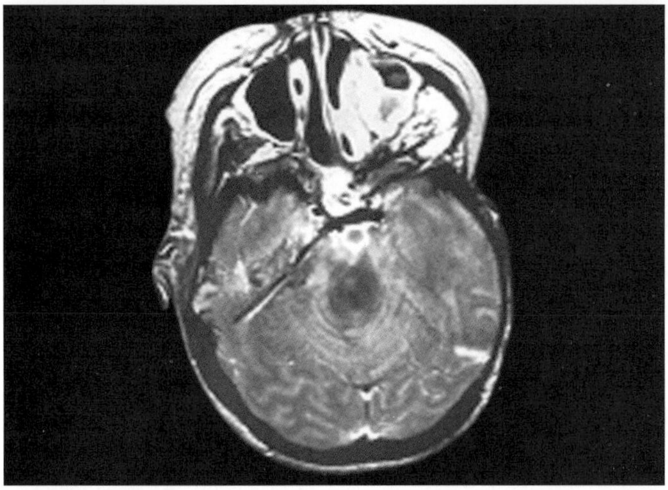

Fig. 9.8: Magnetic resonance imaging (MRI) showing tumor invasion of skull base, foramen lacerum, and posterior aspect of cavernous sinus of a 39-year-old woman with adenocarcinoma of the skull base.

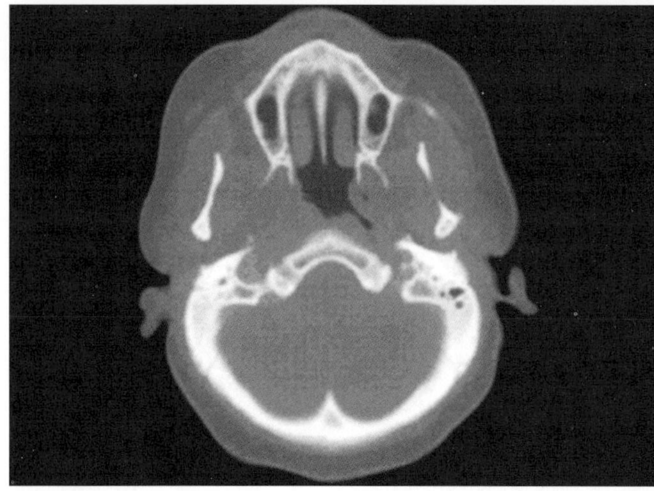

Fig. 9.9: Preoperative computed tomography (CT) showing partial destruction of the right side of the skull base from a patient with right nasopharyngeal squamous cell carcinoma extending from the tonsillar pillar into the parapharyngeal space and eroding through the foramen ovale and into the temporal bone.

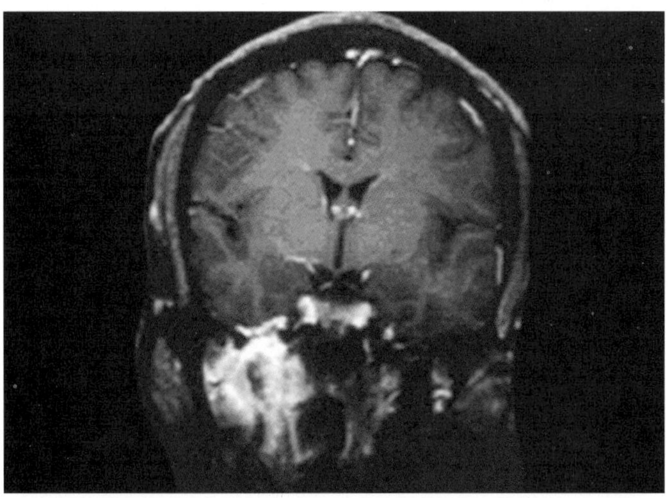

Fig. 9.10: Magnetic resonance showing portion of the nasopharyngeal tumor increasing the size and decreasing the definition of parapharyngeal space, suggesting aggressive neoplasm.

body tumor, or thyroid carcinoma.[46] Biopsy may be used appropriately to rule out other lesions and in patients who are not surgical candidates prior to instituting palliative radiation therapy.[8] Glomus tumors are discussed in greater detail elsewhere in this book.

HISTOLOGY

Chondrosarcomas may arise from pluripotent mesenchymal cells involved in the embryogenesis of the skull base and temporal bone. Alternatively, metaplasia of mature fibroblasts has been implicated as an inciting mechanism in the development of chondosarcomas.[50,51]

Primary chondrosarcoma develops de novo in normal bone (Fig. 9.11A). Most temporal bone chondrosarcomas appear to arise in this manner. Rarely, there are secondary chondrosarcomas that arise from pre-existing cartilaginous tumors or abnormalities. Chondrosarcoma has been reported in association with Paget's disease, Maffucci syndrome, osteocartilagenous exostoses, Ollier disease, and osteochondromas.[52,53]

Osteosarcoma is thought to arise from immature bone-forming cells or through neoplastic differentiation of other mesenchymal cells into osteoblasts. Histologically, a tumor is considered to be an osteosarcoma if it demonstrates malignant spindle cells producing osteoid in various stromal backgrounds (Fig. 9.11B). Subtypes are based on the predominant characteristic of the cells and stroma and include osteoblastic, chondroblastic, fibroblastic, small cell, and telangiectatic.[18-21]

TREATMENT

Rarity of the disease poses challenges not only with the development of a uniform classification but also with management strategies. The Pittsburgh Grading System is used commonly (Fig. 9.12). Despite technological advances, skull base surgery continues to be complex. It requires operative efforts between a patient and an extensive team of professionals. The goal of management is to be curative;

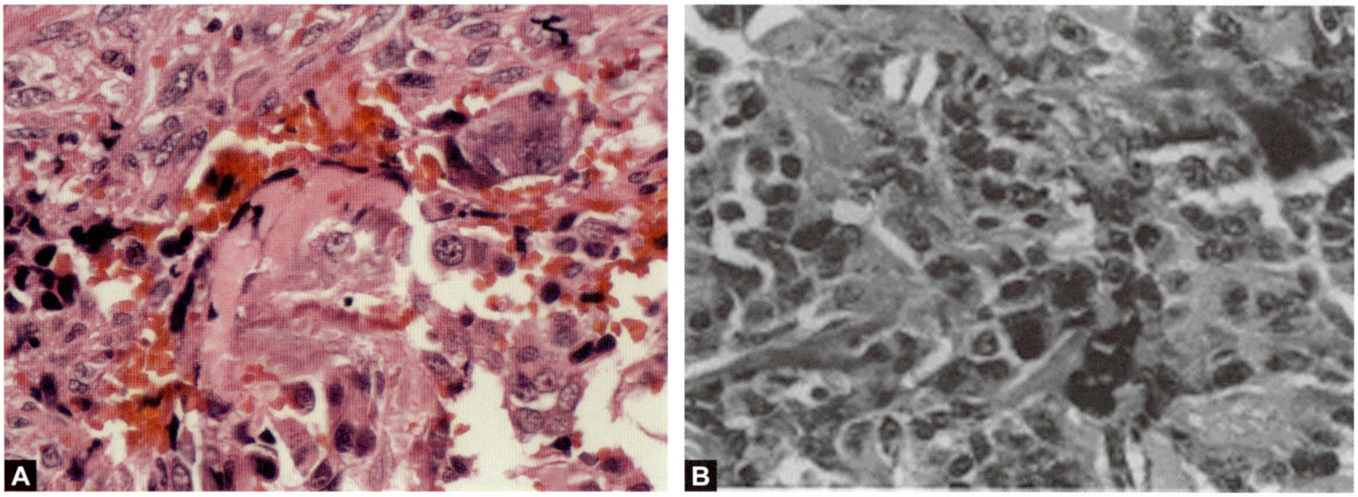

Figs. 9.11A and B: (A) Histology chondrosarcoma of the temporal bone showing chondroid matrix with increased cellularity and binucleate cells. High-grade chondrosarcomas are characterized by high cellularity, prominent nuclear atypia, and mitosis. (B) Histology of an osteogenic sarcoma resected from one of our patients shows high-grade, anaplastic, pleomorphic spindle cells, large hyperchromatic nuclei with osteoid production.

University of Pittsburgh Tumor Lymph Node Metastasis Staging System

T STATUS

T1-Tumor limited to the external auditory canal wilhout bony erosion or evidence of soft tissue extension.

T2-Tumor with limited external auditory canal bony erosion (not full-thickness) or radiographic finding consistent with limited (<0.5 cm) soft tissue involvement.

T3-Tumor eroding osseous external auditory canal (full-thickness) with limited (<0.5 cm) soft tissue involvement, or tumor involving middle ear or mastoid, or patients presenting with facial paralysis.

T4-Tumor eroding cochlea, petrous apex, medial wall of the middle ear, carotid canal, jugular formen, or dura, or with extensive (>0.5 cm) soft tissue involvement.

N STATUS

Involvement of lymph nodes is a poor prognostic finding and automatically places patient in advanced stage (i.e., stage III [T1, N1] or stage IV [T2, T3, and T4, N1] disease).

M STATUS

Distant metastasis indicates poor prognosis and immediately places patient in stage IV.

Fig. 9.12: The Pittsburgh Grading System.

yet, due to the nature of the temporal bone, complete excision of tumor, whether piecemeal or en bloc, is often difficult once the tumor extends beyond the external auditory canal.[8]

A few articles have reviewed the role of radiotherapy as single modality therapy. Kang et al.[54] concluded that radiotherapy alone was not inferior to combined surgery and radiotherapy for disease-specific survival, but they found that local control was worse when radiotherapy alone was used (Figs. 9.13A to C). Advances in skull base techniques proved its current role as primary therapy, using radiotherapy as a postoperative adjuvant. The combination of these two modalities has improved overall survival for patients who have temporal bone cancer.[55,56]

Currently, radiotherapy is recommended for T2 and higher staged tumors.[6,57-59] Other indications for postoperative radiotherapy include recurrent tumors, positive margins, perineural spread, positive lymph nodes, or extracapsular spread.[56] Intensity modulated radiotherapy allows the radiation oncologist the ability to adequately treat the tumor site and minimize dose to surrounding structures, especially the temporal lobe and brainstem. Dosages vary widely in the literature. Pfreundner et al.[4] recommended 54 to 60 Gy in patients with negative margins and a minimum of 66 Gy with positive margins. Prabhu et al.[60] gave doses between 60 and 66 Gy for patients with negative margins and doses between 68 and 72 Gy for patients with positive or close margins.

Only a few isolated studies have examined the role of chemotherapy for temporal bone cancers.[61-63] Nakagawa et al.[61] described a series of 25 patients with primary SCCa of the ear canal and middle ear. Six patients (T2: 1 patient; T3: 3 patients; T4: 2 patients) received preoperative chemotherapy followed by surgery and radiotherapy. Five of these six patients achieved mean survival of 60 months. Chemotherapy and radiotherapy alone were used in 7 patients with T4 disease; 3 of these 7 patients had no evidence of disease at mean of 31.6 months.

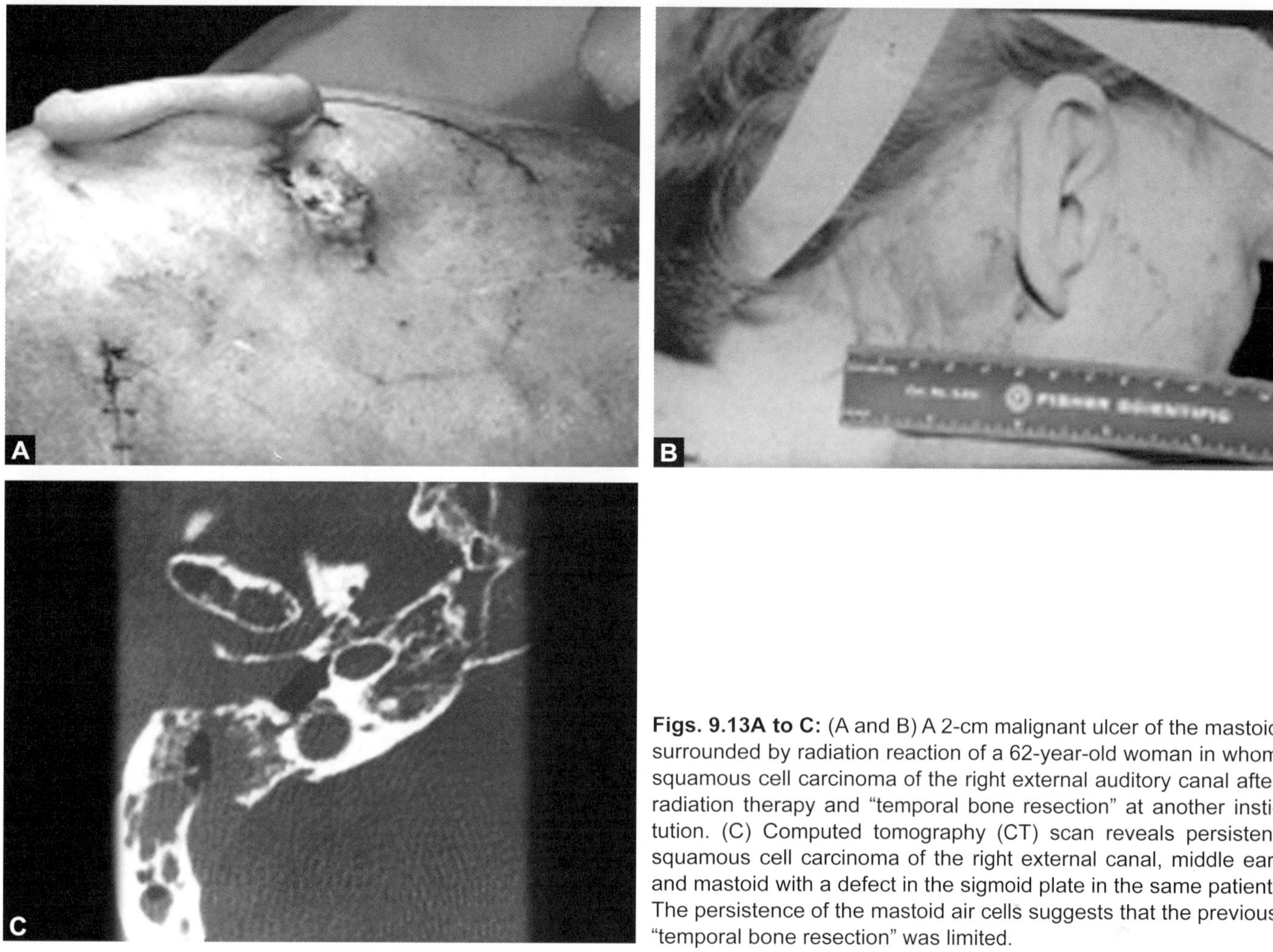

Figs. 9.13A to C: (A and B) A 2-cm malignant ulcer of the mastoid surrounded by radiation reaction of a 62-year-old woman in whom squamous cell carcinoma of the right external auditory canal after radiation therapy and "temporal bone resection" at another institution. (C) Computed tomography (CT) scan reveals persistent squamous cell carcinoma of the right external canal, middle ear, and mastoid with a defect in the sigmoid plate in the same patient. The persistence of the mastoid air cells suggests that the previous "temporal bone resection" was limited.

In a pilot study, Shiga et al.[62] described a series of 14 patients with SCCa of the temporal bone, of whom 9 had stage IV disease and were treated with concomitant chemoradiotherapy. Their chemotherapy regimen included docetaxel, cisplatin, and 5-fluorouracil (TPF). Eight of nine patients achieved complete response. These investigators concluded that the use of concomitant chemotherapy with TPF was safe and effective as a treatment of patients with cancer of the temporal bone.[62]

Intra-arterial chemotherapy has been proposed and tested in a few patients. Sugimoto et al.[63] published a small series of five patients with T3 and T4 SCCa of the temporal bone who were treated with radiotherapy and intra-arterial chemotherapy consisting of cisplatin and thiosulfate. Three patients obtained a complete response and had mean survival of 28 months.

For extensive disease of the middle ear or involvement of the pneumatized spaces, TTBR may provide better oncologic control. In the original description of the procedure by Graham et al., the vascular and neural structures of the petrous apex are included with the resection.[16] The goal of the procedure is en bloc removal of the tumor without tumor transgression, providing tumor-free margins.[8]

TTBR is a formidable procedure, which commonly requires 18–24 hours, and is associated with substantial blood loss (although the author [RTS] has performed one case successfully without transfusion in a Jehovah's witness). It should be performed only as a curative operation in patients who are physiologically and psychologically prepared to tolerate the procedure and a prolonged recovery. Paralysis of cranial nerves VI–XII is planned, and the patient and family must be thoroughly informed before this method is chosen. If the tumor encroaches upon the internal carotid artery, preoperative balloon test occlusion should be performed to determine the perfusion capacity of the contralateral side. This will help determine whether the patient is able to tolerate the resection of the internal carotid artery or will require intracranial bypass surgery.[8].

Treatment approaches for chondrosarcoma have evolved throughout the years and include combinations of surgical debulking, complete surgical excision, radiation, and chemotherapy. Although most studies report a treatment bias, the paucity of patients with chondrosarcoma of the temporal bone makes it impossible to perform prospective trials that could lead to definitive treatment conclusions. Anecdotal protocols are common. Due to a concern that surgical debulking violates tumor boundaries and oncologic principles, the concept of total en bloc resection with total gross removal of disease has been suggested as the preferred surgical procedure when removing chondrosarcoma of the skull base and temporal bone.[8]

Treatment of osteogenic sarcoma has varied widely, and follow-up was inconsistent or not reported in nearly one-third of the cases. Consequently, treatment protocols for temporal bone osteosarcoma have to be extrapolated from series reporting osteosarcomas located in the head, neck, and other body sites. Authors including Sataloff et al.[41, 16] and Sharma et al.[15] support radical resection of temporal bone osteosarcoma with the use of adjuvant radiation and chemotherapy.

SURGICAL TECHNIQUES

Partial Temporal Bone Resection

Sleeve Resection

Lesions in the ear canal lateral to the bony cartilaginous junction may be amenable to a sleeve resection. With this technique, a medial incision is used to assure that the bony cartilaginous junction is not involved. A lateral incision encompasses the lesion, surrounding skin and underlying cartilage. The specimen is removed, and reconstruction may involve a split thickness thin graft or other techniques.

Partial Temporal Bone Resection and Lateral Temporal Bone Resection

Partial temporal bone resection (PTBR) refers to removal of the bony and cartilaginous external auditory canal. The term often is used interchangeably with lateral temporal bone resection (LTBR) (Fig. 9.14).

Lesions that extend medially to the bony cartilaginous junction without involvement of the tympanic membrane or annulus may be treated with a lateral PTBR or LTBR. Tumors of the periauricular skin that extend into the auditory canal and the parotid gland immediately adjacent to, adhering to, or superficially invading the temporal bone but not invading the middle ear space or aerated spaces of the mastoid also may be treated with LTBR. Occasionally, such surgery may be appropriate for tumors in other locations (Figs. 9.15A and B). Following a complete mastoidectomy that is extended well into the zygomatic root, an en bloc resection of the bony external auditory canal and skin is performed. The specimen usually includes the entire bony and cartilaginous external auditory canal wall with the tympanic membrane. The medial resection plane includes the tympanic membrane, malleus and incus, and the most lateral resection margin includes at least the conchal and tragal cartilage surrounding the external auditory meatus. When appropriate, parotidectomy and selective neck dissection may be included. A split thickness skin graft with bolster often is used for closure.

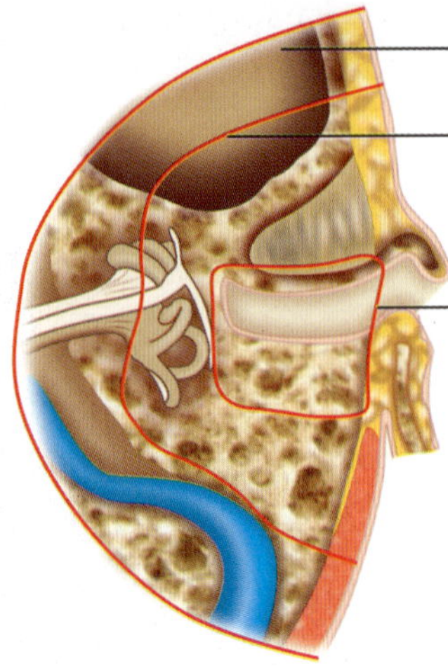

Fig. 9.14: Typical limits of lateral, subtotal, and total temporal bone resection.

Piecemeal Removal

In prior years, temporal bone cancers were handled with piecemeal removal. This operation essentially was a large mastoidectomy in which the surgeon drilled through tumor and removed it as well as possible. Results were poor, and this approach is not recommended.

Subtotal Resection

Tumors that invade the middle ear or aerated spaces of the mastoid bone have been treated traditionally with a STBR combined with parotidectomy and selective neck dissection. STBR removes the temporal bone lateral to the internal carotid artery, and inferiorly to the jugular foramen, leaving only the petrous apex. A temporal

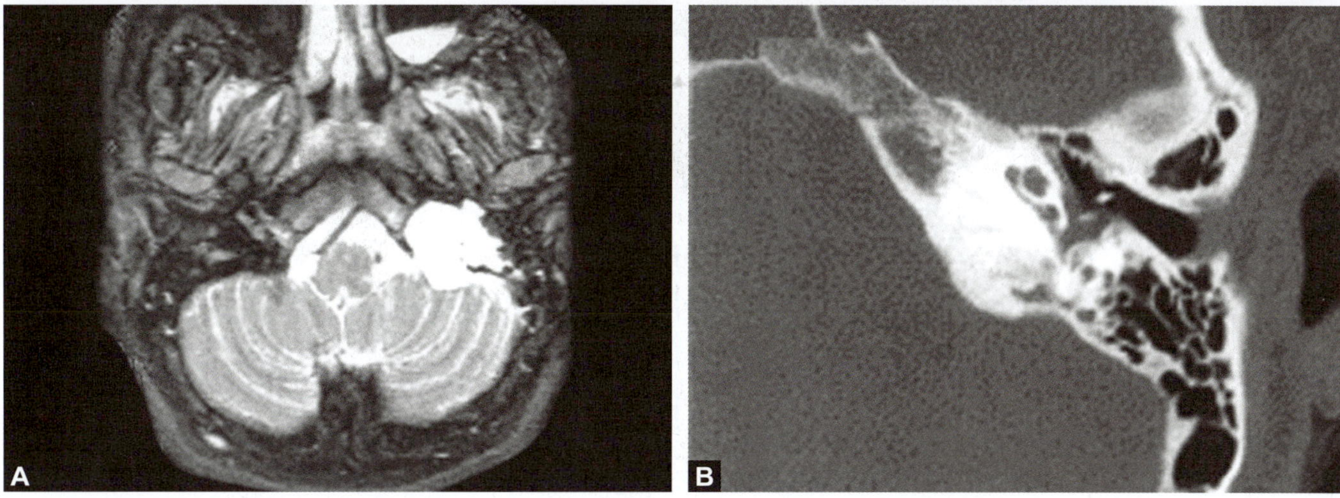

Figs. 9.15A and B: (A) A magnetic resonance imaging (MRI) of a 66-year-old woman with a stage IV, poorly differentiated adenocarcinoma in the jugular foramen with nonspecific enhancement of the seventh and eighth cranial nerves in the internal auditory canals, geniculate ganglion, and descending portion of the nerve. (B) A computed tomography (CT) showing destruction within the left temporal bone of same patient. This patient was prepared for total en bloc temporal bone resection with middle and posterior fossa craniotomy, although only a modified resection was required. The tumor was removed in its entirety with margins using an extended subtotal resection without total temporal bone resection.

craniotomy is performed to allow access to the internal auditory canal (IAC) and define the intracranial margin of the tumor resection. Tumor may be resected if it involves dura only, but if it extends into brain parenchyma, most surgeons consider the tumor inoperable. The temporal lobe is identified superiorly, and the posterior fossa is uncovered posteriorly. The great vessels are controlled in the neck, and a total parotidectomy is performed. The facial nerve is identified within the parotid gland and may be preserved. The mandibular condyle is sectioned, and bone is divided from the middle fossa superiorly, internal carotid artery (ICA) (preserved) anteroinferiorly, and the IAC medially. The jugular bulb and sigmoid sinus are unroofed with a mastoidectomy. The ICA is skeletonized anterior to the jugular bulb, and is exposed in its vertical and horizontal petrous segments. Piecemeal removal of residual tumors may be necessary after this resection, and tumor usually is seen during this approach and often is violated.

Total Temporal Bone Resection

The goal of surgery is en bloc resection of the temporal bone "without seeing tumor".[59] This procedure is appropriate for fully informed patients with tumors traditionally considered unresectable and lethal, who have no metastatic disease, are in good health, and are willing to accept the formidable morbidity and mortality to achieve a chance of cure. Occasionally, there also may be a role for STBR. Using traditional approaches less extensive than TTBR, it may be extremely difficult or impossible not to violate a tumor margin, especially if tumor size is underestimated by imaging studies.

A partial mastoidectomy to expose the sigmoid sinus, e.g. may expose air cells in continuity with the middle ear or mastoid tumor. Carotid artery dissection necessarily comes in close contact with the anterior extension of middle ear tumors. Even with a large resection, some piecemeal resection may be necessary, especially in the occipital condyle, clivus, carotid canal, or cavernous sinus.[60,61] The senior author (RTS) has made some previously unreported changes in his protocol: (1) the procedure has been extended to include the cavernous sinus and clivus in selected cases; (2) preoperative carotid artery screening is performed with temporary balloon occlusion rather than a Silverstein clamp; (3) the carotid artery is occluded below the ophthalmic artery by our interventional radiologist within a few days before the definitive resection; and (4) carotid artery bypass grafting, if necessary, should be from the contralateral internal carotid artery to the ipsilateral internal carotid artery with the graft passing across the head, removing this life-sustaining graft from the surgical field. Because much of the external carotid artery system is sacrificed during this operation, and because substantial manipulation is required to extract the temporal bone, risk to a graft based on the ipsilateral carotid artery is excessively high.

Technique for Total Temporal Bone Resection

TTBR is performed in two stages. The first stage used to involve placement of a Silverstone or Kindt clamp around the internal carotid artery that was occluded over 3 days with the patient awake. In recent years, this procedure has been abandoned in favor of preoperative balloon occlusion and Xenon flow studies. Surgery also used to involve division of the internal carotid artery intracranially below the ophthalmic artery. Now, the carotid artery is occluded in this region by the interventional radiologist using coils, shortly before surgery. It is important to establish that the patient will be able to tolerate resection of the internal carotid artery system before proceeding with surgery. If that is not the case, intracranial bypass from the other carotid artery may be performed. A bypass from the ipsilateral side should not be used because of risk to the graft during the extensive manipulation required for a TTBR. All of our patients have sustained deep vein thrombosis despite precautions. Consequently, a Greenfield filter also is placed preoperatively. We also often place a ventriculoperitoneal shunt preoperatively. In selected cases, when there is question as to the adequacy of venous outflow, a catheter is placed in the venous system and occluded later with the patient awake to be certain that the patient will tolerate resection of intracranial sinuses and the jugular system.[64]

Definitive resection occurs as a second stage. The operation includes:

1. Adequate padding. Intraoperative decubitus ulceration can occur.
2. A temperature probe and temperature control blanket are required.
3. A Swan-Ganz catheter, arterial monitoring catheter, central venous catheter, and peripheral venous catheters. All IV sites are monitored every 30 minutes during the procedure. Unrecognized infiltration from an IV line can result in compartment syndrome and loss of a limb.
4. A lumbar spinal drain if a ventriculoperitoneal shunt has not been placed.
5. A Foley catheter and nasogastric tube.
6. Intermittent compression stockings and other thrombophlebitis prophylaxis measures.
7. Perioperative steroids and antibiotics.
8. Tracheotomy.
9. The patient's head is shaved and placed in the Mayfield tongs (Fig. 9.16).
10. The ipsilateral eye is protected with ointment and Frost stitches, and the contralateral eye is protected.

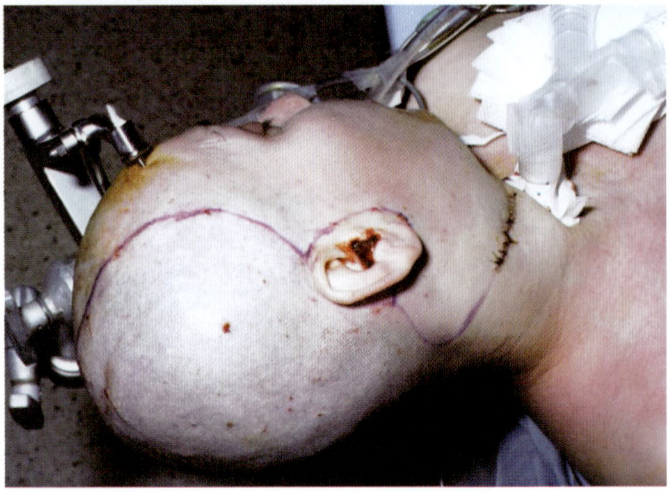

Fig. 9.16: This figure illustrates part of the second stage of the definitive resection. After placement of adequate padding, temperature probe and blanket, Swan-Ganz catheter, arterial monitoring catheter, central venous catheter, peripheral venous catheter, lumbar spinal drain, Foley catheter, nasogastric tube, tracheotomy, the patient's shaved head is placed in Mayfield tongs.

11. The head, neck, abdomen and leg are prepared and draped. Fascia lata may be harvested later in the case, as well as muscle.
12. The incision is designed to optimize preservation of the blood supply to the flaps, allow adequate excision of the lesion being treated, and facilitate primary wound closure when possible.
13. If the patient's internal carotid artery has not already been occluded preoperatively, it is occluded intracranially at this point. Delaying this maneuver until later in the procedure during early cases resulted in embolism of clot that occurred following carotid occlusion in the neck performed before intracranial occlusion.
14. The facial and neck flaps are elevated.
15. The upper neck is dissected and the carotid sheath is exposed. If required, neck dissection and parotidectomy are performed. The great vessels are identified in the neck, and the carotid artery and jugular vein are occluded and divided.
16. A craniotomy is performed to provide broad exposure of the posterior and middle fossae.
17. The superior petrosal sinus is occluded with bipolar cautery approximately 0.5 cm posterior to the cavernous sinus. Attempts to occlude the superior petrosal sinus closer to the cavernous sinus result in bleeding from the cavernous sinus that is difficult to control.
18. The brain stem is retracted gently in order to visualize the inferior petrosal sinus, jugular foramen and foramen magnum.

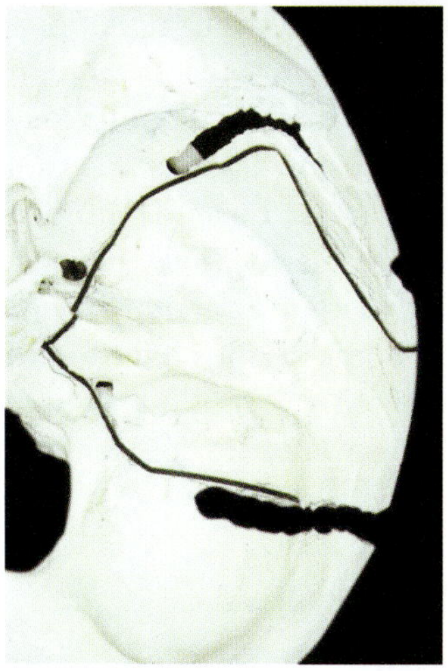

Fig. 9.17: Skull showing the bone cuts and segment of the skull base removed for total temporal bone resection.

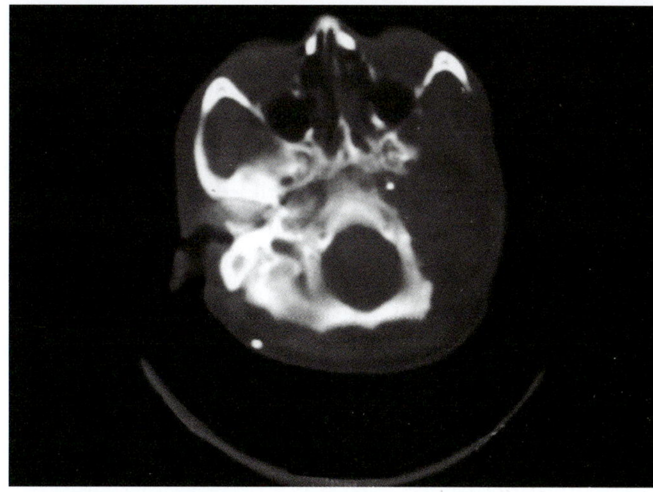

Fig. 9.18: Postoperative computed tomography (CT) scan demonstrating segment of the skull base removed for total temporal bone resection of a 37-year-old woman with osteogenic sarcoma.

19. The anterior lateral bone cut (Fig. 9.17) is made through the lateral skull wall connecting the anterior petrous apex with the neck, the carotid canal just proximal to the cavernous sinus, the superior petrosal sinus, freeing the anterior middle cranial fossa floor. In our original reports, these bone cuts were made with a drill. Since the latter 1980s, the author (RTS) has used a curved chisel. The final bone cuts are made with a chisel extending from posterior to anterior, coursing within an approximately 5 mm of the foramen magnum. The final cut is through the inferior petrosal sinus. The bleeding is controlled with Surgicel (Fig. 9.18).
20. This resection includes the jugular venous system with the sigmoid, superior petrosal and inferior petrosal sinuses, the carotid artery, and cranial nerves VI–XII. If the patient has tolerated the procedure well, the residual facial nerve can be grafted to the brain stem at this time (Fig. 9.19). Experience has shown that attempts to save cranial nerve VI are ill advised.
21. A fascia lata graft is used to close the dura.
22. It is essential that the soft tissue of the eustachian tube be closed with a purse string suture. Failure to perform this maneuver results in cerebral spinal fluid leak through the eustachian tube (since the entire bony eustachian tube has been removed).
23. The wound is closed primarily if possible. The entire external ear has been resected, (Fig. 9.20) and if surrounding skin resection is too extensive to permit primary closure, closure can be accomplished either through Galal relaxing incisions, advancement of the craniotomy flap leaving a secondary defect over intact skull (which may be managed with a skin graft and covered with a wig at the time of discharge), or a free flap (Figs. 9.21A and B).

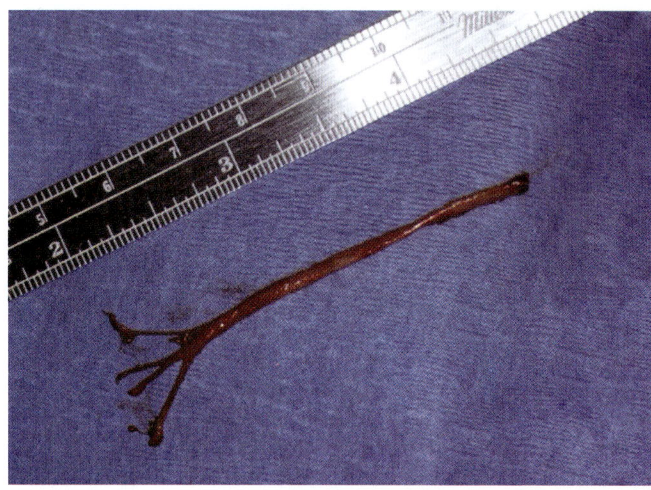

Fig. 9.19: Greater auricular nerve that can be grafted to the brain stem and facial nerve branches after resection of the facial nerve in the temporal bone.

PROGNOSIS

To date, no treatment-control studies have been reported. Most of the many treatment approaches are based on individual experience. In 1994, Prasad and Janecka[65] attempted to gain perspective on the role of surgery in the management of malignant tumors of the temporal bone. They reviewed the available literature and selected 26 publications that had comparable data. From the data analysis of 144 patients, they made the following suggestions: (a) tumors limited to the external auditory canal have a 50% overall cure rate after mastoidectomy or LTBR or STBR; (b) addition of radiation therapy after LTBR does not appear to be advantageous; (c) compared with mastoidectomy and LTBR, STBR improves survival once the tumor involves the middle ear. It may appear that conclusions made from such an in-depth study would hold true, and indeed, multiple authors continue to use their suggestions. However, upon a closer examination, one finds that for each treatment modality the patients' sample size remained small. The staging system they used was limited: tumor confined to the external auditory canal, tumor extended into the middle ear, and tumor invading the petrous apex. Moreover, radiation protocols and techniques have changed. Furthermore, multiple studies (prospective and retrospective) published since 1994 have disputed their conclusions.[8]

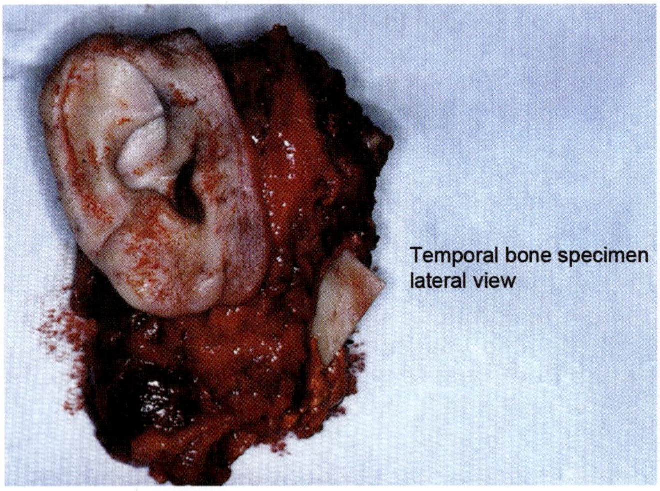

Fig. 9.20: Resection of the entire external ear and surrounding skin, and a portion of the mandible in a patient with osteogenic sarcoma of the temporal bone.

Several factors are associated with decreased survival rates. These include the local extent of the tumor, facial paralysis, positive margins, dural involvement, and lymph node metastasis. Some studies have found that advanced age (< 60–65 years old),[66,67] multiple cranial nerve involvement, moderate-to-severe pain, and female sex may worsen prognosis.[68,69]

CONCLUSION

The optimal management of temporal bone cancer remains unclear because of continued debate regarding staging, the utility of preoperative radiographic evaluation, the value of nonsurgical management with radiation and/or chemotherapy, nomenclature of surgical procedures, and the use of adjuvant radiation. The limited number of cases of temporal bone malignancies at each individual institution precludes definitive conclusions regarding the optimal management protocol.[7]

Total en bloc temporal bone resection can be performed successfully in the hands of an experienced skull base surgical team. This procedure allows resection of extensive, carefully selected, malignant tumors, and maybe appropriate very rarely for histologically benign but biologically aggressive neoplasms. Each new case brings about refinements in technique. Protection against deep vein thrombosis preoperatively has become routine.

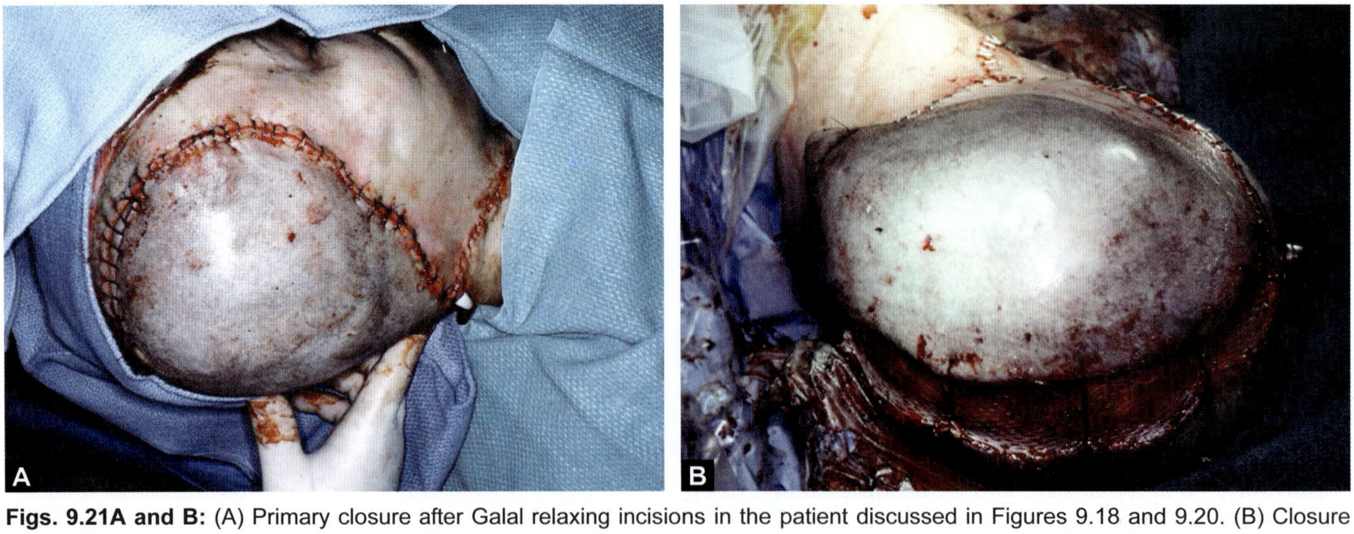

Figs. 9.21A and B: (A) Primary closure after Galal relaxing incisions in the patient discussed in Figures 9.18 and 9.20. (B) Closure accomplished through Galal relaxing incisions and advancement of the craniotomy flap, leaving a secondary defect over intact skull. This can be closed with a skin graft (illustrated) or free flap.

Carotid balloon occlusion testing also has become routine. Experience has shown that it is possible to extend resection beyond the midline, if necessary; and when the inferior aspect of the cavernous sinus is involved, partial resection of the sinus with preservation of nerves is possible. The interest, expertise, and active participation of the operating room nursing team are critical to the success of this surgery. Not only intraoperative nursing participation but also preoperative assessment and postoperative support require special expertise and dedication. Close cooperation and extensive communication among the surgeons, nurses, and consultants are essential.[9] Mortality and morbidity are high, and ideal candidates are young, healthy people with localized disease considered lethal, and regarded traditionally as unresectable. Rarely, intraoperative evaluation and modification to a somewhat less extensive procedure are appropriate. However, in general, patients and the health-care team should be prepared to proceed with the total en bloc resection "without seeing tumor" in order to give these patients with deadly disease at least some chance of cure.

REFERENCES

1. Graham MD, Sataloff RT, Kemink JL, et al. Total en bloc resection of the temporal bone and carotid artery for malignant tumors of the ear and temporal bone. Laryngoscope. 1984;94(4):528-33.
2. Leonetti JP, Smith PG, Kletzker GR, et al. Invasion patterns of advanced temporal bone malignancies. Am J Otol. 1996; 17:438-42.
3. Kenyon GS, Marks PV, Scholtz CL, et al. Squamous cell carcinoma of the middle ear: a 25 year retrospective study. Ann Otol Rhinol Laryngol. 1985;94:273-77.
4. Pfreundner L, Schwager K, Willner J, et al. Carcinoma of the EAC and middle ear. Int J Radiat Oncol Biol Phys. 1999; 44:777-88.
5. Moffat DA, Chiossone-Kerdel JA, Da Cruz M. Squamous cell carcinoma. In: Jackler RK, Driscoll CLW (eds), Tumors of the Ear and Temporal Bone. Philadelphia: Lippincott, Williams, and Wilkins; 2000. pp. 67-83.
6. Moffat DA, Grey P, Ballagh RH, et al. Extended temporal bone resection for squamous cell carcinoma. Otolaryngol Head Neck Surg. 1997;116:617-23.
7. Antonio SM, Hirsch BE. Malignant tumors of the temporal bone. EMedicine. Available from: hrrp://www.emedicine.com/ent/topic476.html [Retrieved on Aug 15, 2007].
8. Sataloff RT, Sataloff J. Hearing Loss. Fourth edition. Boca Raton, FL: CRC Press; 2006. pp. 545-602.
9. Jin YT, Tsai Li C, Chang KC, et al. Prevalence of human papillomavirus in middle ear carcinoma associated with chronic otitis media. Am J Pathol. 1997;150:1327-33.
10. Lim LH, Goh YH, Chan YM, et al. Malignancy of the temporal bone and external auditory canal. Otolaryngol Head Neck Surg. 2000;122(6):882-6.
11. Koch BB, Karnell LH, Hoffman HT, et al. National Cancer Database Report on chondrosarcoma of the head and neck. Head Neck. 2000;22:408-25.
12. Lau DPC, Wharton SB, Antoun NM, et al. Chondrosarcoma of the petrous apex. Dilemmas in diagnosis and treatment. J Laryngol Otol. 1997;111:368-71.
13. Watters GWR, Brookes GB. Chondrosarcoma of the temporal bone. Clin Otolaryngol. 1995;20:53-8.
14. Mark RJ, Sercarz JA, Tran L, et al. Osteogenic sarcoma of the head and neck. The UCLA experience. Arch Otolaryngol Head Neck Surg. 1991;117:761-6.
15. Sharma SC, Handa KK, Panda N, et al. Osteogenic sarcoma of the temporal bone. Am J Otolaryngol. 1997;18(3):220-23.
16. Sataloff RT, Myers DL, Spiegel JR, Roberts BR, Telian S. Total temporal bone resection for osteogenic sarcoma. Ear Nose Throat J. 1988;67:626-51.
17. Goh YH, Chong VFH, Low WK. Temporal bone tumours in patients irradiated for nasopharyngeal neoplasm. J Laryngol Otol. 1999;113:222-8.
18. Nora FE, Unni KK, Pritchard DJ, et al. Osteosarcoma of extragnathic craniofacial bones. Mayo Clin Proc. 1983;58: 268-72.
19. Kassir RR, Rassekh H, Kinsella JB, et al. Osteosarcoma of he head and neck: meta-analysis of nonrandomized studies. Laryngoscope. 1997;107:56-61.
20. Hazarika P, Nayak DR, Sahota JS, et al. Osteogenic sarcoma of the sphenoid bone: an extended lateral skull base approach. J Laryngol Otol. 1995;109:1101-04.
21. Garrington GE, Scofield HH, Cornyn J, et al. Osteosarcoma of the Jaws. Analysis of 56 cases. Cancer. 1967;20(3):377-91.
22. Terzic A, Becker M, Wissmeyer M, et al. 18F-DOPA PET/CT unravels malignant paraganglioma mimicking temporomandibular joint disorder. Dentomaxillofac Radiol. 2011; 40(5):315-9.
23. Chapman DB, Lippert D, Geer CP, et al. Clinical, histopathologic, and radiographic indicators of malignancy in head and neck paraganglioma. Otolaryngol HNS. 2010;143 (4):531-7.
24. Schmahl K, Atamna N, Schonijahn T, et al. Uncommon case of paraganglioma syndrome in combination with malignant paraganglioma. Laryngorhinootologie. 2008;87(2):112-7.
25. Boedeker CC, Neumann HP, Maier W, et al. Malignant head and neck paragangliomas in SDHB mutation carriers. Otolaryngol HNS. 2007;137(1):126-9.
26. Yahsi S, Akpolat N, Karlidag T. Malignant jugular paraganglioma: a case report. Kulak Burun Bogazlhtis Derg. 2004;12(5-6):134-8.
27. Bilinska-Pietraszek E, Mrowka-Kata K, Namyslowski G, et al. Malignant transformation of giant jugular chemodectoma. Otolaryngol Pol. 2002;56(6):717-20.
28. Brewis C, Bottrill ID, Wharton SB, et al. Glomus jugulare tumor with metastases to cervical lymph nodes. J Laryngol Otol. 2000;114(1):67-9.
29. Manolidis S, Shohet JA, Jackson CG, et al. Malignant glomus tumors. Laryngoscope. 1999;109(1):30-4.
30. Athanassopoulou AC, Vlahos LL, Gouliamos AD. MRI features in a malignant glomus jugulare tumour. J Laryngol Otol. 1993;107(11):1066-9.

31. Johnston F, Symon L. Malignant paraganglioma of the glomus jugulare: a case report. Br J Neurosurg. 1993;6(3): 255-9.
32. Bhansali S, Bojrab DI, Zarbo RJ. Malignant paragangliomas of the head and neck: clinical and immunohistochemical characterization. Otolaryngol HNS. 1991;104(1):132.
33. Johnstone PA, Foss RD, Desilets DJ. Malignant jugulotympanic paraganglioma. Arch Pathol Lab Med. 1990;114(9): 976-9.
34. El Fiky FM, Paparella MM. A metastatic glomus jugulare tumor. A temporal bone report. Am J Otol. 1984;5(3): 197-200.
35. Davis JM, Davis KR, Hesselink JR, et al. Malignant glomus jugulare tumor: a case with two unusual radiographic features. J Comput Assist Tomogr. 1980;4(3):415-7.
36. Hoople GD, Bradley WH, Stoner LR, Brewer DW. Histologically malignant glomus jugulare tumor: case report. Laryngoscope. 1958;68(4):670-5.
37. Morton RP, Stell PM, Derrick PP. Epidemiology of cancer of the middle ear cleft. Cancer. 1984;53:1612-7.
38. Moffat DA, Wagstaff SA, Hardy DG. The outcome of radical surgery and postoperative radiosurgery for squamous carcinoma of the temporal bone. Laryngoscope. 2005;115(2):341-7.
39. Chen KTK, Dehner LP. Primary tumors of the external (auricle and auditory canal) and middle ear. I: Introduction and clinicopathological study of squamous cell carcinoma. Arch Otolaryngol. 1978;104:253-9.
40. Wagenfeld DJH, Keane T, van Nostrand AWP, Bryce DP. Primary carcinoma involving the temporal bone: analysis of twenty-five cases. Laryngoscope. 1980;90:912-9.
41. Sataloff RT, Roberts BR, Myers DL, et al. Total temporal bone resection: a radical but life saving procedure. AORN J. 1988;48(5):932-48.
42. Lewis JS. Surgical management of tumor of the middle ear and mastoid. J Laryngol Otol. 1983;97:299-311.
43. Gacek MR, Gacek RR, Gantz, B, et al. Psuedoepitheliomatous hyperplasia *versus* squamous cell carcinoma of the external auditory canal. Laryngoscope. 1998;108:620-3.
44. Moffat DA, Wagstaff SA. Squamous cell carcinoma of the temporal bone. Curr Opin Otolaryngol Head Neck Surg. 2003;11:107-11.
45. Suzuki K, Takahashi M, Ito Y, et al. Bilateral middle ear squamous cell carcinoma and clinical review of an additional 5 cases of middle ear carcinoma. Auris Nasus Larynx. 1999;26:33-8.
46. Glasscock ME. Surgery of glomus tumors of the temporal bone. Paper presented at: Middle Section Meeting. American Laryngological, Rhinological, and Otological Society, Inc., Indianapolis, IN. January 1979.
47. Baker S, Latack JT. Magnetic resonance imaging of the head and neck. Otolaryngol Head Neck Surg. 1986;95:82-9.
48. Levine PA, Paling MR, Black WC, et al. MRI *vs* high resolution CT scanning: evaluation of the anterior skull base. Otolaryngol Head Neck Surg. 1987;96:200-67.
49. Kveton JF, Brackmann DE, Glasscock ME, et al. Chondrosarcoma of the skull base. Otolaryngol Head Neck Surg. 1986;94:23-31.
50. Coltrera MD, Googe PB, Harrist TJ, et al. Chondrosarcoma of the temporal bone. Diagnosis and treatment of 13 cases and review of the literature. Cancer. 1986;58:2689-96.
51. Siedman MD, Nichols RD, Raju UB, et al. Extracranial skull base chondrosarcoma. Ear Nose Throat J. 1989;68:626-32.
52. Brown E, Hug EB, Weber AL. Chondrosarcoma of the skull base. Neuroimaging Clin North Am. 1994;4:529-41.
53. Burkey BB, Hoffman HT, Baker SR, et al. Chondrosarcoma of the head and neck. Laryngoscope. 1990;100:1301-5.
54. Kang HC, Wu HG, Lee JH, et al. Role of radiotherapy for squamous cell carcinoma of the external auditory canal and middle ear. J Korean Soc Ther Radiol Oncol. 2009;27: 173-80.
55. Hahn SS, Kim JA, Goodchild N, et al. Carcinoma of the middle ear and external auditory canal. Int J Radiat Oncol Biol Phys. 1983;9:1003-7.
56. Dean NR, White HN, Carter DS, et al. Outcomes following temporal bone resection. Laryngoscope. 2010;120:1516-22.
57. Gidley PW, Roberts DB, Sturgis EM, et al. Squamous cell carcinoma of the temporal bone. Laryngoscope. 2010;120: 1144-51.
58. Bibas AG, Ward V, Gleeson MJ, et al. Squamous cell carcinoma of the temporal bone. J Laryngol Otol. 2008;122: 1156-61.
59. Ogawa K, Nakamura K, Hatano K, et al. Treatment and prognosis of squamous cell carcinoma of the external auditory canal and middle ear: a multi-institutional retrospective review of 87 patients. Int J Radiat Oncol Biol Phys. 2007;68:1326-34.
60. Prabhu R, Hinerman RW, Indelicato DJ, et al. Squamous cell carcinoma of the external auditory canal: long-term clinical outcomes using surgery and external-beam radiotherapy. Am J Clin Oncol. 2009;32:401-4.
61. Nakagawa T, Kumamoto Y, Natori Y, et al. Squamous cell carcinoma of the external auditory canal and middle ear: an operation combined with preoperative chemoradiotherapy and a free surgical margin. Otol Neurotol. 2006;27: 242-8[discussion: 249]
62. Shiga K, Ogawa T, Maki A, et al. Concomitant chemoradiotherapy as a standard treatment for squamous cell carcinoma of the temporal bone. Skull Base. 2011;21:153-8C.
63. Sugimoto H, Ito M, Yoshida S, et al. Concurrent superselective intra-arterial chemotherapy and radiotherapy for late-stage squamous cell carcinoma of the temporal bone. Ann Otol Rhinol Laryngol. 2011;120:372-6.
64. Sataloff RT, Myers DL. Total temporal bone resection. Caderno Otorinolaringol. 1987;95(5-6):321-32.
65. Prasad S, Janecka IP. Efficacy of surgical treatment for squamous cell carcinoma of temporal bone: a literature review. Otolaryngol Head Neck Surg. 1994;110:270-80.
66. Ruben RJ, Thaler SU, Holzer N. Radiation induced carcinoma of the temporal bone. Laryngoscope. 1977;87:1613-21.
67. Liu FF, Keane TJ, Davidson J. Primary carcinoma involving the petrous temporal bone. Head Neck. 1993;15:39-43.
68. Birzgalis AR, Keith AO, Farrington WT. Radiotherapy in treatment of middle ear and mastoid carcinoma. Clin Otolaryngol. 1992;17:113-6.
69. Manolidis S, Pappas D, Von Doersten P, et al. Temporal bone and lateral skull base malignancy: experience and results with 81 patients. Am J Otol. 1998;19:S1-S15.

CHAPTER

Non-Squamous Cell Carcinoma Tumors of the Temporal Bone

10

Maroun T Semaan, Cameron C Wick, Cliff A Megerian

INTRODUCTION

Malignant and benign neoplasms of the temporal bone present a diagnostic and therapeutic challenge. The clinical presentation varies depending on the anatomic location and extent of the tumor, structures involved, and its biological behavior. The anatomical complexity of the temporal bone and the intimate relationship with vital neural and vascular structures adds to the therapeutic challenge. Apart from being rare, their slow and insidious course often causes a delay in diagnosis and commonly patients present with signs of cranial neuropathies and locally advanced disease. Squamous cell carcinoma (SCC), the most common malignant neoplasm of the temporal bone, will be discussed in a different chapter. Vestibular schwannomas (VS) merit a separate discussion and will not be included in this chapter. The purpose of this chapter is to provide an overview of non-SCC tumors of the temporal bone with emphasis on clinical presentation, diagnostic evaluation and treatment.

ANATOMY

A detailed anatomical description of the temporal bone is beyond the scope of this chapter. The temporal bones are situated at the sides and base of the skull. Each temporal bone includes five parts: the petrous, mastoid, squamous and tympanic bones, and the styloid process. The floor of the middle cranial fossa forms the superior border. Medially, the temporal bone is limited by the cerebellopontine angle (CPA) of the posterior fossa. The external auditory canal and auricle form its lateral border. Inferiorly, the carotid artery begins its intrapetrous course by entering the carotid canal and the internal jugular vein and lower cranial nerves IX, X and XI begin their extracranial course by exiting the jugular foramen.

DIFFERENTIAL DIAGNOSIS

Non-SCC tumors of the temporal bone are listed in Table 10.1. Based on the anatomical site of origin, tumors of the temporal bone can be divided into five anatomical locations (Figs. 10.1 to 10.6): (1) tumors of the middle and lateral temporal bone, (2) tumors of the inferior temporal bone, (3) tumors of the petroclival junction and petrous apex, (4) tumors of the medial temporal surface and (5) tumors of the superior temporal surface.

PARAGANGLIOMAS

Introduction

Paragangliomas (commonly referred to as glomus tumors) are tumors of the paraganglionic tissue. They are slow-growing, usually benign and highly vascular tumors. During embryogenesis, paraganglionic tissue is derived from the migration of neural crest cells in close association with the sympathetic nervous system. Within the head and neck, these cell rests are predominantly distributed throughout the middle ear in close association with Jacobson's nerve [branch of cranial nerve (CN) IX], Arnold's nerve (branch of CN X), the jugular foramen, vagus nerve and carotid body.

Guild coined the term "glomic tissue" for the vascularized ganglionic tissue along the adventitia of the jugular bulb and promontory.[1] Modern pathologic description

Table 10.1: Differential diagnosis of lesions of the temporal bone

Middle and lateral temporal bone	*Inferior temporal bone*	*Petrous apex and petroclival region*	*Medial temporal surface*	*Superior temporal surface*
• Paragangliomas (glomus tympanicum) • Schwannomas of CN VII (mastoid portion) • Adenomas • Adenocarcinomas • Ceruminous adenomas • Adenoid cystic carcinomas • Ceruminous adenocarcinomas • Squamous cell carcinomas • Carcinoid tumors • Leukemia, lymphoma and plasmocytoma • Rhabdosmyoarcoma • Langerhans cells histiocytosis • Metastasis	• Paragangliomas (glomus jugulare and vagale) • Schwannomas of CN IX, X, XI and XII • Meningiomas of jugular foramen • Chondrosarcomas • Osteosarcomas	• Petroclival meningiomas • Schwannomas CN V • Chondrosarcomas • Chordomas • Rhabdosarcomas • Osteosarcomas • Leukemia, lymphomas and plasmocytomas • Metastatic disease	• Schwannomas CN VII and VIII • Meningiomas of IAC and CPA • Endolymphatic sac and duct tumors	• Middle fossa meningiomas • Schwannomas CN VII (Geniculate ganglion) • Hemangiomas (geniculate ganglion)

(CN, cranial nerve; CPA, cerebellopontine angle; IAC, internal auditory canal).

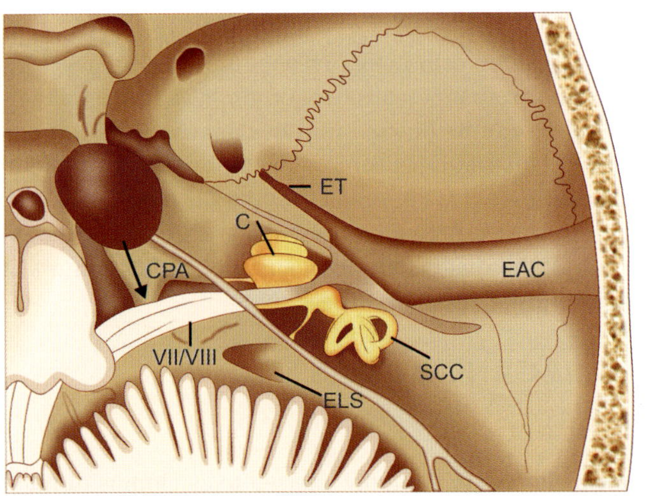

Fig. 10.1: Neoplasm originating in the region of the petroclival junction and petrous apex can involve the CPA by medial and posterior extension. (C, cochlea; CPA, cerebellopontine angle; EAC, external auditory canal; ELS, endolymphatic sac; ET, Eustachian tube; SCC, semicircular canals; VII/VIII, cranial nerves seven and eight complex).

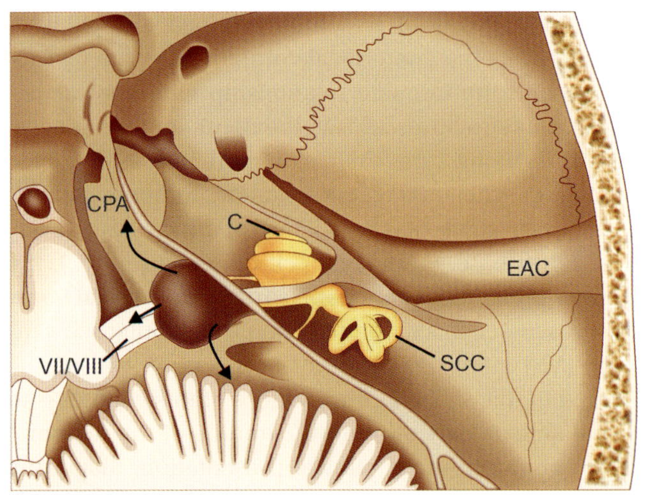

Fig. 10.2: Neoplasms originating from the region of the IAC can involve the CPA by extending medially and anterosuperiorly. (C, cochlea; CPA, cerebellopontine angle; EAC, external auditory canal; SCC, semicircular canals; VII/VIII, cranial nerves seven and eight complex).

reserves the term "glomus tumor" for benign hamartomas of glomus bodies (neuromyoarterial apparatus responsible for thermoregulation) commonly found in the hands and feet. Still, Guild's description of "glomic tissue" in the head and neck has persisted in clinical descriptions of these tumors. Within the temporal bone two types of paragangliomas exist: glomus tympanicum and glomus jugulare. Glomus tympanicum arises from rests of paraganglionic tissue associated with Jacobson's and Arnold's nerves. Glomus jugulare is believed to arise from similar paraganglionic rests within the adventitia of the jugular bulb, intimately associated with CN IX, X and XI.

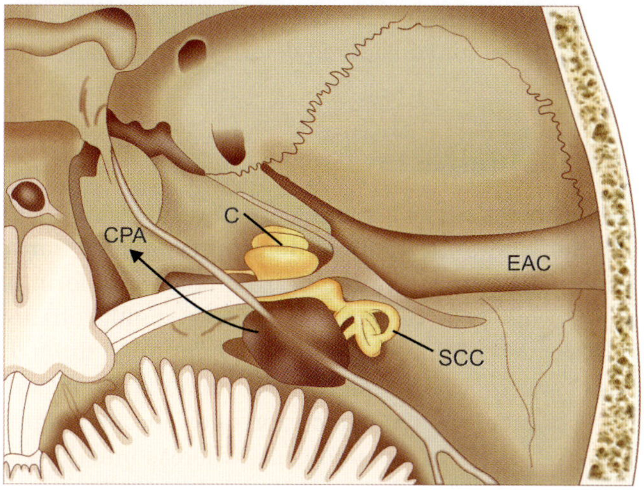

Fig. 10.3: Neoplasms originating from the region of the endolymphatic sac and the posterior petrous ridge can involve the CPA by extending anteriorly. (C, Cochlea; CPA, cerebellopontine angle; EAC, external auditory canal; SCC, semicircular canals).

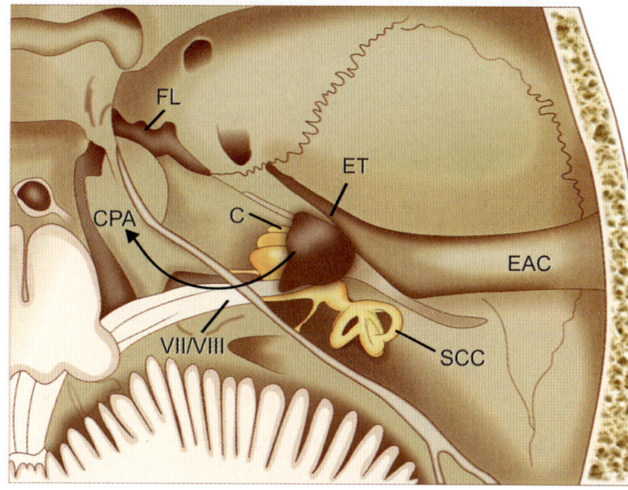

Fig. 10.4: Neoplasms originating from the region of the geniculate ganglion and floor of the middle cranial fossa can spread to the CPA by extending medially and anteriorly. (C, cochlea; CPA, cerebellopontine angle; EAC, external auditory canal; ET, Eustachian tube; FL: foramen lacerum; SCC, semicircular canals; VII/VIII, cranial nerves seven and eight complex).

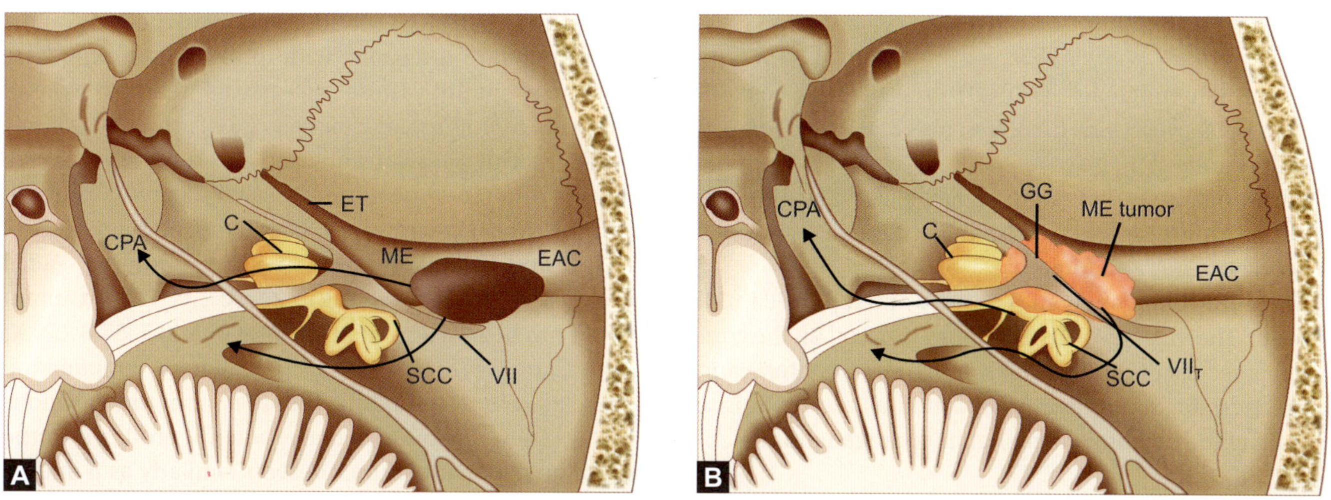

Figs. 10.5A and B: Neoplasms originating from the lateral aspect of the temporal bone, external auditory canal or middle ear can extend to the CPA by spreading medially, posteromedially (via the mastoid and the perilabyrinthine air cell systems) or anteriorly (via the petrous or the infralabyrinthine air cell systems). (C, Cochlea; CPA, cerebellopontine angle; EAC, external auditory canal; ET, Eustachian tube; ME, middle ear; SCC, semicircular canals; GG, geniculate ganglion; VII$_{T,}$ tympanic portion of CN VII).

The incidence of paragangliomas is estimated at 0.012%.[2] No racial predilection has been noted and they commonly occur in the fourth and fifth decades of life.[3] Multicentricity is seen in 3–10%.[4,5] Familial paraganglioma, inherited as an autosomal dominant disorder with genetic imprinting through paternal transmission, occurs in 1/30,000 head and neck tumors.[6] In contrast to the sporadic type, individuals affected by this rare condition develop multiple paragangliomas, often bilateral and at an earlier age. Multicentricity is seen in 30% of cases of familial paragangliomas. The most common association is a carotid body tumor and ipsilateral glomus tympanicum.[5] Recent genetic studies found linkage to two distinct chromosomal loci: 11q13.1 (PGL 2) and 11q22.3-q23 (PGL 1).[6-8] Germline mutations in the genes encoding for the three subunits of the mitochondrial complex II or

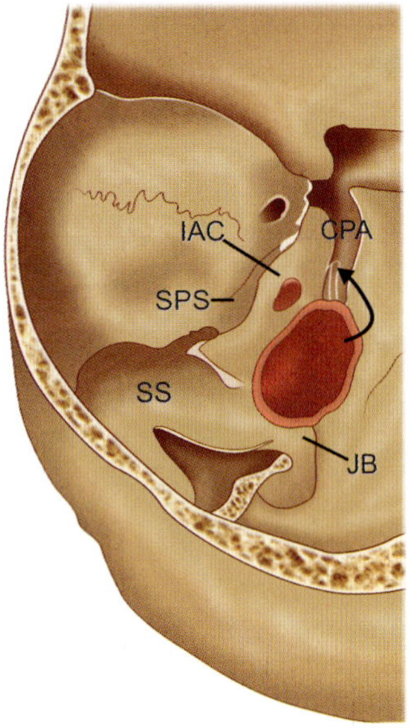

Fig. 10.6: Neoplasms originating from the region of the jugular bulb and lower cranial nerves extend to the CPA by spreading anteriorly and superiorly. (CPA, cerebellopontine angle; IAC, internal auditory canal; JB, jugular bulb; SS, sigmoid sinus; SPS, superior petrosal sinus).

succinate dehydrogenase (SDHD) (an essential component of Krebs cycle)–SDHB, SDHC and SDHD–have been recently found.[9-11]

Paragangliomas spread through pathways of least resistance: air cell tracts, vascular channels, naturally occurring fissures and foramina.

Malignant paragangliomas are rare and reported in 5% of cases.[12] The diagnosis of malignancy is based on the confirmed presence of distant metastasis. Cellular criteria and invasiveness have not been established as a prerequisite for making the diagnosis of malignant paragangliomas.

Pathology

Paragangliomas contain two cell types: the chief and sustentacular cells. The chief cells possess secretory granules that contain catecholamines. They are derivatives of neural crest cells and belong to the diffuse neuroendocrine system (DNES).[13] Only 1–3% of head and neck paragangliomas excrete norepinephrine. Unlike adrenal paragangliomas (pheochromocytoma), extra-adrenal paragangliomas rarely produce epinephrine, as the rate converting enzyme, phenylethanolamine-N-nethyl transferase, is absent.[13,14] On light microscopy (Figs. 10.7A and B), chief cells form clusters (Zellballen) embedded with support cells (sustentacular cells) within an abundant vascular stroma. Mitosis and capsular invasion have been described in a benign variant and are not considered determinant of malignant behavior.

Clinical Manifestations

Paragangliomas may be sporadic or part of an inherited syndrome with an autosomal dominant mode of transmission with genetic imprinting. The hereditary form is characterized by a higher incidence of multicentricity and associated tumors.[15] The genetic imprinting through paternal transmission seen in these tumors is reflected by the absence of phenotypic expression in offspring of females carrying the mutated gene, whereas inheriting a mutated copy from the father results in phenotypic expression with high penetrance.[7,8]

Early stage paragangliomas present with symptoms related to involvement of the middle ear cleft. Pulsatile tinnitus and conductive hearing loss are seen in 98% and 63%, respectively.[16] Glomus tympanicum tend to spread through pathways of least resistance along the peritubal air cells, intrapetrous carotid artery and petrous apex. Glomus jugulare presents with pulsatile tinnitus and cranial neuropathy. These neoplasms tend to spread through the hypotympanic air cells tract, around the jugular bulb, inferior petrosal sinus and carotid artery into the jugular foramen and posterior fossa. The jugular foramen syndrome (Vernet syndrome), characterized by paresis of CN IX, X and XI, may be seen in 50% of tumors.[17] Facial nerve involvement is present in 21–33%.[18-20] Involvement of CN IX has been reported in 4–43%, CN X in 5–57%, CN XI in 4–43% and CN XII in 7–43%.[3,17,19,21] Glomus tympanicum is seen as a retrotympanic red mass on the promontory (Fig. 10.8). Glomus jugulare, when it erodes into the floor of the hypotympanum, presents similarly as a middle ear mass or as an aural polyp if erosion of the tympanic membrane has occurred. Invasion of the middle ear results in conductive hearing loss by encroachment of the neoplasms onto the ossicles.[18] Brown's sign (tumor blanching with positive pressure using pneumatoscopy) or Aquino's sign (cessation of pulsations with compression of the ipsilateral carotid artery) may be seen. As tumor invades into deeper structure, additional cranial neuropathies and cochleovestibular dysfunction ensue.

Diagnosis

It is prudent not to biopsy a vascular middle ear mass, as this may result in profuse bleeding or exsanguination

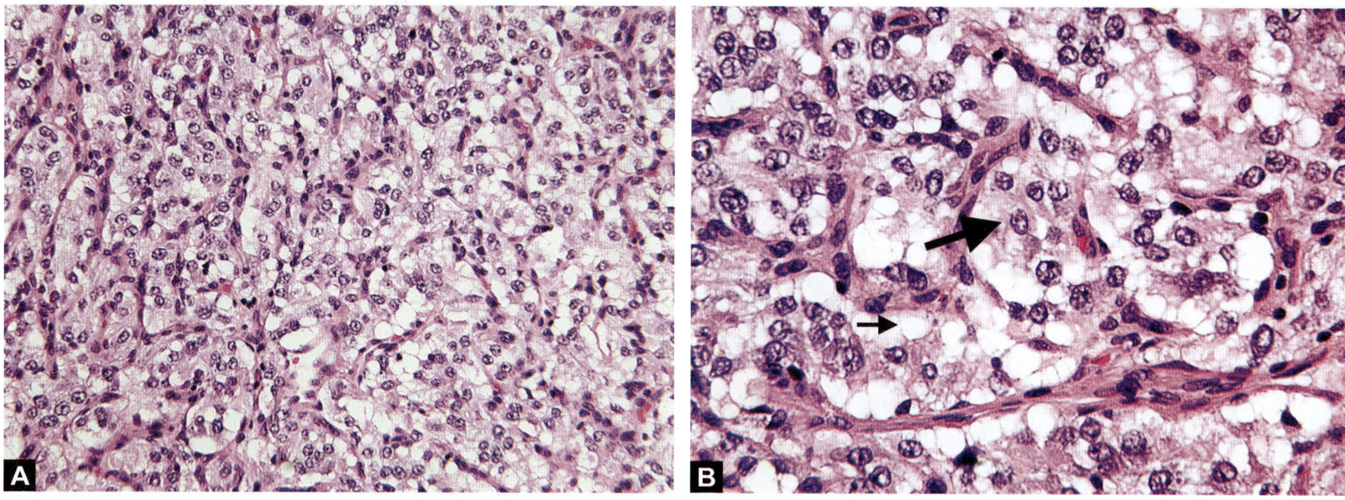

Figs. 10.7A and B: (A) Photomicrograph showing a hematoxylin and eosin (H&E) stain of a glomus jugulare. (B) Photomicrograph showing an hematoxylin and eosin (H&E) stain at a higher magnification of a glomus jugulare showing the nest of chief cells (large black arrow) (Zellballen) with surrounding sustentacular or supportive cells (small black arrow).

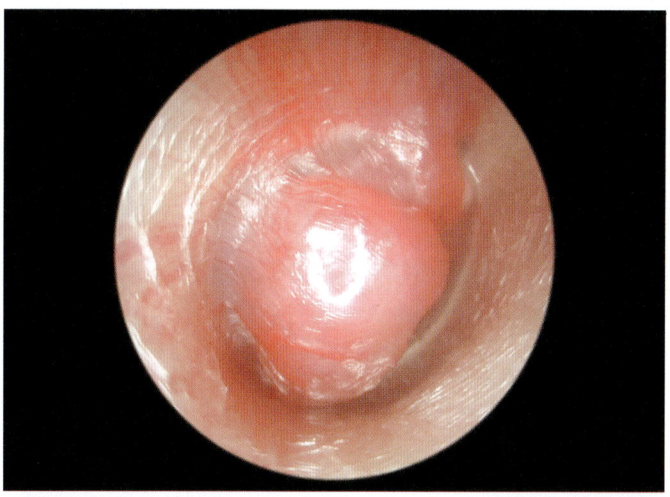

Fig. 10.8: Oto-endoscopic view of a large glomus tympanicum seen as a retrotympanic red mass with expansion of the posterior aspect of the tympanic membrane.

if not properly controlled. An aberrant carotid artery or high-riding, dehiscent jugular bulb may present as a reddish or bluish mass in the hypotympanum, and possibly masquerade as a glomus tumor.

In cases where multicentricity is seen, an appropriate workup should include screening for other adrenal and extra-adrenal tumors and for familial type paragangliomas. A 24-hour urinary vanillylmandellic acid (VMA), plasma catecholamines, and urinary beta-metanephrines or normetanephrines may be obtained as part of the biochemical screening workup.[22] History suggestive of labile hypertension, attacks of headache, anxiety, sweating and flushing may suggest a catecholamine producing tumor. Due to the rarity of functional head and neck paragangliomas, elevated plasma catecholamines should prompt the search for a pheochromocytoma, and perioperative alpha blockade may be indicated to avoid catecholaminergic crisis. Genetic screening is not widely available as a screening tool and remains confined to research laboratory.

The role of neuroradiology in determining the origin, extent and nature of the tumor is of paramount importance. Its role is not only limited to the characterization of the lesion itself, but is essential in differentiating these lesions from vascular anomalies or temporal bone malignant neoplasms. Imaging may also screen for other contralateral or ipsilateral lesions in cases of familial paragangliomas.

On high-resolution computed tomography (HRCT) of the temporal bone, glomus tympanicum in its early phases appears as a well-circumscribed soft tissue mass localized on the promontory. The differential diagnosis of a soft tissue density confined to the promontory includes congenital cholesteatoma, persistent stapedial artery and aberrant carotid artery.[23] Glomus jugulare tumors are associated with an irregular erosive enlargement of the jugular plate (floor of the hypotympanum) and the jugulo-carotid spine, resulting in a pattern described as "moth-eaten" (Figs. 10.9 and 10.10). Depending on its origin, these neoplasms will extend through the skull base to involve the jugular foramen in its neural and vascular compartment and eventually progress intracranially and/or extracranially through cervical extension.[24]

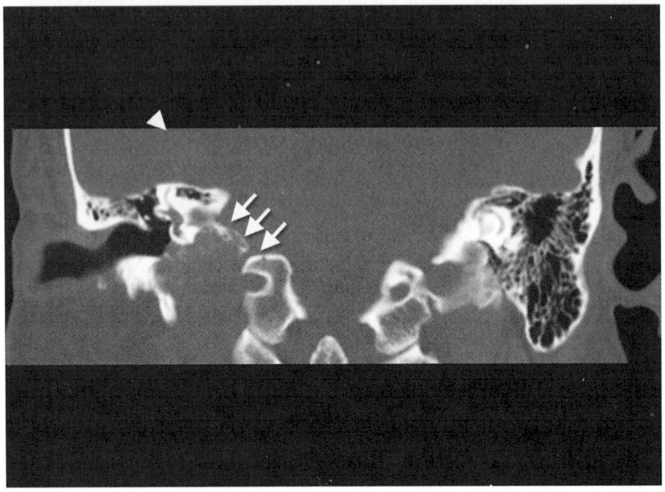

Fig. 10.9: High-resolution computed tomography of the temporal bone, coronal views, demonstrating a glomus jugulare extending toward the posterior fossa. Note the irregular borders, the moth-eaten appearance (small white arrows) and the erosion of the floor of the hypotympanum (arrowhead).

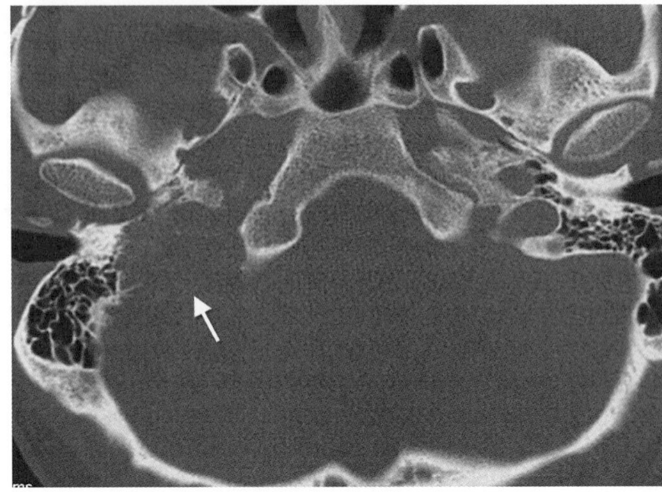

Fig. 10.10: High-resolution computed tomography of the temporal bone, axial views, demonstrating a lesion extending from the jugular bulb into the posterior fossa consistent with a glomus jugulare. Note, the moth-eaten appearance and the irregular borders.

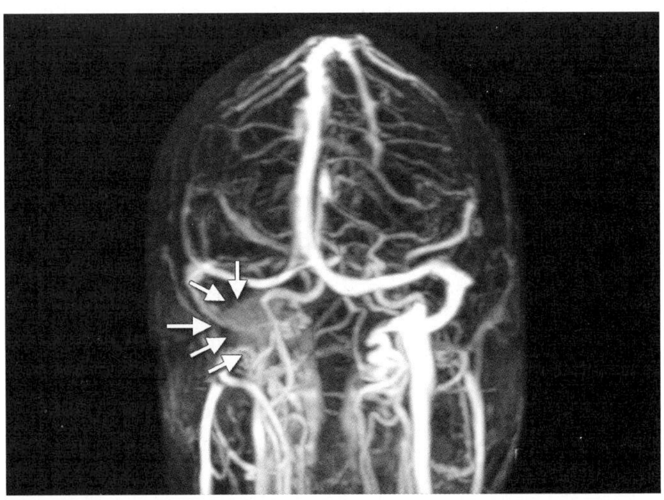

Fig. 10.11: Magnetic resonance venography of a patient with a right glomus jugulare (small white arrows). Note the blush indicative of hypervascularity. The importance of the MRV is in the assessment of the controlateral venous system. This patient has a patent controlateral jugular system.

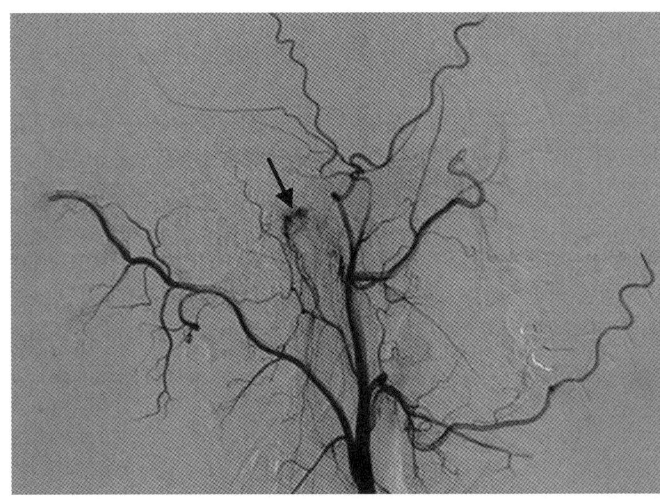

Fig. 10.12: Four-vessel angiography showing a "vascular blush" (black arrow) at the site of a glomus jugulare. The vascular supply appears to originate from the ascending pharyngeal and tributaries of the occipital artery.

Magnetic resonance (MR) weighted images are superior in evaluating tumor vascularity, extension along neural foramina and multicentricity.[25] In addition, magnetic resonance venography (MRV) (Fig. 10.11) is helpful in ensuring intraluminal patency of the jugular vein and retrograde involvement of the venous system as well as the status of the contralateral venous system. On T1 weighted images (T1WI), paragangliomas appear hypointense with a speckled appearance. On gadolinium enhanced T1 images, they demonstrate early and pronounced enhancement. On T2WI, paragangliomas are hyperintense and when larger than 2 cm, they demonstrate a serpentine flow void pattern described as "salt and pepper" appearance.[25,26]

On angiography, paragangliomas exhibit an intense blush or a "bag of worms" appearance. MR angiography may substitute for four-vessels angiography as a tool to evaluate the vascularity of skull base tumors (Fig. 10.12). However, small vascular anomalies and blood feeders are better seen on conventional angiography.[27] Four-vessel angiography is indicated if preoperative embolization is planned. The later may decrease intraoperative blood loss and operative time.[28]

Treatment and Classification of Paragangliomas of the Temporal Bone

Different classification schemes have been described. They are shown in Tables 10.2 to 10.4. They are useful in the selection of the most appropriate treatment approach to tackle these vascular neoplasms. Four treatment modalities currently exist in the management of paragangliomas of the temporal bone: (1) observation, (2) surgery, (3) radiotherapy and (4) limited resection with planned radiotherapy.

Tympanic tumors limited to the middle ear cleft without significant hypo- or retrotympanic extension may be completely excised via a transcanal approach. Tympanomastoid tumors with significant extension into the mastoid or retrofacial air cell tract are removed via a mastoidectomy with an extended facial recess approach. For glomus jugulare tumors limited to the lateral wall of the jugular bulb without extension onto the internal carotid artery (ICA) or neck, a fallopian bridge approach or a combined mastoid-neck approach is used. Glomus jugulare tumors with extension towards the carotid canal or originating from the medial wall of the jugular bulb require an infratemporal fossa type-A approach with resection or packing of the sigmoid sinus and jugular bulb, removal of the posterior bony external auditory canal and tympanic ring, blind closure of the external auditory canal, and at times, limited or complete anterior translocation of the facial nerve (Fig. 10.13A). In tumors involving the lateral wall of the jugular bulb, the proximal sigmoid sinus can be packed extraluminally and the segment involved by the tumor is excised, preserving the medial wall of the vein intact. Bleeding from the inferior petrosal sinus is controlled with packing. Preoperative embolization has been shown to decrease intraoperative bleeding and facilitate neural microdissection.[29] Glomus tumors extending anteriorly towards the carotid canal, petrous apex, petroclival junction and intracranially towards the prepontine cistern can be surgically approached with an infratemporal fossa type-B (Fig. 10.13B). In this approach, exposure of the petroclival area is achieved via a preauricular infratemporal fossa dissection. The parotid and extratemporal facial nerves are retracted inferiorly while proximal and distal osteotomies allow inferior mobilization of the zygomatic arch and temporalis muscle, exposing the infratemporal and temporal fossa. The condyle of the mandible is dislocated and retracted. The Eustachian tube is divided and petrous apicectomy is completed. The intrapetrous ICA is skeletonized, decompressed and anteriorly mobilized. Drilling the petroclival synchondrosis and clivus allows intradural exposure of the prepontine cistern and basilar artery. Additional supratentorial exposure can be obtained by combining a subtemporal craniotomy. The superior petrosal sinus and tentorium are divided with care to avoid injuring the trochlear nerve and tributaries of the vein of Labbé. Although rarely needed in the surgical treatment of glomus tumors, an infratemporal fossa type-C allows access to the cavernous sinus, pterygopalatine fissure and lateral nasopharyngeal wall by removing the pterygoid plates and

Table 10.2: Fisch paraganglioma staging system

Type A	Tumor limited to middle ear
Type B	Tumor limited to the tympanomastoid area with no infralabyrinthine involvement
Type C	Tumor involving the infralabyrinthine compartment of the temporal bone and extending into the petrous apex
Type D1	Tumors with intracranial extension less than 2 cm
Type D2	Tumors with intracranial extension greater than 2 cm

Table 10.3: Glasscock and Jackson paraganglioma staging system

Type I	Small tumor involving the jugular bulb, middle ear and mastoid
Type II	Tumor extending under the internal auditory canal; may have intracranial extension
Type III	Tumor extending into the petrous apex; may have intracranial extension
Type IV	Tumor extending beyond the petrous apex into the clivus or infratemporal fossa; may have intracranial extension

Table 10.4: De La Cruz paraganglioma staging system

Classification	*Surgical approach*
Tympanic	Transcanal
Tympanomastoid	Mastoid-extended facial recess
Jugular bulb	Mastoid-neck
Carotid artery	Infratemporal fossa
Transdural	Infratemporal fossa/intracranial

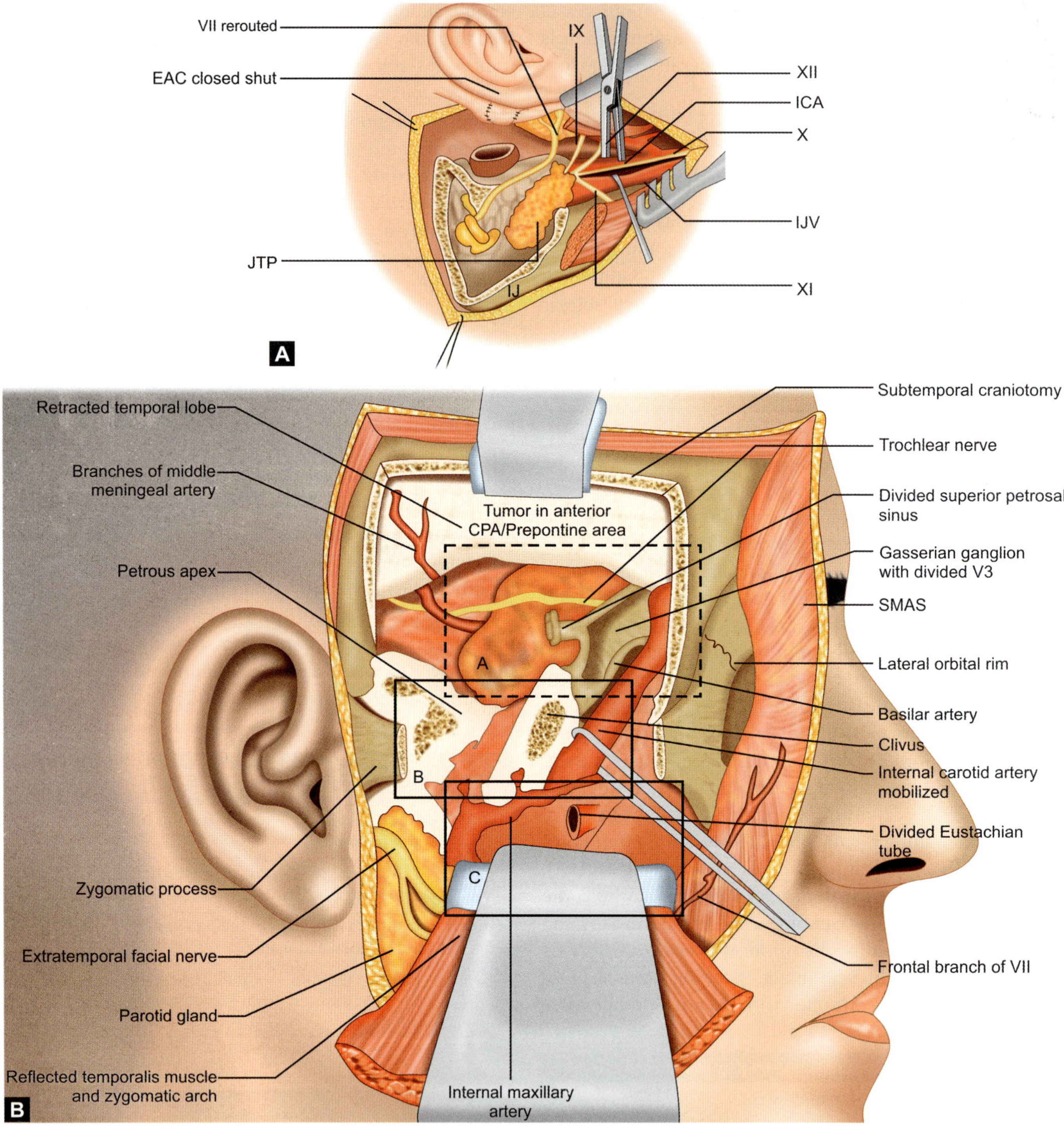

Figs. 10.13A and B: (A) The infratemporal fossa type A approach for removal of large glomus jugulare. Note that the labyrinth is preserved, the EAC has been closed shut and the facial nerve is elevated off the fallopian canal and retracted anteriorly. Vascular control is obtained by performing a neck exploration. Many surgeons advocated against rerouting the facial nerve as this maneuver results in a high incidence of facial paralysis. (B) The infratemporal fossa type-B approach combined with a subtemporal craniotomy for removal of tumors extending towards the anterior ICA, petroclival junction and prepontine cistern. A: subtemporal craniotomy with intracranial exposure. B: anterior petrosectomy with mobilization of the intrapetrous ICA for exposure of the petroclival region. C: exposure of the infratemporal and temporal fossa by retraction and mobilization of parotid gland and extratemporal facial nerve, the mandibular condyle (not shown), the zygomatic arch and temporalis muscle. (EAC, external auditory canal; ICA, internal carotid artery; IJV, internal jugular vein; JTP, jugulotympanic paraganglioma).

extending the surgical dissection further anteriorly. Paragangliomas involving the CPA require a combined extradural and intradural approach, which may require staged procedures.[30] Transpetrous approaches with or without facial nerve rerouting, with or without hearing preservation, with additional craniotomies designed as dictated by tumor extension may be performed for complete tumor excision.[31] These extensive operations are often associated with significant morbidity and increased operative time. For elderly patients or patients in whom extensive surgery is contraindicated, a limited surgical procedure with planned adjuvant radiotherapy affords symptomatic control with minimal comorbidities.[32,33]

Radiotherapy in the form of gamma knife stereotactic radiosurgery (GKRS) or conventional radiotherapy has been used as an adjuvant, as salvage or as the primary treatment of paragangliomas.[32,34-37] Tumor control rates between 70% and 100% have been reported with a low risk of complications. Radiotherapy is currently favored for moribund patients, those with advanced age, bilateral tumors with increased iatrogenic risk of bilateral vagal nerve dysfunction, and in those refusing surgery.[32]

FACIAL NERVE SCHWANNOMAS

Introduction

Facial nerve schwannoma (FNS) are rare, slow-growing benign neoplasms that arise from the nerve sheath of the CN VII. Although FNS may arise anywhere throughout the course of the facial nerve from the CPA to the extratemporal portion, the most common locations are the geniculate ganglion, horizontal and vertical segments.[38] In two separate human temporal bone studies, FNS was noted in 0.8%[39] and 0.07%[40] of specimens. In 1987, a review of the world literature found 248 FNS.[41] FNS originating from the geniculate ganglion tends to extend superiorly toward the middle cranial fossa; however, medial extension toward the internal auditory canal (IAC) and CPA is possible. Tumors originating in the vertical or tympanic segment of the facial nerve involve the mastoid air cells and middle ear cleft.

Pathology

Tumors are generally well-encapsulated with a homogenous tan to gray color that occasionally exhibit areas of cystic degeneration. Microscopically, two histological subtypes exist: Antoni A and Antoni B (Figs. 10.14A and B).[42] Tumor cells are characterized by spindle-shaped nuclei with an abundant cytoplasm with slender eosinophilic processes and indistinct cytoplasmic borders. This appearance is reminiscent of the parent Schwann cell from which they derive. The indistinct cytoplasmic membrane gives the appearance of a seamless uniform stroma background. In Antoni A, the cellular elements form compact intersecting fascicles, creating a dense fibrous palisading background. In Antoni B, the stroma is less dense, characterized by decreased cellularity, increased edema and presence of macrophages. The proportion of Antoni A versus Antoni B histologic subtypes is not correlated with prognostic information. Verocay bodies, seldom present, are a distinctive feature that is formed of parallel rows of tightly spaced parallel nuclei separated by cellular processes (Fig. 10.14C). Schwannomas stain positive with S-100 and neuron specific enolase.[42]

Clinical Manifestations

The most common presenting symptom is slowly progressive facial weakness (73–94%).[41,43] A patient with insidious onset of unilateral facial paralysis, facial twitching, or a "Bell's palsy" that does not resolve after 6–9 months should be considered as having a neoplasm of the facial nerve until proven otherwise. The usual onset is insidious; however, sudden onset and fluctuating or recurrent patterns of facial paresis may occur. An early onset facial palsy in the setting of a tumor involving the IAC or CPA is an indicator that the facial nerve may represent the nerve of origin of the neoplasm. Hearing impairment may be caused by tumor extension toward the middle ear cleft with impingement on the ossicular chain (conductive loss) or by invasion of the otic capsule or compression of the cochlear nerve in the IAC (sensorineural loss).[44] In one study, otic capsule erosion was noted in 29% of cases.[38] Tinnitus and vertigo are reported in 13% and 11%.[41] In FNS originating from the mastoid or tympanic segment of the nerve, extension into the external auditory canal may occur and an aural mass is seen on otoscopy.

Diagnosis

Neurophysiologic Testing

The slowly progressive nature of growth of FNS is manifested by a combination of ongoing neural degeneration and regeneration. The balance between these two neurophysiological phenomena explains the findings seen on electroneuronography (ENoG).[45] In a regenerating nerve, activation of the newly formed fibers results in an

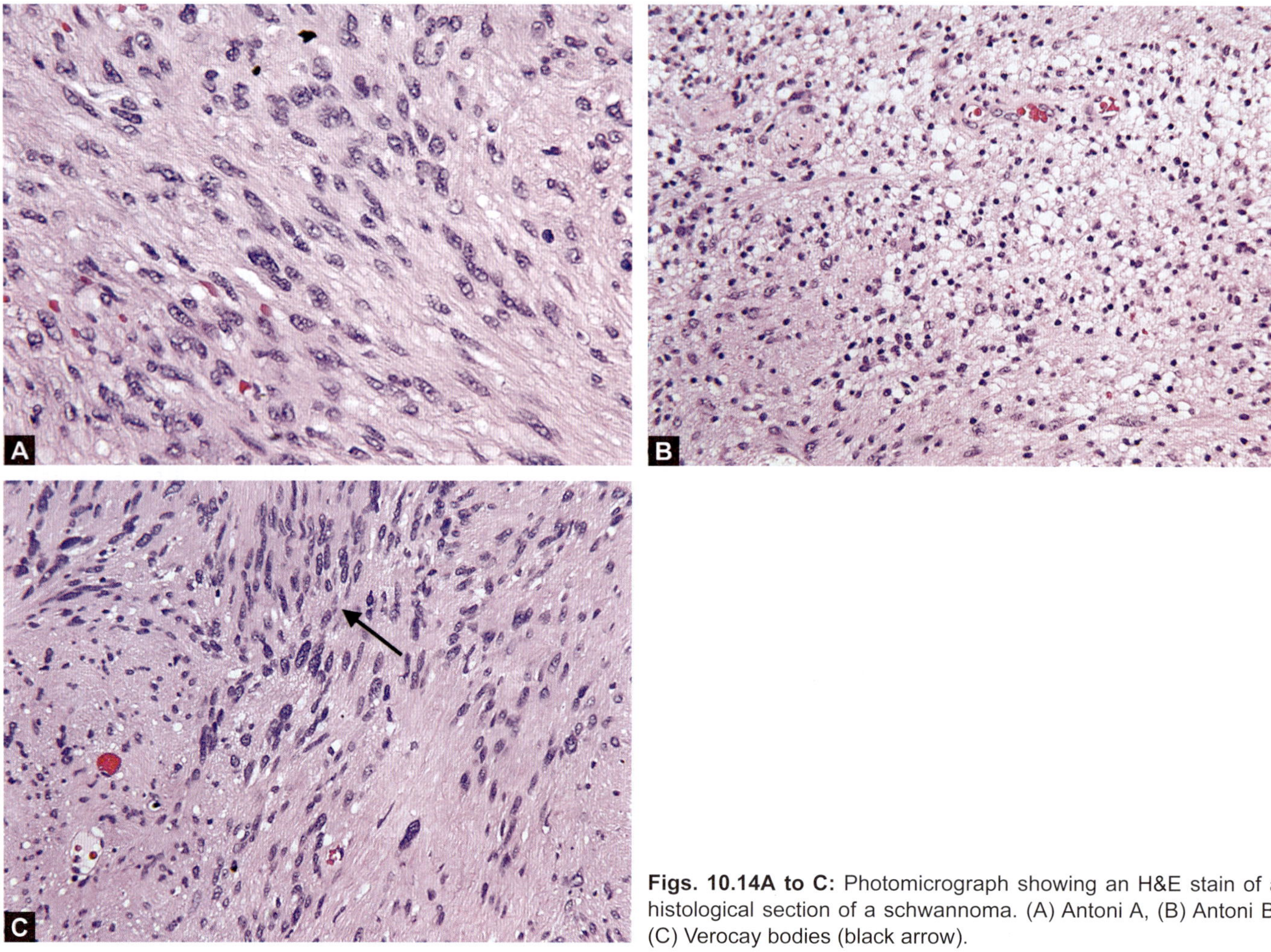

Figs. 10.14A to C: Photomicrograph showing an H&E stain of a histological section of a schwannoma. (A) Antoni A, (B) Antoni B, (C) Verocay bodies (black arrow).

asynchronous sequence. Asynchronous action potentials result in phase cancellation. Hence, the response cannot be recorded on ENoG. On the other hand, if a lesion is causing an ongoing simultaneous degeneration and regeneration, the resultant regenerative summated action potential is "cancelled" by the signal's asynchrony. The latter phenomenon accounts for the finding of ENoG showing more than 90% "degeneration" with a normal voluntary electromyogram (EMG). This is often the case with a slowly growing FNS.

Neuroimaging

Diagnostic imaging is of paramount importance in the evaluation of a patient with atypical "Bell's palsy". HRCT of the temporal bone provides great detail of the bony anatomy and demonstrates an expanded fallopian canal (if FNS involves the mastoid segment) or dilation of the perilabyrinthine facial nerve (if FNS involves the geniculate ganglion). In addition, CT imaging is helpful in the differentiation of FNS from geniculate ganglion hemangioma (GGH). GGH lead to enlargement of the labyrinthine portion of the fallopian canal, and depending on the tumor extent, dilation of the tympanic portion of the nerve may be seen. The soft tissue mass may show intratumoral calcifications and/or bony spicules. Early erosion of the floor of the middle cranial fossa is suggestive of GGH.[46]

On MRI, FNS are iso-hypointense on T1WI and hyperintense in T2WI and enhance with gadolinium (Figs. 10.15A and B). Both enhancement of the labyrinthine portion of the facial nerve and extension into the middle ear with impingement of the ossicular chain are suggestive of FNS.

Treatment

Surgical excision of FNS requires excision of the facial nerve and cable grafting. The best results obtained with cable grafting are House-Brackmann (HB) III. Because of

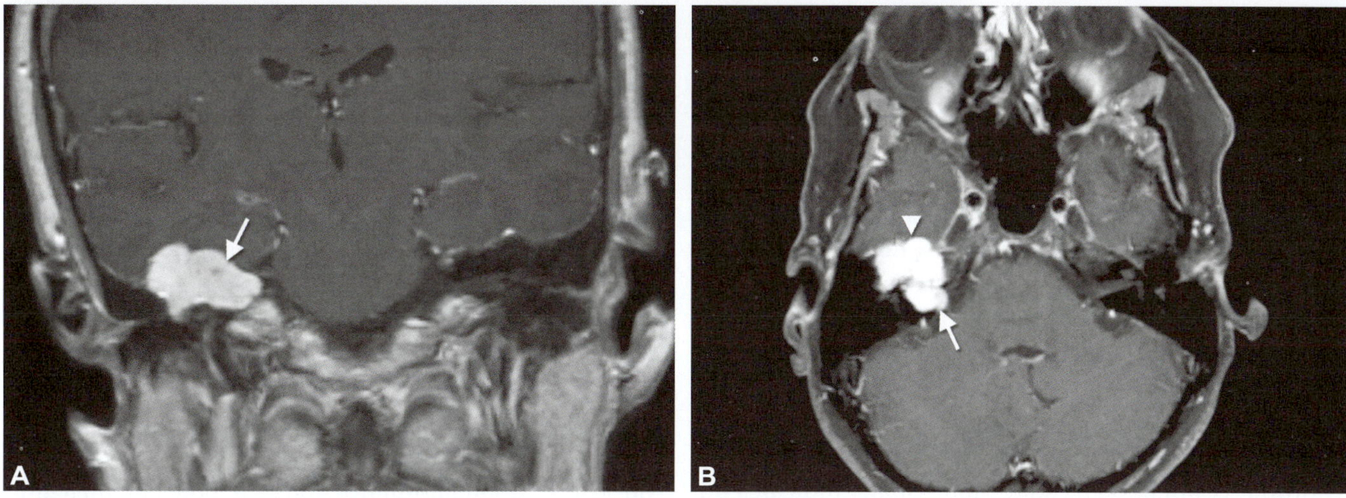

Figs. 10.15A and B: (A) Coronal gadolinium enhanced MR showing a right-sided facial nerve schwannoma centered over the geniculate ganglion. Note the extension towards the flow of the middle cranial fossa (white arrow). (B) Axial gadolinium enhanced MR with fat suppression showing a right-sided facial nerve schwannoma, "dumbbell-shaped" with a component involving the middle cranial fossa (white arrowhead) and a component extending into the internal auditory canal (white arrow).

the insidious growth pattern of these tumors and the less than normal facial nerve outcome with grafting, observation is often recommended if the presenting facial function is good (HB III or less).

The timing for intervention is controversial. Some surgeons intervene when the degree of degeneration exceeds 50% on ENoG, whereas others defer surgical resection until further deterioration of facial function occurs. It is believed that further degeneration may adversely affect the results of cable grafting if longer waiting is advised.[43]

Four treatment modalities have been suggested: (1) excision and grafting, (2) nerve decompression, (3) radiotherapy and (4) observation. Whether cable grafting or hypoglossal-facial nerve anastomosis is performed, the best expected result is HB III. This less than ideal facial nerve outcome after excision and grafting prompted some to attempt facial nerve decompression in patients with good facial function at presentation. Facial nerve decompression can be achieved via a middle fossa (MF) or transmastoid approach, depending on the tumor location. If excision is planned, the translabyrinthine (TL) approach provides good exposure of the intratemporal facial nerve down to the level of the stylomastoid foramen in patients with poor hearing. This approach permits nerve grafting if needed. In patients with "serviceable hearing", the approach chosen depends on the location. For FNS involving the tympanic or mastoid segments, a transmastoid approach is utilized. FNS originating from the geniculate region is best accessed with a MF craniotomy. In a review of 79 FNSs,[47] facial nerve grade was maintained or improved over the follow-up period (mean time = 3.9 years) in 78.9% of the decompression group and 100% of the observation and radiation groups compared to 54.8% of the resection group.

JUGULAR FORAMEN SCHWANNOMAS

Introduction

The jugular foramen is divided into two compartments: pars nervosa (contains CN IX, X and XI) anteromedially and pars venosa (contains jugular bulb and inferior petrosal sinus) posterolaterally. A dural septum separates the glossopharyngeal meatus (CN IX) from the vagal meatus (CN X, XI). The relationship between the opening of the inferior petrosal sinus into the jugular bulb and the cranial nerves rootlets is variable.[29] Jugular foramen schwannomas (JFS) are rare nerve sheath tumors that affect the nerves of the jugular foramen. These tumors originate from CN IX, X and XI. Although the exact incidence is unknown, it is estimated at 2.9 per 10 million people.[48] In comparison to the 2:1 female to male predilection reported in intracranial schwannomas,[49] JFS have an equal sex distribution[50] that slightly favors a male predilection.[51]

Pathology

Like other schwannomas, JFS are well circumscribed, slow-growing benign neoplasms that originate from the transition zone between the central and peripheral myelin[52] of CN IX, X and XI. The exact location of origin may be difficult to determine.

Histologically, JFS may present with a dense Antoni A or hypocellular Antoni B architectural pattern as previously described. Verocay bodies can be seen occasionally.

Clinical Manifestations

The great majority of published literature is limited to small series of patients and often case reports. The classic jugular foramen syndrome (Vernet syndrome) denotes unilateral involvement of CN IX, X and XI. It is clinically manifested by loss of taste in the posterior one-third of the tongue, hemianesthesia of the ipsilateral palate, pharynx and larynx, and weakness of the trapezius, palate, ipsilateral vocal cord and sternocleidomastoid muscle. This syndrome is rarely seen today, and usually indicates an advanced JFS or metastatic lesion. The clinical presentation of JFS is somewhat dependent on their anatomic location. This anatomic location is the basis for the staging system proposed by Kaye et al.[53] Stage A refers to tumors with a predominant intracranial component, stage B is a foraminal tumor located at the jugular foramen, and stage C denotes a tumor with a predominant extracranial growth. A stage D was added to describe dumbbell-shaped tumors with a significant intracranial and extracranial component.[54] Intracranial JFS commonly present with hearing loss, vertigo, ataxia, tinnitus and headache. In tumors with significant extracranial extension, patients may present with a high cervical mass, lower cranial neuropathy and conductive hearing loss. The nerve of origin is often difficult to determine as lesions are large and often blend into multiple cranial nerves. However, isolated or combined involvement of cranial nerves IX, X and XI is often reported.

Diagnosis

Neuroimaging plays an essential role in the diagnostic and preoperative evaluation of a jugular foramen lesion. The three most common lesions of the jugular foramen are glomus jugulare, meningioma and nerve sheath tumors (i.e. schwannoma and neurofibroma).[26,29] Individual signal characteristics may help narrow the differential diagnosis. Contrasted HRCT is invaluable in delineating the bony-tumor relationship. MRI supplements CT images by providing excellent detail of the soft tissue component. In addition, CT angiography or magnetic resonance angiography (MRA) and MRV provide vascular details that are essential to the planning of the surgical treatment. Particular attention is given to the patency of the contralateral sigmoid sinus, transverse sinus and torcular Herophili (confluence of sinuses). The sacrifice of the sole or dominant venous drainage system can have a catastrophic outcome. This is important if intraluminal involvement of the jugular bulb or vein is seen on preoperative imaging. JFS cause a smooth-scalloped enlargement of the jugular foramen with well-defined bone margins.[55] The tumor is usually isodense to surrounding muscles and may show slight enhancement to iodinated contrast. On MR imaging, JFS are hypo- or isointense on T1WI, hyperintense on T2WI and show heterogenous enhancement T1WI with gadolinium (Figs. 10.20 and 10.22). The "dumbbell" appearance is almost pathognomonic to JFS.

Meningiomas do not typically cause enlargement of the jugular foramen, but rather erosion of the cortical bone with occasional calcifications and hyperostosis.[56] On HRCT they are hyperintense and markedly enhance after iodinated contrast. On MR, meningiomas are isointense to brain on T1WI and T2WI. Homogenous enhancement without vascular flow void is seen with gadolinum. A dural tail may be present and suggests the diagnosis.

Paragangliomas result in erosive enlargement of the jugular foramen with irregular bony margin.[26] They may erode the jugulo-carotid spine and extend anteriorly to involve the carotid canal. Superiorly they may involve the middle ear by eroding the floor of the hypotympanum. Their characteristic HRCT and MR findings are described above.

Four-vessel angiography may play a role in the preoperative workup of tumors of the jugular foramen. JFS show minimal to absent tumor blush; meningioma may show a faint tumor blush. Paragangliomas show obvious tumor blush with arteriovenous shunting.

Treatment

Three treatment modalities have been advised for lesions of the jugular foramen: (1) surgery, (2) radiosurgery and (3) observation.

Although the natural history of JFS is unknown, one might extrapolate the biological behavior of VS to JFS. A small tumor detected in a young patient may grow to a very advanced stage after two to three decades, rendering complete tumor removal more laborious. Hence, surgery remains the recommended treatment for a young, healthy patient. Observation is recommended for the moribund patient as other modalities may result in significant morbidity in patients with a short life expectancy. If expectant management is chosen, yearly MRI is recommended to assess the tumor growth and behavior in an individual patient. Stereotactic radiosurgery is generally recommended for patients over the age of 65 and those with surgical contraindications. Unlike surgical removal, the desired outcome in radiotherapy is tumor control and absence of growth (Figs. 10.20 and 10.22). In a large report of 27 patients with JFS treated with GKRS,[57] 15 were treated with GKRS primarily and 12 were treated postoperatively with a mean follow-up of 38.7 months. The mean tumor volume was 13.5 cm^3. The mean marginal dose at 55% isodose line was 14.6 Gy. Tumor regression was seen in 44%, absence of growth in 52%, and progression was noted in 4%. No new cranial neuropathies were reported. In another report of 17 patients with JFS treated over a 10-year period with a mean follow-up of 3.5 years,[58] 8 lesions regressed (47%), one progressed (6%) and the rest remained unchanged (47%). No post treatment complications were reported. The marginal dose utilized ranged between 12 and 18 Gy.

The tumor size and location are important determinants of the surgical approach, as are any preoperative neural deficits. The staging described by Kaye et al.[53] helps provide an algorithm to approach these lesions. Type A lesions (intracranial) are primarily approached using the retrosigmoid approach or a lateral suboccipital craniotomy.[51] Type C lesions (extracranial) have traditionally been removed using the Fisch infratemporal fossa approach. Although the infratemporal fossa approaches (Fisch types A to C) provide excellent exposure to the jugular foramen, recent modifications have aimed to preserve hearing[59] and facial nerve function.[21] In lesions with both an intracranial and extracranial component, a combination of intracranial and extracranial approaches is advised.

GENICULATE GANGLION HEMANGIOMAS

Introduction

Geniculate ganglion hemangiomas are rare vascular malformations that affect the geniculate ganglion. Pulec[60] is credited with the first description of a GGH in 1969. These hemangiomas differ from their pediatric counterpart in that they are often seen in middle-aged individuals and show no clear pattern of involution. They are slow growing and tend to produce facial nerve weakness at early stages.

Pathology

Histologically, they are characterized by a proliferation of small or medium sized vessels, lined by endothelial cells that often appear as cystic spaces filled with blood. In osseous hemangiomas, these proliferating endothelial cells are interspersed within bony trabeculae. The adjacent bone appears "moth-eaten" and bony spicules are occasionally seen.[46] This appearance is not of an invasive nature but rather represents a reactive bony change. Hemangiomas of the geniculate ganglion and the IAC are extraneural tumors that likely originate from the perineural capillary network of the corresponding nerve.[61] Despite their extraneural origin, neural invasion is often seen on histological specimen. This infiltration can be extensive, rendering preservation of the nerve impossible, resulting in nerve transection and subsequent graft placement.[62] Symptoms occur at an early phase even with small sized tumors of both the IAC and the geniculate ganglion.[46] The floor of the MF is almost always dehiscent over the tumor.

Clinical Manifestations

The most common presenting symptom of GGH is progressive facial palsy.[63] The facial nerve paresis may develop even with small sized lesions. The facial palsy may mimic idiopathic facial nerve paralysis or Bell's palsy. Responsiveness to steroid therapy does not exclude the diagnosis as often discontinuation of the steroids is followed by recurrence of the facial weakness. Less frequently, the facial paralysis is acute in onset.[64] Facial twitching and hemifacial spasms may be the presenting symptoms. They are indicative of nerve compression or irritation. Involvement of the greater superficial petrosal nerve may result in epiphora or dry eyes.

Extension into the middle ear results in a conductive hearing loss by disturbance of the ossicular chain. Hemangiomas eroding the otic capsule with creation of a cochlear fistula may cause sensorineural hearing loss. Sensorineural hearing loss may be the presenting symptoms in IAC hemangiomas.[46,65] Hearing loss may be seen at very early stages. Tinnitus is commonly reported.[46,62]

Diagnosis

Audiometry is helpful in delineating the type of hearing loss. In GGH the hearing loss is classically conductive. IAC hemangiomas may present with sensorineural hearing loss.[46,65] In GGH, a cochlear fistula may cause sensorineural hearing loss; however, a fistula may be identified intraoperatively despite a normal preoperative audiogram.[62]

Imaging of the temporal bone is very helpful in differentiating GGH from FNS. The diagnosis of GGH is strongly suggested by HRCT of the temporal bone. Contrasted CT does not necessarily yield much information in terms of delineating the nature of the lesion. The presence of calcifications in an expansile soft tissue density in the region of the geniculate ganglion is usually diagnostic of an "ossifying hemangioma" (Fig. 10.16).[64-66] The absence of bony coverage of the MF is also suggestive of hemangiomas. The absence of calcifications does not exclude the diagnosis. Compared to FNS, these lesions may cause nerve dysfunction even at an early radiographic stage.[46] GGH are iso-hypointense on T1WI, avidly enhance with gadolinium and may have a hyperintense signal on T2WI (Figs. 10.17A and B). Some believe that the presence of heterogenous signal intensity on T2WI may be more suggestive of geniculate hemangioma.[67]

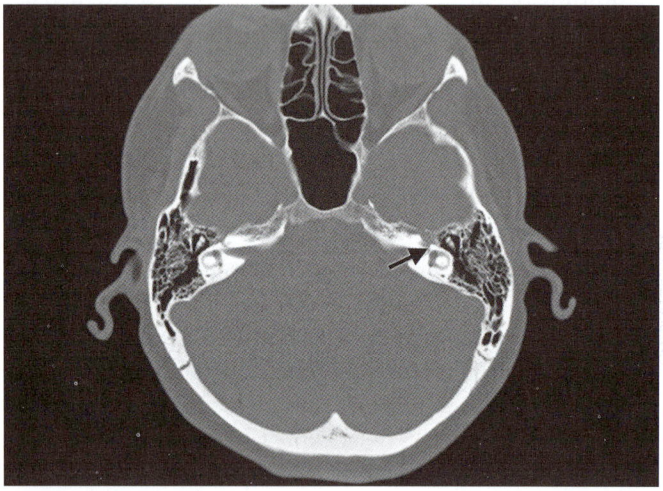

Fig. 10.16: Axial HRCT of the temporal bone demonstrating a left-sided geniculate ganglion hemangioma. Note the granular and "ossifying" appearing of the lesion centered over the geniculate ganglion. The black arrow demonstrates erosion of the apical turn and a cochlear fistula.

Treatment

Surgical resection is the mainstay of therapy for geniculate ganglion and IAC hemangiomas. The decision to intervene depends on the hearing status and the preoperative function of the facial nerve. For lesions localized to the geniculate ganglion with poor hearing, a transmastoid approach will provide adequate exposure for removal of the lesion and grafting of the resected nerve. In the more common situation of patients with preserved hearing, the MF approach provides a better access that allows tumor resection and nerve grafting with hearing preservation. The approach is typically extradural and the dura is easily elevated from the underlying tumor.[46,64] Although the neoplasm is essentially extraneural, excision with preservation of the nerve continuity is not always possible. The surgeon should be prepared to graft the nerve with a greater auricular or sural nerve cable graft. In a review of 19 cases,[63] the facial nerve was preserved in 11 (73%) of 15 patients and was excised and grafted in 4 (27%). Recovery to a HB grade I/II was seen in 8 (72%) of 11 patients in whom the integrity of the facial nerve was preserved. In the surgical group, hearing remained stable in 64% of hearing preservation cases and worsened in 38%. Facial function remained stable in the nonsurgical group.

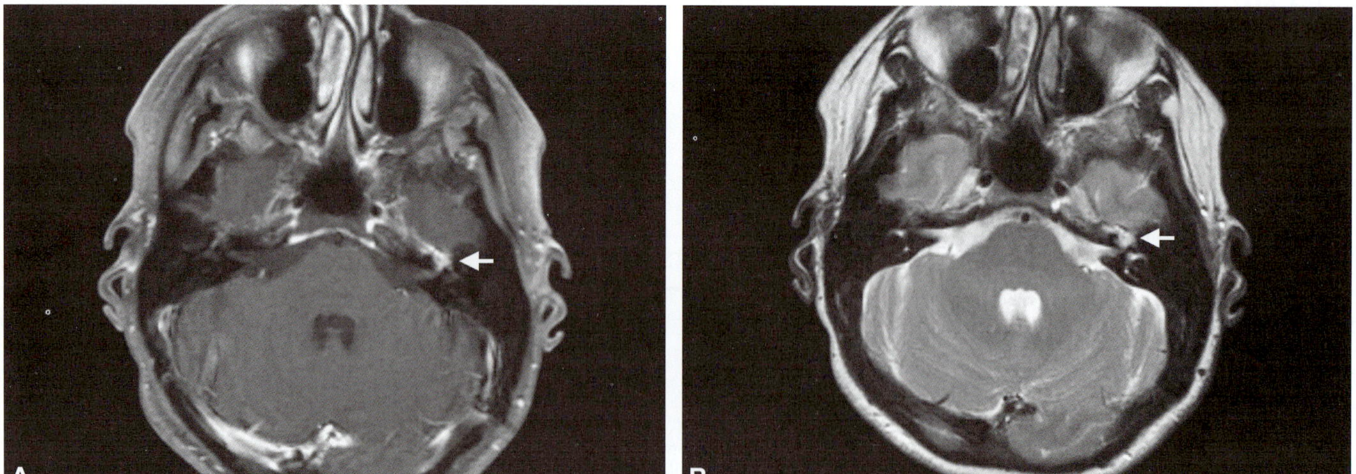

Figs. 10.17A and B: (A) A gadolinium-enhanced axial MRI of the brain demonstrating a left-sided geniculate ganglion hemangioma (white arrow). (B) A T2 weighted MR of the brain demonstrating a left geniculate ganglion hemangioma (white arrow). Note the hyperintense signal typically seen in hemangiomas.

ENDOLYMPHATIC SAC AND DUCT TUMORS

Introduction

Endolymphatic sac tumors (ELST) are rare neoplasms of the temporal bone. Prevalence is unknown. ELST originate from the endolymphatic sac epithelium and are centered over the posterior portion of the petrous bone. They invade the posterior petrous ridge and involve the posterior fossa. In advanced stages, CPA involvement can be seen.

It usually occurs in sporadic forms but may be hereditary in an autosomal dominant manner in the context of von Hippel-Lindau's (VHL) disease.

Pathology

In 1988, Gaffey et al.[68] described low-grade adenocarcinoma of the middle ear and designated them as aggressive papillary middle ear tumors. One year later, Heffner[69] described 20 cases of "adenocarcinoma of the endolymphatic sac" or AES. In 1993, Poe et al.[70] reported bilateral AES in a patient with VHL disease.

Li et al.[71] gave the term ELST to the lesion initially described by Heffner. They tend to behave as a low-grade neoplasm that is locally aggressive and destructive. ELST should be considered in the differential diagnosis of a destructive temporal bone lesion involving the posterior fossa and CPA.

Hematogenous metastasis have not been described; however, "drop metastasis" has been reported.[72] Histologically, they contain cystic and papillary components. The epithelium of the papillary component is lined with a single cell layer of cuboidal or low columnar epithelium (Fig. 10.18).[73] ELST may contain areas of hemosiderin deposits, fibrosis and cholesterol clefts. The cystic component contains a proteinaceous material reminiscent of thyroid colloid. It stains positively with periodic acid-Schiff stain.[69] Thyroglobulin stains are essential to rule out a metastatic thyroid carcinoma. The hypervascularity of the tumor is reflected by an abundant vascular stroma.

Immunohistochemical analysis shows that ELST stain positively with cytokeratin, S-100 and neuron-specific enolase, suggesting a neuroectodermal origin.[74-76] On the other hand, the absence of reactivity to antibodies directed against glial fibrillary acid protein (GLAP) and transthyretin argues against a glial or choroidal origin.[77]

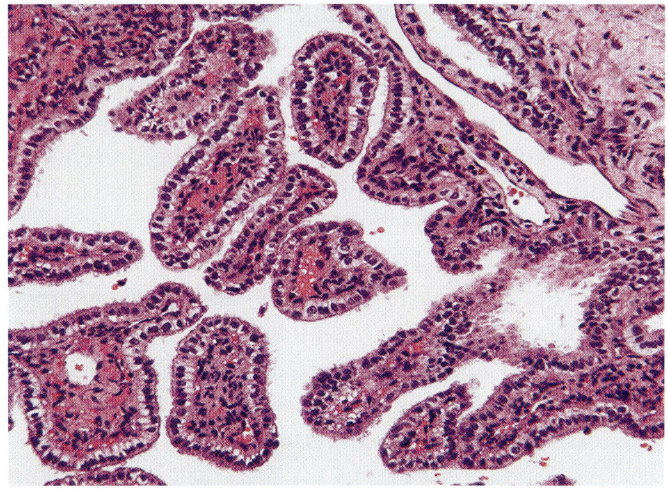

Fig. 10.18: Photomicrograph of an endolymphatic sac tumor showing papillary structures lined with cuboidal cells.

Endolymphatic Sac Tumors and von Hippel-Lindau

von Hippel-Lindau is an autosomal dominant disorder due to a germline mutation of the VHL tumor suppressor gene localized on chromosome 3p25.[78] The prevalence of the disease is estimated to be 1/39,000,[79] and is characterized by an inherited predisposition to visceral (renal cell carcinoma and cysts, pheochromocytoma, pancreatic neuroendocrine tumors and reproductive adnexal cystadenoma) and central nervous system (CNS) neoplasms (cerebellar and brainstem hemangioblastoma, retinal angioma and ELST). ELST has been associated to the Online Mendelian Inheritance in Man in VHL disease (No 193300),[80] and occurs in 11–16% of patients with VHL. Bilateral involvement has been described in 30% of cases of ELST associated with VHL.[81]

The phenotypic expression of VHL occurs with loss of both copies of the tumor suppressor gene. In its hereditary form, a germ-line mutation results in the absence of one allele. The loss of heterozygosity (LOH) or "single-hit" mutation of the second allele results in phenotypic expression.[82] In a study of 3 patients with ELST using fluorescence in-situ hybridization analysis (FISH), LOH was seen in tumor cells but not in normal adjacent cells.[83]

Clinical Manifestations

Endolymphatic sac tumors can occur sporadically or in the context of VHL. If ELST occurs in the context of VHL, associated tumors may be present upon diagnosis. In a study of 121 patients with VHL, 13 patients (11%) showed evidence of 15 ELST on MRI.[84] Sensorineural hearing loss (sudden, fluctuating or progressive), episodic vertigo, aural fullness and tinnitus were commonly described.[84-87] These symptoms are reminiscent of Meniere's syndrome and their combination occurs in 21%.[87] The presence of auditory and vestibular complaints is seen in 59% of VHL patients without evidence of ELST on MRI.[84] Facial weakness is described in 43% of patients.[87] Other cranial neuropathies and headache have been described. In small ELST, obstruction of the endolymphatic duct,[88] overproduction of endolymph, intraductal hemorrhage and neuronal degeneration may cause sudden, fluctuating or progressive hearing loss and vertigo.

Diagnosis

A patient with VHL should be screened for the development of ELST using MRI. Early detection may offer the patient the potential benefit of a hearing preservation approach. Audiometrics should be part of the evaluation. In the great majority of cases, sensorineural hearing loss is present. Conductive loss may be present in tumors invading the middle ear cleft. Vestibular testing may show caloric weakness but is of limited diagnostic value.

Radiological studies are very useful in the evaluation of suspected ELST. The typical finding on HRCT of the temporal bone is a destructive lesion confined to the posterior fossa, often centered over the posterior plate of the petrous bone (Figs. 10.19A and B).[86,89] The lesion shows stippled, reticular, and speculated areas of calcification.[90] In patients with VHL or small (non-detectable) lesions, evidence of intralabyrinthine hemorrhage on non-contrasted HRCT may be the first sign of an image-non-detectable tumor.[83] Large ELST may show otic capsule destruction and neuronal degeneration. Follow-up with repeat MRI is recommended. On T1WI, intralesional foci of hyperintensity are seen in 79% of tumors greater than 3 cm. In tumors less than 3 cm, a circumferential rim of increased intensity is seen on non-enhanced T1WI.[89,90] This rim is likely the result of subacute hemorrhage at the periphery of the tumor. ELST enhance with gadolinium. On T2WI, a heterogenous pattern of intensity is often seen with internal flow void seen in tumors greater than 2 cm.[89] The tumor may spread through the posterior fossa dura into more anteriorly located region, particularly the CPA and jugular foramen.

On four-vessel angiography, ELST are highly vascular. Vascular supply is from the external carotid artery in tumors less than 3 cm, and in tumor greater than 3 cm additional blood supply from the internal carotid artery and posterior circulation is seen.[89]

Recently, a staging system described by Bambakidis et al. offers therapeutic implications (Table 10.5).[72] Stage I tumors are confined to the temporal bone and middle ear cleft, stage II tumors extend to the posterior fossa, stage III tumors are more advanced with MF extension and stage IV tumors are far-advanced lesions extending to the clivus and sphenoid.

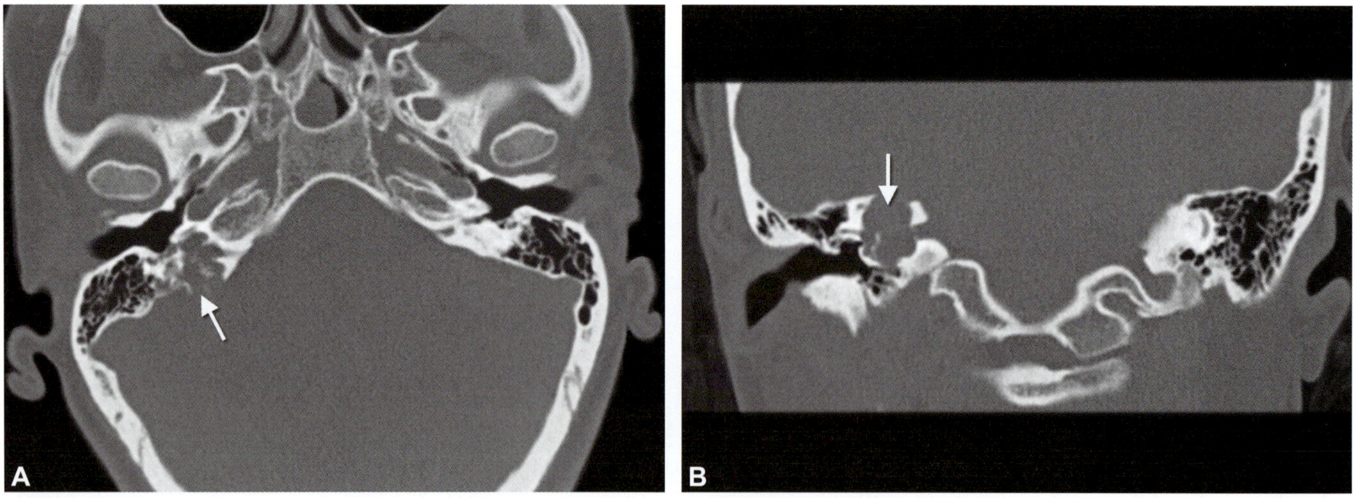

Figs. 10.19A and B: HRCT of the temporal bone with axial views showing an endolymphatic sac tumor (white arrow). Note the destructive pattern, the location along the posterior petrous ridge and the presence of spicules and calcifications. (B) HRCT of the temporal bone, coronal views, showing a destructive lesion invading the otic capsule (white arrow).

Table 10.5: Grading and treatment system for endolymphatic sac tumors*

Grade	*Tumor extent*	*Surgical options*
I	Confined to temporal bone, middle ear cavity, and/or external auditory canal	Hearing preservation with retrolabyrinthine transdural approach (RLTD)
II	Extension into posterior fossa	Extended RLTD approach with labyrinthectomy if hearing poor**
III	Extension in posterior fossa and middle cranial fossa	Sub-temporal craniotomy with petrosectomy**
IV	Extension to clivus and/or sphenoid wing	Staged anterior and posterior fossa techniques**

*Modified from Bambakidis et al.[72]

**Preoperative embolization for grades II-IV and postoperative stereotactic radiosurgery for postoperative residual disease may be adjunctive.

Treatment

The therapeutic modality depends on the size of the lesion, hence the staging, and on the hearing status (Table 10.5). Several reports of tumor removal showed resolution of the vestibular symptoms and stabilization of hearing.[85,87]

In a patient with stage I ELST and good hearing, the tumor may be completely removed through a retrolabyrinthine transdural approach (RLTD) (Fig. 10.20). This approach allows for hearing preservation and tumor removal by excising the dural base and the lip of tumor extending into the ELD.[81,85] The limitations of RLTD are limited access to anteriorly located lesions and decreased angle of exposure in patients with anteriorly displaced sigmoid sinus. Hearing-preservation surgery is particularly important in patients with VHL, with an incidence of bilateral involvement in 30%. In larger lesions extending into the posterior fossa (stage II), hearing may be affected and tumors are removed using a TL approach. The posterior fossa dura is resected and reconstructed. Failure to remove the dural attachment of the posterior fossa, at the site of the endolymphatic sac and the intraductal portion of the tumor, may lead to recurrence.[81,85] In lesions with more significant posterior fossa or MF extension (stage III) and serviceable hearing, a combined approach involving a subtemporal craniotomy with petrosectomy provides good access without violating the hearing end-organ. In extensive lesions involving the petrous apex and CPA (stage IV), a transcochlear approach with complete exenteration of the otic capsule and exposure of the carotid canal may be necessary, or staged anterior and posterior fossa techniques.

When tumors are completely excised recurrence is rare. In small published series,[81,85,87] complete resolution of the vestibular symptoms and stabilization of hearing was possible, if hearing-preservation surgery was done.

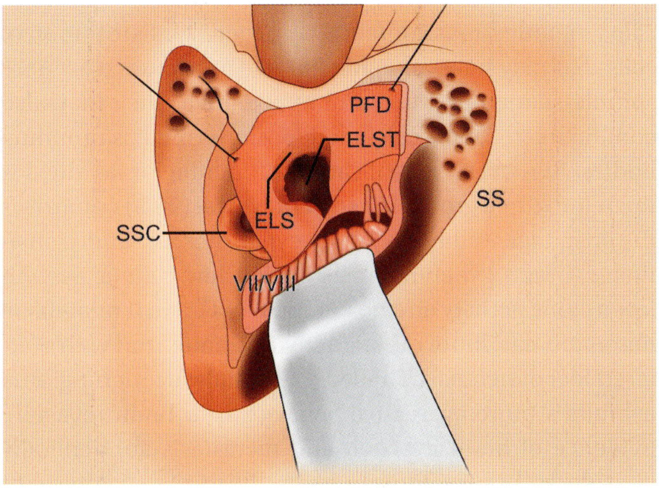

Fig. 10.20: The retrolabyrinthine transdural approach (RLTD) for removal of endolymphatic sac tumors (ELST). Note that the dura is elevated along with the tumor. Residual tumor inside the endolymphatic duct (ELD) can be seen and removed. (ELS, endolymphatic sac; PFD, posterior fossa dura; SS, sigmoid sinus; SSC, superior semicircular canal).

MENINGIOMAS

Introduction

Meningiomas are benign and slow-growing neoplasms that arise from the lining of the arachnoid villi. They account for 13–17% of all intracranial tumors.[91] The CPA is the site of involvement in 8–18% of all intracranial meningiomas.[92] Temporal bone meningiomas are usually the extension of extraaxial intracranial meningiomas into the temporal bone. Meningiomas of the jugular foramen may present as a jugular foramen mass with mastoid and middle ear extension. Isolated IAC meningiomas arising from the dura of the IAC and primary temporal bone meningiomas have been reported but are rare.[93] The peak incidence is in the fourth and fifth decades with a 2:1 female preponderance.[91] Most meningiomas are sporadic but may occur in the context of hereditary disorders such as NF2, Werner syndrome,[94] and Gorlin syndrome.[95]

Pathology

Meningiomas arise from the arachnoidal cap cells located at the tip of the arachnoid villi. Most meningiomas are benign, well-circumscribed tumors. Malignant meningiomas occur in 5% of cases and rarely metastasize to the lung, liver and lymph nodes. Typically these benign lesions displace adjacent neural structures and tend to invade dura and corresponding venous sinuses. Histologically, meningiomas contain a homogenous distribution of cells that may have an epithelial-like appearance or more spindle-shaped and fusiform appearance. They may also contain microscopic calcium deposits termed psammoma bodies. The WHO classification of meningiomas divides them into three groups. Grade I or typical (90%) comprises the histologic subtypes of syncytial, fibrous and transitional. Grade I meningiomas exhibit low cellularity with low mitotic activity and no necrosis. In Grade II or atypical meningiomas, more mitotic activity is noted and with scattered foci of necrosis. Grade III or anaplastic meningioma exhibits a more aggressive behavior with brain invasion. Evidence of brain invasion and metastasis are generally considered as prerequisite to establish the diagnosis of malignancy.

The implication of genetic alterations in the pathogenesis of meningioma has been recently established. Mutations or deletions of NF2 gene on chromosome 22 are seen in 60% of sporadic meningiomas.[96] The deletions of more tumor suppression genes (18p, 1p, 6q, 14q, 18q and 9p)[97,98] and acquisition of pro-oncogenic genes (1q, 9q, 12q, 15q, 17q and 20q)[96-98] may play an important role in the progression of meningioma from a more indolent (Grade I) to a more aggressive subtype (Grade II or III). Most hereditary types of meningioma occur in the context of NF2. The onset of a tumor at an early age and/or the bilateral occurrence of meningiomas must initiate a workup for NF2. Non-NF2-related hereditary meningiomas have also been described.[95]

Anatomic Patterns

Anatomically, meningiomas are best described in relation to the dural surface from which they originate. These lesions may arise from the region of the CPA and IAC, from the adjacent areas of the posterior fossa dura (jugular foramen, petrosal, clival and petroclival) and from the dural cover of the floor of the middle cranial fossa. A simple anatomic classification divides meningiomas into medial to the IAC (superior petrosal sinus, petrosal, clival, petroclival), lateral to the IAC (sigmoid sinus, jugular bulb, superior petrosal sinus), superior to the IAC (midpetrosal), and CPA or IAC meningiomas that are considered when the bulk of the lesion is centered over the CPA or IAC. The relationship to the IAC is of surgical importance as lesions situated superior, posterior and inferior to the IAC have a higher neural preservation rate due to their more accessible location when the retrosigmoid surgical approach is used. Meningiomas arising anterior to the IAC are more challenging to remove as the cranial nerves lay in an unfavorable vantage point.

Meningioma confined to the IAC are rare and are difficult to diagnose preoperatively, even on neuroimaging. This entity is important to recognize, as dural resection is needed for complete tumor removal, which is not usually the case with VS. IAC meningioma may spread toward the cochlea, vestibule and semicircular canals. This lateral spread destroys the inner ear, and in severe cases the tumor may reach the middle ear by traversing the round and oval window. The finding of significant lateral involvement usually favors a meningioma compared to a VS.

Meningiomas arising from the dural surface of the posterior fossa may enlarge to invade the jugular foramen, jugular bulb and sigmoid sinus. Inferiorly, they may extend to involve the lower clivus. Anteriorly, these lesions may wrap around the clivus and present as a petroclival meningioma. Petroclival meningioma may spread to involve the cavum trigeminalis or Meckel's cave and further extend toward the cavernous sinus. Depending on the area involved, they may have a predominant involvement of the middle cranial fossa, posterior cranial fossa or a bi-fossa involvement.

Meningiomas arising from the dural surface of the middle cranial fossa may spread anteriorly to involve Meckel's cave and the cavernous sinus, or inferiorly through the tegmen to involve the middle ear cleft.

Clinical Manifestations

The presenting signs and symptoms depend on the anatomic location and neural involvement. Hearing loss (60–84%), tinnitus (50–70%) and dizziness (76%) are common presenting complaints.[91,99,100]

In a retrospective review of audiometric findings in 25 patients with proven CPA meningiomas,[101] 20% had normal hearing, 12% had low-frequency hearing loss, 36% had a flat loss, 12% had a mid-frequency hearing loss, 20% had profound hearing loss and none had a high-frequency pattern of hearing loss. A delay in diagnosis of 4–6 years has been reported since the onset of the symptomatology.[92,100] Trigeminal neuropathy, facial paresis and lower cranial neuropathy (CN IX, X and XI) are more commonly reported in meningiomas.[99,100,102,103] IAC meningiomas mimic VS and diagnosis may be difficult. Hearing loss, tinnitus and vertigo are seen in 87.5%, 75% and 62.5% of patients, respectively.[93] Meningiomas arising from the jugular foramen comprise 4.3% of posterior fossa meningioma[104] and mimic glomus jugulare tumors. Hearing loss is seen in 78%, tinnitus in 57%, and a middle ear mass in 78%.[102]

Diagnosis

Using neuroimaging modalities, meningiomas can be accurately diagnosed preoperatively in the great majority of cases. In addition to narrowing down the list of differential diagnoses, MR and CT imaging provide a good appreciation of the extent of the lesion and the degree of involvement of critical adjacent neurovascular structures. The information obtained aids in the selection of the appropriate therapeutic approach. For lesions of the CPA, contrasted and non-contrasted MR is superior to CT in delineating the exact nature and extent of the lesion.[105]

On non-contrasted CT,[106-108] meningiomas appear hyperdense or isodense compared to brain tissue. When contrast is used, meningiomas show homogenous enhancement. Schwannomas are hypo- or isodense when compared to adjacent brain tissue and their enhancement pattern is often nonhomogenous. Unlike schwannomas, meningiomas tend not to enlarge involved foramina and frequently demonstrate areas of calcification and hyperostosis. The intralesional calcifications are believed to be calcified psammoma bodies and the observed hyperostosis presents a reactive bone remodeling.

On MR,[109] meningiomas are iso- to hypointense on T1WI and variable on T2WI. When gadolinium is used (Figs. 10.21 and 10.22), meningiomas show homogenous enhancement with enhancement of the adjacent dura known as "dural tail".[110] Calcifications are seen as hypointense signals on T1WI and T2WI. Unlike schwannomas, cystic degeneration is not common. Meningiomas are broad-based (sessile), centered on the dural surface.

Treatment

The goal of surgical intervention is complete removal of the tumor along with a dural margin and drilling of the underlying bone. Hyperostosis may be indicative of meningioma cells invading into the Harversian canal of the underlying bone, a histological finding that may predispose to recurrence without being an indicator of malignancy. The surgeon should make every effort to preserve important neurovascular structures. Intraoperative neurophysiologic monitoring is an integral part of meningioma surgery. The selection of the neural structures to be monitored depends on the location of the lesion and the

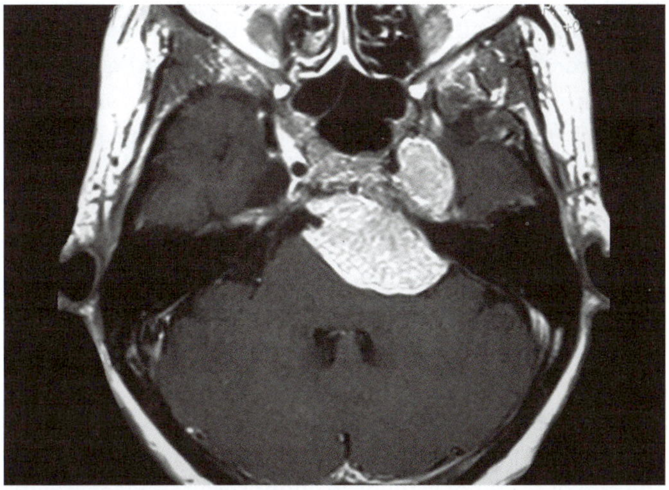

Fig. 10.21: Gadolinium-enhanced MR demonstrates a bi-fossa petroclival meningioma. Note the broad-based attachment.

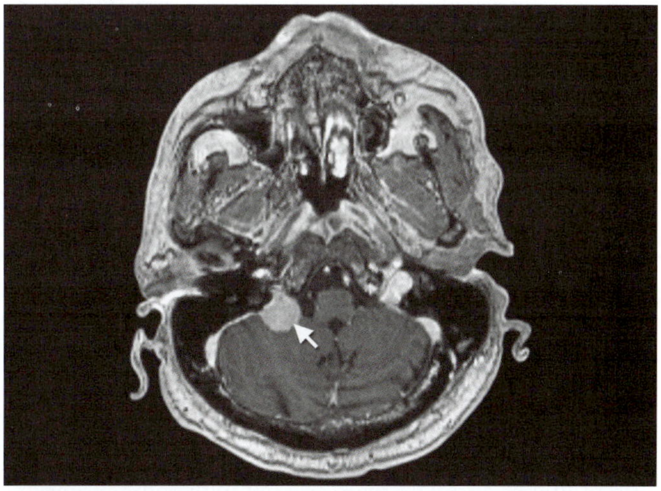

Fig. 10.22: A gadolinium-enhanced MR demonstrating a posterior fossa meningioma extending into the right jugular foramen (white arrow).

degree of preoperative function. When the surgeon is at a disadvantageous vantage point, the risk of neural injury is greater.

Selecting an approach depends on the location and hearing status. A combination of a transpetrous and subtemporal approach affords good exposure for bi-fossa meningiomas such as petroclival meningiomas. A combined retrolabyrinthine (or presigmoid)-subtemporal approach with or without an anterior petrosectomy provides adequate exposure in patients with serviceable hearing. If preoperative hearing is poor, the TL or transcochlear route may be chosen. In meningiomas involving primarily the posterior fossa, a suboccipital or retrosigmoid approach is used.

Involvement of the petrous apex with inferior extension may be best removed using the infratemporal fossa approaches B or C. The goal of microsurgical treatment is complete excision of the lesion, including the dural base, with adequate margins and drilling of the underlying bone. Subtotal excision increases the risk of recurrence.[111] Meningiomas involving the petroclival angle with significant anteromedial extension, the cavernous sinus, and those adherent to the brainstem are often incompletely removed, with a higher risk of recurrence.[112,113]

Microsurgical excision of meningiomas remains the treatment of choice. Two adjunctive therapies may supplement or replace the surgical treatment: external beam radiotherapy and stereotactic radiosurgery. These modalities are usually offered to patients with incompletely resected tumors, recurrence, or malignant lesions and to moribund patients who are not suitable for surgical treatment. In a review of 140 patients with incompletely resected meningiomas[114] treated with external beam radiotherapy, the 5-year progression-free survival rates were 89% and 48% for benign and malignant meningiomas, respectively. In another study[115] comparing 17 patients with incompletely resected meningiomas to historical control, the 8-year progression-free survival rate was 88% for the radiated arm versus 48% for the nonirradiated arm. In 16 patients in whom radiotherapy was administered after the first recurrence, the 8-year progression-free survival rate was 78% in the radiated arm versus 11% in the nonirradiated arm.

In a retrospective review of the use of stereotactic radiosurgery in the treatment of 99 patients with intracranial meningiomas,[116] 43% were treated primarily with this modality and 57% were treated with radiosurgery as an adjunct modality. The average tumor dose was 16 Gy. At 10 years post-treatment, 63% of tumors regressed in size, 32% remained unchanged and 5% progressed. In another review,[117] 62 patients with petroclival meningiomas were treated with stereotactic radiosurgery. In 63% prior microsurgery was performed. The median follow-up time was 37 months. Tumor regression was noted in 23%, growth remained unchanged in 68% and the lesion progressed in 8%. The neurological status improved or remained stable in 87%.

The role of stereotactic radiosurgery continues to be refined. Currently, it is recommended for recurrent disease, incomplete excision or when surgery cannot be offered. Observation is limited to moribund patients with a short life expectancy.

SOFT TISSUE SARCOMAS

Soft tissue sarcomas are rare neoplasms derived from mesenchymal cells. Depending on the specific cell type of origin, different histological variants exist. In the temporal bone, two types are of particular interest and will be discussed: chondrosarcoma and rhabdomyosarcoma (RMS). These two entities differ pathologically, clinically and therapeutically and merit a separate discussion.

Chondrosarcoma

Introduction

Chondrosarcomas of the skull base are rare malignant neoplasms thought to originate from malignant transformation of rests of embryonal chondrocytes that reside at the foramen lacerum. Chondrosarcoma comprises 6% of all skull base lesions, and 75% of all cranial chondrosarcomas occur in the skull base.[118] Embryologically, the chondrocranium (precursor of the skull base) undergoes endochondral ossification whereas the skull vault develops by intramembranous ossification. As the primitive skull base undergoes ossification, an area corresponding to the junction between the petro-occipital, sphenopetrosal, and spheno-occipital synchondrosis remains more or less non-ossified.[119] This area in the skull is confined to the region of the foramen lacerum. As the large majority of posterior fossa chondrosarcomas arise at the convergence of the spheno-occipital, petro-occipital and sphenopetrosal synchondrosis, it is hypothesized that residual endochondral cartilage at the foramen lacerum may be the site of origin of skull base chondrosarcomas.[119,120] First described in 1965,[121] chondrosarcoma of the skull base is a locally aggressive neoplasm. The advent of microsurgery of the skull base and the development of different techniques including endoscopic anterior skull base approaches have improved surgical access to the affected area.

Although most lesions occur de novo, chondrosarcoma has been described arising from nonhereditary enchondromatoses such as Maffucci syndrome and Ollier's disease and in patients with longstanding Paget's disease.[122]

Pathology

Macroscopically, chondrosarcoma appear as lobulated gray-blue masses with a translucent, glistening, cystic surface that may contain yellow to white spicules of calcifications.[120] Histologically, five types have been described: conventional, myxoid, mesenchymal, clear cell and dedifferentiated.[123] Conventional chondrosarcoma is the most common type and comprises 6% of skull base tumors.[120] Histologically, the bone marrow is replaced by hyaline cartilage, cells with plump nuclei, binucleate cells and multinucleated giant cartilage cells. The hyaline component corresponds to neoplastic chondrocytes residing within lacunar spaces and surrounded by a hyaline matrix.[124] With tumor growth, proliferating neoplastic cells gradually separate the bone trabeculae. Scattered calcification and periosteal thickening may be seen. In myxoid chondrosarcoma, the chondroid appearance is predominant. In this subtype, scattered neoplastic chondrocytes are bordered by a frothy mucinous matrix.[120,124] The myxoid subtype may be difficult to differentiate from clival chordomas. Immunohistochemical analysis helps in delineating the two entities. Chordomas are of epithelial origin and stain positively with cytokeratine and epithelial membrane antigen whereas chondrosarcoma stain positive with vimentin and S-100.[125]

Chondrosarcomas can be divided into three grades depending on their degree of differentiation.[126-128] The presence of uniform cellular elements with small dense nuclei, a myxoid appearance and rare mitosis characterizes grade I. The increase in the degree of cellularity, nuclear atypia, and necrosis as well as the number of nuclei and mitosis signals a poorly differentiated type or grade III. Grade II is intermediate. The majority of chondrosarcomas of the skull base are well differentiated and fall into grades I and II.[129] The grading system bears a prognostic significance with five-year survival rates for grade I, II and III of 90%, 81%, and 43%.[128,130]

The central location within the skull base makes a preoperative incisional biopsy difficult, but CT-guided fine-needle aspiration cytology (FNAC) is valuable in the diagnosis of chondrosarcoma. An experienced cytopathologist is essential to the recognition of the different types.[131] Cytopathologic specimens of conventional chondrosarcomas demonstrate large vacuolated cells with eccentric nuclei reminiscent of signet cells along with a chondroid matrix.[132]

Clinical Presentation

Chondrosarcomas affect both sexes equally and are frequently seen between the third and fifth decades.[129,133] Some series favoring male or female predilection have also been published.[129,134] However, all age groups can be affected. A mean delay of 2 years between the onset of symptoms and the diagnosis has been noted.[133,135] The onset of cranial neuropathies in a patient with headache warrants further investigation in the form of neuroimaging. The most common presenting symptoms are headache and diplopia.[118,129,133,136] The latter is due to compression or invasion of the abducens nerve in Dorello's canal. The anterior extension toward the cavernous sinus may lead to involvement of the occulomotor and trochlear nerves. The appearance of additional cranial neuropathies, i.e. facial paresthesias, facial weakness, hearing loss, dysphagia or dysphonia, heralds further progression of the neoplasm and extension toward the posterior fossa, the CPA region, the petrous bone, and the middle cranial fossa.

Diagnosis

The insidious onset of CN dysfunction in a patient complaining of headache warrants further investigation in the form of neuroimaging. Both HRCT of the temporal bone and clival area and MR imaging are essential in the diagnosis of skull base chondrosarcoma. The anatomic location and the radiographic appearance are key elements in the differentiation of lesions involving or extending to the petrous apex.

On HRCT, chondrosarcomas demonstrate irregular bony destruction with scattered areas of calcification referred to as "popcorn pattern". The location lateral to the petroclival synchondrosis is suggestive; however, some chondrosarcomas originate medial to this junction, making their differentiation from clival chordomas more challenging radiographically. Whereas most chondrosarcomas show enhancement on contrasted HRCT, the absence of enhancement does not exclude this diagnosis.

A multitude of benign lesions involving the petrous apex, some also causing bony erosion, may simulate chondrosarcoma. These lesions are cholesterol granuloma, cholesteatoma, petrous apicitis, and carotid aneurysms. Although its differential abilities are less than MRI, HRCT may aid in the specific diagnosis. Bony erosion in chondrosarcoma is typically described as smooth with regular borders. Irregular bony erosion is seen in petrous apicitis, some benign neoplasms (meningiomas and paragangliomas) and most malignant neoplasms and metastases.

On MRI, chondrosarcomas have a low to intermediate signal intensity on T1WI and show heterogenous enhancement on T1WI with gadolinium. On T2WI, chondrosarcomas demonstrate high signal intensity with scattered flow voids corresponding to areas of intratumoral calcifications. Chordomas are typically medially located and extend laterally, inferiorly and superiorly. Their epicenter appears to be the clivus. Chondrosarcomas are usually located lateral to the clivus, with their epicenter at the petroclival region and the area of the foramen lacerum. Cerebral angiography and MRA are helpful in delineating the tumor's relationship to adjacent vascular structures, a key element in the preoperative planning. The histological diagnosis is obtained by an image-guided biopsy. At times, if image-guided biopsy is not a valid option, an exploratory surgery with biopsy at the time of a major extirpative surgery is planned. The downside of this approach is the need for the surgeon to make a major therapeutic decision based on the sole result of the frozen section analysis.

Treatment

Surgery is the mainstay of treatment of skull base chondrosarcoma. Although many approaches have been described to access the central and lateral skull base, lateral approaches have been advocated by many surgeons.[31,118,135,137-140] Transfacial and transpharyngeal approaches do not adequately expose the tumor elements located posterolateral to the intrapetrous carotid artery.[31] The infratemporal fossa type-B approach provides a wide access to the region of the petrous apex and clivus in its upper two-thirds. The provision of excellent tumor exposure is also supplemented by the ability to control the intrapetrous carotid artery.[135,137,140] The addition of a subtemporal craniotomy and/or retrosigmoid craniotomy provides additional exposure. Transpetrous approaches with or without exenteration of the otic capsule (subtemporal-transpetrous, TL and transcochlear) have been utilized.

Transcranial approaches using a fronto-temporal craniotomy with or without pterional craniotomy provide a direct surgical access to the parasellar region. A transfacial or transnasal endoscopic approach coupled with guided navigation has expanded the surgical armamentarium. The most important factor is adequate exposure for gross tumor removal. Although wide excision of uninvolved structures is not necessary, gross tumor removal is important to prevent local recurrence.[137,138,141] The use of adjuvant radiotherapy in the form of proton-beam irradiation or stereotactic radiosurgery has been employed by many centers and appears to result in less local recurrence at the expense of a higher rate of complications.[129,138,141,142] However, large prospective series are lacking due to the rarity of the lesion and the absence of standardized surgical management.

Complications seen may be related to surgical treatment—cerebrospinal fluid leak, iatrogenic cranial neuropathies, vascular injuries or infection—or may be related to radiotherapy—temporal bone osteoradionecrosis, new onset cranial neuropathy and pituitary dysfunction.[138,142]

Rhabdomyosarcoma

Introduction

Rhabdomyosarcoma (RMS) accounts for 5–15% of all childhood neoplasms and for 30% of temporal bone sarcoma.[143,144] It is the most common malignant neoplasm of the temporal bone in childhood. 40% of RMS occur in the head and neck.[145] Commonly affected locations in the head and neck are the orbit, the middle ear, the oral cavity, the nasopharynx and the infratemporal fossa.[146] Most occur before the age of 15 years with an average between 4 and 5 years. In the head and neck, RMS are divided into three categories: orbital (23%), parameningeal (56%) and non-parameningeal (21%).[145] Parameningeal denotes those tumors that develop in proximity to the skull base and adjacent meninges.

Pathology

Rhabdomyosarcoma is a highly aggressive, locally destructive malignant neoplasm of the soft tissue. Distant metastasis is present in 14% at the time of diagnosis with the possibility of distal spread to the lungs, bone, liver and brain.[147] In the temporal bone, it is hypothesized that RMS originates from the malignant transformation of myocytes residing in the stapedial or tensor tympani muscle.

Four histological subtypes have been described: embryonal, alveolar, pleomorphic and botyroid.[148] In the head and neck, embryonal RMS is the most frequently encountered histological subtype (85%), followed by alveolar RMS (15%).[145] Histologically, embryonal RMS is characterized by the presence of elongated, spindle-shaped malignant cells with bipolar processes reminiscent of immature rhabdomyoblasts. A single central nucleus is typically present along with a relatively abundant eosinophilic cytoplasm. Alternating areas of hypercellularity and hypocellularity may be seen. In the hypercellular areas, dense small round blue cells can be predominant, including this neoplasm in the differential diagnosis of tumors with small round blue cells. Numerous mitotic figures are seen. In the hypocellular areas a myxoid-appearing stroma is present.[148] The alveolar subtype shows clusters of cells resembling epithelial cells reminiscent of the pulmonary alveolus with intervening sheets of connective tissue. Striations can be present along with giant and multinucleated cells.[148,149] The primitive appearance of some RMS makes recognition difficult. The addition of immunohistochemical analysis is helpful in differentiating some of these cases. Antibodies directed against actin, sarcomeric actin, desmin, myogenin, and myoD1 can be useful.[149]

Clinical Presentation

In children, RMS mimics all the signs and symptoms of chronic suppurative otitis media.[144,150-153] The prevalence of the infectious disease may result in a delay in diagnosis. The astute physician should have a heightened degree of clinical suspicion in the presence of a middle ear or external auditory canal mass or polyp, unrelenting course despite aggressive antibiotic treatment, and presence of pain associated with cranial neuropathy. Early diagnosis and institution of appropriate multimodality therapy are key elements to a successful outcome. Clinically, RMS can present with earache, middle ear and external auditory canal mass or polyp and intermittent bloody otorrhea. As the tumor invades surrounding structures, additional signs and symptoms develop. Meningeal and CNS involvement portends a worse prognosis and warrants more aggressive therapy.

Diagnosis

On temporal bone imaging, RMS exhibits the characteristics of a locally aggressive neoplasm. On HRCT the lesion is seen as a soft tissue density with infiltrative bony destruction and irregular erosion.[154] The middle ear is commonly affected and different parts of the petrous bone and adjacent areas are involved, depending on the extent of the tumor. The administration of contrast material results in heterogenous enhancement. MRI is helpful in the evaluation of the meningeal and CNS involvement.[155,156] On T1WI, RMS typically has a homogenous appearance isointense to muscle. When gadolinium is administered, enhancement is seen and helps in delineating the soft tissue component. On T2WI, RMS shows a hyperintense signal.

Ultimately, the diagnosis of RMS is made with histological confirmation. Biopsy material may be obtained from an aural polyp or by a myringotomy performed to access the middle ear. On the other hand, tissue can be obtained during a planned mastoidectomy.

Treatment

Rhabdomyosarcoma is a chemosensitive tumor with cure rates approaching 70% when multimodality therapy is used.[157] This is a dramatic improvement from the initial poor results obtained with single modality treatment with an overall 5-year survival of 28%.[158] The results of the studies carried out by the intergroup RMS study (IRS) have increased our understanding of the disease and ultimately affected patients' care by reducing mortality and increasing the disease-free survival and overall survival rates.[147,159-161] Although complete resection is the mainstay of treatment for trunk and extremity RMS, radical surgical resection of parameningeal RMS results in high morbidity and is quite disfiguring. It became evident that the treatment of temporal bone RMS requires multimodality treatment with surgery, radiation and multiagent chemotherapy. In order to predict the tumor behavior and response to treatment in a given individual, classification schemes have been advocated.

The currently used clinical classification scheme is the Intergroup Rhabdomyosarcoma Study (IRS) classification system introduced in 1975.[147] Group I refers to localized disease, group II refers to microscopic residual or regional disease, group III refers to individuals with incomplete resection or biopsy with gross residual disease, and group IV includes patients with metastatic disease at presentation.

The site, histological subtype, IRS stage, patient's age and type of treatment are important prognostic factors.[145,162-165] Parameningeal RMS has a worse prognosis than orbital and non-parameningeal RMS. Embryonal

RMS has a better outcome than the alveolar type. Age greater than 10 years or less than 1 year was associated with a worst outcome.

Prior to the institution of multimodality therapy, the survival rates for IRS clinical groups I, II, III and IV were 0%, 14%, 0% and 0%, respectively.[166] To evaluate and compare the results of multimodality treatment, the IRS conducted a series of studies, IRS I to IV.

IRS-I[147] included 686 patients with RMS or undifferentiated sarcoma followed between 1972 and 1978. The results of IRS-I showed that there was no additional benefit of radiotherapy to combination chemotherapy (vincristine and dactinomycin or VA) for clinical group I (localized disease completely resected). In addition, no benefit was seen in adding low-dose daily oral cyclophosphamide to the combination of radiation and chemotherapy (vincristine and dactinomycin or VA), and no benefit of adding adriamycin to the combination or radiation and chemotherapy (vincristine, dactinomycin and cyclophosphamide or VAC). The 5-year survival for the entire group and parameningeal RMS was 55% and 47%, respectively. IRS-II[161] was conducted between 1978 and 1984 and included 999 patients with RMS. All patients were included after surgical treatment. In IRS clinical group III, the use of radiation and intrathecal chemotherapy increased 5-year survival from 47% to 59%. IRS-III[160] was conducted between 1984 and 1991and included 1,062 patients with RMS. The major difference in the intervention in clinical group III was the reduction in the radiation fields for parameningeal RMS without intracranial extension and the intensification of the chemotherapy regimen. In clinical group III, the results showed increased 5-year survival from 59% to 65%. IRS-IV[159] was conducted between 1991 and 1997 and included 883 patients. For clinical group III, the study compared the efficacy of hyperfractionated radiotherapy to conventional radiotherapy and found no difference.

Currently for parameningeal RMS that includes middle ear RMS, the recommended treatment is surgery for biopsy, followed by radiotherapy and chemotherapy. The timing of treatment is important. For parameningeal RMS with evidence of intracranial extension, radiotherapy should be given concurrently with chemotherapy.[146]

Both chemotherapy and radiotherapy have been associated with complications. The development of long-term side effects from radiotherapy led to the development of trials in Europe where radiotherapy has been excluded from the initial management of low-risk groups and reinstituted in the event of recurrence. Patients with no relapse who did not receive radiotherapy enjoy a long-term disease-free survival without late sequelae.[145] The late sequelae include hormonal dysfunction, cognitive dysfunction, facial growth retardation, hearing loss, and dental and visual problems.[167] The application of this rationale to parameningeal RMS is not currently accepted as these patients are considered a higher-risk group.

HEMATOLOGICAL MALIGNANCIES

Leukemia, lymphoma and plasmocytoma can affect the petrous bone.[168-170] Most commonly, tumor cells infiltrate the temporal bone and its marrow spaces as part of a systemic disease process. Rarely, isolated involvement may be seen. Although all parts of the petrous bone can be affected, involvement of the middle ear and mastoid is a more common finding.

Leukemia is a neoplastic disorder that affects white blood cells and results in the proliferation and accumulation of a large number of immature lymphohematopoietic cells. By the time of diagnosis, leukemic cells have already infiltrated the bone marrow and spread to some extramedullary sites. Based on the particular morphologic and immunophenotypic characteristics of these tumors, different classification schemes have been described. Detailing each subtype is beyond the scope of this chapter. In the temporal bone, symptoms are caused by infiltration and hemorrhage. Rarely, the hyperviscosity caused by the large number of leukocytes in the circulation can present with bilateral hearing loss of acute onset.[171] Leukemic patients may present with middle ear effusion,[168] facial nerve palsy,[172] vertigo, tinnitus and sensorineural hearing loss.[169,173] Infiltration of the cochleovestibular nerve and facial nerve is seen on histopathologic studies of human temporal bones.[168,174] Inner ear involvement is uncommon.[175] In rare instances, the CPA is involved by accumulation of neoplastic granulocytic cells, chloromas, usually seen in patients with acute myelogenous leukemia.[176] The treatment of acute or chronic leukemia involving the temporal bone is medical and the role of surgery is limited to biopsy.

Lymphoma is a neoplastic process that affects the lymphoid system. Hodgkin's lymphoma (HL) is characterized histologically by the presence of Reed-Sternberg's cells in a background of inflammatory stroma. Morphologic and immunophenotypic criteria classify HL into different subsets. The more common non-Hodgkin's lymphoma (NHL) is a heterogenous group of neoplastic disorders of the lymphoid system that lack the characteristic cell type seen in HL. Detailing the different subtypes of HL and NHL is beyond the scope of this chapter. Infiltration of the bone marrow, middle ear and Eustachian tube mucosa is seen in both types of lymphomas.[168,177,178] Patients may present with middle ear effusion, hearing loss and facial paralysis.[179,180] Involvement of the temporal bone is less common with HL.[181] Surgery is limited to biopsy if no other extranodal sites are present. Medical management is the mainstay of treatment.

Plasmocytoma, a monoclonal proliferation of plasma call or plasmacytoid cells, is a variant of multiple myeloma and comprises less than 10% of plasma cell dyscrasias.[182,183] Two clinical forms have been described: solitary plasmacytoma of bone and extramedullary plasmacytoma. Solitary plasmacytoma of bone presents with isolated bone involvement, usually affecting the axial skeleton and the extremities without clinical, radiographic and immunoelectrophoretic evidence of multiple myeloma. Conversion to multiple myeloma usually occurs in more than half of cases over a period of 4–5 years. Extramedullary plasmacytoma presents with a space-occupying lesion that consists of neoplastic proliferation of plasma cells outside the bone marrow, usually the upper aerodigestive tract and paranasal sinuses.[170,182] Temporal bone involvement is rare. HRCT shows a lytic process with occasionally a soft tissue mass.[184,185] Plasmacytoma usually infiltrates the middle ear and mastoid; however, involvement of the otic capsule has been described.[170,185] The diagnosis is based on the presence of extramedullary proliferation of monoclonal plasma cells without evidence of multiple myeloma on bone marrow biopsy. Treatment is usually radiotherapy, and recurrences occur in 25%. Progression into multiple myeloma is uncommon.[186]

Clinically, these lesions can mimic any acute or chronic middle ear and mastoid pathology. Neural involvement in the form of hearing loss, tinnitus, vertigo and facial paralysis is not uncommon. A high index of suspicion, mainly in patients with systemic disease, is necessary for timely diagnosis. A list of adjunctive laboratory tests is often necessary for appropriate diagnosis and treatment is often nonsurgical. Different chemotherapeutic agents are used with or without radiotherapy. Radiotherapy alone is used for extramedullary plasmacytoma and isolated lymphoma.

METASTASIS OF THE TEMPORAL BONE

The temporal bone may harbor metastases from various carcinomatous neoplasms. The most common sites of origin are the breast, lung, kidney, stomach, prostate and melanoma.[187-189] In the temporal bone, metastatic disease commonly affects the petrous apex, followed by the IAC.[187] In a study of 1,354 CPA lesions, the incidence of metastatic disease was 0.2%.[190] Most published series are small and spaced over many years. The most important mechanism of spread is hematogenous seeding of the marrow-rich portion of the temporal bone. If neoplastic cells gain access to the cerebrospinal fluid containing spaces, the IAC and CPA may be the site of involvement, which can be bilateral.[187] Clinically, patients may present during the course of a known malignancy, or rarely the temporal bone may be the revealing site. Hearing loss, facial palsy and vertigo are seen in 60%, 50% and 30%, respectively.[189] The temporal bone may be involved in multiple sites in 20%.[187] Radiographically, metastasis demonstrates a lytic process on HRCT. MRI shows an infiltrative and destructive soft tissue mass with a low signal on T1WI and high on T2WI. Enhancement is usually seen.[156] The petrous apex is commonly involved but other sites may be affected. The destructive process on radiologic studies often exceeds the clinical findings.[188] Prognosis is guarded and treatment is palliative. The role of surgery is limited to tissue confirmation if clinically indicated. Palliative treatment includes chemotherapy with or without radiotherapy as dictated by the nature of the primary lesion.

CONCLUSION

A variety of benign and malignant neoplasms may affect the temporal bone and its vicinity. Symptoms of neoplastic diseases of the temporal bone mimic common chronic otological diseases. Radiographic studies are essential in evaluating patients suspected of having temporal bone neoplasms. The definitive therapeutic modality is dictated by the histological subtype and tailored to the extent of disease and the patient's clinical symptomatology and overall health.

REFERENCES

1. Guild SR. The glomus jugulare, a nonchromaffin paraganglion, in man. Ann Otol Rhinol Laryngol. 1953;62:1045-71; concld.
2. Lack EE, Cubilla AL, Woodruff JM, et al. Paragangliomas of the head and neck region: a clinical study of 69 patients. Cancer. 1977;39:397-409.
3. Alford BR, Guilford FR. A comprehensive study of tumors of the glomus jugulare. Laryngoscope. 1962;72:765-805.
4. Zacks SI. Chemodectomas occurring concurrently in the neck (carotid body), temporal bone (glomus jugulare) and retroperitoneum; report of a case with histochemical observations. Am J Pathol. 1958;34:293-309.

5. Spector GJ, Ciralsky R, Maisel RH, et al. IV. Multiple glomus tumors in the head and neck. Laryngoscope. 1975;85:1066-75.
6. Mariman EC, van Beersum SE, Cremers CW, et al. Fine mapping of a putatively imprinted gene for familial non-chromaffin paragangliomas to chromosome 11q13.1: evidence for genetic heterogeneity. Hum Genet. 1995;95:56-62.
7. Milunsky J, DeStefano AL, Huang XL, et al. Familial paragangliomas: linkage to chromosome 11q23 and clinical implications. Am J Med Genet. 1997;72:66-70.
8. Heutink P, van der Mey AG, Sandkuijl LA, et al. A gene subject to genomic imprinting and responsible for hereditary paragangliomas maps to chromosome 11q23-qter. Hum Mol Genet. 1992;1:7-10.
9. Mhatre AN, Li Y, Feng L, et al. SDHB, SDHC, and SDHD mutation screen in sporadic and familial head and neck paragangliomas. Clin Genet. 2004;66:461-6.
10. Astuti D, Hart-Holden N, Latif F, et al. Genetic analysis of mitochondrial complex II subunits SDHD, SDHB and SDHC in paraganglioma and phaeochromocytoma susceptibility. Clin Endocrinol (Oxf). 2003;59:728-33.
11. Milunsky JM, Maher TA, Michels VV, et al. Novel mutations and the emergence of a common mutation in the SDHD gene causing familial paraganglioma. Am J Med Genet. 2001;100:311-4.
12. Manolidis S, Shohet JA, Jackson CG, et al. Malignant glomus tumors. Laryngoscope. 1999;109:30-4.
13. Gulya AJ. The glomus tumor and its biology. Laryngoscope. 1993;103:7-15.
14. Myssiorek D. Head and neck paragangliomas: an overview. Otolaryngol Clin North Am. 2001;34:829-36, v.
15. McCaffrey TV, Meyer FB, Michels VV, et al. Familial paragangliomas of the head and neck. Arch Otolaryngol Head Neck Surg. 1994;120:1211-6.
16. Green JD, Jr., Brackmann DE, Nguyen CD, et al. Surgical management of previously untreated glomus jugulare tumors. Laryngoscope. 1994;104:917-21.
17. Spector GJ, Ciralsky RH, Ogura JH. Glomus tumors in the head and neck: III. Analysis of clinical manifestations. Ann Otol Rhinol Laryngol. 1975;84:73-9.
18. Brown LA. Glomus jugulare tumor of the middle ear; clinical aspects. Laryngoscope. 1953;63:281-92.
19. Spector GJ, Gado M, Ciralsky R, et al. Neurologic implications of glomus tumors in the head and neck. Laryngoscope. 1975;85:1387-95.
20. Jackson CG, Harris PF, Glasscock ME, et al. Diagnosis and management of paragangliomas of the skull base. Am J Surg. 1990;159:389-93.
21. Pensak ML, Jackler RK. Removal of jugular foramen tumors: the fallopian bridge technique. Otolaryngol Head Neck Surg. 1997;117:586-91.
22. Schwaber MK, Glasscock ME, Nissen AJ, et al. Diagnosis and management of catecholamine secreting glomus tumors. Laryngoscope. 1984;94:1008-15.
23. Lo WW, Solti-Bohman LG. High-resolution CT of the jugular foramen: anatomy and vascular variants and anomalies. Radiology. 1984;150:743-7.
24. Lo WW, Solti-Bohman LG, Lambert PR. High-resolution CT in the evaluation of glomus tumors of the temporal bone. Radiology. 1984;150:737-42.
25. Olsen WL, Dillon WP, Kelly WM, et al. MR imaging of paragangliomas. AJR Am J Roentgenol. 1987;148:201-4.
26. Weber AL, McKenna MJ. Radiologic evaluation of the jugular foramen. Anatomy, vascular variants, anomalies, and tumors. Neuroimaging Clin N Am. 1994;4:579-98.
27. Rodgers GK, Applegate L, De la Cruz A, et al. Magnetic resonance angiography: analysis of vascular lesions of the temporal bone and skull base. Am J Otol. 1993;14:56-62.
28. Murphy TP, Brackmann DE. Effects of preoperative embolization on glomus jugulare tumors. Laryngoscope. 1989;99:1244-7.
29. Lustig LR, Jackler RK. The variable relationship between the lower cranial nerves and jugular foramen tumors: implications for neural preservation. Am J Otol. 1996;17:658-68.
30. Sanna M, Jain Y, De Donato G, et al. Management of jugular paragangliomas: the Gruppo Otologico experience. Otol Neurotol. 2004;25:797-804.
31. Blevins NH, Jackler RK, Kaplan MJ, et al. Combined transpetrosal-subtemporal craniotomy for clival tumors with extension into the posterior fossa. Laryngoscope. 1995;105:975-82.
32. Willen SN, Einstein DB, Maciunas RJ, et al. Treatment of glomus jugulare tumors in patients with advanced age: planned limited surgical resection followed by staged gamma knife radiosurgery: a preliminary report. Otol Neurotol. 2005;26:1229-34.
33. Maniglia AJ, Sprecher RC, Megerian CA, et al. Inferior mastoidectomy-hypotympanic approach for surgical removal of glomus jugulare tumors: an anatomical and radiologic study emphasizing distances between critical structures. Laryngoscope. 1992;102:407-14.
34. Krych AJ, Foote RL, Brown PD, et al. Long-term results of irradiation for paraganglioma. Int J Radiat Oncol Biol Phys. 2006;65:1063-6.
35. Pemberton LS, Swindell R, Sykes AJ. Radical radiotherapy alone for glomus jugulare and tympanicum tumours. Oncol Rep. 2005;14:1631-3.
36. Sheehan J, Kondziolka D, Flickinger J, et al. Gamma knife surgery for glomus jugulare tumors: an intermediate report on efficacy and safety. J Neurosurg. 2005;102 Suppl:241-6.
37. Pollock BE. Stereotactic radiosurgery in patients with glomus jugulare tumors. Neurosurg Focus. 2004;17:E10.
38. O'Donoghue GM, Brackmann DE, House JW, et al. Neuromas of the facial nerve. Am J Otol. 1989;10:49-54.
39. Saito H, Baxter A. Undiagnosed intratemporal facial nerve neurilemomas. Arch Otolaryngol. 1972;95:415-9.
40. Jung TT, Jun BH, Shea D, et al. Primary and secondary tumors of the facial nerve. A temporal bone study. Arch Otolaryngol Head Neck Surg. 1986;112:1269-73.
41. Lipkin AF, Coker NJ, Jenkins HA, et al. Intracranial and intratemporal facial neuroma. Otolaryngol Head Neck Surg. 1987;96:71-9.
42. Wenig B. Atlas of Head and Neck Pathology. Philadelphia: W.B. Saunders; 1993.

43. Kim CS, Chang SO, Oh SH, et al. Management of intratemporal facial nerve schwannoma. Otol Neurotol. 2003;24:312-6.
44. McMenomey SO, Glasscock ME, Minor LB, et al. Facial nerve neuromas presenting as acoustic tumors. Am J Otol. 1994;15:307-12.
45. Preston DC, Shapiro BE. Needle electromyography. Fundamentals, normal and abnormal patterns. Neurol Clin. 2002;20:361-96, vi.
46. Shelton C, Brackmann DE, Lo WW, et al. Intratemporal facial nerve hemangiomas. Otolaryngol Head Neck Surg. 1991;104:116-21.
47. Wilkinson EP, Hoa M, Slattery WH, et al. Evolution in the management of facial nerve schwannoma. Laryngoscope. 2011;121:2065-74.
48. Tan LC, Bordi L, Symon L, et al. Jugular foramen neuromas: a review of 14 cases. Surg Neurol. 1990;34:205-11.
49. Casadei GP, Komori T, Scheithauer BW, et al. Intracranial parenchymal schwannoma. A clinicopathological and neuroimaging study of nine cases. J Neurosurg. 1993;79:217-22.
50. Mazzoni A, Sanna M, Saleh E, et al. Lower cranial nerve schwannomas involving the jugular foramen. Ann Otol Rhinol Laryngol. 1997;106:370-9.
51. Samii M, Babu RP, Tatagiba M, et al. Surgical treatment of jugular foramen schwannomas. J Neurosurg. 1995;82:924-32.
52. Sterkers JM, Perre J, Viala P, et al. The origin of acoustic neuromas. Acta Otolaryngol. 1987;103:427-31.
53. Kaye AH, Hahn JF, Kinney SE, et al. Jugular foramen schwannomas. J Neurosurg. 1984;60:1045-53.
54. Pellet W, Cannoni M, Pech A. The widened transcochlear approach to jugular foramen tumors. J Neurosurg. 1988;69:887-94.
55. Eldevik OP, Gabrielsen TO, Jacobsen EA. Imaging findings in schwannomas of the jugular foramen. AJNR Am J Neuroradiol. 2000;21:1139-44.
56. Macdonald AJ, Salzman KL, Harnsberger HR, et al. Primary jugular foramen meningioma: imaging appearance and differentiating features. AJR Am J Roentgenol. 2004;182:373-7.
57. Zhang N, Pan L, Dai JZ, et al. Gamma knife radiosurgery for jugular foramen schwannomas. J Neurosurg. 2002;97:456-8.
58. Muthukumar N, Kondziolka D, Lunsford LD, et al. Stereotactic radiosurgery for jugular foramen schwannomas. Surg Neurol. 1999;52:172-9.
59. Von Doersten PG, Jackler RK. Anterior facial nerve rerouting in cranial base surgery: a comparison of three techniques. Otolaryngol Head Neck Surg. 1996;115:82-8.
60. Pulec JL. Facial nerve tumors. Ann Otol Rhinol Laryngol. 1969;78:962-82.
61. Gjuric M, Koester M, Paulus W. Cavernous hemangioma of the internal auditory canal arising from the inferior vestibular nerve: case report and review of the literature. Am J Otol. 2000;21:110-4.
62. Isaacson B, Telian SA, McKeever PE, et al. Hemangiomas of the geniculate ganglion. Otol Neurotol. 2005;26:796-802.
63. Semaan MT, Slattery WH, Brackmann DE. Geniculate ganglion hemangiomas: clinical results and long-term follow-up. Otol Neurotol. 31:665-70.
64. Eby TL, Fisch U, Makek MS. Facial nerve management in temporal bone hemangiomas. Am J Otol. 1992;13:223-32.
65. Lo WW, Horn KL, Carberry JN, et al. Intratemporal vascular tumors: evaluation with CT. Radiology. 1986;159:181-5.
66. Curtin HD, Jensen JE, Barnes L, et al. "Ossifying" hemangiomas of the temporal bone: evaluation with CT. Radiology. 1987;164:831-5.
67. Lo WW, Shelton C, Waluch V, et al. Intratemporal vascular tumors: detection with CT and MR imaging. Radiology. 1989;171:445-8.
68. Gaffey MJ, Mills SE, Fechner RE, et al. Aggressive papillary middle-ear tumor. A clinicopathologic entity distinct from middle-ear adenoma. Am J Surg Pathol. 1988;12:790-7.
69. Heffner DK. Low-grade adenocarcinoma of probable endolymphatic sac origin A clinicopathologic study of 20 cases. Cancer. 1989;64:2292-302.
70. Poe DS, Tarlov EC, Thomas CB, et al. Aggressive papillary tumors of temporal bone. Otolaryngol Head Neck Surg. 1993;108:80-6.
71. Li JC, Brackmann DE, Lo WW, et al. Reclassification of aggressive adenomatous mastoid neoplasms as endolymphatic sac tumors. Laryngoscope. 1993;103:1342-8.
72. Bambakidis NC, Rodrigue T, Megerian CA, et al. Endolymphatic sac tumor metastatic to the spine. Case report. J Neurosurg Spine. 2005;3:68-70.
73. Schindler RA. The ultrastructure of the endolymphatic sac in man. Laryngoscope. 1980;90:1-39.
74. Levin RJ, Feghali JG, Morganstern N, et al. Aggressive papillary tumors of the temporal bone: an immunohistochemical analysis in tissue culture. Laryngoscope. 1996;106:144-7.
75. Feghali JG, Levin RJ, Llena J, et al. Aggressive papillary tumors of the endolymphatic sac: clinical and tissue culture characteristics. Am J Otol. 1995;16:778-82.
76. Batsakis JG, el-Naggar AK. Papillary neoplasms (Heffner's tumors) of the endolymphatic sac. Ann Otol Rhinol Laryngol. 1993;102:648-51.
77. Megerian CA, Pilch BZ, Bhan AK, et al. Differential expression of transthyretin in papillary tumors of the endolymphatic sac and choroid plexus. Laryngoscope. 1997;107:216-21.
78. Latif F, Tory K, Gnarra J, et al. Identification of the von Hippel-Lindau disease tumor suppressor gene. Science. 1993;260:1317-20.
79. Neumann HP, Wiestler OD. Clustering of features and genetics of von Hippel-Lindau syndrome. Lancet. 1991;338:258.
80. Sgambati MT, Stolle C, Choyke PL, et al. Mosaicism in von Hippel-Lindau disease: lessons from kindreds with germline mutations identified in offspring with mosaic parents. Am J Hum Genet. 2000;66:84-91.
81. Megerian CA, Haynes DS, Poe DS, et al. Hearing preservation surgery for small endolymphatic sac tumors in patients with von Hippel-Lindau syndrome. Otol Neurotol. 2002;23:378-87.
82. Knudson AG, Jr. Genetics of human cancer. J Cell Physiol Suppl. 1986;4:7-11.
83. Lonser RR, Kim HJ, Butman JA, et al. Tumors of the endolymphatic sac in von Hippel-Lindau disease. N Engl J Med. 2004;350:2481-6.

84. Manski TJ, Heffner DK, Glenn GM, et al. Endolymphatic sac tumors. A source of morbid hearing loss in von Hippel-Lindau disease. Jama. 1997;277:1461-6.
85. Kim HJ, Butman JA, Brewer C, et al. Tumors of the endolymphatic sac in patients with von Hippel-Lindau disease: implications for their natural history, diagnosis, and treatment. J Neurosurg. 2005;102:503-12.
86. Megerian CA, McKenna MJ, Nuss RC, et al. Endolymphatic sac tumors: histopathologic confirmation, clinical characterization, and implication in von Hippel-Lindau disease. Laryngoscope. 1995;105:801-8.
87. Hansen MR, Luxford WM. Surgical outcomes in patients with endolymphatic sac tumors. Laryngoscope 2004;114:1470-4.
88. Hassard AD. Identification of endolymphatic sac tumors. Otolaryngol Head Neck Surg. 1985;93:445.
89. Mukherji SK, Albernaz VS, Lo WW, et al. Papillary endolymphatic sac tumors: CT, MR imaging, and angiographic findings in 20 patients. Radiology. 1997;202:801-8.
90. Ho VT, Rao VM, Doan HT, et al. Low-grade adenocarcinoma of probable endolymphatic sac origin: CT and MR appearance. AJNR Am J Neuroradiol. 1996;17:168-70.
91. Cushing H, Eisenhardt L. Meningiomas: Their Classification, Regional Behavior, Life History, and Surgical End Results. Springfield, IL: Charles C Thomas; 1938.
92. Granick MS, Martuza RL, Parker SW, et al. Cerebellopontine angle meningiomas: clinical manifestations and diagnosis. Ann Otol Rhinol Laryngol. 1985;94:34-8.
93. Nakamura M, Roser F, Mirzai S, et al. Meningiomas of the internal auditory canal. Neurosurgery. 2004;55:119-27; discussion 27-8.
94. Nakamura Y, Shimizu T, Ohigashi Y, et al. Meningioma arising in Werner syndrome confirmed by mutation analysis. J Clin Neurosci. 2005;12:503-6.
95. Gorlin RJ. Nevoid basal-cell carcinoma syndrome. Medicine (Baltimore). 1987;66:98-113.
96. Patel NP, Mhatre AN, Lalwani AK. Molecular pathogenesis of skull base tumors. Otol Neurotol. 2004;25:636-43.
97. Weber RG, Bostrom J, Wolter M, et al. Analysis of genomic alterations in benign, atypical, and anaplastic meningiomas: toward a genetic model of meningioma progression. Proc Natl Acad Sci U S A. 1997;94:14719-24.
98. Simon M, von Deimling A, Larson JJ, et al. Allelic losses on chromosomes 14, 10, and 1 in atypical and malignant meningiomas: a genetic model of meningioma progression. Cancer Res. 1995;55:4696-701.
99. Laird FJ, Harner SG, Laws ER, et al. Meningiomas of the cerebellopontine angle. Otolaryngol Head Neck Surg. 1985; 93:163-7.
100. Matthies C, Carvalho G, Tatagiba M, et al. Meningiomas of the cerebellopontine angle. Acta Neurochir Suppl. 1996; 65:86-91.
101. Baguley DM, Beynon GJ, Grey PL, et al. Audio-vestibular findings in meningioma of the cerebello-pontine angle: a retrospective review. J Laryngol Otol. 1997;111:1022-6.
102. Molony TB, Brackmann DE, Lo WW. Meningiomas of the jugular foramen. Otolaryngol Head Neck Surg. 1992;106: 128-36.
103. Voss NF, Vrionis FD, Heilman CB, et al. Meningiomas of the cerebellopontine angle. Surg Neurol 2000;53:439-46; discussion. 46-7.
104. Roberti F, Sekhar LN, Kalavakonda C, et al. Posterior fossa meningiomas: surgical experience in 161 cases. Surg Neurol. 2001;56:8-20; discussion 20-1.
105. Mikhael MA, Wolff AP, Ciric IS. Current concepts in neuroradiological diagnosis of acoustic neuromas. Laryngoscope. 1987;97:471-6.
106. Valavanis A, Schubiger O, Hayek J, et al. CT of meningiomas on the posterior surface of the petrous bone. Neuroradiology. 1981;22:111-21.
107. Lalwani AK. Meningiomas, epidermoids, and other nonacoustic tumors of the cerebellopontine angle. Otolaryngol Clin North Am. 1992;25:707-28.
108. Robertson WD, Nugent RA, Lapointe JS, et al. Computed tomographic scanning of the cerebellopontine angle and the internal auditory canal. J Otolaryngol. 1982;11:331-9.
109. Lalwani AK, Jackler RK. Preoperative differentiation between meningioma of the cerebellopontine angle and acoustic neuroma using MRI. Otolaryngol Head Neck Surg. 1993;109:88-95.
110. Tokumaru A, O'Uchi T, Eguchi T, et al. Prominent meningeal enhancement adjacent to meningioma on Gd-DTPA-enhanced MR images: histopathologic correlation. Radiology. 1990;175:431-3.
111. Adegbite AB, Khan MI, Paine KW, et al. The recurrence of intracranial meningiomas after surgical treatment. J Neurosurg. 1983;58:51-6.
112. Thomas NW, King TT. Meningiomas of the cerebellopontine angle. A report of 41 cases. Br J Neurosurg. 1996;10: 59-68.
113. Thedinger BA, Glasscock ME, Cueva RA. Transcochlear transtentorial approach for removal of large cerebellopontine angle meningiomas. Am J Otol. 1992;13:408-15.
114. Goldsmith BJ, Wara WM, Wilson CB, et al. Postoperative irradiation for subtotally resected meningiomas. A retrospective analysis of 140 patients treated from 1967 to 1990. J Neurosurg. 1994;80:195-201.
115. Miralbell R, Linggood RM, de la Monte S, et al. The role of radiotherapy in the treatment of subtotally resected benign meningiomas. J Neurooncol. 1992;13:157-64.
116. Kondziolka D, Levy EI, Niranjan A, et al. Long-term outcomes after meningioma radiosurgery: physician and patient perspectives. J Neurosurg. 1999;91:44-50.
117. Subach BR, Lunsford LD, Kondziolka D, et al. Management of petroclival meningiomas by stereotactic radiosurgery. Neurosurgery. 1998;42:437-43; discussion 43-5.
118. Kveton JF, Brackmann DE, Glasscock ME, et al. Chondrosarcoma of the skull base. Otolaryngol Head Neck Surg. 1986;94:23-32.
119. Lau DP, Wharton SB, Antoun NM, et al. Chondrosarcoma of the petrous apex. Dilemmas in diagnosis and treatment. J Laryngol Otol. 1997;111:368-71.
120. Richardson MS. Pathology of skull base tumors. Otolaryngol Clin North Am. 2001;34:1025-42, vii.

121. Tucker WN. Cancer Of The Middle Ear; A Review Of 89 Cases. Cancer. 1965;18:642-50.
122. Noel G, Feuvret L, Calugaru V, et al. Chondrosarcomas of the base of the skull in Ollier's disease or Maffucci's syndrome—three case reports and review of the literature. Acta Oncol. 2004;43:705-10.
123. Barnes L, Kapadia SB. The biology and pathology of selected skull base tumors. J Neurooncol 1994;20:213-40.
124. Neff B, Sataloff RT, Storey L, et al. Chondrosarcoma of the skull base. Laryngoscope. 2002;112:134-9.
125. Ishida T, Dorfman HD. Chondroid chordoma versus low-grade chondrosarcoma of the base of the skull: can immunohistochemistry resolve the controversy? J Neurooncol. 1994;18:199-206.
126. Ishida T, Kikuchi F, Machinami R. Histological grading and morphometric analysis of cartilaginous tumours. Virchows Arch A Pathol Anat Histopathol. 1991;418:149-55.
127. Kreicbergs A, Slezak E, Soderberg G. The prognostic significance of different histomorphologic features in chondrosarcoma. Virchows Arch A Pathol Anat Histol. 1981;390: 1-10.
128. Evans HL, Ayala AG, Romsdahl MM. Prognostic factors in chondrosarcoma of bone: a clinicopathologic analysis with emphasis on histologic grading. Cancer. 1977;40: 818-31.
129. Rosenberg AE, Nielsen GP, Keel SB, et al. Chondrosarcoma of the base of the skull: a clinicopathologic study of 200 cases with emphasis on its distinction from chordoma. Am J Surg Pathol. 1999;23:1370-8.
130. Finn DG, Goepfert H, Batsakis JG. Chondrosarcoma of the head and neck. Laryngoscope. 1984;94:1539-44.
131. Kay PA, Nascimento AG, Unni KK, et al. Chordoma. Cytomorphologic findings in 14 cases diagnosed by fine needle aspiration. Acta Cytol. 2003;47:202-8.
132. Tunc M, Ekinci C. Chondrosarcoma diagnosed by fine needle aspiration cytology. Acta Cytol. 1996;40:283-8.
133. Watters GW, Brookes GB. Chondrosarcoma of the temporal bone. Clin Otolaryngol Allied Sci. 1995;20:53-8.
134. Crockard HA, Cheeseman A, Steel T, et al. A multidisciplinary team approach to skull base chondrosarcomas. J Neurosurg. 2001;95:184-9.
135. Coltrera MD, Googe PB, Harrist TJ, et al. Chondrosarcoma of the temporal bone. Diagnosis and treatment of 13 cases and review of the literature. Cancer. 1986;58:2689-96.
136. Volpe NJ, Liebsch NJ, Munzenrider JE, et al. Neuro-ophthalmologic findings in chordoma and chondrosarcoma of the skull base. Am J Ophthalmol. 1993;115:97-104.
137. Brackmann DE, Teufert KB. Chondrosarcoma of the skull base: long-term follow-up. Otol Neurotol. 2006;27: 981-91.
138. Sekhar LN, Pranatartiharan R, Chanda A, et al. Chordomas and chondrosarcomas of the skull base: results and complications of surgical management. Neurosurg Focus. 2001; 10:E2.
139. Megerian CA, Chiocca EA, McKenna MJ, et al. The subtemporal-transpetrous approach for excision of petroclival tumors. Am J Otol. 1996;17:773-9.
140. Sekhar LN, Schramm VL, Jr., Jones NF. Subtemporal-preauricular infratemporal fossa approach to large lateral and posterior cranial base neoplasms. J Neurosurg. 1987; 67:88-99.
141. Oghalai JS, Buxbaum JL, Jackler RK, et al. Skull base chondrosarcoma originating from the petroclival junction. Otol Neurotol. 2005;26:1052-60.
142. Krishnan S, Foote RL, Brown PD, et al. Radiosurgery for cranial base chordomas and chondrosarcomas. Neurosurgery. 2005;56:777-84; discussion 77-84.
143. Kraus DH, Saenz NC, Gollamudi S, et al. Pediatric rhabdomyosarcoma of the head and neck. Am J Surg. 1997;174: 556-60.
144. Jaffe BF, Fox JE, Batsakis JG. Rhabdomyosarcoma of the middle ear and mastoid. Cancer. 1971;27:29-37.
145. Stevens MC. Treatment for childhood rhabdomyosarcoma: the cost of cure. Lancet Oncol. 2005;6:77-84.
146. Wharam MD, Jr. Rhabdomyosarcoma of Parameningeal Sites. Semin Radiat Oncol. 1997;7:212-16.
147. Maurer HM, Beltangady M, Gehan EA, et al. The Intergroup Rhabdomyosarcoma Study-I. A final report. Cancer. 1988; 61:209-20.
148. Newton WA, Soule EH, Hamoudi AB, et al. Histopathology of childhood sarcomas, Intergroup Rhabdomyosarcoma Studies I and II: clinicopathologic correlation. J Clin Oncol. 1988;6:67-75.
149. Nakhleh RE, Swanson PE, Dehner LP. Juvenile (embryonal and alveolar) rhabdomyosarcoma of the head and neck in adults. A clinical, pathologic, and immunohistochemical study of 12 cases. Cancer. 1991;67:1019-24.
150. Devaney KO, Boschman CR, Willard SC, et al. Tumours of the external ear and temporal bone. Lancet Oncol. 2005; 6:411-20.
151. Ruymann FB. Rhabdomyosarcoma in children and adolescents. A review. Hematol Oncol Clin North Am. 1987;1: 621-54.
152. Verma PL, Marwaha AR. Embryonal rhabdomyosarcoma of the middle ear and mastoid. J Laryngol Otol. 1972;86: 67-71.
153. Potter GD. Embryonal rhabdomyosarcoma of the middle ear in children. Cancer. 1966;19:221-6.
154. Latack JT, Hutchinson RJ, Heyn RM. Imaging of rhabdomyosarcomas of the head and neck. AJNR Am J Neuroradiol. 1987;8:353-9.
155. Maroldi R, Farina D, Palvarini L, et al. Computed tomography and magnetic resonance imaging of pathologic conditions of the middle ear. Eur J Radiol. 2001;40:78-93.
156. Jackler RK, Parker DA. Radiographic differential diagnosis of petrous apex lesions. Am J Otol. 1992;13:561-74.
157. Raney RB, Anderson JR, Barr FG, et al. Rhabdomyosarcoma and undifferentiated sarcoma in the first two decades of life: a selective review of intergroup rhabdomyosarcoma study group experience and rationale for Intergroup Rhabdomyosarcoma Study V. J Pediatr Hematol Oncol. 2001;23: 215-20.

158. Sutow WW, Lindberg RD, Gehan EA, et al. Three-year relapse-free survival rates in childhood rhabdomyosarcoma of the head and neck: report from the Intergroup Rhabdomyosarcoma Study. Cancer. 1982;49:2217-21.
159. Crist WM, Anderson JR, Meza JL, et al. Intergroup rhabdomyosarcoma study-IV: results for patients with nonmetastatic disease. J Clin Oncol. 2001;19:3091-102.
160. Crist W, Gehan EA, Ragab AH, et al. The Third Intergroup Rhabdomyosarcoma Study. J Clin Oncol. 1995;13:610-30.
161. Maurer HM, Gehan EA, Beltangady M, et al. The Intergroup Rhabdomyosarcoma Study-II. Cancer. 1993;71:1904-22.
162. Meza JL, Anderson J, Pappo AS, et al. Analysis of prognostic factors in patients with nonmetastatic rhabdomyosarcoma treated on intergroup rhabdomyosarcoma studies III and IV: the Children's Oncology Group. J Clin Oncol. 2006;24:3844-51.
163. Joshi D, Anderson JR, Paidas C, et al. Age is an independent prognostic factor in rhabdomyosarcoma: a report from the Soft Tissue Sarcoma Committee of the Children's Oncology Group. Pediatr Blood Cancer. 2004;42:64-73.
164. Breneman JC, Lyden E, Pappo AS, et al. Prognostic factors and clinical outcomes in children and adolescents with metastatic rhabdomyosarcoma--a report from the Intergroup Rhabdomyosarcoma Study IV. J Clin Oncol. 2003;21:78-84.
165. Simon JH, Paulino AC, Smith RB, et al. Prognostic factors in head and neck rhabdomyosarcoma. Head Neck. 2002;24:468-73.
166. Schuller DE, Lawrence TL, Newton WA. Childhood rhabdomyosarcomas of the head and neck. Arch Otolaryngol. 1979;105:689-94.
167. Paulino AC, Simon JH, Zhen W, et al. Long-term effects in children treated with radiotherapy for head and neck rhabdomyosarcoma. Int J Radiat Oncol Biol Phys. 2000;48:1489-95.
168. Okura SI, Kaga K. Temporal bone pathology of leukemia and malignant lymphoma with middle ear effusion. Auris Nasus Larynx. 1994;21:1-7.
169. Paparella MM, Berlinger NT, Oda M, et al. Otological manifestations of leukemia. Laryngoscope. 1973;83:1510-26.
170. Panosian MS, Roberts JK. Plasmacytoma of the middle ear and mastoid. Am J Otol. 1994;15:264-7.
171. Harada T, Namiki S, Kawabata I. Acute profound sensorineural hearing loss as the initial manifestation of acute leukemia--report of a case. Auris Nasus Larynx. 2000;27:359-62.
172. Zappia JJ, Bunge FA, Koopmann CF, et al. Facial nerve paresis as the presenting symptom of leukemia. Int J Pediatr Otorhinolaryngol. 1990;19:259-64.
173. Kurtz JE, Andres E, Veillon F, et al. Hearing loss due to acute leukemia. Am J Med. 2000;109:509-10.
174. Zechner G, Altmann F. The temporal bone in leukemia. Histological studies. Ann Otol Rhinol Laryngol. 1969;78:375-87.
175. Berlinger NT, Koutroupas S, Adams G, et al. Patterns of involvement of the temporal bone in metastatic and systemic malignancy. Laryngoscope. 1980;90:619-27.
176. Gokcan MK, Batikhan H, Calguner M, et al. Unilateral hearing loss as a presenting manifestation of granulocytic sarcoma (chloroma). Otol Neurotol. 2006;27:106-9.
177. Nicolaides A, McFerran DJ, Croxson G. Non-Hodgkins lymphoma of the temporal bone. J Laryngol Otol. 1988;102:928-31.
178. Takahara T, Sando I, Bluestone CD, et al. Lymphoma invading the anterior eustachian tube. Temporal bone histopathology of functional tubal obstruction. Ann Otol Rhinol Laryngol. 1986;95:101-5.
179. Lang EE, Walsh RM, Leader M. Primary middle-ear lymphoma in a child. J Laryngol Otol 2003;117:205-7.
180. Merkus P, Copper MP, Van Oers MH, et al. Lymphoma in the ear. ORL J Otorhinolaryngol Relat Spec. 2000;62:274-7.
181. Paparella MM, el-Fiky FM. Ear involvement in malignant lymphoma. Ann Otol Rhinol Laryngol. 1972;81:352-63.
182. Wax MK, Yun KJ, Omar RA. Extramedullary plasmacytomas of the head and neck. Otolaryngol Head Neck Surg. 1993;109:877-85.
183. Abemayor E, Canalis RF, Greenberg P, et al. Plasma cell tumors of the head and neck. J Otolaryngol. 1988;17:376-81.
184. Ruenes R, Palacios E. Plasmacytoma of the petrous temporal bone. Ear Nose Throat J. 2003;82:672.
185. George JC, Caldemeyer KS, Kreipke DL, et al. Solitary plasmacytoma of the mastoid bone presenting as coalescent mastoiditis. Arch Otolaryngol Head Neck Surg. 1994;120:1393-4.
186. Yetiser S, Talas D, Akkaya A, et al. Plasmacytoma of the temporal bone: management with a combination of surgery and radiotherapy. Acta Otolaryngol. 2001;121:915-8.
187. Streitmann MJ, Sismanis A. Metastatic carcinoma of the temporal bone. Am J Otol. 1996;17:780-3.
188. Adams GL, Paparella MM, el-Fiky FM. Primary and metastatic tumors of the temporal bone. Laryngoscope. 1971;81:1273-85.
189. Schuknecht HF, Allam AF, Murakami Y. Pathology of secondary malignant tumors of the temporal bone. Ann Otol Rhinol Laryngol. 1968;77:5-22.
190. Brackmann DE, Bartels LJ. Rare tumors of the cerebellopontine angle. Otolaryngol Head Neck Surg. 1980;88:555-9.

CHAPTER

11

Cholesteatoma

Eric E Smouha, Emily Stucken, Dennis Bojrab

INTRODUCTION/BACKGROUND

Cholesteatoma (keratoma) is a growth of keratinizing squamous epithelium originating from the external layer of the tympanic membrane or ear canal skin that invades the middle ear cleft.[1] Cholesteatoma has two components—the matrix, or epithelial sac, and the acellular keratin debris contained within it. The cholesteatoma matrix consists of an inner layer of keratinizing squamous epithelium and an outer layer of subepithelial connective tissue ("perimatrix"). The matrix is biologically active: the epithelial layer continually produces keratin, and the subepithelial layer contains mesenchymal cells that can produce proteolytic (collagenolytic) enzymes that can erode bone.[2] Cholesteatoma can also become secondarily infected, leading to purulent discharge.

Cholesteatomas can be congenital or acquired. Acquired cholesteatomas, which are far more frequent, can arise by three mechanisms: retraction of the tympanic membrane ("primary acquired cholesteatoma," the most common type) (Fig. 11.1), epithelial migration from the edges of a tympanic membrane perforation ("secondary acquired cholesteatoma") (Fig. 11.2), or squamous metaplasia. Congenital cholesteatomas are epithelial rests that become entrapped in the middle ear cleft during embryogenesis.[3] They appear as a keratin sac behind an intact tympanic membrane (Fig. 11.3).

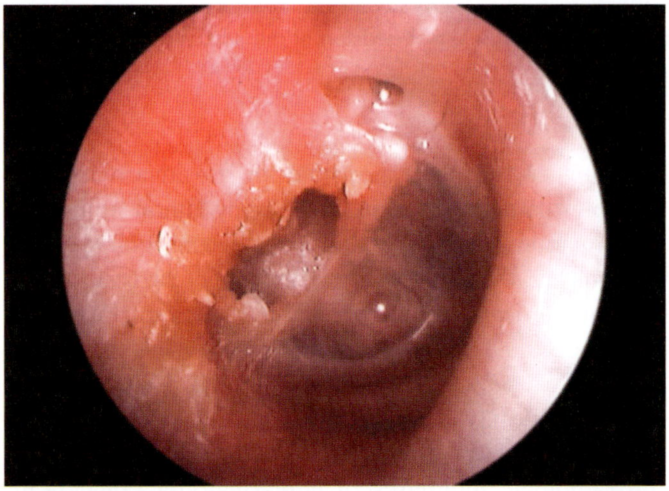

Fig. 11.1: Primary acquired cholesteatoma (arising from retraction pocket of tympanic membrane and pars flaccida).

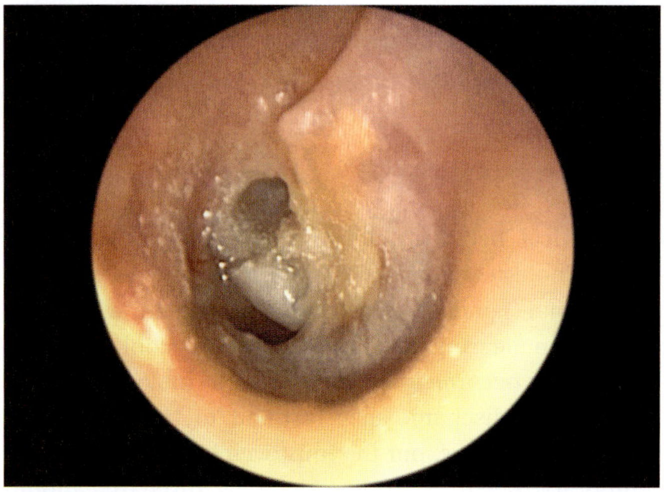

Fig. 11.2: Secondary acquired cholesteatoma (arising from tympanic membrane perforation).

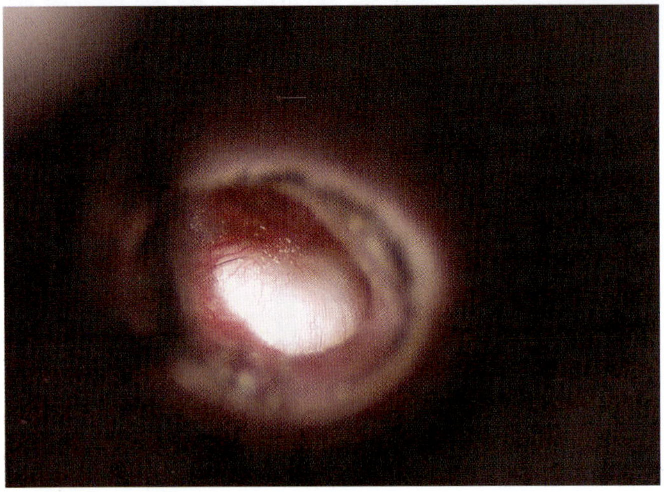

Fig. 11.3: Congenital cholesteatoma (epithelial rest behind intact tympanic membrane).

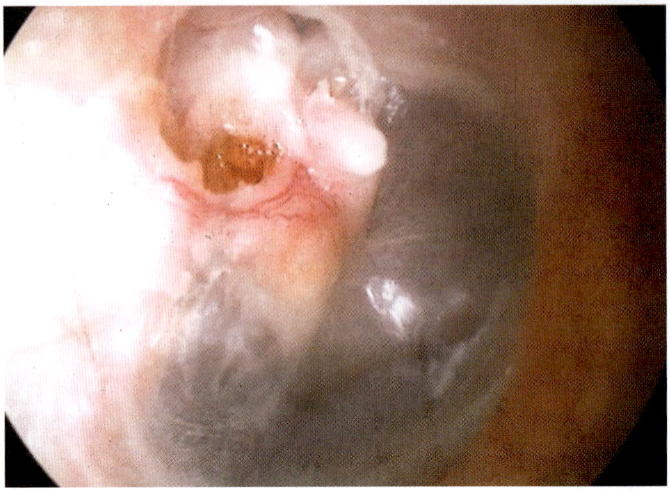

Fig. 11.4: Erosion of scutum (lateral bony wall of attic) by cholesteatoma.

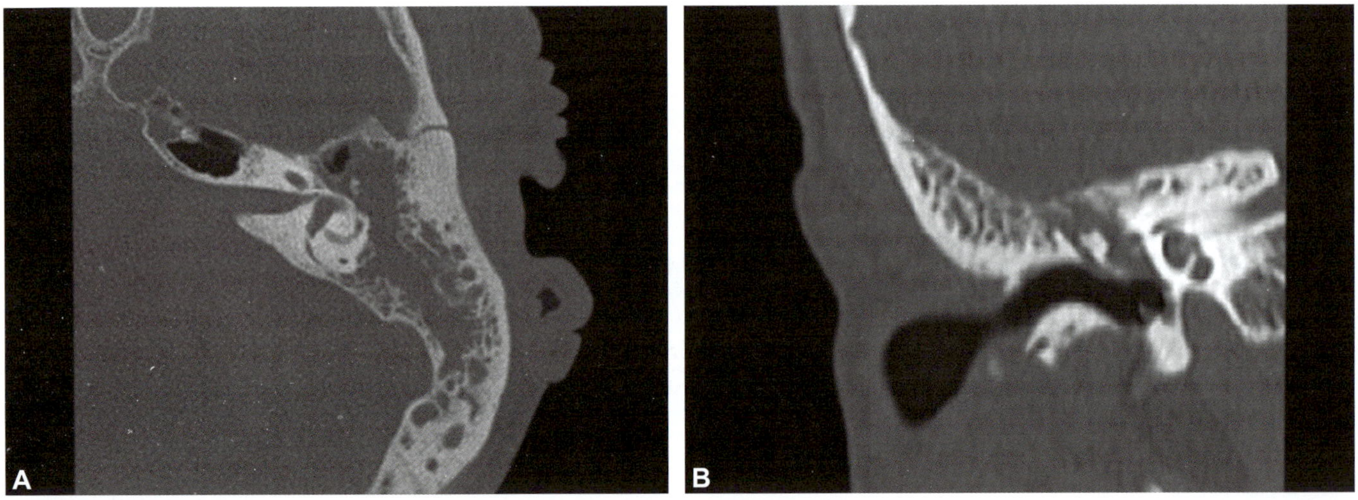

Figs. 11.5A and B: CT, coronal and axial, showing bony destruction within the mastoid and erosion of the scutum and ossicles by cholesteatoma.

PATHOGENESIS

The clinical behavior of cholesteatoma can vary over time.[4] Cholesteatoma may grow insidiously at first, and can attain a significant size without causing any symptoms other than hearing loss. Over time, the cholesteatoma will usually become infected, leading to malodorous discharge. The discharge may respond to treatment with antibiotic eardrops, but the improvement is usually only temporary. Recurrent or persistent ear discharge should make one suspect cholesteatoma, even when the lesion is not clinically evident.

Bone erosion is responsible for the invasive nature of cholesteatoma.[5] Erosion of the bony lateral wall of the epitympanum ("scutum") occurs early as the cholesteatoma expands into the attic (Fig. 11.4). Erosion of the ossicles (the lenticular process of the incus and the superstructure of the stapes) occurs as the cholesteatoma grows into the middle ear, and causes conductive hearing loss. Erosion of the bony septations of the mastoid appears as "coalescence" on CT radiographs; this finding, plus scutum erosion, are the radiologic hallmarks of cholesteatoma (Figs. 11.5A and B). Erosion of bony partitions between the mastoid air cell system and inner ear and intracranial structures permits

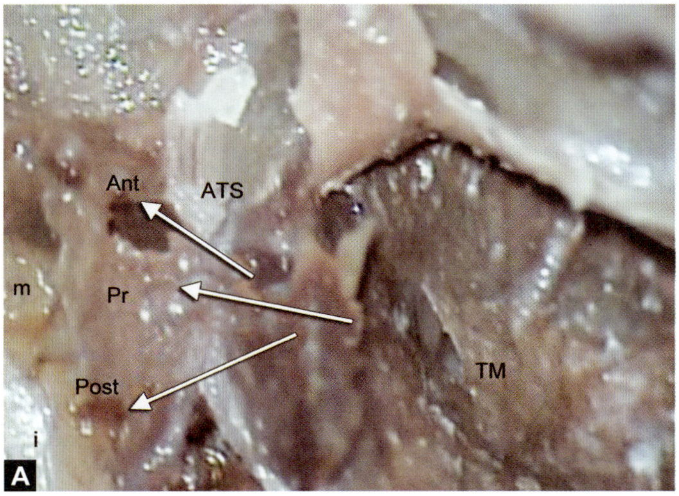

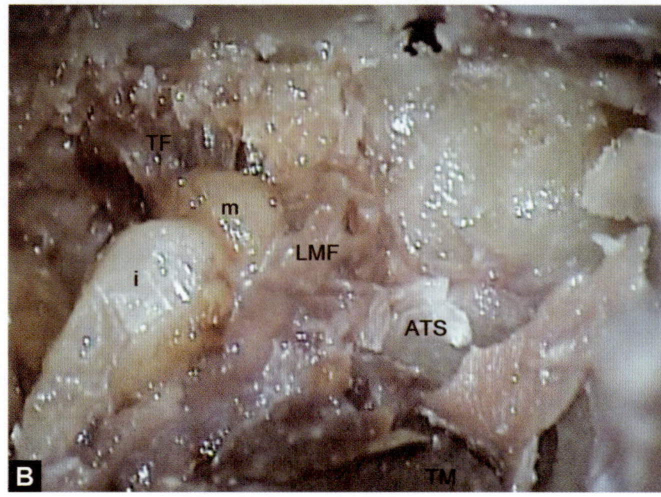

Figs. 11.6A and B: The tympanic membrane (TM), right ear, and the epitympanic spaces of von Troeltsch: Prussak's space (Pr), anterior (Ant) and posterior (Post) spaces. These mucosal pouches are lateral to the body of the incus (i) and malleus (m). (B) The epitympanic diaphragm, as viewed from above, in a cadaver dissection of the right ear. The epitympanic diaphragm bisects the attic into a lower part, containing the epitympanic pouches of von Troeltsch, and an upper part. (m, head of malleus; i, body of incus; TM, tympanic membrane; ATS, anterior tympanic spine; TF, tensor fold; LMF, lateral malleal fold).

complications to occur ("complications" are defined as spread of disease outside of the pneumatized portions of the temporal bone, and include suppurative (coalescent) mastoiditis, labyrinthitis, facial nerve paralysis, petrositis, and intracranial infections).

The anatomic patterns of growth of cholesteatoma are determined by the mucosal partitions of the middle ear and attic.[6,7] A one-cell-thick layer of low cuboidal epithelium lines the middle ear promontory and attic and envelops the ossicles in the same way that the mesentery envelops the intestines. The mucosal folds form the epitympanic spaces of von Troeltsch, which divide the attic into three spaces: a lateral epitympanic space (or Prussak's space) situated between the scutum and the malleus head and incus body, the anterior epitympanic space demarcated posteriorly by the bony "cog," and the posterior epitympanic space medial to the incus and malleus and leading posteriorly to the aditus ad antrum (Fig. 11.6A). The suspensory ligaments and mucosal folds form a horizontal partition called the epitympanic diaphragm that bisects the attic into lower and upper components. Once the cholesteatoma sac grows into the upper attic, it has free access to the mastoid via the aditus. There is a natural break in the epitympanic membrane posteriorly and medial to the incus, termed the tympanic isthmus; by this route middle ear cholesteatomas arising from the pars tensa can reach the upper attic and grow to fill the mastoid (Fig. 11.6B).

CLINICAL FINDINGS: SYMPTOMS AND SIGNS

Diagnosis of Cholesteatoma

Cholesteatoma is diagnosed clinically by physical examination. Most patients will present with a complaint of either hearing loss (unilateral, progressive), or drainage from the ear, which is often malodorous. Some cases are asymptomatic and only detected on physical exam.

On otoscopy, cholesteatoma appears as a retraction pocket of the pars flaccida or pars tensa, with keratin debris. The microscope is a very useful adjunct to the otoscope for judging the depth of a tympanic membrane retraction and for allowing cleaning of the ear and gentle probing of the sac contents. If the ear is draining and the canal is filled with pus it should be suction-debrided and the patient re-examined at a future date when the ear is dry. If an inflammatory polyp is present, it may be cauterized with silver nitrate and debrided with cup forceps in a cooperative patient (the polyp is usually insensate). A polyp arising from the pars flaccida almost always signifies an attic cholesteatoma.

The patterns of growth of cholesteatoma have been classified as follows:

1. Epitympanic (attic) cholesteatomas (Fig. 11.7A) arise from the pars flaccida and grow upward. These may be subdivided into lateral epitympanic cholesteatomas, if they involve only Prussak's space, posterior

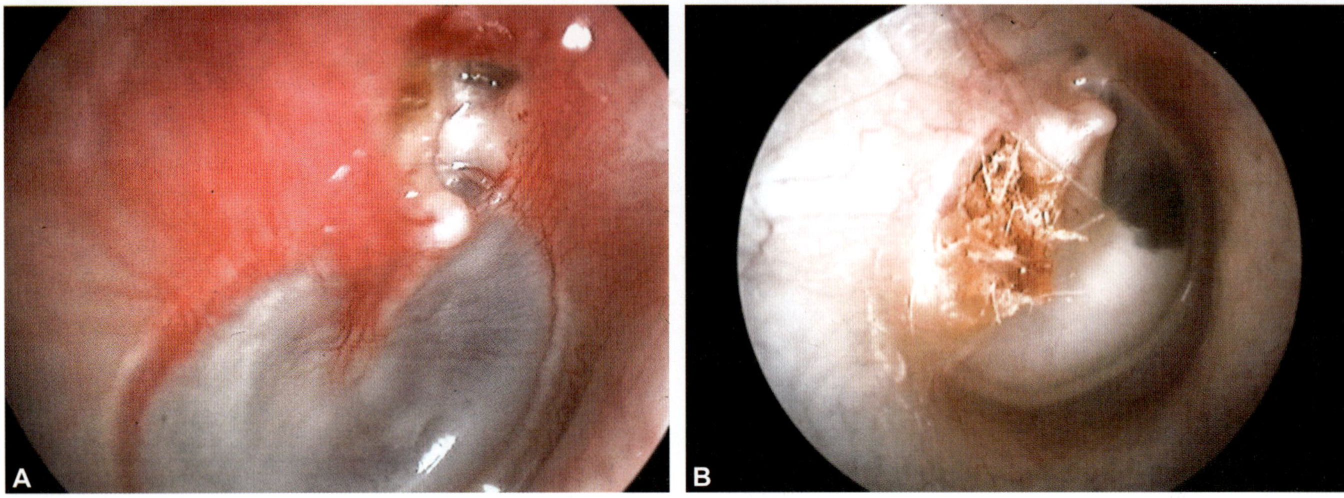

Figs. 11.7A and B: (A) Epitympanic (attic) cholesteatoma. (B) Mesotympanic (middle ear) cholesteatoma.

epitympanic cholesteatomas, if they grow medial to the incus to involve the posterior epitympanic space and mastoid, and anterior epitympanic cholesteatomas if they grow anteriorly to fill the space medial to the cog

2. Mesotympanic (middle ear) cholesteatomas (Fig. 11.7B) arise from the pars tensa and grow medially along the lenticular process and stapes superstructure. They may then grow upward toward the posterior epitympanum or backward into the sinus tympani, and they may fill the entire middle ear. (Tos has further divided middle ear cholesteatomas into sinus cholesteatomas, posterosuperior quadrant retractions that fill the sinus tympani, and tensa cholesteatomas, that are diffuse retractions of the eardrum into the middle ear space.[8])
3. "Holotympanic" cholesteatomas involve the middle ear, epitympanum, and mastoid. These are epitympanic cholesteatomas that have grown down into the middle ear space, or middle ear cholesteatomas that have grown up into the attic
4. Congenital cholesteatomas begin in the middle ear cleft, usually in the anterosuperior quadrant attached to the tensor tympani tendon and processus cochleariformis, but may enlarge in all directions. Infrequently, the congenital cholesteatoma may arise from the stapedial tendon

EVALUATION: LABORATORY, OTOLOGIC, AND NEUROTOLOGIC TESTING

Audiometry should be performed on every patient with cholesteatoma, and preferably when the ear is dry. Audiometry will usually show a conductive or mixed hearing loss, although in some cases the hearing can be surprisingly good. The degree of hearing loss does not necessarily reveal the status of the ossicular chain. Maximal conductive hearing loss implies erosion of the ossicles, but normal hearing does not necessarily signify an intact ossicular chain, however, because the cholesteatoma itself can conduct sound.

Additional testing does not routinely need to be performed. Electronystagmography may be obtained if the patient has vertigo.

EVALUATION: RADIOLOGIC IMAGING

CT scanning is useful for demonstrating the extent of the disease, the size of the mastoid, and the presence of any anatomic complications such as lateral semicircular canal fistula, fallopian canal erosion, tegmen erosion, or sigmoid sinus exposure. On CT, cholesteatoma will appear as a circumscribed mass of soft tissue density, with erosion of the surrounding trabecular bone (*see* Fig. 11.5). Erosion of the scutum is commonly seen in cholesteatoma but is not an essential finding. Erosion of the ossicles is also commonly seen. Postobstructive opacification of the mastoid air cells is also common, and may make it difficult to judge the true posterior extent of the disease.

MRI is generally not useful in the initial diagnosis of cholesteatoma, but may be helpful for detecting recurrence, as discussed under "Prognosis" below.

HISTOLOGY

Cholesteatoma consists histologically of acellular keratin debris, contained within a layer of keratinocytes ("matrix") enveloped by a layer of connective tissue subepithelium ("perimatrix"). The keratinocyte layer is indistinguishable from normal skin. The subepithelial layer may contain areas of inflammation. Sudhoff and Tos[8] have discovered, in sinus cholesteatoma, proliferating keratinocytes within epithelial cones growing toward the underlying stroma through focal discontinuities of the basement membrane in areas of intense subepithelial inflammation. This finding may help to explain the transition from retraction pocket to active and expanding cholesteatoma.

TREATMENT: MEDICAL AND SURGICAL

Cholesteatoma has no medical treatment. The treatment of cholesteatoma is surgical, and while surgery is mandatory, it is not always definitive. The capacity for recurrence is an important feature of cholesteatoma that reflects its invasive nature. Recurrence is the regrowth of disease after adequate surgical extirpation. The significant rate of recurrence makes the management of cholesteatoma daunting for the surgeon and frustrating for the patient. Indeed, in the best hands, recurrence rates of up to 30% in adults and up to 70% in children have been reported.[9,10]

The goals of cholesteatoma surgery are as follows:

1. Complete extirpation of the disease
2. Reconstruction of the middle ear
3. Prevention of recurrence

The operation should be dictated by the extent of the disease in the middle ear cleft and by the size of the mastoid. The status of the ossicular chain and the presence of complications will also determine what surgical procedure is needed.

Disease confined to the middle ear (mesotympanic cholesteatoma) can be dealt with by tympanoplasty alone. Disease confined to the attic can be removed via atticotomy. Disease that extends to the mastoid will require a mastoidectomy. A mastoidectomy can be performed with preservation of the posterior bony canal wall [canal wall up (CWU), intact canal wall, or closed cavity mastoidectomy], or the canal wall can be taken down (canal wall down (CWD), modified radical mastoidectomy, or open cavity mastoidectomy). The Bondy operation is a type of CWD procedure which is done in a retrograde or "inside-out" fashion, and which attempts to avoid the middle ear.

The CWU mastoidectomy preserves the posterior bony canal wall and thereby results in a normal ear canal and tympanic membrane. This heals more rapidly, does not require water precautions, and readily permits the use of a hearing aid. The disadvantage of the closed cavity is that it leaves a place for residual cholesteatoma to hide and a potential space for recurrent cholesteatoma to form. Because of this increased tendency for residual cholesteatoma, a second-stage operation is often recommended after CWU mastoidectomy.[11] The CWD mastoidectomy exteriorizes the mastoid space, so that residual disease can be detected early and recurrence should (theoretically) not occur, but carries the penalty of creating a cavity that may develop mucositis, and require periodic cleaning and constant water avoidance.

Tympanoplasty

Tympanoplasty refers to removal of disease from the middle ear and reconstruction of the tympanic membrane and ossicular chain if necessary (*see* Chapter 12 for more complete discussion). Tympanoplasty can be coupled with mastoidectomy, as determined by the extent of the disease.

Tympanoplasty alone can be used to remove cholesteatoma that is confined to the middle ear. This is possible in most cases of congenital cholesteatoma that are detected early, when they are well encapsulated and confined to the anterior–superior quadrant of the middle ear (congenital cholesteatomas that are detected later are widespread, and will require atticotomy or mastoidectomy, no different from acquired cholesteatoma). A tympanomeatal flap can be raised, and the superior limb of the incision is extended anteriorly to gain additional exposure. Detaching the tympanic membrane from the manubrium mallei and umbo will result in an inferiorly-pedicled tympanomeatal flap, with good surgical access to the anterosuperior mesotympanum and adjacent attic. By sharply lysing the enveloping mucosa, the cholesteatoma can be grasped with a cup forceps and removed in toto. If the capsule is broken, the lesion will have to be removed piecemeal, and a middle ear mirror or microendoscope should be used to inspect for residual. Because congenital cholesteatoma arises anatomically from the area where the tensor tympani tendon attaches to the neck of the malleus, residual disease should be sought for in this area.

Tympanoplasty is also appropriate for acquired cholesteatomas that are confined to the middle ear. The commonest example is retraction pocket cholesteatoma of the pars tensa. These lesions usually form in the posteriosuperior quadrant and initially travel medially along the axis of the lenticular process and stapes superstructure. Erosion of the lenticular process is common, and if a myringostapediopexy forms, the hearing may remain good. Eventually the sac will extend posteriorly to the sinus tympani, or superiorly to the attic by travelling medial to the incus body. The tympanic isthmus is a natural dehiscence of the epitympanic diaphragm, a route which may allow these lesions to reach the upper attic, where they become generalized ("holotympanic") cholesteatomas that require tympanomastoidectomy (*see* Fig. 11.6B).

Secondary acquired cholesteatomas, which arise from invagination of tympanic membrane surface epithelium through a perforation, may remain confined to the middle ear space for a long time. Discovering epithelial ingrowth through a perforation is an absolute indication for surgery. If left untreated, these lesions eventually behave as aggressively as any other mature cholesteatoma.

Tympanoplasty surgery for cholesteatoma is done through the bony ear canal (Fig. 11.8). A postauricular or transmeatal incision can be used, depending on the exposure provided by the natural meatus. Endaural incisions, as historically described by Lempert, can be used to expand the transmeatal exposure; sometimes a simple vertical cut through the thick skin of the incisura will permit a 7.5 or 8 mm speculum to be inserted. The canal (tympanomeatal) incision itself has many variations, but in general, radial cuts are made at 6 and 12 o'clock and connected by a circular cut through the posterior canal skin. The skin is elevated until the annulus is encountered. When a deep retraction pocket is present, the tympanic membrane epithelium will travel posterior to the lip of the bony annulus (Fig. 11.8A). Incising the tympanic membrane epithelium at this point will make the retraction pocket very difficult to retrieve. A better strategy is to lift the fibrous annulus away from the bone, then remove the bony lip with curet or diamond drill until the sac is exteriorized and can be delivered outward with a blunt instrument, such as a whirlybird or hockey-stick dissector. In some cases, the sac will extend posteriorly into the sinus tympani, and exteriorization might require a bony canaloplasty and removal of the bony lip as far back as the mastoid segment of the facial nerve. The sinus tympani can be very deep in certain individuals, and even this much exposure might result in a partly blind dissection. The sac might be very thin, especially if not filled with keratin, and it is important to try to remove it as a continuous sheet because residual disease might be hard to retrieve from a deep sinus tympani. An angled endoscope or mirror should routinely be used to make sure the sinus is clear at the end of the dissection.

Once the posterior part of the cholesteatoma sac is cleared, the inferior part should be dissected until the normal middle ear space is encountered. Inferiorly, these lesions may fill the round window niche and extend to the hypotympanic cells, and these regions may be difficult to clear until the bony exposure is extended by removing the inferior tympanic rim. Superiorly, extension to the attic may require a partial atticotomy by removing the scutum with a drill or curet. Anteriorly, the diseased portion of the tympanic membrane should be excised by making an incision along the malleus manubrium. If additional exposure is needed, the drum should be lifted off the malleus by incising the investing mucosa. Medially, the sac should be elevated off the promontory mucosa. Preserving the mucosal layer will help prevent later adhesive otitis, but this is not always possible.

Disease that adheres to the stapes superstructure, footplate, tympanic segment of facial nerve, and the sulcus between the facial nerve and stapes can be quite challenging to remove. The epithelial layer should be peeled away from these structures using a sharp instrument and patient dissection. At times, the attachment of the stapes superstructure to the footplate is partially eroded and can be detached and removed; some surgeons advocate using a laser to evaporate the superstructure. Dissecting disease from a mobile footplate is always challenging; a free edge should be sought and the matrix gently lifted away. A fractured or perforated footplate should be immediately repaired with a fascia graft. The facial nerve should also be cleared of disease. The fallopian canal is dehiscent in at least 30% of cases, usually along its inferior border facing the stapes superstructure, and so the best strategy is to work in a superior to inferior direction, starting on the dorsum of the nerve where the bony covering is likely to be intact, and lifting the matrix away from the exposed portion of the nerve. The sulcus between the facial nerve and stapes footplate can be a special challenge, especially if the nerve is bare and prolapsed over the footplate.

Following the complete removal of disease, reconstruction of the tympanic membrane and ossicular chain can be addressed. Cartilage is a valuable material for repairing a retracted tympanic membrane; because of its stiffness, cartilage will resist reretraction. The major drawback of cartilage is that it is opaque and may mask residual disease. The cartilage may be harvested from the cimbum concha or tragus, trimmed to the size of the tympanic membrane defect, and left attached to a larger piece of perichondrium. It is placed in an underlay fashion with respect to the remaining drum, concave side outward, with the perichondrium draped over the bony rim

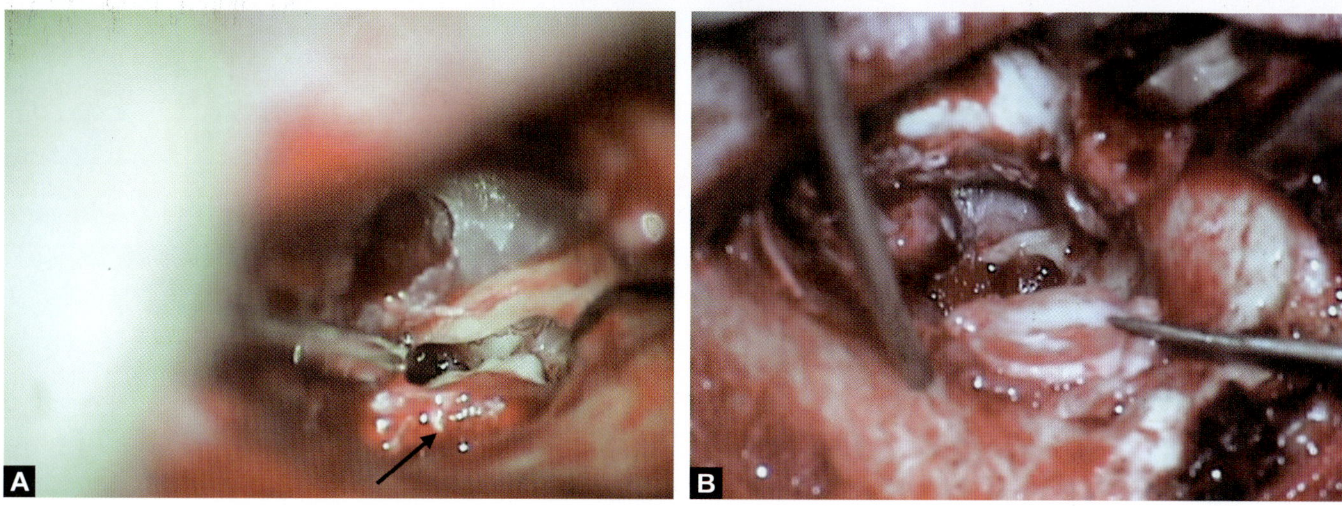

Figs. 11.8A and B: (A) Dissection of mesotympanic cholesteatoma via tympanoplasty approach, left ear. Tympanomeatal flap has been elevated, and sac is shown (arrow) covering stapes and filling sinus tympani. (B) Cartilage graft to posterosuperior quadrant, after excision of cholesteatoma sac.

(Fig. 11.8B). Prior to closure of the drum, the middle ear may be packed with gelatin (Gelfoam) or hyaluronic acid gel (Merogel). If the middle ear mucosa was stripped, a sheet of thin silicone (Silastic) sheeting might help prevent adhesions.

Ossicular reconstruction may be performed primarily or, if there is significant inflammation, delayed to a later stage. There are many options, and the choice of reconstruction depends on the surgical findings, ossicular geometry, condition of the middle ear, and experience and preference of the surgeon. Native or prosthetic material may be used. When the stapes superstructure is present, the tympanic membrane graft can be apposed to the capitulum forming a myringostapediopexy ("Type 3 reconstruction"). For cases of simple erosion of the lenticular process with an intact stapes superstructure (common), the incus may be removed, sculpted, and interposed between malleus neck and stapes capitulum, or a joint-type prosthesis (Applebaum or Krauss) may be placed. Alternatively, ionomeric cement may be used to bridge a small defect, or a wedge of cartilage may be interposed. In cases of absent stapes superstructure, the incus may be removed and sculpted to fit between the stapes footplate and malleus neck, or a total ossicular prosthesis ("TORP") may be used; there are many available variants that are crafted from hydroxyapatite, titanium, or other synthetic bio-inert materials.

Many ears with this type of disease have a retracted malleus with some inherent stiffness to the ossicular chain. In these situations, the tympanic membrane may be removed from the malleus, the incus is removed, the tensor tympani is sectioned and the malleus is laterally displaced. Then a partial prosthesis is placed from the capitulum of the stapes to the undersurface of the malleus or footplate to malleus reconstruction with a total prosthesis from footplate to malleus is utilized. The tympanic membrane reconstruction repaired in the usual fashion.

In cases of fixed stapes footplate, reconstruction should be deferred at least until there is no inflammation, or indefinitely. A hearing aid is an available option for rehabilitating conductive hearing loss, or a bone-anchored hearing device in a troublesome cavity.

Atticotomy

As previously discussed, the attic is comprised of three pouches, which are formed by the membranous folds: the lateral epitympanic space, or Prussak's space, and the anterior and posterior epitympanic spaces.[7] The attic is bisected in the transverse plane by the epitympanic diaphragm, which forms an incomplete partition dividing the attic into an upper and lower division.

Disease in the anterior and posterior epitympanic spaces that has travelled medial to the ossicles usually requires removal of the incus and head of the malleus. However, disease that remains in the plane lateral to the malleus and incus can sometimes be excised without removing the ossicles. Exteriorizing the epitympanic spaces usually involves removing the scutum, and frequently the scutum has already been eroded by the disease.

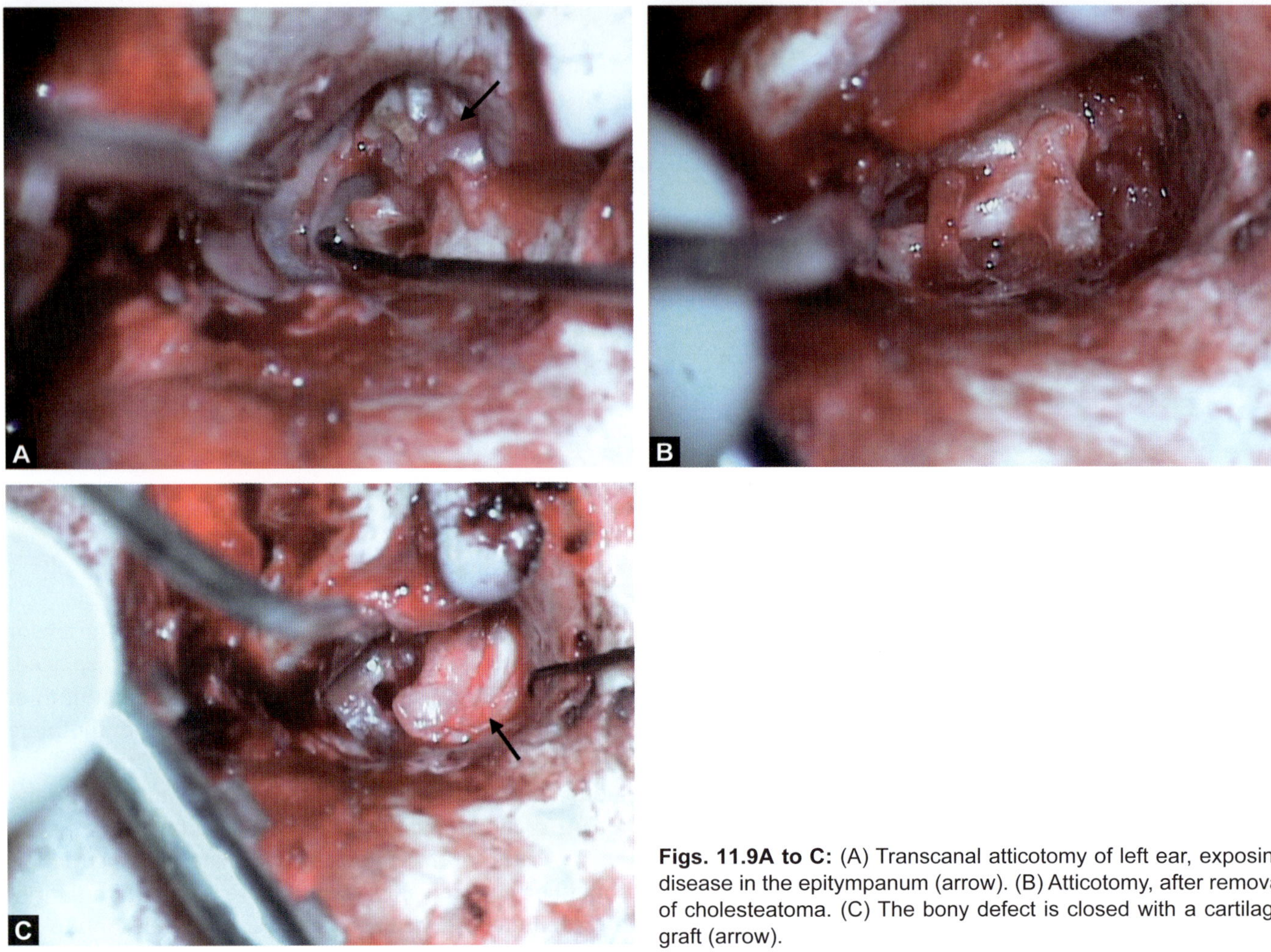

Figs. 11.9A to C: (A) Transcanal atticotomy of left ear, exposing disease in the epitympanum (arrow). (B) Atticotomy, after removal of cholesteatoma. (C) The bony defect is closed with a cartilage graft (arrow).

This procedure is a transcanal atticotomy. Alternatively, Prussak's space can be accessed through a transmastoid atticotomy.

The transcanal atticotomy is performed through a postauricular incision. Within the canal, tympanomeatal incisions are created and the flap is elevated away from the scutum superiorly. Exteriorization of the attic retraction requires first performing a bony canaloplasty, and then removing the anterior tympanic spine with curette and diamond drill. The scutum is then thinned down to eggshell thickness with a diamond bur, and the last layer of bone is removed with a curet, exposing the cholesteatoma sac (Fig. 11.9A). The superior, anterior, and posterior margins of the sac should be visualized (if the posterior limit is not well seen, an atticoantrotomy or Bondy mastoidectomy should be performed). The sac contents are decompressed, and the matrix is lifted away from the malleus and incus, and its attachment to the superior end of the tympanic membrane is sharply divided (Fig. 11.9B). If the sac progresses medial to the ossicles, the incus and malleus head will have to be removed to ensure complete excision. The scutum defect is then reconstructed with a graft of cartilage (Fig. 11.9C) with the overlying perichondrium draped over the bony edges, and the tympanomeatal and conchomeatal skin flaps are rearranged over this.

Scutum reconstruction is important to prevent disease recurrence. When a transcanal atticotomy procedure is performed, a potential space is created where cholesteatoma can reform. If the atticomy defect is excessively large, it may be preferable to create an open mastoid cavity, as described below, than to attempt to close the bony defect with cartilage.

Another way of managing disease in the attic is through a transmastoid atticotomy. This method is desirable in situations where a relatively large attic cholesteatoma develops behind a relatively small scutum defect. In this technique, a CWU mastoidectomy is performed (*see* below), and the attic is opened from behind, by drilling forward from the mastoid into the zygomatic root cells. The advantage of the transmastoid atticotomy over the transcanal atticotomy is that the bony scutum is a more rigid barrier against recurrence than cartilage.

CWU (Intact Canal Wall) Mastoidectomy

The CWU mastoidectomy is favored when the mastoid is well developed, because taking the CWD might result in a large, troublesome cavity. When combined with a transmastoid atticotomy and facial recess opening, the CWU approach provides access to all areas of the mastoid and middle ear. In cases where there is no clear preference for CWU or CWD, the CWU procedure can be performed as the initial approach, and can be converted to CWD during surgery if the exposure proves to be limited. The most troublesome areas for surgical exposure are the anterior epitympanic space, the sinus tympani, and the hypotympanum. At the time of surgery, the surgeon can accurately determine the extent of the disease and may take the CWD if needed to remove the entire disease.

The method of CWU mastoidectomy is as follows. The meatus should be inspected first using microscope and speculum. The ear canal and postauricular skin are injected with 1% lidocaine with epinephrine through a small-gauge needle to provide hemostasis and hydroplane dissection. The opening of the cholesteatoma sac in the pars flaccida or pars tensa can be inspected and probed to see where the disease tracks. A tympanomeatal flap is elevated to determine the extent of middle ear disease. The integrity of the incus and stapes can be determined at this point, and the incudostapedial joint can be separated to prevent vibrational trauma to the cochlea from the drill.

A postauricular incision is made and carried down to the avascular plane lateral to the temporalis fascia and mastoid periosteum. An incision is made in the mastoid periosteum along the linea temporalis and a counter-incision is made toward the mastoid tip. The periosteum is then elevated, exposing the mastoid cortex and bony ear canal. The canal skin is then separated from the bone until the tympanomeatal incision is reached. The auricle can then be retracted forward with self-retaining retractors, providing a good view of the mastoid cortex, ear canal, and middle ear.

A cutting drill is used with constant suction and irrigation to create cuts in the cortical bone just inferior to the temporal line and parallel to the posterior bony meatus, with the deepest point at MacEwen's triangle. A triangle of cortical bone is removed and progressively enlarged and deepened, removing the cellular bone until the mastoid antrum is entered. The internal landmarks of the mastoidectomy are the tegmen superiorly, the posterior canal wall anteriorly, and the sigmoid sinus posteriorly – these structures should be skeletonized by removing all the cellular bone. The Korner septum is a thin plate of bone at the tympanosquamous junction that forms the lateral wall of the antrum.

Depending on the extent of the disease, the cholesteatoma may fill the mastoid antrum (Fig. 11.10A) and it may also involve the pneumatized spaces of the mastoid down to the tip. Usually the cholesteatoma sac must be incised and its contents (debris) delivered before the deeper structures can be identified (Fig. 11.10B). The lateral semicircular canal, a dome-shaped structure of dense ivory bone at the base of the antrum, is the most important landmark, because it has a constant anatomic relationship to the facial nerve and stapes, and it defines the position of the facial recess.

The attic should be opened by creating a transmastoid atticotomy, following the tegmen forward toward the zygomatic root (Figs. 11.10A and B). The bone over the incus should be thinned to an eggshell and opened with a curet to avoid drilling on the incus. The posterior bony canal is thinned down to the level of cortical bone but not fenestrated. The amount of anterior exposure that can be gained depends on the height of the attic, i.e. the distance between the tegmen tympani and the superior aspect of the bony canal.

The atticotomy will expose the incus and malleus head. If the incus and malleus are encased in cholesteatoma, the incus is detached from the stapes and malleus and removed, and the malleus head is cut with a malleus nipper, leaving the manubrium. Occasionally, the sac remains lateral to the malleus and incus and the ossicles can be preserved.

The anterior epitympanum is accessed by removing the "cog," the bony bridge found anterior to the head of the malleus that divides the epitympanic space into posterior and anterior compartments. The cog can be perforated with a small diamond bur or curet. The anterior epitympanic space is capacious, roughly equal in volume to the posterior epitympanic space, and if disease is present there the canal wall will probably have to be removed to obtain adequate exposure.

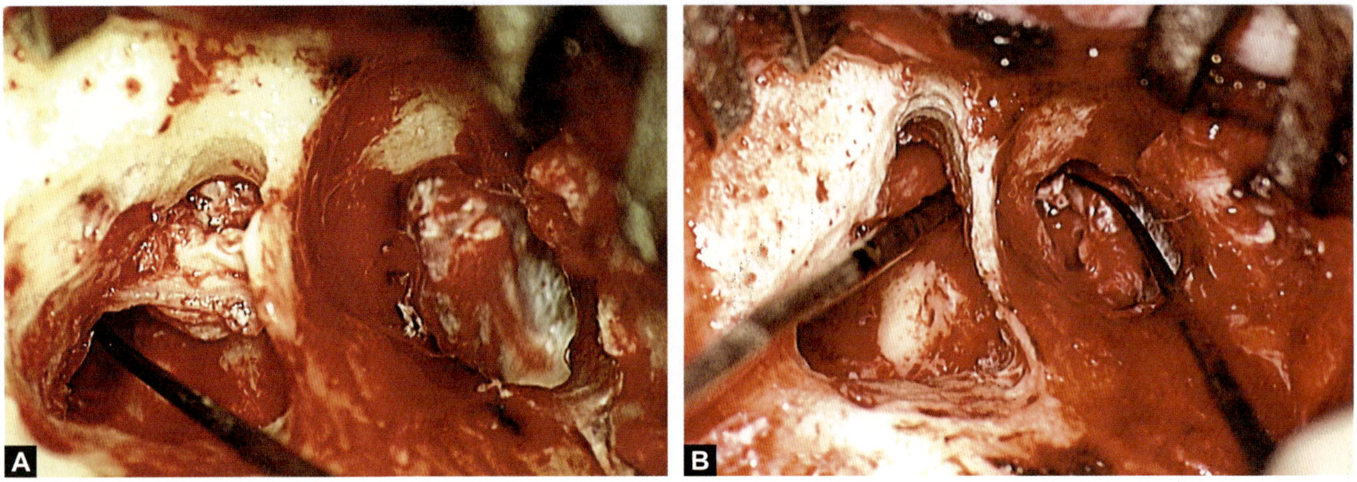

Figs. 11.10A and B: (A) Canal wall up mastoidectomy, right ear, exposing disease in the antrum, attic, and superior middle ear. (B) Excision of cholesteatoma via CWU mastoidectomy.

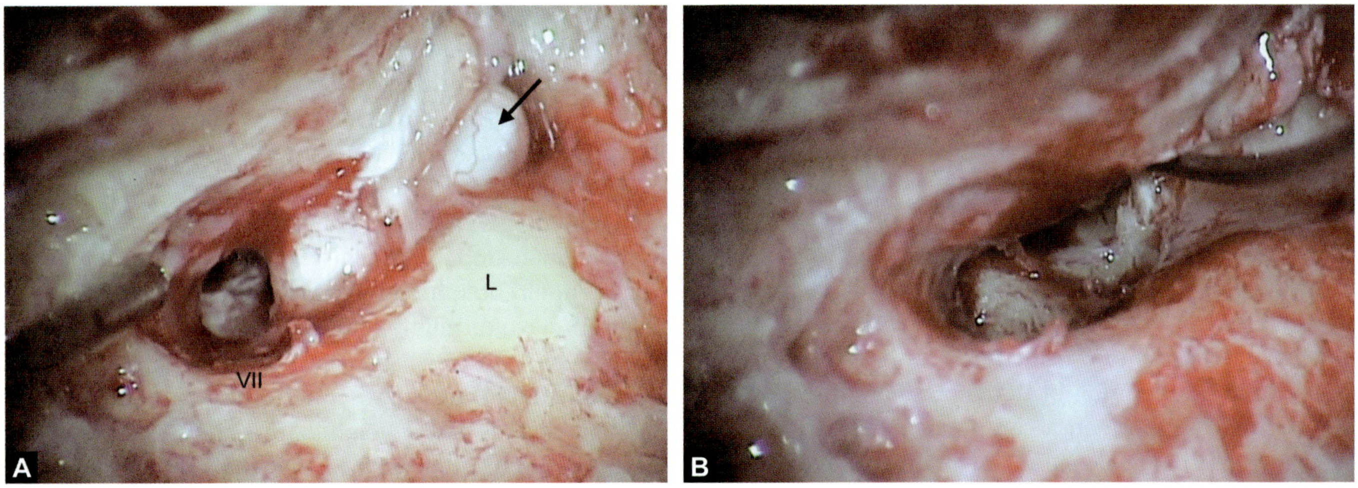

Figs. 11.11A and B: (A) Canal wall up mastoidectomy with facial recess approach, left ear. The cholesteatoma can be seen filling the aditus (arrow) and facial recess opening. L, lateral semicircular canal; VII, facial nerve. (B) After removing the cholesteatoma, the middle ear structures can be seen through the facial recess. The instrument is touching the stapes.

The middle ear is accessed from the mastoid through the facial recess approach (also called "posterior tympanotomy"). The facial recess is a triangular space bounded by the facial nerve medially, the chorda tympani nerve laterally, and the incus buttress superiorly. The mastoid segment (vertical portion) of the facial nerve is located at the level of the lateral semicircular canal and is encased in dense labyrinthine bone (Fig. 11.11A). Superiorly, the incus points to the facial nerve. Inferiorly the mastoid segment of the facial nerve terminates at the digastric ridge.

The facial recess is opened by drilling inferior to the fossa incudus with a small diamond bur, just lateral to the plane of the lateral semicircular canal. The facial recess opening is widened in a direction parallel to the facial nerve, and deepened in an anteromedial direction toward the middle ear. Once the middle ear is entered, the pyramidal process and round window niche will be identified. The facial recess opening can be enlarged medially by drilling the bone anterior to the facial nerve, and by drilling laterally to the tympanic annulus. It can be enlarged superiorly by removing the incus buttress and inferiorly by transecting the chorda tympani.

An adequate facial recess opening allows the surgeon to clear disease from the middle ear under direct vision (Fig. 11.11B). The middle ear will also be visualized directly by raising the tympanomeatal flap. By tilting the operating table, the surgeon can work on either side of the posterior bony canal wall to access all parts of the middle ear.

CWD Mastoidectomy

The CWD procedure is favored in certain situations: when the disease is extensive or cannot be completely removed, when the mastoid is small and sclerotic, when the patient cannot be relied upon for follow-up, when the canal wall is eroded by the disease, when the disease is recurrent, when dealing with a complication such as lateral semicircular canal fistula, and when removing cholesteatoma from an only hearing ear.

By creating an open cavity, CWD mastoidectomy provides an unobstructed view of the middle ear and mastoid. It carries a lower rate of residual and recurrent disease than CWU surgery, it results in a cavity may be prone to drainage and may require periodic cleaning in the office, and this can be problematic for children and for unreliable patients.

The CWD procedure can be planned in advance, or can be converted from CWU during the surgical procedure if the exposure is restricted. It can be performed from behind forward, or by following the disease from the attic back ("inside-out" or retrograde mastoidectomy). A CWD mastoidectomy can be performed in conjunction with tympanoplasty and ossicular reconstruction, or without entering the middle ear at all. In cases of destructive middle ear disease, a "radical mastoidectomy" can be performed, with removal of the middle ear contents.

The CWD mastoidectomy begins with the CWU procedure described above. Once the mastoid landmarks are identified, the canal wall can be taken down with a cutting burr, beginning in the attic where the bony canal meets the tegmen, and progressively lowering the bone toward the mastoid segment (vertical portion) of the facial nerve. The landmarks for the mastoid segment of the facial nerve are the lateral semicircular canal above and the digastric groove below. A smaller diamond bur is used when the facial nerve is approached. As an alternative, the facial recess can be opened first, and then the canal wall can be taken down en bloc. The latter approach has the advantages that (1) the facial nerve is identified early and thus protected from surgical trauma; (2) the facial ridge is maximally lowered, resulting in a more manageable cavity; (3) the bony canal wall can be removed quickly with rongeur once the facial nerve is visualized; and (4) the canal wall bone can be saved and used later for cavity obliteration.

If the mastoid is well developed, it is important to exenterate all the air cells so that only cortical bone remains. Leaving pockets of cellular bone will result in postoperative mucositis and drainage. Measures that can be taken to reduce the size of the mastoid are described below. If the mastoid is diploic, it may not be necessary to remove all the marrow-containing spaces. Often the cavity can be sculpted into a round, well-beveled shape, using a diamond bur to polish the bleeding edges. If the mastoid is sclerotic, the disease-containing spaces can be opened, and the remaining bone can be contoured to result in a round, compact cavity.

The CWD mastoidectomy can also be performed in a front-to-back, or "inside-out," fashion. This method is suitable when it has been decided in advance that a CWD is necessary, such as in a sclerotic mastoid with disease localized to the attic and antrum. This "inside-out" or "retrograde mastoidectomy" has been well described by Dornhoffer[12] in which the disease is followed from its origin in the middle ear or epitympanum, to its posterior limit in the mastoid, and a limited portion of the posterior canal wall is removed, with the mastoid is opened only as far as needed to expose the disease. The resulting canal wall defect is repaired with a cartilage graft harvested from the cimbum concha to result in a closed cavity. The Bondy operation, a variant of CWD described below, can also be performed in an inside-out fashion.

Creating a manageable cavity after CWD mastoidectomy requires four steps: (1) beveling the cavity edges; (2) lowering the facial ridge; (3) amputating the mastoid tip; and (4) creating an adequate meatoplasty (Fig. 11.12).[13] Paying careful attention to these steps will result in a compact but well aerated cavity that can be inspected and cleaned in the office without difficulty.

Beveling the edges of the cavity is performed by drilling away the margins of cortical bone above the tegmen, behind the sigmoid sinus, and anteriorly where the epitympanum meets the middle ear (supratubal recess). The tegmen has a rounded contour, like the bottom of a boat, and it turns upward laterally toward the squamosa. The retrosigmoid air cells, which can be very well developed, should be removed to prevent areas that can be inaccessible in the postoperative cavity. The anterior canal wall bone should then be smoothed with a diamond drill, as that it becomes confluent with the anterior wall of the anterior epitympanum, while avoiding entry into the temporomandibular joint.

Lowering the facial ridge is essential for creating a round confluent cavity between the mastoid and middle

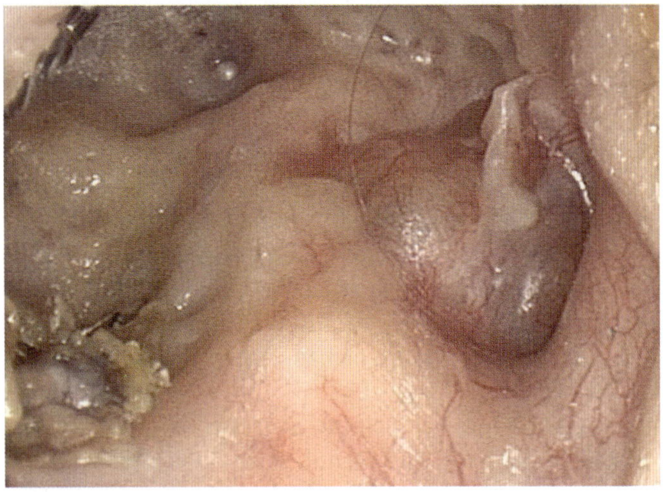

Fig. 11.12: Canal wall down mastoidectomy, right ear, showing beveled bony edges, lowered facial ridge, and amputated mastoid tip.

ear, thus avoiding a dependent mastoid bowl that will collect debris that requires frequent cleaning. At surgery, the mastoid (vertical) segment of the facial nerve should be followed inferiorly from the lateral semicircular canal to the stylomastoid foramen, and skeletonized, leaving only a thin bony covering. It is also important to remove the triangle of bone that separates the mastoid from the hypotympanum, bringing the floor of the ear canal to the level of the mastoid tip. Also, when the middle ear is entered, the bone anterior to the facial nerve should be removed, in order to gain maximal access to the sinus tympani.

Amputating the mastoid tip is important to eliminate dependent cells that can develop mucositis or harbor recurrence. The mastoid tip is bisected by the digastric groove, and large burr can be used to remove the entire bone lateral to the digastric. Beveling the cortical edges, lowering the facial ridge and removing the triangle of bone between the hypotympanum and mastoid, and amputating the mastoid tip allow the soft tissues to collapse medially, resulting in a smaller cavity.

Performing an adequate meatoplasty ensures that the cavity will bewell aerated and accessible for postoperative inspection and cleaning. The meatoplasty consists of three steps: lengthening the incisions at 6 and 12 o'clock through skin and cartilage, excising a crescent of conchal cartilage from behind to widen the meatal opening, and placing stay sutures from the conchal perichondrium to the mastoid periosteum in order to stretch the meatus open. The surgeon has the option of thinning the subcutaneous tissue of the conchomeatal flap prior to closure, which will result in a wider meatus with a skin-lined cavity, or leaving a pedicle of fibromuscular tissue attached to the conchomeatal flap, which can be used to partially obliterate the sinodural angle and result in a smaller cavity.

The Bondy Operation (Retrograde or Inside-Out Mastoidectomy)

The Bondy operation is variation of CWD mastoidectomy. It can be defined as a transcanal atticoantromy, and is ideal for attic-antral cholesteatoma in a compact mastoid. The principle of the Bondy operation is the exteriorization of attic-antral disease to create a "safe" ear while sparing the middle ear hearing mechanism.[14] Bondy first described this procedure in 1910, prior to the advent of microscopes and antibiotics, realizing that some patients with good preoperative hearing and limited cholesteatoma could avoid radical mastoidectomy.[15]

The object of the Bondy operation is to expose the disease in the attic by removing the scutum, then follow the disease back to the mastoid antrum. The middle ear space is avoided unless it contains disease. The procedure is usually done through a postauricular incision, although an endaural approach can also be performed.

From a postauricular approach, the cortical bone is first removed with a cutting or coarse diamond bur until the lateral edge of the tegmen is skeletonized. The tegmen is then followed medially until the scutum is thinned down to an egg shell. A curet can then be used to complete the atticotomy, so as to avoid drilling directly on the malleus and incus. Using the drill, the tegmen is then followed posteriorly until the antrum is exposed (Fig. 11.13A). The cavity that is formed is created in a round shape, paralleling (and enlarging) the curve of the posterior canal wall and beveling the posterior bony edges. The posterior and inferior limits of drilling are defined by the extent of the disease, creating a round, well-beveled cavity with smooth bony contours. The posterior canal wall is removed down to the level of the facial ridge. The tympanic membrane and the intact ossicular chain can be preserved if the disease allows (Fig. 11.13B). At the end of the procedure, the tympanomeatal flap can be redraped over the facial ridge and a temporalis fascia graft can be draped over the medial wall of the cavity. The conchomeatal skin flap is laid onto the lateral bony edges, and a modified meatoplasty is done by lengthening the incisural and tragal-antitragal incisions, and scoring the conchal cartilage from behind.

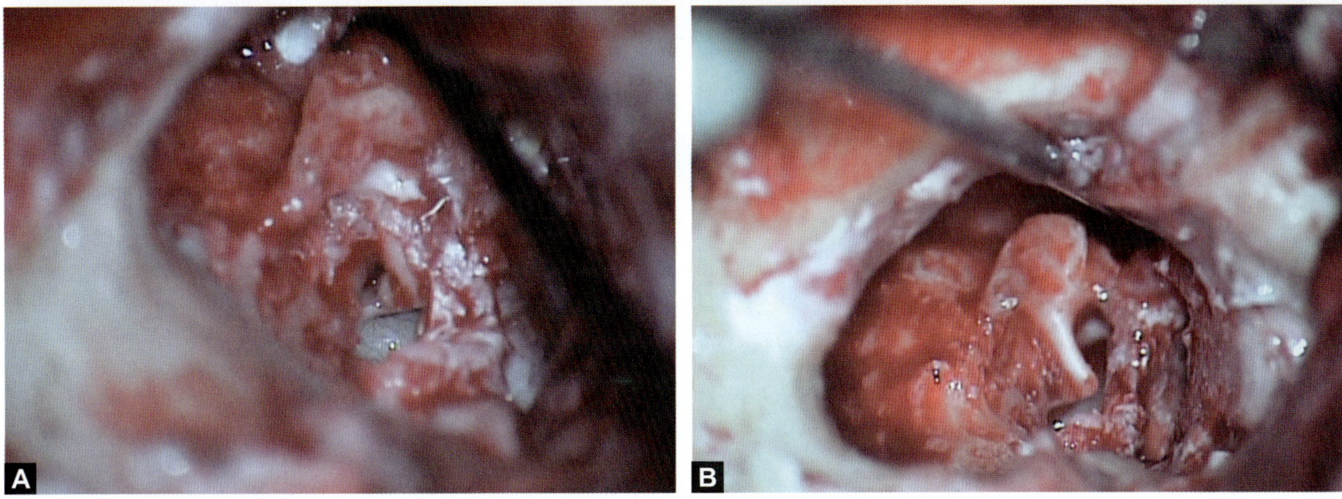

Figs. 11.13A and B: (A) Bondy mastoidectomy, right ear, with exposure of disease in attic, antrum, and superior middle ear. (B) Bondy mastoidectomy completed, with disease removed and preservation of ossicular chain and tympanic membrane.

Surgical Decision-Making: When to Take Down the Canal Wall

The decision to take the CWD can be made before or during the surgical procedure. A CWD procedure should be selected preoperatively if the mastoid is sclerotic, if the canal wall has been breached by cholesteatoma, if the patient has a giant cholesteatoma, if the cholesteatoma is recurrent, or if the patient is unreliable for follow-up.

In many cases, however, there are no absolute criteria for CWD, and the decision for CWU /CWD can be made during surgery, as guided by the anatomy and the extent of disease. The surgeon can begin with a CWU operation, and take the CWD if the exposure proves to be inadequate or if the complete removal of the disease is not certain.

The CWU mastoidectomy can provide access to all areas of the mastoid, epitympanum, and middle ear, and by widely opening the attic and facial recess and removing the incus and malleus head, it is possible to visualize all these regions. However, the intact bony canal wall is a barrier that can make the exposure difficult, and there is a chance that residual disease will remain hidden in the anterior epitympanic space, hypotympanum, or the sinus tympani. A small endoscope or mirror can be useful to inspect these problematic areas, but in cases with poor visualization or limited access, the canal wall will have to be removed. Atelectasis of the posterior mesotympanum may also favor a CWD procedure, because the posterior tympanic membrane will often recollapse into the middle ear space postoperatively, leading to recurrence.

Cavity Reconstruction

Cavity reconstruction may be undertaken after CWD mastoidectomy in a large mastoid cavity to avoid post-operative mucositis and retention of debris. A general word of caution is not to bury disease underneath a flap or partial obliteration, because this can grow silently and cause problems years later.

Reconstruction of the canal wall in mastoid surgery is not a new concept, and different techniques have been tried over many years in an effort to decrease cavity size and prevent recurrent disease. The musculoperiosteal flap, described by Palva,[16] which uses temporalis muscle and fibrous tissue pedicled to the conchomeatal skin, is a simple and readily accessible means of decreasing cavity size by partial obliteration. By lengthening the vertical incisions through the meatal skin and cartilage, the Palva flap can be directed posteriorly and superiorly to close the sinodural angle. The use of bone pate[17] is also a popular means of reducing cavity size, but this material often shrinks back in the weeks after the surgery and carries the risk of placing infected material in the cavity. Mercke[18] and later Gantz[19] described the en bloc removal and replacement of the bony canal wall, using bone chips to obliterate the mastoid cavity, with recurrence rate of 1.5% at 4 years mean follow-up, however, a high rate of wound infection and the continued need for second look operation have limited the popularity of this approach.

Our preferred technique is a modification of the reimplanted canal wall. When creating a CWD, the bony canal

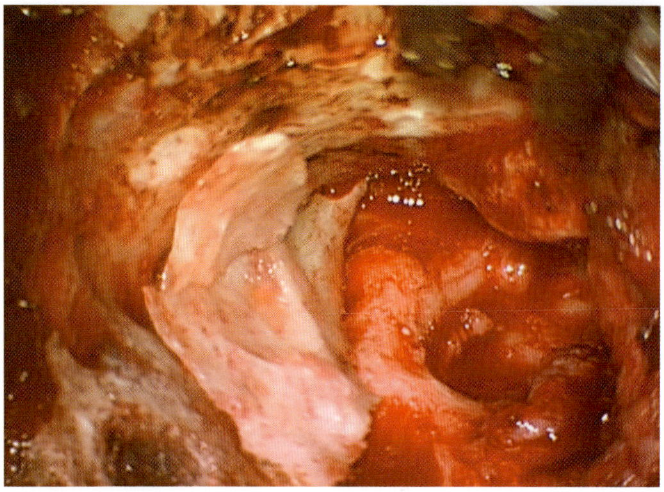

Fig. 11.14: The bony canal wall can be denuded of epithelium and re-implanted across the sinodural angle at the end of the procedure, so as to close off most of the mastoid cavity.

wall is removed en bloc, by opening the facial recess and creating vertical bony cuts with a small diamond bur at the superior and inferior attachments. The bone is then denuded of all epithelium, and reimplanted across the sinodural angle at the end of the procedure, so as to close off most of the mastoid cavity (Fig. 11.14). Temporalis fascia is draped over the medial wall of the antrum and attic and onto the bare bone: laterally, the bone is covered by the conchomeatal skin flap. The attic is left open, to minimize the chance of recurrence.

PROGNOSIS

Results of Surgery

The outcome measures for cholesteatoma surgery are freedom from recidivistic disease, serviceable hearing, and a dry, trouble free ear. Recidivism, discussed in the following section, continues to be a challenge, even in the most experienced hands. Published reports from large series cite rates of recidivistic disease between 20% and 50%, and most surgeons acknowledge that the rate is higher in children.

The hearing outcomes after cholesteatoma surgery vary widely, and depend a great deal on the status of the middle ear at the time of surgery. An intact ossicular chain is occasionally encountered. Preservation of an intact ossicular chain can often be achieved, and will usually result in a good hearing outcome, but this should not compromise the complete removal of the disease. Residual cholesteatoma will usually result in worse hearing than complete removal and primary ossicular repair.

In most cases of cholesteatoma, however, the ossicular chain is eroded at the time of surgery. The most common pattern is erosion of the lenticular process of the incus, followed by erosion of the stapes superstructure. This will result in ossicular discontinuity, with a large (~55 dB) conductive hearing loss unless the ossicular chain is repaired (note that the preoperative hearing status may be better because the cholesteatoma itself may conduct sound). Ossicular reconstruction may be undertaken at the primary procedure, or delayed until a later stage. Native or prosthetic material may be used. A type 3 reconstruction ("myringostapediopexy," or drum on stapes head) is simple to perform when the incus is eroded and the stapes superstructure is present. There can usually be done at the initial surgery, and usually results in hearing between 0 and 30 dB air-bone gap. Additional techniques of ossicular reconstruction are discussed in detail in the chapter on tympanoplasty.

A dry, trouble-free ear is also an important surgical goal. The CWU operation strives to achieve this in every case, by creating a closed mastoid cavity behind an intact tympanic membrane. Postoperative otorrhea after CWU mastoidectomy is rare, and should raise the suspicion of recurrent cholesteatoma. The CWD operation, if properly performed, should result in a dry cavity in the majority of patients. Case selection is important - CWD is favored in a sclerotic mastoid where the mucosal surface area is small. Adherence to good surgical technique will result in a low incidence of a postoperative draining cavity. This includes aggressively beveling the cortical bony edges (resulting in a shallow mastoid bowl), amputating the mastoid tip, lowering the facial ridge (to avoid creating a partition between the mastoid bowl and the external meatus), and, most importantly, performing a good meatoplasty. Cavity obliteration techniques, described above, will also limit the size of the cavity and the propensity for postoperative drainage.

Recidivism: Recurrent and Residual Disease

Cholesteatoma can regrow even after adequate surgery. There are two mechanisms by which cholesteatoma can reform. Recurrence is the regrowth of disease by the reformation of a retraction pocket. Residual disease is disease left behind by the surgeon. "Recidivism" refers to the sum of recurrent and residual disease. Recidivistic disease will continue to progress and enlarge unless treated surgically, so early detection usually leads to better results. We advise patients to return every 6 months after cholesteatoma surgery for routine surveillance, but this is not always achievable because patients move away, become noncompliant, or their medical insurance changes.

Recidivistic disease is usually detected clinically, and is heralded by recurrent infection (otorrhea) or declining hearing, although some cases will recur silently and be only detected on physical examination. Otomicroscopy is essential for examining the ear in the office setting. After CWU surgery, recurrent cholesteatoma will appear as an attic retraction with squamous debris, and may present with otorrhea. Gently probing an attic defect with a blunt hook may reveal the recurrence. Residual disease will appear as a white mass behind the eardrum, and may cause worsening hearing. Residual disease in the mastoid may not manifest itself clinically until it is quite large.

CT scanning may be helpful to detect residual disease. CT will reveal a nodular soft tissue density within the mastoid cavity. However CT cannot differentiate cholesteatoma from hyperplastic mucosa, granulation tissue, or fibrous tissue that may normally fill the postoperative cavity, and so this method lacks specificity. Non-echo planar diffusion-weighted MRI scanning may be the best tool for detecting residual disease noninvasively. Cholesteatoma will appear bright on nonecho planer diffusion-weighted images, and the test has a very high sensitivity and specificity.[20] However, it is expensive and time consuming and may be difficult to perform in children without sedation. Also the cholesteatoma must be of adequate size in order to be visualized which generally is at least 5 mm in diameter and this MRI technique is generally not adequate in disease that is lacey, lining the mastoid cavity with a thin layer of epithelium. In cases where the clinical suspicion of recurrence is high, surgical exploration is warranted.

Second-stage (or "second look") procedures is often recommended after CWU surgery to search for residual disease.[11] Some surgeons advise this procedure routinely, while others reserve this for difficult or extensive cases in which the chance of recurrence is felt to be higher than average. Second-stage surgery may be performed between 6 months and 2 years after the initial operation - there is no consensus on the timing (note that residual disease is present immediately postoperatively, whereas recurrent disease may occur years after the original operation). The second operation also allows the opportunity for ossicular reconstruction in a stable middle ear without inflammatory disease, and so some surgeons routinely postpone ossiculoplasty until the second stage.

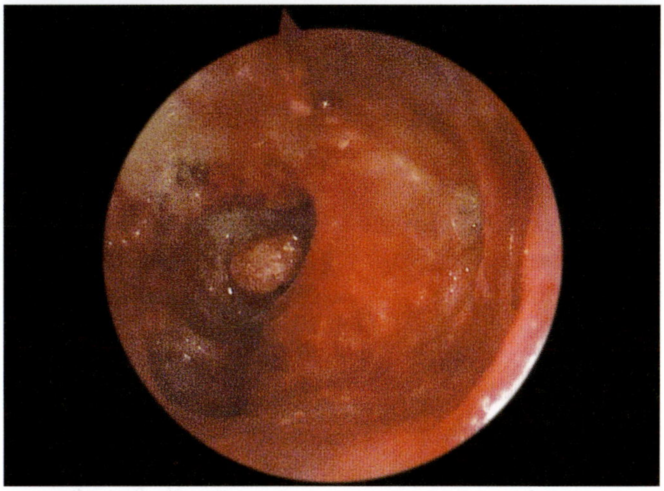

Fig. 11.15: A residual cholesteatoma in CWU mastoidectomy can be identified and removed endoscopically, using a 2.7 mm, 30° endoscope through a postauricular stab incision. (CWU, canal wall up).

The endoscope can be a valuable adjunct during the second-stage operation. A short 2.7 mm diameter, 30° rigid telescope is ideal for this application. After lifting the tympanomeatal flap, the endoscope can be used to look up in the attic and back in the sinus tympani to spot residual disease. The endoscope can also be passed into the mastoidectomy cavity through a postauricular stab incision, and a residual cholesteatoma can be removed through this route if it is well encapsulated (Fig. 11.15). This procedure can be performed under local anesthesia in a cooperative patient.

Residual or recurrent cholesteatoma in a CWU mastoidectomy will require conversion to CWD if the lesion is large, erosive, or invasive. Revision mastoidectomy is performed through a postauricular approach, using the original incision. Fibrous adhesions may be present, and there may be more bleeding than in a primary case. A periosteal incision is made outside of the original bony cavity. The cholesteatoma matrix should be sharply dissected away from the undersurface of the periosteal flap. Once the mastoid cavity is entered, the neocortical bone is removed with a coarse diamond drill and the contents of the sac are debulked. The matrix is dissected away from the bony margins of the cavity. The cholesteatoma is delivered from back to front. The anterior epitympanum might need to be exteriorized by opening the zygomatic root cells. The portion of the sac in the attic should be traced to its origin.

In the case of recurrent cholesteatoma, the disease usually reforms from a new attic retraction pushing through a scutal defect, and if this is so the canal wall will almost certainly have to be taken down. The attachment of the sac to the tympanic membrane margin can be cut with a Bellucci scissors. If the disease pushes down into the middle ear, part of the eardrum will have to be removed and the ossicular chain may have to be separated and the incus removed.

Residual cholesteatoma in a CWD cavity is not common. A well-circumscribed residuum in the mastoid cavity or attic can usually be detected and treated in the office setting. The mucosal envelope is incised with a sharp pick (this can often be performed without anesthesia), and the sac is exteriorized and removed with a cerumen curet. If the mucosal edges are adequately marsupialized, the lesion will rarely recur. Residual cholesteatoma in the middle ear space will usually require a tympanoplasty operation in the operating room. Residual disease around the stapes will often cause worsening hearing and may require ossiculoplasty.

Recurrent cholesteatoma after CWD mastoidectomy is less common, and should theoretically not occur in an open cavity. The usual cause is failure to create an open, self-aerating cavity at the original surgery, leaving a high facial ridge or inadequate meatoplasty behind which cholesteatoma may reform. These cases usually present with fetid drainage and retained squamous debris, and the anatomic limitations of the cavity are usually evident on office examination. Surgical revision is necessary. As with revision mastoidectomy after CWU, the original incision is used, the periosteum is incised behind the original mastoidectomy boundary, and the soft tissue is lifted away from the cavity. The goal of revision surgery is to create a round confluent cavity. The bony margins should be aggressively beveled, and the mastoid tip removed if still present. The facial ridge should be lowered, skeletonizing the mastoid portion of the facial nerve and removing the dense hypotympanic bone inferiorly that forms a partition between the middle ear and mastoid. The zygomatic root cells should be opened as well to ensure exteriorization of the anterior epitympanum. All the disease is dissected from the medial wall of the mastoid and attic, and any remaining mastoid air cells are exenterated with a coarse diamond bur to prevent postoperative mucositis. An adequate meatoplasty is essential in these cases to prevent membranous partitions and allow postoperative surveillance and cavity cleaning.

Complications of Surgery

The consent process for cholesteatoma surgery should include a discussion of the common surgical risks as well as the uncommon but significant surgical complications. By percentages, the commonest risk associated with cholesteatoma surgery is the risk of recurrence, which is between 10% and 50% even in experienced hands. This exposes the patient to the chance of needing more than one operation, and this reality should be discussed with the patient up front. The second most common risk of surgery is that of worsened hearing or persistent hearing loss. Cholesteatoma is an erosive and inflammatory condition, and functional preservation of the ossicular chain and middle ear space is not always possible. This too might require a second surgical operation, to perform a middle ear reconstruction at a later opportunity, when the disease is not present.

The less common but significant risks of cholesteatoma surgery involve injury to the inner ear, facial nerve, dura, or central nervous system. In discussing these risks with the patient it is important to weigh the probability of a surgical complication (low, in experienced hands) against the risk of a complication resulting from untreated disease. Labyrinthitis can result from uncapping a labyrinthine fistula, or from spread of middle ear inflammation through the oval or round windows. Labyrinthitis can lead to vertigo and permanent sensorineural hearing loss. Facial nerve paralysis can occur if the nerve is physically injured by the surgeon, or if inflammation spreads to the nerve through a dehiscence in the bony fallopian canal. The prognosis depends on the degree of injury. A patient who awakens from surgery with facial paralysis should be immediately re-explored, and once the site of injury is identified it should be repaired with a graft from the great auricular nerve. Delayed facial paralysis will usually recover without intervention.

Dural exposure during surgery is common, especially at the tegmen mastoideum that can have an irregular contour. Focal dural exposure is common and rarely leads to any functional consequences unless it involves a broad area, allowing a brain herniation to develop, or if infection tracks intracranially from the epidural space. A dural tear will result in cerebrospinal fluid (CSF) leakage, and this needs to be repaired immediately with a tissue graft, using temporalis fascia or perichondrium against the dura, followed by a cartilage or split calvarial bone graft against the tegmen. A persistent or occult CSF leak can result in meningitis. A tear in the sigmoid sinus can sometimes result in significant blood loss. Brisk venous bleeding can be controlled initially with digital pressure against the site or a nonresorbable pack of oxidized cellulose (Surgicel); definitive control can usually be obtained with gelatin-thrombin packing. The latter should be placed extraluminally, by wedging it against the bony margins, so as to avoid permanently occluding the venous flow.

Additional complications of surgery include persistent inflammation from a draining cavity (mucositis), which may require repeated visits to the office to control, meatal stenosis, and tinnitus.

Complications of the Disease

Cholesteatoma usually grows indolently, but spread of inflammation outside of the middle ear cleft constitutes a medical complication that might require urgent surgery. Classically these complications are referred to as "aural" (intratemporal) and "intracranial" (extratemporal). The aural complications of cholesteatoma are: mastoiditis, petrositis, facial paralysis, and labyrinthitis. The intracranial complications of cholesteatoma include meningitis, epidural abscess, subdural abscess, septic thrombophlebit is of the lateral venous sinus, otitic hydrocephalus, and brain abscess.

Mastoiditis refers to coalescence of the mastoid air cells by liquefactive necrosis of the separated bone. Clinically, this is heralded by fever, purulent otorrhea, and protrusion of the auricle caused by a postauricular subperiosteal abscess. Radiologically, the diagnosis is confirmed on CT by the presence of coalescence (loss of the bony septations), erosion of the outer cortex, and a dome-like lucency in the subcutaneous soft tissues. The treatment remains surgical, incising, and draining the subperiosteal collection of pus, and performing a mastoidectomy to remove the cholesteatoma and the pus within the mastoid. Acute coalescent mastoiditis may occur in the absence of cholesteatoma, after an incompletely treated acute otitis media. When cholesteatoma is present, the sac usually causes a blockade between the middle ear and mastoid air cells ("attic-antral block") that allows pus to collect in the mastoid cells with no egress. This causes liquefactive necrosis of the cortical bone, allows the abscess to "point" within the postauricular soft tissues (rarely, the abscess can form in the preauricular soft tissues through the zygomatic root cells, or in the deep spaces of the neck through the digastric ridge, named "Bezold's abscess").

Petrositis is defined as the spread of inflammation to the petrous apex. This classically results in Gradenigo's syndrome, the triad of otorrhea, retrobulbar headache, and abducens palsy. Petrositis usually arises in the setting of chronic otitis media, and treatment consists of drainage of the petrous apex, either through a transmastoid, infracochlear route, or if anatomically possible through the sphenoid sinus. In the presence of cholesteatoma, a mastoidectomy is inevitable.

Labyrinthitis implies spread of inflammation to the inner ear, either through a labyrinthine fistula, or through the oval or round window. Toxic (serous) labyrinthitis is manifested by vertigo and sensorineural hearing loss, and is treated with antibiotics in addition to surgical removal of the disease. Sensorineural hearing loss may not fully recover. Suppurative labyrinthitis is an otologic emergency, treated with antibiotics, steroids, and urgent surgery. If the suppurative infection spreads to the inner ear, a dead ear may result despite treatment. Suppurative labyrinthitis can occur concurrently with bacterial meningitis, which can be either a cause or an effect of the inner ear infection.

Labyrinthine fistula most common occurs in the lateral semicircular canal. Fistula presents clinically with vertigo elicited by tragal pressure, and on examination the fistula sign can be demonstrated with a pneumatic otoscope, impedance bridge, or cupped had over the ear meatus causing a deviation of the eyes away and toward the affected ear with positive and negative pressure. Some fistulas are asymptomatic, however, and the labyrinthine erosion is often but not always demonstrated by preoperative CT. In the presence of a known fistula, cholesteatoma surgery should be done cautiously, leaving the matrix in place over the lateral semicircular canal until all other disease is removed. In the noninfected ear, the matrix can either be removed, and the fistula immediately sealed with periosteum, or left in place and a CWD mastoidectomy performed to exteriorize the matrix. In an infected cavity, it is better to leave the matrix and perform a CWD because uncapping the fistula can lead to a dead ear.

Facial nerve paralysis is a dire complication of cholesteatoma and can occur by two mechanisms. Direct spread of infection to the facial nerve causes acute facial paralysis. This condition should be treated urgently with antibiotics, steroids, and surgical decompression of the nerve. The prognosis is good if the treatment is delivered quickly, within a day of the onset of paralysis. Subacute or chronic facial nerve palsy arises from pressure against the exposed nerve by the cholesteatoma sac. This is treated by surgical removal of the disease. The prognosis is good if the treatment is administered early, but poor if the paresis is longstanding and fibrosis of the nerve has occurred. Surgical decompression of the facial nerve is done by debulking the cholesteatoma sac contents, and then carefully lifting the matrix away from the nerve sheath. It is likely in these cases that the bony covering of the nerve will be absent and so due caution is advised. The facial nerve stimulator-monitor is advantageous in these cases, first to locate the nerve that is enveloped in disease, second to provide real-time feedback to the surgeon while dissecting the disease from the bare nerve, and finally to stimulate the nerve at the end of the procedure across the area of injury to estimate the degree of conduction block.

SUMMARY

Cholesteatoma is an invasive disease of the middle ear cleft that can cause infection, hearing loss, and intra- and extratemporal complications. The treatment is surgical, although a high rate of recidivism persists despite technical advances. Early detection, thorough surgical removal, and careful postoperative surveillance will produce the best long-term outcomes.

REFERENCES

1. Schuknecht HF. Pathology of the ear, 2nd edn. Philadelphia, PA: Lea &Febiger; 1993. pp.204-6.
2. Abramson M. Collagenolytic activity in middle ear cholesteatoma. Ann Otol Rhinol Laryngol. 1964;78:112-24.
3. Michaels L. Origin of congenital cholesteatoma from a normally occurring epidermoid rest in the developing middle ear. Int J Pediatr Otorhinolaryngol. 1988;15(1):51-65.
4. Semaan MT, Megerian CA. The pathophysiology of cholesteatoma. Otolaryngol Clin N Am. 2006;39:1143-59.
5. Abramson M, Moriyama H, Huang CC. Histology, pathogenesis, and treatment of cholesteatoma. Ann Otol Rhinol Laryngol Suppl. 1984;112:125-8.
6. Palva T, Ramsay H, Northrop C. Color atlas of the anatomy and pathology of the epitympanum. Basel, Switzerland: Karger; 2001.
7. Smouha EE, Bojrab DI. Cholesteatoma. New York, NY: Thieme; 2011. pp. 3-7.
8. Sudhoff H, Tos M. Pathogenesis of sinus cholesteatoma. Eur Arch Otorhinolaryngol. 2007;264:1137-43.
9. Yung M, Jacobsen NL, Vowler SL. A 5-year observational study of the outcome in pediatric cholesteatoma surgery. Otol Neurotol. 2007;28:1038-40.
10. Stankovic M. Follow-up of cholesteatoma surgery: open versus closed tympanoplasty. ORL J Otorhinolaryngol Relat Spec. 2007;69:299-305.
11. Sheehy JL, Brackmann DE, Graham MD. Cholesteatoma surgery: residual and recurrent disease: a review of 1,024 cases. Ann Otol Rhinol Laryngol. 1977;86:451-62.
12. Dornhoffer JL. Retrograde mastoidectomy with canal wall reconstruction: a follow-up report. Otol Neurotol. 2004; 24:653-60.
13. Sheehy JL. Cholesteatoma surgery: canal wall down procedures. Ann Otol Rhinol Laryngol. 1988;97:30-35.
14. Sanna M, Facharzt AA, Russo A, et al. Modified Bondy's technique: refinements of the surgical technique and long term results. Otol Neurotol. 2009;30:64-9.
15. Bondy G. TotalaufmeisselungmitErhaltung von Trommelfell und Gehorknochelchen. Monatsschr Ohrenheilk. 1910: 15–23
16. Silvola J, Palva T. Pediatric one-stage cholesteatoma surgery: long term results. Int J Pediatr Otorhinolaryngol. 1999;5(49 Suppl 1):S87-90.
17. Roberson JB, Mason TP, Stridham KR. Mastoid obliteration: autogenous cranial bone pate reconstruction. Otol Neurotol. 2003;24:132-140.
18. Mercke U. The cholesteatomatous ear one year after surgery with obliteration technique. Am J Otol. 1987; 8:534-6.
19. Gantz BJ, Wilkinson EP, Hansen MR. Canal wall reconstruction tympanomastoidectomy with mastoid obliteration. Laryngoscope. 2005;115:1734-40.
20. De Foer B, Vercruysse JP, Bernaerts A, et al. Detection of postoperative residual cholesteatoma with non-echo-planar diffusion-weighted magnetic resonance imaging. Otol Neurotol. 2008;29(4):513-17.

CHAPTER

12

Tympanoplasty and Ossiculoplasty

Dennis I Bojrab, Emily Z Stucken, Eric E Smouha

DEFINITIONS

The goal of successful tympanoplasty is to create a mobile tympanic membrane or graft with an aerated, mucosa-lined middle ear space and a sound conduction mechanism between the mobile membrane and the inner ear fluids.[1] Many techniques have been developed and employed successfully since the modern era of tympanoplasty began in 1952 with Wullstein and Zollner, then followed by Shea, Hough, Storrs, Herrmann, Austin, Sheehy, Glasscock, Tos, and others. We will describe the most popular techniques employed today.

The technique of tympanoplasty may be utilized for tympanic membrane perforations, adhesive otitis media, chronic suppurative otitis media, tympanosclerosis (with possible middle ear fixation), retraction pockets, cholesteatoma, or conductive hearing loss. These conditions are examples of irreversible middle ear disease, where the middle ear does not return to a normal state after appropriate medical treatment. Mastoid surgery may be helpful to either remove the disease or to provide exposure through a posterior tympanotomy approach. Often times, there will be some degree of ossicular discontinuity as a result of the disease process, and ossiculoplasty will be necessary to reconstruct the hearing apparatus. This may be performed concurrent with tympanoplasty or may be undertaken in a staged fashion.

EVALUATION

As with all of medicine, a thorough history and holistic approach to the medical condition helps to define the extent of the disease process and the best treatment options for the patient. It is important to understand the time course of the current ear-related medical condition and the status of the opposite ear. The function of the Eustachian tube is an important determinant of success; this may be influenced by palatal disease, obesity, sleep apnea, smoking, allergy or gastric reflux. These factors should be addressed preoperatively if possible. Chronic sinus disease or immunoglobulin deficiency may cause a chronic infectious and/or inflammatory condition. When possible these conditions are medically treated. A history of prior otologic surgery, general health, pain, and vestibular symptoms should also be noted.

A careful evaluation of the diseased ear is paramount for treatment planning. Microscopic evaluation is necessary with mechanical debridement; medical treatment and debridement may be necessary several times in the office before final treatment recommendations may be made, as discussed below.

Otomicroscopic examination will reveal the size and location of a tympanic membrane perforation or retraction, the presence of middle ear polyps, granulation tissue, cholesteatoma, tumors, masses, atelectasis, tympanosclerosis, or erosion of the ossicular chain. Perforations are divided into central or marginal. Central perforations maintain a margin of tympanic membrane remnant around the circumference of the perforation (Fig. 12.1). Typically, these perforations only intermittently drain and are not associated with cholesteatoma. Marginal perforations involve the periphery of the tympanic membrane (Fig. 12.2). These may involve mucosal integration into the perforation or squamous epithelial ingrowth that can lead to

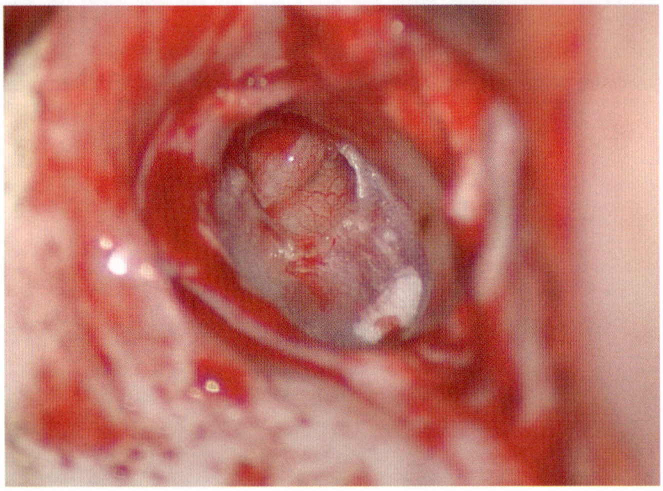

Fig. 12.1: Central perforation in a right ear.

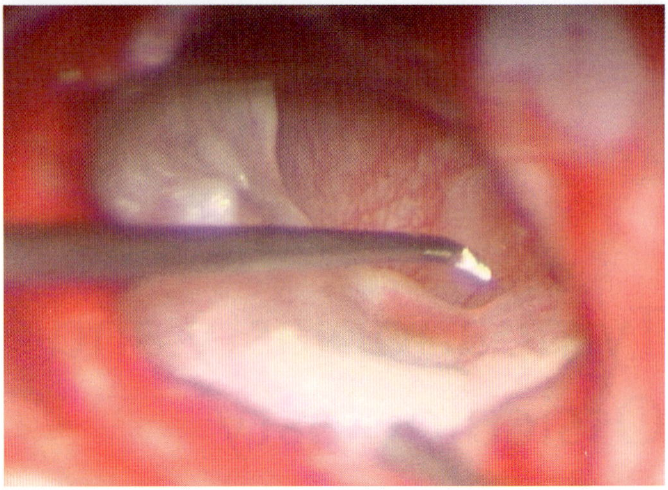

Fig. 12.2: Anterior marginal perforation in a right ear.

cholesteatoma. One may also assess the size of the middle ear cleft with relative distance of the tympanic membrane to the promontory or degree of retraction of the ossicular chain. All of this information helps to determine the success of an operation.

The location of the tympanic membrane perforation is an important technical factor. Because the anterior canal bulge often limits visualization of the anterior sulcus, anterior perforations usually demand a postauricular approach. Anterior perforations also often lack a sufficient rim of healthy epithelium, and so a means must be found to suspend the graft to coapt it to the remaining healthy mucosa. This might require packing the Eustachian tube with gelfoam, using stiffer material such as cartilage in a cantilever fashion, or everting the anterior canal skin to create a larger surface on which to graft.

The size of the perforation is a predictive factor, as very large perforations are more difficult to repair than small perforations. Large perforations imply a chronically diseased ear with a poor capacity for spontaneous healing. These cases in particular demand that the ear be dry and the middle ear mucosa be healthy before the surgery, and that granulation tissue, scar, and tympanosclerosis be excised during the operation. Small perforations are technically easier to close. Perforations <10% of the drum area can often be closed with a simple fat myringoplasty in the office setting. The use of Merogel has recently been advocated in these cases.

All patients should receive preoperative audiologic evaluation with air and bone pure tone thresholds and speech discrimination scores. This information helps the surgeon predict the status of the ossicular chain and the potential for hearing improvement. The presence of sensorineural loss may indicate potential inner ear involvement of chronic otitis media or cholesteatoma such as labyrinthine or cochlear fistulae. Preoperative audiometry is also important for medicolegal documentation. Audiometric results should be confirmed with tuning fork tests by the surgeon. Eustachian tube function testing has not proved beneficial in determining the true condition of the Eustachian tube or predicting the success of an operation.

In patients who present with active otorrhea (the "wet ear"), measures should be taken to dry the ear before undertaking surgery. (We acknowledge that there are published reports stating that active otorrhea does not alter outcome, however, this is not common experience and at the very least surgery is technically easier in a dry, noninflamed field). When a patient first presents with a draining ear, the ear should be suctioned thoroughly, and the patient should be started on antibiotic-containing eardrops such ofloxacin or ciprofloxacin. Steroids may help relieve inflammation as well. These are broad-spectrum antibiotics and generally cover the common organisms that lead to drainage, including gram-negative rods and staph. The patient should be seen periodically in follow-up and the ear suctioned until it is dry. Stagnant pus may prevent the medication from reaching the middle ear mucosa, where it needs to exert its effect.

In cases of chronic, refractory otorrhea, a gram stain and culture may be helpful. Fungal organisms may overgrow an ear that has received long-term antibiotics, and antifungal therapy may be needed. Lotrisone lotion may be used once a day for a week then re-examination and otomicroscopic office cleaning be performed to check on the progress of the infection. Clotrimazole cream (applied b.i.d. to the ear canal with cotton stick applicator) is effective, as are 2% acetic acid rinses (which may be painful in a perforated ear). Cresylate should be avoided in the presence of a perforation because it can be caustic to the middle ear mucosa. Use of combination powders such as CSTF (chloromycetin, sulfa, tinactin, and Fungizone) are quite effective for fungal and bacterial mixed infections. Methicillin-resistant staph aureus (MRSA) has become increasingly prevalent, and this organism may colonize even a dry ear. Systemic therapy is not routinely necessary, as the local concentration of topically administered antibiotics is very high and may overcome in vitro resistance. Aminoglycoside-containing drops are often effective when quinolones fail, although there is a theoretical risk of inner ear toxicity despite years of safe use in inflamed ears.

In an ear that contains cholesteatoma, efforts at drying the ear may fail because the infection may be deep seated. In these cases, surgery may be the only effective intervention.

Age is an important factor in selecting tympanoplasty surgery in children. Younger children with chronic suppurative otitis media or post-tympanostomy perforations have a higher rate of surgical failure than older children or adults after tympanoplasty surgery. Their tendency to have recurrent otitis media places them at risk for reperforation, even after initially successful result. The maturation of Eustachian tube function is most certainly an underlying factor. There is no strictly defined cut-off, but delaying surgery until age 6–8 years old is reasonable. The status of the opposite ear is important; freedom from acute otitis or serous otitis for at least 1 year is a good predictor of success.

Smoking compromises the results of most surgical procedures, and in tympanoplasty, where a patent microcirculation is essential for healing, smoking cessation should be encouraged preoperatively.

NORMAL ANATOMY AND THE HEALING PROCESS

The normal tympanic membrane has an external layer of stratified squamous epithelium, a medial surface lined with flat respiratory epithelium, and two fibrous layers—one radial and one longitudinal—attached to the fibrous annulus between the two epithelial layers. Vascular elements are located within the fibrous layer. When a tympanic membrane spontaneously heals without grafting, the perforation is often closed by the squamous epithelium before fibrous elements develop. There may be an absence of the fibrous layers resulting in lack of the tensile strength, elasticity, blood supply, and resistance to future perforations. Such areas are referred to as monomeric or dimeric and are composed of either the squamous layer alone or the squamous layer juxtaposed with the mucous membrane layer.

The healing process after grafting appears to be initiated by angiogenesis within the tympanic membrane remnant, especially at the margin of the perforation. During healing, the graft material acts as a scaffold for epithelialization. The freshened edges at the margins of a perforation are the source of migrating epithelium. Fascia is composed of fibroblasts in a collagen matrix. Its low metabolic rate and its extracellular matrix permit it to persist until it becomes vascularized.

Many donor materials have been used for grafting the tympanic membrane since the 1950s. Today the most widely used is true fascia from the temporalis muscle, though other tissues utilized include areolar tissue, perichondrium and perichondrium with cartilage, fat tissue, periosteal tissue, allograft tympanic membranes, and prepared collagen materials from cadaveric specimens. Historically, full and partial thickness skin grafts and vein grafts were used, but did not have the same degree of success.

OSSICULOPLASTY

Ossicular chain reconstruction (OCR) should only be undertaken in the absence of middle ear disease such as infection, granulation and scar tissue, retraction of the tympanic membrane and/or cholesteatoma. OCR may be performed at the time of tympanoplasty with or without mastoidectomy, or may be delayed to a second stage operation to allow for the creation of a healthy middle ear environment.

Wullstein's original classification scheme breaks tympanoplasty into five subtypes.[2] Type I tympanoplasty (myringoplasty) involves reconstruction of a tympanic membrane defect with a completely intact ossicular chain. Type II tympanoplasty is performed when there is some degree of ossicular discontinuity (most commonly erosion of the incus), and involves reconstruction of an eardrum in the setting of a reconstructed ossicular chain. Type III

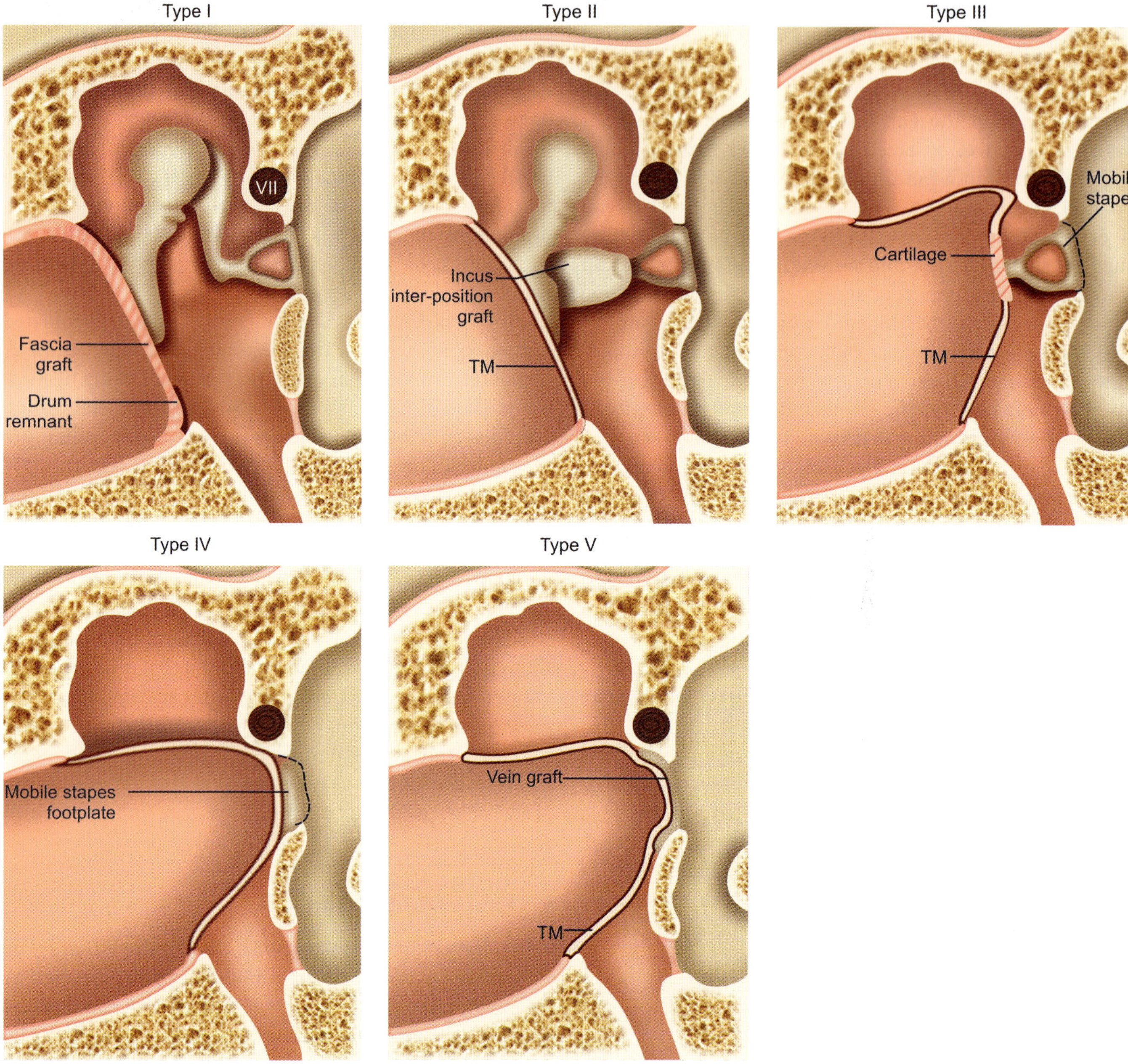

Fig. 12.3: Type I–V tympanoplasty.

tympanoplasty (myringostapediopexy) grafts the eardrum directly to a mobile stapes superstructure, and type IV tympanoplasty (cavum minor) involves grafting the tympanic membrane directly to a mobile stapes footplate and shielding the round window niche from external sound. Finally, the type V tympanoplasty involves removal of a fixed stapes footplate/superstructure and replacement with a fat or vein graft combined with obstruction of the round window niche (Fig. 12.3).[3]

Acoustic Mechanics

The normal human middle ear couples sound energy from the lower impedance of air in the ear canal through the tympanic membrane and ossicles to the relatively high impedance of fluid within the cochlea. The tympanic membrane also isolates the oval window from the round window, preventing phase cancellation of incoming sound. The middle ear mechanism (tympanic membrane and ossicular chain) acts as an impedance-matching transformer to maximize energy transfer from the vibrations of air (sound) in the external auditory canal to the fluids of the inner ear. The acoustic transformation theory states that this occurs by three lever systems: the tympanic membrane lever, the ossicular lever, and the hydraulic lever.[4] As a result of these three lever systems, the acoustic transformer theory predicts a middle ear gain of approximately 27–34 dB.[5] Implied in this transformer theory is the expectation that this gain is independent of frequency. Further investigations indicate that the acoustic transformer theory should be modified and that middle ear sound transmission is actually frequency dependent because of ossicular coupling, acoustic coupling, and stapes-cochlear input impedance.[6]

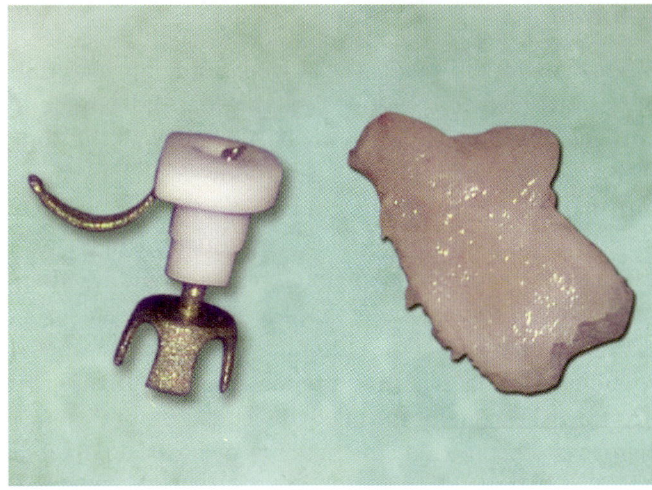

Fig. 12.4: Titanium-hydroxyapatite prosthesis and incus autograft.

Tympanic Membrane Lever Effect

The anatomy of the tympanic membrane and the bony and fibrous tympanic annulus provide a mechanical advantage. Sound energy is directed toward the center of the tympanic membrane so that the manubrium receives the greatest amount of energy. This amplifies the energy and provides a twofold gain in sound pressure at the malleus.[3]

Ossicular Lever Effect

The anatomy of the ossicles affords another mechanical advantage. The malleus and incus work as a unit, but the manubrium of the malleus is 1.3 times longer than the long process of the incus and thus there is a 1.3 to 1 sound energy increase.[7]

Hydraulic Lever Effect

The ratio between the surface area of the tympanic membrane and the area of the stapes footplate allows for an increase in sound pressure proportional to the ratio of the areas. This average ratio gain is calculated to be 20.8 to 1.[8]

Ossicular Coupling and Acoustic Coupling

Ossicular coupling refers to the sound pressure gain that occurs through the actions of the tympanic membrane and the ossicular chain. This gain is frequency dependent. The mean middle ear gain is approximately 20 dB at 250 and 500 Hz, reaching a maximum of about 25 dB around 1 kHz and then decreasing about 6 dB per octave at frequencies above 1 kHz.[9]

The tympanic membrane moves differently depending on the frequency of the vibration presented. The entire tympanic membrane moves in one phase when exposed to low frequency sound energy. At higher frequencies, the tympanic membrane divides into smaller vibrating portions that vibrate in different phases. There is also slippage of the ossicular chain at the higher frequencies above 1–2 kHz. In addition, some energy is lost because of the forces needed to overcome the stiffness and mass of the tympanic membrane and ossicular chain.[5]

Movement of the tympanic membrane produces sound pressure in the middle ear that is transmitted to the oval and round windows. Acoustic coupling is due to the difference in sound pressures acting on these areas. The pressure at each window is different because of the small distance between windows and the varying orientation of each window relative to the tympanic membrane. In normal ears, the difference in pressures between the oval and round windows (acoustic coupling) is negligible. With the reconstructed ear, the difference may become significant and may affect hearing.

History of Prosthesis Development in OCR

OCR has evolved with technological advances over the past 60 years. Many materials have been used for ossicular substitution or reconstruction (Fig. 12.4). The ideal prosthesis should be made of material that is biocompatible, maintains its shape, has the correct rigidity for acoustic properties and is cost-effective.

Autografts

The first materials used in OCR were autograft materials such as ossicles, bone, and cartilage. Mastoid bone and cartilage have been shown to be unstable in the long term, as they lose rigidity and resorption occurs.[10–13] Incus and malleus grafts demonstrated no evidence of bone erosion and little resorption and therefore have been ideal middle ear reconstruction materials until today. There are instances where the ossicles are too diseased to be utilized in reconstruction, either from chronic otitis media or cholesteatoma, or the remaining length of the ossicles is not long enough for the needed reconstruction. Though there is no cost in using the patient's own ossicle, there is a cost for shaping the material with the drill bits necessary for sculpting the ossicles.

Homografts

For years, homografts were used in ears lacking a suitable autograft. These implants may have been harvested incus or malleus bones treated with irradiation or alcohol solutions then sold to the institution from various bone banks, or these ossicles were preshaped into struts of various lengths for reconstructive needs. Since 1986, homograft materials have been rarely used because of the risk of disease transmission (e.g. HIV and Creutzfeldt-Jakob disease).[14]

Alloplasts

Because of the disadvantages of autograft and homograft implants, synthetic materials or alloplasts have become popular. The history of synthetic implants is referenced in other articles and will not be covered here.[15-17] Alloplastic materials that have been used include polyethylene tubing, Teflon, Silastic tubing, stainless steel, titanium, gold, high-density polyethylene sponge (HDPS), bioglasses, and bioceramics. These materials have been fashioned into either total or partial replacement prostheses. The partial design will fit from an intact stapes superstructure to the tympanic membrane or malleus. Total reconstructive prostheses fit from the footplate of the stapes to the undersurface of the tympanic membrane or the malleus.

Prosthesis Design

There have been a number of advances in prosthetic design including improved biocompatibility to decrease extrusion, greater ease of use at the time of surgery, lighter weight while maintaining rigid design, the provision of an acoustically reliable mechanism for the efficient transfer of sound, and a more firm attachment of the prosthesis to the available middle ear structures. The ideal prosthesis should have the appropriate weight, provide an acoustically reliable mechanism for the transfer of sound while allowing the incorporation of existing ossicles, and be stable in the middle ear environment. The differences we noted in frequency-specific hearing improvement demonstrate that the mass of the prosthesis does not play a significant role in outcome.[18] Factors other than the prosthesis design – namely, surgical technique, middle ear fibrosis, tympanic membrane retraction, and cholesteatoma – are often more important in determining hearing results after ossiculoplasty.

Prosthesis Weight

A lightweight and rigid prosthesis minimizes sound impedance while maximizing sound energy transfer.

Prosthesis Extrusion

Prosthesis extrusion is more likely related to the status of the middle ear than to the prosthesis material. Extrusion may result from recurrent middle ear disease with retraction of the tympanic membrane from Eustachian tube dysfunction or adhesive middle ear disease with scar tissue formation. Some prostheses such as the older HDPS implants are designed to be covered by cartilage, as they will erode through the tympanic membrane. Newer hydroxyapatite prosthesis have a more rounded and smooth head design that is biocompatible with the mucosal layer of the tympanic membrane, though some surgeons still elect to cover this with cartilage.

Prosthesis Mechanics

A prosthesis should have its center of mass perpendicular to its intended line of movement. The center should be directly over the footplate of the stapes to provide a maximal resultant force vector in the intended direction of sound transmission. Sometimes the angulation of the stapes superstructure makes the reconstruction difficult; in these instances, even with an intact superstructure, the best results may be obtained using a total prosthesis from the footplate to the malleus or tympanic membrane. Flexibility of the head attachment may be important in some middle ear situations in order to adjust the head of the prosthesis to fit to the malleus or the undersurface of

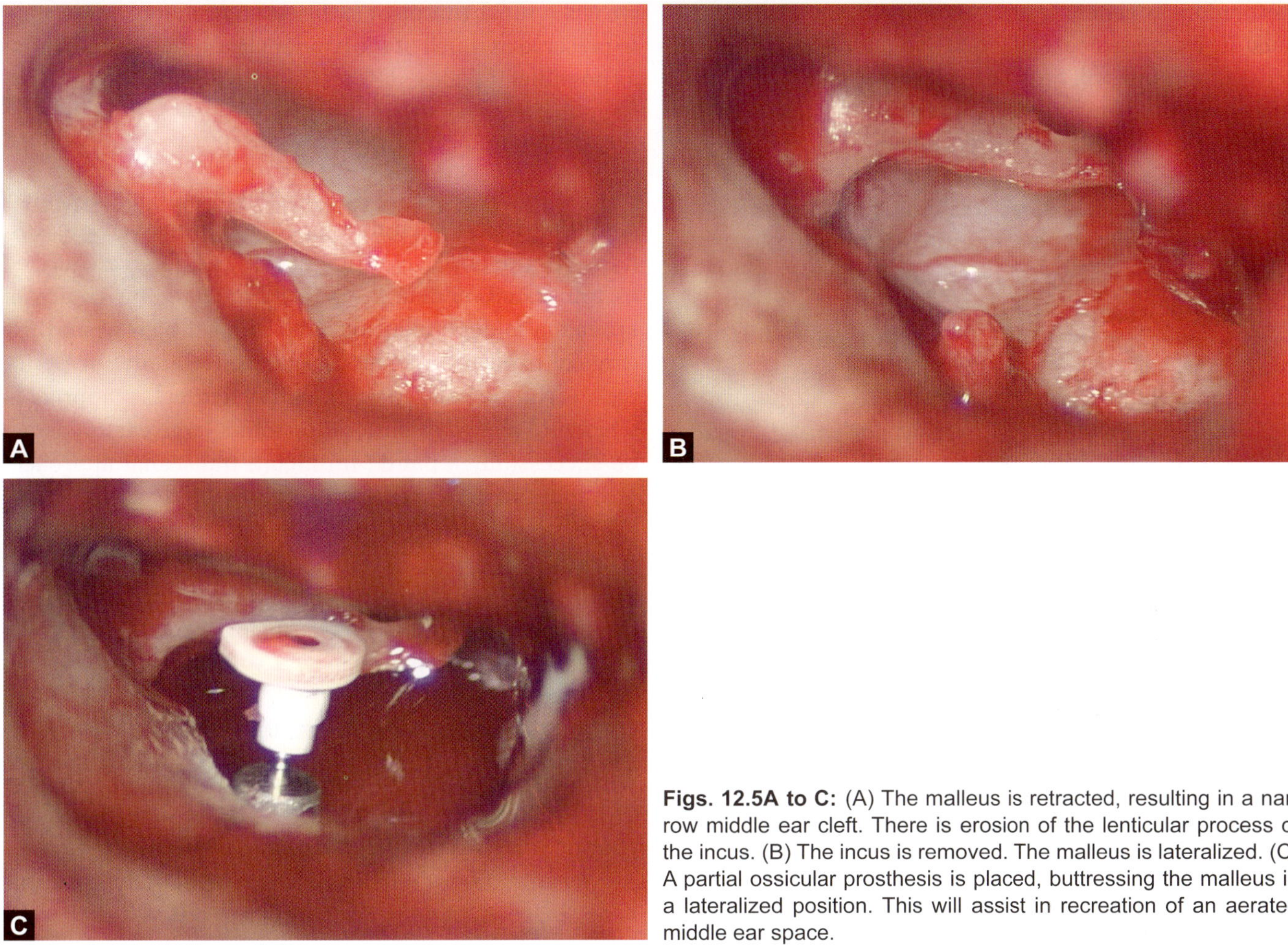

Figs. 12.5A to C: (A) The malleus is retracted, resulting in a narrow middle ear cleft. There is erosion of the lenticular process of the incus. (B) The incus is removed. The malleus is lateralized. (C) A partial ossicular prosthesis is placed, buttressing the malleus in a lateralized position. This will assist in recreation of an aerated middle ear space.

a conical or angled tympanic membrane. Several studies have demonstrated that maintaining a malleus (when possible) results in reduced extrusion rates and improved postoperative air-bone gap closure.[19-21] The importance of incorporating the capitulum in reconstruction is less clear.[22] In cases of a retracted or narrow middle ear cleft, a prosthesis may be used to help recreate an aerated middle ear space (Figs. 12.5A to C).

Prosthesis Slippage

Prosthesis slippage is always a concern because it may compromise a good result. Slippage may occur at the point of attachment to the malleus, the stapes superstructure, or the stapes footplate. Therefore, if the malleus is present, it is beneficial to engage the prosthesis firmly under the malleus neck, using either a groove in the head of the hydroxyapatite prosthesis or a titanium hook to reach under the malleus. At the attachment to the capitulum of the stapes, a claw or bell over the structure helps to keep the prosthesis from slipping. There are times when the stapes superstructure is fragile, or is angled inferiorly toward the promontory, and the best reconstruction would be to reconstruct the hearing mechanism with a total prosthesis from the malleus or tympanic membrane directly to the footplate. If there is no superstructure of the stapes present, then the prosthesis should fit comfortably onto the footplate and slippage can be minimized if necessary with a footplate shoe or wider base of the implant.

SURGICAL TECHNIQUE: TYMPANOPLASTY

Myringoplasty

Myringoplasty is a technique confined to the tympanic membrane without middle ear surgery and may be performed through the ear canal. Surgical repair of acute perforations is generally not necessary. These perforations must be examined carefully under a microscope because occasionally one will find under-turned epithelium. If this is the case, then microscopic eversion of the under-turned epithelium is performed in the office. At times, a paper patch will be beneficial in this situation to aid in the repair. The patch is applied after freshening the edges of the tympanic membrane perforation with a fine right-angled hook, needle or silver nitrate. Various materials have been used as a patch, with the most common being cigarette paper or rice paper that has been cut to 3 mm circular size. The patch is placed dry or with minimal saline. The patient is then examined in 2–3 weeks and the patch removed to check for healing. One may repeat this again if epithelial migration has begun, but has not completely healed the perforation.

In the case of a small nonhealing perforation, it may be necessary to take the patient to surgery, where a graft myringoplasty may be done through the ear canal by freshening the margins of the perforation then placing a fat, fascia, or alloderm graft through the perforation in a dumbbell fashion.

Tympanoplasty

The goal of successful tympanoplasty is to create an intact, mobile tympanic membrane with an aerated mucosa-lined middle ear space, and a continuous sound conduction mechanism between the mobile membrane and the inner ear fluids.

Tympanoplasty may be performed utilizing the underlay, overlay, and the over-under techniques. The most common graft material is fascia, but perichondrium, perichondrium with cartilage, periosteum, and areolar tissue have all been described. The benefits of each technique will be discussed.

Tympanosclerotic plaques are patches of hyalinized (calcified) scar that replace portions of the fibrous layers of the tympanic membrane following periods of inflammation from chronic otitis media. There are varying degrees of this process. If the process is minimal and is not obstructing the middle ear cleft, then we choose to keep this in place as it adds some structure and rigidity to the reconstruction. The underside of the tympanosclerosis is scored with a right-angled hook to stimulate some bleeding that seems to help the repair; the graft is placed medial to the tympanosclerotic plaque. For patients in whom the tympanosclerosis is very thick (frequently along the anterior and superior margin of the tympanic membrane), we will remove this prior to the reconstruction, attempting to preserve as much of the tympanic membrane epithelium as possible.

Evolution of Techniques

A review of the literature reveals that many tympanoplasty techniques have been developed and employed successfully. Tympanoplasty approaches can be categorized as transcanal, endaural, or postauricular. The choice of approach is dependent on the size of the canal and the surgical exposure—a small canal and an anterior perforation will usually require a postauricular approach, whereas a posterior perforation and a large ear canal can be successfully repaired through a transcanal approach. The graft can be placed under or over the tympanic membrane remnant and annulus, as well as under or over the malleus. We will describe the various techniques and approaches commonly used in the past, and a personal evolution of technique for the majority of cases utilizing the over-under tympanoplasty.[1]

Underlay (Undersurface) Technique

The underlay or undersurface technique employs the use of grafting material medial to or under the remnant of tympanic membrane, typically under the malleus when the perforation extends to that area.[1] Most of the time this is approached from a postauricular incision. Temporalis fascia is harvested free from underlying muscle and overlying areolar tissue (1.5 cm by 2.0 cm size) early in the procedure and placed on a cutting block to dry. In the case of cholesteatoma or retraction pocket where the surgeon desires to use perichondrium or cartilage, the graft is harvested from a posterior tragal incision, or from the cymba concha through the postauricular wound. Vascular strip incisions are then made from behind at the tympanomastoid and tympanosquamous suture lines down to about 4–5 mm from the annulus (Figs. 12.6A to D). The free edges of the perforation are prepared using a right-angled hook, and in some instances a fine scissor is used to resect the perforation margins.[1] The intent is to separate the outer cutaneous layer from any under-turned epithelium or to separate the inner mucosal layer from the external tympanic membrane epithelium. This develops a fresh edge for healing. Then a tympanomeatal flap is raised to enter the middle ear space. We use 8 mm discs of absorbable material (Gelfoam) that have been soaked in saline then dried to pack the Eustachian tube and middle

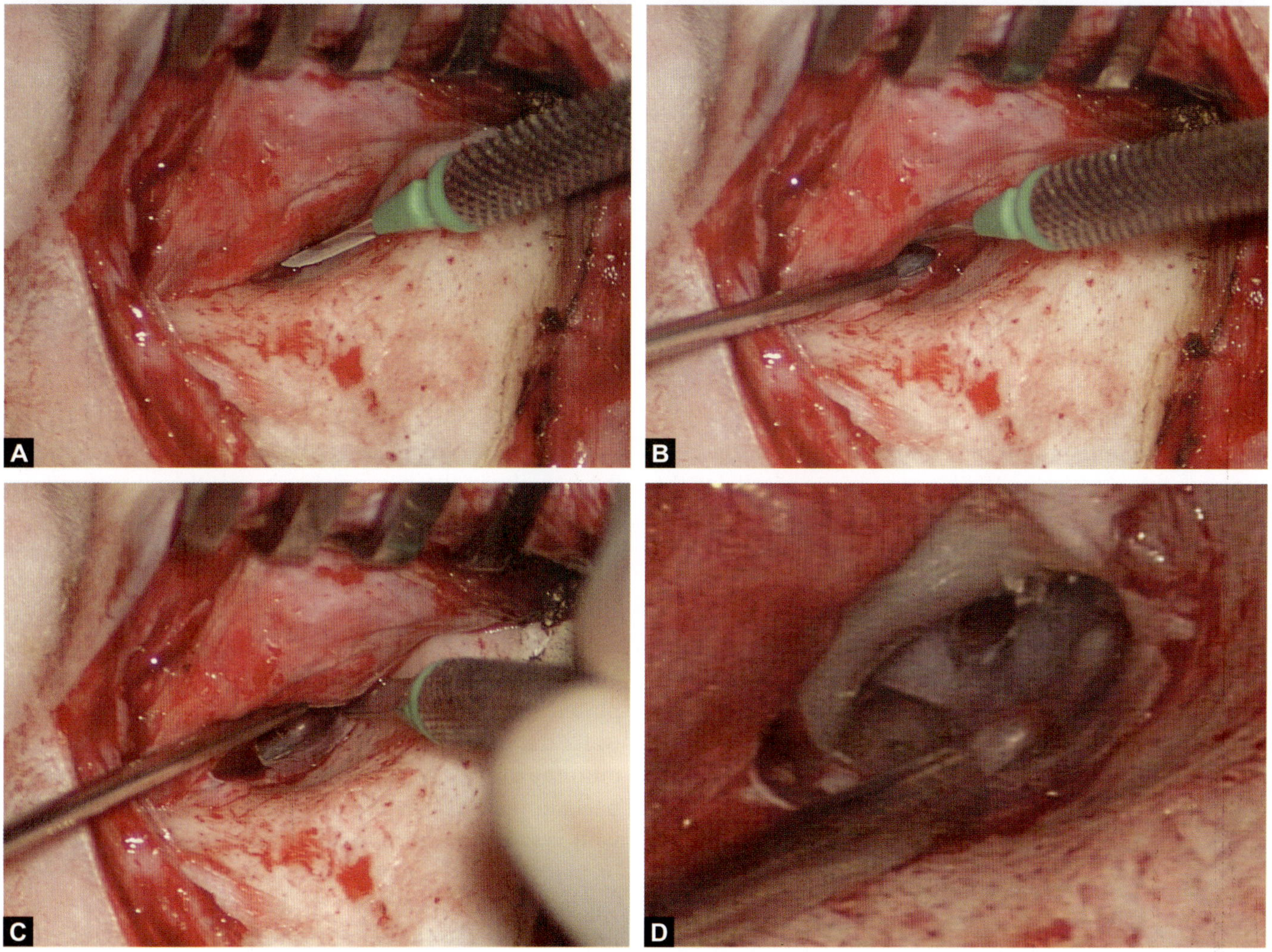

Figs. 12.6A to D: (A) The posterior canal skin is elevated but kept tethered to the tympanomastoid and tympanosquamous suture lines. (B) The canal skin is incised and the distance from the tympanic membrane is visualized. Adjustments can be made to assure that the medial extent of the canal incisions is 4–5 mm from the annulus. (C) The vascular strip incisions are then made from behind along the tympanomastoid and tympanosquamous suture lines and connected about 4–5 mm from the annulus. (D) The vascular strip is reflected anteriorly, providing exposure to the tympanic membrane and middle ear space.

ear cleft. The fascia graft is trimmed to the proper size, then placed under the remnant of tympanic membrane and usually the malleus. The tympanomeatal flap is replaced into its normal position. Often the tympanomeatal skin can be advanced and rotated to cover much of the area of the perforation. Saline soaked Gelfoam packing is placed lateral to the tympanic membrane-graft interface. The postauricular incision is sutured into place and the vascular strip tissue is placed back into its anatomic position, making sure to evert the skin into the ear canal. This is held into place with an absorbable sponge or polyethylene sponge soaked with an antibiotic suspension. The patient is instructed to use the antibiotic suspension 2–3 times per day to keep the packing moist. The lateral ear canal is cleaned about 5–7 days postoperatively, leaving some tympanic membrane absorbable sponge in place for another week or two. The integrity of the graft is then checked and all of the external packing material removed at that time.

Overlay Technique

The overlay technique was practiced in the 1960s and is occasionally used today, depending on the training of the surgeon, the location of the perforation, and the extent of anterior canal wall overhang that may obscure adequate view of the tympanic membrane. The exposure is generally from a postauricular incision and the temporalis fascia is harvested using the same technique as with all tympanoplasty surgeries.

Removal of canal skin and de-epithelialization of the tympanic membrane remnant: The skin and periosteum are dissected from the bony canal in a lateral to medial direction along a broad front until the fibrous annulus is reached. Removal of the canal skin medial to the anterior canal bulge may require blind dissection because this bulge often obscures vision of the anterior meatal recess. Once the skin is elevated to the level of the annulus, a plane is developed between the skin of the canal with the tympanic membrane remnant and the annulus and fibrous layer of the tympanic membrane. Working in a plane parallel to the annulus, the skin of the canal and tympanic membrane remnant are removed. Beginning superiorly and anteriorly, the skin of the canal and tympanic membrane remnant can often be removed in continuity by using a fine alligator forceps. It is important that all remaining squamous epithelial components be completely removed from the drum remnant.

Drilling of ear canal: Drilling of the bony canal is routine in all lateral graft procedures, as it enlarges the field of surgery and allows satisfactory graft placement. Drilling begins laterally and posteriorly with removal of the spine of Henle and tympanosquamous suture line. The posterior wall of the temporal mandibular joint represents the anterior wall of the bony canal. It is most prominent in the midportion of the bony canal in both the superior to inferior and medial to lateral planes. It is important not to violate the joint when drilling the bony canal wall anteriorly, and also not to violate the air cells posteriorly. Final medial dissection just lateral to the annulus completely exposes the anterior sulcus and converts the acute anterior meatal angle into an obtuse angle. This is critical to prevent postoperative blunting.

Grafting with fascia and replacement of the canal skin: Once the middle ear and Eustachian tube have been filled with Gelfoam, dried fascia is cut into an oval shape with a superior slit. The graft is placed under the manubrium with the slit edges overlapping around the manubrium to secure the graft. The remainder of the graft is spread onto the anterior canal wall and the lateral wall of the epitympanum. The fascia is gently hydrated with saline.

The canal skin is trimmed of any irregular edges and replaced over the bony canal. Medially, the skin is positioned to overlap the fascia graft by 1–2 mm, which helps promote epithelialization of the drum and prevent anterior blunting. The canal is then packed with Gelfoam. Retractors are removed and the vascular strip skin replaced into anatomic position.

With this technique, marked bony and soft tissue dissection is necessary. Blunting of the anterior canal wall and tympanic membrane is possible, with the formation of cholesteatoma pearls and conductive hearing loss. In the hands of surgeons experienced with this technique, these complications become minimal.

Over-Under Tympanoplasty Technique

Indications for over-under tympanoplasty: By combining the benefits of the two previously mentioned techniques, the over-under tympanoplasty has become the preferred technique in tympanoplasty surgery. This technique places the fascia graft lateral to the malleus but medial to the fibrous and bony annulus. In the situation of a very medial annulus inferiorly or a lateral promontory, the graft may be placed medial to the anterior annulus and placed onto the lateral surface of the inferior bony canal wall. The remnant of tympanic membrane is then laid onto the graft and held into position with an absorbable packing material. In the case of a marginal perforation, with no remnant of tympanic membrane, the graft may be placed onto the medial bony canal wall and the medial ear canal skin (with freshened margins) is elevated and placed onto the lateral surface of the fascia graft. This allows excellent exposure to the anterior middle ear space and prevents medialization of the graft to the promontory. Ossicular reconstruction may be performed directly to the undersurface of the malleus if present. Over-under tympanoplasty has become a preferred technique for perforations that abut the malleus, large or near total perforations, cases of significant malleus retraction (making the classic underlay technique impractical), significant anterior tympanosclerosis, or anterior middle ear cholesteatoma (Figs. 12.7A and B).[1]

This technique is rarely described but commonly used by many otologic surgeons. Austin in 1972 stated that the graft may be secured either over or under the malleus tip, depending on the ease of positioning the graft, and then some of the skin covering the malleus is dissected and replaced on the graft surface. Glasscock, Wehrs, and Hough also made similar inferences when describing underlay grafting in particular situations, usually with significant retraction of the malleus, large perforations,

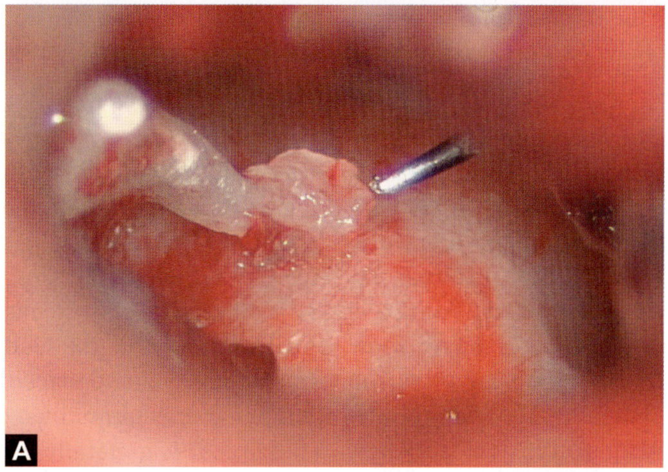

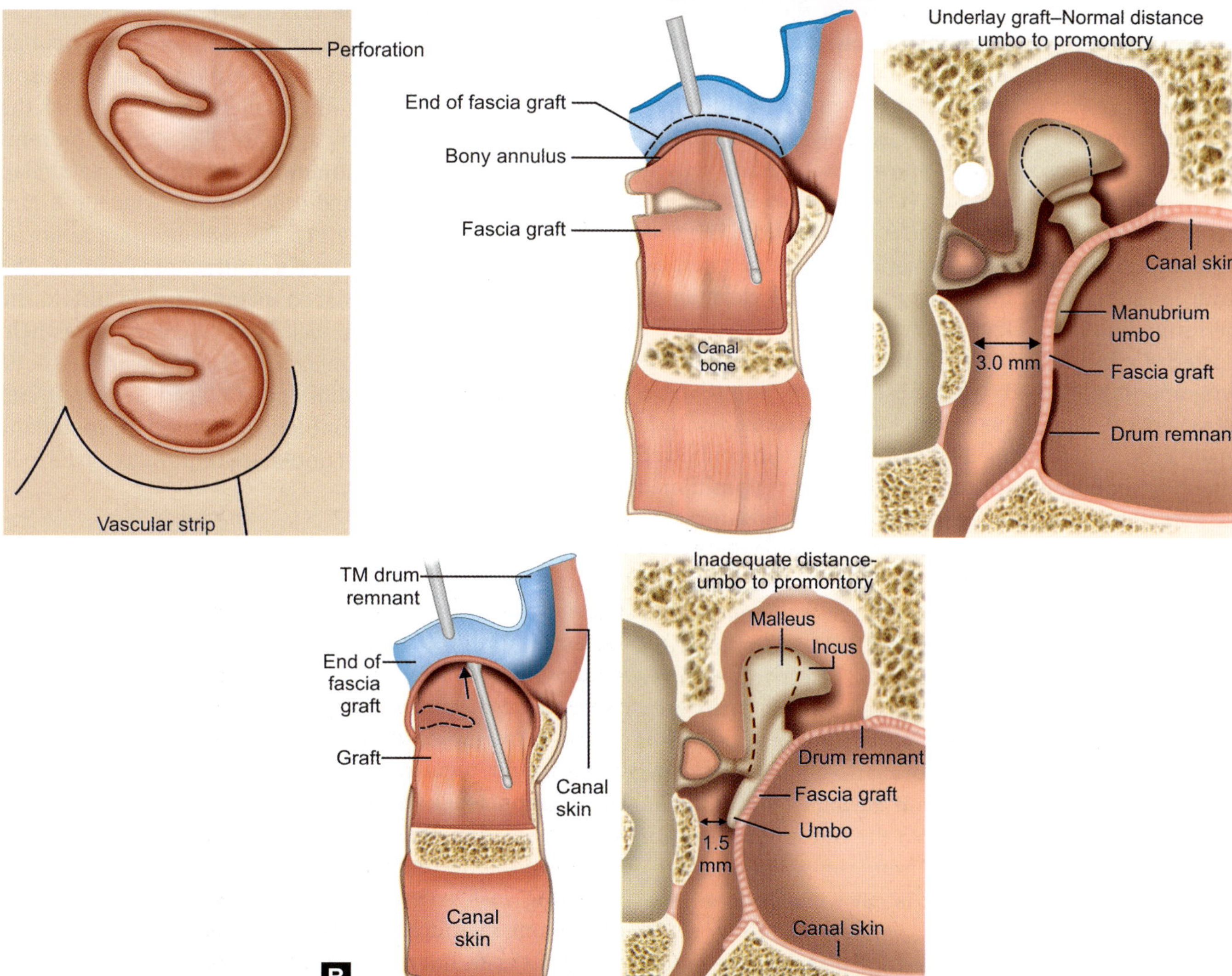

Figs. 12.7A and B: (A) Intraoperative view of a retracted middle ear space in a right ear. Note that the malleus is adherent to the promontory, creating a narrow middle ear cleft. This configuration is an indication for an over-under tympanoplasty. (B) In cases of significant malleus retraction the underlay technique does not allow for proper placement of the fascia graft. This problem is overcome by using the over-under technique.

or anterior middle ear disease. The refined technique and results have been described in book chapters and articles by Bojrab, Kartush, and others.[1]

Surgical technique of the over-under tympanoplasty: Patients undergo the usual preparation and positioning for ear surgery. The ear is injected with lidocaine-HCL 1% with 1:100,000 epinephrine in a subdermal plane along the postauricular incision site. Afour-quadrant external ear canal injection is also performed. The ear speculum is placed into the ear canal and then pulled back to show the bony cartilaginous junction site where the lidocaine solution is slowly injected, blanching the skin of the posterior canal wall (vascular strip skin). A postauricular incision is made and carried down to the layer of the temporalis fascia. This avascular plane is followed to the posterior ear canal soft tissue and then carried to the mastoid tip. A retractor is placed and a fascia graft is harvested and set on a cutting block. The graft is cleaned under the microscope to remove any medial muscle tissue or lateral areolar tissue (Figs. 12.8A to E). Using a bovie electrocautery, a T incision is made from the root of the zygoma along the linea temporalis, with a vertical limb incision to the mastoid tip. Periosteal elevation is performed with an elevator to the Spine of Henle. The posterior canal skin is elevated but kept tethered to the tympanomastoid and tympanosquamous suture lines as described above. The vascular strip incisions are then made from behind along these suture lines and connected about 4–5 mm from the annulus. A retractor is positioned to hold the vascular strip skin forward, allowing good visualization of the tympanic membrane and pathology of the ear.

The margins of the perforation are freshened with a right-angled hook (Figs. 12.9A and B). A tympanomeatal flap is created about 4–5 mm lateral and parallel to the annulus and the middle ear is entered (Fig. 12.10). Next the tympanic membrane is elevated off the malleus (Fig. 12.11). This is done by scoring the periosteum of the malleus with a fine needle and elevating the tympanic membrane off of the malleus to the umbo. At the umbo there is a fibrous extension from the middle layer of the tympanic membrane that is cut with a fine scissors (Figs. 12.12A to E).

The middle ear is inspected for disease and cholesteatoma; granulation tissue and diseased middle ear mucosa are dealt with at this time. Ossicular chain abnormalities are noted and planned reconstruction is considered for treatment. If a mastoidectomy is required to remove disease in the mastoid then an intact canal mastoidectomy with possible facial recess approach is employed.

Grafting technique: The parchment-like fascia graft is trimmed into an appropriate size for the perforation. For a near total perforation, the graft is trimmed into a tongue shape of approximately 10 mm in diameter and 15–20 mm in length. For smaller central perforations, a smaller graft is fashioned. Gelfoam packing is the author's preferred packing material. The Gelfoam is hydrated then pressed into a thin layer and placed onto the cutting block. With an 8 mm ear speculum, pledgets are cut and separated. The middle ear is generally packed with one 8-mm Gelfoam into the Eustachian tube and one 8-mm Gelfoam into the middle ear. Anterior to the malleus, an additional half (8-mm) Gelfoam is placed into the middle ear. The fascia graft is placed lateral to the malleus but medial to the anterior and inferior bony annulus (Fig. 12.13). The remnant of tympanic membrane and tympanomeatal flap skin are replaced and held into position with the 8-mm Gelfoam pledgets (Fig. 12.14). The retractors are removed and the postauricular wound is sutured into position. The vascular strip skin is replaced making sure to unfold the skin onto the bony canal wall. The vascular strip is held into position with Gelfoam packing soaked in an antibiotic suspension. A mastoid dressing is placed overnight and removed the next day. Antibiotic ear drops are used daily to keep the packing moist until pack removal is performed in the office in 1 week.

Cartilage Tympanoplasty

The cartilage graft has been utilized in certain tympanoplasties for over 40 years. Situations that may benefit from the use of cartilage with or without perichondrium are scutal defects, repair of posterior retraction pockets, total tympanoplasties, recurrent retracted middle ear clefts, and recurrent perforations after previous failed tympanoplasties. Although similarly used as fascia for reconstruction, the rigid quality of cartilage tends to resist resorption and retraction. The anticipation of conductive hearing loss when using cartilage to reconstruct the tympanic membrane is of concern, but most reports state that there is not a statistically significant difference in advanced tympanic membrane reconstruction.[1] There are various cartilage grafting techniques utilized; the authors prefer to use a perichondrial-cartilage graft technique. The graft is generally harvested from a posterior tragal

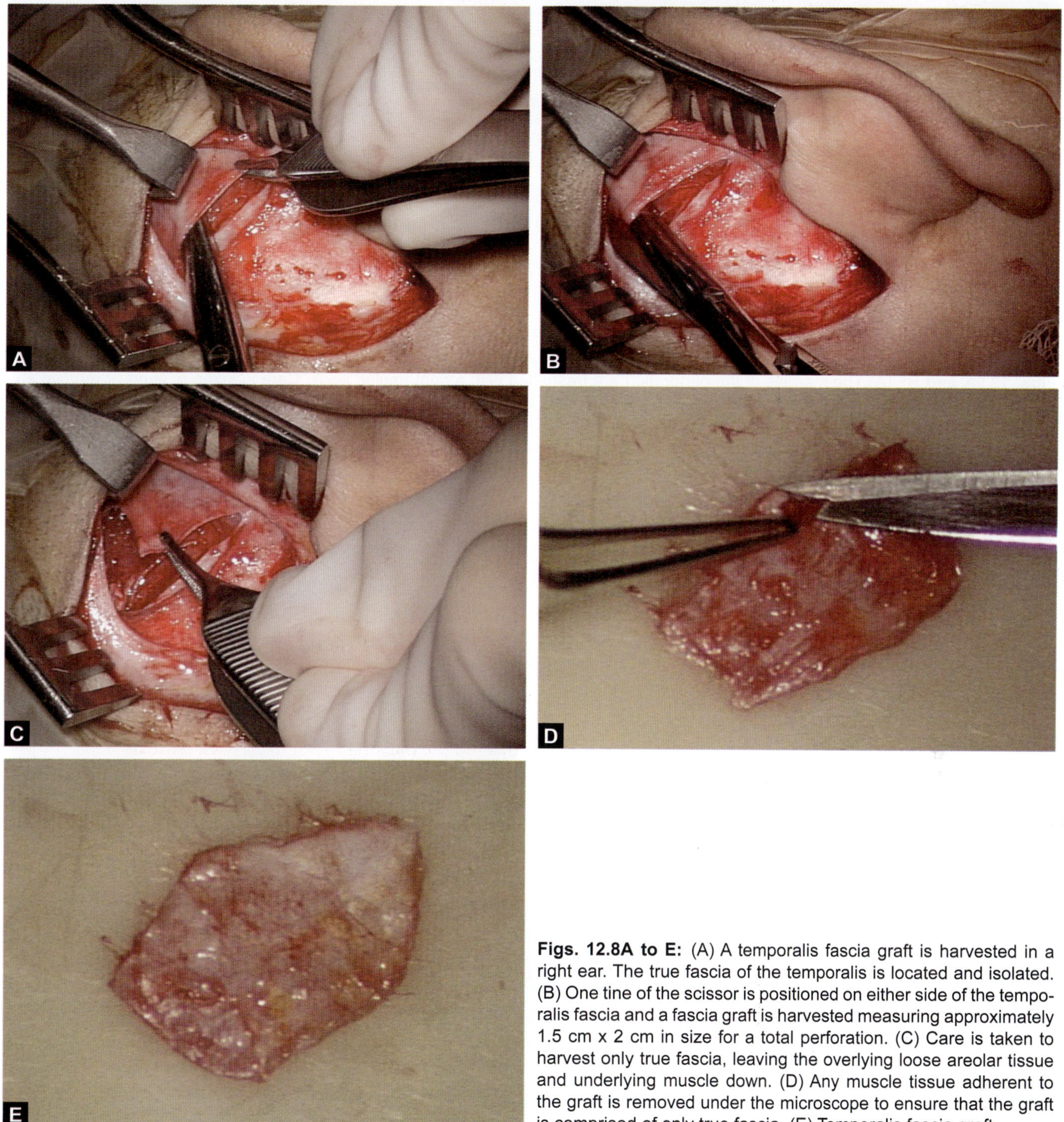

Figs. 12.8A to E: (A) A temporalis fascia graft is harvested in a right ear. The true fascia of the temporalis is located and isolated. (B) One tine of the scissor is positioned on either side of the temporalis fascia and a fascia graft is harvested measuring approximately 1.5 cm x 2 cm in size for a total perforation. (C) Care is taken to harvest only true fascia, leaving the overlying loose areolar tissue and underlying muscle down. (D) Any muscle tissue adherent to the graft is removed under the microscope to ensure that the graft is comprised of only true fascia. (E) Temporalis fascia graft.

incision, keeping perichondrium adherent to the posterior surface of the tragal cartilage and maintaining the lateral dome of the cartilage. The anterior perichondrium is dissected free from the cartilage in situ and left in the tragus site. A suitable graft can also be harvested from the cymba concha, if a postauricular incision is used. The cartilage is trimmed from the perichondrium to the appropriate size for the grafting (Figs. 12.15A to K). The

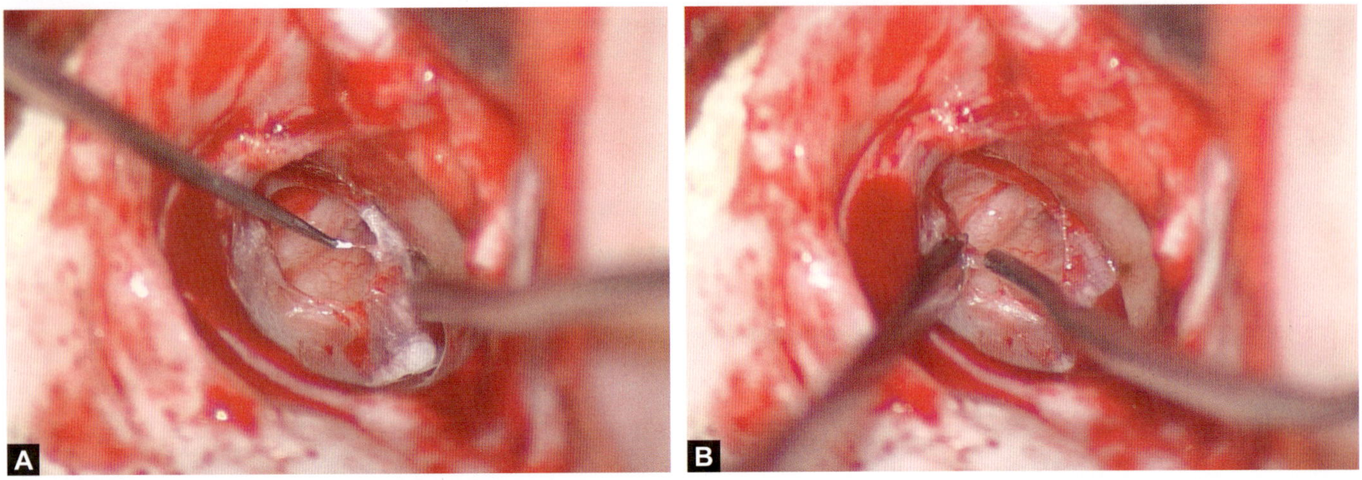

Figs. 12.9A and B: (A) The margins of the perforation are freshened with a right-angled hook. Care is taken to evert or remove any under-turned epithelium. (B) A fine scissor may be used to remove under-turned epithelium.

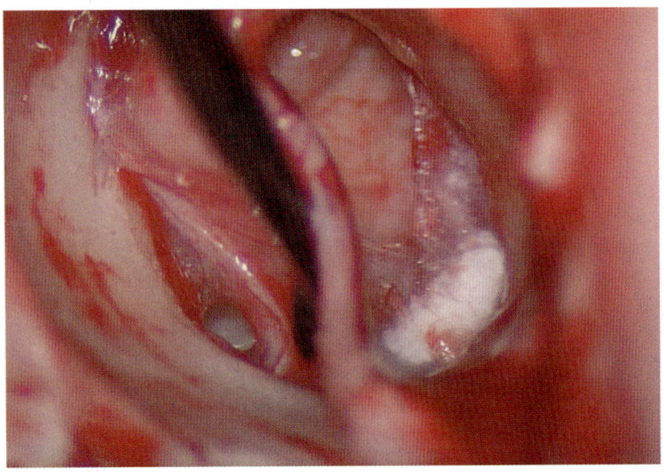

Fig. 12.10: The annulus is lifted with the tympanomeatal flap, and the middle ear is entered.

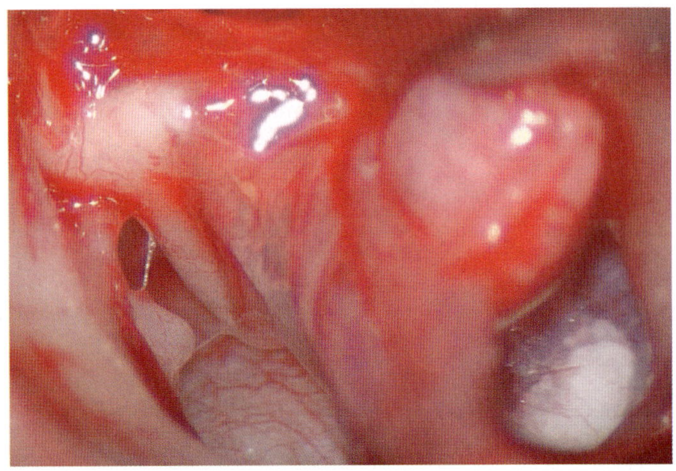

Fig. 12.11: The tympanic membrane remnant is reflected forward to provide a view of the ossicular chain.

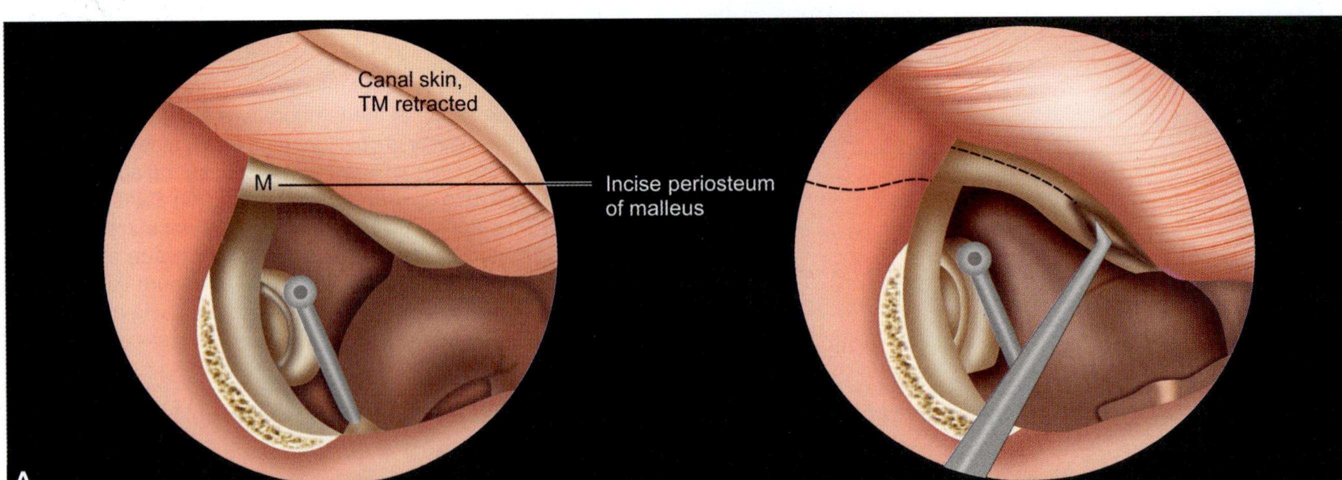

Fig. 12.12A: (A) The periosteum of the malleus is incised with a curved needle.

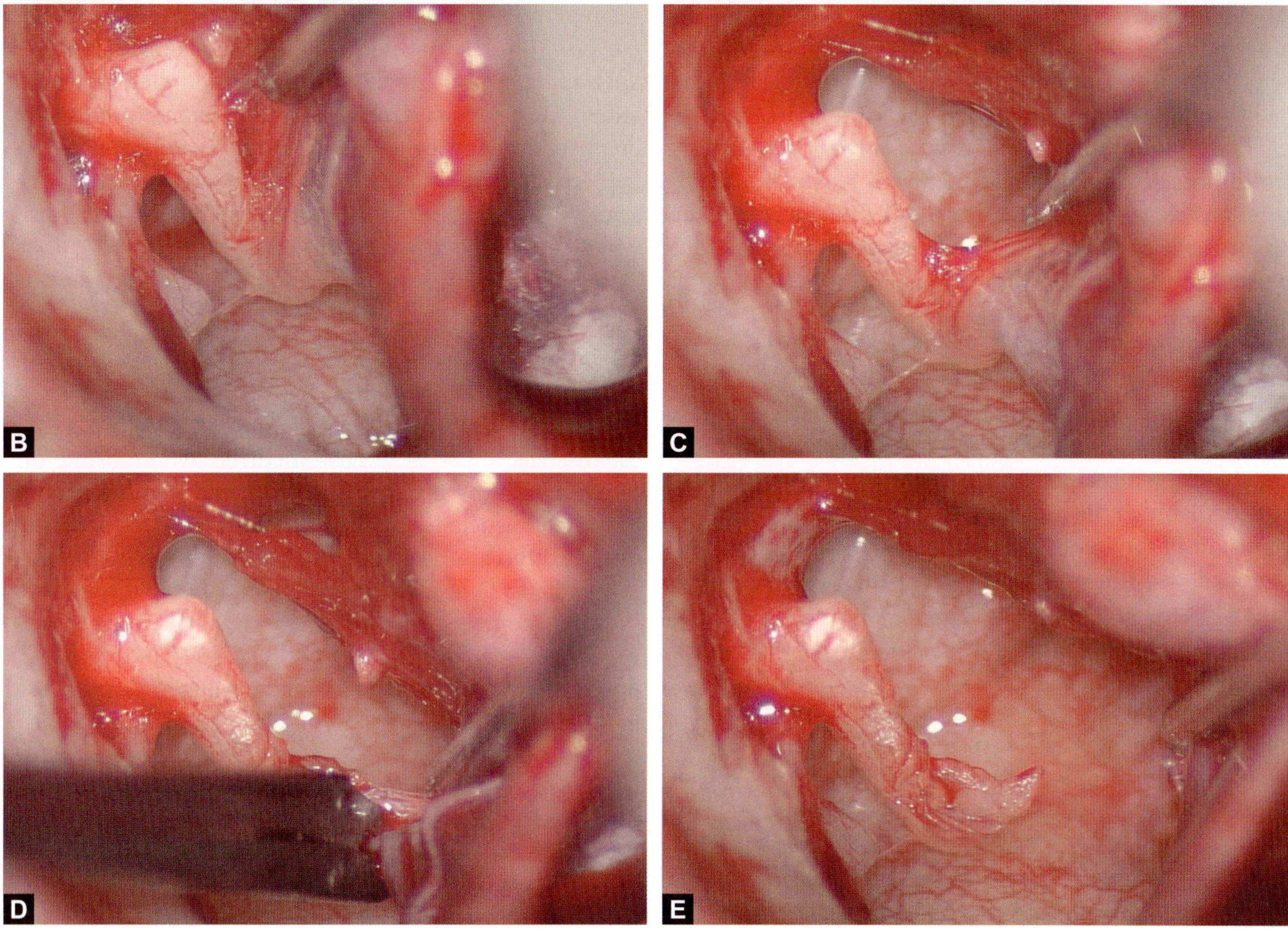

Figs. 12.12B to E: (B) The periosteum of the malleus has been incised with a curved needle and is carefully elevated off of the long and short processes of the malleus. (C) Fibrous extension from the middle layer of the tympanic membrane to the umbo. (D) The fibrous extension to the umbo is cut with a fine scissor. (E) The malleus has been freed from the tympanic membrane, providing excellent exposure for graft placement.

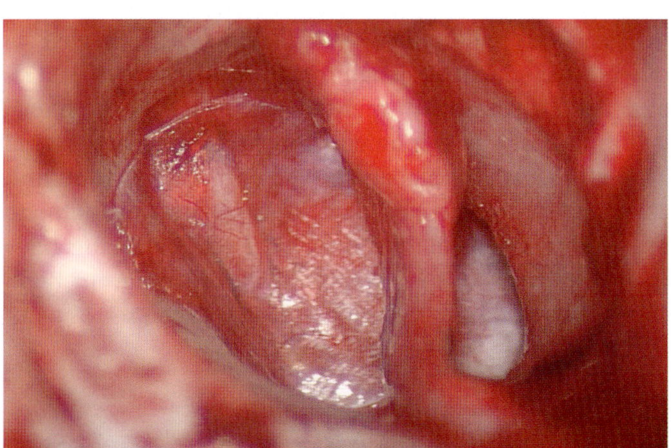

Fig. 12.13: The fascia graft is placed medial to the annulus and tympanic membrane remnant, and lateral to the malleus.

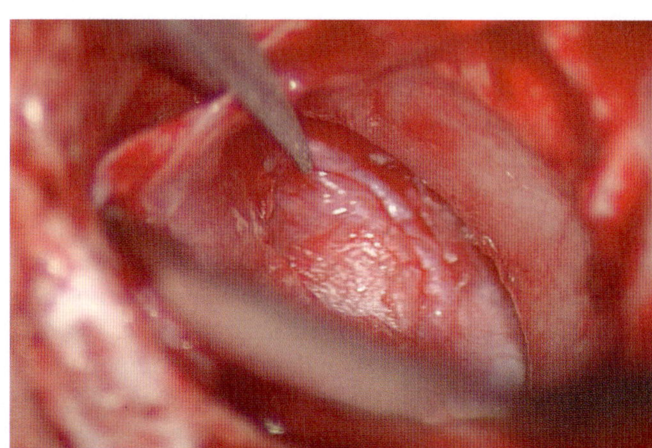

Fig. 12.14: The tympanic membrane remnant is laid down over the fascia graft.

perichondrium is used like fascia with the cartilage on the undersurface of the perichondrium facing the middle ear cleft (the perichondrium is the actual graft that replaces the tympanic membrane, while the cartilage serves as scaffolding that provides stiffness to prevent retraction). The authors generally use a semicircular block of cartilage to reconstruct defects of the scutum, but a scored or hinged piece of cartilage may also be used to reconstruct the entire tympanic membrane area.

SURGICAL TECHNIQUE: OSSICULOPLASTY

Situations encountered in middle ear surgery are variable, and the surgeon should have a number of options for OCR available in his toolkit. The most common situation is erosion of the incus. Frequently the lenticular process is eroded and not making contact with the head of the stapes. There are several potential options for repair: removing, sculpting, and repositioning the incus between stapes and malleus, using a bridging implant, such as an Applebaum or Krauss prosthesis, placing an interposition graft of cartilage or bone between the long process and the stapes head, or simply cementing the incus to the stapes head if the gap is small. For larger gaps between incus and stapes, a sculpted incus interposition or alloplastic partial prosthesis are the best options, described below. In cases of canal wall down mastoidectomy, where the middle ear space is lowered to the level of the facial ridge, a type 3 reconstruction (applying the drum directly to the stapes head) offers a reliable method of repair with a predictable hearing result in the 10 to 25 dB range. Alternatively, the surgeon may use a small perichondrial-cartilage graft to fit onto the capitulum of the stapes, increasing the vibratory unit to the stapes. Another option is to lateralize the malleus and use an alloplastic prosthesis to bridge the distance and increase the size of the middle ear cleft with excellent hearing results.

In cases where the stapes superstructure is absent, a "total" repair, forming a columella from the drum or malleus neck to stapes footplate, is needed. In this situation, the available options are sculpted incus interposition autograft or various prostheses, discussed below.

The malleus handle is an important component of ossicular reconstruction. In most cases of chronic ear disease with or without cholesteatoma, the malleus manubrium can be preserved along with its attachment to the tensor tympani tendon. This is true even when the head of the malleus is removed, or when the umbo is tilted toward the promontory. The neck of the malleus forms a lateral anchor point for the total prosthesis or sculpted incus, and allows for a secure repair with little chance of migration or misalignment. In cases where the manubrium of the malleus cannot be preserved, the tympanic membrane graft will have to be draped over the top of a total prosthesis, which is also effective but less secure.

Autografts

When possible, the patient's own ossicle is used for reconstruction of the hearing mechanism (Figs. 12.16A to C). Since the surgeon must use one or two drill bits to sculpt the ossicle, there is a cost incurred when using this technique. If the incus is well preserved, the dimensions of the reconstruction may be 2–4 mm when drilled as an interposition graft between the stapes superstructure and the malleus. One must know the way to use the incus in order to complete the reconstruction—a notch should be created near the tip of the incus body to engage the malleus neck, and a well should be drilled on the cut end of the long process to accommodate the capitulum of the stapes (Fig. 12.16C, top, left). In the situation where a total reconstruction is necessary (footplate to the malleus), then one may achieve 4–6 mm of reconstruction by drilling a notch in the articular facet to coapt against the malleus neck and whittling the body so that the tip will rest on the footplate without touching the bony margins of the oval window niche (Fig. 12.16C, top, right).

Alloplasts

Today most manufactured implants are made of titanium with and without hydroxyapatite. Both partial and total designs feature implants with fixed lengths as well as others with adjustable-length titanium shafts (Figs. 12.17A and B). As previously mentioned, the authors believe it is important to minimize slippage both at the lateral aspect against the malleus or tympanic membrane and also medially at the capitulum of the stapes or footplate area. Therefore, all of the authors' preferred implants have a groove in the hydroxyapatite head or a titanium hook (Fig. 12.17) to fit under the malleus and secure the implant in place.

Universal Prosthesis

The concept of a "universal" prosthesis is advantageous in that a single prosthesis may be used for multiple

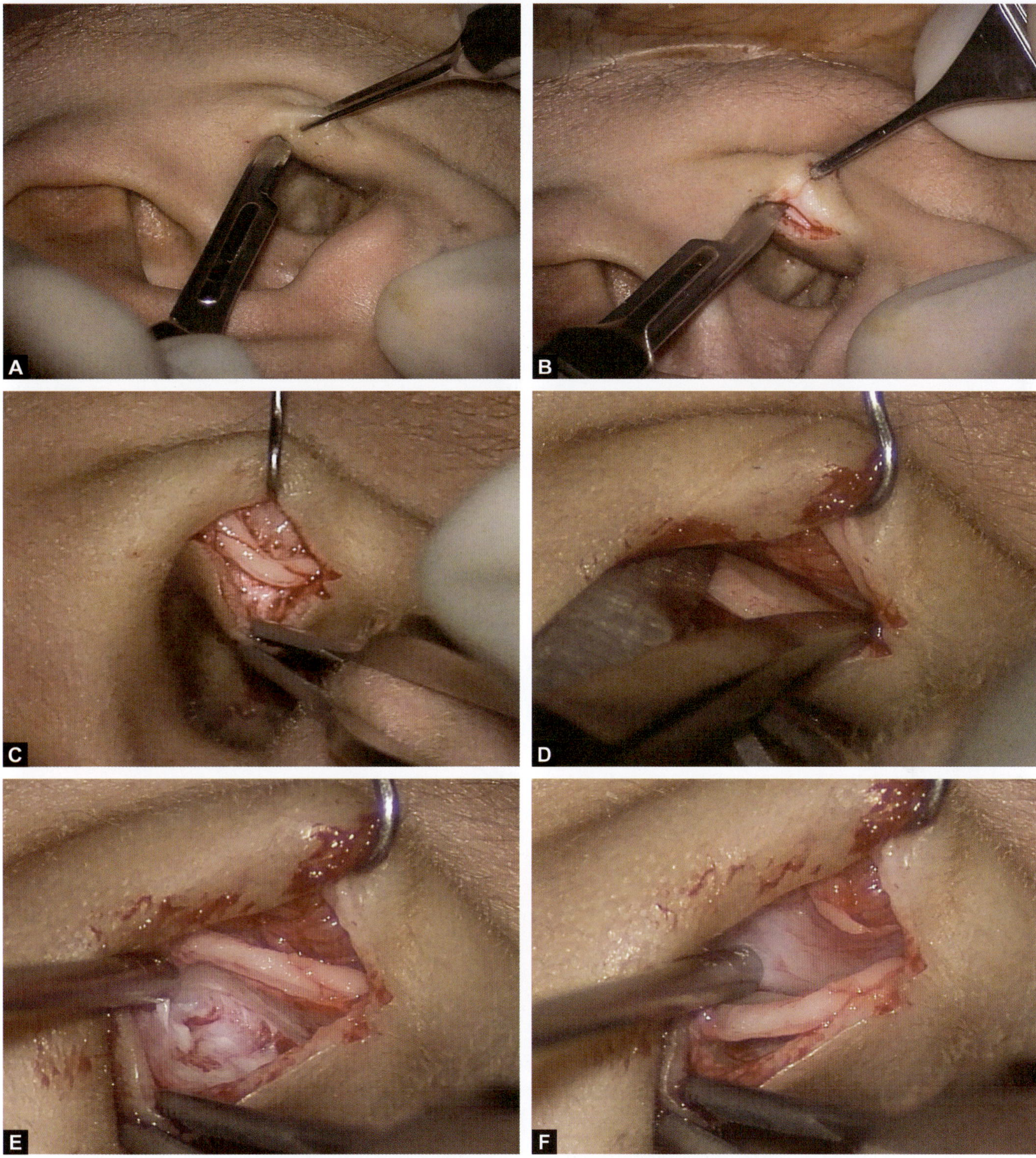

Figs. 12.15A to F: (A) The cartilage graft is harvested from a posterior tragal incision. (B) An incision is made through skin and cartilage. (C) The cartilage has been incised without breaching the anterior perichondrium. (D) A subperichondrial plane of dissection is developed on the anterior surface of the tragal cartilage. (E) A supraperichondrial plane of dissection is developed on the posterior surface of the tragal cartilage. (F) The tragal cartilage is isolated. The posterior perichondrium remains adherent to the cartilage. The anterior perichondrium is left in situ.

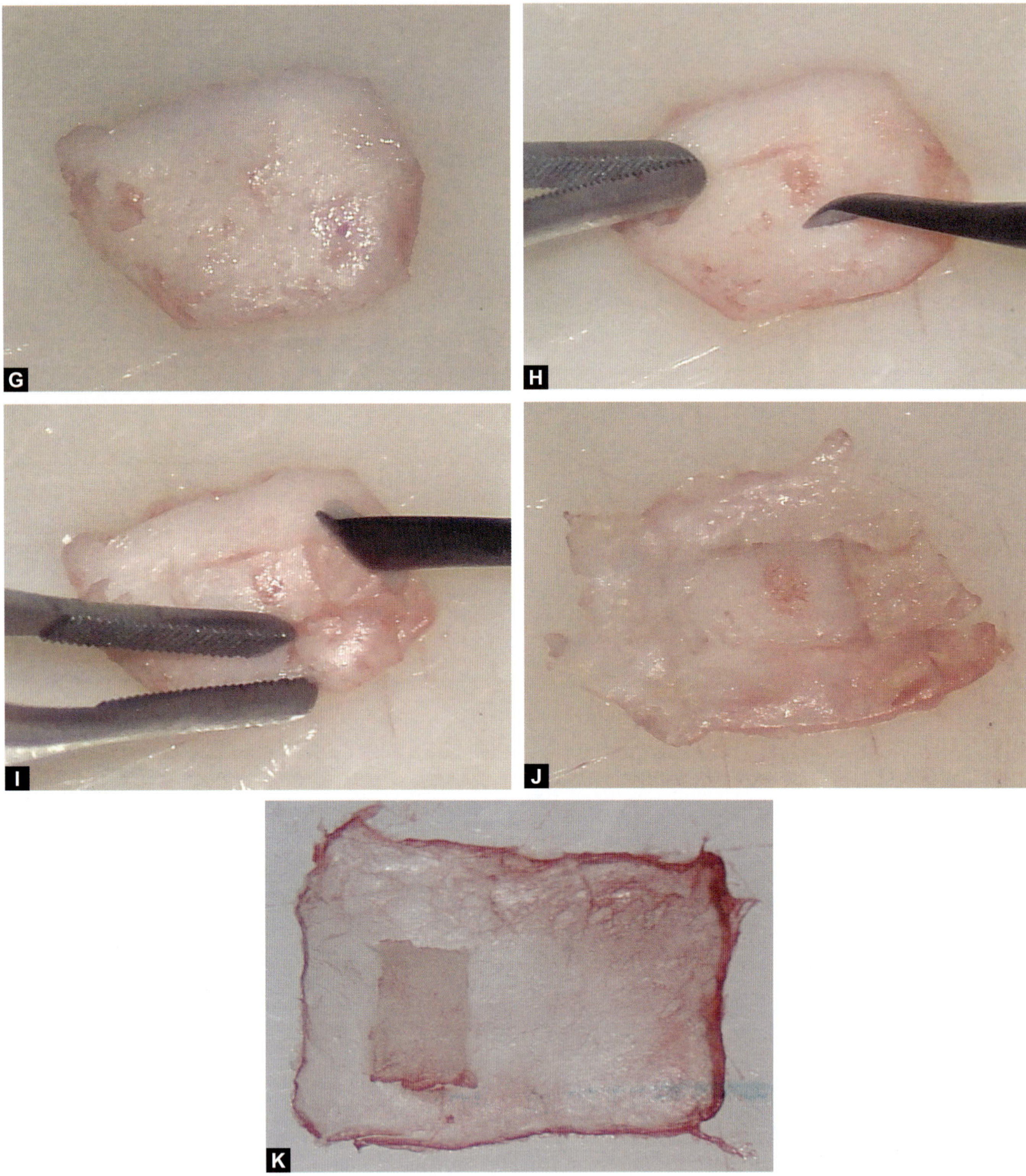

Figs. 12.15G to K: (G) The tragal perichondrial-cartilage graft is harvested. (H and I) The cartilage may be trimmed from the perichondrium to provide a composite graft with appropriately-sized cartilaginous and perichondrial elements. (J) The completed graft includes a central island of cartilage with surrounding perichondrium. (K) In this case, the graft was fashioned to provide cartilage support for a scutal defect; the remaining perichondrium was used as a pliable tympanic membrane graft.

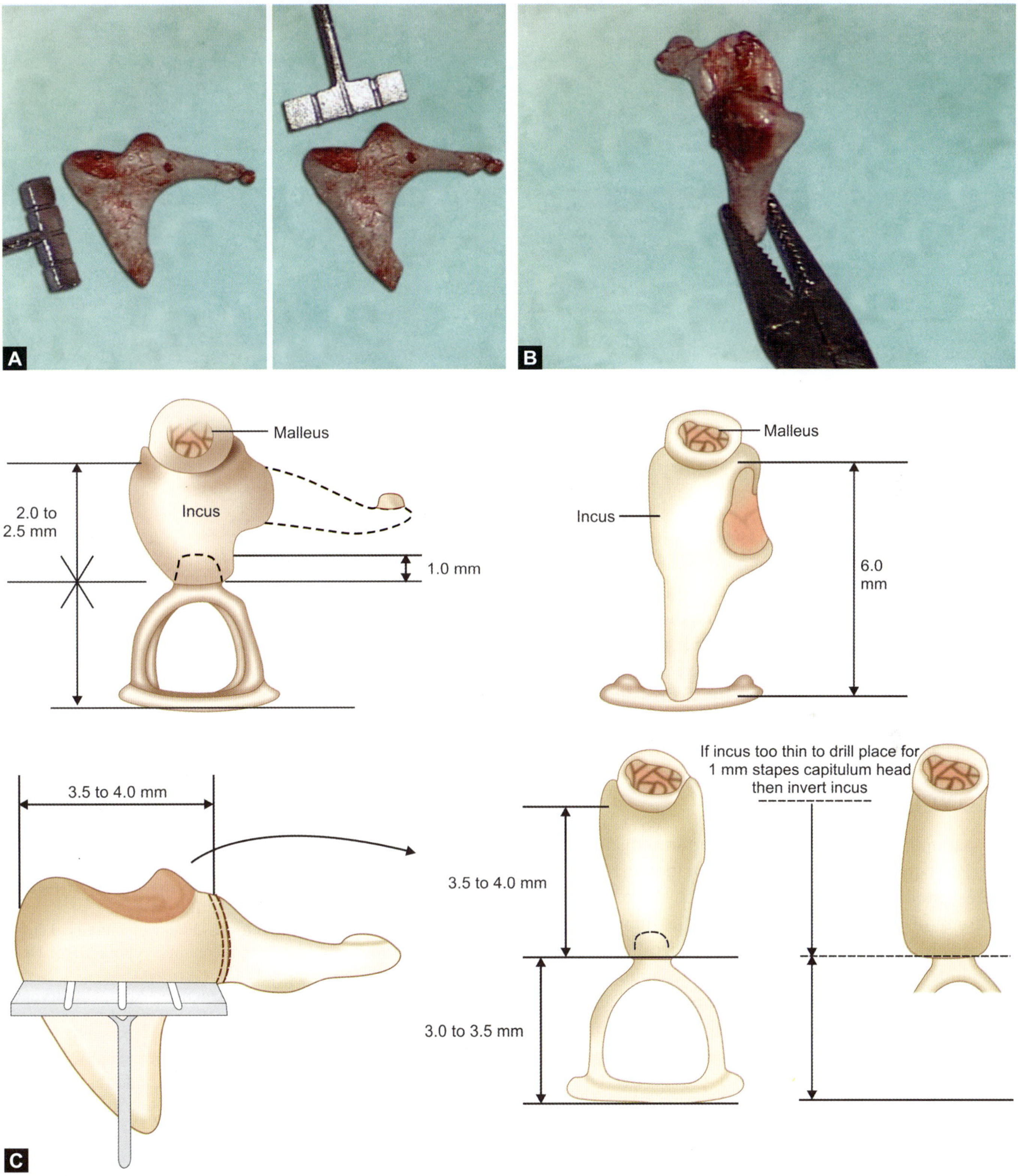

Figs. 12.16A to C: (A) Dimensions of the incus. (B) Profile of the incus. Note that depending on the amount of erosion that has occurred, the incus may be too narrow to properly drill a support for the stapes capitulum. (C) Incus shaping to create an interposition autograft.

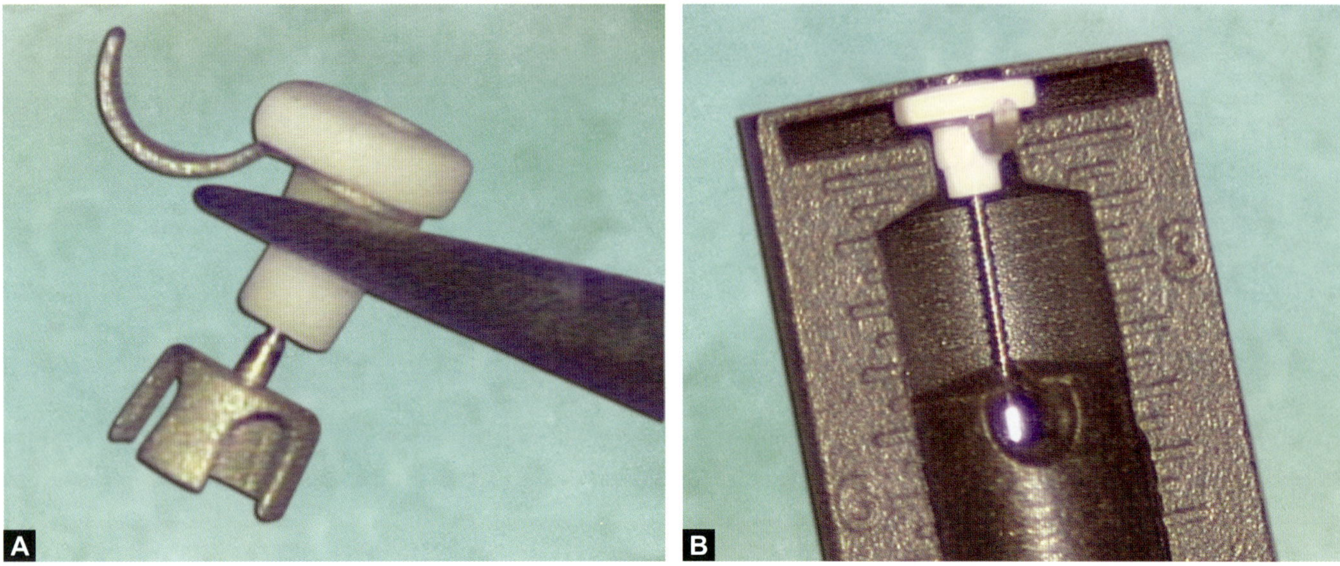

Figs. 12.17A and B: (A) For partial ossicular reconstruction, an adjustable-length prosthesis is trimmed to 2.5–4 mm in length. (B) For total ossicular reconstruction, a prosthesis 4–6 mm in length is appropriate.

reconstructive conditions. In 1988, the Bojrab Universal Prosthesis was designed to be used as a total prosthesis, partial prosthesis, incus sleeve, and incus to footplate prosthesis in its various conformations. The design has been used with hydroxyapatite, Hapex with a hydroxyapatite head, Flex-hydroxyapatite and hydroxyapatite head, and HDPS and hydroxyapatite head. The hydroxyapatite head used in each design features a groove to fit under the malleus if present.

CONCLUSION

Tympanoplasty surgery has been performed successfully to treat tympanic membrane perforations, retractions, cholesteatoma, and other middle ear disease. Though a variety of approaches and techniques have been described, the authors most commonly utilize the over-under technique. This technique is reliable in repairing the majority of tympanic membrane perforations and is appropriate to use for many challenging middle ear situations. Both incus autografts and alloplastic prostheses are commonly used to reconstruct the ossicular chain. The choice of prosthesis is generally an intraoperative decision that is dependent on the presence of usable ossicular stock as well as surgeon preference. Ultimately, any technique that provides a mobile tympanic membrane and an aerated middle ear space can be coupled with a sound conducting mechanism to provide a good outcome for the patient.

REFERENCES

1. Smouha E, Bojrab DI. Tympanoplasty: indications and technique. In: Cholesteatoma. New York, NY: Thieme; 2011. pp. 15-28.
2. Wullstein H. The restoration of the function of the middle ear, in chronic otitis media. Ann Otol Rhinol Laryngol. 1956;65(4):1021-41.
3. Goode RL, Killion M, Nakamura K, et al. New knowledge about the function of the human middle ear: development of an improved analog model. Am J Otol. 1994:15: 145-54.
4. Gan RZ, Dyer RK, Wood MW, Dormer KJ. Mass loading on the ossicles and middle ear function. Ann Otol Rhinol Laryngol. 2001;110:478-85.
5. Merchant SN, Tavicz ME, Puria S, et al. Analysis of middle ear mechanics and application to diseased and reconstructed ears. Am J Otol. 1997;18:139-54.
6. Murakami S, Gyo K, Goode RL. Effect of increased inner ear pressure on middle ear mechanics. Otolaryngol Head Neck Surg. 1998;118:703-8.
7. Austin, DF. Ossicular reconstruction. Arch Otolaryngol. 1971;94:525-35.
8. Zollner F. The principles of plastic surgery of the sound conduction apparatus. J Laryngol Otol. 1955;69:637-52.
9. Lesser TH. Mechanics and material in middle ear reconstruction. Clin Otolaryngol. 1991;16:29-32.
10. Smyth G. Long term results of middle ear reconstructive surgery. J Laryngol Otol. 1971;85:1227-30.
11. Merchant SN, Nado JB Jr. Histopathology of ossicular implants. Otolaryngol Clin North Am. 1994;27:813-33.
12. Merchant SN, Ravicz ME, Puria S, et al. Analysis of reconstructed ears. Am J Otol. 1997;18:139-54.

13. Schuknecht HF, Shi SR. Surgical pathology of middle ear implants. Laryngoscope. 1985;95:249-58.
14. Glasscok ME III, Jackson CG, Knox GW. Can acquired immunodeficiency syndrome and Creutzfeldt-Jakob disease be transmitted via otologic homografts? Arch Otolaryngol Head Neck Surg. 1988;114:1252-5.
15. Smouha E, Bojrab DI. Ossicular chain reconstruction. In: Cholesteatoma. New York, NY: Thieme; 2011. pp.29-45.
16. Bojrab DI, Causse JB, Battista RA, et al. Ossiculoplasty with composite prostheses: overview and analysis. Otologic Clin N Am. 1994;27(4):759-76.
17. Bojrab DI, Babu S. Ossiculoplasty I. In: Middle ear and mastoid surgery. New York: Thieme; 2004. Chapter 19, pp. 151-8.
18. Hahn Y, Bojrab DI. Outcomes following ossicular chain reconstruction with composite prostheses: hydroxyapatite-polyethylene vs. hydroxyapatite-titanium. Ear Nose Throat J. 2013;92(6):250-52.
19. Fisch U. Reconstruction of the ossicular chain. HNO. 1978; 26:53-6.
20. Albu S, Babighian G, Trabalzini F. Prognostic factors in tympanoplasty. Am J Otol. 1998;19:136-40.
21. Dornhoffer J, Gardner E. Prognostic factors in ossiculoplasty: a statistical staging system. Otol Neurotol. 2001;22: 299-304.
22. Goldenberg R, Driver M. Long term results with hydroxyapatite middle ear implants. Otolaryngol Head Neck Surg. 2000;122:635-42.

CHAPTER 13

Complications of Temporal Bone Infection

Daniel Jethanamest, Simon I Angeli

INTRODUCTION

Complications arising from underlying infections within the temporal bone can represent a broad spectrum of presentations and acuity. Otitis media commonly plays a role as the initial infection, with associated sequelae limited to the confines of the middle ear such as tympanic membrane perforation, atelectasis, and hearing loss. However, acute infections or acute progression of chronic infections can spread through the pneumatized spaces and other anatomic channels of the temporal bone, directly involving or seeding adjacent critical structures.

Complications of temporal bone infection beyond the middle ear may be classified by their location with respect to intracranial spaces, by their chronicity, or by their order or degree of complexity. First-order complications would include mastoiditis, facial palsy in acute otitis media, labyrinthine fistula, and serous labyrinthitis that result from direct or adjacent involvement by the initial infection. These complications typically have a clear presentation and diagnosis, can be treated with directed local measures within the temporal bone, and generally have a better prognosis. Second-order complications usually result from the further unhalted progression of one of the first-order entities and can be more challenging to diagnose. Second-order complications may require a more urgent and specialized intervention but may be challenging to recognize because they sometimes present with more subtle findings.

Modern trends have been influenced by advancements in imaging detection and a broader arsenal of antibiotic therapy, particularly in children when less invasive management is often sufficient in selective cases. Whether it be mastoidectomy for acute mastoiditis in the pediatric population or neurosurgical intervention for brain abscesses, many authors have offered case reports or small case series with some success in conservative management, though unfortunately the rarity of many of these complications has prohibited thorough investigation and comparison of various management strategies.[1,2] Clinicians must carefully review the individualized risks and benefits of each management choice in each case of infectious complication.

MASTOIDITIS

The term mastoiditis is broad and in theory every episode of acute otitis media (AOM) is accompanied by some degree of mastoiditis if the middle ear is contiguous with the mastoid antrum. Currently no defined clinical or diagnostic criteria exist in the literature defining acute mastoiditis, which typically implies the presence of otitis media with associated clinical examination signs surrounding the mastoid or radiologic and/or surgical findings. The entity of complicated mastoiditis generally refers to the development of some structural change or bony erosion involving the mastoid air cell system. Suppurative infections within the middle ear extending into the mastoid create inflammatory changes within the mucosa and eventual breakdown of thin bony borders. This can first manifest solely within the mastoid itself as an acute coalescent mastoiditis, with the loss of the normal bony septations and architecture, or external to the mastoid such as in a subperiosteal abscess or postauricular fistula formation.

Most studies of incidence have focused on the pediatric population in which this complication is most common. In a study reviewing the incidence of acute mastoiditis in children under the age of 14, as defined by hospital discharge information from several European countries, Canada, Australia, and the United States, the incidence ranged from 1.2 to 4.2 cases per 100,000 person years.[3] A separate review of 399 children in Norway noted that patients <2 years of age had a higher relative incidence than those between the ages of 2–16.[4] Multiple studies have suggested a greater predominance in males. The introduction of pneumococcal conjugate vaccines has reduced invasive pneumococcal infections in general including AOM, though in retrospective observational studies no decrease in the admissions for acute mastoiditis was seen in the years after introduction of the heptavalent conjugate vaccine.[5,6]

In a review of acute mastoiditis in children including 63 studies with reported culture information, *Streptococcus pneumoniae* was the most frequently cultured pathogen in 43% of cultures on average. In 36% of cultures on average, no growth of pathogens was found.[7] Other common pathogens including *Haemophilus influenzae, Streptococcus pyogenes, Proteus mirabilis, Staphylococcus aureus, Pseudomonas aeruginosa* and anaerobes can also be isolated, and many cases represent polymicrobial infections.[8–10] In addition to acute instances, many patients may develop coalescence after a chronic period of infection with or without the presence of cholesteatoma.

Acute coalescent mastoiditis can present with new or persistent pain over the mastoid during or after an episode of otitis media. Often the time course to develop coalescence requires some latent period of ongoing infection, whether a chronic stage or prolonged AOM, with mastoiditis presenting a week or more after the initial onset. In addition to signs associated with otitis media, postauricular local findings including protrusion of the pinna (Fig. 13.1), erythema, edema, or tenderness can be observed, on average in >80% of patients.[7] In some cases masked mastoiditis can be witnessed after some period of treatment, when persistent infection continues within the spaces of the mastoid bone though the signs and symptoms of the initial acute middle ear infection have resolved.[11]

Laboratory markers such as C-reactive protein (CRP) and white blood cell (WBC) counts are usually elevated.[12] In one study of 308 children with acute mastoiditis, those with complications were noted to present with a higher grade fever, absolute neutrophil count and CRP in comparison to children with uncomplicated disease.[8] Radiologic examination with computed tomography (CT) scan can be utilized to confirm the presence of bony destruction or coalescence. CT review must also include evaluation for associated second-order intracranial and extracranial complications progressing from mastoiditis. Some debate also exists, particularly in the pediatric population, whether radiologic imaging is required for all patients with a clinical suspicion of acute mastoiditis. Though CT scans may include risks of radiation exposure and in some cases anesthetics, the risks of missing intracranial complications with associated high morbidity and possible mortality must also be considered. In studies evaluating presenting symptoms and clinical signs to distinguish patients with intracranial complications, no markers could be found to guide the use of selective imaging and it is known that some patients with acute mastoiditis without initial imaging proceed to develop more severe intracranial complications during conservative management.[13,14] Magnetic resonance imaging (MRI) may be reserved for cases with suspected intracranial complications after CT scan.

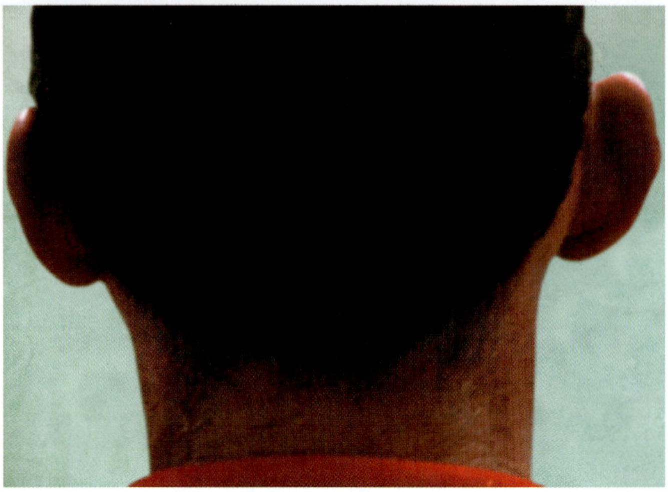

Fig. 13.1: Protruding pinna. In the examination of a patient with right-sided acute mastoiditis from posteriorly, protrusion of the pinna on the right side in relation to the unaffected left side can be noted, in association with soft tissue edema and inflammation in the postauricular region.

The treatment of mastoiditis includes medical and surgical components. Though it is the most common complication of AOM, controversy exists over the criteria for and degree of surgical intervention in these cases. Simple mastoidectomy with aspiration of the middle ear via myringotomy with or without tympanostomy tube placement, culture of middle ear purulence, and intravenous (IV) antibiotic therapy would constitute the historical standard treatment combination. However, the use of mastoidectomy in cases of acute mastoiditis, particularly in the pediatric population, varies greatly within the literature, as more recent literature has suggested approaches relying upon antibiotics alone or in combination with myringotomy while reserving mastoidectomy for cases with evidence of poor response. Improvement in signs and symptoms within 48 hours is a commonly used outline for surgical decision making. Rates of mastoidectomy in the pediatric population have been reported to vary from 9% to 88%, though the definition of acute mastoiditis also varies between studies.[4,9,12,15,16] The significant risk of delaying treatment for poor responders to conservative management is progression of coalescent mastoiditis to highly morbid and potentially life-threatening intracranial complications, which is weighed against the risk of a cortical mastoidectomy and anesthetic risks. In cases with associated cholesteatoma, if the patient is healthy and stable enough to tolerate the procedure, removal of cholesteatoma may be performed in the same setting as mastoidectomy.

SUBPERIOSTEAL AND BEZOLD'S ABSCESS

The most common progression of acute mastoiditis is to subperiosteal abscess formation. This is most often in the lateral direction from the mastoid cortex with associated fluctuance in the postauricular region and possible bogginess or bulging of the posterior wall of the external auditory canal. Though the lateral site is most frequent, suppurative extension can less commonly follow a direct route from the mastoid and epitympanum to the zygomatic root, or seed this region via venous drainage. The standard approach to treatment of any site of subperiosteal abscess includes the same elements as in acute mastoiditis with the additional incision and drainage of the subperiosteal abscess overlying the mastoid. Similarly to the management of acute mastoiditis, some authors have proposed less invasive management in pediatric cases such as needle aspiration or incisional drainage without mastoidectomy.[17,18] In some reviews, a small subset of conservatively managed patients have been found to require repeated procedures, eventual mastoidectomy, or additional treatments for progressing intracranial complications, which are weighed against the risks of abscess drainage and simple mastoidectomy for patients who may have otherwise responded to antibiotics.

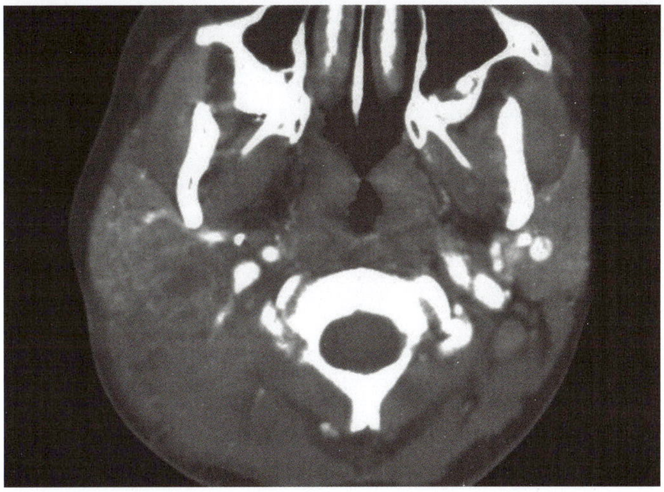

Fig. 13.2: Bezold's abscess. Contrast enhanced axial CT reveals a medially placed rim-enhancing small abscess just medial and below the mastoid tip in this case.

First described by Friedrich von Bezold in the late 1800s, Bezold's abscess refers to the medial extension of mastoiditis through the cortex of the mastoid tip and into the soft tissues of the neck.[19] Though mastoiditis is more common in children, young patients have not fully developed the pneumatization of the mastoid tip air cells, making deep medial extension of purulence in this route more common in older children and adults. As the infection spreads from the digastric ridge and mastoid tip through the deep spaces of the neck, initial signs and symptoms may be subtle. Once suspected, imaging that incorporates the neck spaces from the skull base through the mediastinum should be obtained. Contrast-enhanced CT imaging reveals typical signs of abscess formation with rim enhancement in a location medial to the mastoid process (Fig. 13.2). Untreated progression of early collections can lead to significant enlargement and tracking through deep neck spaces prominently seen on clinical examination (Figs. 13.3 and 13.4). Treatment for the associated mastoiditis and Bezold's abscess includes IV antibiotics, mastoidectomy with removal of the mastoid tip with direct neck exploration and drainage. In this particular route of spread of temporal bone infection, careful assessment and monitoring of the airway must be considered, with tracheostomy an option for any compromise.

PETROUS APICITIS

The petrous apex of the temporal bone is less commonly involved but can be a deeper site of spread in complicated

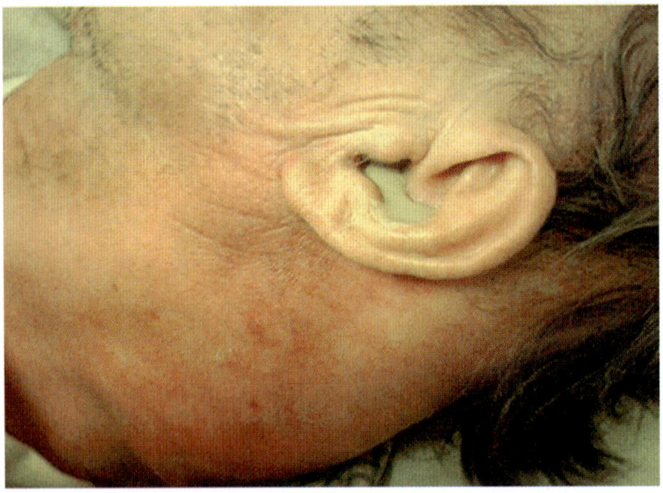

Fig. 13.3: Neck abscess. Untreated or late presentation of an otogenic neck abscess reveals an erythematous and prominent fluctuant bulge within the neck in association with purulent otorrhea.

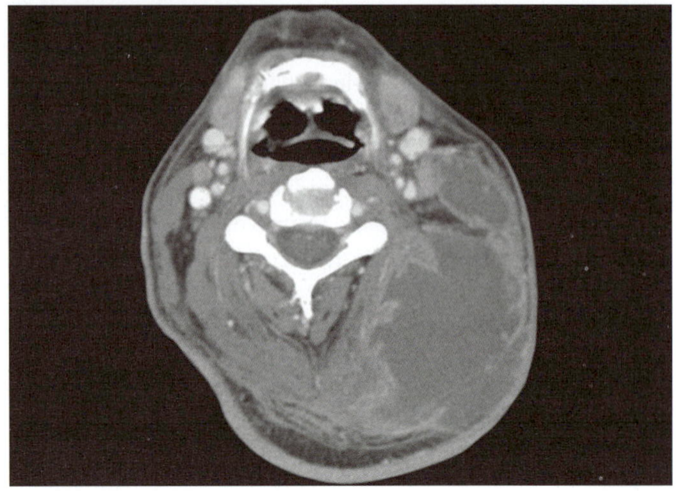

Fig. 13.4: Neck abscess CT. The CT scan with contrast for the same patient reveals the extensive collection within the neck spaces that has spread inferiorly from the mastoid.

infections. This anatomic site displays variability in development of air cells, with approximately 35% of temporal bones displaying pneumatization, and can differ not only between patients but also asymmetrically between the two sides of the same individual.[20] The apex may have varying degrees of pneumatization, be sclerotic or contain bone marrow. The lower rate of air cell tract communication between the mastoid and this region as well as limited space for coalescence may account for the decreased incidence of petrous apicitis in comparison to mastoid coalescence.

In 1904 Giuseppe Gradenigo reported on the finding of abducens palsy in association with retro-orbital pain he postulated to be trigeminal in origin, in the setting of acute or chronic otitis media (COM).[21] This triad of physical examination findings is now referred to as Gradenigo's syndrome. The involvement of the sixth cranial nerve was speculated soon after by a young anatomist, Primo Dorello, to be due to edema in a limited, narrow bony canal now known as Dorello's canal. The majority of patients, even in Gradenigo's original series, do not have the full triad so clinicians should not hesitate to suspect this complication in the absence of a finding.

The diagnosis of petrous apicitis, or petrositis, can be suspected by clinical presentation, though this can vary significantly and diagnosis is best confirmed with radiological work-up. As the petrous apex is a separate compartment from the mastoid and middle ear, some cases may develop recurrence of symptoms even after mastoidectomy. In these instances, infection within the deeper petrous apex has not completely cleared though the more lateral sites may have completely responded. CT and MRI are often both used as complementary studies for this anatomic region. The bony detail of a CT aids in the assessment of whether any bony erosion or opacification is present within the region and depicts their relative location to intracranial structures. When opacified spaces are seen, complimentary T1, T2, and diffusion weighted MRI sequences can help narrow the differential diagnosis, which can include acute infection, bone marrow, cholesterol granuloma, epidermoid/cholesteatoma, and neoplasm.

Treatment of petrositis includes IV antibiotics with central nervous system (CNS) penetration and mastoidectomy with exenteration of infected petrous apex cells. The development of air cell tracts varies among individuals and approaches to the petrous apex must be carefully chosen, though infection often delineates a route between the mastoid and petrous apex. In a radical mastoidectomy cavity, peritubal air cells between the carotid artery and basal turn of the cochlea can be accessed. Other possible approaches include dissection through the subarcuate fossa, supralabyrinthine cell tract, supracochlear, transmeatal-infralabyrinthine approach as well as, in the modern era, endoscopic endonasal approaches to the petrous apex. The combination of medical and surgical interventions has been the traditional treatment choice for this entity. Some case reports have noted successful treatment with antibiotics in combination with tympanostomy tube insertion alone, reserving further surgical decompression for patients failing to respond to conservative management, though the rarity of this complication makes treatment comparisons challenging.[22–24] Abducens palsy recovery is variable and has been reported to occur over weeks to months after treatment.

FACIAL PARALYSIS

With its intricate course within the temporal bone, the facial nerve is anatomically adjacent at various points to coalescent or complicated infections. Nevertheless, the incidence of facial palsy complicating otitis media in the antibiotic era is low, ranging from 0.04% to 0.16%.[25,26] In the pediatric population, acute otitis media and mastoiditis can often lead to facial palsy, while in adults COM and cholesteatoma are more likely causes of facial dysfunction. The facial nerve is often dehiscent, most commonly in the tympanic segment, where it may be vulnerable to surrounding unresolved infections.

The pathophysiology of facial palsy in the setting of infection is not well defined. Possible hypotheses include inflammatory edema with entrapment and compression causing ischemia, direct intraneural involvement by infectious organisms or toxins at dehiscent sites, surrounding bony osteitis with adjacent erosion and reactivation of latent herpes virus.

In the setting of acute infection, palsy can be either sudden or gradual and generally has a good prognosis if promptly treated. In one study of children presenting to an emergency department with facial palsy, 22.4% were attributed to infectious causes and among those, AOM-related cases showed shorter recovery times than non-AOM infections.[27] Alternatively, in cases of COM with cholesteatoma that involve the facial nerve, prognosis for improvement is poorer than AOM or COM without cholesteatoma.[25]

Clinical assessment of the patient including neurologic examination is indicated, including careful documentation of the degree of facial nerve dysfunction over time. Temporal bone CT can be obtained to evaluate for sites of dehiscence in cases of COM with or without cholesteatoma, as well as to rule out possible intracranial complications of infection. Electrodiagnostic testing may aid in determining prognosis.[28]

Determining the infectious setting during which facial palsy occurs will guide treatment planning. In cases of acute infection, treatment with antibiotic therapy for otitis media and myringotomy with aspiration for culture is recommended. In a review of 37 patients with facial palsy due to AOM with varying treatment regimens, 92% recovered to a HB grade I or II.[29] In the 12 patients undergoing surgical facial nerve decompression, the authors questioned and ultimately recommended against the routine decompression of the facial nerve. In the small group of patients, they felt electrical testing was prognostic and independent of surgical intervention. Corticosteroids are often utilized in facial palsy, though no clear evidence for or against them in the setting of otitis media exists.

Mastoidectomy, however, is indicated for unresolving infections, coalescence, or other complications. In cases of COM particularly with cholesteatoma, however, surgical exploration is recommended within a short time frame. In these cases, a likely localized site of cholesteatoma or infective granulation against the nerve is the site of involvement and should be cleared and decompressed to remove active infection. If cholesteatoma significantly involves the facial nerve, we favor leaving cholesteatoma matrix on the nerve and creating an open cavity rather than radical exenteration of matrix and nerve fibers.

LABYRINTHITIS

Involvement of the perilymphatic space by infection causing labyrinthitis can be categorized in a number of ways depending on the foreign substrate. Serous labyrinthitis can evolve from viral-induced mechanisms unrelated to ear disease or potential bacterial toxins from otitis media. The development of suppurative labyrinthitis is less common and can be due to either tympanogenic sources or meningogenic. In addition, COM may involve cholesteatoma or granulation tissue that causes a disruption in the otic capsule, predisposing that ear to the subsequent entry of infection.

Symptoms of labyrinthitis include acute onset of vertigo, tinnitus, and hearing loss, often with nausea and vomiting. Serous labyrinthitis may have a more gradual onset in some cases while suppurative labyrinthitis is often closely associated with meningitis and bilateral involvement. No specific radiologic study is required though signs of active labyrinthitis can be seen on imaging, which also aids in ruling out other intracranial complications and assessing delayed pertinent sequelae such as cochlear ossification.

Patients diagnosed with labyrinthitis may be very ill at presentation and should be admitted and have myringotomy with or without tube placement to clear middle ear infection and obtain cultures. Lumbar puncture with cerebrospinal fluid (CSF) studies in the evaluation for meningitis should be performed. Imaging may reveal enhancement within the vestibule and labyrinth

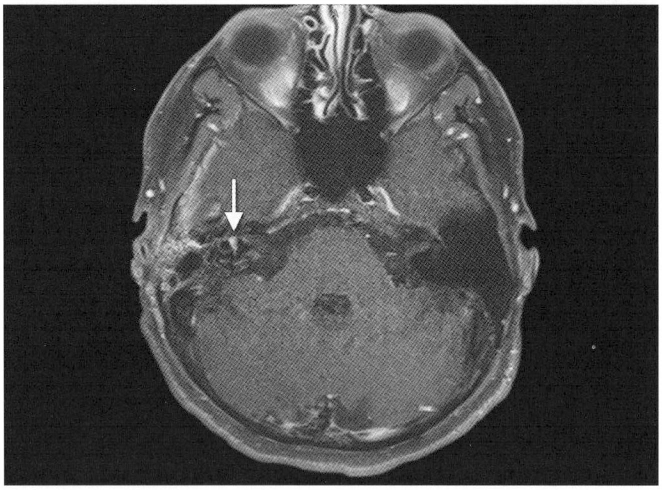

Fig. 13.5: Labyrinthitis MRI. T1-weighted MRI postgadolinium axial view in this patient after mastoidectomy for ongoing otitis media and right-sided acute mastoiditis with symptoms of profound hearing loss reveals enhancement in the right vestibule (white arrow) and labyrinth as seen in comparison to the nonenhancing contralateral side.

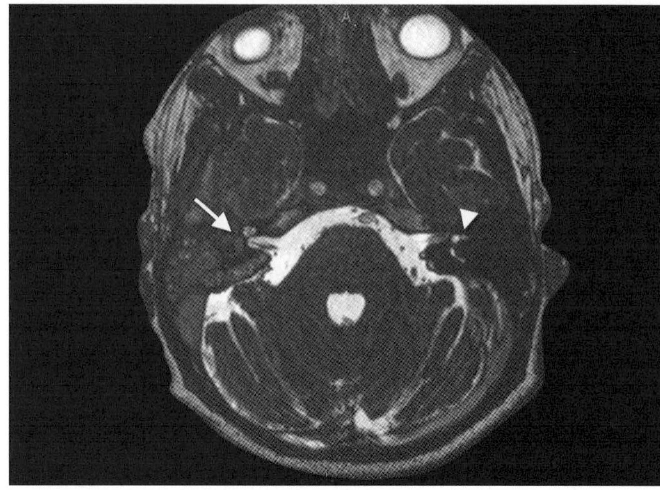

Fig. 13.6: Labyrinthitis MRI CISS. Constructive interference in steady state (CISS) gradient echo sequence of the same patient provides good resolution and reveals a lack of signal in the right vestibule and semicircular canals (white arrow) in contrast to the normal high signal expected as in the unaffected contralateral side (white arrowhead).

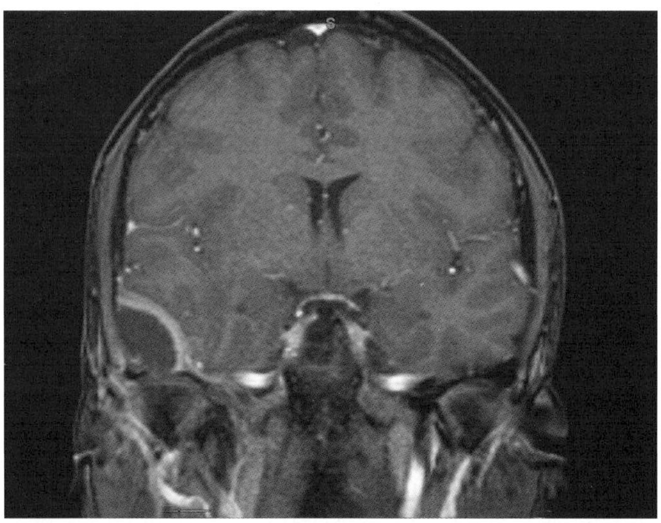

Fig. 13.7: Epidural abscess MRI. Contrast enhanced T1-weighted MRI in coronal section reveals and right-sided low signal collection with surrounding enhancement and medial concave displacement of the dura and brain. T2-weighted images show a similar appearance with high T2 signal of the fluid collection.

(Figs. 13.5 and 13.6). If no other complications such as coalescence are present, mastoidectomy is not necessary and IV antibiotics with good CSF penetration are given. Labyrinthectomy is not routinely performed and may be reserved only for cases in which the infection and meningitis fail to resolve or recur after appropriate medical treatment. It may also be pursued if cholesteatoma or granulation has caused significant erosion or entry to the vestibule. Labyrinthine fistulas treatment depends upon the extent of invasion by cholesteatoma and associated risk of inner ear disruption. In shallow fistulas of the semicircular canals in which endosteum is not exposed, removal of granulation and cholesteatoma matrix can be achieved. However, when fistulas extend deeply with involvement of the membranous vestibule or cochlea, the matrix may be left in place with exteriorization.

EXTRADURAL/EPIDURAL ABSCESS

Infections crossing the boundaries of the skull base may cause abscess formation along the lateral surface of the dura, without deeper extension. These usually occur at sites with discontinuity of bony boundaries such as in dehiscent tegmen sites, though less commonly spread of infection may traverse intact bone hematogenously.

Patients with an epidural abscess share the same symptoms as mastoiditis, accompanied by generalized headache. Typically CSF studies will be normal. Imaging with CT or MRI should clearly outline the abscess site and can assess the surrounding mastoid infection and possible sites of continuity. A fluid collection with rim enhancement within the epidural space displacing dura and brain in concave fashion is seen as in Figure 13.7. A coronal image from the temporal bone CT of the same patient (Fig. 13.8) at this time shows opacification of the middle ear consistent

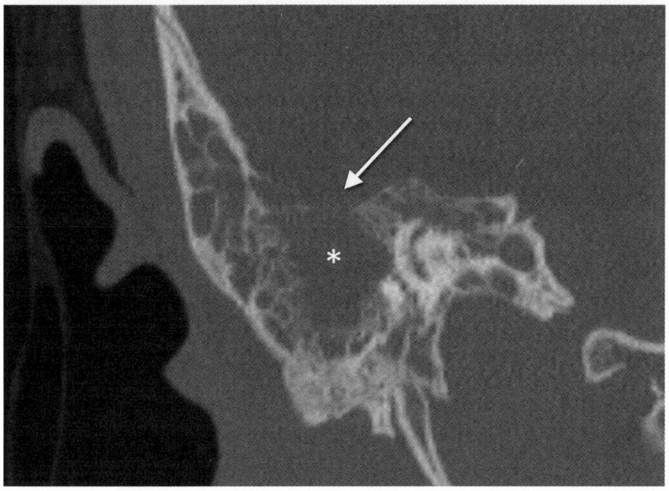

Fig. 13.8: Epidural abscess CT. A coronal CT section of the same patient reveals an opacified mastoid with some coalescence (asterisk) and a tegmen defect (white arrow) corresponding to the site of epidural abscess seen on MRI.

with AOM as well as a site of likely tegmen dehiscence correlating with the site of epidural abscess development. The treatment of this condition includes admission with IV antibiotics with good CNS penetration. A mastoidectomy to clear infection is performed and the sites of suspected bony defects carefully explored to drain the abscess. Care is taken in dissection of granulation tissue that often develops at these sites as it can be very adherent to the dura, which should be kept intact throughout.

OTITIC MENINGITIS

Bacterial meningitis evolving from an otogenic infection can produce significant morbidity and mortality. It is the most common intracranial complication of suppurative otitis media and its incidence in one study of adults was 0.42 per 100,000 per year.[30] In a multicenter study of 223 cases of acute mastoiditis, seven patients developed meningoencephalitis, and it was the most common intracranial complication of mastoiditis in that series.[10] Patients with temporal bone infection and meningitis often have a second or multiple concurrent complications. The mortality rate in modern series has ranged from 3% to 9%.[30,31]

Symptoms of meningitis include irritability, somnolence, fever, headaches, photophobia, nausea, and neck stiffness. Assessment should include lumbar puncture and CSF analysis. Patients with completely normal CSF findings with nuchal rigidity and fever in the setting of otitis should also be examined for possible retropharyngeal infection or abscess in the setting of petrositis. Head and temporal bone CT are utilized to rule out hydrocephalus, other intracranial complications such as abscess formation, and any anatomic sites of predisposition to this episode of meningitis or future recurrent episodes. Evaluation for anatomic abnormalities such as tegmen defects, meningoceles, and anomalies of the inner ear should be completed as these patients would be at risk for recurrent meningitis.

Treatment of bacterial meningitis should be initiated without delay to prevent severe neurologic sequelae and possible mortality. Blood cultures and CSF sampling prior to initial dosing of IV antibiotics with CNS penetration is preferred when possible. Antimicrobial treatment can then be directed by culture results. For confirmed cases of *H. influenzae* and *Neisseria meningitides* meningitis, prophylactic treatment of close contacts with rifampin may be considered, especially when high-risk individuals live within the household of the close contacts. Myringotomy with or without tympanostomy tube and aspirate culture is completed for cases with otitis media. In acute mastoiditis, mastoidectomy can be completed once the meningitis is well controlled by medical treatment, or if the meningitis is not improving. In cases secondary to COM, mastoidectomy and clearance of disease is performed once the patient is stable enough to tolerate the procedure. Any surgical exploration should include careful observation for CSF fistulas and abscess formation. Corticosteroids have been recommended to reduce neurologic sequelae in bacterial meningitis of any etiology, particularly when given at the onset of antibiotic therapy in pneumococcal meningitis.[32] In a recently updated systematic review of the literature, evidence for improved neurologic outcomes was found, although no reduction in overall mortality was seen.[33] Subgroup analysis revealed that corticosteroid use reduced severe hearing loss in children with meningitis due to *H. influenza* but not in children with meningitis due to other infectious species.

OTOGENIC LATERAL SINUS THROMBOSIS

Otologic infections that involve extradural surfaces around the sigmoid portion of the lateral venous sinus can lead to phlebitis and thrombus formation. This is a rare complication of otitis media but can be associated with significant morbidity and mortality. Progression of thrombus

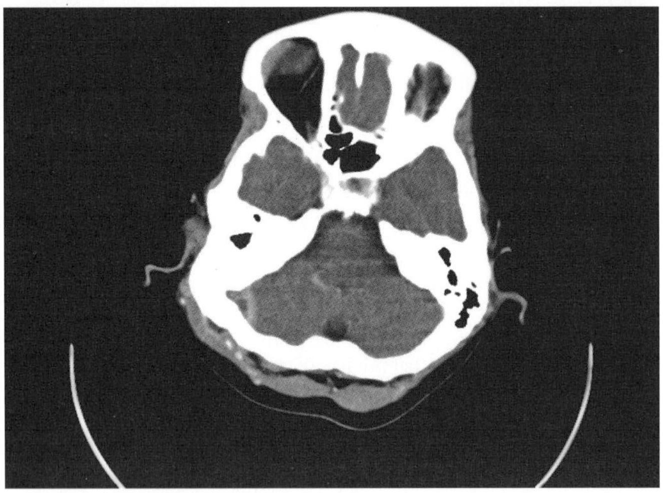

Fig. 13.9: Delta sign. An initial axial CT of the right temporal bone reveals opacification of mastoid cells with some decalcification of the bone overlying the sigmoid sinus, indicating possible granulation and involvement of the venous sinus. On contrast enhanced axial CT view, the right sigmoid sinus displays the class empty delta sign: a triangular rim of enhancement with low attenuation center corresponding with the thrombus.

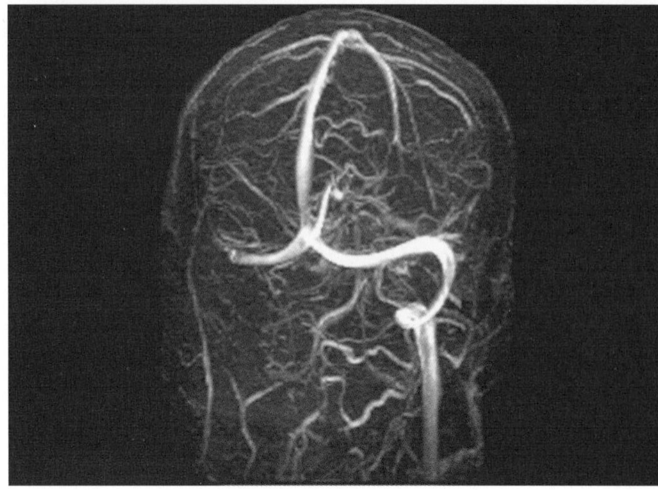

Fig. 13.10: Lateral sinus thrombosis MRV. Magnetic resonance venography (MRV) can be performed with or without contrast administration, and provides excellent visualization of flow within the venous sinus system. In this MRV, a lack of flow is noted distal to the junction of the transverse and sigmoid sinus in continuity with the jugular bulb and internal jugular vein on the right side.

leads to hydrocephalus and cavernous sinus thrombosis. In the preantibiotic era, mortality was nearly 100% and has ranged from 0% to 25% in the modern era.[34-36] Thrombus may completely occlude the venous system, become infected, propagate intraluminally, or release septic emboli into the blood stream.

The presentation of lateral sinus thrombosis can vary greatly from a relatively asymptomatic patient to florid sepsis with emboli. Symptoms include headache, malaise, "picket fence" spiking fevers, chills and symptoms of increased intracranial pressure such as vision changes, nausea, vomiting, and confusion. The manifestation of these symptoms differs from patient to patient, and at times appears to simply represent otitis media. It has been speculated that in locales with good antibiotic availability and frequent use for otitis media, the initial otologic complaints may fade by the time of presentation and neurologic symptoms predominate with just a history of resolved otitis.[34] Upon examination patients may exhibit Griesinger's sign—edema and tenderness over the posterior portion of the mastoid, representing the septic thrombosis of the mastoid emissary vein that is in continuity with the sigmoid sinus. This should not be confused with the more anterior bulging of the postauricular soft tissues and posterior-superior external auditory canal seen in cases of subperiosteal abscess, which may also cause proptosis of the pinna. Queckenstedt's test (or Tobey-Ayer test) was historically used to confirm suspected sinus thrombosis. The test begins with a lumbar puncture and monitoring of CSF pressure at baseline. The internal jugular vein on the suspected side is then compressed and measurement of CSF pressure change recorded, followed by release of the vein and repeating the sequence for the contralateral internal jugular vein. Occlusion of a patent vein should increase CSF pressure and failure to do so on the affected side with a good response on the unaffected side would be positive, indicating the presence of thrombosis. This maneuver has since been avoided as it is unreliable and adds unwarranted risks, including possible brain herniation.

Multiple modalities of imaging can detect sinus thrombosis. CT with contrast may reveal the empty "delta sign," in which triangular high attenuation is seen in the peripheral rim of the sinus on axial section, with a low attenuation center representing thrombus, though this sign is not always present (Fig. 13.9). MRI is a more sensitive modality to detect flow and thrombus, with increased T1 and T2 signal intensity seen at the site of thrombus, and magnetic resonance venography (MRV) would be the most accurate modality to observe flow deficiency (Fig. 13.10).

Treatment for thrombosis with IV antibiotics in combination with mastoidectomy, drainage of infection, dissection and clearance of granulation tissue around the affected sinus extradurally has been well described.

Surgical management of the thrombosed sinus itself has been debated. Conservative management includes needle aspiration of the sinus, with consideration for a very small opening into the sinus in the absence of flow to drain any frank purulence only. Prior recommendations to incise the sigmoid sinus and proceed with complete thrombectomy have become controversial, with many modern small series showing no additional benefit in removing the clot.[37,38] One contemporary series argues that strict conservative management may not always apply in the modern era of antibiotic resistance, and described a small series of tailored aggressive surgical management with either venous sinus resection or Fogarty catheter embolectomy of thromboses.[39] Antibiotic coverage for at least 4–6 weeks is often recommended.

Anticoagulation for the thrombosis has been controversial within the literature. Anticoagulation is utilized in attempts to prevent further thrombosis and obstruction with venous infarction, though has associated risks itself including bleeding, thrombocytopenia, and interactions with other medications. Experience with anticoagulation for sinus thrombosis arising from causes other than temporal bone infection, such as prothrombotic states or trauma, in the medical literature has been extrapolated to otogenic cases and has found benefit in the use of anticoagulation. In a series of nine patients with otogenic sigmoid sinus thrombosis in whom six patients received anticoagulation, Bradley and colleagues observed no persistent sepsis and embolization, though patients were heterogeneously treated and some patients lost to follow-up.[40] The authors recommended selective use of anticoagulation rather than routinely in these patients. In a case series and review of the pediatric literature, Sitton and colleagues found 19 cases treated with anticoagulation, with 4 patients suffering a complication of anticoagulation, which were either postoperative bleeding or hematoma formation.[41] All but three of those patients had complete resolution of symptoms, although 16 patients had partial thrombus or persistent occlusion at follow-up. Authors have suggested selective use in patients with higher risk such as those with extensive thrombosis beyond the sigmoid sinus, neurologic changes, underlying prothrombotic states, or septic emboli. Prevention of thrombus progression and symptomatic improvement may be goals of anticoagulation but the finding of recanalization is not necessary. Due to the rarity of otogenic thrombosis, no clear evidence exists to date. Patients should undergo serial imaging to monitor thrombus progression or resolution. Initially proposed in the preantibiotic era, internal jugular vein ligation for the prevention embolization is now rarely required, reserved for uncontrolled instances of septic embolization or direct spread of suppuration into the neck.

OTITIC HYDROCEPHALUS

Suppurative ear infections can lead to increased intracranial pressure in the absence of focal neurologic signs and normal CSF analysis without intracranial abscess, mass effect, edema, or meningitis. Otitic hydrocephalus refers to this uncommon condition when associated with any middle ear or mastoid disease. Though previously described, this condition was first referred to as otitic hydrocephalus by C.P. Symonds in 1931.[42] Its pathophysiology is not well understood, but has been suspected to be related to decreased CSF absorption from arachnoid granulations, and some have argued that a degree of thrombosis of the venous sinuses, particularly the superior sagittal sinus, must be involved.[43,44] Though a high correlation of sinus thrombosis with this entity has been found, some cases without any signs of thrombosis have been reported, and patients with lateral sinus thrombosis do not necessarily exhibit increased pressures. Variations in dominance of venous sinus flow and possible biochemical phenomenon related to the sinus epithelium rather than mechanical flow obstruction may contribute.

Generic symptoms of increased intracranial pressure including intermittent nausea, headache, somnolence, and vision changes can be observed in addition to otologic symptoms, though the increased intracranial pressure may occur in delayed fashion after the onset of ear disease. Physical examination may include papilledema, less commonly lateral rectus palsy with diplopia, and elevated CSF opening pressure on lumbar puncture. Radiologic work-up is aimed at ruling out the other intracranial complications of otologic disease covered in this text, particularly intracranial abscess formation and sinus thrombosis. MRV is useful to assess complete or partial thrombosis of the sinuses. Close monitoring of the patient and treatment of the otologic source should be completed. Visual symptoms should be carefully monitored in conjunction with ophthalmological consultation. Treatment is similar to that for lateral sinus thrombosis with additional interventions to address increased intracranial pressure medically with corticosteroids and diuretics such as acetazolamide and dexamethasone. Resolution of increased pressures may require months of treatment and in severe cases may be required neurosurgical and ophthalmological interventions such as CSF shunts or optic nerve sheath fenestration.

SUBDURAL EMPYEMA

Subdural empyema refers to the development of purulent fluid within the space between the dura mater and arachnoid or pia mater. This is a rare complication overall and more commonly associated with infections other than otogenic sources, such as sinusitis, trauma, or neurosurgical procedures. It is associated with a high mortality rate and morbidity from neurologic sequelae.

Patients may present similarly to the other intracranial complications with fever, otorrhea and signs of otogenic infection in combination with signs and symptoms of increased intracranial pressure, neurological decline, or possibly seizures. Contrast-enhanced CT scan will reveal a rim-enhancing low-attenuation collection, though the pus is slightly hyperdense to CSF characteristics, in the subdural space over a cerebral convexity and possible effacement of cerebral sulci. In cases where imaging is obtained early in the development of disease, a small fluid collection may be subtle and its location relative to the dura not immediately clear.[45] MRI is superior in delineating the purulent fluid from surrounding brain, CSF, and laterally displaced dura. MRI with gadolinium contrast reveals intense meningeal enhancement around the empyema.

Treatment of subdural empyema requires urgent neurosurgical intervention in addition to IV antibiotics with CNS penetration. Typically a craniotomy or burr hole is required for drainage of the purulent collection. If the patient is stable and can tolerate the procedure, mastoidectomy and any associated procedures to clear the otologic infection can be undertaken in the same setting.

BRAIN ABSCESS

Abscess formation within the brain parenchyma can occur with surrounding encephalitis as a complication of temporal bone infections. Spread of infection is suspected to be due to retrograde spread in venous thrombophlebitis, causing accumulation of purulence and eventual capsule formation in either the cerebrum, typically in the temporal lobe, or in the cerebellum. Case series in the literature conflict as to whether children or adults more commonly develop these abscesses.[46,47]

The clinical presentation of otogenic brain abscess may include fever, neurologic change in mental status, headache, seizures, and papilledema. A generalized progression of symptoms may correlate with pathological changes: (1) initial cerebritis is related to a clinical encephalitic stage with fever, headache, and drowsiness; (2) localization and early abscess formation initially may be silent; (3) expansion of the initial fluid collection may trigger focal neurological deficits, mental status changes, and increased intracranial pressure; and (4) rupture of the abscess may produce abrupt, rapid neurological deterioration and possible mortality. Imaging work-up with and without contrast should be obtained with CT and MRI, which reveal regions of cerebritis in early formation and mass effect and rim enhancement for well-formed collections. MRI is more sensitive in evaluating for early abscess, though CT may be useful for the bony detail in assessing the otologic source.

The classic treatment for brain abscesses involves IV antibiotics and neurosurgical drainage, often through an open craniotomy or image-guided approach with aspiration through a burr hole. Mastoidectomy and clearance of the otologic source has been suggested to follow either in the same setting or at a second stage. In one review from India of 36 patients with intracranial abscess, all patients were treated with neurosurgical drainage and mastoidectomy during the same setting and the authors recommended concurrent procedures as a safe and cost-effective option.[48] As with other intracranial complications, more conservative or less invasive management trends have been found in more modern literature and remain controversial. In a pediatric series of patients with intracranial abscess formation, one out of seven patients with intraparenchymal abscess was treated with mastoidectomy and medical therapy without neurologic sequelae, similar to the other six undergoing surgical drainage of the abscess.[49] A separate case series of adults and children with intracranial complications noted five brain abscesses: all of which were treated with IV antibiotics and tympanomastoidectomy without the need for neurosurgical intervention.[46] In a review of the literature on all brain abscesses including those not of otogenic origin, which includes only retrospective reviews, patients with smaller abscesses (<2.5 cm), good initial Glasgow Coma Scale scores (>12) and in whom the micro-organism is likely isolated appeared to be better candidates for medical treatment alone.[50] In addition to the infection, brain edema and control or prophylaxis for seizures should be treated medically.

REFERENCES

1. Jung TT, Alper CM, Hellstrom SO, et al. Panel 8: Complications and sequelae. Otolaryngol Head Neck Surg. 2013; 148(4 Suppl):E122-43.

2. Osborn AJ, Blaser S, Papsin BC. Decisions regarding intracranial complications from acute mastoiditis in children. Curr Opin Otolaryngol Head Neck Surg. 2011;19(6):478-85.
3. Van Zuijlen DA, Schilder AG, Van Balen FA, et al. National differences in incidence of acute mastoiditis: relationship to prescribing patterns of antibiotics for acute otitis media? Pediatr Infect Dis J. 2001;20(2):140-44.
4. Kvaerner KJ, Bentdal Y, Karevold G. Acute mastoiditis in Norway: no evidence for an increase. Int J Pediatr Otorhinolaryngol. 2007;71(10):1579-83.
5. Daniel M, Gautam S, Scrivener TA, et al. What effect has pneumococcal vaccination had on acute mastoiditis? J Laryngol Otol. 2013;127(Suppl 1):S30-34.
6. Choi SS, Lander L. Pediatric acute mastoiditis in the post-pneumococcal conjugate vaccine era. Laryngoscope. 2011; 121(5):1072-80.
7. van den Aardweg MT, Rovers MM, de Ru JA, et al. A systematic review of diagnostic criteria for acute mastoiditis in children. Otol Neurotol. 2008;29(6):751-7.
8. Bilavsky E, Yarden-Bilavsky H, Samra Z, et al. Clinical, laboratory, and microbiological differences between children with simple or complicated mastoiditis. Int J Pediatr Otorhinolaryngol. 2009;73(9):1270-73.
9. Geva A, Oestreicher-Kedem Y, Fishman G, et al. Conservative management of acute mastoiditis in children. Int J Pediatr Otorhinolaryngol. 2008;72(5):629-34.
10. Luntz M, Brodsky A, Nusem S, et al. Acute mastoiditis - the antibiotic era: a multicenter study. Int J Pediatr Otorhinolaryngol. 2001;57(1):1-9.
11. Holt GR, Gates GA. Masked mastoiditis. Laryngoscope. 1983; 93(8):1034-7.
12. Groth A, Enoksson F, Hultcrantz M, et al. Acute mastoiditis in children aged 0-16 years - a national study of 678 cases in Sweden comparing different age groups. Int J Pediatr Otorhinolaryngol. 2012;76(10):1494-1500.
13. Luntz M, Bartal K, Brodsky A, et al. Acute mastoiditis: the role of imaging for identifying intracranial complications. Laryngoscope. 2012;122(12):2813-17.
14. Mallur PS, Harirchian S, Lalwani AK. Preoperative and postoperative intracranial complications of acute mastoiditis. Ann Otology Rhinol Laryngol. 2009;118(2):118-23.
15. Psarommatis IM, Voudouris C, Douros K, et al. Algorithmic management of pediatric acute mastoiditis. Int J Pediatr Otorhinolaryngol. 2012;76(6):791-6.
16. Chesney J, Black A, Choo D. What is the best practice for acute mastoiditis in children? Laryngoscope. 2014;124(5): 1057-8.
17. Psarommatis I, Giannakopoulos P, Theodorou E, et al. Mastoid subperiosteal abscess in children: drainage or mastoidectomy? J Laryngol Otol. 2012;126(12):1204-8.
18. Bakhos D, Trijolet JP, Moriniere S, et al. Conservative management of acute mastoiditis in children. Arch Otolaryngol Head Neck Surg. 2011;137(4):346-50.
19. Pappas DG. Friedrich von Bezold (1842-1908). Ear Nose Throat J. 1996;75(12):760-61.
20. Virapongse C, Sarwar M, Bhimani S, et al. Computed tomography of temporal bone pneumatization: 1. Normal pattern and morphology. AJR. 1985;145(3):473-81.
21. Matis GK, de ASDO, Chrysou OI, et al. Giuseppe Gradenigo: Much more than a syndrome! Historical vignette. Surg Neurol Int. 2012;3:122.
22. Kong SK, Lee IW, Goh EK, Park SE. Acute otitis media-induced petrous apicitis presenting as the Gradenigo syndrome: successfully treated by ventilation tube insertion. Am J Otolaryngol. 2011;32(5):445-7.
23. Burston BJ, Pretorius PM, Ramsden JD. Gradenigo's syndrome: successful conservative treatment in adult and paediatric patients. J Laryngol Otol. 2005;119(4):325-9.
24. Marianowski R, Rocton S, Ait-Amer JL, et al. Conservative management of Gradenigo syndrome in a child. Int J Pediatr Otorhinolaryngol. 2001;57(1):79-83.
25. Makeham TP, Croxson GR, Coulson S. Infective causes of facial nerve paralysis. Otol Neurotol. 2007;28(1):100-103.
26. Redaelli de Zinis LO, Gamba P, Balzanelli C. Acute otitis media and facial nerve paralysis in adults. Otol Neurotol 2003;24(1):113-17.
27. Wang CH, Chang YC, Shih HM, et al. Facial palsy in children: emergency department management and outcome. Pediatr Emerg Care. 2010;26(2):121-5.
28. Angeli SI, Chiossone E. Surgical treatment of the facial nerve in facial paralysis. Otolaryngol Clini N Am. 1997;30(5): 683-700.
29. Telischi FF, Chandler JR, May M, Schaitkin B. Infection: otitis media, cholesteatoma, necrotizing external otitis, and other inflammatory disorders. In: May M, Schaitkin B (eds), The facial nerve. New York: Thieme; 2000. pp. 383-91.
30. Ibrahim SI, Cheang PP, Nunez DA. Incidence of meningitis secondary to suppurative otitis media in adults. J Laryngol Otol. 2010;124(11):1158-61.
31. Kangsanarak J, Navacharoen N, Fooanant S, et al. Intracranial complications of suppurative otitis media: 13 years' experience. Am J Otol. 1995;16(1):104-9.
32. Odio CM, Faingezicht I, Paris M, et al. The beneficial effects of early dexamethasone administration in infants and children with bacterial meningitis. N Engl J Med. 1991; 324(22):1525-31.
33. Brouwer MC, McIntyre P, Prasad K, et al. Corticosteroids for acute bacterial meningitis. Cochrane Database Syst Rev. 2013;6:CD004405.
34. Bales CB, Sobol S, Wetmore R, et al. Lateral sinus thrombosis as a complication of otitis media: 10-year experience at the children's hospital of Philadelphia. Pediatrics. 2009;123(2):709-13.
35. Seven H, Ozbal AE, Turgut S. Management of otogenic lateral sinus thrombosis. Am J Otolaryngol. 2004;25(5):329-33.
36. Garcia RD, Baker AS, Cunningham MJ, et al. Lateral sinus thrombosis associated with otitis media and mastoiditis in children. Pediatr Infect Dis J. 1995;14(7):617-23.
37. Ropposch T, Nemetz U, Braun EM, et al. Management of otogenic sigmoid sinus thrombosis. Otol Neurotol. 2011; 32(7):1120-23.
38. Ropposch T, Nemetz U, Braun EM, et al. Low molecular weight heparin therapy in pediatric otogenic sigmoid sinus thrombosis: a safe treatment option? Int J Pediatr Otorhinolaryngol. 2012;76(7):1023-26.

39. Manolidis S, Kutz JW, Jr. Diagnosis and management of lateral sinus thrombosis. Otol Neurotol. 2005;26(5):1045-51.
40. Bradley DT, Hashisaki GT, Mason JC. Otogenic sigmoid sinus thrombosis: what is the role of anticoagulation? Laryngoscope. 2002;112(10):1726-9.
41. Sitton MS, Chun R. Pediatric otogenic lateral sinus thrombosis: role of anticoagulation and surgery. Int J Pediatr Otorhinolaryngol. 2012;76(3):428-32.
42. Lenz RP, McDonald GA. Otitic hydrocephalus. Laryngoscope. 1984;94(11 Pt 1):1451-4.
43. Sadoghi M, Dabirmoghaddam P. Otitic hydrocephalus: case report and literature review. Am J Otolaryngol. 2007; 28(3):187-90.
44. Tomkinson A, Mills RG, Cantrell PJ. The pathophysiology of otitic hydrocephalus. J Laryngol Otol. 1997;111(8):757-9.
45. Rich PM, Deasy NP, Jarosz JM. Intracranial dural empyema. Br J Radiol. 2000;73(876):1329-36.
46. Wanna GB, Dharamsi LM, Moss JR, et al. Contemporary management of intracranial complications of otitis media. Otol Neurotol. 2010;31(1):111-17.
47. Sennaroglu L, Sozeri B. Otogenic brain abscess: review of 41 cases. OtolaryngolHead Neck Surg. 2000;123(6):751-5.
48. Kurien M, Job A, Mathew J, et al. Otogenic intracranial abscess: concurrent craniotomy and mastoidectomy – changing trends in a developing country. Arch Otolaryngol Head Neck Surg. 1998;124(12):1353-6.
49. Isaacson B, Mirabal C, Kutz JW, et al. Pediatric otogenic intracranial abscesses. Otolaryngol Head Neck Surg. 2010; 142(3):434-7.
50. Arlotti M, Grossi P, Pea F, et al. Consensus document on controversial issues for the treatment of infections of the central nervous system: bacterial brain abscesses. Int J Infect Dis. 2010;14(Suppl 4):S79-92.

CHAPTER 14

Otosclerosis

Alicia M Quesnel, Michael J McKenna

INTRODUCTION

Otosclerosis is a disease of abnormal bone remodeling that is localized to the otic capsule[1] and occurs only in man. Most commonly, otosclerosis causes a conductive hearing loss, but may also present with mixed or sensorineural hearing loss. The bony pathologic changes in otosclerosis occur only in the otic capsule, unlike other metabolic bone disorders, such as Paget's disease or osteoporosis. It is among the most common causes of acquired conductive hearing loss, and the clinical prevalence is approximately 0.3%[2,3] (although a large range has been reported in the literature). The incidence of otosclerosis seen on temporal bone specimens, however, is significantly higher at 8% to 12%.[4] The prevalence varies significantly by gender and race. The incidence is twofold higher in women than in men, suggesting a role of female hormones in its development or progression. The disease is much more prevalent in Caucasians than in Asians, Native Americans, and Africans. Patients typically present between the late teen years to 45 years old. Otosclerosis is bilateral in most patients, with clinical symptoms ultimately developing in both ears in approximately 85%. In about 20–30% of patients, a sensorineural component of hearing loss develops in addition to the conductive loss.

PATHOGENESIS

Histopathology

Stapes ankylosis as a cause of deafness was first reported by Valsalva in 1704. In 1857, Toynbee reported osseous ankylosis of the stapes to be one of the most common causes of deafness, and von Troltsch in 1867 described the pathologic findings as sclerosis.[5] Adam Politzer is credited as clearly describing bony proliferation as the cause of stapes ankylosis and hearing loss in this condition, which stood in contradistinction to previous theories that dry catarrhal inflammation of the middle ear led to fixation of the stapes.[6] In 1893, Politzer began gaining worldwide acceptance of this pathologic basis of the condition, and in 1901, he coined the term otosclerosis.[7]

Since the establishment of otosclerosis as a primary disorder of the otic capsule bone, many authors have contributed to the description of the pathologic findings in otosclerosis. This has been accomplished through the study of meticulously prepared and carefully sectioned human temporal bones. The histopathologic findings in otosclerosis consist of islands of new bone formation, bone resorption, and vascular proliferation in characteristic locations throughout the otic capsule (Figs. 14.1A and B). Lesions begin with resorption of bone around blood vessels, creating an enlargement of the perivascular spaces. Connective tissue is deposited in these spaces, and there may be increased cellularity consisting of fibroblasts, histiocytes, and osteoclasts. When this appearance dominates, the lesion is referred to as "otospongiotic." Deposition of immature woven bone then proceeds, which becomes mature lamellar bone. This causes a thickening of structures and often results in very dense mineralized bone, which is called "sclerotic." Frequently, the temporal bone from a patient with otosclerosis will contain otospongiotic, otosclerotic, and mixed foci, representing the various stages of the disease.[8]

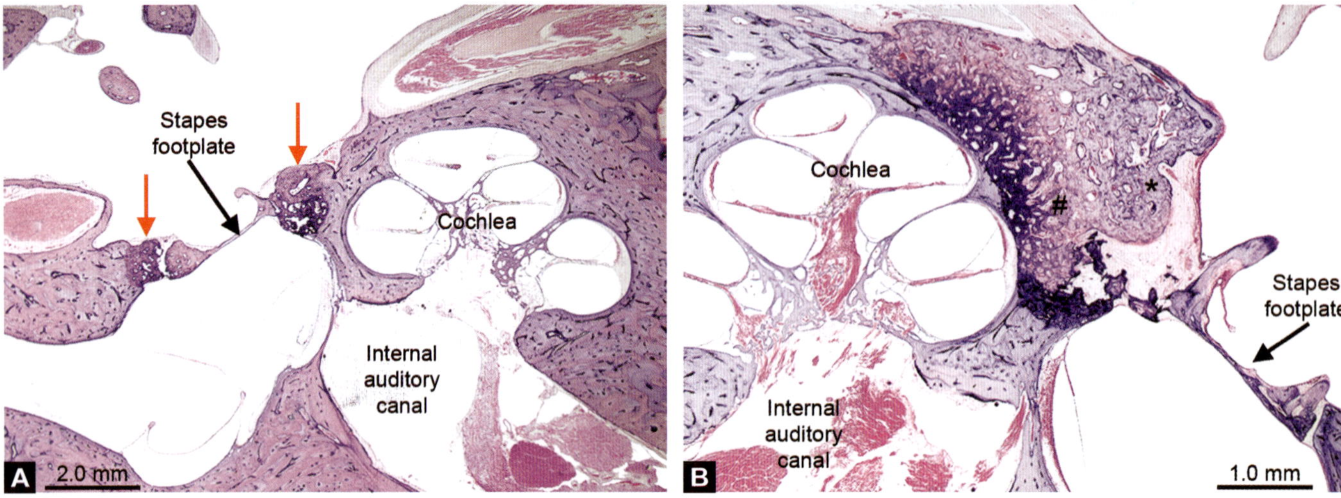

Figs. 14.1A and B: Histopathology of otosclerosis in temporal bone specimens. (A) Patient with small foci of otosclerosis both anterior to the footplate and posterior to the footplate (arrows). The anterior focus can be seen fixing the footplate. (B) Patient with more extensive otosclerosis. There are areas of otosclerotic bone (*), with more dense bone and small fibrous spaces, and areas of otospongiotic bone (#), with larger vascular channels and osteocytes present.

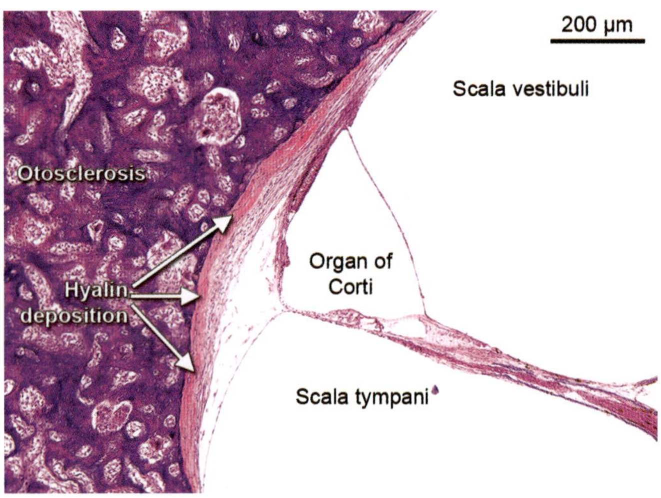

Fig. 14.2: Otosclerosis involving the endosteal layer of the cochlea, with associated hyaline deposition in the spiral ligament.

The most common site of involvement in the temporal bone is the area anterior to the oval window. In fact, 96% of temporal bones from patients with clinical otosclerosis have a focus of otosclerosis anterior to the oval window.[9] The fissula ante fenestra, which is an embryologic remnant of fibrous tissue anterior to the oval window, was initially thought to be the site of origin of otosclerosis due to this predilection. Identification of specimens in which the foci of otosclerosis lies anterior to the oval window, but separate from the fissula ante fenestrum, however, does not support this theory.[2,10] Other sites of involvement for otosclerosis include the round window niche in 30%, the area posterior to the oval window in 12%, around the cochlea in 12%, the posterior and anterior walls of the internal auditory canal in 5% each, and around the semicircular canals in 2.4%.[8]

The development of otosclerosis at the anterior margin of the oval window may initially result in posterior impaction of the footplate at the posterior stapedovestibular joint. This results in a small conductive hearing loss.[11] True bony ankylosis of the stapes footplate may then ensue, causing a larger conductive hearing loss, usually > 30 dB.

Sensorineural hearing loss in otosclerosis may develop when foci of otosclerosis invade the endosteal layer of the cochlea (Fig. 14.2). This results in hyalin deposition in the spiral ligament adjacent to pericochlear otosclerotic foci, and has been shown to correlate with sensorineural hearing loss.[12,13] There are likely additional mechanisms for sensorineural hearing loss in otosclerosis, including release of toxic cytokines, such as tumor necrosis factor alpha.[14] Cytokines may reach the fluid spaces within the cochlea from a remote lesion of otosclerosis by diffusion through a network of interconnected canalicular channels.[15]

Pathophysiology

The normal otic capsule bone is unique in its extremely low rate of bone turnover and remodeling, at a rate of 0.13% per year compared to 10% per year in the general skeleton.[16] Osteoprotegerin has been identified as a local factor that restricts bone remodeling in the otic capsule. It is a competitive inhibitor of the receptor activator of nuclear factor KB (RANK) ligand. RANK ligand, which is located on osteoblasts, stimulates osteoclast-mediated bone resorption when it binds to RANK receptor on an osteoclast.[17,18] Osteoprotegerin knockout mice develop abnormal bone remodeling in the otic capsule and hearing loss, suggesting a role of osteoprotegerin pathway in the pathophysiology of otosclerosis.[18]

Etiology

There is evidence to support both genetic and environmental factors in the development of otosclerosis. There is a clear hereditary component to the etiology of otosclerosis, with about 50% of patients reporting a family member who is also affected. Most studies support an autosomal dominant transmission with variable penetrance. A null mutation in the COL1A1 gene, which codes for type I collagen and is also mutated in mild forms of osteogenesis imperfect, has been associated with clinical otosclerosis.[19] Ten separate loci, labeled OTSC1 through OTSC10, have been identified by genetic linkage analyses.

There is considerable evidence that the measles virus plays a role in the development of otosclerosis, perhaps in patients who are genetically susceptible. In specimens from patients with otosclerosis, the following evidence has been reported: (1) measles-like structures have been seen on electron microscopy, (2) measles RNA has been isolated with reverse transcription polymerase chain reaction amplification, (3) measles antigens have been identified immunohistochemically,[20] and (4) elevated levels of antimeasles IgG has been found in perilymph.[21,22]

CLINICAL FINDINGS: SYMPTOMS AND SIGNS

Symptoms

Patients with otosclerosis most commonly present with progressive hearing loss, which may be unilateral or bilateral. Patients with unilateral hearing loss from otosclerosis often seek evaluation when they notice difficulty in hearing background noise and difficulty that occurs when the affected ear is toward the speaker. Patients most commonly present when thresholds reach the 30–50 dB range in the mid frequencies, but there is variation depending on whether symptoms are unilateral or bilateral and the complexity of hearing needs for each patient. Paradoxically, some patients with otosclerosis report improved hearing in noisy environments. This is the result of increased signal-to-noise ratio with conductive hearing loss and the tendency for raised voices in noisy environments and is termed paracusis of Willis.

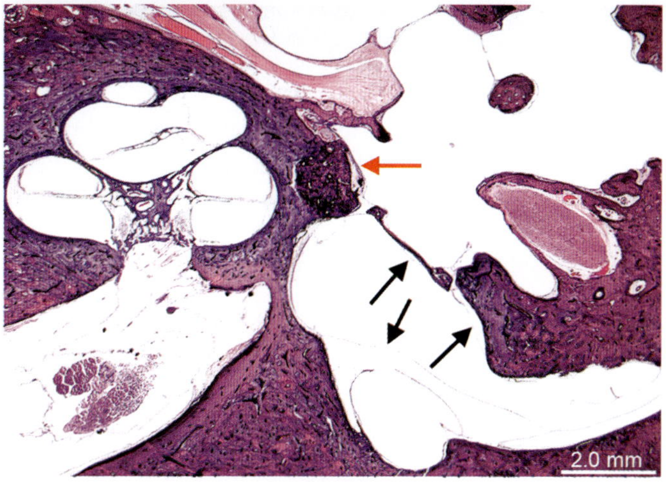

Fig. 14.3: Temporal bone specimen from a patient with both Meniere's disease and otosclerosis. The red arrow indicates a focus of otosclerosis. The saccular membrane (solid arrows) can be seen contacting the undersurface of the footplate, which would put this ear at risk for sensorineural hearing loss with fenestration of the footplate causing disruption of the saccular membrane.

Tinnitus is present in 65% of patients with otosclerosis,[23] and often resolves with surgical correction of the conductive hearing loss.[24]

Vestibular symptoms occur in 10% to 30% of patients with otosclerosis, and range from unsteadiness to rotatory vertigo to benign paroxysmal positional vertigo.[25] Vestibular symptoms are more common in patients with mixed hearing loss and elevated bone thresholds. Vestibular nerve degeneration with reduced counts of scarpa's ganglion neurons is seen in patients with otosclerosis with vestibular symptoms as compared to otosclerosis patients without vestibular symptoms or controls.[26] In any patient with both otosclerosis and vestibular symptoms, the clinician should perform a careful history to elicit any features suggestive of concomitant Meniere's syndrome. Stapedectomy is contraindicated in otosclerosis patients with Meniere's syndrome due to the significantly increased risk of profound sensorineural hearing loss (Fig. 14.3).

Signs

Patients with otosclerosis have normal-appearing tympanic membranes on otoscopy and otomicroscopic examination.

Table 14.1: Differential diagnosis for otosclerosis (i.e. causes of conductive hearing loss with normal otoscopy)
Malleus head fixation
Chronic otitis media leading to ossicular discontinuity, such as incus long process erosion
Tympanosclerosis causing ossicular fixation, including stapes footplate fixation
Traumatic subluxation or dislocation of the ossicles
Third window syndrome (e.g. superior semicircular canal dehiscence) causing a pseudoconductive hearing loss

In fact, this normal appearance will help eliminate other possible causes of progressive conductive hearing loss from the differential diagnosis (Table 14.1). The tympanic membrane is normally mobile on pneumatic otoscopy. A reddish hue to the promontory when viewed through the tympanic membrane, called Schwartze's sign, is seen in a minority of patients. Increased blood flow over the promontory as measured by Doppler flowmetry has been reported in patients with Schwartze's sign, and may suggest more active disease.[27]

Tuning fork examination is critical if otosclerosis is suspected. The typical conductive hearing loss is confirmed by the Rinne and Weber tests. The Rinne test should demonstrate bone conduction hearing better than air conduction hearing, which is referred to as a negative Rinne test. The Weber test demonstrates lateralization of the sound to the ear with the worse conductive hearing loss. Most clinicians use the 512 Hz tuning fork, which results in a negative Rinne when there is at least a 25 dB conductive hearing loss. The 256Hz tuning fork can be used to identify mild conductive hearing loss of 20 dB* or more, and may identify early otosclerosis. The 1024 Hz tuning fork can confirm a conductive hearing loss of at least 30 dB with the Rinne test.

Although otosclerosis is considered a localized disease of the temporal bone, some patients with otosclerosis have slightly blue-colored sclera of the eyes on careful inspection. Blue sclera is characteristically seen in patients with type I osteogenesis imperfecta, which results from mutations encoding type I collagen and causes pathologic lesions in the temporal bone consistent with otosclerosis.[28] There is also an association between otosclerosis and osteoporosis. A retrospective study has shown a nearly fourfold higher incidence of osteoporosis in female patients with otosclerosis compared to a control group of women without otosclerosis.[29]

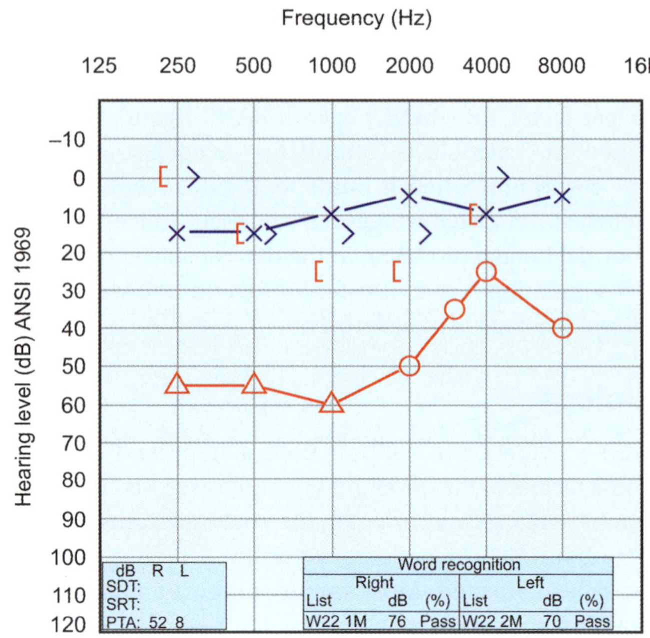

Fig. 14.4: Typical audiogram with Cahart's notch. In the right ear, a large air–bone gap is demonstrated with elevation of the bone threshold at 2000 kHz, called the Cahart's notch. Word recognition scores of "pass" in both ears indicate normal speech discrimination.

EVALUATION: AUDIOLOGY, RADIOLOGY, AND HISTOLOGY

Audiologic Testing

The characteristic audiogram for otosclerosis demonstrates a moderate conductive hearing loss with a Cahart's notch and normal word recognition score (Fig. 14.4). The Cahart's notch refers to an artifactual elevation of the bone threshold at 2000 Hz that results from an alteration in the resonance of the otic capsule with an ankylosed stapes. The notch disappears after stapedectomy. Clinicians estimate that 20 to 30% of patients develop a mixed hearing loss, although the sensorineural component may not be present at the time of initial audiologic evaluation. Presentation with pure sensorineural hearing loss, termed *cochlear otosclerosis*, is exceedingly rare.[30] Otosclerosis should only be considered the cause of pure sensorineural hearing loss if other etiologies, such as a retrocochlear lesion, have been ruled out and: (1) there is evidence of the typical conductive or mixed loss in the contralateral ear, (2) there is a convincing family history of otosclerosis, (3) there is a strong Schwartze's sign,[31] and/or (4) there is evidence of

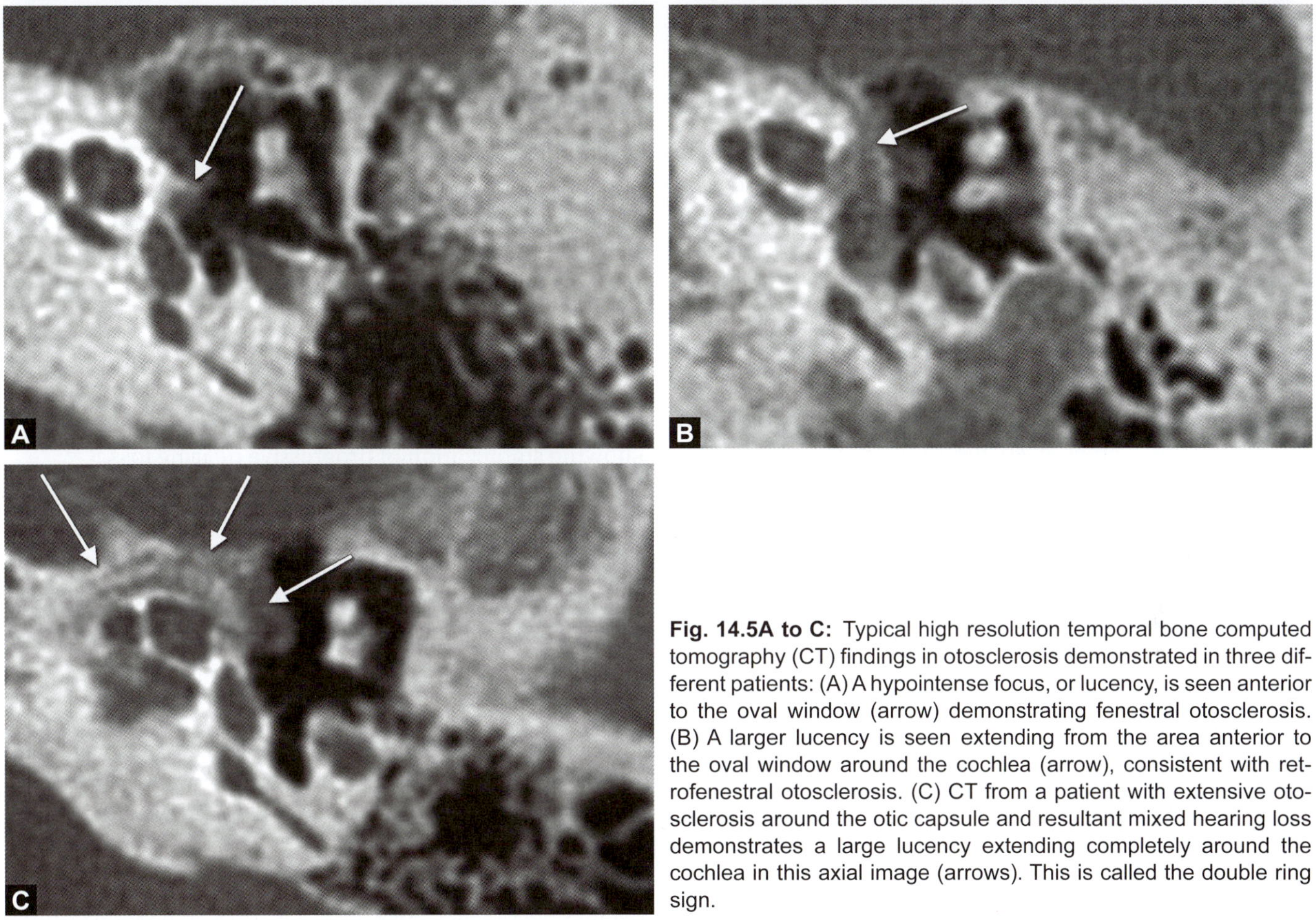

Fig. 14.5A to C: Typical high resolution temporal bone computed tomography (CT) findings in otosclerosis demonstrated in three different patients: (A) A hypointense focus, or lucency, is seen anterior to the oval window (arrow) demonstrating fenestral otosclerosis. (B) A larger lucency is seen extending from the area anterior to the oval window around the cochlea (arrow), consistent with retrofenestral otosclerosis. (C) CT from a patient with extensive otosclerosis around the otic capsule and resultant mixed hearing loss demonstrates a large lucency extending completely around the cochlea in this axial image (arrows). This is called the double ring sign.

otosclerosis on computed tomography (CT). CT provides the most valuable radiographic evidence to confirm that otosclerosis is the cause of sensorineural hearing loss.

Tympanometry is usually normal, although cases with rigid stapes fixation may result in type A_s tympanogram, indicating stiffness of the ossicular chain. Abnormal tympanometry, such as type B tympanogram (flat immittance) or type C tympanogram (indicating negative pressure in the middle ear), suggests another etiology of conductive hearing loss or coexistence of otosclerosis with another pathology. Acoustic reflex testing is typically abnormal or absent, which confirms that the conductive hearing loss is of middle ear origin. This is important because patients with semicircular canal dehiscence and other third window syndromes may present with conductive hearing loss, mimicking otosclerosis.[32] Laser Doppler vibrometry measurements of umbo velocity may help confirm the diagnosis of otosclerosis, but is not routinely performed as it does not suffice a definitive diagnostic tool.[33]

Radiologic Imaging

High-resolution CT of the temporal bone is the most useful radiologic imaging test for otosclerosis because of the detailed bony structure that can be depicted. Very thin slice imaging (0.5–0.6 mm collimation), which is used in most modern temporal bone protocols, helps increase the sensitivity for detecting pathologic lesions around the stapes footplate, cochlea, and labyrinth. An otosclerotic focus appears as a lucency, or hypodense area, on CT. When this is located anterior to the oval window or around the footplate, this is termed fenestral otosclerosis. When the area of lucency extends around the cochlea, this is termed retrofenestral otosclerosis, and suggests more extensive otosclerosis that is often associated with a mixed hearing loss. Very advanced otosclerosis that surrounds the otic capsule can appear as a double ring sign, in which there is a complete circular lucency surrounding the cochlea (Figs. 14.5A to C).

The diagnosis of otosclerosis can be confirmed by CT imaging with a high sensitivity. CT is accurate in identifying cases of otosclerosis, in which the diagnosis is suggested by clinical evaluation and confirmed by intraoperative surgical findings, >90% of the time.[34,35] The ability of CT to identify small, subtle otosclerotic foci that can be seen on histologic sections of temporal bones with otosclerosis may be more limited. The extension of an otosclerotic foci through the pericochlear bone to the endosteal layer of the cochlea can be identified on CT, though CT may underestimate extension to the endosteal layer.[36] This distinction may be important in consideration of medical therapy for progressive sensorineural hearing loss related to otosclerosis. Direct extension of the otosclerotic focus to the cochlear endosteal layer has been associated with hyalin deposition in the spiral ligament and sensorineural hearing loss[12,13] (*see* Fig. 14.2).

Active foci of otosclerosis can be appreciated as areas of enhancement on magnetic resonance imaging (MRI) of the temporal bones with gadolinium contrast. This is presumably related to the highly vascular structure of active otospongiosis, which allows pooling of the contrast. However, given the lack of signal in the normal dense temporal bone on both T1- and T2-weighted MRI, CT is much more sensitive for the diagnosis of otosclerosis.[37,38]

Histology

Histologic examination of the removed portion of the stapes footplate (when a stapedectomy rather than a small fenestra stapedotomy is performed) can confirm the diagnosis of otosclerosis. However, a removed stapes footplate specimen may fail to demonstrate otosclerosis due to fracture of the footplate such that the otosclerotic focus is left attached to the otic capsule or lack of direct involvement of the stapes footplate. Since otosclerosis is a disease of the otic capsule, which is not removed or biopsied during life, more complete examination of the extent of otosclerotic lesions is performed through histopathologic processing of postmortem donated temporal bone specimens (*see* Fig. 14.1).

TREATMENT

Medical Management

Medical treatment of otosclerosis remains controversial, as high-quality evidence to support definite benefit is still lacking. There is a wide variation in practice patterns with the use of medical therapies. Medications that inhibit osteoclast recruitment and activation have been utilized in the treatment of otosclerosis. Shambaugh and Scott first introduced sodium fluoride as a treatment for otosclerosis in the 1960s.[39] Since then multiple retrospective studies and one blinded prospective study have shown minimal reduction in progression of hearing loss due to otosclerosis in patients treated with fluoride.[40,41] Bisphosphonates are more potent inhibitors of bone remodeling and have subsequently become a standard treatment for other metabolic bone diseases, such as osteoporosis. Bisphosphonates remain at this time the most promising medical treatment for otosclerosis, with several clinical studies showing stabilization of progressive hearing loss.[42–44]

Amplification with hearing aids is another option for hearing rehabilitation for patients with otosclerosis. Speech discrimination is usually well preserved in otosclerosis, which enables successful amplification in these patients.

Surgical Management

Surgical management with stapedectomy is a well established and highly successful procedure for correcting the conductive hearing loss due to otosclerosis. Patients become candidates for stapedectomy when the conductive hearing loss exceeds approximately 25 dB at multiple frequencies. Most surgeons consider a negative Rinne tuning fork test (i.e. when bone conduction is better than air conduction) with a 512 Hz tuning fork a prerequisite for surgical candidacy. Concerns with operating on patients with smaller degrees of conductive hearing loss include failure to achieve a noticeable benefit to the patient even with successful surgery, and creation of a floating footplate during surgery due to incomplete fixation of the stapes footplate. For patients with bilateral disease, the ear with worse hearing should be operated on first. If a successful hearing result remains stable postoperatively for at least 6 months, the patient may choose to undergo stapedectomy on the second side.

Patients with Meniere's syndrome in the ear to be operated on are at significant risk of a severe sensorineural hearing loss postoperatively. In Meniere's syndrome, the wall of the saccule may become so distended that it adheres to the undersurface of the stapes footplate or approaches the footplate (*see* Fig. 14.5). This increases the risk of direct injury to the saccule, which may result in sensorineural hearing loss via mechanical trauma or

Table 14.2: Contraindications for stapedectomy

Absolute contraindications	*Relative contraindications*
Meniere's disease in the ear to be operated	Meniere's disease in the contralateral ear
Ear to be operated is the only hearing ear (unless patient has far advanced otosclerosis and receives minimal benefit from a hearing aid)	Concomitant chronic otitis media or severe Eustachian tube dysfunction in the ear to be operated
Ear to be operated is the only balancing ear	Significant concomitant sensorineural hearing loss that would necessitate the use of hearing aids after successful stapedectomy
Active infection (surgery should be delayed until resolved)	Occupation in which safety is dependent on balance (e.g. airplane pilot and roofing contractor)
Tympanic membrane perforation (perforation should be managed first)	Occupation that is dependent on tasting skills (e.g. chef and sommelier)

mixing of endolymphatic and perilymphatic fluid in the vestibule. Operating on an only hearing ear or an only balancing ear is contraindicated. Table 14.2 summarizes other conditions, in which observation or a hearing aid may be a better choice.

Outcomes for stapedectomy surgery are impressive, with up to 94% of patients achieving closure of the air-bone gap to within 10 dB.[45] Most modern series report at least significant hearing improvement (i.e. closure of the air bone gap within 20 dB) in 90% of patients, and closure within 10 dB in >80% of patients.[46-49] Although the stapedectomy technique has evolved over the past several decades, including the modern use of small fenestra stapedotomy with or without tissue grafts and introduction of lasers for fenestration, results have remained essentially unchanged, though excellent.

The immediate potential complications from stapedectomy include a 1-2 % of anacusis, dysequilibrium or vertigo (which rarely persists long term), change in taste (due to manipulation of the chorda tympani nerve), tympanic membrane perforation, and facial nerve injury (which is extremely rare). If there is an initially good hearing result, followed by sensorineural hearing loss in the week after surgery, the possibility of a granuloma, labyrinthitis, or pneumolabyrinth should be considered. Long term, there is some risk of recurrent hearing loss,

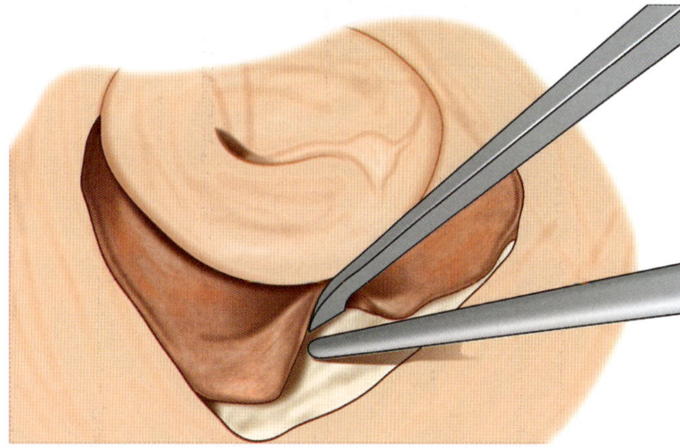

Fig. 14.6: A triangular tympanomeatal flap is created, with the longest portion of the flap overlying the area of the scutum that will be removed for exposure.

most commonly due to lateralization of the prosthesis with incus erosion. This can be addressed with revision stapedectomy.

Surgical Technique

Stapedectomy can be performed under either local or general anesthesia. Local anesthesia has the advantages of enabling monitoring of vestibular symptoms and hearing improvement with placement of the prosthesis, and reduced postanesthesia recovery time. General anesthesia assures the patient will remain still during the critical parts of the procedure, and many patients elect this due to anxiety about being awake during a surgical procedure.

A head holder, rather than standard flat headrest, is used to allow positioning of the patient's head relative to the shoulders and body. Positioning the head in a head-hanging position with an open angle between the operative ear and shoulder is helpful. Local injection of epinephrine with or without lidocaine in the external ear canal improves hemostasis. A triangular tympanomeatal flap incision in made in the medial posterior bony external canal wall skin, so that longest portion of the skin is centered in the area of the scutum where bone will be removed. The tympanomeatal flap is elevated from lateral to medial, until the annulus is encountered, taking care not to tear the delicate skin (Fig. 14.6). The annulus is elevated in a 180° fashion, so that the tympanomeatal flap can be folded anteriorly providing wide exposure of the middle ear space. The bony annulus and scutum is removed with a stapes curette until the facial nerve can be easily identified superiorly and the pyramidal eminence

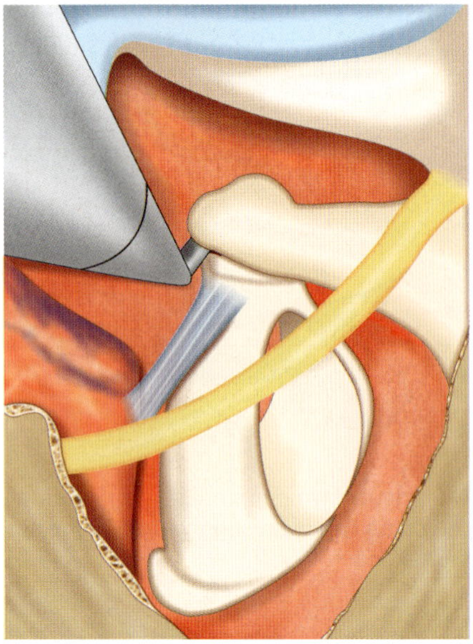

Fig. 14.7: The incudostapedial joint is separated with a joint knife. Note that the incudostapedial joint is positioned medial to the lenticular process of the incus. The exact joint location can be appreciated by gentle palpation of the incus and observation of the differential motion of the incus versus the fixed stapes at the incudostapedial joint.

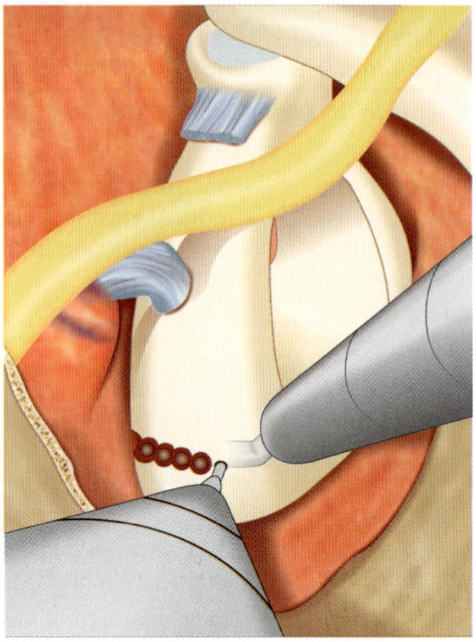

Fig. 14.8: The posterior crus of the stapes is transected with a laser. When possible, the anterior crus of the stapes is similarly transected with the laser. The stapes suprastructure is then down-fractured and removed.

can be seen posteriorly. This ensures adequate exposure. The ossicular chain is then palpated, confirming fixation of the stapes. The malleus and incus should be palpated at this time to confirm normal mobility, as rarely malleus fixation can coexist with otosclerosis. The round window niche is inspected for patency, and any concern for complete round window obliteration should be noted in the operative note. Given the inability to accurately identify complete obliteration with the surgical microscope, the stapedectomy may be performed even if concerns for round window obliteration exist. This will often still result in hearing improvement, but revision stapedectomy should not be attempted if there is no improvement in such a case.

Next, the incudostapedial joint is separated with a joint knife (Fig. 14.7). The posterior crus of the stapes is transected with a laser, traditionally a potassium titanyl phosphate (KTP), argon, or carbon dioxide (CO_2) laser (Fig. 14.8). One advantage of the KTP laser has been its convenient application using a handheld fiberoptic cable, in which the tip can be precisely directed at a target. Recent technology has enabled use of the CO_2 laser via a handheld fiber that utilizes layers of mirrors to propagate the CO_2 laser energy. The CO_2 wavelength is readily absorbed in water, and therefore the CO_2 laser has the theoretical advantages of less thermal energy spread and less collateral tissue damage. Improved hearing outcomes in stapedectomy with use of the CO_2 laser compared to the KTP laser has been suggested by some studies, but not demonstrated definitively.[50]

When possible, the anterior crus of the stapes is transected, and the stapes suprastructure is downfractured and removed. A measuring stick is used to determine the appropriate length of the stapes prosthesis, which should extend into the vestibule by 0.2 mm. Next, the footplate is fenestrated with the laser by creating a "rosette" pattern of laser spots that results in a 0.8 mm diameter fenestra (Fig. 14.9). The ash is then gently cleared away with a straight pick, typically revealing a completed fenestra. When the footplate is thick enough that the laser does not readily penetrate it, a micro-otologic drill with a small hand piece can be used at a low speed to complete the fenestration. The stapes prosthesis is brought into position, with the piston inserted into the fenestra and the "loop" placed around the long process of the incus. For most traditional stapes prostheses, the loop is then crimped around the long process of the incus to hold it securely in position (Fig. 14.10). In the last decade, stapes prostheses with a loop made from a heat-activated nickel titanium memory shape alloy have become more popular. These prostheses can be "crimped" into position using the heat of the laser at a lower setting, which results in a secure fixation to

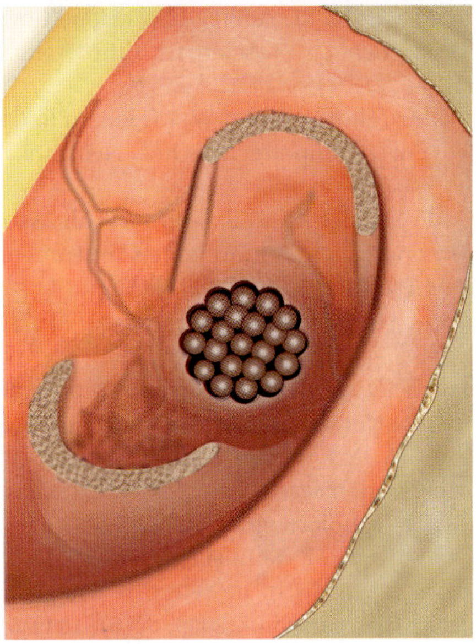

Fig. 14.9: The fenestra in the stapes footplate is created by making a series of laser spots in the central footplate in a rosette pattern. The ash is then cleared away to reveal the fenestra.

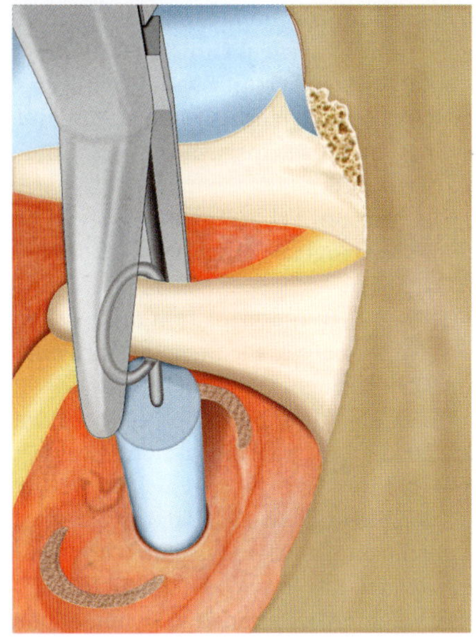

Fig. 14.10: The prosthesis is crimped into position by pressing the anterior limb of the hook of the prosthesis around the long process of the incus. The prosthesis should be securely fastened to the incus, and is confirmed by palpation of the incus or malleus after crimping.

the incus and avoids the technical challenge of manually crimping the prosthesis. Results with the self-crimping memory shape alloy prostheses have been equivalent to those with the traditional manually crimped platinum or stainless steel prostheses.[48]

The tympanomeatal flap is then unfurled and laid back into position along the bony posterior canal wall. Packing material is left in the medial external auditory canal to hold the flap in position, and removed 1 week later.

Postoperatively, patients are instructed to refrain from auto-insufflation of the ear or Valsalva maneuvers (i.e. heavy lifting or straining), to avoid airplane flights, and to keep the ear dry for two weeks. Scuba diving and sky diving are relatively contraindicated for life after a stapedectomy due to the potential development of a perilymph fistula with inadequate pressure equalization of the middle ear.

SUMMARY

Otosclerosis is a disease of abnormal bone remodeling of the otic capsule, which most commonly presents with conductive hearing loss due to fixation of the stapes footplate. Measles virus infection may play a role in the pathophysiology of otosclerosis, and there is a clear hereditary component with multiple genetic loci identified. Traditionally, the evaluation includes otoscopy, tuning fork examination, and audiometry, but there may be a role for CT imaging in diagnosis and management. Treatment options include observation, amplification with hearing aids, medical therapies such as fluoride or bisphosphonates, and surgery. Stapedectomy surgery for otosclerosis typically results in excellent hearing outcomes, and is generally well tolerated by patients with minimal recovery time.

REFERENCES

1. Wang PC, Merchant SN, McKenna MJ, et al. Does otosclerosis occur only in the temporal bone? Am J Otol. 1999;20(2):162-5.
2. Hall JG. Otosclerosis in Norway, a geographical and genetical study. Acta Otolaryngol Suppl. 1974;324:1-20.
3. Pearson RD, Kurland LT, Cody DT. Incidence of diagnosed clinical otosclerosis. Arch Otolaryngol. 1974; 99(4):288-91.
4. Guild SR. Histologic otosclerosis. Ann Otol Rhinol Laryngol. 1944;53:1045-71.
5. Mudry A. First descriptions of the ankylosis of the stapes. Otol Neurotol. 2010;31(7):1177.
6. Politzer A. Ueber primare Erkrankung der knochernen Labyrinthkapsel. Zeitschr Ohrenheil. 1893;25:309.
7. Mudry A. Adam Politzer (1835-1920) and the description of otosclerosis. Otol Neurotol. 2006;27(2):276-81.
8. McKenna MJ, Merchant SN. Disorders of bone. In: Merchant SN, Nadol JB Jr (eds), Schuknecht's pathology of the ear, 3rd edn. Shelton, CT: People's Medical Publishing House; 2010.
9. Schuknecht HF, Barber W. Histologic variants in otosclerosis. Laryngoscope. 1985;95(11):1307-17.

10. Bretlau P. Relation of the otosclerotic focus to the fissula ante-fenestram. J Laryngol Otol. 1969;83(12):1185-93.
11. Cherukupally SR, Merchant SN, Rosowski JJ. Correlations between pathologic changes in the stapes and conductive hearing loss in otosclerosis. Ann Otol Rhinol Laryngol. 1998;107(4):319-26.
12. Parahy C, Linthicum FH, Jr. Otosclerosis and otospongiosis: clinical and histological comparisons. Laryngoscope. 1984; 94(4):508-12.
13. Kwok OT, Nadol JB, Jr. Correlation of otosclerotic foci and degenerative changes in the organ of Corti and spiral ganglion. Am J Otolaryngol. 1989;10(1):1-12.
14. Adams JC. Clinical implications of inflammatory cytokines in the cochlea: a technical note. Otol Neurotol. 2002; 23(3):316-22.
15. Zehnder AF, Kristiansen AG, Adams JC, et al. Osteoprotegerin in the inner ear may inhibit bone remodeling in the otic capsule. Laryngoscope. 2005;115(1):172-7.
16. Sorensen MS, Frisch T, Bretlau P. Dynamic bone studies of the labyrinthine capsule in relation to otosclerosis. Adv Otorhinolaryngol. 2007;65:53-8.
17. Stankovic KM, McKenna MJ. Current research in otosclerosis. Curr Opin Otolaryngol Head Neck Surg. 2006;14(5): 347-51.
18. Zehnder AF, Kristiansen AG, Adams JC, et al. Osteoprotegrin knockout mice demonstrate abnormal remodeling of the otic capsule and progressive hearing loss. Laryngoscope. 2006;116(2):201-6.
19. McKenna MJ, Kristiansen AG, Bartley ML, Rogus JJ, Haines JL. Association of COL1A1 and otosclerosis: evidence for a shared genetic etiology with mild osteogenesis imperfecta. Am J Otol. 1998;19(5):604-10.
20. McKenna MJ, Mills BG. Immunohistochemical evidence of measles virus antigens in active otosclerosis. Otolaryngol Head Neck Surg. 1989;101(4):415-21.
21. Chole RA, McKenna M. Pathophysiology of otosclerosis. Otol Neurotol. 2001;22(2):249-57.
22. Niedermeyer HP, Arnold W. Otosclerosis: a measles virus associated inflammatory disease. Acta Otolaryngol. 1995; 115(2):300-3.
23. Gristwood RE, Venables WN. Otosclerosis and chronic tinnitus. Ann Otol Rhinol Laryngol. 2003;112(5):398-403.
24. Sobrinho PG, Oliveira CA, Venosa AR. Long-term follow-up of tinnitus in patients with otosclerosis after stapes surgery. Int Tinnitus J. 2004;10(2):197-201.
25. Grayeli AB, Sterkers O, Toupet M. Audiovestibular function in patients with otosclerosis and balance disorders. Otol Neurotol. 2009;30(8):1085-91.
26. Saim L, Nadol JB, Jr. Vestibular symptoms in otosclerosis—correlation of otosclerotic involvement of vestibular apparatus and Scarpa's ganglion cell count. Am J Otol. 1996; 17(2): 263-70.
27. Nakashima T, Sone M, Fujii H, et al. Blood flow to the promontory in cochlear otosclerosis. Clin Otolaryngol. 2006; 31(2):110-5.
28. Santos F, McCall AA, Chien W, Merchant S. Otopathology in osteogenesis imperfecta. Otol Neurotol. 2012;33(9): 1562-6.
29. Clayton AE, Mikulec AA, Mikulec KH, et al. Association between osteoporosis and otosclerosis in women. J Laryngol Otol. 2004;118(8):617-21.
30. Schuknecht HF. Myths in neurotology. Am J Otol. 1992; 13(2):124-6.
31. Shambaugh GE, Jr. Clinical diagnosis of cochlear (labyrinthine) otosclerosis. Laryngoscope. 1965;75(10):1558-62.
32. Merchant SN, Rosowski JJ, McKenna MJ. Superior semicircular canal dehiscence mimicking otosclerotic hearing loss. Adv Otorhinolaryngol. 2007;65:137-45.
33. Jakob A, Bornitz M, Kuhlisch E, et al. New aspects in the clinical diagnosis of otosclerosis using laser Doppler vibrometry. Otol Neurotol. 2009; 30(8): 1049-57.
34. Lagleyre S, Sorrentino T, Calmels MN, et al. Reliability of high-resolution CT scan in diagnosis of otosclerosis. Otol Neurotol. 2009;30(8):1152-9.
35. Shin YJ, Fraysse B, Deguine O, et al. Sensorineural hearing loss and otosclerosis: a clinical and radiologic survey of 437 cases. Acta Otolaryngol. 2001;121(2):200-4.
36. Quesnel AM, Moonis G, Appel J, et al. Correlation of computed tomography with histopathology in otosclerosis. Otol Neurotol. 2013;34(1):22-8.
37. Virk JS, Singh A, Lingam RK. The role of imaging in the diagnosis and management of otosclerosis. Otol Neurotol. 2013;34(7):e55-60.
38. Sakai O, Curtin HD, Hasso AN, et al. Otosclerosis and dysplasias of the temporal bone. In: Som PM, Curtin HD (Eds.), Head and neck imaging. St. Louis, MO: Elsevier; 2011. Pp. 1231-41.
39. Shambaugh GE, Jr, Scott A. Sodium fluoride for arrest of otosclerosis: theoretical considerations. Arch Otolaryngol. 1964;80:263-70.
40. Bretlau P, Causse J, Causse JB, et al. Otospongiosis and sodium fluoride: a blind experimental and clinical evaluation of the effect of sodium fluoride treatment in patients with otospongiosis. Ann Otol Rhinol Laryngol. 1985;94 (2 Pt 1):103-7.
41. Cruise AS, Singh A, Quiney RE. Sodium fluoride in otosclerosis treatment: review. J Laryngol Otol. 2010;124(6): 583-6.
42. Kennedy DW, Hoffer ME, Holliday M. The effects of etidronate disodium on progressive hearing loss from otosclerosis. Otolaryngol Head Neck Surg. 1993;109(3 Pt 1): 461-7.
43. Brookler K. Medical treatment of otosclerosis: rationale for use of bisphosphonates. Int Tinnitus J. 2008;14(2):92-6.

44. Quesnel AM, Seton M, Merchant SN, et al. Third-generation bisphosphonates for treatment of sensorineural hearing loss in otosclerosis. Otol Neurotol. 2012;33(8): 1308-14.
45. Vincent R, Sperling NM, Oates J, et al. Surgical findings and long-term hearing results in 3,050 stapedotomies for primary otosclerosis: a prospective study with the otology-neurotology database. Otol Neurotol. 2006;27(8 Suppl 2): S25-47.
46. Wiet RJ, Battista RA, Wiet RM, et al. Hearing outcomes in stapes surgery: a comparison of fat, fascia, and vein tissue seals. Otolaryngol Head Neck Surg. 2013;148(1): 115-20.
47. Kisilevsky VE, Dutt SN, Bailie NA, et al. Hearing results of 1145 stapedotomies evaluated with Amsterdam hearing evaluation plots. J Laryngol Otol. 2009;123(7):730-36.
48. Fayad JN, Semaan MT, Meier JC, House JW. Hearing results using the SMart piston prosthesis. Otol Neurotol. 2009; 30(8):1122-7.
49. Gerard JM, Serry P, Gersdorff MC. Outcome and lack of prognostic factors in stapes surgery. Otol Neurotol. 2008; 29(3):290-94.
50. Vincent R, Bittermann AJ, Oates J, et al. KTP versus CO_2 laser fiber stapedotomy for primary otosclerosis: results of a new comparative series with the otology-neurotology database. Otol Neurotol. 2012;33(6):928-33.

CHAPTER

15

Tumors of the Middle Ear

Alan G Micco, Qiu Zhong

INTRODUCTION

Tumors of the middle ear represent a diverse group of pathologic entities with widely different pathogenesis, biology, and clinical findings. Glomus tumors, or paragangliomas, are the most common tumor of the middle ear followed by adenomas. Tumors in the middle ear are not necessary confined to the middle ear, and may extend to other portions of the temporal bone, skull base, or intracranially. Middle ear tumors can be primary lesions or part of a systemic process such as lymphoma or leukemia. Systemic processes with middle ear involvement will not be discussed in this chapter. Cholesteatomas, commonly found as masses in the middle ear, are covered in detail in a separate chapter.

GLOMUS TUMORS

Glomus tumors, also known as paragangliomas, are the most common tumor of the middle ear. Glomus tumors of the temporal bone arise from glomus bodies, or paraganglia, which are small (<1.5 mm) masses of tissue composed of clusters of epithelioid (chief) cells within a network of capillary and precapillary caliber vessels. The number seems to increase until the fourth decade of life and then seems to decline. Glomus bodies develop from the neural crest and are believed to function as chemoreceptors. Based on the presence of catecholamines and neuropeptides, glomus bodies are included in the amine precursor uptake and decarboxylase system, which has more recently been referred to as the diffuse neuroendocrine system. They likely play a role as neuromodulators or monitors of vascular activity; however, their role is unclear in the temporal bone.[1]

Histologically, glomus tumors have a thin capsule and are composed of round or polygonal epithelioid cells arranged in compact cell nests or trabecular patterns (Zellballen appearance) (Fig. 15.1). Spindle-shaped supporting cells are found peripheral to the chief cell nests. The chief cells have centrally located nuclei with finely clumped chromatin and a moderate amount of eosinophilic, granular cytoplasm. Glomus tumors appear similar histologically to a variety of tumors, including meningioma, nerve sheath tumor, hemangiopericytoma, adult rhabdomyoma, melanoma, sarcoma, and metastatic carcinoma. Immunohistochemical staining typically confirms the neuroendocrine nature of the chief cells with diffuse, strong positivity for neuron-specific enolase, synaptophysin, and/or chromogranin, and usually negative staining

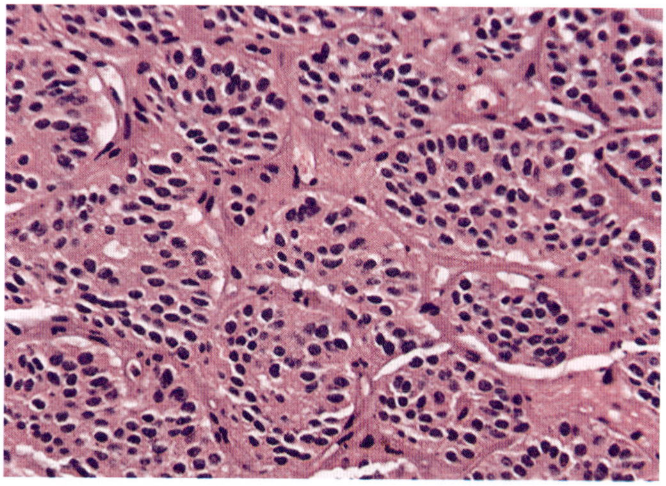

Fig. 15.1: Glomus tumor with Zellballen appearance—round or polygonal epithelioid cells arranged in compact cell nests or trabecular patterns.

for keratins. Ultrastructurally, chief cells contain dense core neurosecretory granules (100–200 nm), which are the sites of catecholamine storage. Supporting cells are negative for neuroendocrine markers but may be S-100 or glial fibrillary acidic protein-positive.[2]

Glomus tympanicum tumors originate from the glomus bodies that lie along the Jacobson's nerve (tympanic branch of cranial nerve IX), and the Arnold's nerve (auricular branch of cranial nerve X). In contrast, glomus jugulare tumors originate from the glomus bodies located in the adventitia of the dome of the jugular bulb or the hypotympanum with secondary invasion of the jugular bulb. There are several classification systems of glomus tumors proposed, but the most widely accepted are the one proposed by Fisch and Mattox (Table 15.1) and the one developed by Glasscock and Jackson (Table 15.2).

Glomus tumors are found more commonly in females with a female-to-male ratio of 3-6:1. Glomus jugulare tumors have also been noted to be more common on the left side. Most tumors occur in patients aged 40–70 years, but cases have been reported in patients as young as 6 months and as old as 88 years.

Most cases of glomus tumors are sporadic; however, the identification and study of "paraganglioma syndromes" (PGLs) have attracted attention in the last several years. There are four different types of PGLs, and to date, three of four PGLs have been characterized on a molecular genetic basis. PGL 1 is associated with mutations of the succinate dehydrogenase subunit D *(SDHD)* gene, PGL 3 is caused by *SDHC* gene mutations, and PGL 4 is caused by *SDHB* gene mutations. The mitochondrial SDH complex catalyzes the oxidation of succinate to fumarate in the Krebs cycle and also feeds electrons to the respiratory chain ubichinone pool.[3] PGL 1 and 4 have been shown to carry high risk of head and neck glomus tumors. The role of transmission is autosomal dominant. In patients with mutations of the *SDHD* gene (PGL 1), however, there is maternal imprinting. This means that the risk of manifestation of the disease phenotype is increased only if the mutation is inherited through the paternal line. Maternal transmission does not increase the risk of glomus tumor development.[3] Multicentric tumors are found in 3–10% of sporadic cases and in 25–50% of familial cases.

Although the chief cells of glomus tumors have neurosecretory granules that store catecholamines, only a small percentage of tumors are actively secreting (1–4%). Glomus jugulare tumors are much more likely than glomus tympanicum tumors to secrete catecholamines. In addition to catecholamines, tumors may also secrete somatostatin, vasoactive intestinal polypeptide, calcitonin, and neuron-specific enolase. Patients who exhibit adrenergic or dopaminergic symptoms such as flushing, frequent diarrhea, headaches, poorly controlled hypertension, orthostasis, palpitations, or excessive diaphoresis should have serum catecholamine levels measured and 24-hour collection of urine for analysis of vanillylmandelic acid and metanephrine.

Approximately 10% of head and neck glomus tumors (including carotid body tumors and glomus vagale in addition to glomus tympanicum and glomus vagale tumors) have been cited as malignant.[4] Of the group, glomus tympanicum and jugulare tumors have the lowest rate of malignancy (2–4%). Interestingly, there are no histopathologic or immunohistochemical features that indicate the malignant potential of the primary tumor.[5,6] Only the presence of local metastases in cervical lymph nodes or systemic metastases can confirm the diagnosis of a malignant glomus tumor. Distant metastases are most frequently detected in the bones, lung, and liver.[4] If metastasis is present, a node dissection with postoperative radiation therapy is necessary in the absence of systemic disease. The 5-year survival is 72%.[7]

Due to their slow rate of growth, the time lapse between onset of symptoms and the actual diagnosis of glomus

Table 15.1: Fisch and Mattox classification of glomus tumors

Type	*Description*
A	Tumors limited to the middle ear cleft
B	Tumors limited to tympanomastoid compartment of the temporal bone
C	Tumor extends in the infralabyrinthine region towards petrous apex
D	Tumor with <2 cm intracranial extension

Table 15.2: Glasscock and Jackson classification of glomus tympanicum tumors

Grade	*Description*
I	Tumors limited to the promontory
II	Tumors completely filling the middle ear cleft
III	Tumors filling the middle ear cleft and extending into the mastoid
IV	Tumors filling the middle ear cleft, extending into the mastoid or filling the external auditory canal, and may extend to involve the internal carotid artery

tumor can be years. The most common symptoms are pulsatile tinnitus and conductive hearing loss when the tumor is confined to the middle ear cavity. Additional symptoms may vary depending on the extent and location of the tumor. Tumors that grow beyond the tympanic membrane may present with otorrhea or hemorrhage. Tumor involvement of the inner ear can produce vertigo and sensorineural hearing loss. Jugular foramen syndrome, also known as Vernet syndrome, occurs when tumor growth around the jugular foramen affects cranial nerves IX, X, and XI and causes symptoms such as dysphonia, dysarthria, aspiration, and dysphagia. Villaret syndrome is a rare combination of jugular foramen syndrome with Horner syndrome. Patients with tumors that involve the carotid canal and the sympathetic plexus present with Horner syndrome (miosis, ptosis, anhydrosis, and enophthalmos). Tumors with significant erosion of the middle ear and mastoid may develop facial nerve weakness or paralysis. Tumors with intracranial extension may produce headaches and elevated intracranial pressure. Ataxia and brain stem symptoms may also develop. Involvement of the dural sinuses may mimic sinus thrombosis.

On otoscopic examination of a middle ear glomus tumor, a characteristic reddish-blue pulsatile mass can frequently be seen medial to the inferior tympanic membrane. The Brown sign refers to blanching of the mass with positive pressure during pneumatic otoscopy, correlating to the highly vascular nature of these tumors. Another helpful physical examination finding is the Aquino sign, which refers to a reduction in tumor pulsation with ipsilateral carotid artery compression. Tumors that grow through the tympanic membrane will appear like a hemorrhagic aural polyp on otoscopy. Due to the highly vascular nature of these tumors, transcanal biopsy of the apparent polyp should be avoided before imaging studies can rule out a glomus tumor. Tuning fork and audiometric examination will frequently show a conductive hearing loss and, less commonly, a sensorineural hearing loss.

Imaging studies are essential modalities in the diagnosis and treatment planning of glomus tumors. High-resolution CT scans (HRCTs) of the temporal bone with contrast should be the first study ordered when a temporal bone glomus tumor is suspected (Figs. 15.2A and B). It provides detailed information on tumor extension and relevant anatomy for surgical planning. When the bony partition between the jugular fossa and the hypotympanum is intact, a HRCT can accurately identify the tumor origin. Conversely, when the bony partition is eroded by tumor, it may be difficult to differentiate between a glomus jugulare tumor and glomus tympanicum tumor. MRI/MRA can be considered in addition to HRCT, especially in cases of large tumors with possible intracranial extension. Glomus tumors have a characteristic "salt and pepper" appearance on T2-weighted images, reflecting vascular flow voids. HRCTs are more sensitive than MRIs in detection of smaller tumors. More recently ^{111}indium octreotide, a radioisotope somatostatin analogue, has been used to selectively identify glomus tumors. These highly sensitive studies can be used to evaluate for multiple tumors and recurrent or metastatic disease.[8,9]

Complete surgical excision is the primary treatment modality for glomus jugulare and glomus tympanicum

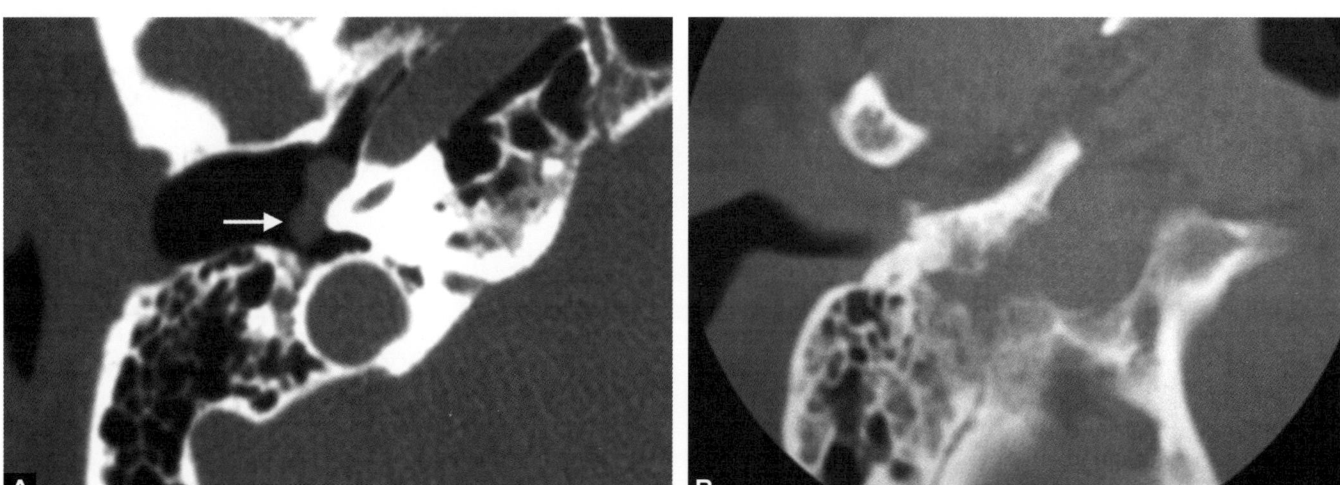

Figs. 15.2A and B: CT images of (A) glomus tympanicum; note the soft tissue mass arising from the cochlear promontory (arrow); and (B) glomus jugulare, a large destructive mass involving skull base and extending into the mastoid.

tumors. Patients with secreting tumors can be medically treated with adjunctive α- and β-blockade. Large glomus tumors should be evaluated preoperatively with four-vessel angiography. Angiography is combined with embolization preoperatively to decrease surgical blood loss and avoid surgical morbidity. Angiography of the intracranial circulation evaluates patency of the circle of Willis for determining adequate cerebral perfusion if unilateral carotid blood flow is interrupted for temporary control or for permanent ligation and sacrifice. This is commonly done with a balloon occlusion test. Surgical resection of glomus tumors frequently results in lower cranial nerve dysfunction, requiring anticipation of postoperative rehabilitation. Resection of larger-sized tumors frequently results in postoperative voice, swallowing, articulation, and facial weakness/paralysis problems.

Radiation therapy and stereotactic radiosurgery, in addition to or in place of surgery, sometimes must be considered in the treatment of glomus tumors. Radiation is most often reserved for tumors with extensive intracranial or skull base involvement, multiple or bilateral tumors with potential postoperative debility from cranial nerve dysfunction, and poor risk patients. Radiation therapy may result in shrinkage of the tumor, but there is rarely total resolution.[10] The main advantage of radiation therapy is avoidance of the morbidity of surgery for larger tumors while offering a high probability (96–100%) of tumor control.[11] Radiation therapy is not favored as a primary treatment by some, because persistent tumor may result in subsequent malignant degeneration and metastases,[7] especially in younger patient populations.

In certain situations, in place of treatment, only observation with serial imaging studies is used to follow tumor growth. This approach may be most appropriate in the elderly, in a setting of multiple medical problems, or in those patients with multiple tumors who are at risk of severe debility due to cranial nerve dysfunction after surgery. Rapid tumor enlargement is unlikely, as recent studies reveal a relatively slow growth pattern, with a median growth rate of 1 mm per year and a median tumor doubling time of 4.2 years.[12]

ADENOMAS

Adenomas are the second most common benign tumor of the middle ear, arising from middle ear epithelium. Adenomas are infrequently reported in the literature, mostly in small case series or case reports, either because of low prevalence or low rate of discovery. Previous terms used to describe this tumor included *ceruminoma, ceruminous adenoma, monomorphic adenoma,* and *carcinoid tumor.*[13] The pathogenesis of these benign lesions is unknown. Histology reveals benign glandular proliferation, suggestive of reactive hyperplasia; however, in most reported cases there is no prior history of otitis media or chronic inflammation (Fig. 15.3).

There is no age or sex predilection for middle ear adenomas. The most common presenting symptoms are aural fullness, progressive hearing loss, and tinnitus. Vertigo and facial paralysis have been occasionally reported in cases involving large adenomas. Physical examination usually reveals a whitish mass in the middle ear with an intact tympanic membrane; however, in rare cases the adenoma may extend through the tympanic membrane or into the mastoid. Radiographically there is soft tissue mass in the middle ear without bony erosion.

Surgical excision is the treatment of choice for middle ear adenomas, and histological examination is required for definitive diagnosis. Adenomas usually peel off the bony walls of the middle ear but may entrap and destroy the ossicles. Recurrence is uncommon with complete excision. Grossly, middle ear adenomas are usually white, gray, or reddish-brown in color. They may be grossly vascular and relatively well circumscribed, but they are not encapsulated. The histologic architectural patterns of middle ear adenomas may be solid, glandular, or trabecular. The tumor cells are uniform and may be cuboidal or cylindrical. They have a moderate amount of acidophilic cytoplasm and may assume a plasmacytoid appearance. Nuclei are

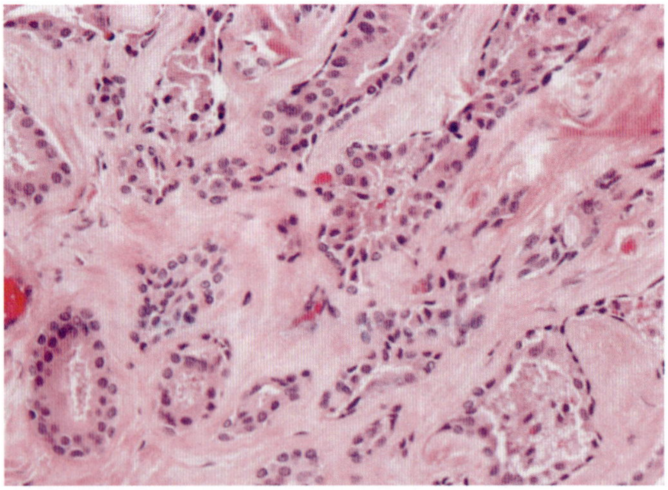

Fig. 15.3: Adenoma with benign glandular proliferation. Surrounding the epithelial cells are myoepithelial cells with slightly smaller nuclei and less conspicuous cytoplasm.

round to oval with a "salt and pepper" chromatin pattern and inconspicuous nucleoli. Moderate to marked nuclear pleomorphism can occur. The tumors can produce mucin, which is positive on periodic acid–Schiff, Alcian blue, and mucicarmine stains. Papillary features are not present in a middle ear adenoma and suggest a papillary adenocarcinoma (aggressive papillary tumor).[14]

HEMANGIOMAS

Hemangiomas are benign vascular tumors found commonly in the head and neck region. They are the most common tumors of infancy. Hemangiomas are characterized by phases of proliferation and involution as defined by a rapid proliferation of blood vessels in the first year of life, followed by gradual regression of the vascular component with replacement by fibrofatty tissue. This growth pattern differentiates these lesions from vascular malformations that are always present at birth, grow in proportion to the body, and do not have an involution period. Glucose transporter isoform 1 and placenta-associated vascular antigens (Fc-gamma-receptor II, merosin, and Lewis Y antigen) are highly expressed in the endothelial cells of infantile hemangiomas during both the proliferative and involution phase.[15] These markers are not expressed in normal dermal or subcutaneous capillaries, nor are they expressed in other types of vascular tumors.

Histopathology varies according to the stage of the hemangioma. In early proliferation, hemangiomas are characterized by nonencapsulated masses and dense cords of mitotically active, plump endothelial cells in close association with pericytes (Fig. 15.4). Few, small-caliber lumina are present. Special stains reveal well-developed basement membranes around primitive vessels. Mast cells are present in varying numbers in all stages. As the hemangioma proliferates, the vascular lumina enlarge. An increase in apoptotic endothelial cells and a decrease in plump, mitotically active endothelial cells herald the involution phase. As involution progresses, the endothelial cells continue to mature and assume a flatter appearance. The vascular lumina continue to enlarge until few mature ecstatic vessels remain. The proliferating endothelial cell mass may be replaced with fibrofatty tissue. Varying degrees of epidermal atrophy, scar tissue, and loss of elastic tissue can be seen in late involuting lesions.

Although hemangiomas of the head and neck involving the skin and airway are well documented and characterized in the literature, hemangiomas of the temporal bone middle ear are rarely reported. Excluding the middle ear, hemangiomas of the temporal bone are most frequently found at the geniculate ganglion, the internal auditory meatus, and the origin of the chorda tympani.[16,17] To date there are <15 cases of middle ear hemangiomas reported in the literature.[16,18,19] Patients may be asymptomatic or may present with aural fullness, conductive hearing loss, pulsatile tinnitus, or recurrent otitis media. Otologic examination may show a reddish polypoid retrotympanic mass that can be confused for a glomus tumor, adenoma, or aberrant vasculature. On CT, the hemangiomas appear as soft tissue densities with or without bony or ossicular erosion and sometimes contain ossifications. On MRI, these tumors show moderate or intermediate T1 signal and as a high T2 signal. Angiography shows a vascular blush similar to glomus tumors; however, the intravascular contrast associated with hemangiomas persists late into the venous phase, whereas in glomus tumors the contrast dissipates earlier. The radiologic features of middle ear hemangiomas, therefore, can resemble many other middle ear lesions and are by no means pathognomonic.

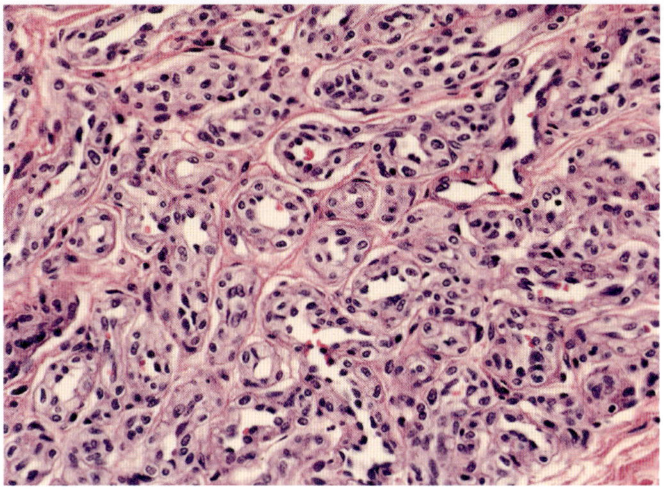

Fig. 15.4: Hemangioma in the proliferative phase with plump endothelial cells.

Surgical excision is usually the treatment reported in the literature; however, this is biased as the definitive diagnosis of hemangioma is based on histopathology. Surgery may not be necessary in pediatric patients due to the natural course of hemangioma involution.[16] Once a tissue diagnosis is made to exclude malignant lesions, it can be treated expectantly or surgically. If growth of a middle ear hemangioma appears to be causing complications refractory to conservative therapy, then early surgical excision may be indicated.

RHABDOMYOSARCOMA

Sarcomas of the temporal bone are exceedingly rare; however, they are the most common primary malignancy of the temporal bone in children. Rhabdomyosarcoma (RMS) is the most common type, accounting for 30% of sarcomas of the temporal bone and 4–7% of all temporal bone malignancies. It is a neoplasm of primitive mesenchyme expressing skeletal muscle differentiation. RMS cells tend to have variable differentiation along the myogenesis pathway and may appear as strap cells or myotubes that sometimes contain muscle cross-striations. RMS cells may demonstrate positive immunohistochemical results for muscle-specific markers, such as myoglobin, actin, and desmin. Soderberg described the first case of middle ear RMS in 1933.[20]

Ninety percent of patients with middle ear RMS are <10 years of age at time of diagnosis, and 5% are <1 year old. The median age is 5 years (range, 0–20 years). There is a male preponderance with a male:female ratio of 1.7:1.[21]

There are numerous classification schemas of RMS based on histology, with great overlap and controversy (Table 15.3). Broadly speaking, there are four major types: embryonal, botryoid (considered by some to be a variant of embryonal), pleomorphic (or anaplastic in some classification systems such as the International Classification of RMS), and alveolar.[22] Embryonal RMS tumors contain dense condensations of rhabdomyoblasts amid foci with a loose myxoid stroma (Fig. 15.5A). The botryoid type is so named due to the resemblance of the gross specimen to a bunch of grapes (*botryos,* Greek for cluster of grapes). The cambium layer is characteristic of botryoid tumors, containing a condensation of loose tumor cells below an epithelial surface. Pleomorphic RMS tumors arise almost exclusively in the soft tissues of adults and comprise part of the spectrum of lesions known as "malignant fibrous histiocytoma". They form spindle cell lesions with a whorled or storiform pattern and contain cells with enlarged, hyperchromatic nuclei (Fig. 15.5B). In the rare pleomorphic RMS seen in the pediatric age group, there is usually another component, so that this category currently is not used for pediatric subtyping and has been subsumed into the anaplastic and spindle cell subtypes. Lastly, the alveolar type of RMS is defined by the alveolar structure formed by the fibrous septa of these neoplasms. These fibrous septa are composed of collagenous fibrovascular tissue that forms a scaffold suspending attached rhabdomyoblasts and circumscribing central clusters of tumor cells that appear to float in alveolar spaces (Fig. 15.5C). The histopathologic variants of RMS pursue markedly different biologic courses. Embryonal subtypes (botryoid, spindle cell) are the most common form of RMS (70%) and the type most frequently found in the head and neck region (83%), as well as the middle ear (93%), with a superior survival rate (3-year failure-free survival of 83% for all tumor locations), whereas alveolar variants are often seen in the extremities and metastasize early in the course of disease, with a poorer survival rate (3-year failure-free survival of 66% for all tumor locations).[21,23] This stark difference in survival makes it critically important to accurately diagnose variants of RMS so that the biologic course of disease can be predicted and appropriate therapeutic response made.

The clinical presentation of RMS of the middle ear and mastoid is similar to that of chronic suppurative otitis media; patients may present with chronic otorrhea and otalgia that is refractory to antibiotic therapy. Otologic examination findings include purulent and blood-stained otorrhea, aural polyps, granulation tissue, and possible mastoid swelling. The most common neurologic feature of RMS is facial nerve involvement and may indicate a malignant process. Radiographic imaging of the temporal bone shows a soft tissue mass in the middle ear and mastoid cavity with surrounding bony erosion. Tissue biopsy analysis is critical to establish the correct diagnosis in a timely manner.

Formed in 1972, the Intergroup Rhabdomyosarcoma Study (IRS) Committee [later called the Intergroup Rhabdomyosarcoma Study Group (IRSG)] designed and conducted four consecutive clinical trials that defined the

Table 15.3: Characteristics of rhabdomyosarcoma subtypes

RMS subtypes	*Prevalence in middle ear rhabdomyosarcoma (%)*[21]	*Most commonly affected age group*	*Most commonly affected anatomic regions*	*Prognosis*
Embryonal/botryoid	92	children	Head and neck, bladder, vagina, prostate and testicles	Intermediate to superior
Pleomorphic/anaplastic	6	adults	Lower extremities	Poor
Alveolar	2	all age groups	Trunk and extremities	Poor

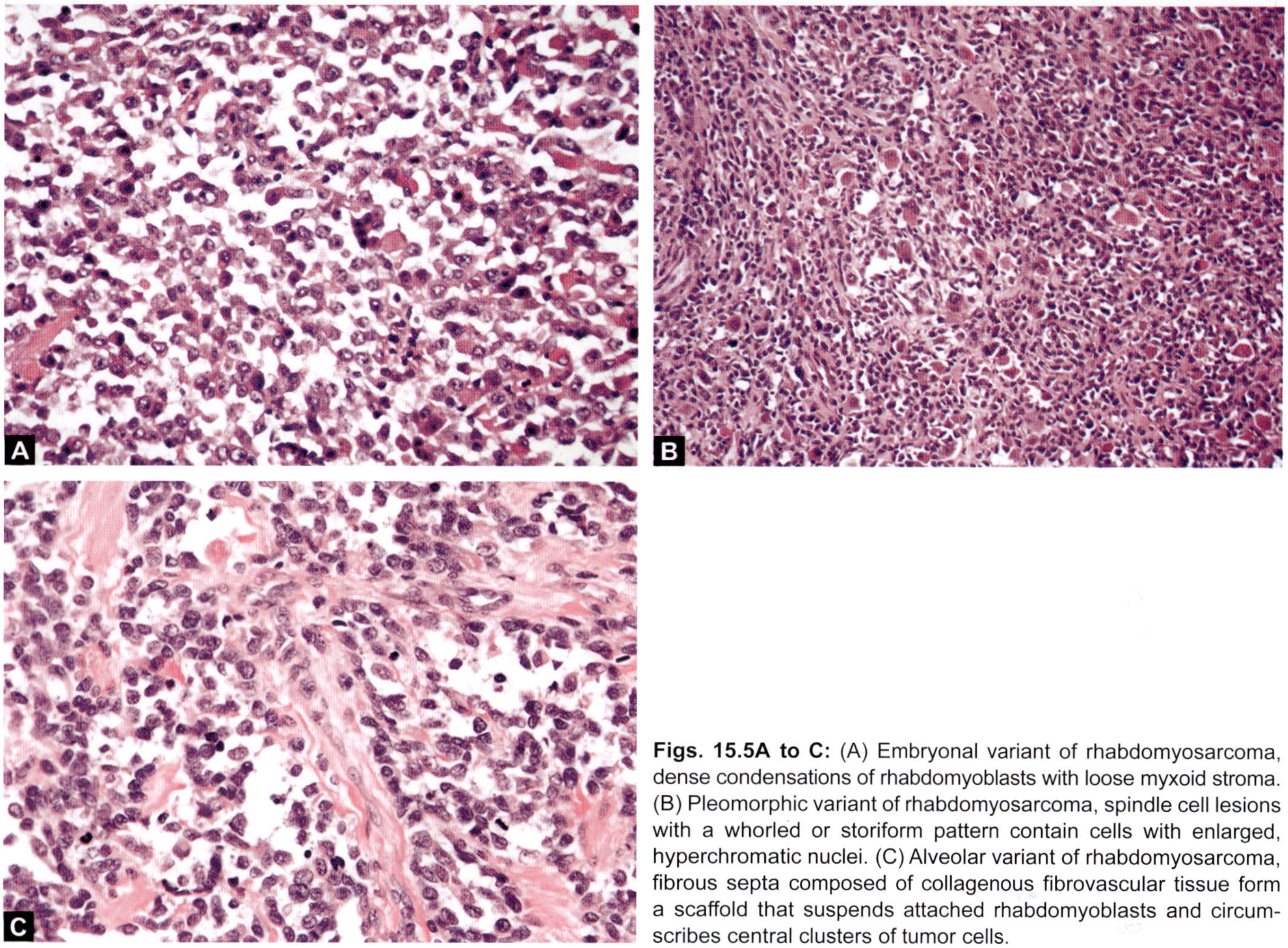

Figs. 15.5A to C: (A) Embryonal variant of rhabdomyosarcoma, dense condensations of rhabdomyoblasts with loose myxoid stroma. (B) Pleomorphic variant of rhabdomyosarcoma, spindle cell lesions with a whorled or storiform pattern contain cells with enlarged, hyperchromatic nuclei. (C) Alveolar variant of rhabdomyosarcoma, fibrous septa composed of collagenous fibrovascular tissue form a scaffold that suspends attached rhabdomyoblasts and circumscribes central clusters of tumor cells.

components of multimodality therapy associated with the favorable outcome for pediatric RMS. The anatomic diversity of primary sites for RMS has complicated the development of treatment. In determining optimal treatment, the IRSG has observed that patients with tumors in favorable anatomic sites, including the orbit, genitourinary tract (nonbladder, prostate), and nonparameningeal head and neck sites, can be successfully treated with less intensive systemic chemotherapy. In addition, the IRSG has identified treatment guidelines for each anatomic site with regard to local control, including the timing and extent of surgery and the timing, dose, and fields for radiation therapy. Tailoring the components of multimodality therapy to the anatomic site of RMS has improved survival and decreased side effects. Analysis of the extensive data collected from the IRSG has also described the clinical features, treatment, and outcome of pediatric middle ear RMS. A large-scale review of the four IRSG studies to date has shown that middle ear RMS commonly presents as an invasive, unresectable tumor that rarely metastasizes to regional lymph nodes. Survival of patients has improved from 33% in IRS-I to 72% in IRS-IV.[21] Because < 5% of middle ear RMS were grossly resected at diagnosis, improvements in surgical techniques were unlikely to have contributed to increased local control. Progressively more intensive chemotherapy was used during the successive IRSG trials, particularly dose escalation of alkylating agent. The IRSG trials have also been notable for significant standardization in the timing, dose, and fields for radiation therapy. Most likely, advances in chemotherapy and radiation algorithms as well as supportive services have led to the improved survival rates.

TERATOMA AND DERMOID

Teratomas are a group of tumors that contain all three germ layers (ectoderm, mesoderm, endoderm). They occur in 1:4000 births, with approximately 1–3.5% affecting the head and neck. Three theories have been proposed for the origin of teratomas. Acquired implantation suggests that skin or mucous membrane with its associated mesodermal component has been traumatically implanted into deeper tissues. Congenital inclusion theorizes that incomplete closure of embryogenic fusion lines results in the capture of germ layers into ectopic areas. The third theory proposes that totipotential rest cells from two or three germ layers become isolated and begin independent growth in a disorganized manner.

True teratomas are composed of all three germ layers with differentiation to the extent of identifying structures such as teeth and hair within them. Teratomas of the middle ear are exceedingly rare, with <10 cases reported in the literature.[24] While true teratomas are wholly benign lesions, there has been at least one report of a middle ear teratoma with immature elements,[25] thereby posing a oncogenic risk. Head and neck teratomas, including those of the middle ear, are tumors of neonates and infants. It is rare to find these tumors in older children. A cranial nerve palsy may lead to the discovery of a middle ear or temporal bone teratoma. CT may reveal a soft tissue mass with calcifications and both solid and cystic components. Complete surgical excision should be the definitive treatment of middle ear teratomas. Surgery will ensure that the tumor will not continue to grow and endanger adjacent structures and ensure that an unsuspected immature or malignant component is not contained within the lesion.

Dermoid cysts, a type of teratoma, are composed of only ectodermal and mesodermal derivatives. A keratinizing squamous epithelium is typically present along with dermal derivatives including hair follicles, smooth muscle, and sweat and sebaceous glands. While they are the most common teratoma of the head and neck, dermoids of the middle ear and temporal bone have only been reported in isolated case reports.[26,27] Approximately one-third of dermoids are diagnosed at birth and many are not discovered until the adolescent years. Patients may be asymptomatic with an incidental finding of retrotympanic mass or may present with otorrhea, serous effusion, and hearing loss. Clinically and radiographically, dermoids are difficult to distinguish from cholesteatomas. Definitive diagnosis can only be made on tissue pathology. Complete surgical excision will prevent recurrence.

CHORISTOMA

A choristoma is a mass of mature, normal tissue that is located in an area where it is not normally found. Middle ear choristomas are rare, and when found, usually consist of salivary tissue. Neural and sebaceous gland tissue has also been reported in the literature.[28,29] Salivary choristomas of the middle ear show a clear left-sided predominance and a higher incidence in females (male-to-female ratio, 1:1.7). The age at diagnosis ranges from 3 to 52 years.[30,31]

Although the etiology of salivary gland choristoma in the middle ear is not well understood, it is believed to involve an aberration in embryologic development. The major salivary glands develop from oral epithelial buds that migrate into the underlying mesenchyme. The minor salivary glands, on the other hand, arise from oral endoderm and ectoderm that eventually become the ducts and acini that are distributed throughout the oropharynx. One theory postulates that the development of salivary gland choristoma is similar to the development of congenital cholesteatoma, with ectodermal cells that are destined to develop into salivary tissue becoming trapped in the temporal bone during development and later proliferating in the middle ear.[32]

Common presenting symptoms of salivary gland choristoma in the middle ear include otorrhea, tinnitus, and conductive hearing loss. In addition, most patients have some degree of ossicular abnormalities, usually involving both the incus and stapes, followed in frequency by the malleus. Our patient displayed all these clinical features except for otorrhea and tinnitus. Choristomas have been reported to be closely associated with the facial nerve and facial nerve abnormalities such as aberrant course of the nerve and nerve dehiscence. Close association of a choristoma with the facial nerve may make complete resection difficult.

Recurrence is unlikely with complete surgical excision. Facial nerve monitoring during biopsy and surgical excision should be utilized to reduce the risk of facial nerve damage during exploratory tympanotomy. If complete resection cannot be achieved without significant risk to the facial nerve, then biopsy to confirm the diagnosis followed by observation is adequate as the mass has very little growth potential.

REFERENCES

1. Gulya AJ. The glomus tumor and its biology. Laryngoscope. 1993;103(11 Pt 2 Suppl 60):p7-15.
2. Kliewer KE, et al. Paragangliomas: assessment of prognosis by histologic, immunohistochemical, and ultrastructural techniques. Hum Pathol. 1989;20(1):29-39.
3. Boedeker CC, et al. Malignant head and neck paragangliomas in SDHB mutation carriers. Otolaryngol Head Neck Surg. 2007;137(1):126-9.
4. Lee JH, et al. National Cancer Data Base report on malignant paragangliomas of the head and neck. Cancer. 2002; 94(3):730-7.

5. Boedeker CC, Ridder GJ, Schipper J. Paragangliomas of the head and neck: diagnosis and treatment. Fam Cancer. 2005;4(1):55-9.
6. Persky MS, et al. Combined endovascular and surgical treatment of head and neck paragangliomas—a team approach. Head Neck. 2002;24(5):423-31.
7. Manolidis S, et al. Malignant glomus tumors. Laryngoscope. 1999;109(1):30-34.
8. Kwekkeboom DJ, et al. Octreotide scintigraphy for the detection of paragangliomas. J Nucl Med. 1993;34(6):873-8.
9. Hammond SL, et al. Indium In-111 pentetreotide scintigraphy: application to carotid body tumors. J Vasc Surg. 1997;25(5):905-8.
10. Cole JM, Beiler D. Long-term results of treatment for glomus jugulare and glomus vagale tumors with radiotherapy. Laryngoscope. 1994;104(12):1461-5.
11. Evenson LJ, et al. Radiotherapy in the management of chemodectomas of the carotid body and glomus vagale. Head Neck. 1998;20(7):609-13.
12. Jansen JC, et al. Estimation of growth rate in patients with head and neck paragangliomas influences the treatment proposal. Cancer. 2000;88(12):2811-6.
13. Mills, SE, Fechner EF. Middle ear adenoma: a cytologically uniform neoplasm displaying a variety of architectural patterns. Am J Surg Pathol. 19848:677-85.
14. Berns S, Pearl G. Middle ear adenoma. Arch Pathol Lab Med. 2006;130(7):1067-9.
15. Leon-Villapalos J, Wolfe K, Kangesu L. GLUT-1: an extra diagnostic tool to differentiate between haemangiomas and vascular malformations. Br J Plast Surg. 2005;58(3):348-52.
16. Hecht DA, Jackson CG, Grundfast KM. Management of middle ear hemangiomas. Am J Otolaryngol. 2001;22(5):362-6.
17. Kojima H, Yaguchi Y, Moriyama H. Middle ear hemangioma: a case report. Auris Nasus Larynx. 2008;35(2):255-9.
18. Nouri H, et al. Capillary hemangioma of the middle ear: one case report and review of the literature. Case Rep Otolaryngol. 2012;2012:305172.
19. Pistorio V, et al. Capillary haemangioma of the middle ear: a rare lesion difficult to evaluate. Acta Otorhinolaryngol Ital. 2011;31(2):109-12.
20. Soderberg F. Rhabdomyome epipharynge ayant envahi l'oreille et les meninges. Acta Otolaryngol. 1933;18:453-9.
21. Hawkins DS, et al. Improved outcome for patients with middle ear rhabdomyosarcoma: a children's oncology group study. J Clin Oncol. 2001;19(12):3073-9.
22. Parham DM. Pathologic classification of rhabdomyosarcomas and correlations with molecular studies. Mod Pathol. 2001;14(5):506-14.
23. Crist WM, et al. Intergroup rhabdomyosarcoma study-IV: results for patients with nonmetastatic disease. J Clin Oncol. 2001;19(12):3091-102.
24. Devaney KO, Rinaldo A, Ferlito A. Teratoma of the middle ear: a real entity or a non-entity? Acta Otolaryngol. 2005; 125(2):122-4.
25. Navarro Cunchillos M, et al. Middle ear teratoma in a newborn. J Laryngol Otol. 1996;110(9):875-7.
26. Vrabec JT, Schwaber MK. Dermoid tumor of the middle ear: case report and literature review. Am J Otol. 1992;13(6): 580-1.
27. Farris PE, Meyerhoff WL, Vuitch F. Congenital dermoid cyst of the middle ear. Skull Base Surg. 1998;8(2):77-80.
28. Gyure KA, Thompson LD, Morrison AL. A clinicopathological study of 15 patients with neuroglial heterotopias and encephaloceles of the middle ear and mastoid region. Laryngoscope. 2000;110(10 Pt 1):1731-5.
29. Nelson EG, Kratz RC. Sebaceous choristoma of the middle ear. Otolaryngol Head Neck Surg. 1993;108(4):372-3.
30. el-Naggar AK, et al. Tumors of the middle ear and endolymphatic sac. Pathol Annu. 1994;29 (Pt 2):199-231.
31. Namdar I, Smouha EE, Kane P. Salivary gland choristoma of the middle ear: role of intraoperative facial nerve monitoring. Otolaryngol Head Neck Surg. 1995;112(4): 616-20.
32. Peron DL, Schuknecht HF. Congenital cholesteatomata with other anomalies. Arch Otolaryngol. 1975;101(8):498-505.

CHAPTER 16

Sensorineural Hearing Loss

Andrea Vambutas

INTRODUCTION

Sensorineural hearing loss (SNHL), colloquially referred to as "nerve deafness," often may be the result of pathology in various proteins of the cochlea, rather than of the auditory nerve itself. SNHL affects 28 million Americans, and approximately 2–3 infants per 1000 delivered are born deaf or hard of hearing. Afflicted individuals range from newborns to the elderly. Early identification and rehabilitation of SNHL is critical for better expressive language development in infants,[1] and preservation of speech discrimination scores[2] and recent studies also show that cognitive decline and dementia are associated with SNHL.[3,4] Etiologies for SNHL are extensive, and although clear identification of the etiology may not be possible in the older individual, in children, in many cases, we are able to identify the underlying pathology causing the hearing loss. Studies on SNHL are published on a daily basis, thus our understanding grows exponentially; what we previously ascribed to idiopathic etiologies diminish at a similar rate.

SNHL refers to a defect in the auditory pathway that may involve the cochlea, the internal auditory canal (IAC), or the central auditory pathway. Defects in any of these areas can result in SNHL, as the audiogram alone cannot distinguish the site of the lesion. Use of ancillary testing, as described below, can be particularly useful to distinguish cochlear from retrocochlear (medial, or behind, the cochlea). Identifying whether a SNHL is of cochlear or retrocochlear origin is critical, not only in identifying risk to the patient, but also in choosing the appropriate rehabilitative strategy for the patient.

PATHOGENESIS

SNHL may arise from number of different etiologies. Damage of the auditory hair cells, supporting cells, spiral ganglion cells, and other cell types may arise from a variety of factors. Gene mutations, trauma, inflammation, tumors, structural abnormalities, and altered ion homeostasis such as in endolymphatic hydrops, all may result in SNHL.

SNHL of genetic origin more commonly affects both ears, and is divided into nonsyndromic and syndromic types. The percentage of SNHL ascribed to genetic causes evolved and expanded in the past several decades, in large part due to the discovery of nonsyndromic genes that are associated with SNHL. Connexin 26, an ion channel of the inner ear, represents one of the most common gene mutations to cause nonsyndromic SNHL.[5] The discovery of mutations in connexin 26 shifted our characterization of the percent of hearing loss attributed to genetic causes, especially because of the high prevalence of carriers of this gene.[6] Although there are clear examples of adult onset genetic SNHL, and genetic associations in presbycusis, the majority of clinical genetic testing in SNHL is performed in children. Inheritance of connexin 26 and other genes that cause SNHL may be autosomal recessive or dominant, although over 90% is inherited by autosomal recessive transmission, explaining why the majority of deaf infants are born to hearing parents. The nomenclature used to distinguish autosomal dominant, recessive and sex-linked nonsyndromic genes is DFNA, DFNB, and DFN, respectively. To complicate interpretation further, some genes may be associated with both nonsyndromic and syndromic SNHL. Mutations in the myosin

Table 16.1: Genes included in the otoscope panel

Autosomal recessive, nonsyndromic		*Autosomal dominant, nonsyndromic*		*X-linked nonsyndromic*	*Micro-RNA and mitochondrial*
CDH23	MYO7A	ACTG1	KCNQ4	POU3F4	miR-96
CLDN14	MYO15A	CCDC50	MYH14	PRPS1	miR-182
COL11A2	OTOA	COCH	MYH9		miR-183
ESPN	OTOF	COL11A2	MYO1A		MT-RNR1
ESRRB	PCDH15	CRYM	MYO6		MT-TS1
GIPC3	PJVK	DFNA5	MYO7A		
GJB2	PTPRQ	DIAPH1	POU4F3		
GJB3	RDX	DSPP	SLC17A3		
GJB6	SLC26A4	EYA4	TECTA		
GPSM2	SLC26A5	GJB2	TMC1		
GRXCR1	STRC	GJB6	TJP2		
HGF	TECTA	GRHL2	WFS1		
ILDR1	TMC1				
LHFPL5	TMIE				
LOXHD1	TMPRSS3				
LRTOMT	TPRN				
MARVELD2	TRIOBP				
MYO3A	USIC				
MYO6	WHRN				

*Also included are Usher (CDH23, CLRN1, GPR98, MYO7A, PCDH15, USH1C, USH1G, WHRN) and Pendred (SLC26A4) syndrome genes.

genes may affect hair cell function, as the myosins have been characterized to be expressed in the stereocilia of the inner and outer hair cells of the cochlea.[7] Myosin 7a mutations are associated with Usher's syndrome;[8] however, nonsyndromic mutations may occur as well. As research progresses, it is entirely possible that other highly prevalent genes accounting for hearing loss will be identified. One significant recent advance in this area is development of a panel test of 66 different genes involved in nonsyndromic SNHL, Usher's syndrome, and Penred's syndrome, now commercially referred to as the otoscope panel[9] (Table 16.1).

Syndromic SNHL, although less common than nonsyndromic, has the particular advantage of having a clinically distinguishable phenotype concomitant with the SNHL. Prior to the advent of more sophisticated genetic testing, the percentage of congenital SNHL ascribed to a genetic etiology was largely based on identification of syndromic features. Some of the more common, classic syndromic SNHL syndromes that we can readily identify clinically include Waardenburg's syndrome, Usher's syndrome, Alport's syndrome, Jervell–Lange-Nielson's syndrome, branchio-oto-renal syndrome, and Pendred's syndrome. These syndromes, with their clinical manifestations, inheritance patterns and responsible genetic mutation, are summarized in Table 16.2. Waardenburg's patients are readily identifiable, with a white forelock, premature graying of the hair or presence of heterochromic irises. Notably, this syndrome is incompletely penetrant, so not all afflicted with this autosomal dominant syndrome will demonstrate the same clinical features. Usher's syndrome has come to be recognized as comprising half of the "deaf-blind" community of patients. The classic described finding is retinitis pigmentosa; however, an electroretinogram may detect abnormality as many as 5 years prior to clinical detection. These patients may have vestibular findings as well. Minor interventions, such as use of sunglasses, may help to delay some of the incurred visual losses.[10] Alport's syndrome, a type IV collagen disease, is comprised of SNHL and progressive glomerulonephritis of the kidneys. The

Table 16.2: Genetic sensorineural hearing loss

Syndrome	*Gene/protein*	*Inheritance*	*Clinical manifestations in addition to SNHL*
Waardenburg	PAX3, MITF, EDN3, EDNRB, SOX10, SNAI2[58]	AD	Heterochromic Irises, white forelock, premature greying
Usher	MYO7A, USH1C, USH1G, USH2A,	AS	Blindness, vestibular
Alport	COL4A3-6[59]	AS	Glomerulonephritis
Jervell–Lange-Nielsen	KCNQ1, KCNE1[60, 61]	AS	Long Q-T
Branchio-oto-renal	EYA	AS	Pits along sternocleidomastoid, Renal anomalies
Pendreds	SLC26A4	AS	Enlarged Vestibular Aqueduct
MELAS	A3243G tRNA(Leu(UUR))	Mitochondrial	Mitochondrial myopathy, encephalopathy, lactic acidosis, stroke-like episodes
Muckle–Wells	NLRP3	AD	Periodic fevers, skin rashes, uveitis

site of lesion in Alport's is the stria vascularis of the cochlear and glomerular basement membrane in the kidney. Symptomatology is worse in affected males than females. Jervell–Lange-Nielsen's syndrome, an autosomal recessive hearing loss syndrome, is important to identify as these patients have cardiac conduction delays, manifested by a long Q–T interval. Certain common medications can further prolong this interval (i.e. Zofran) and result in cardiac arrest. Therefore, for all patients undergoing cochlear implantation to rehabilitate, their SNHL should have a preoperative electrocardiogram if the etiology of their hearing loss is unknown. Branchio-oto-renal syndrome may be associated with either sensorineural or conductive hearing loss. These patients are readily identified by pits along the anterior border of the sternocleidomastoid, and they also have renal abnormalities. Some of the more newly described genetic syndromes associated with SNHL belong to two areas: mitochondrial disorders and autoinflammatory disorders. Mitochondrial syndromic SNHL includes MELAS syndrome. MELAS syndrome, exclusively transmitted by maternal mitochondrial DNA, includes findings of short stature, SNHL, blindness, diabetes, cardiac conduction defects, and convulsions.[11,12] Temporal bone histopathology demonstrates atrophy of both the stria vascularis and spiral ganglion cells in these patients.[13] CADASIL, a similar microangiopathy inherited by autosomal dominant transmission, is even rarer than MELAS, but may present as a sudden sensorineural hearing loss (SSNHL) in the context of recurrent strokes, migraine, and dementia.[14] Autoinflammatory disorders are equally rare, but would be classified as syndromic SNHL, based on clinical findings of SNHL, transient skin rashes, periodic fevers, and recurrent uveitis and eventual renal involvement. These diseases are part of the cryopyrin-associated periodic syndrome (CAPS), which is characterized by the dysregulation of Interleukin-1 and other related pro-inflammatory cytokines. Muckle–Wells' syndrome is the most common of this family of rare disorders, and is inherited in an autosomal dominant fashion.[15] NOMID (neonatal onset multisystem inflammatory disease) syndrome is part of the CAPS family of diseases; however, as the name implies, it is usually identified in infants. For each of these syndromes, Table 16.2 shows their inheritance pattern, responsible genetic defect, and clinical findings other than SNHL.

Lesions or altered anatomy anywhere along the central auditory pathway can result in a central neural hearing loss. Tumors of the IAC, inferior colliculus, and auditory cortex all can result in clinical hearing loss, as the central auditory pathway courses through all of these areas to transmit information from the cochlea to the auditory cortex in the contralateral (and a significantly smaller percentage of fibers to the ipsilateral) temporal lobe. Axial and coronal MRI scans are shown in Figure 16.1, with the regions of the central auditory pathway labeled. The images shown demonstrate the importance of examining the entire auditory pathway, as this patient derived little benefit from a left cochlear implant because of gliosis in his right auditory cortex. Similarly, congenitally narrow IACs cause hearing loss. Rehabilitation of hearing in these narrow IAC cases is typically unsuccessful or results in limited functional gain with a cochlear implantation. Use

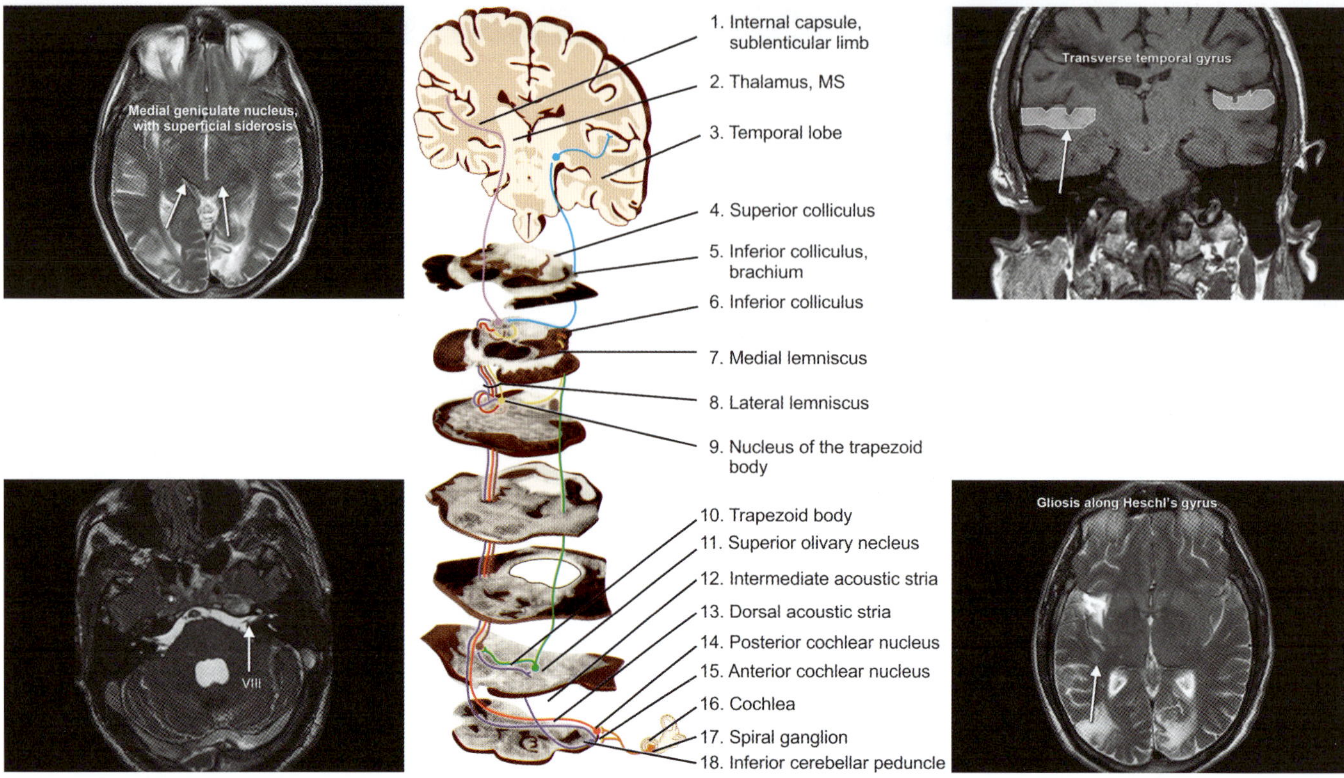

Fig. 16.1: Composite MRI sections and drawing of the central auditory pathway of a patient that received a left cochlear implant. The patient had a prior history of multiple cerebrovascular accidents (CVAs). He derived little benefit from his cochlear implant despite normal cochlear anatomy, normal IAC anatomy, and measurable unaided thresholds of hearing in both ears prior to his implant. His MRI demonstrates gliosis of his right auditory cortex at Heschl's gyrus (white arrow). (IAC, internal auditory canal).

of T2 MRI scanning is essential in the assessment for cochlear implantation of these narrow IACs to demonstrate the presence of two nerve bundles on axial imaging,[16] although the relative loss of CSF surrounding the neural bundles can make visualization difficult and erroneously fail to identify the auditory nerve in the IAC. Examples of normal IAC anatomy and presumptive absent auditory nerve are shown in Figures 16.2A to C. Any lesion affecting the central auditory pathway is significantly more difficult to manage for several reasons. Interventions targeting the central auditory pathway are not appropriate for cochlear implantation for rehabilitation. Moreover, the tonotopic organization afforded by the cochlea is not present in the auditory nerve.

Malformations of the inner ear have been shown to be clearly associated with the presence of SNHL. Most commonly, enlarged vestibular aqueduct is an abnormality identified in imaging evaluation of SNHL (as seen in Figure 16.3). Although more frequently unilateral and sporadic, bilateral cases also exist, and when bilateral, are commonly associated with Pendred's syndrome. Interestingly, it has been unclear how this malformation causes SNHL, as the abnormality is not within the cochlea. It was hypothesized that the hearing loss in Pendred's results from arrested inner ear development, as multiple subtle malformations may be detected in these patients.[17] We now know that enlarged vestibular aqueduct syndrome is caused by mutations in SLC26A4, a gene that encodes pendrin. This gene is required for homeostasis of hearing, and is expressed not only in the endolymphatic sac, but in the stria vascularis of the cochlea, and therefore may provide some explanation as to why this structural abnormality gives rise to SNHL.[18]

Enlargement of the vestibular aqueduct results in a variable, progressive SNHL. It has long been recognized that minor head trauma may result in progression of the hearing loss,[19] which has resulted in many physicians restricting patients with enlarged vestibular aqueducts from participating in contact sports. In some cases of enlarged vestibular aqueduct, concurrent cochlear malformations may be identified. Mondini malformations range from the more favorable 1.5 turns of the cochlea to the less favorable common cavity malformation with incomplete partition (Fig. 16.4). In cases where the cochlea is relatively well formed, outcomes with cochlear implantation are quite good. Conversely, in patients with a common cavity malformation,

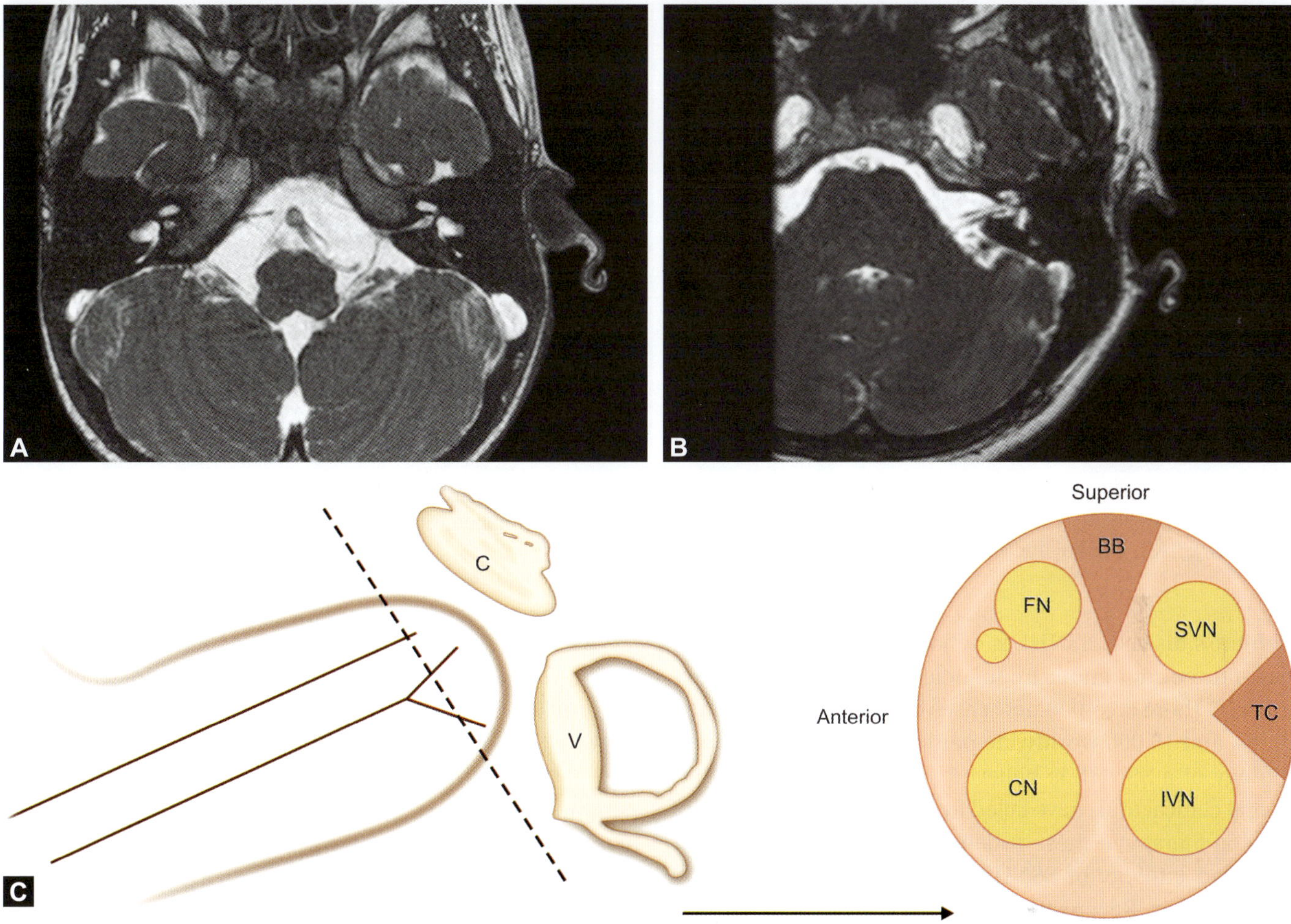

Figs. 16.2A to C: Composite MRI images and drawing in the axial plane demonstrating that in the normal internal auditory canal (IAC), 2 nerve bundles should be observed on T2 imaging, the anterior VIIIth nerve, and the posterior vestibular nerves. In the sagittal plane, all four nerves in the IAC can be visualized. The upper image shows a congenitally narrow IAC, whereas the lower image shows the expected configuration of the IAC. (FN, facial nerve; CN, cochlear nerve; IVN, inferior vestibular nerve; SVN, superior vestibular nerve; BB, bill's bar; TC, transverse crest).

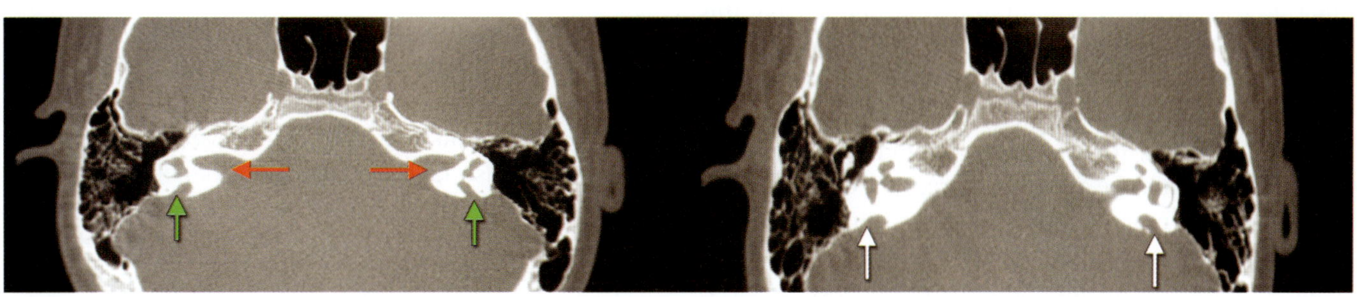

Fig. 16.3: An axial CT scan shows bilateral enlarged vestibular aqueducts in (red arrows). Note the perpendicular orientation to the IAC shown in (green arrows). (IAC, internal auditory canal).

it is unclear where the neural elements lie within this cavity and which areas represent which frequencies, so obviously results with implantation are worse.

Immune-mediated SNHL is the resultant hearing loss in cases where presumptive inflammation exists within the inner ear. This disease process preferentially affects adults, although pediatric and adolescent disease also exists; however, it is significantly more difficult to both identify and manage. Three separate types of immune-mediated SNHL exist: SSNHL, autoimmune inner ear disease (AIED), and

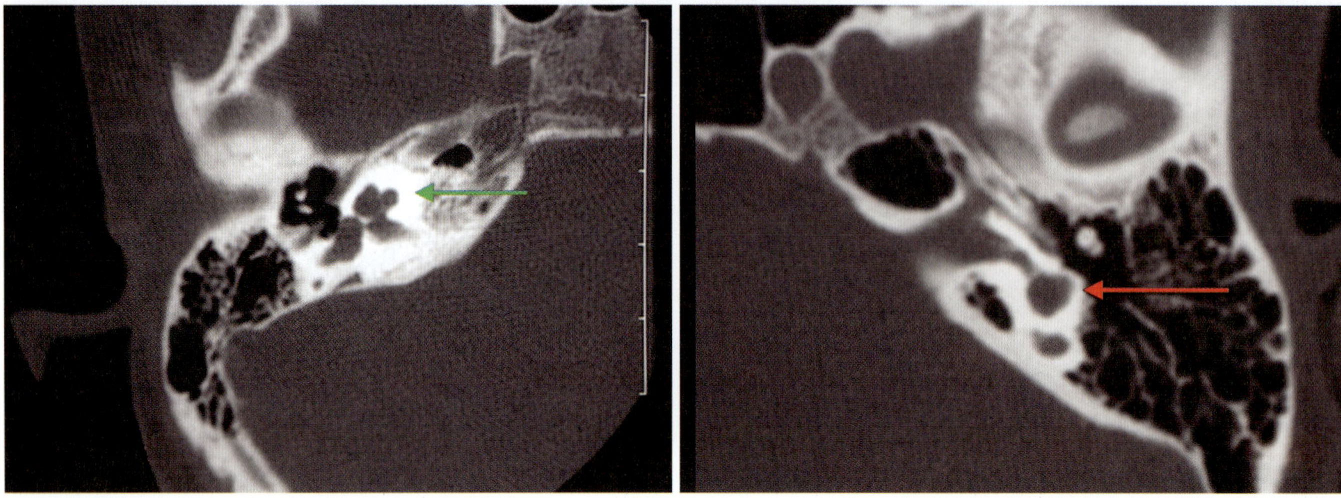

Fig. 16.4: An axial CT scan shows the spectrum of Mondini malformations that may be detected: on the left, a well formed, 1.5 turn, Mondini malformation is seen (green arrow). On the right, a common cavity malformation with an incomplete partition to the IAC is seen (red arrow). (IAC, internal auditory canal).

Meniere's disease. SSNHL is defined as a sudden hearing loss at three contiguous frequencies evolving in three days or less.[20] There are 4000 new cases of SSNHL in the United States, and 15,000 worldwide per year. The most common etiology of a SSNHL is believed to be viral. Despite this, several clinical trials have failed to demonstrate any utility of antiviral therapy in these patients.[21,22] Interestingly, another proposed etiology of SSNHL is vascular compromise of the inner ear. Recent investigations have suggested that SSNHL may be an index event, preceding myocardial infarction, and thereby supporting the vascular theory.[23]

The gold standard for treatment of SSNHL has been corticosteroids.[24,25] Of those treated, approximately 60% of those treated are responsive to steroids.[24] Unfortunately, 40% fail to derive benefit from oral steroids. For this reason, and because systemic steroids may have significant deleterious side effects, in the past decade many otolaryngologists began administering corticosteroids intratympanically. Initially, reports suggested that intratympanic steroid therapy may be a salvage therapy for those who did not respond to oral steroids.[26,27] More recently, however, investigators have sought to determine whether intratympanic steroids were an alternative to oral steroids. In 2011, the results of a National Institutes of Health-sponsored clinical trial determined that intratympanic steroid therapy was comparable to oral steroids.[28] Several small studies have found the combination of oral and intratympanic achieved the best benefit over either route alone.[29] Further studies are necessary to validate this observation.

AIED patients are patients with bilateral fluctuating SNHL, triggered by unknown stimuli, which initially responds to steroid therapy. The hearing loss may affect either ear, sequentially or simultaneously, typically evolving in over 3 days but <90 days.[30,31] Thirty percent of patients with AIED may have a systemic autoimmune disease as well, although there is no enrichment of any one systemic autoimmune disease seen with AIED. Maintenance of hearing with steroids can be accomplished in the short term,[31] although of the 60–70% of AIED patients who are initially steroid responsive, only 14% remain so after 34 months.[32] Therapy for AIED patients who cannot continue on steroids or are refractory to steroids remains limited. Methotrexate has been shown to be beneficial in a small series of patients; however, a large prospective trial failed to confirm these findings.[30] Animal studies demonstrated the potential efficacy of Etanercept, a tumor necrosis factor (TNF) antagonist, in AIED;[33] however, recent human clinical trials also failed to confirm a beneficial effect of this therapy.[34,35] TNF may play a role in steroid sensitive AIED, as patients with high plasma levels of TNF are more likely to respond to corticosteroid therapy and these levels normalize following corticosteroid therapy.[36] For patients who do not respond to corticosteroids, few therapeutic alternatives exist. We recently identified that these steroid refractory patients express high levels of interleukin-1β, which became the rationale for use of an interleukin-1 antagonist in a recent phase I clinical trial.[37]

SNHL may also be a manifestation of systemic disease. Certain autoimmune diseases deserve special mention. Sarcoidosis may manifest with SNHL and uveitis. Sarcoid may also cause leptomeningeal or dural enhancement, and mimic tumor development.[38] Diagnosis may be made by an angiotensin-converting enzyme level, and possibly by biopsy of the affected area. Cogan's syndrome is characterized by interstitial keratitis, Meniere's-like attacks, vasculitis, and in a small percent of patients, aortic insufficiency.[39] Given that fever may be included among the symptoms during the clinical presentation,[40] it is possible that Cogan's syndrome and Muckle-Wells' disease may be related. Cogan's syndrome has been reported in a patient with familial Mediterranean fever, a disease in the same family as Muckle-Wells.[41] In addition to the SNHL associated with autoimmune diseases, there are some infectious diseases that should not be forgotten. Lyme disease has been reported to cause SNHL, tinnitus, and vertigo. In addition, other cranial nerves may be affected in Lyme disease, and the patient may report temporomandibular joint discomfort, otalgia, and neck pain. Interestingly, electrocochleography studies may be positive.

Environmental factors may also influence hearing thresholds. Noise exposure, allergen exposure, and smoking may all influence hearing. The best characterized environmental factor provoking hearing loss is noise exposure.[42] Although occupational noise exposure is the risk that most otolaryngologists refer to, use of personal listening devices for music also poses significant risk.[43] Allergen exposure may indirectly affect hearing. In atopic patients, exposure to the causative allergen can result in endolymphatic hydrops, which clearly affects hearing.[44,45] Smoking or second-hand smoke may also adversely affect hearing.[46] Finally, opiate abuse may also cause an irreversible SNHL.[47]

CLINICAL FINDINGS

One of the most important parameters to establish in the clinical evaluation of SNHL is the duration, symmetry, and stability of the hearing loss. Stable symmetric SNHL of lengthy duration requires amplification, as there is rarely opportunity for medical intervention for correction of the hearing loss. Conversely, recent onset (sudden) SNHL may be ameliorated by rapid medical intervention to reverse the hearing loss. New onset tinnitus, aural fullness, or vertigo should alert the clinician to a potential change in hearing. Asymmetric SNHL should be carefully examined, even if it is not sudden in clinical presentation. In these instances, the clinician should further investigate the etiology of the asymmetry prior to recommendations for rehabilitation.

Concomitant symptoms of hyperacusis, depression, anxiety, dementia, or auditory hallucinations may be present. Although not a direct result of the SNHL, these symptoms are important to identify, as they may adversely affect the motivation of the patient to pursue aural rehabilitation. Appropriate referrals to neurology and psychiatry may ultimately improve the patient's compliance with auditory rehabilitation as well.

EVALUATION

Audiometric testing: The majority of older children and adults can be tested by a conventional audiogram. By convention, red circles are used to demonstrate the right ear, and blue "Xs" are used for the left ear. The degree of hearing loss may be divided into mild (25–40 dB), moderate (40–60 dB), severe (60–80 dB), and profound (over 80 dB). Acoustic reflexes are typically present in SNHL of mild or moderate degree; however, they are typically absent once the hearing loss is >60 dB on average, or if the hearing loss is conductive. Otoacoustic emissions are typically absent in the presence of hearing loss (either conductive or SNHL); however, they may still be present in a mild SNHL, or in cases of auditory neuropathy. Use of bone conduction thresholds and masking can distinguish SNHL from conductive hearing loss or mixed hearing loss: marks of "< , >" show unmasked bone and "[,]" show masked bone. One issue to be aware of is in a unilateral profound SNHL, the bone line will not be superimposed on the air threshold line, as crossover occurs, also referred to as a shadow curve. This does not indicate a mixed hearing loss. An example of this shadow curve is shown in Figure 16.5. Absence of speech discrimination is almost never observed if part of the hearing loss is attributed to a conductive pathology. Notably, in some young children with unilateral or asymmetric hearing loss, special consideration should be given to interpretation of the audiogram. These young children, even with mild to moderate SNHL, often are unable to understand/comply with masking tasks. As such, some audiologists will obtain unmasked bone thresholds. It is critically important for the physician to recognize this and not draw the conclusion that the observed hearing loss is conductive, as shown in Figure 16.6. The CT scan of this young child is seen in Figure 16.3.

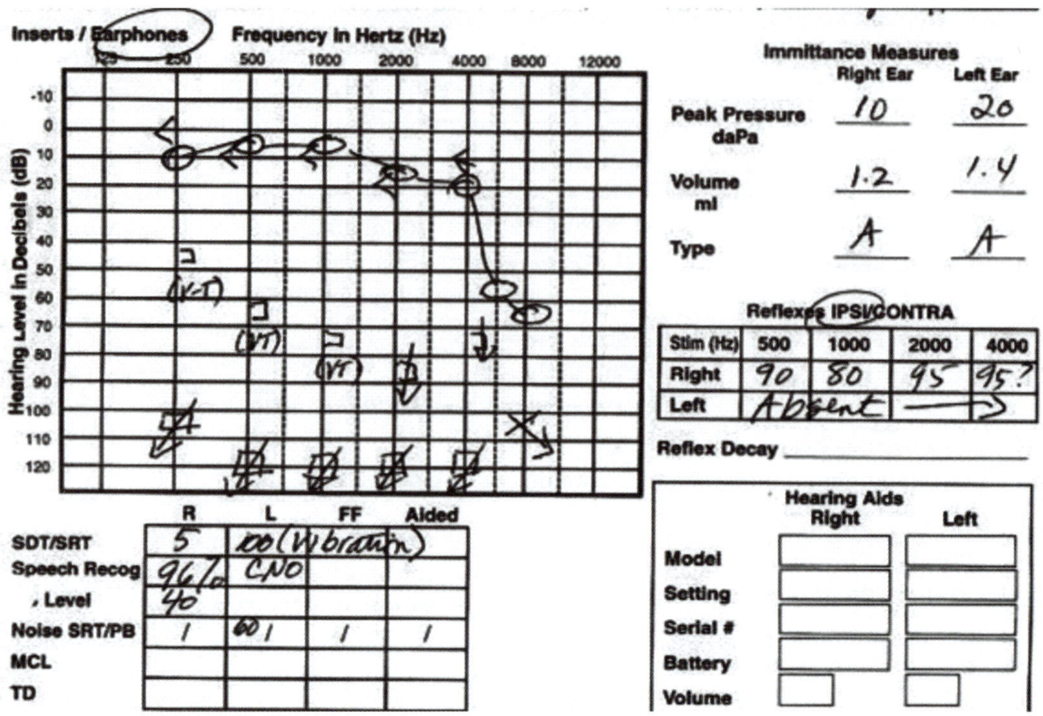

Fig. 16.5: An audiogram of a profound, unilateral, sensorineural hearing loss is seen. Note the absence of measurable speech discrimination and ']' masked bone marks are not superimposed on the air threshold marks demonstrating the presence of a shadow curve. VT, vibrotactile.

Infants, Young Children, and Cognitively Impaired Older Children and Adults

Audiometric testing in this cohort presents more difficulties and requires audiologists familiar with testing these individuals. Young children, ages up to 3 years, typically require sound field audiometry. The otolaryngologist must be cognizant that this type of testing does not exclude a unilateral hearing loss. Although otoacoustic emissions (OAEs) are a useful adjunctive test in these children, absent OAEs in the context of middle ear pathology do not exclude the possibility of a concurrent SNHL. Confirmation of SNHL or detection of SNHL in infants may be accomplished by ABR (automated brainstem response testing). In this test, objective thresholds of hearing may be obtained in each individual ear, up to approximately 102 dB. ABR has some limitations however. ABR requires sedation in the older infant and young child (typically 6 months of age and above). ABR does not test higher cortical function, or how we process the information. ABR is particularly useful in the diagnosis of auditory neuropathy. Here, the auditory nerve is the source of pathology. Patients typically have normal otoacoustic emissions; however, they have a variable SNHL on an audiogram, speech delays, and may have other neurologic or cognitive pathology. ABR classically shows an inverted polarity on wave I, which is pathognomonic for auditory neuropathy[48]

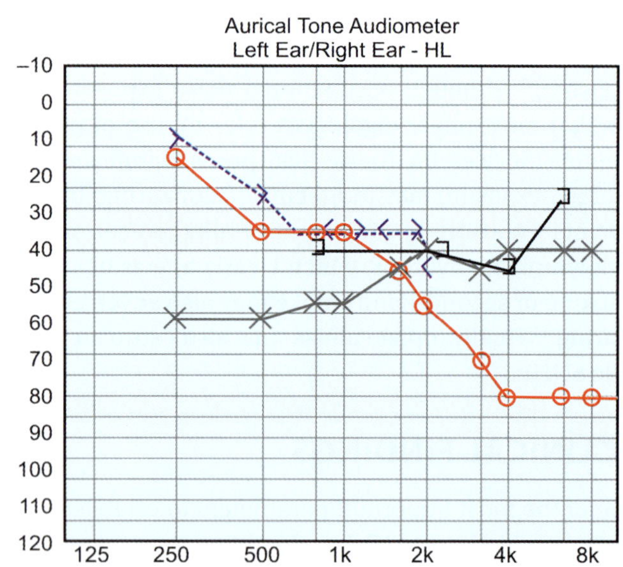

Fig. 16.6: An audiogram of a 4-year-old child referred for a conductive hearing loss. On close examination, the audiogram shows unmasked bone thresholds. The CT scan of this patient is shown in Figure 16.3.

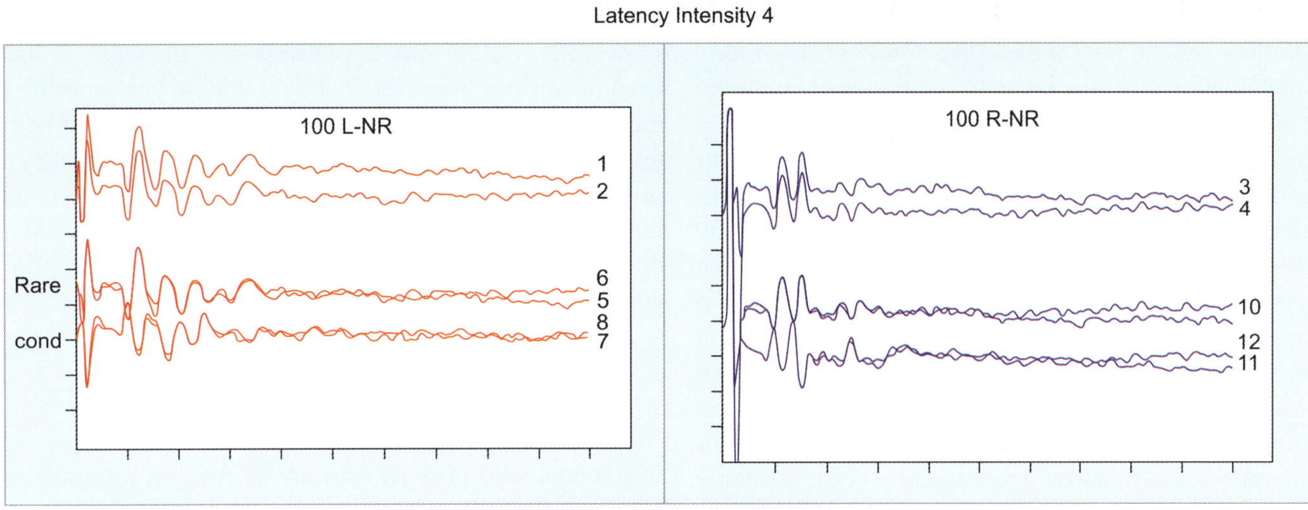

Insert Phone Dly: 0.90 msec

Sensitivity and Sweep Time Per Division

1	0.31 uV	1.5 msec	2	0.31 uV	1.5 msec	3	0.31 uV	1.5 msec	4	0.31 uV	1.5 msec	5	0.31 uV	1.5 msec	6	0.31 uV	1.5 msec
7	0.31 uV	1.5 msec	8	0.31 uV	1.5 msec	9	0.31 uV	1.5 msec	10	0.31 uV	1.5 msec	11	0.31 uV	1.5 msec	12	0.31 uV	1.5 msec

Wave	Flect	Date	Time	Remarks	Wave	Flect	Date	Time	Remarks
1	Cz-A1	07/25/2007	13:02	100L	2	Cz-A1	07/25/2007	13:02	
3	Cz-A2	07/25/2007	13:04	100R	4	Cz-A2	07/25/2007	13:05	
5	Cz-A1	07/25/2007	13:02	100L	6	Cz-A1	07/25/2007	13:02	
7	Cz-A1	07/25/2007	13:03	100L CON	8	Cz-A1	07/25/2007	13:03	
9	Cz-A2	07/25/2007	13:04	100R	10	Cz-A2	07/25/2007	13:05	
11	Cz-A2	07/25/2007	13:05	100R CON	12	Cz-A2	07/25/2007	13:06	

Fig. 16.7: An ABR evaluation of a child with auditory neuropathy. The classic finding of a wave I inversion, with inversion of the polarity is seen (rarefaction vs. condensation).

(Fig. 16.7). Auditory neuropathy is associated with hyperbilirubinemia and prematurity.[49] Some studies suggest that in some infants this condition may improve over time, and therefore cochlear implantation should be approached slowly and cautiously in this population.[50] Presumptive unilateral auditory neuropathy, with present OAEs and an absent ABR, is a unique observation that requires special attention. In these cases, the most likely pathology is a narrow IAC. In these cases, the OAEs may be present in the young child and as the child ages, the OAE disappears.

EVALUATION

The type of evaluation undertaken for SNHL is largely based on the clinical scenario in which it arises. Here we will describe several different patient types with SNHL.

Congenital Sensorineural Hearing Loss

Congenital SNHL (meaning present at birth) may be divided into bilateral/symmetric or unilateral asymmetric. For those with bilateral, symmetric SNHL, it is most prudent to investigate genetic etiologies first. The advantage to this approach is that in the event a genetic etiology is identified, no sedation and no radiation exposure are required. Simple blood testing may identify the etiology of the SNHL. In the event the etiology is not identified, then imaging can be obtained. In the event the hearing loss is asymmetric or unilateral, it is more likely that a structural or anatomic abnormality of the cochlea may be present. For the evaluation of children with an asymmetric SNHL, especially if not present at birth or worsening after birth, the most common abnormality identified is a structural abnormality of the inner ear, such as an enlarged vestibular aqueduct. In these instances, earlier identification of an enlarged vestibular aqueduct, or other inner ear malformations, may allow parents to take appropriate measures to prevent further progression of hearing loss by preventing minor head trauma (i.e. use of a bicycle helmet to prevent head trauma). Noncontrast CT scan imaging of the temporal bone, in the axial and coronal planes, can detect enlarged vestibular aqueducts. CT scanning of the temporal bones, in slices as close as 0.5 mm, in the axial, coronal, and sagittal planes provides superior imaging of the inner ear. Criteria to call the vestibular aqueduct enlarged are controversial; originally reported to be equal to or >1.5 mm from anterior to posterior, mid-fundus by Valvesori, newer criteria suggest >0.9 mm mid-fundus and 1.9 mm at the operculum.[51] Furthermore, although historically imaged by CT scan, newer concerns over radiation exposure and the risk of developing a malignancy[52] may eventually change the test of choice to MRI. The disadvantage to MRI scanning in children is the frequent need for sedation, whereas often CT scans may be able to be performed unsedated in the cooperative preschooler or school-aged child. The concern about CT scanning will need to be counterbalanced by the requirement of sedation, for MRI in particular, as the use of N-methyl-D-aspartate receptor antagonists in some sedation agents has been linked to long-term neurodegeneration and impairment of cognition in some infants and young children.[53] In the event radiographic studies demonstrate normal inner ear anatomy; genetic testing can be undertaken following radiographic studies if the etiology of the SNHL is not identified.

Since the advent of newborn hearing screening, many of the congenital hearing impairments may now be identified at birth, rather than the first school screening, or first evaluation of delayed speech. Historically, part of the evaluation of SNHL was to perform TORCH titers to identify perinatal infectious causes of SNHL. TORCH titers are comprised of Toxoplasma IgG, Rubella IgG, Cytomegalovirus (CMV) IgG, Herpes Simplex IgG, type 1 and 2. Although all of these congenital infections may result in chronic sequelae or fatal infections, testing is of limited utility as IgM expression is limited in duration, CMV is ubiquitous, and serum IgG to CMV in toddler-aged children or older is not necessarily indicative of congenital infection. Identification of IgM antibodies to CMV in cord blood is indicative of congenital CMV infection. Given that identification of congenital SNHL is significantly earlier because of universal newborn hearing screening initiatives, early TORCH titer testing in the newborn nursery by the neonatologist may have a significantly higher yield than later testing by the otolaryngologist.

Once an infant or child is identified with a SNHL, it is important that the child undergo evaluations of their vision, and their kidneys. A high prevalence of ocular abnormalities has been detected in children with SNHL.[54] It was originally argued that the inner ear and the kidneys develop around the same time, and therefore an in utero insult was the most likely explanation for the high concurrence of otic and renal involvement, such as in branchio-oto-renal, and Alport's syndromes, for example. Interestingly, the primordia of the ear and kidney do not develop at the same time, calling this hypothesis into question. It has become obvious, however, that a number of key genes play important regulatory functions in the development of both the inner ear and kidney, thus explaining the relationship of these two organs. Genes involved in branchio-oto-renal and Townes-Brock are expressed at different times in the developing inner ear and the kidney during morphogenesis, arguing against a single in utero insult.[55]

Adult Onset SSNHL, Asymmetric and Progressive SNHL

In patients who present with an SSNHL, an asymmetric SNHL, or a rapidly progressive SNHL, imaging studies are essential to exclude retrocochlear pathology as the etiology of the SNHL. Appropriate imaging for these types of hearing loss is an MRI of the IACs with gadolinium. Approximately 2% of patients with SSNHL are found to have a vestibular schwannoma as the etiology of their SSNHL; however, approximately 20% of patients with vestibular schwannoma report SSNHL in their clinical history.[56] Additionally, lesions that affect any portion of the central auditory pathway may result in either a sudden or asymmetric SNHL. Especially in the older adult, stroke may result in acute SNHL as well as focal deficits.

HISTOLOGY

Unfortunately, one of the greatest limitations to identification of the etiology of SNHL is the inability to obtain a histopathologic diagnosis. Much of what we have learned about etiologies of SNHL has come from histopathology of the temporal bone. We are currently in crisis as few temporal bone histopathology laboratories and registries remain. Those still in existence are in jeopardy of closure because of fiscal constraints. Although we have entered an age of molecular biology and genetic diagnosis, failure to correlate molecular signatures of disease with histopathology of the temporal bone will similarly result in an incomplete understanding of the etiopathogenesis of SNHL.

TREATMENT

The majority of treatment efforts are for rehabilitation rather than correction of SNHL. The majority of interventions for SNHL are the use of amplification through hearing aids.

For newborns who fail the newborn hearing screen, fitting an infant with amplification by 6 months of age results in better expressive language development than fitting after the age of 6 months.[1]

In the classroom setting, additional adjunctive measures are often employed. Preferential classroom seating for patients with asymmetries of hearing can position the better-hearing ear closer to the teacher. FM systems reduce the signal-to-noise ratio and preferentially deliver the teacher's voice to the hearing impaired student. Newer technologies include use of CART (communication access real-time translation) captioning technologies for older high school and college age students with hearing-impairment. This technology provides real-time captioning of not only the teacher's voice but also of the classmates, so the hearing-impaired student may participate in discussions without missing vital information put forth by colleagues.

Access to rehabilitative technologies has remained challenging. State-run early intervention programs provide hearing aids and services to infants and toddlers identified with hearing loss through age 3. If, however, a child is identified late or develops a progressive sensorineural hearing loss, the onus of paying for hearing aids is transferred to the parents. Many insurance carriers do not cover hearing aid costs. Although some provide limited coverage, this often will not exceed a fraction of the cost, despite full coverage for cochlear implants by many insurance carriers. As school budgets continue to shrink, access to assistive devices such as FM systems, CART services, teachers of the deaf and speech-language pathologists becomes increasingly more challenging.

Continued auditory stimulation has remained the guiding principle of improved performance with both hearing aids and cochlear implants. Adults with symmetric and asymmetric SNHL may experience declining speech discrimination in the absence of binaural amplification.[2,57] Similarly, cognitive decline in older adults has been linked to SNHL.[4] These observations provide the rationale for rehabilitation of hearing at any age of detection.

PROGNOSIS

The prognosis for SNHL is clearly contingent on the underlying etiology of the SNHL. Identification of the etiology is beneficial for the patient and family to understand the stability of the SNHL, whether other organs may be affected, and the prognosis with various interventions.

REFERENCES

1. Yoshinaga-Itano C. Early intervention after universal neonatal hearing screening: impact on outcomes. Ment Retard Dev Disabil Res Rev. 2003;9(4):252-66.
2. Silman S, Gelfand SA, Silverman CA. Late-onset auditory deprivation: effects of monaural versus binaural hearing aids. J Acoust Soc Am. 1984;76(5):1357-62.
3. Lin FR, Ferrucci L, Metter EJ, et al. Hearing loss and cognition in the Baltimore Longitudinal Study of Aging. Neuropsychology. 2011;25(6):763-70.
4. Lin FR, Yaffe K, Xia J, et al. Hearing loss and cognitive decline in older adults. JAMA Intern Med. 2013;173(4): 293-9.
5. Zelante L, Gasparini P, Estivill X, et al. Connexin26 mutations associated with the most common form of non-syndromic neurosensory autosomal recessive deafness (DFNB1) in Mediterraneans. Hum Mol Genet. 1997;6(9):1605-9.
6. Green GE, Scott DA, McDonald JM, et al. Carrier rates in the midwestern United States for GJB2 mutations causing inherited deafness. JAMA. 1999;281(23):2211-6.
7. Mhatre AN, Li Y, Atkin G, Maghnouj A, Lalwani AK. Expression of Myh9 in the mammalian cochlea: localization within the stereocilia. J Neurosci Res. 2006;84(4):809-18.
8. Liu XZ, Walsh J, Mburu P, Kendrick-Jones J, et al. Mutations in the myosin VIIA gene cause non-syndromic recessive deafness. Nat Genet. 1997;16(2):188-90.
9. Shearer AE, DeLuca AP, Hildebrand MS, et al. Comprehensive genetic testing for hereditary hearing loss using massively parallel sequencing. Proc Natl Acad Sci USA. 2010;107(49):21104-9.
10. Fahim AT, Daiger SP, Weleber RG. Retinitis Pigmentosa Overview. In: Pagon RA, Adam MP, Bird TD, Dolan CR, Fong CT, Stephens K (eds), Gene reviews. Seattle, WA: University of Washington, Seattle; 1993.
11. Onishi H, Inoue K, Osaka H, et al. Mitochondrial myopathy, encephalopathy, lactic acidosis and stroke-like episodes (MELAS) and diabetes mellitus: molecular genetic analysis and family study. J Neurol Sci. 1993;114(2):205-8.
12. Rosenthal EL, Kileny PR, Boerst A, et al. Successful cochlear implantation in a patient with MELAS syndrome. Am J Otol. 1999;20(2):187-90; discussion 90-1.
13. Takahashi K, Merchant SN, Miyazawa T, et al. Temporal bone histopathological and quantitative analysis of mitochondrial DNA in MELAS. Laryngoscope. 2003;113(8): 1362-8.
14. Phillips JS, King JA, Chandran S, et al. Cerebral autosomal dominant arteriopathy with subcortical infarcts and leukoencephalopathy (CADASIL) presenting with sudden sensorineural hearing loss. J Laryngol Otol. 2005;119(2): 148-5.
15. Hoffman HM, Mueller JL, Broide DH, et al. Mutation of a new gene encoding a putative pyrin-like protein causes familial cold autoinflammatory syndrome and Muckle-Wells syndrome. Nat Genet. 2001;29(3):301-5.
16. Govaerts PJ, Casselman J, Daemers K, et al. Cochlear implants in aplasia and hypoplasia of the cochleovestibular nerve. Otol Neurotol. 2003;24(6):887-91.

17. Valvassori GE, Clemis JD. The large vestibular aqueduct syndrome. Laryngoscope. 1978;88(5):723-8.
18. Choi BY, Kim HM, Ito T, et al. Mouse model of enlarged vestibular aqueducts defines temporal requirement of Slc26a4 expression for hearing acquisition. The Journal of clinical investigation. 2011;121(11):4516-25.
19. Jackler RK, De La Cruz A. The large vestibular aqueduct syndrome. Laryngoscope. 1989;99(12):1238-42; discussion 42-3.
20. Hughes GB, Freedman MA, Haberkamp TJ, et al. Sudden sensorineural hearing loss. Otolaryngol Clin N Am. 1996; 29:393-405.
21. Stokroos RJ, Albers FW, Tenvergert EM. Antiviral treatment of idiopathic sudden sensorineural hearing loss: a prospective, randomized, double-blind clinical trial. Acta Otolaryngol. 1998;118(4):488-95.
22. Tucci DL, Farmer JC Jr, Kitch RD, et al. Treatment of sudden sensorineural hearing loss with systemic steroids and valacyclovir. Otol Neurotol. 2002;23(3):301-8.
23. Ciccone MM, Cortese F, Pinto M, et al. Endothelial function and cardiovascular risk in patients with idiopathic sudden sensorineural hearing loss. Atherosclerosis. 2012; 225(2):511-6.
24. Wilson WR, Byl FM, Laird N. The efficacy of steroids in the treatment of idiopathic sudden hearing loss: a double-blind clinical study. Arch Otolaryngol (Chicago, IL : 1960). 1980;106(12):772-6.
25. Stachler RJ, Chandrasekhar SS, Archer SM, et al. Clinical practice guideline: sudden hearing loss. Otolaryngol Head Neck Surg. 2012;146(3 Suppl):S1-35.
26. Ho HG, Lin HC, Shu MT, et al. Effectiveness of intratympanic dexamethasone injection in sudden-deafness patients as salvage treatment. Laryngoscope. 2004;114(7):1184-9.
27. Plontke SK, Lowenheim H, Mertens J, et al. Randomized, double blind, placebo controlled trial on the safety and efficacy of continuous intratympanic dexamethasone delivered via a round window catheter for severe to profound sudden idiopathic sensorineural hearing loss after failure of systemic therapy. Laryngoscope. 2009;119(2): 359-69.
28. Rauch SD, Halpin CF, Antonelli PJ, et al. Oral vs intratympanic corticosteroid therapy for idiopathic sudden sensorineural hearing loss: a randomized trial. JAMA. 2011; 305(20):2071-9.
29. Battaglia A, Burchette R, Cueva R. Combination therapy (intratympanic dexamethasone + high-dose prednisone taper) for the treatment of idiopathic sudden sensorineural hearing loss. Otol Neurotol. 2008;29(4):453-60.
30. Harris JP, Weissman MH, Derebery JM, et al. Treatment of corticosteroid-responsive autoimmune inner ear disease with methotrexate: a randomized controlled trial. JAMA. 2003;290:1875-83.
31. Niparko JK, Wang NY, Rauch SD, et al.; AIED study group. Serial audiometry in a clinical trial of AIED treatment. Otol Neurotol. 2005;26:908-17.
32. Broughton SS, Meyerhoff WE, Cohen SB. Immune mediated inner ear disease: 10-year experience. Semin Arthritis Rheum. 2004;34:544-8.
33. Satoh HFG, Billings PB, Firestein GS, et al. Tumor necrosis factor alpha, an initiator, and etanercept, an inhibitor of cochlear inflammation. Laryngoscope. 2002;112: 1627-34.
34. Cohen S, Shoup A, Weisman MH, Harris J. Etanercept treatment for autoimmune inner ear disease: results of a pilot placebo-controlled study. Otol Neurotol. 2005;26: 903-7.
35. Matteson EL, Choi HK, Poe DS, et al. Etanercept therapy for immune-mediated cochleovestibular disorders: a multicenter, open-label, pilot study. Arthritis Rheum. 2005;53: 337-42.
36. Svrakic M, Pathak S, Goldofsky E, et al. Diagnostic and prognostic utility of measuring tumor necrosis factor in the peripheral circulation of patients with immune-mediated sensorineural hearing loss. Arch Otolaryngol Head Neck Surg. 2012;138(11):1052-8.
37. Pathak S, Goldofsky E, Vivas EX, et al. IL-1beta is overexpressed and aberrantly regulated in corticosteroid nonresponders with autoimmune inner ear disease. J Immunol. 2011;186(3):1870-79.
38. Shah R, Roberson GH, Cure JK. Correlation of MR imaging findings and clinical manifestations in neurosarcoidosis. AJNR Am J Neuroradiol. 2009;30(5):953-61.
39. Haynes BF, Kaiser-Kupfer MI, Mason P, et al. Cogan syndrome: studies in thirteen patients, long-term follow-up, and a review of the literature. Medicine. 1980;59(6):426-41.
40. Gluth MB, Baratz KH, Matteson EL, et al. Cogan syndrome: a retrospective review of 60 patients throughout a half century. Mayo Clin Proc. 2006;81(4):483-8.
41. Zenone T, Puget M. Cogan's syndrome in a patient with familial Mediterranean fever. Clinical and experimental rheumatology. 2012;30(1):141.
42. Azizi MH. Occupational noise-induced hearing loss. Int J Occup Environ Med. 2010;1(3):116-23.
43. Punch JL, Elfenbein JL, James RR. Targeting hearing health messages for users of personal listening devices. Am J Audiol. 2011;20(1):69-82.
44. Gibbs SR, Mabry RL, Roland PS, et al. Electrocochleographic changes after intranasal allergen challenge: A possible diagnostic tool in patients with Meniere's disease. Otolaryngol Head Neck Surg. 1999;121(3):283-4.
45. Noell CA, Roland PS, Mabry RL, et al. Inhalant allergy and Meniere's disease: Use of electrocochleography and intranasal allergen challenge as investigational tools. Otolaryngol Head Neck Surg. 2001;125(4):346-50.
46. Lalwani AK, Liu YH, Weitzman M. Secondhand smoke and sensorineural hearing loss in adolescents. Arch Otolaryngol Head Neck Surg. 2011;137(7):655-62.
47. Friedman RA, House JW, Luxford WM, et al. Profound hearing loss associated with hydrocodone/acetaminophen abuse. Am J Otol. 2000;21(2):188-91.

48. Berlin CI, Bordelon J, St John P, et al. Reversing click polarity may uncover auditory neuropathy in infants. Ear Hearing. 1998;19(1):37-47.
49. Berlin CI, Hood LJ, Morlet T, et al. Multi-site diagnosis and management of 260 patients with auditory neuropathy/dys-synchrony (auditory neuropathy spectrum disorder). Int J Audiol. 2010;49(1):30-43.
50. Attias J, Raveh E. Transient deafness in young candidates for cochlear implants. Audiol Neuro-otol. 2007;12(5):325-33.
51. Gopen Q, Zhou G, Whittemore K, et al. Enlarged vestibular aqueduct: review of controversial aspects. Laryngoscope. 2011;121(9):1971-8.
52. Slovis TL. The ALARA concept in pediatric CT: myth or reality? Radiology. 2002;223(1):5-6.
53. Rappaport B, Mellon RD, Simone A, et al. Defining safe use of anesthesia in children. N Engl J Med. 2011;364(15):1387-90. PubMed PMID: 21388302.
54. Mafong DD, Pletcher SD, Hoyt C, et al. Ocular findings in children with congenital sensorineural hearing loss. Arch Otolaryngol Head Neck Surg. 2002;128(11):1303-6.
55. Izzedine H, Tankere F, Launay-Vacher V, et al. Ear and kidney syndromes: molecular versus clinical approach. Kidney Int. 2004;65(2):369-85.
56. Sauvaget E, Kici S, Kania R, et al. Sudden sensorineural hearing loss as a revealing symptom of vestibular schwannoma. Acta Otolaryngol. 2005;125(6):592-5.
57. Silverman CA, Silman S, Emmer MB, et al. Auditory deprivation in adults with asymmetric, sensorineural hearing impairment. J Am Acad Audiol. 2006;17(10):747-62.
58. Pingault V, Ente D, Dastot-Le, et al. Review and update of mutations causing Waardenburg syndrome. Hum Mutat. 2010;31(4):391-406.
59. Kashtan CE. Alport syndrome. An inherited disorder of renal, ocular, and cochlear basement membranes. Medicine. 1999;78(5):338-60.
60. Schulze-Bahr E, Wang Q, Wedekind H, et al. KCNE1 mutations cause Jervell and Lange-Nielsen syndrome. Nat Genet. 1997;17(3):267-8.
61. Neyroud N, Richard P, Vignier N, et al. Genomic organization of the KCNQ1 K+ channel gene and identification of C-terminal mutations in the long-QT syndrome. Circ Res. 1999;84(3):290-97.

CHAPTER

17

Presbycusis

Selena E Heman-Ackah, Steven K Juhn

INTRODUCTION

Presbycusis is one of the most common conditions affecting the aging population. Also commonly referred to as age-related hearing loss, presbycusis may be defined that occurs as a function of a variety of contributing factors that progresses with in the geriatric population. The hearing loss associated with age-related hearing loss is characteristically high frequency with deficits in speech discrimination. The prevalence of age-related hearing loss increases with age. The etiology of age-related hearing loss is multifactorial with oxidative injury, noise exposure, heredity, and otologic injury (i.e. ototoxins and otologic disease) as major contributing factors. Presbycusis has a wide potential impact not only on the individual but on society as a whole, making prevention, early diagnosis and treatment of critical importance in circumventing this potential impact. This chapter will give an overview of the current state of knowledge regarding etiology, diagnosis, treatment, and prevention of age-related hearing loss as well as briefly highlight future therapies on the horizon for the treatment and prevention of age-related hearing loss.

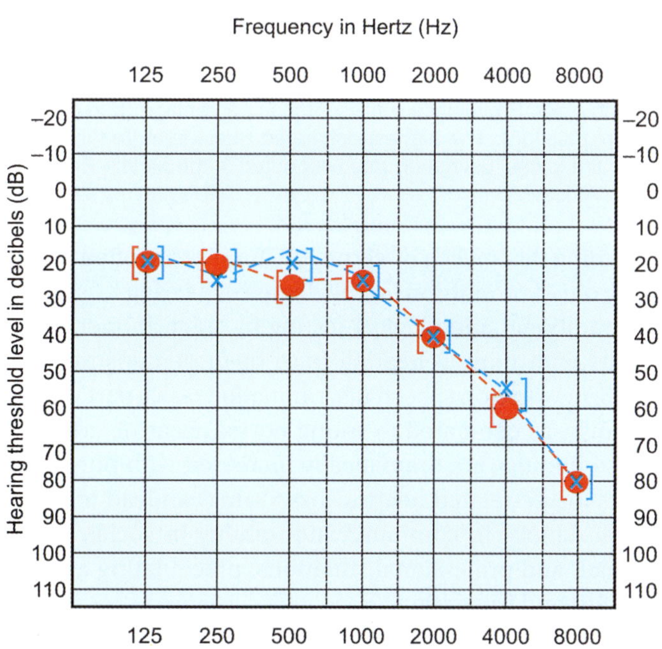

Fig. 17.1: Pure tone audiogram characteristic of presbycusis. This audiogram depicts the characteristic pattern of hearing loss encountered in patient with presbycusis. Sensorineural hearing loss typically begins in the region at and above 2000 Hz.

DEFINITION OF PRESBYCUSIS

Presbycusis may be defined as any sum of conditions and exposures that lead to the development and progression of hearing loss with aging. Age-related hearing loss is characterized by high-frequency sensorineural hearing loss that progressively increases with aging. Figure 17.1 depicts an audiogram characteristic of moderately advanced age-related hearing loss. As can be seen in Figure 17.1, individuals with age-related hearing loss tend to develop losses within the 2000 to 4000 Hz range earlier in the process. As such, individuals tend to experience difficulty with understanding the voiceless consonants of speech (i.e. c [k], ch [tʃ], f [f], k [k], p [p], s [s], sh [ʃ], t [t], th [θ]). For example, patients with presbycusis may experience difficulty discriminating the words "bash", "bath", "bat", "back", "batch", and "bass". Because of this, patients often experience difficulty with understanding speech, particularly in ambient conditions. The complaints that patients present with

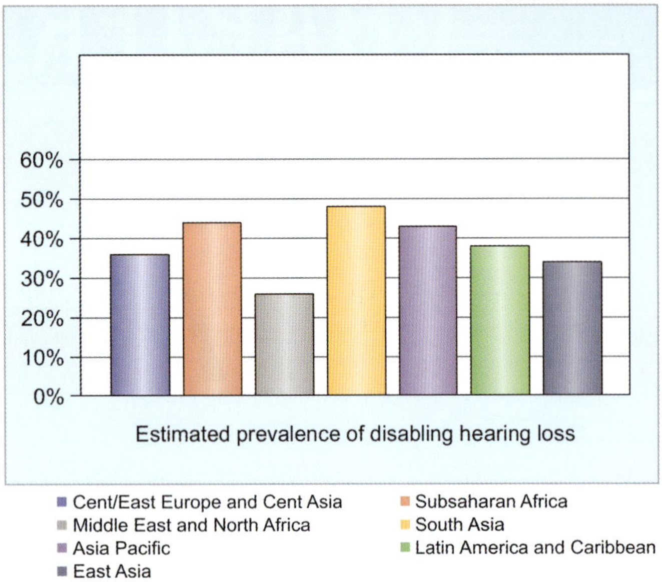

Fig. 17.2: WHO 2012 estimates of disabling hearing loss in individuals 65 years and over by region. This graph depicts the estimated prevalence of age-related hearing loss in individuals age 65 and older. Prevalence is presented in percentage (persons per 100 population). The highest estimated rate was noted in South Asia; the lowest estimated rate was noted in the Middle East and North Africa.

regarding this speech discernment in noise are often seemingly out of proportion for the degree of hearing loss noted on traditional audiological testing in quiet. In fact, older adults with normal hearing have been demonstrated to perform worse on speech discrimination tasks, particularly in noise, as compared to young normal hearing adults.[1-4] These findings are dramatically increased with pure-tone shifts in age-related hearing loss.[1,4] This can lead to significant deficits in communication ability in social, recreational, and professional situations, precipitating a sense of angst and frustration.

EPIDEMIOLOGY

Presbycusis or age-related hearing loss is one of the most common conditions affecting the aging population. Within the United States, presbycusis is among the top three most common condition affecting the aging population.[5,6] It is the most common communication disorder affecting the geriatric population.[5] Table 17.1 presents recently published prevalence rates for age-related hearing loss.[6-9] Within the United States, for individuals over the age of 65 years, the prevalence of age-related hearing loss ranges from 35% to 50%.[6-8] By age 75 years, the prevalence increases to 40% to 65%. By age 80 years, the prevalence

Table 17.1: US prevalence of presbycusis with increasing age

Age of population	*Prevalence*
65 years of age or greater	35–50%
75 years of age or greater	40–65%
85 years of age or greater	Over 80%
100 years of age or greater	Approximately 90%

increases to approximately 80%, and at 100, the prevalence is approximately 90%.[6-9] Similar prevalence rates have been reported internationally.

In a review of 42 population-based studies in 2012, the World Health Organization (WHO) released estimates of disabling hearing loss rates in individuals over the age of 65. The WHO defined disabling hearing loss as hearing loss >40 dB in the better hearing ear.[10] The estimated prevalence of disabling hearing loss in individuals aged 64 years and older by international region is presented in Figure 17.2. With the exception of the Middle East and North Africa region, all estimated prevalence rates fall between 30% and 50% for individuals 65 years of age and over. The highest prevalence rates for disabling hearing loss in adults over 65, according to this review, were noted in South Asia. Interestingly, on review of United States prevalence alone, racial differences in prevalence have been reported.[11] When comparing individuals who classify themselves as black and white, statistically significant differences in the rates of hearing loss, defined as pure tone average in speech frequencies of >25 dB in the better hearing ear were noted. Overall prevalence of hearing loss in black males age 70 and older was noted as 48.3% (95% confidence interval: 36.3–60.3) versus 71.5% (95% confidence interval: 64.8–78.3) in white males ($p = 0.002$). Similar, prevalence differences were found among females age 70 years and older ($p = 0.03$): black females 39.8% (95% confidence interval: 20.6–59.1) versus white females 59.0% (95% confidence interval: 51.3–66.8). These findings are consistent with previous reports within the literature regarding a decreased prevalence of age-related hearing loss in black individuals.[12-14] This is believed by some to be secondary to a hypothesized protective effect of increased melanin, particularly within the stria vascularis.[15-17]

Economic status has been noted to be correlated with the presentation of age-related hearing loss. This may be related to the multifactorial etiology of age-related hearing loss and the fact that undertreated otologic disease and systemic disease may contribute to hearing loss. Thus, individuals with improved socioeconomic status may have access to more preventive care and therapeutic treatment preventing the onset or progression of hearing loss. According to the WHO study, greater overall increased income was correlated with a decreased prevalence of age-related hearing loss.[10] Similar findings were reported by Lin et al. in a review of presbycusis prevalence in the United States.[11]

Genders have been found to impact the presentation of presbycusis. The male population appears to be more affected by age-related hearing loss as compared to their female counterparts. This has been identified in a number studies based both on self-reported subjective measures and objective audiometric data.[1,18-20] In a data analysis of the National Health and Nutritional Examination Survey 2005–2006 cycle hearing assessment among 717 adults age 70 and older, a statistically significant difference in the rate of presbycusis (defined as speech frequency pure tone average of >25 dB in the better hearing ear) was noted in males as compared to females (69.8% and 58.2%, respectively).[11]

Etiology

As presbycusis represents the sum of life influences that precipitate the presentation of hearing loss with aging, there are a number of factors that have been associated with the development of presbycusis. Gates poignantly describes presbycusis as "a mixture of acquired auditory stresses, trauma, and otologic diseases superimposed upon an intrinsic, genetically controlled, aging process".[21] The etiology of presbycusis is influenced by genetics (up to 50% have significant family history), cardiovascular health (in turn influenced by smoking and diabetes), history of noise exposure, as well as ototoxic exposure and otologic disorders.[22]

Aging and Oxidative Injury

In a landmark article by Denham Harman in 1956, the free-radical theory of aging was introduced.[23] Since that time, free radical damage has been implicated as an etiologic factor in various organ systems, including the ophthalmologic, integumentary, and hepatic systems.[24-27] Similarly, oxidative stress has been hypothesized to be an integrally involved etiological factor in the development of presbycusis via free radical (reactive oxygen species and reactive nitrogen species) associated mitochondrial dysfunction.[28] Various findings have been identified in animal studies to support this theory. Increased markers of oxidative stress have been noted to be increased in the cochlea of aged CBA/J mice.[29] Mice missing the gene encoding Cu/Zn superoxide dismutase, a critical enzyme in the reduction of reactive oxygen species and maintenance of oxidative balance show premature presbycusis.[30,31] Similarly, overexpression of mitochondria-localized catalase that eliminates reactive oxygen species has been demonstrated to be protective against age-related threshold shift.[32] It is postulated that with the accumulation of mitochondrial DNA mutation, oxidative phosphorylation is impaired and expression of antioxidant enzymes is altered, leading to further increase in reactive oxygen species in the cochlea.[33] Human temporal bone studies support these findings. Various deletions within the mitochondrial genome have been noted in human temporal bone tissue.[34-38] A correlation has been identified between the extent of age-related threshold shifts and mitochondrial DNA deletions. [34,37]

Noise

Noise exposure is a well-established risk factor for hearing loss.[14] Noise exposure not only contributes to oxidative stress and the production of reactive oxygen species that mediates short-term injury but also may contribute to long-term damage. Hearing loss from noise exposure, also known as noise-induced hearing loss, may take the form of transient threshold shifts or long-term acoustic changes. Everyday noise exposure can cause hearing loss and may accelerate the process that leading to presbycusis. Table 17.2 presents the current National Institute for Occupational Safety and Health (NIOSH) and Occupational Safety and Health Administration (OSHA) guidelines for noise exposure. To put these noise level exposures into perspective, Table 17.3 provides a list of commonly and less commonly encountered noises with associated noise levels. It is interesting to note that listening to high power headphones on a near maximum level for a period of 1 hour in the gym or on a long commute, attending a concert, or using the snow blower for over 30 minutes may exceed the current NIOSH recommendations for noise exposure. It is easy to see how simple life experiences may contribute to noise damage over time.

Remarkably, recent studies have demonstrated that the effect of noise-induced hearing loss may extend long after the exposure has stopped.[39] Noise damage occurs even with temporary or no immediate hearing loss, which is believed to contribute to accelerated presbycusis. This

Table 17.2: National Institute for Occupational Safety and Health (NIOSH) and Occupational Safety and Health Administration (OSHA) recommended permissible noise exposure levels

Permissible noise level exposure		
	Sound level	
Hours per day	*NIOSH (dB)*	*OSHA (dB)*
8	85	90
6	86	92
4	88	95
3	89	97
2	90	100
1.5	92	102
1	94	105
0.5	97	110
0.25	100	115
0	112	

Table 17.3: Commonly and less commonly encountered environmental sounds

Environmental sounds	
Stimulus	*Sound level (dB)*
Rustling leaves	20
Whisper at 6 ft	30
Residential area at night	40
Quiet office	50
Normal conversation	60–65
Car noise	70
City traffic	85
Lawnmower	90
Subway train at 200 ft	95
Hand drill	95–100
Snowmobile	100
Motorcycle	100
Power mower	105
Jackhammer	110
Power saw	110
Sandblaster	115
Maximum volume ear buds	85–115
Ambulance siren	120
Loud concert	100–125
Pneumatic riveter	125
Jet engine	140
0.22 Caliber riffle	145
12 Gauge shotgun	165
0.357 Caliber revolver	170–175

Purple: Within the cautionary range for limited noise exposure.
Gray: Within the cautionary range for immediate noise injury.

is supported by findings in animal models of hearing loss demonstrating permanent neuronal losses in the spiral ganglion correlated with accelerated age-related hearing loss[40-42] and loss of synaptic terminal between inner hair cells and spiral ganglion neurons.[41,43] In clinical studies, presbycusis has been found to be more severe in individuals thought to have suffered cochlear damage in their youth from noise exposure.[39]

It is important to note that presbycusis can develop in patients without a history of excessive noise exposure. Additionally, the shape and progression of hearing loss may differ in individuals with significant noise exposure. Gates et al. found that in subjects with noise induced threshold shifts, there is a reduced progression of hearing loss at 3, 4, and 6 kHz and accelerated hearing loss at the surrounding frequencies, particularly 2 kHz, with age, which is the reverse of that seen in individuals without previous significant noise exposure.[39] Not only does noise exposure contribute to the development of presbycusis, it also impacts the character of threshold shifts associated with presbycusis.

Hereditary Factors

Heredity is an important factor in age-related hearing loss. A strong familial association has been implicated in presbycusis. This familial association implying potential genetic susceptibility to age-related hearing loss.[44,45] Approximately 30–50% of variance in presbycusis is attributed to the effects of genes.[45,46] Various candidate genes have been proposed; however, there currently is no widely accepted genetic etiology that has been identified. The multifactorial nature of the etiology of presbycusis poses a challenge in the identification of genetic contribution to this disease process in clinical studies.

Additional Etiological Factors

As presbycusis represents the progression of hearing loss with aging, various additional factors have been identified that affect the development and progression of presbycusis. Table 17.4 describes additional etiological factors that have been proposed in the development of age-related

Table 17.4: Factors contributing to presbycusis

Factor	*Exposures*
Environmental	• Noise • Low socioeconomic status
Chemical exposures	• Toluene • Trichloroethylene • Styrene
Otologic disease	• Otosclerosis • Chronic otomastoiditis • Temporal bone trauma • Meniere's
Medications	• Aminoglycosides • Platinum-based chemotherapeutic agents • Loop diuretics • Phosphodiesterase type 5 inhibitors • Salicylate
Habitual	• Tobacco* • Alcohol abuse*
Systemic disease	• Renal failure • Diabetes • Cardiovascular disease • Immunodeficiency
Protective factors	• Estrogen • High bone mineral density • Caloric restriction* • Aldosterone

*Conflicting reports in the literature.

hearing loss.[5,7,40-43,47-70] One major contributing factor is otologic disease. In theory, any otologic condition that precipitates hearing loss throughout life will contribute to the progression of age-related hearing loss. Studies in the literature have highlighted the etiologic contribution of otosclerosis, chronic otitis, Meniere's and temporal bone trauma or head trauma to the presentation of age-related hearing loss.[54,71,72] In addition to otologic disease, ototoxins have been described as a contributing factor in the etiology of age-related hearing loss, namely aminoglycosides (e.g. gentamicin and streptomycin), platinum-based chemotherapeutic agents (e.g. cisplatin and carboplatin), high-dose loop diuretics, and salicylate and phosphodiesterase type 5 inhibitors (e.g. sildenafil, vardenafil, and tadalafil).[65-70,73,74] Additionally, toxic exposures to heavy metals (e.g. lead and mercury) and solvents (e.g. toluene, styrene, and xylene) have been implicated as potential contributing factors for age-related hearing loss.[59-62]

Tobacco and alcohol abuse have been proposed as etiologic factors in presbycusis; however, there are conflicting reports within the literature in this regard.[55,63,64] In multiple studies, cardiovascular disease and diabetes have been associated with the progression of presbycusis.[5,47,49,56,57,75,76] Additionally, renal failure and impaired immune function may play a contributing role.[53,58]

A number of factors have been found to be protective against the progression of age-related threshold shift. Hormonal function, including aldosterone and estrogen, have been found to protective against age-related changes in hearing.[48,77] Higher levels of bone mineral density have been correlated with decreased rate of change in hearing with age.[55] Additionally, caloric restriction may play a preventive role.[7,52] Further study would be required to fully elucidate these effects.

Impact of Presbycusis

The impact of age-related hearing loss is not limited to merely the ability of an individual to hearing and comprehend speech. The impact of presbycusis is far reaching. It not only impacts the individual from a psychosocial perspective and potentially increases the progression of dementia, but it also has a significant public health impact internationally.

Psychosocial Impact

The psychosocial impact of presbycusis has been well established. With progression, presbycusis typically precipitates difficulty with speech discrimination and word understanding, particularly in ambient situations. This translates to difficulty participating in conversation at a busy restaurant or understanding the punch line of a joke at a family gathering. Although this may seem minor, for many individual this can produce significant embarrassment and frustration. Social isolation and anxiety in social situation have been described in association.[78,79] In countless patients, this progresses to decreased autonomy and depression, significantly impacting their activity level and social interconnectivity.[79-85] This has been associated with a significant decline in overall quality of life reported by individuals affected by presbycusis.[86,87]

Association with Dementia

The association between dementia and age-related hearing loss has been described for decades within the literature. However, our understanding of the impact that presbycusis plays on the progression of dementia has evolved significantly. Within the mid-1980s, various publications revealed the significant correlation between hearing impairment in the elderly and the progression of dementia.[80,88,89] Global functional decline also has been noted in association with age-related hearing loss, shy of the clinical diagnosis of dementia within this population.[78,90,91] A direct positive correlation between degree of hearing loss and cognitive decline has been noted on both verbal and nonverbal cognitive testing in numerous reports in the literature.[55,80,92-97] More recently, this association has been further quantified. Among individuals free of prevalent dementia or mild cognitive impairment, impact of degree of hearing loss was quantitatively associated with decline in cognitive function. It was noted that a 25 dB hearing loss produces a decline equivalent to an age difference of 6.8 years on test of executive function.[98,99] Additional study is require to further investigate this potential causative relationship.

Public Health Impact

Presbycusis poses a significant public health concern internationally. The percentage of the population over the age of 65 is projected to grow internationally over the new few decades.[100] As such, the prevalence of age relating hearing loss will increase precipitously. According to the WHO hearing loss is one of the six leading contributors to the burden of disease in industrialized countries (WHO, 2000). Based upon the WHO 2012 Hearing Loss Estimate, adults make up 91% of individuals internationally with disabling hearing loss, accounting for 328 million of 360 million total individuals internationally affected (disabling hearing loss defined as ≥40 dB of hearing loss).[10] Adults over the age of 64 years make up more than half of all adults with hearing loss.[101] It is projected by 2025 that there will be 1.2 billion people over 60 years of age worldwide, with >500 million individuals who will suffer significant impairment from presbycusis.[102] Presbycusis may contribute to early undesired retirement and decreased workforce participation, creating a significant economic impact.

Pathophysiology

Pathophysiological changes have been noted in various components of the auditory system in association with age-related hearing loss. Traditionally, presbycusis was believed to be a disorder of the peripheral auditory system, namely the cochlea. Schuknecht developed a classification system that highlights the cochlear changes that have been noted in association with age-related hearing.[103,103a]. Figures 17.3A to D depicts audiograms that would accompany four of the classic classifications of presbycusis proposed by Schuknecht. Sensory presbycusis is characterized by slowly progressive, bilateral steep down-sloping high-frequency hearing loss associated with loss of cochlear hair cells, particularly at the basal turn of the cochlea. Neural presbycusis is characterized by decline in speech discrimination associated with spiral ganglion cell loss. Metabolic presbycusis is characterized by flat hearing loss attributed to atrophy within the stria vascularis. Mechanical presbycusis is associated with a gradual descending pattern of hearing loss presumed to occur as a function of stiffening of the basilar membrane. The most common form encountered is mixed presbycusis that encompasses flat, sloping, or high-frequency hearing loss and is associated with a combination of hair cell, spiral ganglion, and strial losses.[104] In addition to the histopathologic changes described within the Schuknecht classification system, various cochlear changes have been described in association with aging, including loss of outer hair cells and support cells, changes in hair cell stereocilia, vascular changes in the stria vascularis, decreased synapses, particularly at the basal turn, and loss of nerve fibers and ganglion cells.[105-110] In addition to the previously proposed peripheral histopathology related to age-related hearing loss, recent evidence supports a central component to age-related hearing loss, citing the fact that auditory performance in elderly individuals is largely impacted by decreased spiral ganglion cells, decreased central plasticity, central auditory processing disorder, as well as increased incidence of central nervous system disease and cognitive decline.[22,111] Central presbycusis likely represents a component of the overall presentation of presbycusis rather than an isolated entity in and of itself.[112] Further study is required to better characterize the central component of presbycusis.

Clinical Evaluation

The clinical evaluation of patients present with age-related hearing loss often begins with the primary care provider. Primary care providers, including gerontologists, are typically charged with the responsibility of coordinating the care of elderly patients. Referral for audiometric evaluation should be included in the routine evaluation of the geriatric patients. This appears as one of the goals of the United States National Institutes of Health (NIH) Healthy People 2020 (ENT-VSL-5: increase the number of persons

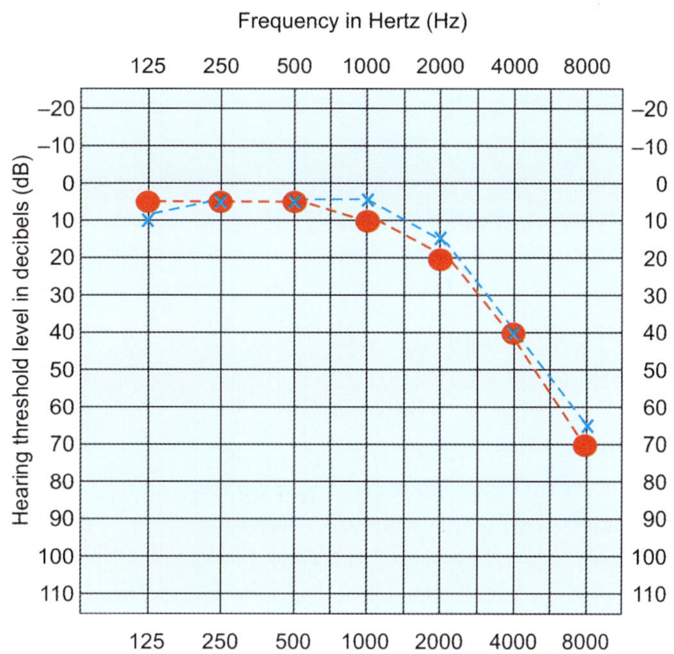

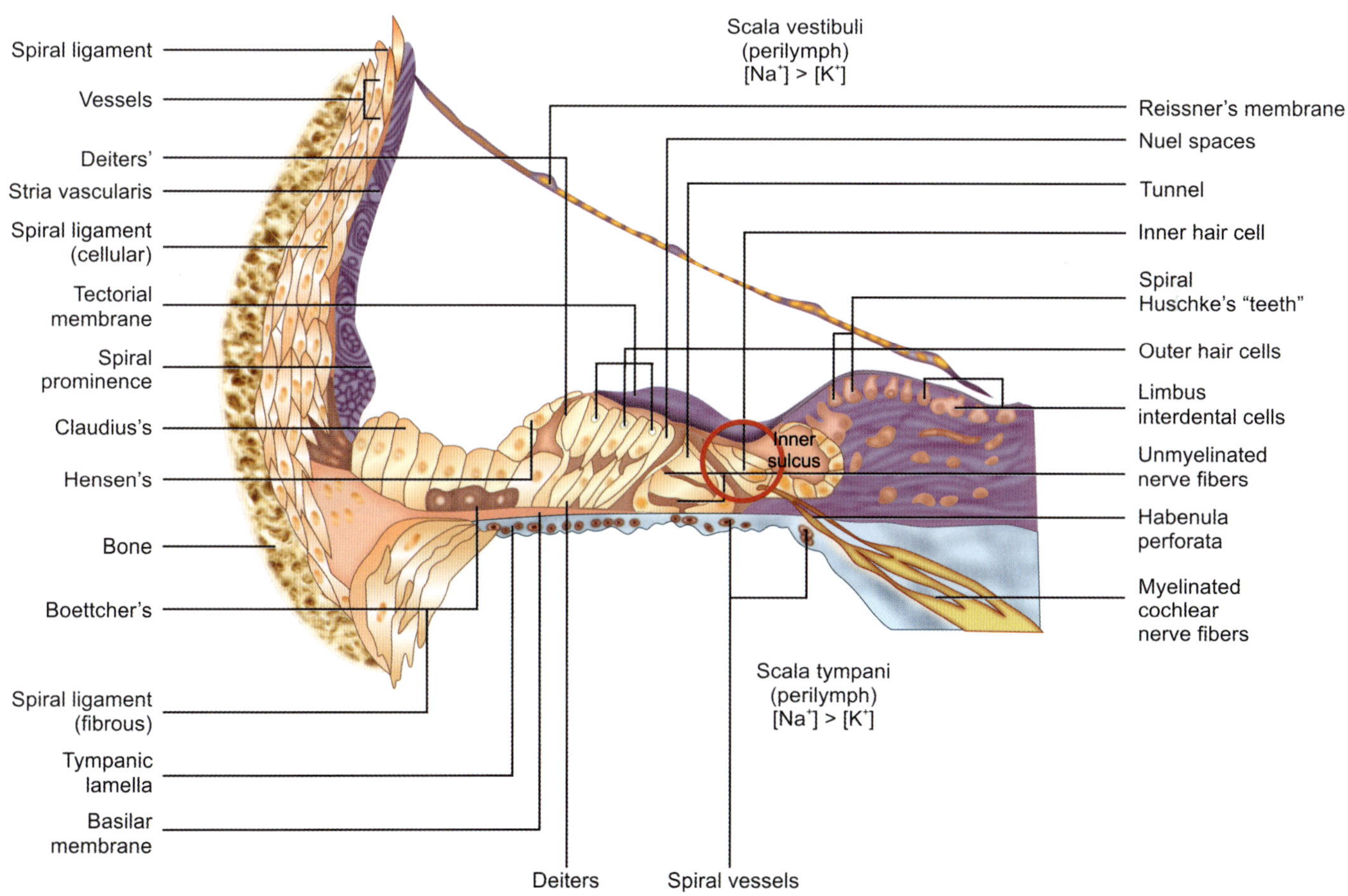

Fig. 17.3A: Pure tone audiogram characteristic of the various classes of presbycusis described by Schuknecht with illustration of proposed region of cochlear involvement. (A) Sensory presbycusis. The audiogram depicts the typical shape of hearing loss associated with sensory presbycusis, which is postulated to be secondary to hair cell loss.

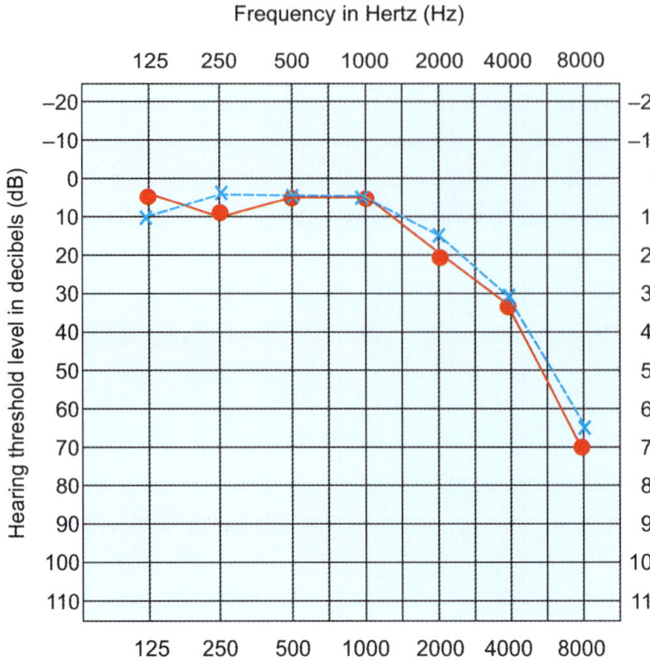

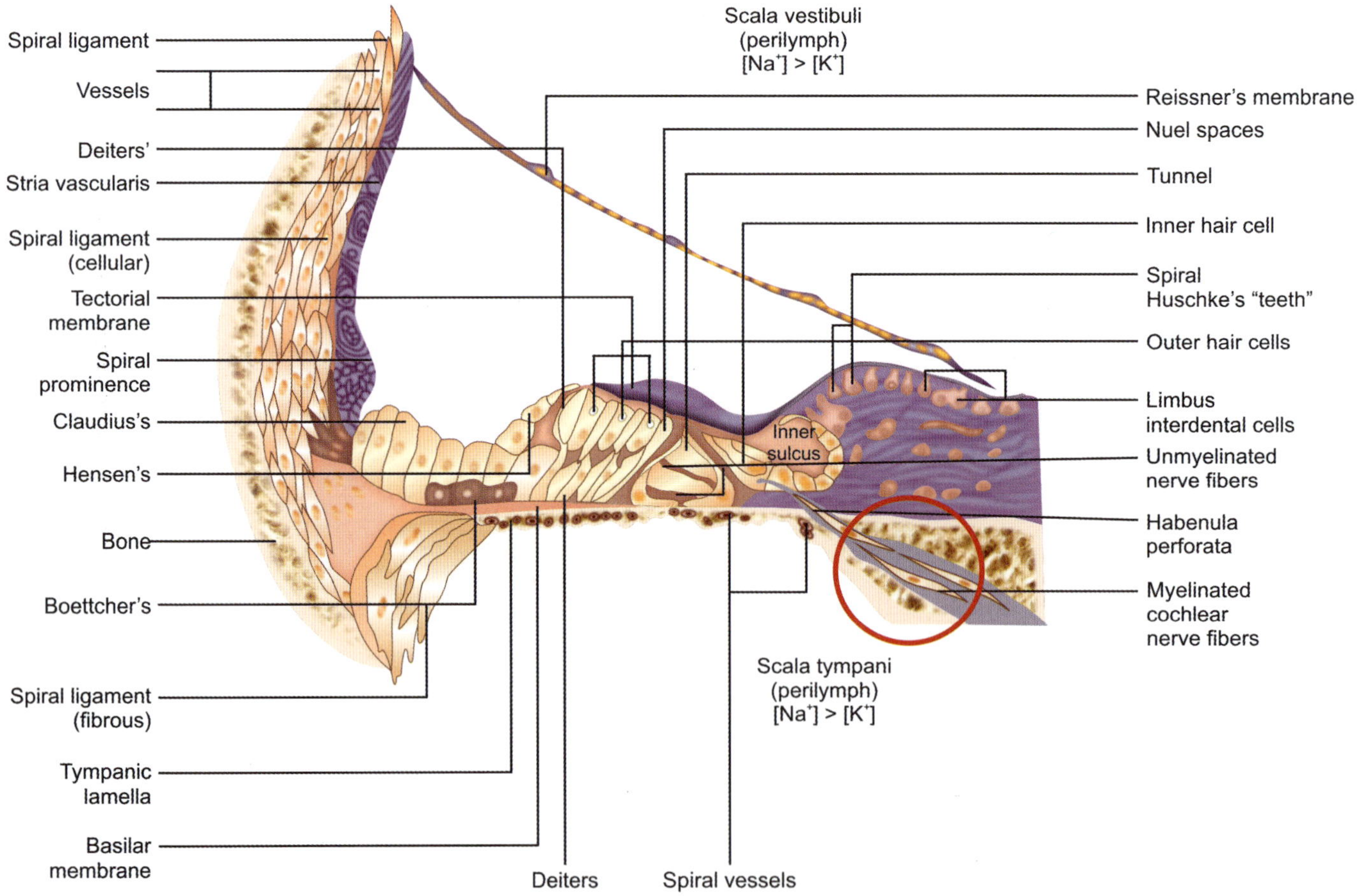

Fig. 17.3B: Neural presbycusis. The audiogram depicts the typical high frequency of hearing loss associated with neural presbycusis that is postulated to be secondary to loss of spiral ganglion cells. The key change noted with neural presbycusis is decline in speech discrimination.

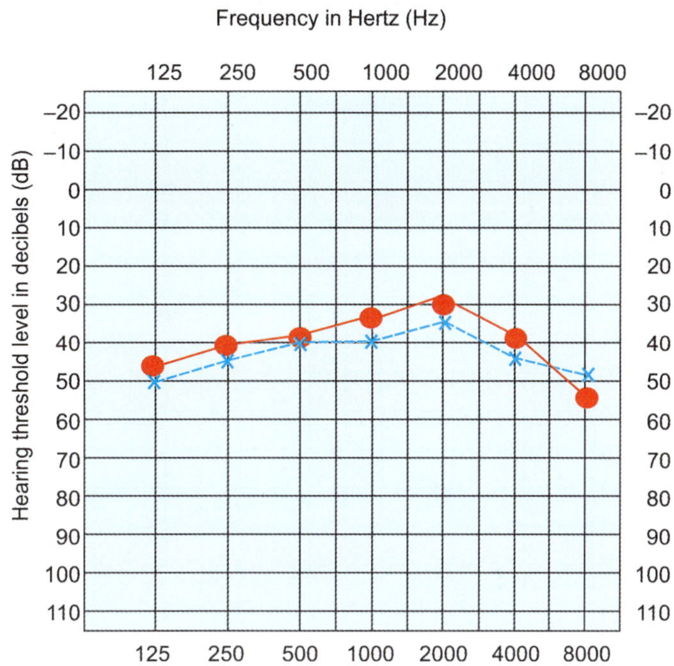

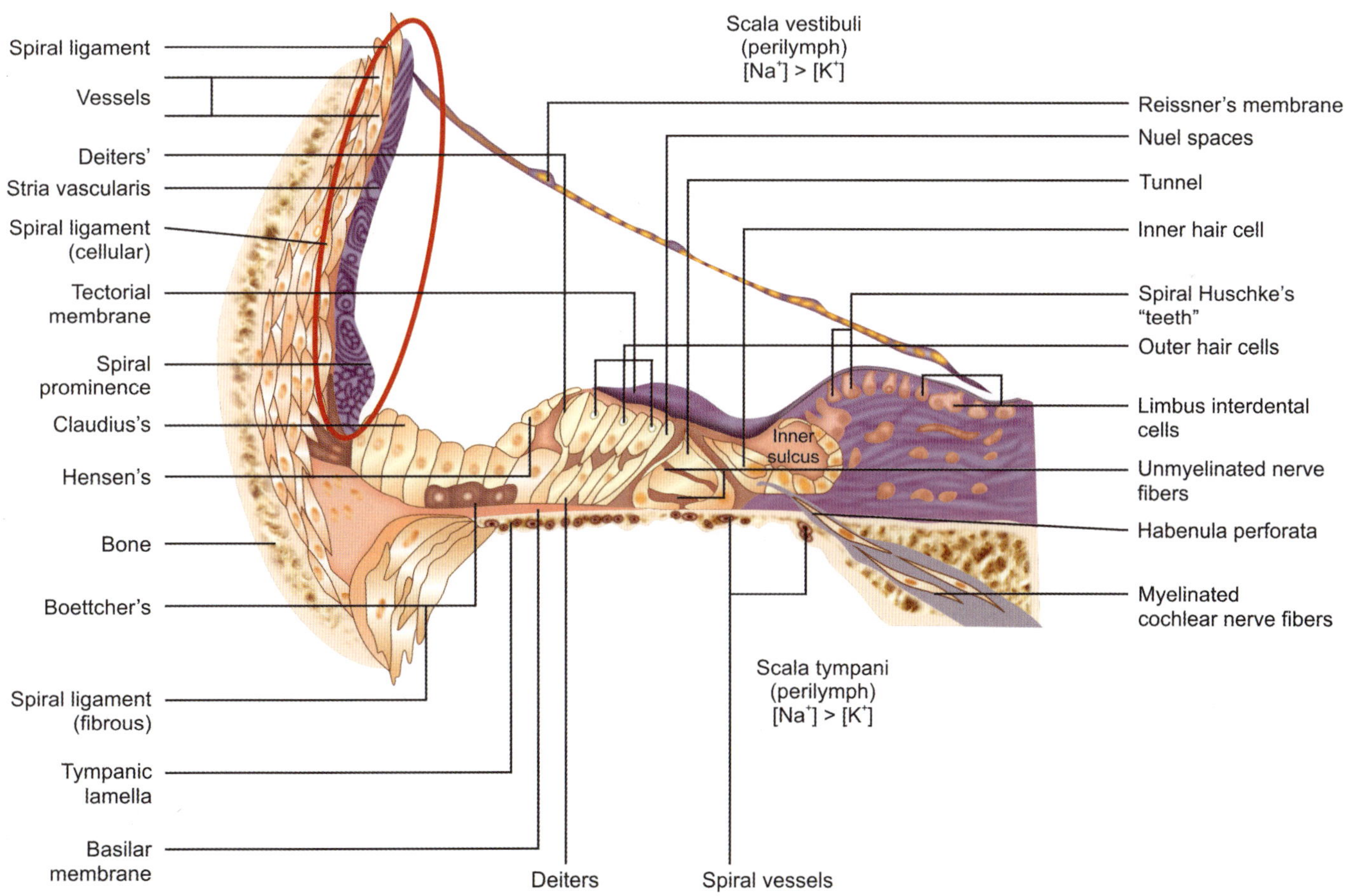

Fig. 17.3C: Metabolic presbycusis. The audiogram depicts the typical flat hearing loss associated with metabolic presbycusis that is postulated to be secondary to atrophy within the stria vascularis.

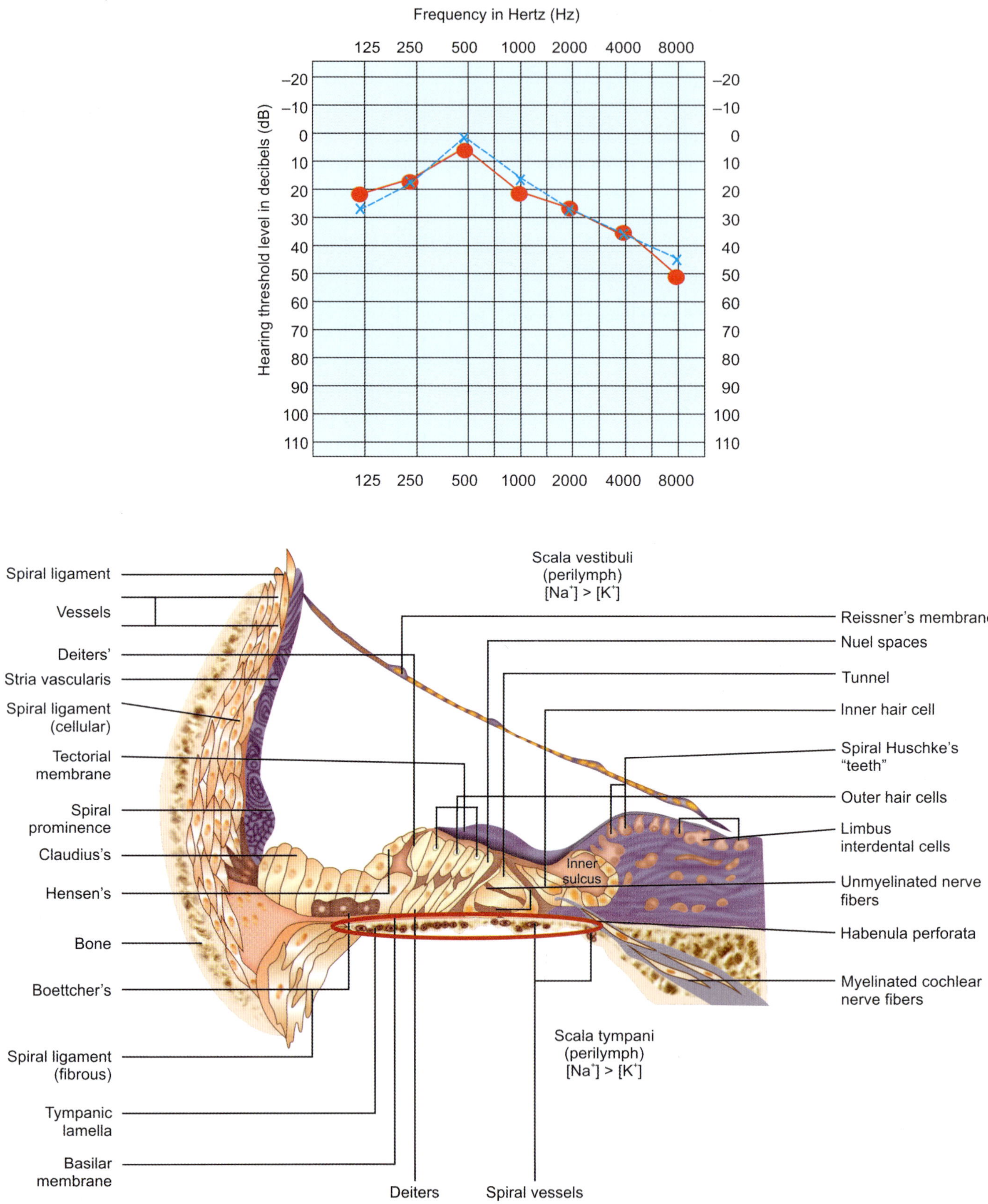

Fig. 17.3D: Mechanical presbycusis. The audiogram depicts the typical gradual sloping shape of hearing loss associated with mechanical presbycusis that is postulated to be secondary to stiffening of the basilar membrane.

who are referred by their primary care physician or other health care provider for hearing evaluation and treatment).[113] It is essential to realize that individuals with early presbycusis may minimize their symptoms. Patients with presbycusis may initially be reluctant to admit that they are experiencing hearing loss. Alternatively, some individuals view hearing loss as a normal process of aging "like wrinkles" or perceive it as something that they suffer through. Therefore, regardless of patient report among the geriatric population, referral for audiometric evaluation should be made at least every 5 years. This is in accordance with the NIH Healthy People 2020 objective ENT-VSL-4 that aspires to increase the proportion of persons who have had hearing examination on schedule, which is suggested as within a 5-year period.[113]

On clinical presentation, patients typically present with high-frequency sensorineural hearing loss accompanied by decline in speech discrimination and speech understanding. Patients may report particular difficulty understanding conversation in ambient conditions. They may report complaints or their family may report that they complain that other tend to mumble or slur their words. Individuals with presbycusis often report that men's voices are easier to hear and understand than women's and children's.

A major related complaint of patients with presbycusis is associated tinnitus. As the hearing loss progresses, tinnitus tends to progress as well. The tinnitus may present as intermittent, but typically becomes constant with progression of hearing loss.

The clinical evaluation of patient should include a complete head and neck examination with cranial nerve evaluation and otologic evaluation. Audiometric evaluation should be performed, including pure tone audiometry, speech discrimination, tympanometry, and acoustic reflexes. Typical findings are of high-frequency sensorineural hearing loss that is symmetric. Imaging of the temporal bone or skull base is typically not indicated with normal otologic examination and characteristic audiometric findings. If asymmetric hearing loss or otologic abnormalities, are noted, clinical discretion should direct imaging.

Prevention

The key to prevention of age-related hearing loss is avoidance of factors that can promote or accelerate its progression. Adequate treatment of potentially contributing otologic disease should be employed. Ototoxins should be avoided when possible. Potential contributing comorbidities should actively and aggressively be managed to prevent associated threshold shifts.

Prevention of noise trauma is a major component of prevention of age-related hearing loss. Patients should avoid excessive noise exposure. When noise exposure is unavoidable (e.g. occupational requirements or recreation), adequate noise protective equipment should be utilized to dampen noise exposures. Inserted ear plugs provide approximately 15–25 dB of sound attenuation. Alternatively, noise protection ear muffs provide approximately 20–30 dB of sound attenuation. For individuals with high acoustic professional demand with significant noise exposure (i.e. musicians, music teachers, recording engineers or sound crew members), high fidelity hearing protection or musicians ear plugs are recommended. These customized ear plugs reduce sound levels presented to the ear while maintaining clear and nature sound without a muffled character as experienced with traditional ear plugs. The level of attenuation too is customizable.

MANAGEMENT

The mainstay of management of age-related hearing loss is environmental optimization and auditory rehabilitation. Auditory rehabilitation takes many forms, ranging from simple assistive devices to cochlear implantation. Currently there are no medical therapies available for the treatment or prevention of age-related hearing loss. This presents a significant opportunity for future research and development.

Environmental Optimization

Patients with presbycusis, whenever possible, should make modifications to their environment to optimize their auditory milieu. This may take the form of turning off televisions or decreasing the volume of background music during dinner conversations or sitting in a favorable location to facilitate face to face conversation to allow not only lip reading but also the use of nonverbal cues (i.e. facial expression and gestures) to augment speech understanding. If comfortable, individuals may request speakers to speak more slowly as comprehension of rapid speakers is commonly impaired in individuals with presbycusis.

Auditory Assistive Devices

Hearing assistive devices are nonprescription, nonpersonalized aids that augment environmental sounds or provide alternatives to challenging acoustic situation. These aids include such devices as telephone amplifiers, television amplifiers, alarm clocks with vibrators, frequency-modulation transmitters, doorbell signalers, and modified smoke detectors. These devices are of great benefit to patient with age-related hearing loss, but are limited in their ability to assist in the most challenging of communication situations.

Hearing Aids

Hearing aids represent the mainstay of treatment for age-related hearing loss. Hearing aids are typically recommended for sound amplification in individuals with hearing thresholds within the speech frequencies of 40 dB or greater. In selective cases where employment or educational demands are unusually demanding, losses of < 40 dB may derive benefit from amplification.

Currently available hearing aids are mainly digital, although analog devices remain on the market. Recent advances in hearing aid technology have leaned to the development of enhanced features to improve sound appreciation and functionality, including noise suppression technology, telephone coils, and multiple programming modes optimized for quiet, noise, or music appreciation. These features are accessible manually or in some cases with automatic smart technologies.

Unfortunately, hearing aids are not covered by many healthcare plans and for countless patients the cost of the devices is prohibitive. Within the United States, < 25% of patients affected by presbycusis who would benefit from hearing aids use them.[114,115] Amongst individuals with presbycusis who do not use hearing aids, 76% indicate that the cost is a significant reason for not using hearing aids and 64% simply state that they cannot afford hearing aids.[116] Conversely, in health systems where hearing aids are a covered benefit, elder hearing-impaired hearing aid use is >60%.[117] As hearing aid use has been reported to improve quality of life,[118] increasing hearing aid availability provides a significant opportunity to improve public health internationally.

Hearing aid use does require a period of cognitive adaptation. Unfortunately, for some patients intermittent use causes dissatisfaction secondary to lack of complete adaptation to the hearing aid device. In a study of hearing aid use among individuals 70 years and older, use of 5 hours or greater was reported in only 19.1% of individuals.[11] The rate of use was noted to be dependent upon the degree of hearing loss, with reported use rates of 3.4% for individuals with mild hearing loss, 40% for individuals with moderate hearing loss, and 76% for individuals with severe hearing loss.[11] These data are similar to previous reports within the literature of underuse or abandonment of hearing aids of (25% underuse and 40% abandonment).[119,120] The most commonly reported reasons for abandoning hearing aid use or underusing the technology are problems with fit, understanding the operation of the device, and unmet expectations.[115,119,121-124] Thus, adequate education and establishment of realistic expectations are critical to hearing aid acceptance, adaptation and use.

Cochlear Implants

For patients with severe to profound bilateral hearing loss, cochlear implantation may be an option. Cochlear implantation is recommended for patients who do not derive benefit from hearing aid use and meet certain criteria for speech discrimination testing (i.e. score 50% or less on sentence recognition testing in their worse hearing ear and 60% or less in the bilateral best aided conditions). However, criteria for cochlear implantation are continually evolving and broadening to encompass individuals with a greater degree of residual hearing. Within the geriatric population, the procedure is typically performed in the outpatient setting unless precluded by medical comorbidities. It is well tolerated with low surgical morbidity and high rates of success and with noted improvement in quality of life.[125-130] Interestingly, unlike hearing aids, cochlear implantation is covered by most healthcare plans.

CONCLUSION

Presbycusis (or age-related hearing loss) is a common condition affecting the aging population. With the rapidly increasing aging population, presbycusis is becoming an increasingly important public health concern. It represents the sum of cumulative damage to the auditory system that progresses with aging. As such its etiology is multifactorial, including oxidative injury associated with aging, noise exposure, ototoxin exposure, environmental toxin exposures, otologic disease, and injury from systemic disease. Various histopathologic changes have been noted in association with presbycusis, including diffuse cellular loss. The typical clinical presentation of presbycusis is of high-frequency sensorineural hearing loss. Difficulty with speech understanding in ambient conditions and tinnitus are also commonly associated. Audiometric evaluation should be performed to confirm diagnosis. Preventive actions should be employed to prevent otologic insult throughout life. Management options include environmental modifications, hearing assistive devices, hearing aids, and cochlear implants.

REFERENCES

1. Gordon-Salant S. Hearing loss and aging: new research findings and clinical implications. J Rehabil Res Dev. 2005; 42:9-24.
2. Humes LE, Dubno JR. Factors affecting speech understanding in older adults. In: Gordon-Salant S, Frisina R (eds), The aging auditory system. New York: Springer; 2009.
3. Gordon-Salant S, Yeni-Komshian GH, Fitzgibbons PJ. Recognition of accented English in quiet and noise by younger and older listeners. J Acoust Soc Am. 2010;128:3152-60.
4. Gordon-Salant S, Yeni-Komshian GH, Fitzgibbons PJ. Recognition of accented English in quiet by younger normal-hearing listeners and older listeners with normal hearing and hearing loss. J Acoust Soc Am. 2010;128:444-55.
5. Frisina ST, Mapes F, Kim S, et al. Characterization of hearing loss in aged type II diabetics. Hear Res. 2006;211:103-13.
6. Yueh B, Shapiro N, MacLean CH, et al. Screening and management of adult hearing loss in primary care: scientific review. JAMA. 2003;289:1976-85.
7. Seidman MD. Effects of dietary restriction and antioxidants on presbycusis. Laryngoscope. 2000;110:727-38.
8. Parham K, McKinnon BJ, Eibling D, et al. Challenges and opportunities in presbycusis. Otolaryngol Head Neck Surg. 2011;144:491-5.
9. Mao Z, Zhao L, Pu L, et al. How well can centenarians hear? PLoS ONE. 2013;8(6):e65565.
10. World Health Organization. WHO global estimates of prevalence of hearing loss. Mortality and Burden of Diseases and Prevention of Blindness and Deafness. Geneva: World Health Organization, 2012.
11. Lin FR, Thorpe R, Gordon-Salant S, et al. Hearing loss prevalence and risk factors among older adults in the United States. J Gerontol A Biol Sci Med Sci. 2011; 66A: 682-590.
12. Cooper JC Jr. Health and Nutrition Examination Survey of 1971-75: part I. Ear and race effects in hearing. J Am Acad Audiol. 1994;5:30-36.
13. Helzner EP, Cauley HA, Pratt SR, et al. Race and sex differences in age-related hearing loss: the Health, Aging and Body Composition Study. J Am Geriatr Soc. 2005;53: 2119-27.
14. Agrawal Y, Platz EA, Niparko JK. Prevalence of hearing loss and differences by demographic characteristics among US adults: data from the National Health and Nutrition Examination Survey, 1999–2004. Arch Intern Med. 2008; 168:1522-30.
15. Riley PA. Melanin. Int J Biochem Cell Biol. 1997;29:1235-9.
16. Ohlemiller KK, Rice ME, Lett JM, et al. Absence of strial melanin coincides with age-associated marginal cell loss and endocochlear potential decline. Hear Res. 2009;249: 1-14.
17. Murillo-Cuesta S, Contreras J, Zurita E, et al. Melanin precursors prevent premature age-related and noise-induced hearing loss in albino mice. Pigment Cell Melanoma Res. 2010;23:72-83.
18. Garstecki DC, Erler SF. Older adult performance on the communication profile for the hearing impaired: gender difference. J Speech Lang Hear Res. 1999;42:785-96.
19. Uchida Y, Nakashima T, Ando F, et al. Prevalence of self-perceived auditory problems and their relation to audiometric thresholds in a middle-aged to elderly population. Acta Otolaryngol. 2003;123:618-26.
20. Stevens G, Flaxman S, Brunskill E, et al. Global and regional hearing impairment prevalence: an analysis of 42 studies in 29 countries. Eur J Pub Health. 2011; 1-7.
21. Gates GA, Mills JH. Presbycusis. Lancet. 2005;366: 1111-20.
22. Parham K, Lin FR, Coelho DH, et al. Comprehensive management of presbycusis: central and peripheral. Otolaryngol Head Neck Surg. 2013;148:537-9.
23. Harman D. Aging: a theory based on free radical and radiation chemistry. J Gerontol. 1956;11:298-300.
24. Beatty S, Koh H, Phil M, et al. The role of oxidative stress in the pathogenesis of age-related macular degeneration. Surv Ophthal. 2000;45:115-34.
25. Justilien V, Pang JJ, Renganathan K, et al. SOD2 knockdown mouse model of early AMD. Invest Ophthal Vis Sci. 2007; 48:4407-20.
26. Lu CY, Lee HC, Fahn HJ, et al. Oxidative damage elicited by imbalance of free radical scavenging enzymes is associated with large-scale mtDNA deletions in aging human skin. Mutat Res. 1999;423:11-21.
27. Sanz N, Diez-Fernandez C, Alvarez A, et al. Age-dependent modification in rate hepatocyte antioxidant defense systems. J Hepatol. 1997;27:525-34.
28. Kidd AR III, Bao J. Recent advances in the study of age-related hearing loss: a mini-review. Gerontology. 2012;58: 490-96.
29. Jiang H, Talaska AE, Schacht J, et al. Oxidative imbalance in the aging inner ear. Neurobiol Aging. 2007; 28: 1605-12.
30. McFadden SL, Ding D, Reaume AG, et al. Age-related cochlear hair cell loss is enhanced in mice lacking copper/ zinc superoxide dismutase. Neurobiol Aging. 1999; 20: 1-8.
31. Keithley EM, Canto C, Zheng QY, et al. Cu/Zn superoxide dismutase and age-related hearing loss. Hear Res. 2005;209: 76-85.
32. Someya S, Xu J, Kondo K, et al. Age-related hearing loss in C57BL/6J mice is mediated by Bak-dependent mitochondrial apoptosis. Proc Natl Acad Sci USA. 2009;106:19432-7.
33. Wang CH, Wu SB, Wu YT, Wei YH. Oxidative stress response elicited by mitochondrial dysfunction: implication in the pathophysiology of aging. Exp Biol Med. 2013;238:450-60.
34. Bai U, Seidman MD, Hinojosa R, Quirk WS. Mitochondrial DNA deletions associated with aging and possibly presbycusis: a human archival temporal bone study. Am J Otolaryngol. 1997;18:449-53.
35. Fischel-Ghadsian N, Bykhovskaya Y, Taylor K, et al. Temporal bone analysis of patient with presbycusis reveals high frequency of mitochondrial mutations. Hear Res. 1997;110: 147-54.
36. Maykaryan A, Nelson EG, Hinojosa R. Detection of mitochondrial DNA deletions in the cochlea and its structural elements from archival human temporal bone tissue. Mut Res. 2008;640:38-45.
37. Maykaryan A, Nelson EG, Hinojosa R. Quantification of the mitochondrial DNA common deletion in presbycusis. Laryngoscope. 2009;119:1184-9.

38. Maykaryan A, Nelson EG, Hinojosa R. Major arc mitochondrial DNA deletions in cytochrome c oxidase-deficient human cochlear spiral ganglion cells. Acta Otolaryngol. 2010;130:780-7.
39. Gates GA, Schmid P, Kujawa SG, et al. Longitudinal threshold changes in older men with audiometric notches. Hear Res. 2000;141:220-28.
40. Kujawa SG, Liberman MC. Acceleration of age-related hearing loss by early noise exposure: evidence of a misspent youth. J Neurosci. 2006;26:2115-23.
41. Kujawa SG, Liberman MC. Adding insult to injury: cochlear nerve degeneration after 'temporary' noise-induced hearing loss. J Neurosci. 2009;29:14077-85.
42. Lin HW, Furman AC, Kujawa SG, et al. Primary neural degeneration in the guinea pig cochlea after reversible noise-induced threshold shift. J Assoc Res Otolaryngol. 2011;12:605-16.
43. Bao J, Ohlemiller KK. Age-related loss of spiral ganglion neurons. Hear Res. 2010;264:93-7.
44. Christensen K, Frederiksen H, Hoffman HJ. Genetic and environmental influences on self-reported reduced hearing in the old and oldest old. J Am Geriatr Soc. 2001;49:1512-7.
45. McMahon CM, Kifley A, Rochtchina E, et al. The contribution of family history to hearing loss in an older population. Ear Hear. 2008;29:578-84.
46. Gates GA, Couropmitree NN, Myers RH. Genetic associations in age-related hearing thresholds. Arch Otolaryngol Head Neck Surg. 1999;125:654-9.
47. Fowler PD; Jones NS. Diabetes and hearing loss. Clin Otolaryngol Allied Sci. 1999; 24: 3-8.
48. Hultcrantz M, Simonoska R, Stenberg AE. Estrogen and hearing: a summary of recent investigations. Acta Otolaryngol. 2006;126:10-14.
49. Uchida Y, Sugiura S, Ando F, et al. Diabetes reduces auditory sensitivity in middle-aged listeners more than in elderly listeners: a population-based study of age-related hearing loss. Med Sci Monit. 2010;16:PH63-8.
50. Cruickshank KJ, Nondahl DM, Tweed TS, et al. Education, occupation, noise exposure history and the 10-year cumulative incidence of hearing impairment in older adults. Hear Res. 2010;264:3-9.
51. Poortinga W. The prevalence and clustering of four major lifestyle risk factors in an English population. Prev Med. 2007;44:124-8.
52. Torre P 3rd, Mattison JA, Fowler CG, et al. Assessment of auditory function in rhesus monkeys (*Macaca mulatta*): effects of age and calorie restriction. Neurobiol Aging. 2004;25:945-54.
53. Iwai H, Lee S, Inaba M, et al. Correlation between accelerated presbycusis and decreased immune function. Exp Gerontol. 2003;38:319-25.
54. Danielidis V, Tsimpiris N, Balatsouras DG, et al. Short-term pathophysiologic changes and histopathologic findings of the auditory pathway after closed head injury, using a rabbit model. Audiol Neurootol. 2007;12:145-54.
55. Helzner EP, Cauley JA, Pratt SR, et al. Hearing sensitivity and bone mineral density in older adults: the Health, Aging and Body Composition Study. Osteoporosis Int. 2005;16: 1675-82.
56. Picciotti P, Torsello A, Wolf FI, et al. Age-dependent modifications of expression level of VEGF and its receptors in the inner ear. Exp Gerontol. 2004;39:1253-8.
57. Torre P 3rd, Cruickshanks KJ, Klein BE, et al. The association between cardiovascular disease and cochlear function in older adults. J Speech Lang Hear Res. 2005;48:473-81.
58. Antonelli AR, Bonfioli F, Garrubba V, et al. Audiological findings in elderly patient with chronic renal failure. Acta Otolaryngol Suppl. 1990;476:54-68.
59. Johnson AC, Nylen PR. Effect of industrial solvents on hearing. Occup Med. 1995;10:623-40.
60. Fuente A, McPherson B. Organic solvents and hearing loss: the challenge for audiology. Int J Audiol. 2006;45:367-81.
61. Fuente A, McPherson B, Munoz V, et al. Assessment of central auditory processing in a group of workers exposed to solvents. Acta Otolaryngol. 2006;126:118-94.
62. Morata TC, Johnson AC, Nylen P, et al. Audiometric findings in workers exposed to low level of styrene and noise. J Occup Environ Med. 2002;44:806-14.
63. Brant LJ, Gordon-Salant S, Pearson JD, et al. Risk factors related to age-associated hearing loss in speech frequencies. J Am Acad Audiol. 1996;7:152-60.
64. Itoh A, Nakashima T, Arao H, et al. Smoking and drinking habits as risk factors for hearing loss in the elderly: epidemiological study of subjects undergoing routine health checks in Aichi, Japan. Public Health. 2001;115:192-6.
65. Stypulkowski, PH. Mechanisms of salicylate ototoxicity. Hear Res. 1990;46:113-45.
66. Mills JH, Matthews LJ, Lee FS, et al. Gender-specific effects of drugs on hearing levels of older persons. Ann NY Acad Sci. 1999;884:381-8.
67. Chen Y, Huang WG, Zha DJ, et al. Aspiring attenuates gentamicin ototoxicity: from the laboratory to the clinic. Hear Res. 2007;226:178-82.
68. Lee FS, Matthews LJ, Mills JH, et al. Analysis of blood chemistry and hearing levels in a sample of older persons. Ear Hear. 1998;19:180-90.
69. Rybak LP, Whitworth CA, Mukherjea D, et al. Mechanisms of cisplatin-induced ototoxicity and prevention. Hear Res. 2007;226:157-67.
70. Selimoglu E. Aminoglycoside-induced ototoxicity. Curr Pharm Des. 2007;13:119-26.
71. Howarth A, Shone GR. Ageing and the auditory system. Postgrad Med J. 2006;82:166-71.
72. Rosenhall U, Hederstierna C, Idrizbegovic E. Otological diagnoses and probable age-related auditory neuropathy in 'younger' and 'older' elderly persons. Int J Audiol. 2011;50:578-81.
73. Snodgrass AJ, Campbell HM, Mace DL, et al. Sudden sensorineural hearing loss associated with vardenafil. Pharmacotherapy. 2010;30:112.
74. Barreto MA, Bahmad F Jr. Phosphodiesterase type 5 inhibitors and sudden sensorineural hearing loss. Braz J Otorhinolaryngol. 2013;79:727-33.
75. Diniz TH, Guida HL. Hearing loss in patient with diabetes mellitus. Braz J Otorhinolaryngol. 2009;75:573-8.
76. Ren J, Zhao P, Chen L, et al. Hearing loss in middle-aged subjects with type 2 diabetes mellitus. Arch Med Res. 2009; 40:18-23.

77. Tadros SF, Frisina ST, Mapes F, et al. Higher serum aldosterone correlates with lower hearing thresholds: a possible protective hormone against presbycusis. Hear Res. 2005;209:10-18.
78. Cacciatore F, Napoli C, Abete P, et al. Quality of life determinants and hearing function in an elderly population: Osservatorio Geriatrico Campano Study Group. Gerontology. 1999;45:323-8.
79. Bernabei V, Morini V, Moretti F, et al. Vision and hearing impairments are associated with depressive-anxiety syndrome in Italian elderly. Aging Ment Health. 2011;15: 467-74.
80. Uhlmann RF, Larson EB, Rees TS, et al. Relationship of hearing impairment to dementia and cognitive dysfunction in older adults. JAMA. 1989;261:1916-19.
81. Kalayam B, Meyers MB, Kakuma T, et al. Age at onset of geriatric depression and sensorineural hearing deficits. Biol Psychiatry. 1995;38:649-58.
82. Heine C, Browning CJ. Communication and psychosocial consequences of sensory loss in older adults: overview and rehabilitation directions. Disabil Rehabil. 2002;24:736-73.
83. Dalton DS, Cruickshanks KJ, Klein BE, et al. The impact of hearing loss on quality of life in older adults. Gerontologist. 2003;43:661-8.
84. Kramer SE, Kapteyn TS, Kuik DJ, et al. The association of hearing impairment and chronic diseases with psychosocial health status in older age. J Aging Health. 2008;14:122-37.
85. Mohlman J. Cognitive self-consciousness - a predictor of increased anxiety following first-time diagnosis of age-related hearing loss. Aging Ment Health. 2009;13:246-54.
86. Li-Korotky HS. Age-related hearing loss: quality of care for quality of life. Gerontologist. 2012;52:265-71.
87. Ciobra A, Bianchini C, Pelucci S, Pastore A. The impact of hearing loss on the quality of life of elderly adults. Clin Interv Aging. 2012;7:159-63.
88. Uhlmann RF, Larson EB, Koepsell TD. Hearing impairment and cognitive decline in senile dementia of the Alzheimer's type. J Am Geriatr Soc. 1986;34:207-10.
89. Weinstein BE, Amsel L. Hearing loss and senile dementia in the institutionalized elderly. Clin Gerontologist. 1986;4: 3-15.
90. Herbst KG, Humphrey C. Hearing impairment and mental state in the elderly living at home. BMJ. 1980;281:903-5.
91. LaForge RG, Spector WD, Sternberg J. The relationship of vision and hearing impairment to one-year mortality and functional decline. J Aging Health. 1992;4:126-48.
92. Ohta RJ, Carlin MF, Harmon BM. Auditory acuity and performance on the mental status questionnaire in the elderly. J Am Geriatr Soc. 1981;29:476-8.
93. Peters CA, Potter JF, Scholer SG. Hearing impairment as a predictor of cognitive decline in dementia. J Am Geriatr Soc. 1988;36:981-6.
94. Lindenberger U, Baltes PB. Sensory functioning and intelligence in old age: a strong connection. Psychol Aging. 1994;9:339-55.
95. Gussekloo J, de Craen AJ, Oduber C, et al. Sensory impairment and cognitive functioning in oldest-old subjects: the Leiden 85+ Study. Am J Geriatr Psychiatry. 2005; 13: 781-6.
96. Tay T, Wang JJ, Kifley A, et al. Sensory and cognitive association in older persons: findings from an older Australian population. Gerontology. 2006;52:386-4.
97. Valentijn SA, van Boxtel MP, van Hooren SA, et al. Change in sensory functioning predicts change in cognitive functioning: results from a 6-year follow-up in the Maastricht Aging Study. J Am Geriatr Soc. 2005;53:374-80.
98. Lin FR. Hearing loss and cognition among older adults in the United States. J Gerontol. 2011;66A:1131-6.
99. Lin FR, Ferrucci L, Metter EJ, et al. Hearing loss and cognition in the Baltimore Longitudinal Study of Aging. Neuropsychology. 2011;25:763-70.
100. Kinsella K, Wan H. U.S. Census Bureau, International Population Reports, P95/09-1, An Aging World: 2008, U.S. Government Printing Office, Washington, DC, 2009.
101. Schiller JS, Lucas JW, Ward BW, Peregoy JA. Summary health statistics for U.S. adults: National Health Interview Survey, 2010. National Center for Health Statistics. Vital Health Stat. 2012;10(252):46.
102. Sprinzl GM, Riechelmann H. Current trends in treating hearing loss in elderly people: a review of the technology and treatment options—a mini-review. Gerontology. 2010;56:351-8.
103. Schuknecht HF. Further observation on the pathology of presbycusis. Arch Otolaryngol. 1964;80:369-82.
103a. Ramadan HH, Schuknecht HF. Is there a conductive type of presbycusis? Otolaryngol Head Neck Surg. 1989;100: 30-4.
104. Schuknecht HF, Gacek MR. Cochlear pathology in presbycusis. Ann Otol Rhinol Laryngol. 1993;102:1-16.
105. Nadol JB Jr. Electron microscopic findings in presbycusis degeneration of the basal turn of the human cochlea. Otolaryngol Head Neck Surg. 1979;87:818-36.
106. Suga F, Lindsay JR. Histopathological observations of presbycusis. Ann Otol Rhinol Laryngol. 1976;85:169-84.
107. Felder E, Schrott-Fischer A. Quantitative evaluation of myelinated nerve fibres and hair cells in cochleae of humans with age-related high-tone hearing loss. Hear Res. 1995;91:19-32.
108. Scholtz AW, Kammen-Jolly K, Felder E, et al. Selective aspects of human pathology in high-tone hearing loss of the aging inner ear. Hear Res. 2001;157:77-86.
109. Nelson EG, Hinojosa R. Presbycusis: a human temporal bone study of individuals with flat audiometric patterns of hearing loss using a new method to quantify stria vascularis volume. Larngoscope. 2003;113:1672-86.
110. Nelson EG, Hinojosa R. Presbycusis: a human temporal bone study of individuals with downward sloping audiometric patterns of hearing loss and review of the literature. Laryngoscope. 2006;116:1-12.
111. Gates GA, Gibbons LE, McCurry SM, et al. Executive dysfunction and presbycusis in older persons with and without memory loss and dementia. Cogn Behav Neurol. 2010; 23:218-23.
112. Humes LE, Dubno JR, Gordon-Salant S, et al. Central presbycusis: a review and evaluation of the evidence. J Am Acad Audiol. 2012;23:635-66.

113. National Institutes of Health. Healthy People 2020: Hearing and other sensory or communication disorders. http://www.healthypeople.gov/2020/topicsobjectives2020/objectiveslist.aspx?topicId=20. (Last accessed 31 January 2014.)
114. Kochkin S, MarkeTrak V. Twenty-five year trends in the hearing health market. Hear Rev 2009; 16: 21-31.
115. Popelka MM, Cruickshanks KJ, Wiley TL, et al. Low prevalence of hearing aid use among older adults with hearing loss: the Epidemiology of Hearing Loss Study. J Am Geriatr Soc. 1998; 46: 1075-8.
116. Henkel, G. Managed correctly, hearing aid dispensing augments the bottom line. ENT Today. December 1, 2009. http://www.enttoday.org/details/article/496241/Managed_Correctly_Hearing_Aid_Dispensing_Augments_the_Bottom_Line.html. (Last accessed 31 January 2014.)
117. Corna LM, Wade TJ, Streiner DL, et al. Corrected and uncorrected hearing impairment in older Canadians. Gerontology. 2009;55:468-76.
118. Tsakiropoulou E, Konstantinidis I, Vital I, et al. Hearing aids: quality of life and socio-economic aspects. Hippokratia. 2007;11:183-6.
119. Gates GA, Cooper JC Jr, Kannel WB, et al. Hearing in the elderly: the Framingham cohort, 1983-1985, part I—basic audiometric test results. Ear Hear. 1990;11:247-56.
120. Hannratty B, Lawlor DA. Effective management of the elderly hearing impaired: a review. J Public Health Med. 2000;22:512-17.
121. Kochkin S, MarkeTrak V. Why my hearing aids are in the drawer: the consumers' perspective. Hearing J. 2000;53: 34-42.
122. Ovegard A, Ramstrom AB. Individual follow-up of hearing aid fitting. Scand Audiol. 1994;23:57-63.
123. Smeeth L, Fletcher AE, Ng E, et al. Reduced hearing ownership, and use of hearing aids in elderly people in the UK. Lancet. 2002;359:1466-70.
124. McCormack A, Fortnum H. Why do people fit with hearing aids not wear them? Int J Audiol. 2013;52:360-68.
125. Poissant SF, Beaudoin F, Huang J, et al. Impact of cochlear implantation on speech understanding, depression, and loneliness in the elderly. J Otolaryngol Head Neck Surg. 2008;37:488-94.
126. Coelho DH, Yeh J, Kim JT, Lalwani AK. Cochlear implantation is associated with minimal anesthetic risk in the elderly. Laryngoscope. 2009;119:355-8.
127. Budenz CL, Cosetti MK, Coelho DH, et al. The effects of cochlear implantation on speech perception in older adults. J Am Geriatr Soc. 2011;59:446-53.
128. Sanchez-Cuadro I, Lassaletta L, Perez-Mora RM, et al. Is there an age limit for cochlear implantation? Ann Otol Rhinol Laryngol. 2013;122:222-8.
129. Lenarz M, Sonmez H, Joseph G, et al. Cochlear implant performance in geriatric patients. Laryngoscope. 2012;122: 1361-5.
130. Lin FR, Chien WW, Li L, et al. Cochlear implantation in older adults. Medicine (Baltimore) 2012; 91: 229-41.

CHAPTER

18

Occupational Hearing Loss

Robert T Sataloff

INTRODUCTION

Hearing loss due to occupational noise exposure is our most prevalent industrial malady and has been recognized since the Industrial Revolution. There are millions of employees with occupational hearing loss (OHL) in American industry. Our neglect of hearing loss, especially OHL, has resulted in human and economic consequences that affect virtually every American household. This is especially regrettable because noise-induced hearing loss is almost always preventable at relatively little cost.

Although legislative and legal developments over the last few decades have catapulted the problem of OHL to national prominence, elimination of this occupational disease has been technologically possible for many years. The delay in addressing the issue effectively has been caused by legislative, economic, and political resistance, as well as by a paucity of scientific information adequate to formulate reasonable standards for hearing conservation and noise control programs. Most occupational diseases and injuries are covered in workers' compensation legislation. However, OHL has been included only recently in these laws, and it is still excluded in some states. The principle behind workers' compensation legislation is reimbursement for lost wages. Because hearing loss is not visible and usually does not interfere with earning power, it has been neglected despite its impact on living power.

Legislation was delayed not only by industrial lobbying from a few companies that did not want to spend money for noise control or hearing conservation, but also because the relationship between noise and hearing was difficult to establish. This information is critical to writing a reasonable standard that will protect the vast majority of exposed workers and will be scientifically and economically feasible to implement and enforce.

Prevention of noise-induced hearing loss is relatively simple and inexpensive. Although the obvious and most desirable solution is to reduce noise from machinery and the environment to intensities below damaging levels, this is often impractical, costly, or scientifically impossible. However, properly worn personal hearing protection in association with audiometric monitoring is inexpensive and extremely effective in preventing hearing loss. Many major industries now have comprehensive hearing conservation programs that include noise surveys to identify hazardous noise, audiometric testing programs to detect hearing loss from all causes (not just noise), medical diagnosis of all abnormal audiograms, follow-up for any abnormalities, retraining and monitoring of all testing personnel, audiometric monitoring for the effective use of ear protection, and medico-legal services. Among the many additional benefits of such a program is recognition of nonnoise-induced, curable hearing loss, such as otosclerosis, as well as early diagnosis of serious causes of hearing loss such as acoustic neuromas.

Physicians are called on to consult in occupational otologic problems. When rendering a judgment, it is no longer acceptable to conclude that a person has OHL simply because he/she works in a noisy plant. The differential diagnosis is lengthy, and a diagnosis of OHL must be established on the basis of positive evidence. Not only are there potentially staggering sums of money involved (leading to a natural increase in spurious claims of noise-induced hearing loss), but there are also many serious causes of

Modified in part from Sataloff RT, Sataloff J. Hearing loss, 4th edn. New York, NY: Taylor and Francis; 2005.

hearing impairment that may mimic OHL. It is our medical (and medico-legal) obligation to detect them. In order to establish a diagnosis of OHL, one must have at least a history of adequate exposure to noise levels sufficient to explain the hearing loss, an audiogram, ideally a complete audiogram (air conduction, bone conduction, and discrimination), consistent with noise-induced hearing loss, relative stability of the hearing level after the subject is removed from noise exposure, absence of other causes of hearing loss, and other data. The differential diagnosis includes many other causes. Even the typical "4000-Hz dip" audiogram that shows maximum hearing loss between 3000 and 6000 Hz can be caused by many conditions other than noise.

FEDERAL REGULATION OF OHL

Occupational Safety and Health Act Legislation

The federal government showed its concern for the large numbers of workers with OHL by establishing the Occupational Safety and Health Act (OSHA) Noise Regulation mandating some hearing conservation measures in essentially every plant in the United States that produced 85 dBA or more of noise for 8 hour daily. The government also emphasized its interest in federal workers' compensation regulations for hearing loss, and this has been the impetus for many states that have passed legislation to include OHL in their workers' compensation statutes. A conservative estimate of the potential cost of compensation for hearing loss in workers exceeds 20 billion dollars. This helps make it the number one environmental and medico-legal problem in the United States. The number of claims remains high, spurred by layoffs and economic difficulties. However, insurance companies and workers' compensation funds are not prepared to bare the brunt of this potentially explosive problem. A few companies, such as E.I. DuPont which has had a hearing conservation program for >60 years, established voluntary hearing safety programs and have virtually no OHL in their employees.

The history of the OSHA Noise Regulation and of the Hearing Conservation Amendment is complex, as with most other important regulations and laws. Comparatively little valid and reliable scientific data were available on which to base a noise standard. Practical measures, politics, economics, and numerous other factors played important roles in determining the final regulation. Discussion and review of the most important features of OSHA's requirements are detailed elsewhere.[1] The most recent final OSHA ruling, complete details of which are listed in the Federal Register, Vol. 67, No. 126, July 1, 2002, details the requirements for recording hearing loss. The register contains Occupational Safety and Health Administration Regulation 29 CFR 1904, Occupational Injury and Illness Recording and Reporting Requirements, Final Rule, which became effective January 1, 2003. It requires the reporting of hearing losses that have a minimum of a 10 dB shift in hearing acuity for the average of 2000, 3000, and 4000 Hz when compared with baseline (known as a Standard Threshold Shift) resulting in hearing thresholds over 25 dB.

Development of a Noise Standard

Comprehensive understanding of the nature of OHL has been hindered by the difficulties associated with scientific studies in an industrial setting. A brief review of old literature and an in-depth discussion of more comprehensive and more recent studies highlights the complexities of the problem and the clinical and scientific findings that form the basis for the guidelines set forth in this chapter.

In 1952, James H. Sterner conducted an opinion poll among a large number of individuals working with noise and hearing investigating the maximum intensity level of industrial noise that they considered safe to hearing[2] (Fig. 18.1). The wide range of estimates demonstrated clearly the lack of agreement even among knowledgeable individuals and the futility of any attempt to establish meaningful guidelines by means of such polls.

In 1954, the Z24-X-2 Subcommittee of American Standards Association (now ANSI) published its exploratory

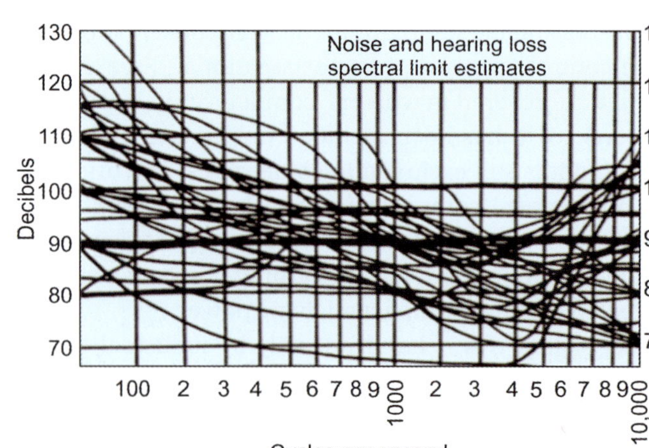

Fig. 18.1: Estimates of "safe" frequency intensity levels.

report on the relations of hearing loss to noise exposure.[3] On the basis of available data, they could not establish a "line" between safe and unsafe noise exposure. They presented questions that required answers before criteria could be formulated, including: (a) What amount of hearing loss constitutes a sufficient handicap to be considered undesirable? (b) What percentage of workers should a standard be designed to protect? The report emphasized the need for considerably more research before "safe" intensity levels could be determined.

Many authors between 1950 and 1971 proposed damage risk criteria, only some of which were based on stated protection goals. Articles are referenced in Table IX of NIOSH's Criteria for Occupational Exposure to Noise.[4] All these reports had limitations that precluded the adoption of any one of them as a basis for the establishment of standards. In 1973, Baughn[5] published an analysis of 6835 audiograms from employees in an automobile stamping plant, with employees divided into three groups on the basis of estimated intensity of noise exposure. Its validity as the basis for a national noise standard was seriously questioned by Ward and Glorig[6] and others because of shortcomings of nonsteady-state noise exposures, vague estimates of noise dosage, auditory fatigue, and test room noise. Baughn's raw data were never made available to the Secretary of Labor's Advisory Committee for Noise Standard despite a formal request from that group.

A study by Burns and Robinson[7] avoided many of the deficiencies of previous studies but was based on a very small number of subjects exposed to continuous steady-state noise, particularly in the 82–92 dBA range. The study included workers who "change position from time to time using noisy hand tools for fettling, chipping, burnishing, or welding"—hardly continuous or steady state. Their report admitted to the inclusion of workers exposed to nonsteady-state levels under 90 dBA. In fact, some workers were included whose noise exposures varied by 15 dBA. The oft-quoted Passchier-Vermeer report[8] was not based on an actual field investigation but was rather a review of published studies up to 1967. Some of these studies addressed the validity of measuring sound levels in dBA; none was really designed to be used as the basis for a noise standard.

As early as 1970, interested individuals from industry, labor, government, and scientific organizations discussed the concept of an interindustry noise study. The project was started in 1974 for the stated purpose of gathering data on the effect of steady-state noise in the range of 82–92 dBA. While the results of such a study would obviously be of interest to those involved in noise regulation, the basic purpose of the study was scientific rather than regulatory. The detailed protocol has been published[6] and will not be repeated here. Some of the important points were: (a) Clear definitions of the temporal and spectral characteristics of the noise. (b) Noise exposures had to fall between 82 and 92 dBA, with no subject exceeding a 5-dBA range (later modified to a 6-dBA range). (c) Noise environment had to be steady state throughout a full shift, with few, if any, sharp peaks of impact noise. (d) Subjects, both experimental and control, had to include men and women. (e) No prior job exposure to noise over 92 dBA for experimentals and 75 dBA for controls. (f) Minimum of 3 years on present job. (g) All audiometric testing, noise measurement, equipment calibration, otological examinations, histories, and data handling had to be done in a standardized manner, as detailed in the protocol. (h) The original raw data had to be made available to all serious investigators upon request at the conclusion of the study. Hearing levels were measured in 155 men and 193 women exposed to noise levels ranging from 82 to 92 dBA for at least 3 years, with a median duration of ~15 years; they were also measured in 96 men and 132 women with job exposure that did not exceed 75 dBA. Noise exposure was considered steady state in that it did not fluctuate >3 dB from the midpoint as of the time of the first audiogram. As many subjects as possible were re-examined 1 year later and 2 years later.

Jobs involving some 250,000 employees were examined to find the 348 experimental subjects who met the criteria of the inter-industry noise study as of the time of entry. Within the range of 82–92 dBA, differences in noise intensity had no observable "effect" on hearing level. That is, the hearing levels of workers at the upper end of the noise intensity exposure were not observably different from the hearing levels of workers at the lower end of the noise exposure. Age was a more important factor than duration on the job in explaining differences in hearing level within any group. Comparisons between experimental and control subjects were made on an age-adjusted basis.

Differences between women exposed to 82–92 dBA and their controls were small and were not statistically significant. Differences between men exposed to 82–92 dBA and their controls were small and were not statistically significant at 500, 1000, and 2000 Hz. Levels in the noise-exposed group significantly exceeded those in the control group at 3000, 4000, and 6000 Hz by 6–9 dB. At 8000 Hz, differences again became not significant.

There was no real evidence of a difference between noise-exposed workers and their controls with respect to the changes in hearing level during the course of follow-up 1 and 2 years after initial audiograms. Changes were negligible for both groups.

It is important to note that the studies discussed and the regulations promulgated to date concern themselves with exposure to continuous noise. More recent research demonstrated that intermittent exposure to noise results in different effects on hearing.[9] Although it may produce marked, high frequency, sensorineural hearing loss, intermittent noise does not have the same propensity to spread to the speech frequencies even after many years of exposure, as happens with continuous noise exposure.

Disability and Impairment

Methods for compensating people with OHL vary from jurisdiction to jurisdiction.[1] An essential part of a compensation act is the manner of calculating how much compensation an employee should receive for a specific amount of hearing loss. It is first necessary to distinguish among impairment, disability, and handicap. Impairment is a medical concept meaning a deviation from normal. Disability and handicap involve many nonmedical factors and include a concept of loss of ability to earn a daily livelihood, "loss of living power" or reduction of the individual's enjoyment of daily living. Hearing impairment contributes to a disability, but many other factors are involved. Compensation is awarded for disability.

CHARACTERISTICS OF OHL

Audiometric Features

OHL is a specific disease due to repetitive injury with established symptoms and objective findings. The diagnosis of OHL cannot be reached reliably solely on the basis of an audiogram showing high-frequency sensorineural loss and a patient's history that he/she worked in a noisy plant. Accurate diagnosis requires a careful and complete history, physical examination, and often laboratory, imaging, and special audiologic studies. Numerous entities such as acoustic neuroma, labyrinthitis, ototoxicity, viral infections, acoustic trauma (explosion), head trauma, hereditary hearing loss, diabetes, presbycusis, autoimmune and genetic causes must be ruled out, as they are responsible for similar hearing loss in millions of people who were never employed in noisy industries.

The American College of Occupational Medicine Noise and Hearing Conservation Committee promulgated a position statement on the distinguishing features of occupational noise-induced hearing loss.[10,11] This statement summarized the accepted opinions of the medical community regarding diagnosis of OHL. The American Occupational Medicine Association (AOMA) Committee defined occupational noise-induced hearing loss as a slowly developing hearing loss over a long time period (several years) as the result of exposure to continuous or intermittent loud noise. The committee stated that the diagnosis of noise-induced hearing loss is made clinically by a physician and should include study of the noise exposure history. It is also distinguished OHL from acoustic trauma, an immediate change in hearing resulting from a single exposure to a sudden burst of sound, such as an explosive blast. The committee recognized that the principle characteristics of occupational noise-induced hearing loss are as follows:

1. It is always sensorineural affecting the hair cells in the inner ear
2. It is almost always bilateral. Audiometric patterns are usually similar bilaterally
3. It almost never produces a profound hearing loss. Usually, low-frequency limits are 40 dB and high-frequency limits 75 dB
4. Once the exposure to noise is discontinued, there is no substantial further progression of hearing loss as a result of the noise exposure
5. Previous noise-induced hearing loss does not make the ear more sensitive to future noise exposure. As the hearing threshold increases, the rate of loss decreases
6. The earliest damage to the inner ears reflects a loss at 3000, 4000, and 6000 Hz. There is always far more loss at 3000, 4000, and 6000 Hz than at 500, 1000, and 2000 Hz. The greatest loss usually occurs at 4000 Hz. The higher and lower frequencies take longer to be affected than the 3000–6000 Hz range
7. Given stable exposure conditions, losses at 3000, 4000, and 6000 Hz will usually reach a maximal level in 10–15 years
8. Continuous noise exposure over the years is more damaging than interrupted exposure to noise, which permits the ear to have a rest period.

Since that time, the criteria have been updated twice.[12,13] The most recent guidance statement from the American College of Occupational and Environmental Medicine is considerably more extensive.[13] It includes a list of characteristics and additional consideration associated with noise-induced hearing loss. In summary, the current list of characteristics of noise-induced hearing loss includes the following:

1. It is always sensorineural, affecting primarily the cochlear hair cells
2. It is typically bilateral
3. The first audiometric sign is "notching" between 3000 Hz and 6000 Hz with recovery at 8000 Hz
4. Noise exposure alone usually does not produce hearing loss >75 dB in the high frequencies and 40 dB in the lower frequencies
5. Hearing loss due to noise increases most rapidly during the first 10–15 years of exposure
6. Ears previously exposed to noise are not more sensitive to future noise exposure
7. There is no conclusive evidence that hearing loss due to noise progresses once the noise exposure has been discontinued
8. The risk of noise-induced hearing loss is low at exposures below 85 dBA TWA but increases as exposures rise above this level
9. Continuous noise exposure is more damaging than intermittent noise exposure
10. Hearing protectors provide less attenuation than suggested by the noise reduction rating. Hearing protectors should be selected to reduce exposure to < 85 dBA TWA
11. The presence of a temporary threshold shift (TTS) is a risk indicator for permanent threshold shift (PTS) if hazardous noise exposures continue.

Additional considerations discussed include the following:

1. Unilateral sources of noise such as sirens and gunshots can produce asymmetric hearing loss, as can situations in which the work involves fixed placement of the affected ear relative to a noise source
2. Exposures to very intense and frequent impulse/impact noise added to steady-state noise may be more harmful than steady-state noise of the same A-weighted energy exposure alone
3. Exposure to ototoxic agents may act in synergy with noise to cause hearing loss
4. Individual susceptibility to the auditory effects of noise varies widely
5. Causes of hearing loss other than noise must be considered
6. Noise-induced hearing loss may cause "significant morbidity" in some workers
7. Early detection and intervention are essential to prevention of OHL
8. Age correction of audiograms allows age standardization, permitting comparison of hearing loss rates among working populations. OSHA permits but does not require the use of an age correction procedure
9. Assessment of hearing loss requires review of previous audiograms, noise exposure records, hearing protection data, and clinical history to assist in the diagnosis.

Sensorineural Hearing Loss

Habitual exposure to occupational noise damages the hair cells in the cochlea causing a sensory hearing loss. No damage to the outer or middle ear (conductive loss) can be caused by routine daily exposure to loud industrial noise. Ultimately, some of the nerve fibers supplying the damaged hair cells may also become damaged from many causes and result in a neural loss of hearing, as well.

Bilaterality of OHL

Both ears are equally sensitive to TTS and PTS (hearing loss) due to most free-field occupational noise exposure; and, therefore, damage is equal or almost equal in both ears. If an employee working in a very noisy environment develops substantial one-sided sensorineural hearing impairment, it is essential to find the cause and to rule out an acoustic neuroma, which commonly presents as unilateral sensorineural hearing loss. In weapons and range fire, the ear nearest the stock (left ear in a right-handed rifle shooter) sustains damage before and to a somewhat greater degree than the other ear; however, a loss will generally be present to some degree bilaterally.

The 4000-Hz Audiometric Dip

Occupational noise-induced hearing loss is not only sensorineural and usually bilateral but it also has a characteristic frequency distribution known as the 4000-Hz dip. Figure 18.2 shows a composite audiogram of the classic progress of many cases of OHL. This pattern is common in hearing loss caused by gunfire; and exposure to continuous noise, such as in weaving mills, some metal plants, etc., also produces this pattern in which the earliest damage occurs between 3000 and 6000 Hz. Some noise sources, such as papermaking machines, can damage the 2000-Hz frequency somewhat before the higher frequencies, while noise exposures to chipping and jackhammers, for example,

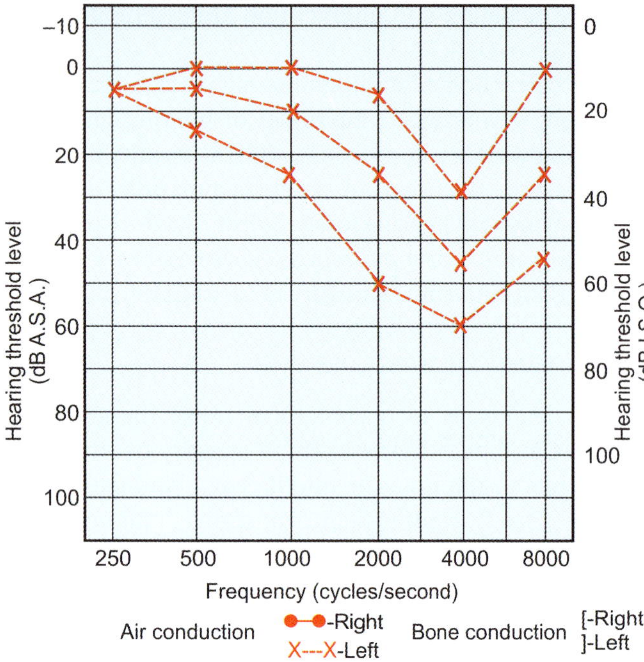

Fig. 18.2: Series of audiometric curves showing a "classic" progressive loss that may be found in employees with excessive noise exposure.

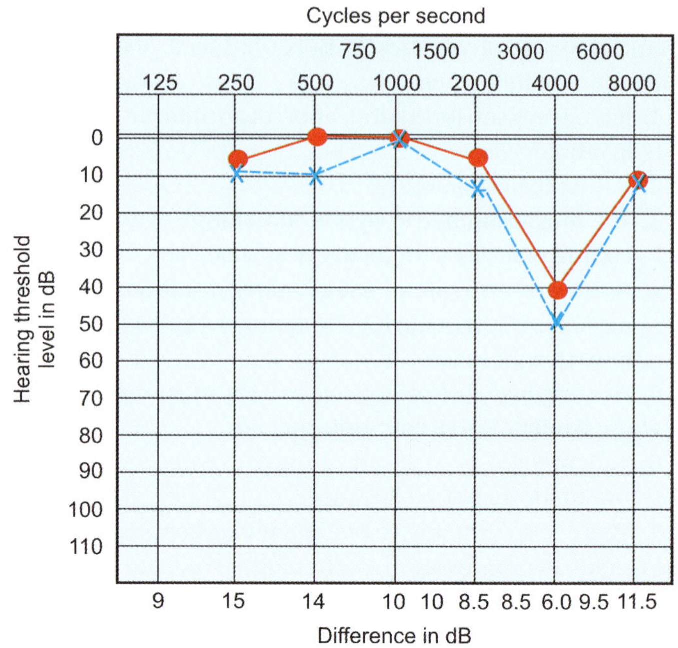

Fig. 18.3: Typical 400-Hz dip. In this audiogram, and in all other audiograms in this chapter, bone conduction equals air conduction. ●—●, right; X – – X, left.

characteristically damage the higher frequencies severely before affecting the lower ones. However, in general, frequencies below 3000 Hz are almost never damaged by occupational noise without earlier damage to the higher frequencies.

It has been known for many years that prolonged exposure to high-intensity noise results in sensorineural hearing loss that is greatest between 3000 and 6000 Hz. In such cases, the classic audiogram shows a 4000-Hz dip in which hearing is better at 2000 and 8000 Hz (Fig. 18.3). Unfortunately, the fact that noise produces this 4000-Hz dip has led some physicians to assume that any comparable dip is produced by noise. This error can lead to misdiagnosis and can result in undesirable medical and legal consequences.

Although there are numerous hypotheses that attempt to explain the 4000 Hz dip in noise-induced hearing loss,[14–17] its pathogenesis remains uncertain. However, it is known that in most cases this loss affects hearing between 4000 and 6000 Hz initially and then spreads to other frequencies.[18,19] Frequencies higher than those usually measured clinically may be tested on special audiometers and are helpful in diagnosing noise-induced hearing loss in selected cases.[20] This hearing loss may result from steady state or intermittent noise, although the intensities required to produce comparable hearing losses differ,[21] and controversy exists as to the nature of the actual cochlear damage.[21–24] Other types of acoustic trauma, such as from blast injuries, may result in other audiometric patterns or in a 4000-Hz dip, but they will not be considered in this discussion. Head trauma may produce the same audiometric pattern.

Discrimination Scores

In almost all cases of OHL in which the high frequencies are affected (even severely), the discrimination scores are good (>85%) in a quiet room. If patients have much lower discrimination scores, another cause in addition to OHL should be suspected.

Gradual Hearing Loss with Early Onset

In addition to having the characteristics of a bilateral sensorineural hearing loss with a 4000 Hz dip, OHL begins early with noise exposure and progresses gradually. Sudden deafness is not caused by noise to which a patient is exposed regularly at his/her job. There are, of course, incidents of unilateral sudden deafness due to acoustic trauma from an explosion or similar circumstance. Other causes must be sought in sudden deafness in one or both ears regardless of occupational noise exposure.

OHL characteristically develops during the first few years of exposure and may worsen over the next 12–15 years of continued exposure, but the damage does not continue to progress rapidly or substantially with additional exposure beyond 12–15 years. Rarely, an employee working in consistent noise will have good hearing for 4 or 5 years and then develop progressive hearing loss from occupational causes. Employees who retire after age 60 and develop additional hearing loss without continued noise exposure generally should not attribute this to their past jobs.[25] The same pertains to employees who wear hearing protectors effectively and either develop hearing loss or have additional hearing loss. Accurate diagnosis is important because some such hearing losses occur from etiologies that are amenable to treatment.

Asymptotic Hearing Loss

Another characteristic of OHL is that specific noisy jobs produce a maximum degree of hearing loss. This has been called asymptotic loss. For example, employees using jackhammers develop severe high frequency, but minimal low frequency, hearing losses. Employees working for years in 92 dBA generally do not have >20-dB losses in the low frequencies and once they reach a certain degree of high-frequency hearing loss, little additional loss occurs. Many employees exposed to weaving looms experience a maximum of 40-dB loss in the speech frequencies, but they rarely have greater losses. This is believed to be due to the hearing impairment itself protecting the ear from further damage. For example, if someone with a 35-dB hearing loss is exposed to a 95-dB sound, he hears only 60 dB (in the absence of loudness recruitment), and little or no additional noise-induced hair cell damage occurs. If an employee shows a loss much greater than is typical for similar exposure, the otologist should suspect other causes.

LIMITATIONS OF THE AUDIOGRAM

We already have noted that an audiogram showing a 4000-Hz dip is not sufficient evidence to make a diagnosis of noise-induced hearing loss. A thorough investigation must be considered to establish the true cause of the hearing loss whenever there is any question regarding etiology. It is not always possible to ascribe a hearing loss to noise or to completely rule out other causes. However, if the patient's noise exposure has been sufficient, and if investigation fails to reveal other causes of hearing loss, a diagnosis of noise-induced hearing loss can be made with reasonable certainty in the presence of supportive audiometric findings.

Other Causes of the 4000-Hz Dip

Viral Infections

It is well known that viral upper-respiratory infections may be associated with hearing loss, tinnitus, and aural fullness. This fullness is frequently due to inner-ear involvement rather than middle-ear dysfunction. Viral cochleitis also may produce either temporary or permanent sensorineural hearing losses, which can have a variety of audiometric patterns, including a 4000-Hz dip (Fig. 18.4).[26] In addition to viral respiratory infections as causes of sensorineural hearing loss, rubella, measles, mumps, cytomegalic inclusion disease, herpes, and other viruses have been implicated (Fig. 18.5).

Skull Trauma

Severe head trauma that results in fracture of the cochlea usually produces profound hearing loss or total deafness. However, lesser trauma to the inner ear may produce concussion-type injury that may be manifested audiometrically as a 4000-Hz dip. Human temporal bone pathology in such cases is similar to that seen in noise-induced hearing loss.[27] Similar findings can also be produced by experimental temporal-bone injury.[17]

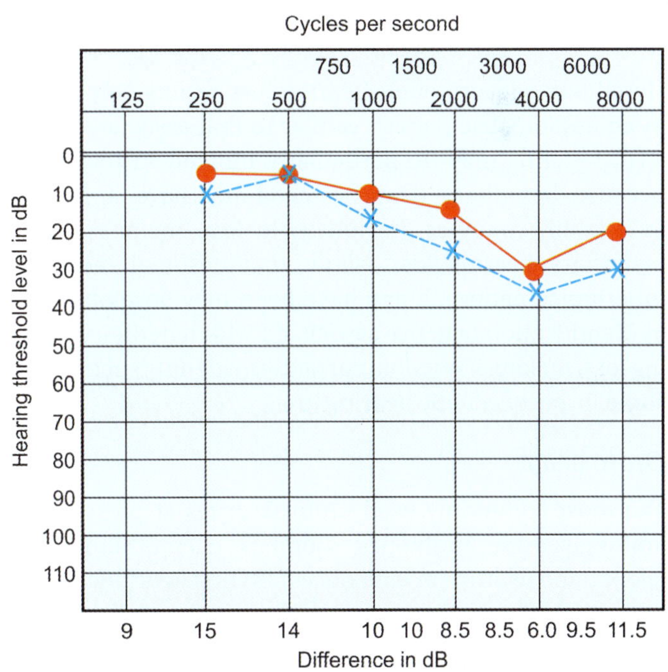

Fig. 18.4: Audiogram of a 51-year-old woman who developed sudden hissing tinnitus and a feeling of fullness in her ears during a typical head cold. She had no other ear problems and no noise exposure. The audiogram remained unchanged during a 2-year observation period. ●—●, right; X – – X, left.

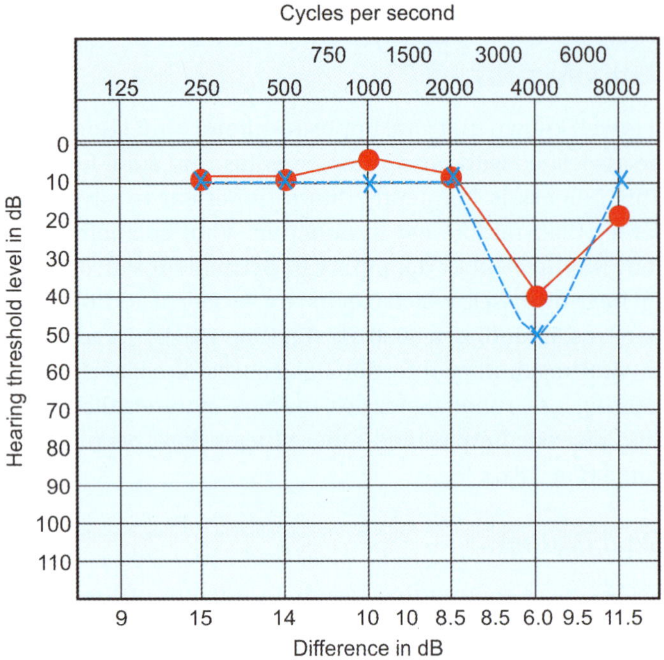

Fig. 18.5: Audiogram of a 24-year-old woman who developed tinnitus and a feeling of fulleness in her ears during an attack of herpetic "cold sores" not associated with an upper-respiratory illness. Electronystagmography showed right-sided weakness. Examination showed decreased sensation in the distribution of the second cervical and glossopharyngeal nerves. ●—●, right; X – – X, left.

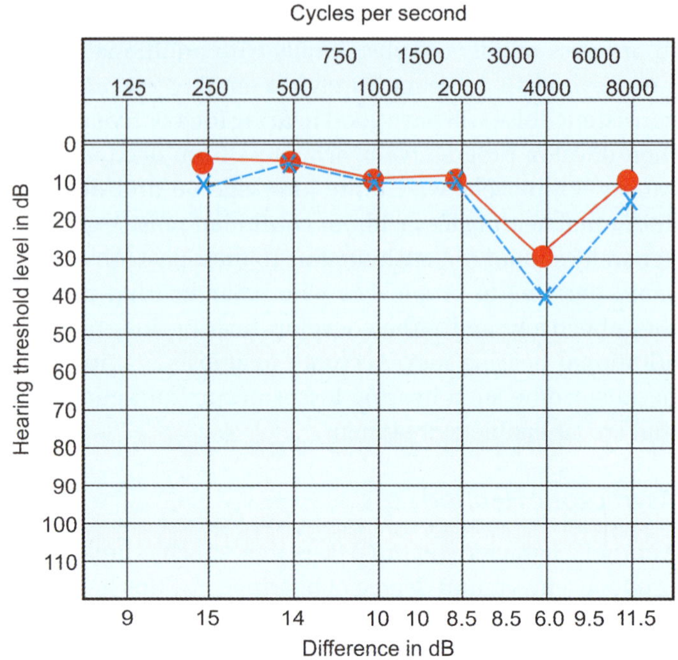

Fig. 18.6: Audiogram of a 54-year-old woman who developed bilateral high-pitched tinnitus 2 weeks after beginning an oral diuretic for mild hypertension. Electronystagmography showed nght-sided weakness. Examination showed decrease sensation in the distribution of the second cervical and glossopharyngeal nerves. ●—●, right; X – – X, left.

Hereditary (Genetic) Hearing Loss

Hereditary sensorineural hearing loss results commonly in an audiometric pattern similar to that associated with OHL.[28-30] This may be particularly difficult to diagnose, because hereditary deafness need not have appeared in a family member previously; in fact, many cases of hereditary hearing loss follow an autosomal recessive inheritance pattern. There have been new developments in identification of genes associated with hereditary hearing loss, making it possible currently to identify specifically some forms of genetic hearing loss.

Ototoxicity

The most commonly used ototoxic drugs at present are aminoglycoside antibiotics, diuretics, chemotherapeutic agents, and aspirin (in high doses).[1] When toxic effects are seen, high-frequency sensorineural hearing loss is most common, and profound deafness may result, although a 4000-Hz dip pattern may also be seen (Fig. 18.6).[24]

Unlike damage caused by the other ototoxic drugs listed above, aspirin-induced hearing loss usually is only temporary, recovering after cessation of the medication.

Acoustic Neuroma

Eighth-nerve tumors may produce any audiometric pattern, from that of normal hearing to profound deafness, and the 4000-Hz dip is not a rare manifestation of this lesion (Figs. 18.7 and 18.8).[31] In these lesions, low speech discrimination scores and pathological tone decay need not be present and cannot be relied on to rule out retrocochlear pathology. Nevertheless, asymmetry of hearing loss should arouse suspicion even when a history of noise exposure exists. There are several cases in which patients were exposed to loud noises producing hearing losses that recovered in one ear but not in the other because of underlying acoustic neuromas.

Sudden Hearing Loss

Each year, clinicians see numerous cases of sudden sensorineural hearing loss of unknown origin. Although the hearing loss is usually unilateral, it may be bilateral; and it may show a 4000-Hz dip. This audiometric pattern may also be seen in patients with sudden hearing loss due to inner-ear membrane breaks[32,33] and barotrauma.[34,35]

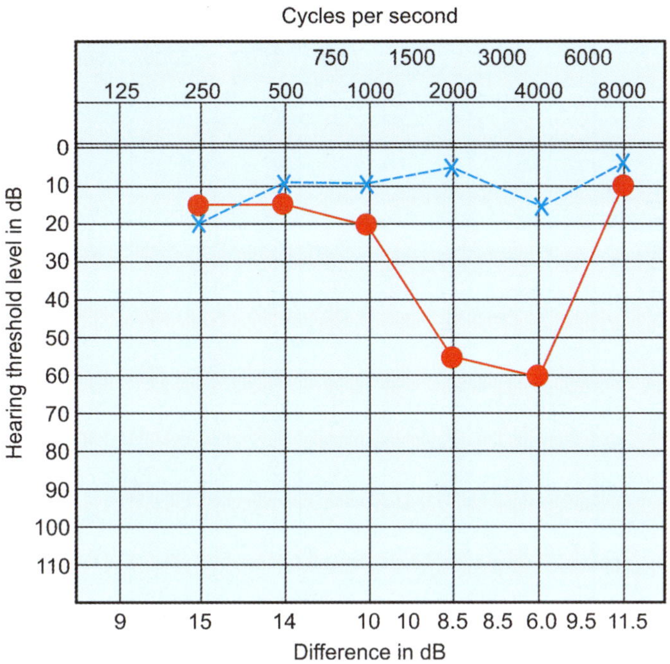

Fig. 18.7: Audiogram of a 28-year-old male machinery worker with a 6-month history of intermittent tinnitus and right-sided hearing loss but without vertigo. Speech discrimination in the right ear was 88%. Electronystagmography showed reduced right-vestibular function. A 1-cm neuroma was removed through the right middle fossa. ●—●, right; X – – X, left.
Courtesy of: MD Graham.[28]

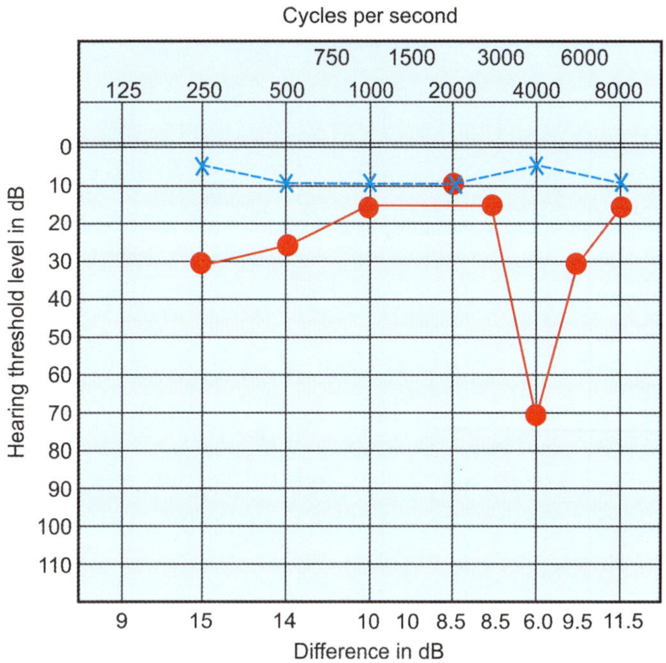

Fig. 18.8: Audiogram of a 40-year-old woman with a 1-year history of tinnitus and right-sided hearing loss that was especially apparent when she used the telephone. Speech discrimination in the right ear was 88%. Electronystagmography revealed absent right caloric responses. A 1.5 cm acoustic neuroma was removed through a translabyrinthine approach. ●—●, right; X – – X, left.
Courtesy of: MD Graham.[28]

Multiple Sclerosis

Multiple sclerosis can also produce sensorineural hearing loss that may show almost any pattern and may fluctuate from severe deafness to normal threshold levels. An example demonstrating a variable 4000-Hz dip is shown in Figure 18.9.

Other Causes

A variety of other causes may produce audiograms similar to those seen in noise-induced hearing loss. Such conditions include bacterial infections such as meningitis, systemic toxins,[36] and neonatal hypoxia and jaundice. Figure 18.10 illustrates one such sensorineural hearing loss that resulted from kernicterus because of Rh incompatibility.

NOISE EXPOSURE HISTORY

It is important to recall that sound of a given frequency spectrum and intensity requires a certain amount of time to produce hearing loss in most subjects. Although the necessary exposure varies from person to person, a diagnosis of noise-induced hearing loss requires a history of sufficient noise exposure. Guidelines for estimating how much noise is necessary to cause hearing loss in most people have been established by the scientific community and the federal government and are reviewed in this chapter. However, a reasonable assessment of a patient's occupational noise exposure cannot be obtained solely from his/her history, especially if compensation is a factor.

Patients who have worked for many years without hearing protection with weaving looms, papermaking machines, boilers, sheet metal, riveters, jackhammers, chippers, and the like, nearly always have some degree of OHL. However, many other patients have marked hearing losses that could not possibly have been caused by their minimal exposures to noise. Many patients working in industry can claim that they have been exposed to a great deal of noise. It is essential, especially in compensation cases, to get more accurate information by obtaining from the employer, if possible, a written work history and time-weighted average of noise exposure. If a physician does not have first-hand knowledge of the noise exposure in a patient's job, definitive diagnosis generally should be delayed until such information is made available.

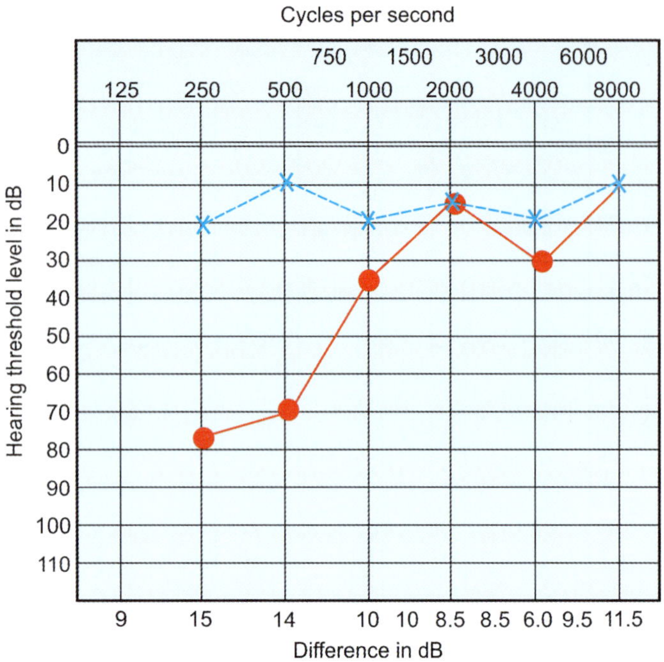

Fig. 18.9: Audiogram of a 20-year-old woman with fluctuating sensorineural hearing loss due to multiple sclerosis. Brainstem evoked-response audiometry showed conduction slowing between the cochlear nucleus and the superior olivary nucleus. ●—●, right; X – – X, left.
Courtesy of: MD Graham.[28]

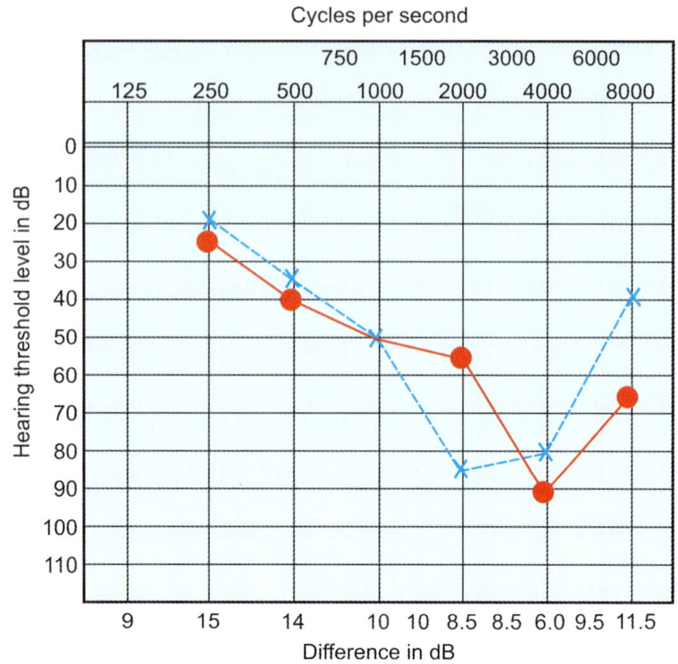

Fig. 18.10: Audiogram of a 1-year-old boy had sever neonatal jaundice with kernicterus as a result of Rh incompatibility, ●—●, right; X – – X, left.
Courtesy of: MD Graham.[28]

Some publications[6,9] have perpetuated the idea that exposures to <90 dBA can produce handicapping hearing losses in the speech frequencies. A critical review of the most quoted publications[37-38] reveals that all these reports contain serious shortcomings casting considerable doubt on their conclusions. The Inter-industry Noise Exposure studies are the best conducted and monitored research projects relating hearing loss and noise exposure, but even these authors emphasize the need for additional valid and reliable research.

The 85- and 90-dBA noise exposure levels designated by OSHA are the levels at which initiation of a hearing conservation program and use of hearing protection are recommended. They are not necessarily the levels at which hearing becomes impaired in the speech frequencies even after years of exposure. Individuals who have handicapping hearing loss in their speech frequencies and are habitually exposed to <90 dBA probably have hearing losses from other causes. These losses have developed regardless of their jobs. It is important to find the specific causes for their hearing losses rather than make misleading, unjustified, and hasty diagnoses of OHL.

The term biological hypersensitivity to noise is often misused and requires clarification. Many physicians and attorneys have attributed patients' substantial sensorineural hearing loss to hypersensitivity to noise, even though the exposure was to 85 dBA or less. There is no basis for such an opinion. Prolonged exposure to this type of noise level will not cause handicapping hearing loss in the speech frequencies. Biological hypersensitivity to noise does not mean that individuals exposed to mild levels <90 dBA can sustain substantial hearing losses, but rather that in a group of employees habitually exposed to very loud noise (>95 dBA) without hearing protectors, a few will have little or no hearing loss (so-called "hard ears"), most will have a fair amount of loss, and a few will sustain substantially greater losses because they are hypersensitive.

Many years of otologic studies and clinical experience have demonstrated certain symptoms and findings that are characteristic of OHL. For instance, we know that employees do not suffer total or very severe sensorineural deafness in the speech frequencies even if they work for years in the loudest industrial noise areas. Several explanations have been proposed for this observation, for example: "the nerve-deafened ear acts as a hearing protector" and "what you do not hear does not hurt you". Even when noise exposure is very high and undoubtedly a contributing cause, all patients with severely handicapping losses in the speech frequencies should be studied carefully to find the underlying etiology.

Otologic history should include use, duration, and effectiveness of hearing protection, type of noise exposure (including continuous or intermittent), dosage of exposure (daily hours and years), and presence of recreational noise exposure such as target practice, trap shooting, hunting, snow-mobile use, motorcycling, chain saw or power-tool use, etc. Recreational exposure may contribute to noise-induced hearing loss. Employees should be advised to use hearing protectors during recreational exposure to loud noise. Infrequent exposures and intermittent exposures are far less hazardous than continuous daily exposures. It seems that if the ear has sufficient rest periods, damage to the speech frequencies is minimized.

HISTOPATHOLOGY OF NOISE-INDUCED HEARING LOSS

Histologic studies of human inner ears damaged by noise reveal diffuse degeneration of hair cells and nerves in the second quadrant of the basal turn of the cochlea - the area sensitive to 3000–6000 Hz sounds (Figs. 18.11 to 18.13).[24] Similar findings have been demonstrated in cochlear hair cells and first-order neurons in experimental animals exposed to loud noises, as discussed subsequently. Further experimental studies in rodents have shown noise-induced injury to the stria vascularis as well,[39] but there is some question as to the applicability of this finding to clinical medicine.

Comprehensive discussion of the histopathology of noise-induced hearing loss is beyond the scope of this chapter. The subject is controversial, and many questions remain unanswered. However, certain recent observations are of particular clinical interest and worthwhile reviewing, particularly those of Spoendlin of Innsbruck, Austria.[40]

The psychophysical effects of sound stimulation at various intensities include the following:

1. Adaptation is an immediate and rapidly reversible threshold shift proportional to the sound intensity at the frequency of stimulation
2. TTS is pathological, metabolically induced fatigue. Its development and recovery are proportional to the logarithm of exposure time. It reverses slowly over a period of hours
3. PTS, such as from OHL, develops by exposure to excessive noise for sufficiently long period of time

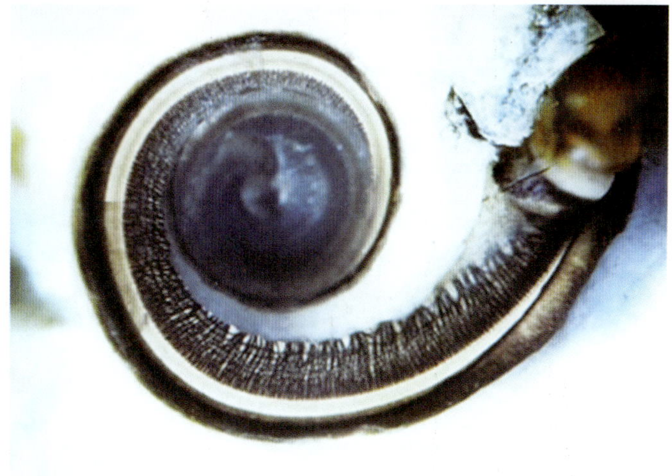

Fig. 18.11: Anterolateral view of the left cochlea from a 17-year-old female car accident victim. Most of the vestibular portion of the membranous wall of the cochlea. Reissner's membrane, and the tectorial membrane have been removed for surface preparations. At 12 o'clock, a part of Reissner's membrane is still in situ, and at 9 o'clock, a portion of the spiral ligament is arching over the scala vestibule. By courtesy of Lars-Göran Johnsson, Karolinska Institute, Helsinki, Finland.

The extended exposure time results in the destruction and eventual loss of the cells of the organ of Corti. Two mechanisms appear to be involved in this process:

1. In high-intensity noise exposure, there may be direct mechanical destruction
2. In exposure to moderately intense noise, there is a metabolic decompensation with subsequent degeneration of sensory elements

If a cochlea is examined shortly after even short-term exposure to extremely intense noise, it may show entire absence of the organ of Corti in the epicenter of the injured area. Moving laterally from the epicenter, the hair cells are swollen and severely distorted with cytoplasmic organelle displacement. More laterally, the cells reveal bending of sensory hairs. Further from the epicenter, but still in the area of damage, one finds only slight distortion of the outer hair cells. In addition to sensory damage, dislocation of the tympanic lamina cells, disruption of the heads of the pillar cells, holes in the basilar membrane, and other findings may be seen.

After exposure to moderately intense acoustic stimuli, the nuclei of outer hair cells become extremely swollen. Swelling is also seen in the terminal unmyelinated portion of the afferent nerve fibers to the inner hair cells. This pathological condition of afferent nerve fibers may be seen in hypoxia, as well. In both instances, it appears

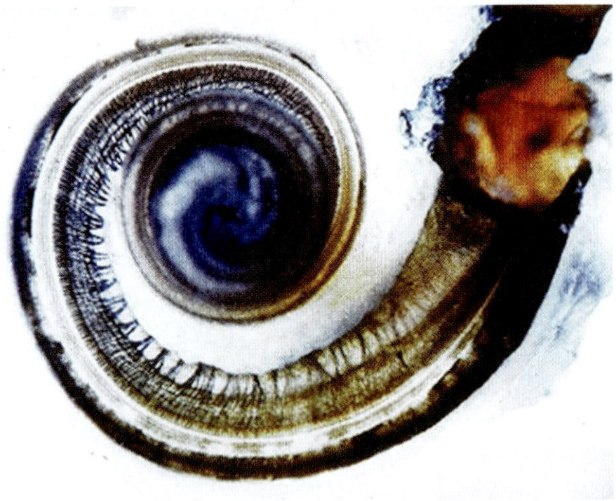

Fig. 18.12: The left cochlea of a 76-year-old male cancer patient with hypertension and generalized arteriosclerosis. Note the patchy degeneration of the organ of Corti in the lower basal turn and the nerve degeneration. Paraformaldehyde 11-hour postmortem, OsO4. By courtesy of Lars-Göran Johnsson, Karolinska Institute, Helsinki, Finland.

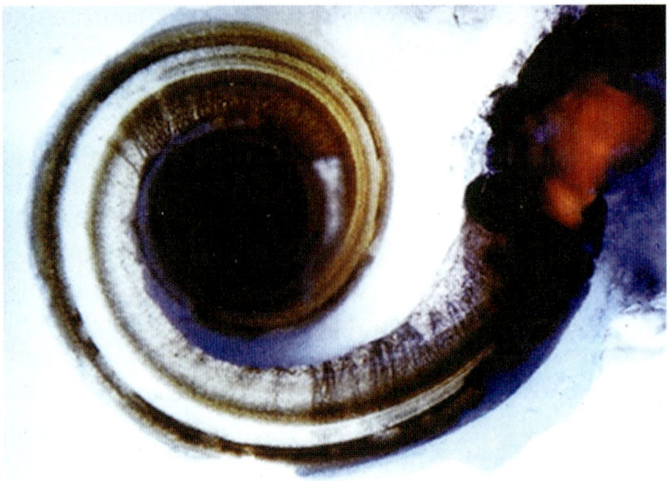

Fig. 18.13: The left cochlea from a 59-year-old male patient who had worked in noisy surroundings and had been an enthusiastic hunter. There is a total loss of hair cells and nerve fibers in the middle of the basal turn. Note in the upper basal turn the presence of nerve fibers in an area where no organ of Corti remains. Paraformaldehyde 8-hour postmortem, OsO_4. By courtesy of Lars-Göran Johnsson, Karolinska Institute, Helsinki, Finland.

to result from metabolic derangement. Degeneration of mitochondria and alteration of the synaptic vesicles may be observed in the efferent nerve endings of the outer hair cells after long exposure.[41]

TTS appears to cause only an increase in number and size of lysosomes, primarily in the outer hair cells, a finding probably also related to increased metabolic activity.

The localization of damage depends on the type of noise exposure. Exposure to white noise, multifrequency noise encountered under most industrial circumstances, usually produces damage in the upper basal turn of the cochlea, the 3000–6000-Hz frequency range in humans. Narrow-band noise causes damage in different areas depending on the frequency of the noise; the extent of the damage increases with increasing intensity of the center frequency. These observations are true for continuous noise; impulse noise results in much more variability in site of damage. The rise time of the impulse appears to be an important factor in the amount of hearing damage. Histologically, square-noise impulses appear to produce less damage than impulses with a gradual rising time of 25 ms.[40] The practical implications of this finding remain unclear.

The histological progression of cochlear injury over time is also of interest. Some of the mechanically or metabolically induced structural changes are reversible, whereas others progress to degeneration. Metabolically induced changes such as swollen nuclei in the outer hair cells and swollen nerve endings usually reverse, although scattered degeneration occurs. Severe distortion of cells often leads to degeneration and membrane ruptures, which may result in the disappearance of the organ of Corti in the area of injury. In places where the organ of Corti is completely destroyed, the cochlear neurons undergo slow, progressive retrograde degeneration over months. Eventually, 90% of the cochlear neurons associated with the injured area disappear, including their spiral ganglion cells of origin. This retrograde neural degeneration usually is not observed when only outer hair cells are missing.[42] No significant neural degeneration has been noted in adjacent areas. Thus, although histopathological changes progress even after acoustic stimulation has stopped, significant degeneration occurs only in regions where substantial hair cell destruction (hence, substantial hearing loss) has already occurred. Consequently, progressive histological changes do not imply progressive clinical hearing deterioration.

Histologically, maximal damage to the cochlea secondary to noise exposure is never total. Even under laboratory circumstances, there are always some sensory elements preserved in the cochlea. Moreover, for each exposure intensity, a "saturation damage" occurs after a certain time.The time interval is short for high-intensity noise exposure and longer for low-intensity noise exposure. Additional exposure to noise of the same intensity does not produce additional observable damage beyond this "saturation damage" limit. This histological finding corresponds to asymptotic hearing loss. Moreover, even under laboratory conditions, there is a great variability in the cochlear damage produced by controlled noise exposure, especially following stimulation by moderately intense noise or impulse noise. These are the conditions encountered most commonly in an industrial environment. This histological and experimental evaluation corresponds to the biological variability (hard ears and soft ears) observed in industrial populations.

COFACTORS ASSOCIATED WITH OHL

Nonoccupational Noise Exposure

Habitual exposure to loud rock-and-roll and amplified music can produce hearing damage between 2000 and 8000 Hz. Occasional exposure, however, can be annoying to unaccustomed listeners, but it does not cause substantial hearing damage in most cases. Household noises such as vacuum cleaners, fans, air conditioners, etc., generally do not damage hearing even though they may be disturbing.

Exposure to ultrasonic noise, such as in certain commercial cleaners, does not affect hearing in the usually recorded frequencies (up to 8000 Hz). Community noises such as trolley cars, airplanes, noises from industrial plants, sirens, etc., also usually do not cause hearing damage, although very loud noises such as sirens may cause hearing loss to an ear that is close to the sound source.

Aspirin

Limited research exists that investigates the interaction of aspirin and noise exposure on hearing loss. A study by Carson et al.[43] explored the interaction of different aspirin doses and presence of noise on the hearing of rats. Permanent hearing losses and hair cell damage were noted in all animals exposed to the noise condition; however, a greater amount of hair cell loss was observed in the animals with the highest dose of aspirin. Although some animal studies, like the one mentioned earlier, have shown a relationship between noise-induced hearing loss and aspirin, its interaction on human hair cells and hearing loss is unknown at this time.

Smoking

Research studies have implicated smoking as a cofactor that may affect the degree and risk of OHL. Past experiments investigating the correlation of smoking and high-frequency noise-induced hearing loss illustrate a higher risk of hearing loss.[44–48] One study revealed that current smokers had an increased rate of hearing loss by a ratio of 1.39:1 with an increase in the trend based on the number of packs smoked per day.[44] However, the results of these investigations have been inconsistent regarding the exact role smoking plays in OHL, in some part because of poor controls of noise exposure levels in participants. Some studies have suggested that smoking, by itself, does not increase the risk of OHL; however, when coupled with elevated blood pressure and other cardiovascular risk factors, those workers have a higher risk of hearing loss.[49,50]

Industrial Solvents

Another group of cofactors has been the topic of experimental research in both humans and animals. Industrial solvents such as toluene, styrene, xylene, trichloroethylene, and carbon disulfide, by themselves or in mixtures, have been implicated in affecting the inner ear both with and without the presence of noise. A review of audiograms and electronystagmography (ENG) results for workers in a paint and varnish plant revealed that 42% of those exposed to industrial solvents had high-frequency hearing losses when compared with 5% in the age-matched control group; 47.5% of that same group demonstrated abnormal ENGs, vs. 5% in the control group.[51] In investigating the effects of styrene and styrene plus noise exposure, Sliwinska-Kowalska et al.[52] found that exposure to the styrene increased the risk of hearing loss in humans; in addition, the styrene plus noise exposed group had two to three times higher odds of developing hearing loss. Both of these studies support the conclusion that exposure to some industrial solvents can increase the risk of high-frequency hearing loss. More research is needed to investigate other industrial solvents and their possible effect on workers and their hearing.

NONORGANIC HEARING LOSS

Owing to the compensation and legal factors involved in OHL, some individuals present with nonorganic hearing loss in alleged noise-induced loss cases. The diagnosing physician needs to be aware of possible nonorganic components including functional hearing loss, functional overlay, and malingering.

Functional or psychogenic hearing loss results from the influence of psychological or emotional factors resulting in an inability to hear when the peripheral mechanism may be essentially normal. Patients with extreme anxiety or emotional conflicts may outwardly manifest their mental disturbances by converting it into hearing loss or other conversion disorders. Conversion disorders are an involuntary response, escaping from the extreme emotions that cannot be faced voluntarily. A component of functional hearing loss can also be noted in addition to actual organic, peripheral hearing loss. When this is evident, it is called functional overlay. Careful history taking and accurate audiometry will assist in the diagnosis of these nonorganic components.

Unlike functional hearing loss, malingering is the intentional misrepresentation of one's hearing, usually for monetary or emotional gain. Individuals have been known to misrepresent their hearing for financial gain, to avoid work environments such as military deployment, to evade responsibility, or for purposes of gaining attention. Functional overlay also can exist in malingering hearing losses. Most malingerers are revealed by their inconsistent test results. In cases of unilateral malingering, the shadow curve that should be present due to interaural sound transmission is often absent. For other cases, the pure tone average is not consistent with the speech reception threshold. To try to find the malingerer's true thresholds, a number of techniques are useful in audiology. An ascending method of test presentation decreases people's ability to estimate loudness; this is also reduced if smaller 1–2 dB steps are used instead of the traditional 5 dB steps. Physiological measures such as otoacoustic emissions and auditory brainstem response also can be helpful in determining normal hearing, as can other special tests.

PREVENTION AND HEARING PROTECTORS

When it is not possible to reduce noise levels by treatment of the source, the problem may sometimes be solved by covering surrounding surfaces with acoustically absorbent materials, by the use of noise barriers, or by moving either the offending noise source or the persons exposed to another location. When it is impractical to attain enough noise reduction by these means, personal protective devices must be used. All factors considered, hearing protectors usually provide immediate, effective protection against OHL.

An effective personal protective device serves as a barrier between the noise and the inner ear where noise-induced damage to hearing may occur. Hearing protectors usually take the form of either earmuffs, which are worn over the external ear and provide an acoustical seal against the head; canal caps that supply an acoustical seal at the entrances of the external ear canal; and earplugs or inserts that offer an acoustical seal in the outermost portion of the ear canal. Hearing protectors need to be fitted individually and chosen expertly. The protection afforded by a hearing protector depends on its design and on several physiological and physical characteristics of the wearer. Assessing, recommending, and monitoring effective hearing protection requires considerable training and skills.

The professional responsible for hearing protection must be familiar with the various ways sound energy may reach the inner ears, different types of hearing protection, various anatomical configurations of external auditory canals, the real meaning of noise reduction ratings for various ear protectors, appropriate hearing protectors designed for specific noise environments, the effects of ear protectors on communication in noise, ear protector management for people with ear infections, and many other important factors. These are discussed in details in Chapter 17 of Sataloff and Sataloff.[1]

CASE REPORTS

Chiefly because of OSHA requirements and greater emphasis on worker's compensation for OHL, hundreds of thousands of employees will ultimately be referred to otologists for consultations. Physicians must provide expert advice on matters such as employing people with possible safety and communication problems, managing numerous otologic problems and determining whether hearing loss is because of occupational noise or some other cause. The general characteristics of OHL described can help guide physicians to a reasonably accurate diagnosis. In order to illustrate some of the numerous problems that have arisen in managing claims for OHL, it may be helpful to review a series of actual cases that have come to workers' compensation court for adjudication. The histories are abstracted and the findings of plaintiff's and defense's experts are abbreviated, but included in each case are important features that illustrate both justified and unjustified contentions.

In all these cases, the physical aspects of the otologic examination revealed no abnormalities unless specifically stated in the case report. Appropriate complete physical examination, blood studies, and other examinations were performed with no abnormalities found unless specifically stated in the report.

Case Report 1

A 63-year-old pipefitter, employed by a shipbuilding company for 40 years, had 10 years' exposure to chippers and ship "scraping" noise. Hearing loss developed gradually over many years, most pronounced after chipping exposure. He denied tinnitus, vertigo, and gunfire exposure. Audiometry (Fig. 18.14) showed bilateral sensorineural hearing loss with fairly good residual hearing at 10,000 and 12,000 Hz, discrimination between 82% and 88%, and good speech reception. These findings are characteristic of OHL due to prolonged exposure to intense noise such as chipping, and the history is consistent with the diagnosis. If presbycusis or hereditary deafness were factors, the highest frequencies would be more seriously involved and the discrimination score might be worse.

Case Report 2

A 67-year-old railroad brakeman had worked for 35 years and retired 2 years ago. About 7 years prior to this otologic examination, he had been examined for hearing loss by an otologist, who concluded, on the basis of the patient's history of working with excessive noise and vibration, that the patient had "sensorineural hearing loss due to prolonged exposure to noise and vibration". Only two audiograms were available (Fig. 18.15), one taken in 1974, 5 years prior to retirement, and one in 1981, 2 years after retirement. Note the rather late onset of hearing loss and the progressive nature of the condition even over the past 4 or 5 years. This employee had been working in the same noise environment for many years, yet he did not notice the hearing loss until a few years prior to retirement. These factors help indicate that the diagnosis is presbycusis rather than OHL. This is further substantiated by the fact that measurements revealed that this patient's exposure did not exceed 87 dBA, and he had not been exposed to the especially loud noises occasionally found in railroad employment.

Case Report 3

A 65-year-old railroad machinist worked around diesel engines for 25 years. He said he had been exposed to roaring diesel train engines for many years and that his hearing loss started many years ago and gradually got worse. He had occasional vertigo but no tinnitus. He denied any family history of hearing loss and was in good health. The audio-logic studies showed a flat mixed hearing loss in both ears of 60 dB, slightly worse in the higher frequencies. The bone conduction threshold was reduced but slightly better than the air conduction in the lower frequencies.

The otologist who first evaluated this patient diagnosed nerve deafness due to occupational exposure to diesel engines.

A later examination by another otologist showed the same audiologic findings but noted excellent bone conduction when a 500-Hz tuning fork was applied to the upper teeth. Discrimination was excellent. The diagnosis was otosclerosis with sensorineural as well as conductive hearing loss. In many older patients, bone conduction tests on the mastoid are not necessarily good indications of actual sensorineural function. Occupational noise did not cause this patient's hearing loss.

Case Report 4

A 36-year-old man began work in a paper mill in 1976. His occupation often involved exposure to noise levels in excess of 95 dBA throughout the workday. He also had a history of exposure to firearms, discharging a shotgun 200–300 times annually. He is left-handed. In addition, he listened to loud music daily. Serial audiograms revealed development between 1976 and 1984 of an obvious dip at 4000 and 6000 Hz. Despite continued exposure to the same occupational and extracurricular noise sources, there is no evidence of significant deterioration after approximately his first 10 years on the job (Fig. 18.16). This is typical of OHL.

Case Report 5

A 45-year-old man gave a complex history of having been evaluated by four otologists. The patient claimed that he had been hit in September 1981 on the right side of his face by a landloader. He was not dazed or unconscious, and there was no bleeding or visible trauma; but he could not hear with his right ear immediately after the incident and had been unable to hear since. He denied any hearing loss prior to the accident and also denied any familial hearing loss. In April 1982, an otologist performed a stapedectomy and the patient's hearing subjectively improved. He developed recurrent vertigo postoperatively. However, audiograms performed shortly after the surgery showed no evidence of hearing improvement compared with preoperative thresholds. The otologist stated that surgery was for otosclerosis and that, in his opinion, the otosclerosis had no relation to the accident. Another otologist who

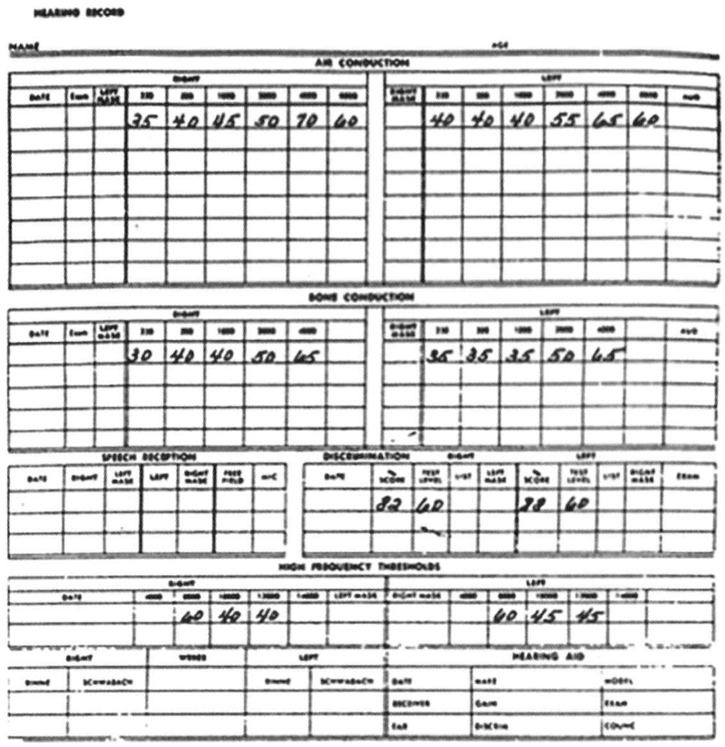

Fig. 18.14: Audiogram of a 63-year-old pipefitter showing bilateral sensorineural hearing loss with fairly good hearing at 10,000 and 12,000 Hz (not shown) and discrimination between 82% and 88% and good speech reception.

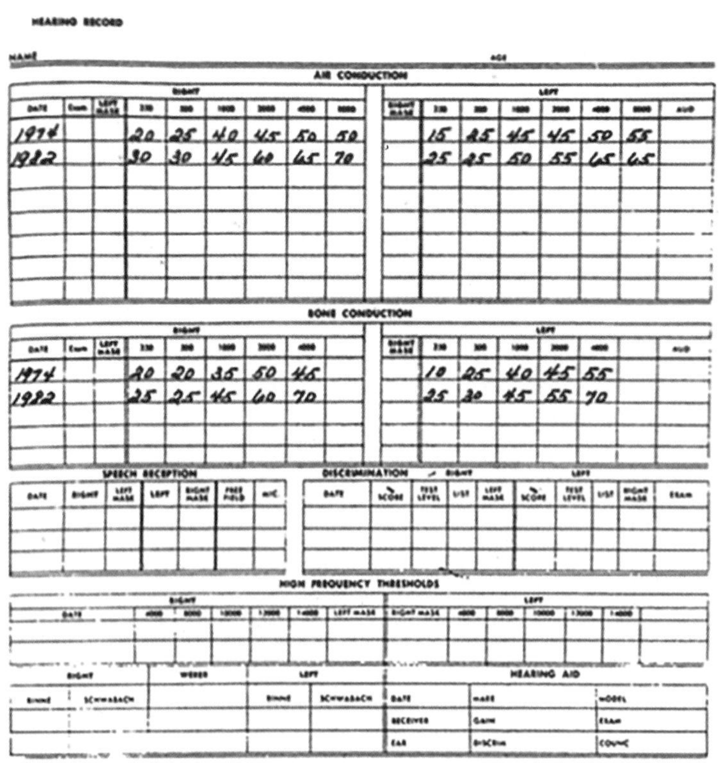

Fig. 18.15: Audiogram of a 67-year-old railroad brakeman showing late onset of hearing loss and the progressive nature of the condition even after the retirement.

NAME :

	RIGHT EAR AIR CONDUCTION								LEFT EAR AIR CONDUCTION						
DATE	500	1000	2000	3000	4000	6000	8000		500	1000	2000	3000	4000	6000	8000
10/76	5	5	5	10	20	40			5	5	10	10	25	25	
8/81	5	0	5	10	50	35			5	5	0	30	65	75	
8/82	5	10	5	20	50	30	30		5	5	5	20	55	35	25
8/83	5	0	5	30	55	35	40		10	10	10	20	35	30	20
7/84	0	0	0	20	40	65	30		5	5	10	10	50	30	20
1/85	0	5	0	35	60	65	25		0	0	10	25	50	25	10
1/86	0	0	0	25	70	50	25		0	0	0	20	50	15	10
2/87	5	0	0	20	70	80	25		0	0	5	25	50	20	10
8/87	5	0	0	25	65	65	20		5	5	0	15	40	30	20
9/88	0	0	0	25	65	60	20		0	0	0	25	35	25	20
9/89	5	5	5	30	70	70	30		5	5	5	30	35	20	15
11/90	0	0	0	25	65	65	30		0	0	0	25	40	20	10
5/91	5	0	0	25	65	60	25		0	0	0	25	40	20	10

Fig. 18.16: Case 4 shows a typical case of asymptotic occupational hearing loss, reaching maximum level in approximately 10 years.

examined the patient because of his persistent vertigo agreed that the vertigo was postoperative and that the diagnosis was otosclerosis, not related to the accident. The patient underwent unsuccessful right revised stapes surgery in an attempt to resolve his vertigo and restore his hearing. At the request of the plaintiff's attorney, another otologist examined this patient in March 1983. Remarks from his report are as follows: "It is apparent from reviewing the records that the patient had a dormant otosclerosis which has been activated and aggravated by the head injury suffered [in 1981]. It is my opinion that without this trauma the otosclerosis would have remained dormant for many years".

In April 1984, another otologic evaluation was performed and the audiologic findings revealed conductive hearing loss with no sensorineural involvement on the right side, excellent bone conduction and discrimination, and a good chance of improving this patient's hearing and clearing up his other symptoms. The difference of interpretation of the etiology of this otosclerotic process is an important issue for otologists. There is no question that all otologists have seen otosclerosis progress to this degree and in this manner without being aggravated by trauma. The contention that trauma could produce this sudden aggravation of otosclerosis has not been substantiated by any valid and reliable otologic study. An otologist may form an opinion that this could have happened, but in order for such an opinion to carry weight or be defensible, it is important that it be creditably based on scientific studies and accepted by the medical community.

Case Report 6

A 65-year-old diabetic man worked in a noisy cannery for >40 years, using hearing protectors only in the last 10 years. His ears had drained intermittently over a 40-year period, most severely in the left ear for the last 7 years. Otologic examination revealed a large left perforation, with scarring and thickening of the residual tympanic membrane. Audiometry of the left ear revealed better bone conduction than air conduction. Bone conduction was excellent by Weber's test. Audiometry of the right ear revealed sensorineural hearing loss. Discrimination scores were good bilaterally. Serial audiograms from 1975 to 1981 showed progressive deterioration of hearing in the left ear. One otologist diagnosed right-sided occupational sensorineural hearing loss and left-sided mixed hearing loss due to occupational exposure with superimposed infection. Another otologist, basing his opinion on the most recent (1981) audiogram, claimed the entire hearing loss was due to occupational noise exposure. At the deposition, it became evident that the deterioration of hearing in the left ear between 1975 and 1981 was not a result of cannery noise, because the worker had worn hearing protection and had not been exposed to loud noise in that time period. Good discrimination scores helped indicate that a large portion of the hearing loss present before 1978 was attributed to occupational noise exposure, although superimposed chronic otitis, tympanosclerosis, and presbycusis were contributory. It was determined that the actual amount of noise exposure that warranted compensation should be determined by the 1975 audiogram.

Case Report 7

A 57-year-old dye caster and screw conveyor operator worked in a machine shop for many years. In 1979, while working around a screw conveyor, he was subjected to an extremely loud sound for ~30 s. He had no discomfort, but his wife noted marked hearing loss that evening. His physician diagnosed "vascular accident resulting from intense noise exposure" and prescribed medication.

The consulting otologist noted disparity in hearing tests taken before and after the incident and expressed the following opinion: "The cause and effect relationship between the loud noise exposure and sudden hearing loss is real, particularly in view of the fact that he has had normal hearing previously". He advised studies to rule out the possibility of other "disease processes".

The employee put in a claim for OHL compensation because of deafness produced by loud noise, particularly in his left ear. Studies revealed the presence of a left acoustic neuroma that was confirmed operatively. It is important to note that all studies, including a CT scan, had missed this small tumor. It was diagnosed only because of the otologist's insistence that the patient undergo a myelogram or air-contrast CT scan. Currently, a MR would be used. An estimated 11% of acoustic neuromas can present as "sudden deafness".[53]

Case Report 8

A 50-year-old employee had worked since 1969 in a plant making tires. His annual audio-grams showed normal hearing until 1973, when annual testing of his hearing was discontinued. He gave a vague history of a "press explosion" in 1975 with some ringing in his right ear, but he did not complain of hearing loss. The explosion was not confirmed either at the plant or in any medical records. In 1976, he had fullness in his right ear that was diagnosed by his otologist as "Eustachian tube blockage due to a temporomandibular joint problem". In 1976, he developed hearing loss and tinnitus in his right ear, causing the otologist to rule out an acoustic neuroma based on normal calorics, tomograms, and posterior fossa myelograms. In 1979, a myringotomy was done for right-ear blockage. In 1981, he had two vertigo attacks and his otologist diagnosed Meniere's disease. The employee retired in 1981 because of physical disabilities. In 1983, he applied for workers' compensation for hearing loss after being examined by his otologist and audiologist. His otologist's report included the following.

The patient shows a bilateral sensorineural hearing loss, which appears to be worse on the right side. The Weber test lateralized to the left ear as would be expected with this audiometric configuration. Speech discrimination is reduced in both ears. Based on the long time history of noise exposure in his occupation, it is very likely that a significant amount of the current hearing loss is probably related to noise.

The otologist representing the defense during litigation demonstrated clearly that:

1. The employee actually was not exposed to noise exceeding 88 dBA during his work and generally worked at much lower levels, chiefly in the loading department
2. He worked for at least 4 years at the same job before developing any hearing loss.
3. The hearing loss started and became severe in his right ear long before the left ear became involved
4. The hearing loss continued to get worse even after he retired in 1981.

The real cause for his hearing loss was probably related to his generalized arteriosclerosis, hypertension, peripheral vascular disease, and long-standing diabetes. In February 1981, he had transient cerebral ischemia attacks, arterial insufficiency of the left leg with occlusion of the left femoral artery, and stenosis of the common iliac artery, treated surgically. The employee's otologist and audiologist were apparently unaware of the patient's diabetes and peripheral vascular problems and surgery. Their impression of his job-related noise exposure, which they obtained from his history, was inaccurate. They were not aware that his actual noise exposure was not capable of producing his hearing loss. There is no question that this hearing loss was neither caused nor aggravated by the worker's job.

CALCULATING HEARING IMPAIRMENT

The ultimate test for determining hearing disability is the ability to understand speech; however, speech audiometry has certain limitations for practical use, so pure-tone audiometry is used. The most commonly used frequencies for calculating hearing impairment used to be 500, 1000, and 2000 Hz. More recently, 3000 Hz also has been included, in accordance with the recommendations of the American Academy of Otolaryngology—Head and Neck Surgery (AAO-HNS). A so-called "low fence" has been determined, below which a hearing loss is considered insufficient to warrant compensation. There is a difference of opinion as to precisely where this low fence should be. The Committee on Hearing and Bio-Acoustics (CHABA) had recommended that the low fence be placed at 35 dB. The AAO-HNS recommends that the low fence be maintained at 25 dB. Each state has its own method of paying disability, using its own formula and providing a method for measuring and calculating binaural hearing impairment. The hearing level for each frequency is the number of decibels at which the listener's threshold of hearing lies above the standard audiometric 0 for that frequency. The hearing level for speech is a simple average of the hearing levels at the frequencies 500, 1000, 2000, and 3000 Hz.

Despite the OSHA and other legislation enacted to help prevent OHL, noise-induced hearing impairment still occurs. Otolaryngologists are called upon frequently to evaluate claimants who allege that they have suffered work-related hearing impairment. Physicians are involved not only in confirming or refuting the presence of hearing loss, but also in diagnosing its cause and helping to determine the degree to which it may have impacted a person's life or caused disability. Fortunately, for everyone concerned, physicians do not have to depend on individual experience and unsubstantiated opinion to make such judgments. The medical and scientific community has accepted nationally (and in some cases internationally) standards to guide such judgments so that they can be as valid, reliable, fair, and consistent as possible across individuals, geographical locations and even organ systems. All physicians involved with evaluations of impairment and disability should be familiar with the AMA Guides to the Evaluation of Permanent Impairment[54] in order to be able to comply with the standard of care as reviewed previously.[55]

It is important to understand the Guides in historical context in order to appreciate the value of this dynamic book and its importance as a scientific compendium. In the United States, physicians from all specialties have been developing and refining the Guides for more than half a century. The AMA established an ad hoc committee in 1956 that led to a publication in the *Journal of the American Medical Association* (*JAMA*) in 1958 called "A Guide to the Evaluation of Permanent Impairment of the Extremities and Back".[56] By 1970, a total of 13 such Guides had appeared in *JAMA*. They were collected as a compendium in 1971, and published as the first edition of the Guides.[57] The value and importance of the Guides became apparent, and great effort has been devoted toward revising and improving the book. In 1981, the AMA established 12 expert panels in preparation for the second edition which was published in 1984. The third (1988), fourth (1993), fifth (2000), and sixth (2008) editions all contained important changes, many of which are summarized in the introductory chapters of each edition. However, the most striking changes were promulgated throughout the sixth edition, to which I was privileged to be contributing editor for the otolaryngology chapter. I had followed the process for many years through my father Joseph Sataloff, MD, who was a contributor or chapter editor for otolaryngology for the second through fifth editions, and I also serve as the AAO-HNS's Advisory Committee Representative to the AMA for Evaluation of Permanent Impairment. This editorial reviews some of the perspective gained through these activities which has proven valuable. It is hoped that the insights summarized briefly herein will assist clinicians, attorneys, and others in understanding the genesis of the Guides, and the importance of their proper application.

As scientific knowledge and methodology expand and our knowledge base grows, it is essential for physicians and scientists to incorporate new knowledge and allow our practices to evolve. The Guides has been strikingly successful in this regard, especially the most recent edition. It warrants discussion because it has some fundamental differences from the first five editions with which all otolaryngologists should be familiar. Each new edition has been changed in order to incorporate the latest scientific research and practice. The first five editions provided the best available information for evaluating permanent impairment, but they had some shortcomings that were acknowledged by most of the scientific community, including by those involved in writing the Guides. The sixth edition incorporates a radical paradigm shift to a simplified, function-based, internally consistent model of disablement that has rectified many of the concerns about earlier editions. The new approach involves using the internationally accepted International Classification of Functioning, Disability and Health (ICF).[58] The latest edition of the Guides also focuses more directly on diagnosis using evidence-based medicine when possible; simplicity to optimize inter-rater and intra-rater reliability; functionally based ratings percentages; and consistent conceptual and methodological approaches and ratings across organ systems.

The ICF model is a comprehensive classification for describing and measuring health and disability in individuals and populations. It assesses bodily functions and structures (including impairments), activity (including activity limitations), and participation in life situations (including participation restrictions). It relates the health condition of an individual to environmental and personal factors. This internationally accepted approach is new to the sixth edition to the Guides, and it represents a major improvement toward which contributors to the Guides have been striving for many years. Developing the ICF model was a complex process, and it was not complete at the time of printing the fifth edition. The ICF arose from a worldwide consensus process, was endorsed by the World Health Assembly in 2001,[59] and has been accepted as a member of the World Health Organization family of international classifications. The AMA Guides has now adopted ICF terminology and definitions and used this approach to refine evaluation of impairment, disability and impairment rating in the Guides. This approach has created greater consistency within and between organ systems and established impairment and disability classifications based on the latest available evidence and expert consensus. Emphasis was placed on precision, accuracy, reliability, and validity. However, evaluation of functional impact was enhanced using the five-point scale taxonomy created by the ICF. The approach allows incorporation of information from the history, physical findings, objective test results, functional assessment, and determining the burden of treatment compliance when appropriate.

The revision process for each chapter in the Guides is not only rigorous but also multidisciplinary. For example, contributors to the otolaryngology chapter included not only otolaryngologists but also physicians in other specialties such as occupational and environmental medicine and pulmonology. As an example, all aspects of the otolaryngology chapter were re-examined and researched during the revision process. Literature was searched for new evidence and new consensus opinions, and the content of our chapter was compared with overlapping content in other chapters in order to optimize consistency across organ systems. This revision effort included reviewing the formula used for calculating hearing impairment. The original approach to this problem was published in 1959.[60] That formula used 500, 1000, and 2000 Hz. Based on additional study, the formula was revised to include 3000 Hz in 1979.[61] Higher frequencies are not included because they are not necessary to understand speech. For example, most early telephones used through the 1960s did not transmit through their ear pieces frequencies above 2800 Hz, and speech comprehension on these devices was not problematic. In the 1950s through the early 1970s, many physicians believed that higher frequencies were not needed to understand speech in quiet environments. Since 1979, considerable conjecture and opinion have been promulgated supporting the formula as it stands[62–68] and advocating changes[69] in the formula; and there has been vast experience in applying it for >30 years. After reassessment of available data, the relevant committees of the AAO-HNS, as well as other expert clinicians and the authors of the otolaryngology chapter in the sixth edition of the Guides, have found no credible evidence to support revising the formula again. In addition, the consensus and evidence still indicate that puretone audiometry is the most appropriate test in this population for estimating an individual's ability to hear speech. While other audiometric tests can be used in the diagnostic process, measures such as discrimination score can be manipulated so easily that they cannot be considered a valid standard for routine determination of hearing performance in medical legal settings. Consequently, the AAO-HNS formula remains the basis for the formula in the AMA Guides.

As a result of the exceedingly rigorous scientific process through which the Guides were developed and have evolved, the publication has been recognized and accepted nationally. In nearly all US territories, states, and commonwealths, the AMA Guides is either recommended or mandated for use by Workers' Compensation Law. It is also used for actions involving the Federal Employees Compensation Act, Longshore and Harbor Workers' Compensation Act and Federal Employees Compensation Laws. The AMA Guides to the Evaluation of Impairment is the premier compendium of scientific evidence and expert opinion related to the topic and has been accepted as establishing the standard of care by the American Medical Association and essentially all major specialty societies in the United States (including the AAO-HNS). Physicians involved with patients being assessed for possible noise-induced or other work-related hearing impairment should be not only loosely familiar with the Guides from past editions, but also current on the latest scientific and methodological advances in the most recent edition of this definitive reference.

The following is an example of how to calculate hearing impairment for compensation purposes (AAO-HNS Guidelines, 1979, and AMA Guides, 2008):

1. The average of the hearing threshold levels at 500, 1000, 2000, and 3000 Hz should be calculated for each ear
2. The percent impairment for each ear should be calculated by multiplying by 1.5% the amount by which the above average hearing threshold level exceeds 25 dB (low fence) up to a maximum of 100%, which is reached at 92 dB (high fence)
3. The hearing handicap, a binaural assessment, should then be calculated by multiplying the smaller percentage (better ear) by 5, adding this figure to the larger percentage (poorer ear), and dividing the total by 6

Example 1. Mild Hearing Loss

	500 Hz	1000 Hz	2000 Hz	3000 Hz
Right ear	15	25	45	55
Left ear	20	30	50	60

AAO/Method: 25-dB Fence

1. Right ear: (15 + 25 + 45 + 55)/4 = 140/4 = 35-dB average
2. Left ear: (20 + 30 + 50 + 60)/4 = 160/4 = 40-dB average

Monaural impairment:

3. Right ear: 35–25 = 10 dB × 1.5% = 15%
4. Left ear: 40–25 = 15 dB × 1.5% = 22.5%
5. Better ear: 15 × 5 = 75
6. Poorer ear: 22.5% × 1 = 22.5
7. Total: 97.5 ÷ 6 = 16.25%

Model Legislation Method used to calculate the above loss:

1. Right Ear: (15 + 25 + 45 + 55)/4 = 140/4 = 35-dB average
2. Left Ear: (20 + 30 + 50 + 60)/4 = 160/4 = 40-dB average
3. Better ear threshold = 35 dB = 5%

Example 2. Severe Hearing Loss

	500 Hz	1000 Hz	2000 Hz	3000 Hz
Right ear	80	90	100	110
Left ear	75	80	90	95

AAO/Method: Average Hearing Test Level

1. Right Ear: (80 + 90 +100 +110)/4 = 95 dB (use 92 maximum)
2. Left Ear: [(75 + 80 + 90 + 95)/4] + (340/4) = 85 dB

Monaural Impairment:

3. Right Ear: 92–25 = 67 dB × 1.5% = 100.5% (use 100%)
4. Left Ear: 85–25 = 60 dB ×1.5% = 90%
5. Better Ear: 90 × 5 = 450
6. Poorer Ear: 100 × 1 = 100
7. Total: 550÷6 = 91.7%

New Jersey method used to calculate the above loss:

1. Right Ear: (80 + 90 +100 +110)/4 = 380/4 = 95 dB (use 92 maximum)
2. Left Ear: [(75 + 80 + 90 + 95)/4] + (340/4) = 85 dB
3. Better ear > 81 dB = 100%

SUMMARY

A diagnosis of OHL must be based on specific criteria. Otologists rendering medical diagnoses or legal opinions for patients alleging OHL must be careful to base their opinions on facts. The potential medical, legal, and economic consequences of lesser diligence may be serious. OHL is generally preventable. Ideally, noise should be reduced. When this is not possible, the use of hearing protectors generally provides an effective deterrent to noise-induced hearing damage. Readers interested in this important, complex topic are encouraged to consult additional sources.[1]

REFERENCES

1. Sataloff RT, Sataloff J. Occupational hearing loss, 3rd edn. New York: Taylor & Francis; 2006.
2. Fleming AJ, D'Alonzo CA, Zapp JA. Modern occupational medicine. Philadelphia, PA: Lea & Febiger, 1954.
3. Exploratory Subcommittee Z24-X-2, American Standards Association, The relations of hearing loss to noise exposure, 1954.
4. National Institute for Occupational Safety and Health (NIOSH), Criteria document: Recommendation for an occupational exposure standard for noise, 1972.
5. Baughn WL. Relation between daily noise exposure and hearing loss based on the evaluation of 6,835 industrial noise exposure cases. Wright Patterson AFB OH: Aerospace Medical Research Lab. AMRL-TR-73-53, June 1973.
6. Ward WD, Glorig A. Protocol of inter-industry noise study. J Occup Med. 1975;17:760-70.
7. Burns W, Robinson DS. Hearing and noise in industry. London: Her Majesty's Stationery Office; 1970.
8. Passchier-Vermeer W. Hearing loss due to steady state broadband noise. Report No. 55, Leiden, The Netherlands: Institute for Public Health, Eng., 1968.
9. Sataloff J, Sataloff RT, Yerg A, et al. Intermittent exposure to noise: Effects on hearing. Ann Otol Rhinol Laryngol. 1983; 92(6):623-8.

10. Orgler GK, Brownson PJ, Brubaker WW, et al. American Occupational Medicine Association Noise and Hearing Conservation Committee Guidelines for the Conduct of an Occupational Hearing Conservation Program. J Occup Med. 1987;29:981-2.
11. ACOM Noise and Hearing Conservation Committee. Occupational noise-induced hearing loss. J Occup Med. 1989;31:996.
12. On Oct 27, 2002 the American College of Occupational and Environmental Medicine (ACOEM) reaffirmed these criteria in an evidence-based statement which was published in the Journal of Occupational & Environmental Medicine. 2003;45(6):579-81.
13. Kirchner DB, Evenson E, Dobie RA, et al. Occupational Noise-Induced Hearing Loss. ACOEM Task Force on Occupational Hearing Loss. JOEM. 2012;54(1):106-8.
14. Schuknecht HF, Tonndorf J. Acoustic trauma of the cochlea from ear surgery. Laryngoscope. 1960;70:479-505.
15. Lawrence M. Current concepts of the mechanism of occupational hearing loss. Am Ind Hyg Assoc J. 1964; 25:269-73.
16. Kellerhals B. Pathogensis of inner ear lesions in acute acoustic trauma. Acta Otolaryngol. 1972;73:249-53.
17. Schuknecht HG. Pathology of the ear. Cambridge, MA: Harvard University Press; 1974. pp. 295-7, 300-308.
18. Gallo R, Glorig A. Permanent threshold shift changes produced by noise exposure and aging. Am Ind Hyg Assoc J. 1964;25:237-45.
19. Schneider EJ, Mutchler JE, Hoyle HR, et al. The progression of hearing loss from industrial noise exposure. Am Ind Hyg Assoc J. 1970;31:368-76.
20. Sataloff J, Vassallo L, Menduke H. Occupational hearing loss and high frequency thresholds. Arch Environ Health. 1967;14:832-6.
21. Sataloff J, Vassallo L, Menduke H. Hearing loss from exposure to interrupted noise. Arch Environ Health 1969;17: 972-81.
22. Salmivalli A. Acoustic trauma in regular Army personnel: clinical audiologic study. Acta Otolaryngol (Stockh). 1967;(suppl 22):1-85.
23. Ward WD, Fleer RE, Glorig A. Characteristics of hearing losses produced by gunfire and steady noise. J Audiol Res. 1961;1:325-56.
24. Johnsson L-G, Hawkins JE Jr. Degeneration patterns in human ears exposed to noise. Ann Otol Rhinol Laryngol. 1976;85:725-39.
25. Gates GA, Cooper JC Jr, Kannel WB, et al. Hearing in the elderly: the Framingham cohort, 1983–1985. Part I. Basic audiometric test results. Ear Hear. 1990;11(4):247-56.
26. Sataloff J, Vassallo L. Head colds and viral cochleitis. Arch Otolaryngol. 1968;19:56-9.
27. Igarashi M, Schuknecht HF, Myers E. Cochlear pathology in humans with stimulation deafness. J Laryngol Otol. 1964;78:115-23.
28. Anderson H, Wedenberg E. Genetic aspects of hearing impairment in children. Acta Otolaryngol (Stockh). 1970;69:77-88.
29. Fisch L. The etiology of congenital deafness and audiometric patterns. J Laryngol Otol. 1955;69:479-93.
30. Huizing EH, van Bolhuis AH, Odenthal DW. Studies on progressive hereditary perceptive deafness in a family of 335 members. Acta Otolaryngol (Stockh). 1966;61:35-41, 161-7.
31. Graham MD. Acoustic tumors: selected histories and patient reviews. In: House WF, Luetje CM (eds), Acoustic tumors. Baltimore, MD: University Park Press; 1979. pp. 192-3.
32. Facer GW, Farell KH, Cody DTR. Spontaneous perilymph fistula. Mayo Clin Proc. 1973;48:203-6.
33. Simmons FB. Theory of membrane breaks in sudden hearing loss. Arch Otolaryngol. 1968;88:67-74.
34. Soss SL. Sensorineural hearing loss with diving. Arch Otolaryngol. 1971;93:501-4.
35. Freeman P, Edwards C. Inner ear barotrauma. Arch Otolaryngol. 1972;95:556-63.
36. van Dishoeck HAE. Akustisches Trauma. In: Berendes J, Link R, Zollner F (eds), Hals-Nasen-Ohren-Heilkunde. Band III. Stuttgart: Georg Thieme; 1966. pp. 1764-99.
37. Yerg RA, Sataloff J, Glorig A, et al. Inter-industry noise study. J Occup Med. 1978;20:351-8.
38. Cartwright LB, Thompson RW. The effects of broadband noise on the cardiovascular system in normal resting adults. Am Ind Hyg Assoc J. 1978:653-8.
39. Johnsson L-G, Hawkins JE Jr. Strial atrophy in clinical and experimental deafness. Laryngoscope. 1972;82:1105-25.
40. Spoendlin H. Histopathology of nerve deafness. J Otolaryngol. 1985;14(5):282-6.
41. Spoendlin H, Brun JP. Relation of structural damage to exposure time and intensity in acoustic trauma. Acta Otolaryngol. 1973;75:220-26.
42. Spoendlin H. Primary structural changes in the organ of Corti after acoustic over-stimulation. Acta Otolaryngol. 1971;71:166-76.
43. Carson SS, Prazma J, Pulver SH, et al. Combined effects of aspirin and noise in causing permanent hearing loss. Arch Otolaryngol Head Neck Surg. 1989;115:1070-75.
44. Barone JA, Peters JM, Garabrant DH, et al. Smoking as a risk factor in noise-induced hearing loss. J Occup Med. 1987;29(9):741-6.
45. Thomas GB, Williams CE, Hoger NG. Some non-auditory correlates of the hearing threshold levels of an aviation noise exposed population. Aviat Spac Environ Med. 1981; 9:531-6.
46. Chung DY, Wilson GN, Gannon RP, et al. Individual susceptibility to noise. In: Hamernik RP, Henderson D, Salvi R (eds), New perspectives in noise-induced hearing loss. New York: Raven Press; 1982. pp. 511-19.
47. Drettner B, Hedstrand H, Klockhoff I, et al. Cardiovascular risk factors and hearing loss. Acta Otolaryngol. 1975;79: 366-71.
48. Siegelaub AB, Friedman GD, Adour K, et al. Hearing loss in adults. Arch Environ Health. 1984;29:107-9.
49. Cocchiarella LA, Sharp DS, Persky VW. Hearing threshold shifts, white-cell count and smoking status in working men. Occup Med (Lond). 1995;45:179-85.

50. Starck J, Toppila E, Pyykko I. Smoking as a risk factor in sensory neural hearing loss among workers exposed to occupational noise. Acta Otolaryngol (Stockh). 1999;119:302-5.
51. Sulkowski WJ, Kowalska S, Matyja W, et al. Effects of occupational exposure to a mixture of solvents on the inner ear: a field study. Int J Occup Med Environ Health. 2002;15: 247-56.
52. Sliwinska-Kowalska M, Zamyslowska-Szmytke E, Szymczak W, et al. Ototoxic effects of occupational exposure to styrene and co-exposure to styrene and noise. J Occup Environ Med. 2003;45:15-24.
53. Sataloff RT, Davies B, Myers DL. Acoustic neuromas presenting as sudden deafness. Am J Otol. 1985;6(4):349-52.
54. American Medical Association. Guides to the Evaluation of Permanent Impairment, 6th edn. Chicago, IL: American Medical Association; 2008.
55. Sataloff RT. Evaluating occupational hearing loss: the value of the AMA guides to the evaluation of permanent impairment [editorial]. ENT J. 2014;93(4-5):132-5.
56. American Medical Association. A guide to the evaluation of permanent impairment of the extremities and back. JAMA. 1958;166(suppl):1-122.
57. Guides to the Evaluation of Permanent Impairment. Chicago, IL: American Medical Association; 1971.
58. World Health Organization. International Classification of Functioning, Disability and Health: ICF. Geneva, Switzerland: World Health Organization; 2001.
59. Resolution of the World Health Organization. International classification of functioning, disability and health. 54th World Health Assembly; May 22, 2001.
60. Guide for the evaluation of hearing impairment. J Occup Med. 1959;1(3):167-8.
61. American Academy of Otolaryngology Committee on Hearing and Equilibrium and American Council of Otolaryngology Committee on the Medical Aspects of Noise. Guide for the evaluation of hearing handicap. JAMA. 1979;241: 2055-59.
62. Dobie RA, Sakai CS. Monetary compensation for hearing loss: clinician survey. JOHL. 1998;1(1):73-80.
63. Doerfler LG, Nett EM, Matthews J. The relationships between audiologic measures and handicap: Part One. JOHL. 1998;1(2):103-52.
64. Dobie RA, Sakai CS. Monetary compensation for hearing loss: choice and weighting of frequencies. 1998;1(3): 163-71.
65. Doerfler LG, Nett EM, Matthews J. The relationships between audiologic measures and handicap: part two. JOHL. 1998;1(3):213-35.
66. Sataloff J, Vassallo LA, Sataloff RT. The validity of the AMA impairment formula for hearing loss. JOHL. 1998;1(4): 237-42.
67. Doerfler LG, Nett EM, Matthews J. The relationships between audiologic measures and handicap: part 3. JOHL. 1998;1(4):243-64.
68. Nelson RA. Development of the AMA formula or who built this camel anyway? JOHL. 1999;2(4):145-51.
69. American Speech-Language-Hearing Association. Task Force on the Definition of Hearing Handicap. http://www.asha.org/docs/html/RP1981-00022.html. Accessed August 7, 2012.

CHAPTER

19

Ototoxicity

Karen Jo Doyle, Brent Wilkerson

INTRODUCTION/BACKGROUND

This chapter covers the major classes of pharmaceutical drugs that have been demonstrated to produce hearing loss and/or vestibular loss. Some classes of ototoxic drugs such as salicylates, aminoglycosides, and platinum chemotherapy drugs have been known to produce adverse effects on their inner ear since their discovery but continue to be used because in many clinical settings their efficacy outweighs their potential for toxicity. In other cases, such as the combination of opioid analgesic Vicodin, macrolide antibiotics erythromycin, clarithromycin and azithromycin, the chemotherapy/chemoprevention agent α-difluoromethylornithine (DFMO), and the oral chemotherapy drug imatinib (Gleevec), the drugs were placed into use before their ototoxicities were recognized.

More than a century ago, aspirin was the first drug found to produce hearing loss.[1] In the 1940s reversible hearing loss and tinnitus were observed in patients treated with large doses of aspirin.[2–3] McCabe and Dey studied the effects of 925 mg of aspirin given four times daily for 5 days to volunteers, finding that it produced tinnitus and hearing loss (worse for high frequencies) that increased in severity each day, but were completely reversible within 72 hours of stopping its administration.[4] In similar experiments, Meyers et al. noted that when aspirin was taken by patients with rheumatoid arthritis at doses as high as 6–8 g per day, the hearing loss was flat across frequencies and reached severity of as much as 40–50 dBHL.[5] Again, the hearing loss was completely reversible after discontinuing the drug. These same authors administered high doses of aspirin subcutaneously to squirrels and found no histological abnormalities in the cochlea despite noting 30 dB hearing loss in the animals.[6]

The earliest aminoglycoside antibiotic, streptomycin, was discovered by Schatz in 1943[7] and was used to treat tuberculosis in the first ever randomized clinical trial of a drug.[8] Soon after its introduction streptomycin was documented to cause permanent hearing loss in tuberculosis patients.[9] Other aminoglycoside antibiotics—neomycin, kanamycin, and gentamicin—were introduced in 1949, 1956, and 1963.[10–12] Unfortunately, all aminoglycoside antibiotics demonstrated ototoxic effects.

In 1966, furosemide was the first loop diuretic used in the United States. However, the first report of loop diuretic ototoxicity was in 1965 by Maher and Schreiner, who demonstrated reversible hearing loss in patients with clinical edema treated using ethacrynic acid.[13] Similar ototoxic effects were later noted for furosemide.[14] Permanent hearing loss occurred when loop diuretics were given in patients having renal failure.[15]

The platinum chemotherapy drugs cisplatin, carboplatin, and oxaliplatin are used to treat a large variety of cancers. Cisplatin received full FDA approval in 1978, after the first clinical trial was published in 1972.[16] Early reports acknowledged cisplatin's adverse effects on hearing, but given its chemotherapeutic efficacy the side effect was underemphasized.[17]

PATHOGENESIS

Ototoxic drugs have their effects on different parts of the auditory/vestibular system. The peripheral auditory system (Fig. 19.1) consists of the outer ear, the middle ear,

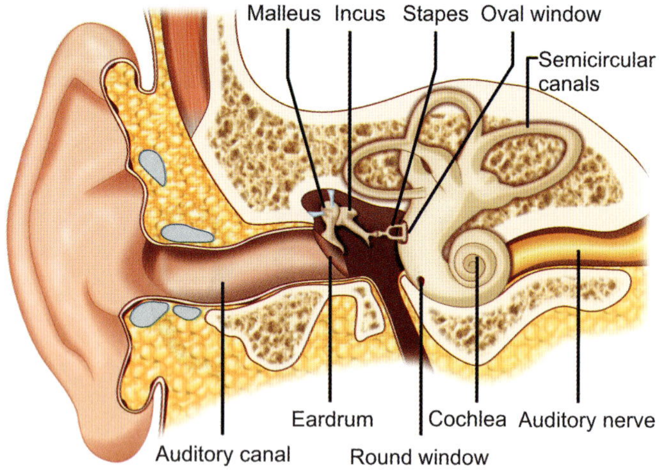

Fig. 19.1: Peripheral auditory system.

the cochlea and auditory nerve, while the central auditory system (Fig. 19.2) consists of brainstem and cortical neural pathways that convey neural signals. The human peripheral vestibular system includes the inner ear structures (in each ear the utricle, saccule and three semicircular canals), vestibular nerves, and central peripheral pathways. An ototoxic medication can have effects on one or more of these components. There has been much investigation of the mechanisms by which different classes of ototoxic drugs produce sensorineural hearing loss.

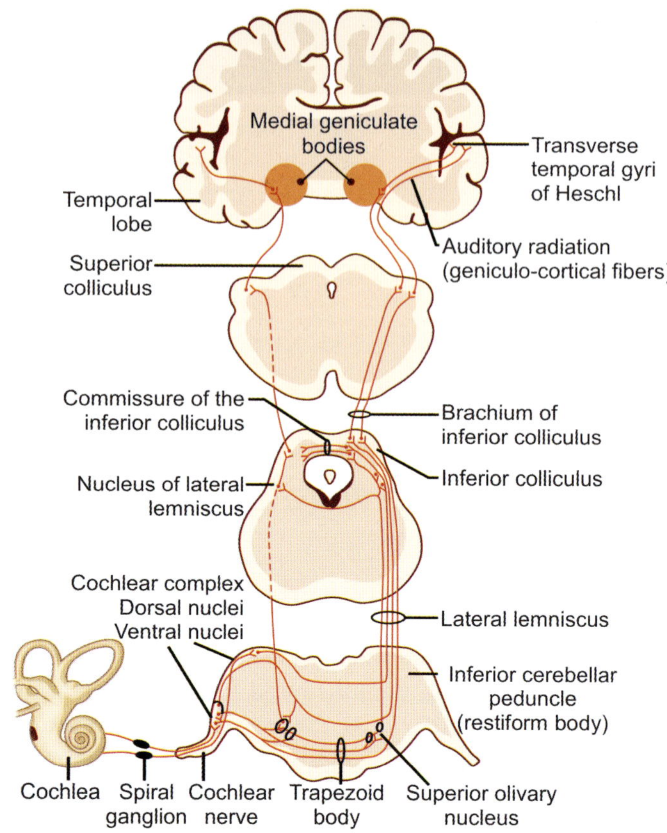

Fig. 19.2: Central auditory system.

Mechanisms of Aminoglycoside Ototoxicity

In aminoglycoside toxicity, aminoglycosides enter hair cells through mechanically sensitive ion channels on the tips of the stereocilia of hair cells.[18] Figures 19.3A and B show the molecular structure of gentamicin and streptomycin. Aminoglycosides produce their ototoxic effects by generation of free radicals within the inner ear, inducing apoptosis of outer hair cells in the cochlea[19,20] and type 1 hair cells in the vestibular system.[21] Research that demonstrates how depletion of free radicals by antioxidants such as glutathione, iron, methionine, and superoxide dismutase reduces aminoglycoside ototoxicity supports this mechanism.[22]

Mechanisms of Cisplatin Ototoxicity

As in aminoglycoside ototoxicity, with cisplatin administration oxygen radicals are generated, followed by outer hair cell apoptosis.[23,24] The molecular structure of the platinum chemotherapy agents cisplatin, carboplatin, and oxaliplatin is shown in Figure 19.4. Outer hair cell loss happens first in the basal cochlea and proceeds apically as damage increases.[25] Damage to supporting cells in the organ of Corti[26] and atrophy of the stria vascularis[27] have been reported with cisplatin. Unlike the aminoglycosides, the platinum chemotherapy agents cause little alteration in the peripheral vestibular system. Pretreatment of experimental animals with the antioxidant D-methionine can prevent some of the loss of inner hair cells that is unique to carboplatin ototoxicity.[28]

Mechanisms of Salicylate Ototoxicity

Aspirin ototoxicity is completely reversible and does not cause gross histopathological changes.[6] Stypulchowski described the effects of salicylates on cochlear potentials in the cat, noting that they decreased the amplitudes of the action potential and summating potential, while increasing the amplitude of the cochlear microphonic.[29] Similarly, salicylates can increase levels of distortion product otoacoustic emissions.[30] However, others have shown that salicylates diminish outer hair cell electromotility and spontaneous otoacoustic emissions.[31–33] Salicylates decrease outer hair cell wall stiffness and motility.[34,35]

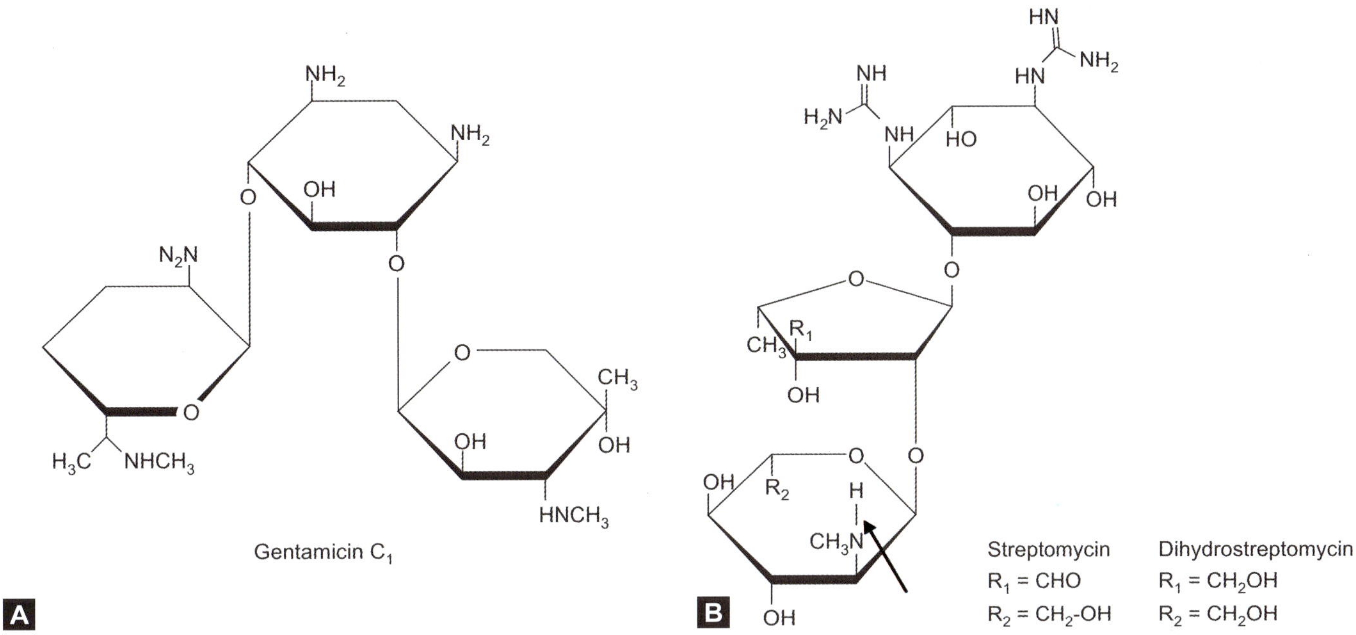

Figs. 19.3A and B: Chemical structures of gentamicin and streptomycin.

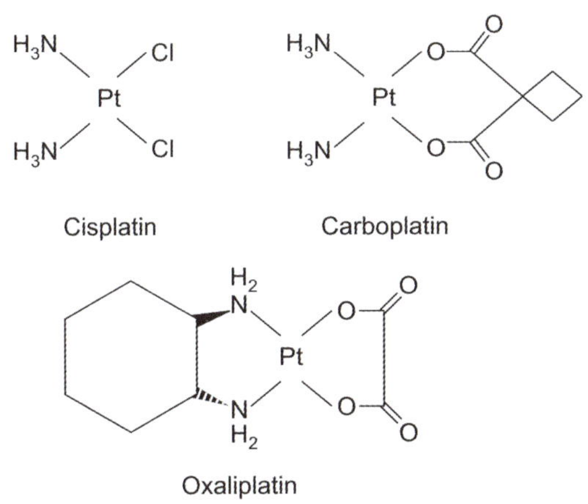

Fig. 19.4: Molecular structures of cisplatin, carboplatin, and oxaliplatin.

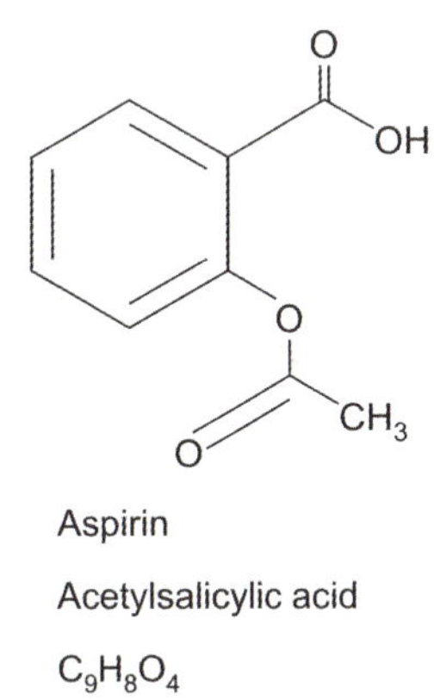

Fig. 19.5: Structure of the aspirin molecule.

Figure 19.5 shows aspirin's molecular structure. Others have found evidence that salicylate directly and reversibly inhibits chloride anions at the anion-binding site of prestin, the motor molecule of the outer hair cells.[36] Still others have produced evidence that salicylate blocks the outer hair cell potassium channel KCNQ4 as an alternate mechanism of salicylate ototoxicity.[37] Salicylate has multiple effects in the central nervous system, and is believed to enhance sound-evoked central auditory activity.[38]

Mechanisms of Loop Diuretic Ototoxicity

Na-K-2Cl cotransporter is also found at the basal plasma membrane of marginal cells of the stria vascularis and is inhibited by the loop diuretics[39] (Fig. 19.6). In animals, administration of loop diuretics reduces the endocochlear potential, which is reversible. The hearing loss produced by loop diuretics is typically reversible in animals.[40]

Mechanisms of DFMO Ototoxicity

DFMO is an irreversible blocker of the enzyme ornithine decarboxylase, the first step in the synthesis of polyamines.[41] The polyamines putrescine, spermidine, and spermine are positively charged molecules that are found in nearly every cell (Fig. 19.7).[42] Very-high-dose oral administration of DFMO causes some hair cell damage in animal models.[43] However, there are no gross histopathological

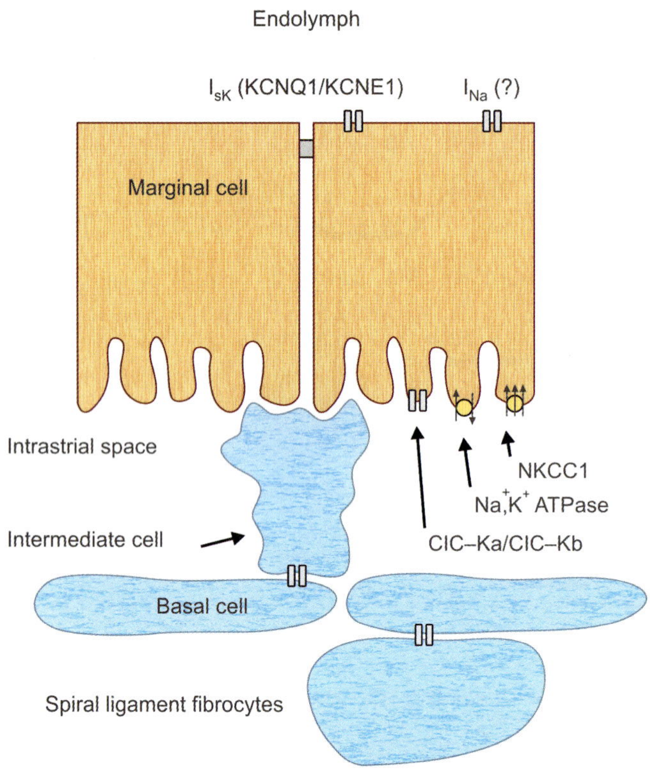

Fig. 19.6: NKCC1 co-transporter on the basal membrane of the marginal cell.

changes in the cochlea when DFMO is given at lower doses subcutaneously for a month in the gerbil, even though mild hearing loss affecting all frequencies tested occurred that was completely reversible after 3 weeks of recovery.[44] Administration of DFMO lowers the endocochlear potential.[45] The intermediate cells of the stria vascularis contain inwardly rectifying K^+ channels (Kir4.1), and similar channels that are found in other tissues such as the heart owe their inward rectification properties to voltage-dependent blockage of these channels by the positively charged polyamines.[46,47] Nie et al. concluded that the reversible hearing loss following administration of DFMO to mice is produced by alteration of intermediate cell Kir4.1 channel inward rectification.[45]

Mechanisms of Hydrocodone/ Acetaminophen Ototoxicity

When taken at much higher than recommended doses, the commonly prescribed combination analgesic hydrocodone and acetaminophen (Vicodin) causes a rapidly progressive and irreversible sensorineural deafness.[48-50] There is only one investigation of the possible mechanism of high-dose Vicodin. Neonatal mouse cultures and auditory cell lines were exposed in vitro to different concentrations of

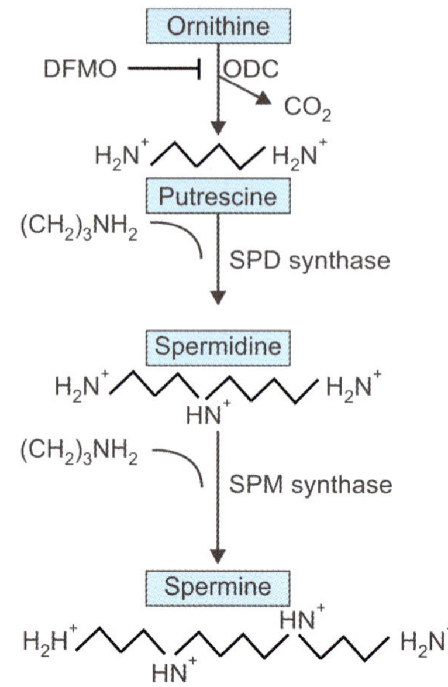

Fig. 19.7: DFMO blocks the enzyme ODC and therefore polyamine synthesis. (DFMO, α-difluoromethylornithine).

acetaminophen alone, hydromorphone (metabolite of hydrocodone) and the combination of the two.[51] Acetaminophen exposure caused cell death that was further potentiated when combined with hydromorphone, while exposure to hydrocodone or hydromorphone alone failed to kill cells. They concluded that acetaminophen was the more likely cause of Vicodin ototoxicity, though the combination was more damaging.

Mechanisms of Macrolide Ototoxicity

Despite numerous clinical reports of hearing loss due to erythromycin and the other macrolide antibiotics, there are no journal articles relevant to pathophysiology. Brummett et al. published an abstract reporting that when erythromycin was infused intravenously in guinea pigs, initially there was an increase in the latency of the fourth wave of the auditory brainstem response.[52] Eventually, the fourth wave disappeared, followed by the third and the second waves. All peaks returned when the drug was discontinued, and there was no change in the action potential. They concluded that erythromycin had a central auditory system site of ototoxic action.

Vinka Alkaloid Mechanisms of Ototoxicity

There are very few cases of ototoxicity related to the use of vincristine and vinblastine, anti-cancer drugs derived from the periwinkle plant, *Vinca rosea*.[53-56] Serafy and colleagues published the only animal studies relevant to vinca alkaloid ototoxicity.[57–58] They found that vinblastine damaged organ of Corti hair cells in rabbits, while vincristine destroyed hair cells as well as spiral ganglion cells.

CLINICAL FINDINGS IN OTOTOXICITY

Aminoglycosides

Aminoglycoside ototoxicity can be identified in one third of treated patients who undergo audiological screening.[59] It manifests as a permanent high-frequency sensorineural hearing loss that progresses from higher frequencies to lower frequencies and is related to the number of doses of drug.[60] Some authors have reported that streptomycin is the most cochleotoxic aminoglycoside, while others have found gentamicin to be more cochleotoxic, though kanamycin and neomycin are usually thought to be the most cochleotoxic aminoglycosides.[61] Kanamycin and amikacin are primarily cochleotoxic, while streptomycin and gentamicin have greater vestibulotoxicity.[62] Genetic predisposition to aminoglycoside ototoxicity via mitochondrial DNA mutations has been discovered due to mutations in mitochondrial 12S ribosomal rRNA.[63] Because aminoglycosides initially produce a relatively asymptomatic high-frequency sensorineural hearing loss and because the incidence of hearing loss is unrelated to serum antibiotic levels, some authors have proposed screening high-frequency audiometric thresholds during treatment periods to identify ototoxicity before it becomes severe.[64]

Cisplatin

Cis-platinum is the most ototoxic drug in that it causes irreversible high-frequency sensorineural hearing loss in approximately 70% of patients receiving it, which is dependent upon cumulative dose of the drug.[65] Tinnitus typically precedes the hearing loss, and the hearing loss first involves the high frequencies but can progress to lower frequencies as therapy continues. Risk factors include young or advanced age, renal insufficiency, coadministration of high-dose vincristine, and cranial irradiation. Children under the age of 5 years are particularly susceptible to cisplatin ototoxicity, having a 40% incidence of hearing loss.[66] Patients with both alleles of Val-GSTP1 may have more glutathione available to protect against cisplatin and are less likely to have the ototoxic hearing loss.[67] Vestibulotoxicity does not typically occur with platinum agents.

Salicylates

Hearing loss due to large doses of salicylates may involve the high frequencies but is usually flat across frequencies, mild to moderate, and reversible after discontinuance of the drug.[4,5] Increasing dosage and duration produces a greater degree of hearing loss for the frequencies 250–8000 Hz.[68]

Loop Diuretics

In humans, every loop diuretic except torsemide has been reported to cause hearing loss, both temporary and permanent. The patients have usually suffered from renal failure and underwent rapid infusion of the diuretic.[69] The hearing loss is often reversible and is typically mild, affecting the middle frequency range.[70–72] Edema of the stria vascularis was found in temporal bone histopathology of patients after loop diuretic ototoxic hearing loss.[73,74]

Macrolide Antibiotics

Erythromycin ototoxicity is reported to present as relatively mild sensorineural hearing loss, flat across frequencies, appearing within days of high-dose intravenous administration, and usually reversible.[75,76] There are, however, individual case reports of irreversible macrolide ototoxicity.[77]

DFMO

At high doses (>1 g/m^2), DFMO causes hearing loss from 250 to 8000 Hz that is often reversible.[78] At low doses used for chemoprevention, DFMO produces at worst a minimal hearing loss that is always reversible.[79,80] Unlike salicylate ototoxicity, the hearing loss from DFMO reverses slowly, over days to months.[79]

Vicodin

The patients described in case reports of Vicodin ototoxicity had rapidly progressive, permanent sensorineural deafness. Fortunately, the patients benefited from cochlear implantation.[44–46] The audiograms presented showed involvement across frequencies, and the patients had no vestibular complaints.[46]

Imatinib (Gleevec)

Imatinib is an oral tyrosine kinase inhibitor used initially to treat chronic myelogenous leukemia that is FDA-approved to treat myelodysplastic diseases, lymphoma as well as other tumors. Only three case reports have linked imatinib to progressive sensorineural hearing loss, irreversible in all cases, moderately severe to severe, and flat across frequencies in two of the three patients, with poor word discrimination (one patient did not undergo audiological evaluation).[81-83] The author of this chapter recently saw a 6-year-old child treated for 8 months with oral imatinib for non-Hodgkin's lymphoma who developed profound deafness during the course of treatment (unpublished observation). The mechanism for the hearing loss associated with Gleevec has not been studied, though tyrosine kinases are present in mammalian auditory neurons and could be the ototoxic target.[83]

Vincristine/Vinblastine

Only a few cases of vinblastine or vincristine ototoxicity have been reported, two of which were at least partially reversible.[53-56]

PREVENTION OF OTOTOXICITY

Because both aminoglycoside and platinum chemotherapy drugs seem to generate reactive oxygen species in the cochlea that lead to killing of outer hair cells via caspase-dependent or caspase-independent cell death mechanisms, a great deal of work has been dedicated to preventing toxicity by administration of antioxidants or chelators to decrease reactive oxygen species.[62] Several antioxidant sulfur-containing compounds (methionine, lipoic acid, N-acetylcysteine, and amifostine) have been shown in animals to protect from cisplatin ototoxicity; their application in human trials is still uncertain because of concerns that these compounds may interfere with the tumoricidal effects of the platinum drugs.[84] One clinical trial has been performed in China, showing that administration of aspirin, an iron chelator and free radical scavenger, reduces gentamicin ototoxicity from 13% to 3%.[85]

Other authors have proposed protection of hair cells by inoculating an adenoviral vector encoding human neurotrophic factor.[86] In vivo inoculation of adenovirus with the Math1 gene inserted into guinea pig cochlear endolymph results in Math1 overexpression in the organ of Corti , new hair cells, and axons extended from the auditory nerve bundle toward the new hair cells.[87] In aminoglycoside-treated mice, delivery of Math1 via adenovirus vector induced recovery of the vestibular neuroepithelium within 8 weeks after treatment.[88]

Another method proposed to prevent ototoxic hair cell damage is to prevent the aminoglycoside molecule from entering the hair cell through the mechano-electrical transducer channels.[89] Huth et al. point out that one could modify the chemical structure of aminoglycosides to widen their diameters by binding inert molecules on sites irrelevant for antimicrobial activity to prevent passage of aminoglycoside molecules through the channel into the hair cells, while ensuring that the molecules could still pass into the bacterial ribosome.[90]

CONCLUSION

In this chapter, we have reviewed the classes of pharmaceutical agents known to confer varying degrees of reversible or permanent hearing loss or vestibular damage in humans. New compounds are constantly being introduced, as well as biological agents for treatment of cancers and inflammatory diseases, some of which may be ototoxic.[91] Clinicians should acquaint themselves with these adverse side effects, and scientists should investigate these agents to identify ways to cure or prevent ototoxicity, and to discover more about the workings of the auditory system.

REFERENCES

1. Muller G. Beitrag zur wirking der salicylasuren natrons beim diabetes melleus. Berl Klink Wochenschrift. 1877;14:29-31.
2. Jager BV, Alway R. The treatment of acute rheumatic fever with large doses of sodium salicylate; with special reference to dose management and toxic manifestations. Am J Med Sci. 1946;211:273-85.
3. Graham JD, Parker WA. The toxic manifestations of sodium salicylate therapy. Q J Med. 1948; 17:153-63.
4. McCabe PA, Dey FL. The effect of aspirin upon auditory sensitivity. Ann Otol Rhinol Laryngol. 1965;74:213-25.
5. Meyers E, Bernstein J, Fostiropolous G. Salicylate ototoxicity: a clinical study. N Engl J Med. 1965;273:587-90.
6. Meyers EN, Bernstein JM. Salicylate ototoxicity. Arch Otolarygol. 1965;82:483-93.
7. Schatz A, Bugie E, Waksman SA. Streptomycin: a substance exhibiting antibiotic activity against gram-positive and gram-negative bacteria. Proc Soc Exper Bio Med. 1944; 55:66-9.
8. Medical Research Council. Streptomycin treatment of pulmonary tuberculosis: A Medical Research Council Investigation. Br Med J. 1948;2:769-82.
9. Hinshaw HC, Feldman WH. Streptomycin in the treatment of clinical tuberculosis: a preliminary report. Proc Mayo Clin. 1945;20:313-18.

10. Waksman SA, Lechevalier HA. Neomycin a new antibiotic active against streptomycin-resistant bacteria, including tuberculosis organisms. Science. 1949;109:305-7.
11. Umezawa H, Ueda M, Maeda K, et al. Production and isolation of a new antibiotic: kanamycin. J Antibiotics. 1957; 10:181-8.
12. Weinstein MJ, Luedemann E, Oden EM, et al. Gentamicin, a new antibiotic complex from *Micromonospora*. J Medicinal Chem. 1963;6:463-4.
13. Maher JF, Schreiner GE. Studies on ethacrynic acid in patients with refractory edema. Ann Intern Med. 1965;62: 15-29.
14. Schwartz GN, David DS, Riggo RR, et al. Ototoxicity induced by furosemide. N Eng J Med. 1970;181:1413-4.
15. Pillay VKG, Schwartz FD, Aimi K, et al. Transient and permanent deafness following treatment with ethacrynic acid in renal failure. Lanet. 1969;1:77-9.
16. Rossof AH, Slayton ER, Perlia CP. Preliminary clinical experience with cis-diamminedichloroplatinum. Cancer. 1972; 30:1451-6.
17. Kovach JS, Moertel CG, Schutt AJ, et al. Phase II study of cis-diamminedichloroplatinum in advanced carcinoma of the large bowel. Cancer Chemother Rep. 1973;57:357-9.
18. Vu AA, Nadaraja GS, Huth ME, et al. Integrity and regeneration of mechanotransduction machinery regulate aminoglycoside entry and sensory cell death. PLoS One. 2013; e54794.
19. Clerici WJ, Hensley K, DiMartino DL, et al. Direct detection of ototoxicant-induced reactive oxygen species generation in cochlear explants. Hear Res. 1996;98:116-24.
20. Hirose K, Hockenberry DM, Rubel EW. Reactive oxygen species in chick hair cells after gentamicin exposure in vitro. Hear Res. 1997;104:1-14.
21. Hawkins JE. Drug ototoxicity. In: WD Keidel, WD Neff (eds), Handbook of sensory physiology. Berlin: Springer Verlag; 1976, pp. 707-48.
22. Song BB, Schact J. Variable efficacy of radical scavengers and iron chelators to attenuate gentamicin ototoxicity in guinea pig in vivo. Hear Res. 1996;94:87-93.
23. Ravi R, Somani SM, Rybak LP. Mechanism of cisplatin ototoxicity: antioxidant system. Pharmacol Toxicol. 1995; 76:386-94.
24. Rybak LP, Whitworth C, Somani S. Application of antioxidants and other agents to prevent cisplatin ototoxicity. Laryngoscope. 1999;109:1740-44.
25. Schweitzer VG, Hawkins JE, Lilly DJ, et al. Ototoxic and nephrotoxic effects of combined treatment with cis-diamminedichloroplatinum and kanamycin in the guinea pig. Otolaryngol Head Neck Surg. 1984;92:38-49.
26. Ramirez-Camacho R, Garcia-Berrocal JR, et al. Supporting cells as a target of cisplatin-induced inner ear damage: therapeutic implications. Laryngoscope. 2004;114:533-7.
27. Meech RP, Campbell KC, Hughes LP, et al. A semiquantitative analysis of the effects of cisplatin on the rat stria vascularis. Hear Res. 1998;124:44-59.
28. Lockwood DS, Ding DL, Wang J, et al. D-methionine attenuates inner hair cell loss in carboplatin-treated chinchillas. Audiol Neurotol. 2000;5:263-6.
29. Stypulkowski PH. Mechanisms of salicylate ototoxicity. Hear Res. 1990;46:113-45.
30. Huang ZW, Luo Y, Wu Z, et al. Paradoxical enhancement of active cochlear mechanics in long-term administration of salicylate. J Neurophysiol. 2005;93:2053-61.
31. Shehata WE, Brownell WE, Dieler R. Effects of salicylate on shape electromotility and membrane characteristics of isolated outer hair cells from guinea pig cochlea. Acta Otolaryngol. 1991;111:707-18.
32. Wier CC, Pasanen EG, McFadden D. Partial dissociation of spontaneous otoacoustic emissions and distortion products during aspirin use in humans. J Acoust Soc Am. 1988; 84:230-37.
33. Long GR, Tubis A. Modification of spontaneous and evoked otoacoustic emissions and associated psychoacoustic microstructure by aspirin consumption. J Acoust Soc Am. 1988;84:1343-53.
34. Lue AJ, Brownell WE. Salicylate induced changes in outer hair cell lateral wall stiffness. Hear Res. 1999;135:163-8.
35. Dieler R, Shehata-Dieler WE, Brownwell WE. Concomitant salicylate-induced alterations of outer hair cell subsurface cisternae and electromotility. J Neurocytol. 1991;20:637-53.
36. Rybalchenko V, Santos-Sacchi J. Cl^- flux through a nonselective, stretch-sensitive conductance influences the outer hair cell motor of the guinea-pig. J Physiol. 2003;547: 873-91.
37. Wu T, Lv P, Kim HJ, et al. Effect of salicylate on KCNQ4 of the guinea pig outer hair cell. J Neurophysiol. 2010;103: 1969-77.
38. Chen GD, Stolzberg D, Lobarinas E, et al. Salicylate-induced cochlear impairments, cortical hyperactivity and re-tuning, and tinnitus. Hear Res. 2013;295:100-13.
39. Wangemann P, Liu J, Marcus DC. Ion transport mechanisms responsible for K^+ secretion and the transepithelial voltage across marginal cells of the stria vascularis in vitro. Hear Res. 1995;84:19-29.
40. Rybak LP, Whitworth C, Scott V. Comparative acute ototoxicity of loop diuretic compounds. Eur Arch Oto-Rhino-Laryngol. 1991;101:1167-74.
41. Sjoerdsma A, Schechter J. Chemotherapeutic implications of polyamine biosynthesis inhibition. Clin Pharmacol Ther. 1984;35:287-300.
42. Tabor CW, Tabor H. Polyamines. Ann Rev Biochem. 1984; 53:749-90.
43. Salzer SJ, Mattox DE, Brownell WE. Cochlear damage and increased threshold in alpha-difluoromethylornithine (DFMO) treated guinea pigs. Hear Res. 1990;46:101-12.
44. Smith MC, Tinling S, Doyle KJ. Difluoromethylornithine-induced reversible hearing loss across a wide frequency range. Laryngoscope. 2004;114:1113-7.
45. Nie L, Feng W, Diaz R, et al. Functional consequences of polyamine synthesis inhibition by α-difluoromethylornithine (DFMO). J Biol Chem. 2005;280:15097-102.

46. Hibino H, Horio Y, Inanobe A, et al. An ATP-dependent inwardly rectifying potassium channel, K_{AB}-2 (Kir4.1), in cochlear stria vascularis of inner ear: Its specific subcellular localization and correlation with the formation of endocochlear potential. J Neurosci. 1997;17:4711-21.
47. Lopatin AN, Nichols CG. [K^+] dependence of polyamine-induced rectification in inward rectifier potassium channels (IRK1, Kir2.1). J Gen Physiol. 1996;108:105-13.
48. Friedman RA, House JW, Luxford WM, et al. Profound hearing loss associated with hydrocodone/acetaminophen abuse. Am J Otol. 2000;21:188-91.
49. Oh AK, Ishiyama A, Baloh RW. Deafness associated with abuse of hydrocodone/acetaminophen. Neurology. 2000; 54:2345.
50. Ho T, Vrabec JT, Burton AW. Hydrocodone use and sensorineural hearing loss. Pain Physician. 2007;10:467-72.
51. Yorgason JG, Kalinec GM, Luxford WM, et al. Acetaminophen ototoxicity after acetaminophen/hydrocodone abuse: evidence from two parallel in vitro mouse models. Otolaryngol Head Neck Surg. 2010;142:814-9.
52. Brummett RE, Hager G, Fox KE, et al. Association for Research in Otolaryngology Midwinter Meeting Abstracts. 1984;36:25.
53. Moss PE, Hickman S, Harrison BR. Ototoxicity associated with vinblastine. Ann Pharmacother. 1997;33:423-5.
54. Lugassy G, Shapira A. Sensorineural hearing loss associated with vincristine treatment. Blut 1990;61(5):320-21.
55. Mahajan SL. Acute acoustic nerve palsy associated with vincristine therapy. Cancer. 1981;24:2404.
56. Yousif H, Richardson SG, Saunders W. Partially reversible nerve deafness due to vincristine. Postgrad Med J. 1990;66: 688-9.
57. Serafy A, Hashash M, State F. The effect of vinblastine sulfate on the neurological elements of the rabbit cochlea. J Laryngol Otol. 1982;96:975-9.
58. Serafy A, Hashash M. The effect of vincristine on the neurological elements of the rabbit cochlear. J Laryngol Otol. 1981;95:49-54.
59. Fausti SA, Henry JA, Helt WJ, et al. An individualized, sensitive frequency range for early detection of ototoxicity. Ear Hear. 1999;20:497-505.
60. Mulheran M, Degg C, Burr S, et al. Occurrence and risk of cochleotoxicity in cystic fibrosis patients receiving repeated high-dose aminoglycoside therapy. Antimicrob Agents Chemother. 2001;45:2502-9.
61. Kalkandelen S, Selimoglu E, Ergogan F, et al. Comparative cochlear toxicities of streptomycin, gentamicin, amikacin and netilmicin in guinea-pigs. J Int Med Res. 2002;30: 406-12.
62. Rybak LP, Ramkumar V. Ototoxicity. Kidney Int. 2007;72: 931-5.
63. Fischel-Ghodsian N. Genetic factors in aminoglycoside toxicity. Ann N Y Acad Sci. 1999;884:99-109.
64. Fausti SA, Henry J, Schaffer HI, et al. High-frequency audiometric monitoring for early detection of aminoglycoside ototoxicity. J Infect Dis. 1992;165:1026-32.
65. Wright CG, Schaefer SD. Inner ear histopathology in patients treated with cis-platinum. Laryngoscope. 1982;92:1408-13.
66. Li Y, Womer RB, Silber JH. Predicting cisplatin ototoxicity in children: the influence of age and the cumulative dose. Eur J Cancer. 2004;40:2445-51.
67. Oldenburg J, Kraggerud SM, Cvancarova M, et al. Cisplatin-induced long-term hearing impairment is associated with specific glutathione-S-transferase genotypes in testicular cancer survivors. J Clin Oncol. 2007;25:708-14.
68. McFadden D, Plattsmier H. Aspirin can potentiate the temporary hearing loss induced by intense sounds. Hear Res. 1983;9:295-316.
69. Wigand MD, Heidland A. Ototoxic side effects of high doses of furosemide in patients with uremia. Postgrad Med J. 1971;47(Suppl):54-6.
70. Heidland H, Wigand ME. The effect of furosemide at high doses on auditory sensitivity in patients with uremia. Klin Wochenschr. 1970;48:1051-6.
71. Boston Collaborative Drug Surveillance Program. Drug-induced deafness: a cooperative study. JAMA. 1973;224: 516-7.
72. Tuzel IH. Comparison of adverse reactions to bumetanide and furosemide. J Clin Pharmacol. 1981;21:615-9.
73. Matz GJ. The ototoxic effects of ethacrynic acid in man and animals. Laryngoscope. 1976;86:1065-86.
74. Arnold W, Nadol JB, Geidauer H. Ultrastructural histopathology in a case of human ototoxicity due to loop diuretics Acta Otolaryngol. 1981;91:391-414.
75. Mintz U, Amir J, Pinkhas J, et al. Transient perceptive deafness due to erythromycin lactobionate. J Am Med Assn. 1973; 226: 1122-3.
76. McGhan LJ, Merchant SN. Erythromycin ototoxicity. Otol Neurotol. 2003; 24: 701-2.
77. Coulston J, Balaratnam N. Irreversible sensorineural hearing loss due to clarithromycin. Postgrad Med J. 2005; 81: 58-9.
78. Croghan MK, Aickin MG, Meyskens FL. Dose-related alpha-difluoromethylornithine ototoxicity. Am J Clin Oncol. 1991; 14:331-5.
79. Pasic TR, Heisey D, Love RR, α-difluoromethylornithine. J Natl Cancer Inst. 1993;85:732-6.
80. Meyskens FL, Gerner EW, Emerson S, et al. Effect of α-difluoromethylornithine on rectal mucosal levels of polyamines in a randomized, double-blinded trial for colon cancer prevention. J Natl Cancer Inst. 1998;90:1212-8.
81. Attili VSS, Bapsy PP, Anupama G, et al. Irreversible sensorineural hearing loss due to Imatinib. Leuk Res. 2008; 32: 991-2.
82. Janssen JJWM, Berendse HW, Schuurhuis GJ, et al. A 51-year-old male CML patient with progressive hearing loss, confusion, ataxia, and aphasia during imatinib treatment. Am J Hematol. 2009;84:679-82.
83. Lin HE, Roberts DS, Kay J, et al. Sensorineural hearing loss following Imatinib (Gleevec) administration. Otolaryngol Head Neck Surg. 2012;146:335-7.
84. Rybak LP, Whitworth CA. Ototoxicity: therapeutic opportunities. Drug Discovery Today. 2005;10:1313-21.
85. Chen Y, Huang WG, Zha DJ, et al. Aspirin attenuates gentamicin ototoxicity: From the laboratory to the clinic. Hear Res. 2007;226:178-82.

86. Yagi M, Magal E, Sheng Z, et al. Hair cell protection from aminoglycoside ototoxicity by adenovirus-mediated overexpression of glial cell line-derived neurotrophic factor. Human Gene Ther. 1999;10:813-23.
87. Kawamoto K, Ishimoto S, Minoda R, et al. Math1 gene transfer generates new cochlear hair cells in mature guinea pigs in vivo. J Neurosci. 2003;23:4395-400.
88. Staeker H, Praetorius M, Baker K, et al. Vestibular hair cell regeneration and restoration of balance function induced by math1 gene transfer. Otology Neurotol. 2007;28: 223-31.
89. Marcotti W, van Netten SM, Kros CJ. The aminoglycoside antibiotic dihydrostreptomycin rapidly enters mouse outer hair cells through the mechano-electrical transducer channels. J Physiol. 2005;567:505-21.
90. Huth ME, Ricci AJ, Cheng AG. Mechanisms of aminoglycoside ototoxicity and targets of hair cell protection. Int J Otolaryngol. 2011; 937861 . doi: 10.1155/2011.937861. Epub 2011 Oct 25.
91. Seaman BJ, Guardiani EA, Brewer CC, et al. Audiovestibular dysfunction associated with adoptive cell immunotherapy for melanoma. Otolaryngol Head Neck Surg. 2012;147:744-9.

CHAPTER 20

Tinnitus

Carol Bauer

INTRODUCTION/BACKGROUND

Subjective tinnitus is an auditory perception without an external acoustic source. The sensation is not a modern malady, and references to tinnitus are found in some of the earliest medical manuscripts.

Tinnitus is a symptom associated with a wide range of etiologies and pathologic mechanisms, from conductive hearing loss secondary to cerumen impaction and otosclerosis, from turbulent blood flow in an intracranial vessel or enhanced blood flow in a glomus jugulare tumor, from acute acoustic trauma with temporary threshold shift to age-related sensorineural hearing loss, from auditory hallucinations to hearing loss secondary to vestibular schwannomas. Tinnitus that occurs in association with sensorineural hearing loss (age-related, noise-induced, related to ototoxins, or otherwise idiopathic) is termed primary tinnitus. Tinnitus that can be linked to a specific cause or organic condition is termed secondary tinnitus. The wide range of causative pathology dictates a thorough evaluation of the tinnitus complaint.

The experience of tinnitus and the impact of tinnitus on daily life is highly individual, and can range from minimal to severe. Fortunately, severely disturbing tinnitus affects <5% of people with tinnitus. The variable nature of the symptom requires all physicians to have a practical plan for evaluation and cost-effective treatment of the patient presenting with tinnitus. Patients that seek treatment for their tinnitus are concerned about what they are hearing, why they hear it and how can it be eliminated or controlled. They benefit the most from a knowledgeable physician, a thorough assessment and good information about their symptom. The general goals for the evaluation and treatment of a patient with tinnitus are: identify and treat associated pathology causing the tinnitus, identify exacerbating and mitigating factors that modulate tinnitus, provide education that improves the patient's understanding of tinnitus, and provide or arrange access to therapies that improve coping skills. It is important to provide reassurance and hope. Current research is making unprecedented strides toward unraveling tinnitus mechanisms and this ultimately will translate into more effective treatments.

Incidence and Prevalence

The prevalence of tinnitus in the adult population is estimated to range from 6% to 19% of adults, depending on the population sampled and the definition of tinnitus used in the survey.[1] The most conservative estimate of tinnitus would indicate that 24 million people in the United States experience tinnitus.[2] Risk factors for tinnitus have been identified from large epidemiological surveys and include nonmodifiable factors of gender (male) and ethnicity (non-Hispanic Whites), and modifiable factors including body mass index ($\geq$30 kg/m^2), hypertension, diabetes mellitus, dyslipidemia, anxiety disorder, noise exposure, and smoking.[3]

Estimates of the range of tinnitus severity vary with the definition used, the survey instrument and the demographic population sampled. Population studies that assess the severity and impact of tinnitus are significantly affected by questionnaire wording and individual variation in subjective tinnitus ratings. The definitions of mild, moderate, or severe tinnitus may not be comparable between different studies. Severe tinnitus is estimated to affect 1–3% of the adult population.[2,4] In the Blue Mountain study, 82% of the study population rated their tinnitus as not annoying to mildly annoying, and 16% as very annoying.[5] The British National Study of Hearing reported tinnitus prevalence of 35%, with 8% rating their tinnitus as moderately to severely annoying and 0.5% reporting tinnitus with a severe negative impact on their ability to lead a normal life.[6]

There are two population-based estimates of the incidence of tinnitus.[2,7] The Beaver Dam study established the overall prevalence at baseline in adults between the ages of 48 and 92 as 8.2%. The tinnitus was rated as moderate in 74% and severe in 18%. A 5-year follow-up examination of the original participants documented a 5-year incidence of tinnitus as 5.7%. In the Blue Mountain study, the 5-year incidence of tinnitus was 18%. Longitudinal studies suggest that for many people tinnitus becomes less bothersome over time. A large longitudinal study reported that nearly 40% of adults with mild tinnitus on initial evaluation had no tinnitus on 5-year follow-up, and only 20% reported progression to moderate/severe tinnitus. Forty-five percent of participants with tinnitus rated as significant at baseline reported no tinnitus at follow-up (43%) or improvement to mild tinnitus (57%).[2] In the Blue Mountain study, 20% of people with tinnitus at baseline reported resolution of the symptom at 5-year follow-up.[7] It is very beneficial to include these data on spontaneous tinnitus improvement when counseling patients with tinnitus. Patients with new onset tinnitus often experience anxiety and distress; reassurance regarding the natural improvement of tinnitus impact over time is an important feature of the tinnitus education and counseling. The observed spontaneous improvement of tinnitus also has significant implications for clinical trials assessing efficacy of tinnitus interventions.

PATHOGENESIS

Objective tinnitus (OT) results from an internal active process that is either mechanical, vascular, or musculoskeletal in origin. OT can be continuous or episodic, pulsatile or nonpulsatile, and variable in character and duration. OT is, by definition, detectable, with or without amplification or auscultation, by an observer. Some internal active physiological processes that generate acoustic percepts are not easily detected by an observer; these are termed somatosounds. Examples of somatosounds include the sounds generated by swallowing, air movement in the presence of a patulous Eustachian tube, and the pulsatile flow of intracranial blood with intracranial hypertension. Examples of mechanical sources of OT include the pulsatile blood flow of a dural arteriovenous fistula and spontaneous otoacoustic emissions. Table 20.1 outlines the causes of pulsatile and nonpulsatile tinnitus. Subjective tinnitus, by definition, cannot be detected or perceived by another person. Subjective tinnitus is the topic of this chapter.

CLINICAL FINDINGS: SYMPTOMS AND SIGNS

Subjective tinnitus is a symptom of a range of otologic and occasionally nonotologic disorders. Evaluation of the

Table 20.1: Tinnitus features

Feature	*Options*	*Implications*
Onset	Sudden vs. gradual	May identify a precipitating factor, such as sudden sensorineural hearing loss
Duration	Less than 3–6 months vs greater than 6 months	Resolution may occur for acute tinnitus; natural habituation occurs over time
Severity	Minimal, mild, moderate, severe, maximal	Management options and extent of intervention linked to severity of tinnitus impact
Laterality/ location	Lateralized vs. central	May implicate a treatable otologic process such as otosclerosis, effusion, or retrocochlear lesion
Pitch	Low vs. high vs. tonal vs. static/white noise	May implicate hydrops (low pitch tinnitus), acoustic trauma (tonal)
Exacerbating factors	Sleep, diet (alcohol, caffeine), allergies, stress	
Modulators	Somatic (temporomandibular joint (TMJ), neck manipulation)	

patient with tinnitus begins with a history and physical examination. Important features of the history include descriptive features of the tinnitus and associated symptoms and sensory deficits (Table 20.2). It is important to recognize the signs and symptoms of specific disorders that can cause tinnitus. Asymmetry of thresholds or speech discrimination, for example, would trigger investigation for a retrocochlear process. Associated symptoms of otalgia, otorrhea and ear fullness would suggest chronic inflammation or infection in the middle ear or mastoid. Tinnitus that occurs in the setting of sudden hearing loss, with or without vertigo, warrants further evaluation with imaging.[8–9]

Descriptive features of the tinnitus will guide further investigation and the subsequent treatment course. The descriptive features discriminate tinnitus that arises from otologic and nonotologic sources. Two critical features that guide treatment are the duration and the severity of the tinnitus.

Table 20.2: Objective tinnitus

- Pulsatile
- Synchronous with pulse
  - Arterial etiologies
  - Arteriovenous fistula or malformation
  - Paraganglioma (glomus tympanicum or jugulare)
  - Carotid artery stenosis
  - Other atherosclerotic disease (subclavian, external carotid)
  - Arterial dissection (carotid, vertebral)
  - Persistent stapedial artery
  - Intratympanic carotid artery
  - Vascular compression of cranial nerve VIII
  - Increased cardiac output (pregnancy, thyrotoxicosis)
  - Intraosseous (Paget's disease, otosclerosis)
- Venous etiologies
  - Pseudotumor cerebri
  - Venous hum
  - Sigmoid sinus and Jugular bulb anomalies
- Asynchronous with pulse
  - Palatal myoclonus
  - Tensor tympani or stapedius muscle myoclonus
- Nonpulsatile
  - Spontaneous otoacoustic emission
  - Patulous Eustachian tube

OTOLOGIC DISORDERS AND TINNITUS

Conductive hearing loss from any etiology (e.g. cerumen impaction, ossicular chain fixation, middle ear effusion) can cause subjective tinnitus that is pulsatile or nonpulsatile in character. Identifying and treating these causes will usually resolve the tinnitus and leave the clinician with a grateful patient.

Sensorineural hearing loss of any magnitude and pattern can cause subjective tinnitus. Interestingly, only 30% of people with age-related sensorineural hearing loss and 50% of people with noise-induced hearing loss have associated tinnitus. It is a rare occurrence to have tinnitus without some auditory deficit or asymmetry. High-frequency audiometry and outer hair cell assessment with otoacoustic emissions will usually detect a functional deficit in patients with "normal" audiograms and tinnitus. Sudden sensorineural hearing loss and Meniere's disease are disorders that nearly always have concomitant tinnitus as a presenting feature.

Nonotologic Disorders and Tinnitus

Vascular causes of tinnitus include dural arteriovenous malformations, arteriovenous fistulas of the head and neck, increased cardiac output with high blood flow, and turbulent blood flow in the cranial venous drainage system.

Muscular causes of tinnitus include myoclonus of the stapedius muscle, the tensor tympani muscle, and the tensor palatine muscles. Rare mechanical causes of acoustic percepts that can be disturbing to patients are the audible breath sounds associated with patulous Eustachian tube and the normal sounds of the Eustachian tube opening and closing with swallowing.

Somatic Tinnitus and Somatic Modulation

Somatic tinnitus is a unique form of tinnitus in which the loudness, laterality, or tonality of the tinnitus can by modulated by somatic manipulation. This form of tinnitus was originally observed in a small group of patients after surgical removal of large vestibular schwannomas. Postoperatively, these patients had the ability to modulate the loudness or tonal character of their chronic tinnitus by exaggerated eye movements, leg motion, or cutaneous stimulation of the hands or face. The presumed mechanism of action for this unusual form of tinnitus is neural sprouting or aberrant reinnervation after auditory deafferentation. Subsequent to these observations, however, a more general form of somatosensory modulation of tinnitus has been recognized in some patients with primary tinnitus, that is, tinnitus not associated with a retrocochlear tumor. In these cases, tinnitus pitch and loudness can be modulated by forceful isometric contraction of the head and neck muscles.

A systematic review of treatments that target somatosensory systems suggests that somatic tinnitus may be a unique subtype that responds to targeted intervention. Levine and colleagues defined somatic tinnitus syndrome as tinnitus that is (1) perceived in the ear and (2) occurs ipsilateral to a somatic trigger and (3) is not associated with any new hearing complaints. Tinnitus that is strongly lateralized to one ear in the presence of symmetric hearing (including symmetric hearing loss) would theoretically have a somatic component by the definition of Levine and colleagues. The authors concluded that somatic tinnitus is often responsive to acupuncture, electric stimulation of the scalp and auricle, trigger point treatment, and treatment of temporomandibular joint dysfunction (TMD).

Typewriter Tinnitus

Typewriter tinnitus is defined by a characteristic sensation. The tinnitus has a staccato quality, similar to a typewriter tapping, popcorn popping, or a Morse code signal. The tinnitus is intermittent and chronic. The percept is often triggered by specific head movements or sounds. Typewriter tinnitus may be confused with tinnitus arising from a muscular source, such as spasm of the tensor tympani or stapedius muscle, or palatal myoclonus. Evidence that typewriter tinnitus is not generated by a myogenic source is illustrated by the history of a patient with typewriter tinnitus that failed to respond to tensor tympani and stapedius muscle transection. Tinnitus resolution was achieved, however, with carbamazepine (Tegretol).[10] Two small case series reported successful treatment with carbamazepine suggesting that typewriter tinnitus may be caused by vascular compression of the auditory nerve ipsilateral to the tinnitus.[11-12]

Temporomandibular Joint Disorders and Tinnitus

The association between TMD and tinnitus is well recognized. Large clinical surveys document an increased prevalence of TMD symptoms in patients with tinnitus compared with the general population, and a higher incidence of tinnitus in individuals with TMD and normal audiometric thresholds compared with controls.[13] The causative relationship, if present, for tinnitus and TMD is speculative at present. Somatic modulation of qualitative features of tinnitus such as loudness, location, and tonality with craniomandibular manipulation is well-documented, although the prevalence of this form of tinnitus is not precisely known.

One third of patients with symptoms of TMD can modulate their tinnitus with jaw movement or pressure to the TMJ.[14] Selected patients with tinnitus and TMD have symptom improvement when the TMD is treated with an occlusal splint.[15] Tinnitus associated with specific head and neck pathology, such as TMD, unilateral facial pain, otalgia, occipital or temporal headaches, may be amenable to interventions that target the somatic dysfunction.

Tinnitus and Comorbid Conditions

People who are bothered by their tinnitus report difficulties with concentration, sleep, daily activities, and social interaction.[16] It is well recognized that affective disorders exacerbate chronic medical illnesses, and the association of tinnitus with depression and anxiety supports this observation. There is some debate, however, regarding the true prevalence of psychologic distress related to tinnitus, and it is unclear if the psychological distress is directly related to the tinnitus or the disruption of activities of daily life.[17-19] Recent National Health Survey data suggest that people who perceive their tinnitus to be at least a moderate problem are more likely to be depressed. Furthermore, being bothered by tinnitus at bedtime increases the odds of depression 2.44 times.[20] Disrupted sleep exacerbates depressive symptoms, impairing coping ability with additional bidirectional interaction with bothersome tinnitus. Clinicians should be aware of these comorbid conditions and query tinnitus patients accordingly.

EVALUATION: LABORATORY, OTOLOGIC, AND NEUROTOLOGIC TESTING

Complete audiometric assessment has primary importance for evaluating the patient with tinnitus. Testing should include pure-tone threshold assessment by air and bone conduction, speech discrimination, and tympanometry. Distortion product otoacoustic emissions are useful when evaluating patients with tinnitus and a normal audiogram with pure tone thresholds <25 dBHL.

Demographic studies have shown the association between tinnitus and systemic diseases (diabetes, hypertension, hypercholesterolemia, and thyroid dysfunction).[3] Tinnitus may occur as one of a constellation of presenting symptoms of systemic infections such as Lyme disease and syphilis and systemic illnesses such as autoimmune disease. Despite the association, the universal underlying cause of tinnitus is hearing loss. Laboratory testing for specific metabolic, infectious, or inflammatory markers is indicated only if there are signs and symptoms that raise suspicions for specific primary causes associated with tinnitus. Routine testing for thyroid dysfunction, autoimmune markers, and viral infections is not indicated. The diagnostic yield of a battery of blood tests when evaluating tinnitus is very low and not justified.

Standardized questionnaires are useful in the primary assessment and follow-up of tinnitus patients (Table 20.3). Most questionnaires assess the functional, emotional, and cognitive factors impacted by tinnitus. Tinnitus can have negative consequences on daily activities such as sleep, concentration ability, and social enjoyment.[16] In some patients, the impairments are related to the underlying hearing loss. Identifying and distinguishing the impact of hearing loss from the associated tinnitus is important for counseling and treatment decisions. It is important to remain cognizant of the potential for serious psychological distress associated with tinnitus. Depression and anxiety are not uncommon comorbid conditions, although prevalence of these psychiatric disorders within the general population of people with nonbothersome tinnitus is not known.

EVALUATION: RADIOLOGIC IMAGING: CT, MRI, PET, ANGIOGRAPHY, ETC.

In the absence of any hearing loss, vertigo or other neural deficits, incidental discovery of a treatable cause such as schwannoma, CNS disease or middle ear and mastoid disease is unusual. Vestibular schwannoma or other incidental pathology was detected on MRI in <2% of cases presenting with the isolated symptom of nonpulsatile tinnitus or tinnitus in combination with hearing loss.[21] The diagnostic yield of CT and MRI for patients with primary tinnitus is low and therefore these studies are not indicated as part of the routine clinical evaluation. Imaging is appropriate when there are signs and/or symptoms that raise suspicions for a specific abnormality, such as unilateral tinnitus, pulsatile tinnitus, asymmetric hearing loss, vertigo, or cranial neuropathy.

Tinnitus Duration

It is important to ascertain the duration that tinnitus has been present and persistent for an individual. Counseling and treatment management strategies should be tailored

Table 20.3: Partial list of validated tinnitus questionnaires with utility for clinical application

Questionnaire	*Author (year)*	*Items*	*Response options*	*Cronback's alpha (α) test retest (r)*
Tinnitus questionnaire	Hallam et al.[69] (1988)	52	3: true, partly true, not true	α: 0.91–0.95 *r*: 0.91–0.94 (6–8 weeks)
Tinnitus severity questionnaire	Axelsson et al.[70] (1989)	10		α: ? *r*: 0.62–0.79 (18 months)
Tinnitus handicap questionnaire	Kuk et al.[71] (1990)	27	100: 0 = strongly disagree, 100 = strongly agree	α: 0.95 *r*: 0.89 (6–8 weeks)
Tinnitus reaction questionnaire	Wilson et al.[72] (1991)	26	5: not at all, a little of the time,..., almost all of the time	α: 0.96 *r*: 0.88
Tinnitus severity index	Meikle et al.[73] (1995)	12	5: never, rarely, sometimes, usually, always	α: >0.87 *r*: na
Tinnitus handicap inventory	Newman et al.[74] (1996)	25	3: yes, sometimes, no	α: = 0.93 *r*: 0.92 (20 days)
Tinnitus functional index	Meikle et al.[75] (2012)	25	10	α: 0.97 *r*: 0.78

as a function of tinnitus duration. At present, there are no widely accepted definitions that delineate acute or new onset tinnitus from chronic, persisting tinnitus. The NHIS-specified time period for a chronic condition is 3 months. Data from clinical trials that include wait-list controls suggest that spontaneous improvement in the intrusiveness or bothersomeness of tinnitus occurs within the first 6 months of onset.[22] The most improvement is seen in younger people with short duration tinnitus.[23] Clinical experience is consistent with these data, with observed improvement in tinnitus distress occurring within the first year of onset. Epidemiological studies report similar time frames for symptom improvement. In the Blue Mountain Study, over half the people reporting severe annoyance from tinnitus at baseline reported only moderate annoyance on follow-up, and 18% with moderate annoyance at baseline reported only mild annoyance on follow-up.[7] Similar findings were reported from the Beaver Dam study surveying 2500 adults over age 48 at baseline and on 5-year follow-up.[2] Tinnitus was defined as significant if it was rated as moderate severity, impacted sleep, or both. Tinnitus was not counted as significant if it was rated as mild in severity and did not interfere with sleep. Nearly half the respondents with significant tinnitus at baseline reported improvement on 5-year follow-up. In the group with improved tinnitus on follow-up, 43% reported no tinnitus and 57% reported only mild tinnitus. These data provide some benchmarks regarding the natural progression (and regression) of tinnitus over time. The factors that promote habituation and adaptation to new onset tinnitus are not known but are important topics that deserve thoughtful investigation.

Tinnitus Severity

The impact of tinnitus on the individual can range from mild or no impact to severe with significant negative impact on daily functioning and emotional well-being. The degree of severity and impact can be assessed using standardized questionnaires, of which several are available that are validated, have good test-retest reliability and are easy to administer (Table 20.3). Questionnaires are useful for organizing tinnitus impact into the domains of emotional, cognitive, and functional distress. Questionnaires facilitate understanding how tinnitus impacts the individual and are an effective way to monitor treatment progress.

PATHOPHYSIOLOGY

Most current theories on the mechanisms responsible for tinnitus hypothesize that the sensation results from central compensation in response to peripheral deafferentation. Variations on this theme involve the specific sites involved in central compensation, ranging from the cerebellum[24] to the auditory cortex,[25] with primary auditory pathway involvement[26] to critical input from nonauditory pathways.[27] Debate is ongoing regarding the neural mechanisms, neurotransmitters, and cell types that are critical to the pathology of tinnitus. Challenges in sorting out these basic science questions have included the heterogeneity of patients with tinnitus and the confounding factor of associated hearing loss. How does one control for genetic factors (there may be a "susceptibility" gene for tinnitus) and acoustic history (accurate historical information on sound exposure is rarely available) that impact the onset, severity, and persistence of tinnitus? Animal models of tinnitus have allowed investigation of tinnitus mechanisms that otherwise would have been impossible.[28]

TREATMENT: MEDICAL AND SURGICAL

Historically, medical treatments for tinnitus were based on empiricism and anecdotal evidence. The earliest records of the pharmacologic treatments for tinnitus are from Egyptian papyrus dating from the sixteenth century BC, recommending treatment of a bewitched ear with infusing a mixture of frankincense and balanites oil. In first century Mesopotamia, tinnitus treatments were organized on the basis of specific characteristics of the tinnitus. There were remedies for left ear tinnitus, right ear tinnitus, and tinnitus that was singing, whispering, or speaking. Masking tinnitus with external sounds dates back millenia, when Hippocrates pondered "why one sound can drive out another sound".[29] Modern pharmacologic treatments typically begun with serendipitous observations of tinnitus improvement, such as the temporary reduction of tinnitus after intravenous injection of lidocaine. [30] Advances in neuroscience, availability of tools for assessing neural correlates of tinnitus, and the development of models for testing tinnitus theories have led to theory-driven clinical trials and treatments.

Current medical treatments for tinnitus include pharmacologic therapy, acoustic-based therapy, counseling and education, cognitive behavioral therapy (CBT), and treatments based on complementary and alternative medicine. Standardized guidelines for the management of tinnitus have recently been developed. The Agency for Healthcare Research and Quality (AHRQ) and the United States Department of Health and Human Services commissioned the McMaster University Evidence-Based Practice Center (EPC) to conduct a comparative effectiveness review of tinnitus evaluation and management.[31] The EPC search strategy yielded nearly 10,000 citations of which 834 (8.6%) passed initial screening. Fifty-one publications of tinnitus treatments were deemed appropriate for inclusion in the review and guideline recommendations. Treatments were categorized as pharmacologic and food supplements, medical therapy, sound (acoustic)-based therapy, and psychological (behavioral) therapies. Included in the analysis were clinical trials evaluating therapies not based on accepted physiology of the ear or tinnitus pathophysiology, detracting from the merit and face validity of the review. Guideline endorsement of specific treatment recommendations were withheld citing various limitations of the selected clinical trials, including insufficient evidence, inconsistent effect sizes, small sample sizes, levels of bias, etc. Two key questions were identified by the EPC as important factors in tinnitus management. First, what are the effective methods that identify patients in need of further evaluation and treatment? Second, what are the prognostic factors, patient characteristics, and symptoms that impact treatment outcomes? No studies were identified that addressed triage strategies for patients with tinnitus. No studies were identified investigating prognostic factors that illuminate the natural history, progression, and regression of tinnitus.

Effective surgical treatments for tinnitus are those that address a specific underlying disorder. Tinnitus that occurs with middle ear effusion and tympanic membrane perforation resolves with treatment of the conductive hearing loss. Curiously, elimination of tinnitus with stapes surgery is successful in only 50% of patients.[32] Tinnitus related to acoustic neuroma will frequently resolve if hearing is preserved after tumor resection.[33]

Surgical treatment for primary tinnitus is limited. Historically, the cochlea and eighth nerve were thought to be the source of tinnitus, and cochlear nerve section for severely disturbing tinnitus was a treatment option. Outcomes were disappointing, with worsening tinnitus in a significant portion of patients. Nearly 50% of patients report unchanged or worse tinnitus after labyrinthectomy performed for vestibular symptoms.[32]

MEDICATIONS FOR TINNITUS

A wide range of drug classes have been investigated for efficacy in modulating tinnitus (Table 20.4). There are currently no medications approved by the Federal Drug Administration to treat tinnitus, and the medications and supplements listed in Table 20.4 have all been used off-label. The majority of clinical trials have not shown any benefit of antidepressants or anxiolytics on the loudness of tinnitus. However, there is evidence that modest improvement in the annoyance and bothersomeness of tinnitus can occur with these medications when the associated depression and anxiety is addressed. High doses of paroxetine may be effective in reducing tinnitus loudness, severity, and impact in patients without major depression or anxiety disorders.[34] Sertraline was more effective than placebo in decreasing tinnitus severity and perceived tinnitus loudness in patients with severe tinnitus.[35] Interestingly, correlation analysis suggested that the clinical improvement was largely related to a direct effect on tinnitus and only 20% of the improvement was attributed to a reduction in depression and anxiety.

There is no role for intratympanic medications in the treatment of tinnitus. There are only three published randomized control trials that have investigated the effect of intratympanic steroids on tinnitus.[36–38] No benefit was demonstrated over placebo. There are no controlled trials investigating intratympanic lidocaine for tinnitus treatment.

GABAERGIC MEDICATIONS FOR TINNITUS

Several lines of scientific evidence and clinical observations suggest that chronic tinnitus may develop because of pathological loss of central inhibition triggered by peripheral deafferentation.[28,39-40] Gamma-aminobutyric acid (GABA) is one of two major inhibitory neurotransmitters widely distributed throughout the auditory pathway. If tinnitus is the result of downregulation of GABA, then potentially GABA-enhancing drugs may be useful to restore homeostasis and alleviate tinnitus. Benzodiazepines are GABA receptor modulators that may improve tinnitus by reducing the perceptual loudness of tinnitus and decreasing distress through anxiolytic action. Although nearly all clinical trials investigating benzodiazepines for tinnitus have been criticized for flawed experimental

Table 20.4: Pharmacologic treatments for tinnitus and evidence for efficacy

Class	*Drug*	*Evidence base*	*Dose*	*Outcome*	*Side effects*
Tricyclic antidepressants	Nortriptyline	Placebo-controlled, double-blind trial (Dobie et al.[76] 1993)	100 mg qhS	Global benefit (0.008) Tinnitus severity (ns) Significant predictors of benefit: female gender, insomnia, absence of cervical muskuloskeletal complaints	Dry mouth, sedation, dizziness, headache, weight gain
	Cyclobenzaprine	Open label pilot study (Coelho et al.[77] 2012) Active vs. wait list control (Vanneste et al.[78] 2012)	30 mg qD	Reduction in THI after 3 months ($p < 0.001$)	Sedation, headache, dizziness, dry mouth
SSRI	Sertraline	Randomized, placebo-controlled, double-blind trail (Zoger et al. [35])	50 mg qD	Improved subjective rating of tinnitus loudness and severity, in patients with depression	Fatigue, dry mouth, increased tinnitus, lightheadedness
	Paroxetine	Randomized, placebo-controlled, double-blind trial (Robinson et al.[34])	10–50 mg qD	Improved tinnitus severity and distress; reduction in tinnitus loudness match (in the 50 mg qD dose group only)	Sedation, dry mouth, sexual dysfunction
Anticonvulsants/ GABA or glutamate modulators	Gabapentin	Single-blind, crossover, placebo-controlled, multidose trial (Bauer and Brozoski[46]) Double-blind, placebo-controlled, single-dose trail (Witsell et al.[79] 2007) Randomized, double-blind, placebo-controlled, single-dose trial (Piccirillo et al.[80] 2007) Randomized, double-blind, placebo-controlled, single-dose trial (Dehkordi et al.[81] 2011)	300–2400 mg	Improved loudness and annoyance in subjects with noise-induced hearing loss[1] Improved severity[2] Improved THI in subjects with normal hearing[3] Improved severity in subjects with hypertension, diabetes, hyperlipidemia[4]	Sedation, nausea, weight gain, sleep disturbance, dizziness, depression
	Carbamazepine	Case reports for paroxysmal staccato tinnitus (Brantberg[82] 2010)	100–400 mg BID		Sedation, dizziness, nausea, dry mouth, anxiety
	Acamprosate	Randomized, double-blind trial (Azevedo et al.[83] 2005; Sharma et al.[84] 2012)	333 mg TID	Tinnitus improvement (NOS) ($p = 0.012$)	Depression, diarrhea, anxiety, lethargy
Anxiolytics	Alprazolam	Crossover, randomized, blinded, placebo-controlled trial (Jalali et al.[42]) Prospective, randomized, placebo controlled, double-blind trial (Johnson et al.[41])	1.5 mg qD	Significant improvement in VAS tinnitus loudness and severity; change in THI (ns)	Sedation, dizziness, tinnitus
Vasodilator/ vasoactive	Cyclandelate	Randomized, blinded, placebo-controlled trail (Oma Hester et al.[85] 1998)	400 mg TID	No significant change in objective loudness match; decreased subjective loudness rating ($p < 0.01$)	Dizziness, headache, nausea, gastric distress
Herbal and supplement	Melatonin	Prospective, randomized, double-blind, crossover trail (Hurtuk et al.[86] 2011) Prospective open-label trail (Megwalu et al.[87] 2006)	3 mg qHS	Improved tinnitus loudness and severity ($p < 0.05$); most effective in men with severe bilateral tinnitus, a history of noise exposure and without depression	Headache, depression, drowsiness, dizziness, irritability
	Gingko biloba	Cochrane Database Systematic Review of three trials (1143 patients) (Hilton et al.[88] 2013)	120– 240 mg qD	Evidence for efficacy is mixed	Headache, gastrointestinal distress, medication interactions

(THI, tinnitus handicap index; VAS, visual Analog Scale).

design, most of the trials do report some level of tinnitus improvement using global assessment ratings.[41–42] There are potential risks associated with chronic benzodiazepine use and caution is warranted when using these drugs in the elderly.

Gabapentin is a chemical analog of GABA. Although chemically similar to GABA, the drug does not significantly interact with GABA receptors nor does it appreciably modulate endogenous GABA levels.[43] Nevertheless, it is used effectively as an adjunctive anti-epileptic to enhance inhibition of neural activity associated with seizures and has also been used to treat other medical conditions similar to tinnitus such as neuropathic pain.[44] Gabapentin was first reported to reduce the loudness of tinnitus is a case report of new onset tinnitus of unknown etiology.[45]

Three controlled trials have investigated the efficacy of gabapentin on tinnitus. Two studies used only a single target dose, did not stratify subjects for tinnitus etiology and included subjects with a range of tinnitus duration. Both studies reported improvement for a subset of subjects. Witsell reported a significant difference ($p = 0.026$) in the number of subjects with improved global tinnitus severity ratings treated with gabapentin compared with placebo.

Piccirillo et al. reported a significant improvement in tinnitus handicap index (THI) score in subjects with normal hearing treated with gabapentin ($p = 0.005$).

A prospective single-blind study of gabapentin enrolled only subjects with moderate to severe chronic tinnitus. Subjects were stratified by etiology of hearing loss, history of acoustic trauma and evidence of acoustic trauma on audiometric testing.[46] The drug was most effective in reducing the loudness and the annoyance of tinnitus in subjects with tinnitus related to acoustic trauma. A significant improvement in tinnitus annoyance was obtained at a drug dose of 900 mg per day in the subjects with tinnitus related to acoustic trauma ($p = 0.015$). There was also a significant improvement in the objective measurement of tinnitus loudness in half the subjects on the 1800 mg and 2400 mg dose. This effect was not seen in the subjects with tinnitus not related to acoustic trauma. These results suggest that gabapentin may be a useful drug for tinnitus treatment in a specific population of patients, and the effective drug dose must be individualized.

Transcranial Magnetic Stimulation

Transcranial magnetic stimulation (TMS) is a noninvasive neuromodulation technique that has been adapted from the neuropsychiatric field and applied to the treatment of acute and chronic tinnitus. Pulsed current is passed through a coiled wire held over the cranium. The current generates a strong magnetic field inducing an electric field which painlessly stimulates the underlying brain area of interest. The affected brain area is either hyperpolarized (excited) or inhibited, depending on the coil size, shape, skull orientation, current pulse characteristics, and stimulation frequency. Low-frequency (<1 Hz) TMS decreases cortical excitation and high frequency (5–20 Hz) increases cortical excitation. The accuracy of targeting the brain area of interest is influenced by the brain size and shape. The depth of penetration of the magnetic field is limited to a few centimeters, although neural changes in subcortical structures may be achieved through interconnected neural circuitry.

Interest in applying TMS to modulate auditory symptoms was sparked after low-frequency stimulation of the left temporoparietal cortex using repeated TMS (rTMS) reduced auditory hallucinations in schizophrenic patients.[47] The treatment subsequently was applied to patients with idiopathic new onset and chronic tinnitus. Although initial reports of rTMS therapeutic efficacy were promising, evidence for clinically significant, long-term improvement in tinnitus distress has not yet emerged. Utilization of appropriate controls has been particularly challenging for trials investigating rTMS as a tinnitus treatment. The placebo effect can be significant and clearly has an impact on clinical trials involving tinnitus.[48,49] It is well known that the placebo response increases with the invasiveness of the intervention, further emphasizing the importance of including appropriate controls in studies of rTMS efficacy for tinnitus management. Development of adequate control conditions in rTMS studies is challenging because the coil stimulation results in audible, tactile, and motor stimulation during activation. The optimum control or sham stimulation parameters have not yet been established.[50]

The optimum site of stimulation for treatment of tinnitus is currently not known. Targets for stimulation have included auditory cortex contralateral to the tinnitus, ipsilateral to the tinnitus, the left temporoparietal cortex, and the association cortex. Techniques for accurately locating the site of coil placement vary between studies and include neuronavigation combined with functional or structural imaging studies, anatomical landmarks, or physiologic markers from electroencephalography. Successful targeting of specific brain loci of interest is consequently influenced by intersubject variability.

Acoustic Therapy

Environmental sounds have been used to mask tinnitus and decrease subjective awareness of the sensation for millennia. Hippocrates is credited with the observation that an external sound can mask or inhibit tinnitus.[29] Itard recognized the value of matching tinnitus with specific masking sounds to obtain relief and improve disturbed sleep.[51] Environmental sounds can also facilitate the natural process of habituation to the tinnitus perception. Habituation is a form of learning in which repeated exposure to a stimulus no longer evokes a response. Most people habituate to meaningless sounds and sensations, including tinnitus. This natural habituation is experienced by over 90% of people with persisting tinnitus; the perception is essentially nonbothersome and does not impact daily life.[6] Emotional reactions to a sensation prevent the normal habituation process. When habituation fails to occur, tinnitus becomes bothersome and disruptive. The negative reaction or response that some people develop to their tinnitus may occur therefore, in part, because of failure to habituate.[52]

Sound therapy has a positive impact on tinnitus for several reasons. Sound therapy provides a mechanism for patients to control their tinnitus. Specific sounds are perceived as soothing and provide tinnitus relief through stress reduction. The strategic selection of sounds that are nonintrusive and blend into the background is critical for decreasing the contrast between perceived tinnitus and the surrounding acoustic environment, thereby fostering a shift of attention away from the tinnitus.

Many tinnitus therapies use sound stimuli as primary or adjunctive treatment. Methods of acoustic stimulation range from broadband environmental enrichment with free-field sound generators to ear level devices that deliver constant low level customized modulated frequencies adapted to the individual's hearing threshold profile. Sound stimulation devices marketed for tinnitus relief range from off-the-shelf white-noise generators to custom devices generating complex amplitude modulated sounds or spectrally modified music. Although the rationale for acoustic stimulation as a tinnitus intervention is supported by current theories of tinnitus mechanisms, there are limited objective data demonstrating positive effects of these devices on tinnitus loudness, intrusiveness, or bothersomeness.

Hearing aids are an ideal technology for providing sound therapy when treating tinnitus associated with hearing loss.[53-54] Amplification improves communication, and consequently reduces the straining to hear phenomenon. Enhancement of ambient sound also provides low-level tinnitus masking and concomitantly reduces awareness of the tinnitus. The consistent stimulation may reverse central auditory pathway changes that occur in response to hearing loss and auditory deprivation. Clinically significant improvement in tinnitus severity has been reported in the large majority of patients fitted with bilateral digital hearing aids.[54-55] The benefit of hearing aids combined with counseling over counseling alone has been demonstrated in a group of chronic tinnitus sufferers.[56] The hearing aid plus counseling group had a 37% improvement in total tinnitus handicap questionnaire (THQ), compared with a 13% improvement in THQ in subjects receiving counseling alone.

Tinnitus retraining therapy (TRT) uses acoustic stimulation combined with directive counseling to facilitate habituation to the tinnitus perception and decrease the emotional reaction to the tinnitus. Acoustic stimulation can be achieved with enrichment of environmental sounds, hearing aids, combination instruments, or most commonly, white noise generators. A prospective randomized trial compared the long-term efficacy of TRT with a control treatment of general counseling and placebo noise generators in subjects with moderate to severe chronic tinnitus for at least 1 year without associated hearing loss.[57] The THI improved for both groups at the 6, 12, and 18 month assessment points compared with baseline. However, the effect size for the improvement with TRT was large (1.13) compared with the moderate effect size (0.78) for the control group. There was a greater improvement in the TRT group for the global assessment of total time distressed, annoyed, or irritated by tinnitus compared with the control group from entry to study completion at 18 months (46% vs. 22%). Finally, on multiple measures of global severity (THI) and intrusiveness, more subjects treated with TRT achieved the benchmark of 50% or better improvement compared to subjects who received the control treatment at the 18 month assessment point. This study demonstrated that general counseling on healthy living and general education about tinnitus results in long-lasting reductions in the global severity of tinnitus and that directive counseling combined with sound therapy results in even greater improvements in these same measures.

A variation of the technique of counseling combined with sound therapy to treat tinnitus uses customized sound therapy to promote habituation, relaxation, and desensitization. Neuromonics is a proprietary structured 6 month tinnitus treatment protocol designed to reduce tinnitus severity and annoyance 60. The protocol treatment involves listening 2–4 hours a day to a broadband auditory stimulus that is spectrally contoured to the individual's hearing loss profile including frequencies up to 12.5 kHz. In theory, the customized high-frequency stimulation is more effective than low- or mid-frequency broadband white noise in reversing the tonotopic central auditory reorganization that occurs in response to hearing loss and auditory deprivation. The stimulus is embedded in music that promotes relaxation, with decreasing audibility of a masking sound to promote desensitization to the tinnitus percept. The sound stimulation device is not combined with amplification and therefore the underlying hearing loss is not addressed.

The promising results of this treatment approach are noteworthy. Large, unbiased, controlled studies examining treatment efficacy for chronic tinnitus with comparison to hearing aid benefits combined with counseling are in order.

Electrical Stimulation

Nonauditory Electric Stimulation

Early attempts to improve tinnitus using electrical stimulation of the face, ear, or neck met with mixed results.[58] Subsequent investigations of somatic modulation have shown promising results in some people. Herraiz et al. hypothesized that transcutaneous electrical stimulation (TENS) of the periauricular region could augment the inhibition of the dorsal cochlear nucleus through somatosensory inputs.[59] Subject selection was restricted to people with an identified somatic trigger that initiated the tinnitus and the ability to modulate the tinnitus with either orofacial movements or postural changes. Subjects were evaluated using a visual analog scale before and after 2 weeks of daily TENS applied to the head or neck area. Nearly half the subjects reported improvement in their tinnitus: 23% reported complete suppression and 23% reported reduced intensity of the sensation. Notably, 59% of subjects with isolated somatic tinnitus improved, compared with only 14% of patients with somatic tinnitus with an associated otologic disorder. In a recent controlled study, Vanneste et al. reported similar improvement.[60] TENS was applied to the C2 region in 240 patients with tinnitus that could be somatically modulated. There was an 18% response rate, with 43% improvement in most and complete suppression of tinnitus in 6%. These studies illustrate the need for further work addressing specific subtypes of tinnitus and tailoring treatments accordingly.

Auditory Electric Stimulation (Cochlear Implants)

Cochlear implantation for rehabilitation of bilateral hearing loss with either single-channel or multichannel devices improves tinnitus in the majority of patients, with a small percentage of patients reporting worse tinnitus after implantation.[32,61] Electrical stimulation of the cochlea for tinnitus control is less effective when the primary indication is for tinnitus, not hearing loss. Outcomes for a series of five patients implanted with a single channel device solely for relief of tinnitus ranged from complete success with elimination of tinnitus to total failure.[62]

Cochlear implantation has recently been investigated for treatment of tinnitus in the challenging clinical setting of sudden hearing loss resulting in single-sided deafness. Traditional options for acoustic stimulation to promote habituation are limited in this situation. Most people with bothersome tinnitus after sudden hearing loss have normal hearing in the contralateral ear. Acoustic stimulation necessarily must be delivered to the "good ear", and this is poorly tolerated in general. Several trials have reported moderate to significant improvement in tinnitus distress with cochlear implantation in the deafened ear.[63] The relative importance of improved communication in this situation is unknown, but likely is significant.[64] Novel mapping and stimulation strategies may be critical for these patients. Recent data on outcomes of implantation for tinnitus related to single-sided deafness suggest that tinnitus suppression is maximal with use of full-length multichannel electrode arrays that access a broader region of the tonotopic map.[65]

Counseling Strategies

Counseling is a well-established tinnitus treatment strategy that has been utilized alone and in combination with other therapies. Counseling can encompass a wide range of approaches, including individual or group-based education, activities-based therapy and CBT. Significant improvements in tinnitus related distress have been demonstrated with CBT. CBT is a form of psychotherapy that helps patients identify and modify maladaptive thoughts and behaviors related to tinnitus and tinnitus distress. CBT includes education, relaxation training, cognitive restructuring, controlled stimulus exposure, and mindfulness-based training. CBT does not modify tinnitus loudness. Comparing CBT to active control treatments (rather than wait list controls) showed a small to moderate effect size.

General Health Strategies

Demographic studies have established tinnitus risk factors that include systemic diseases amenable to modification. These are the same risk factors associated with hearing loss.[66-67] Successful control of hypertension, hyperlipidemia and diabetes likely impacts tinnitus through optimized tissue perfusion and cochlear function. The benefits of general physical activity for decreasing tinnitus also support the approach of maximizing general health status.[68] The association between bothersome tinnitus and psychological distress presents an important opportunity to modify tinnitus distress through effective management of depression and anxiety. Finally, clinical experience suggests that specific ailments such as chronic sinusitis, environmental allergies, and uncontrolled sleep apnea can exacerbate tinnitus loudness and impair an individual's ability to cope with their tinnitus. Clinical investigations of the interaction between tinnitus and other common illnesses are needed.

PROGNOSIS

The prognosis for the majority of people with tinnitus is excellent. There are many effective interventions that decrease the negative impact of tinnitus. Significant advances in auditory neuroscience have advanced the treatment of tinnitus beyond the traditional recommendation instructing the patient to "learn to live with it".

REFERENCES

1. US Department of Commerce. Profiles of General Demographic Characteristics. Washington, DC: US Census Bureau; 2001. http://www.census.gov/prod/cen2000/dpl/2kh00.pdf. Accessed August 16, 2001.
*2. Nondahl DM, Cruickshanks KJ, Wiley TL, et al. Prevalence and 5-year incidence of tinnitus among older adults: the epidemiology of hearing loss study. J Am Acad Audiol. 2002;13:323-31.
*3. Shargorodsky J, Curhan GC, Farwell WR. Prevalence and characteristics of tinnitus among US adults. Am J Med. 2010;123:711-18.
4. Axelsson A, Ringdahl A. Tinnitus—a study of its prevalence and characteristics. Br J Audiol. 1989;23:53-62.
5. Sindhusake D, Mitchell P, Newall P, et al. Prevalence and characteristics of tinnitus in older adults: the Blue Mountains Hearing Study. Int J Audiol. 2003;42:289-94.
6. Coles RR. Epidemiology of tinnitus: (1) prevalence. J Laryngol Otol Suppl. 1984;9:7-15.
7. Gopinath B, McMahon CM, Rochtchina E, et al. Incidence, persistence, and progression of tinnitus symptoms in older adults: the Blue Mountains Hearing Study. Ear Hear. 2010; 31:407-12.
8. Schick B, Brors D, Koch O, et al. Magnetic resonance imaging in patients with sudden hearing loss, tinnitus and vertigo. Otol Neurotol. 2001;22:808-12.
9. Stachler RJ, Chandrasekhar SS, Archer SM, et al. Clinical practice guideline: sudden hearing loss. Otolaryngol Head Neck Surg. 2012;146:S1-35.
10. Mardini MK. Ear-clicking 'tinnitus' responding to carbamazepine. N Engl J Med. 1987;317:1542.
11. Brantberg K. Paroxysmal staccato tinnitus: a carbamazepine responsive hyperactivity dysfunction symptom of the eighth cranial nerve. J Neurol Neurosurg Psychiatry. 2010; 81:451-5.
12. Levine RA. Typewriter tinnitus: a carbamazepine-responsive syndrome related to auditory nerve vascular compression. ORL J Otorhinolaryngol Relat Spec. 2006;68:43-6; discussion 6-7.
13. Chole RA, Parker WS. Tinnitus and vertigo in patients with temporomandibular disorder. Arch Otolaryngol Head Neck Surg. 1992;118:817-21.
14. Rubinstein B, Axelsson A, Carlsson GE. Prevalence of signs and symptoms of craniomandibular disorders in tinnitus patients. J Craniomandib Disord. 1990;4:186-92.
15. Tullberg M, Ernberg M. Long-term effect on tinnitus by treatment of temporomandibular disorders: a two-year follow-up by questionnaire. Acta Odontol Scand. 2006;64: 89-96.
*16. Tyler RS, Baker LJ. Difficulties experienced by tinnitus sufferers. J Speech Hear Disord. 1983;48:150-54.
17. Geocze L, Mucci S, Abranches DC, et al. Systematic review on the evidences of an association between tinnitus and depression. Braz J Otorhinolaryngol. 2013;79:106-11.
18. McFerran DJ, Baguley DM. Is psychology really the best treatment for tinnitus? Clin Otolaryngol. 2009;34:99-101; discussion 2.
19. Ooms E, Meganck R, Vanheule S, et al. Tinnitus severity and the relation to depressive symptoms: a critical study. Otolaryngol Head Neck Surg. 2011;145:276-81.
20. Loprinzi PD, Maskalick S, Brown K, et al. Association between depression and tinnitus in a nationally representative sample of US older adults. Aging Ment Health. 2013; 17:714-17.
21. Vandervelde C, Connor SE. Diagnostic yield of MRI for audiovestibular dysfunction using contemporary referral criteria: correlation with presenting symptoms and impact on clinical management. Clin Radiol. 2009;64:156-63.
22. Nyenhuis N, Zastrutzki S, Weise C, et al. The efficacy of minimal contact interventions for acute tinnitus: a randomised controlled study. Cogn Behav Ther. 2013;42:127-38.
23. Hesser H, Weise C, Rief W, et al. The effect of waiting: A meta-analysis of wait-list control groups in trials for tinnitus distress. J Psychosom Res. 2011;70:378-84.
24. Bauer C, Wisner K, Sybert LT, Brozoski TJ. The cerebellum as a novel tinnitus generator. Hear Res. 2013;295:130-9.
*25. Eggermont JJ. Central tinnitus. Auris Nasus Larynx. 2003;30 Suppl:S7-12.
26. Kaltenbach JA, Zhang J, Finlayson P. Tinnitus as a plastic phenomenon and its possible neural underpinnings in the dorsal cochlear nucleus. Hear Res. 2005;206:200-26.

*References with asterisks refer to critical sources.

27. Rauschecker JP, Leaver AM, Muhlau M. Tuning out the noise: limbic-auditory interactions in tinnitus. Neuron. 2010;66:819-26.
28. Bauer CA, Brozoski TJ. Assessing tinnitus and prospective tinnitus therapeutics using a psychophysical animal model. J of the Assoc for Res in Otolaryngol. 2001;2:54-64.
29. Vernon J. The history of masking as applied to tinnitus. J Laryngol Otol Suppl. 1981:76-9.
30. Bárány R. Die Beeinflussing des Ohrensausens durch intravenous injizierte Lokalanasthetica. Acta Otolaryngol. 1935; 23:201-3.
31. Pichora-Fuller MK, Santaguida P, Hammill A, et al. Evaluation and treatment of tinnitus: comparative effectiveness. Rockville, MD: Agency for Healthcare Research and Quality (US); 2013.
32. House JW, Brackmann DE. Tinnitus: surgical treatment. Ciba Found Symp. 1981;85:204-16.
33. Catalano PJ, Post KD. Elimination of tinnitus following hearing preservation surgery for acoustic neuromas. Am J Otol. 1996;17:443-5.
34. Robinson SK, Viirre ES, Bailey KA, et al. Randomized placebo-controlled trial of a selective serotonin reuptake inhibitor in the treatment of nondepressed tinnitus subjects. Psychosom Med. 2005;67:981-8.
35. Zoger S, Svedlund J, Holgers KM. The effects of sertraline on severe tinnitus suffering—a randomized, double-blind, placebo-controlled study. J Clin Psychopharmacol. 2006; 26:32-9.
36. Topak M, Sahin-Yilmaz A, Ozdoganoglu T, et al. Intratympanic methylprednisolone injections for subjective tinnitus. J Laryngol Otol. 2009;123:1221-5.
37. Araujo MF, Oliveira CA, Bahmad FM, Jr. Intratympanic dexamethasone injections as a treatment for severe, disabling tinnitus: does it work? Arch Otolaryngol Head Neck Surg. 2005;131:113-17.
38. She W, Dai Y, Du X, et al. Treatment of subjective tinnitus: a comparative clinical study of intratympanic steroid injection vs. oral carbamazepine. Med Sci Monit. 2009;15: PI35-9.
39. Shulman A, Strashun AM, Seibyl JP, et al. Benzodiazepine receptor deficiency and tinnitus. Int Tinnitus J. 2000;6: 98-111.
40. Caspary DM, Holder TM, Hughes LF, et al. Age-related changes in GABA(A) receptor subunit composition and function in rat auditory system. Neuroscience. 1999;93: 307-12.
41. Johnson RM, Brummett R, Schleuning A. Use of alprazolam for relief of tinnitus. A double-blind study. Arch Otolaryngol Head Neck Surg. 1993;119:842-5.
42. Jalali MM, Kousha A, Naghavi SE, et al. The effects of alprazolam on tinnitus: a cross-over randomized clinical trial. Med Sci Monit. 2009;15:PI55-60.
43. Taylor CP, Gee NS, Su TZ, et al. A summary of mechanistic hypotheses of gabapentin pharmacology. Epilepsy Res. 1998;29:233-49.
44. Rice AS, Maton S. Gabapentin in postherpetic neuralgia: a randomised, double blind, placebo controlled study. Pain. 2001;94:215-24.
45. Zapp JJ. Gabapentin for the treatment of tinnitus: a case report. Ear Nose Throat J. 2001;80:114-16.
46. Bauer CA, Brozoski TJ. Effect of gabapentin on the sensation and impact of tinnitus. Laryngoscope. 2006;116: 675-81.
47. Hoffman RE, Boutros NN, Hu S, et al. Transcranial magnetic stimulation and auditory hallucinations in schizophrenia. Lancet. 2000;355:1073-5.
*48. Dobie RA. A review of randomized clinical trials in tinnitus. Laryngoscope. 1999;109:1202-11.
*49. Duckert LG, Rees TS. Placebo effect in tinnitus management. Otolaryngol Head Neck Surg. 1984;92:697-9.
50. Loo CK, Taylor JL, Gandevia SC, et al. Transcranial magnetic stimulation (TMS) in controlled treatment studies: are some 'sham' forms active? Biol Psychiatry. 2000;47: 325-31.
51. Stephens SD. The treatment of tinnitus—a historical perspective. J Laryngol Otol. 1984;98:963-72.
52. Hallam RS, Rachman S, Hinchcliffe R. Psychological aspects of tinnitus. In: Rachman S (ed.), Contributions to medical psychology. Oxford: Pergamon Press; 1984:31-53.
53. Saltzman M, Ersner MS. A hearing aid for the relief of tinnitus aurium. Laryngoscope. 1947;57:358-66.
54. Trotter MI, Donaldson I. Hearing aids and tinnitus therapy: a 25-year experience. J Laryngol Otol. 2008;122:1052-6.
55. Surr RK, Montgomery AA, Mueller HG. Effect of amplification on tinnitus among new hearing aid users. Ear Hear. 1985;6:71-5.
*56. Searchfield GD, Kaur M, Martin WH. Hearing aids as an adjunct to counseling: tinnitus patients who choose amplification do better than those that don't. Int J Audiol. 2010;49:574-9.
*57. Bauer CA, Brozoski TJ. Effect of tinnitus retraining therapy on the loudness and annoyance of tinnitus: a controlled trial. Ear Hear. 2011;32:145-55.
58. Shulman A. External electrical tinnitus suppression: a review. Am J Otol. 1987;8:479-84.
59. Herraiz C, Toledano A, Diges I. Trans-electrical nerve stimulation (TENS) for somatic tinnitus. Prog Brain Res. 2007;166:389-94.
60. Vanneste S, Plazier M, Van de Heyning P, et al. Transcutaneous electrical nerve stimulation (TENS) of upper cervical nerve (C2) for the treatment of somatic tinnitus. Exp Brain Res. 2010;204:283-7.
*61. Quaranta N, Wagstaff S, Baguley DM. Tinnitus and cochlear implantation. Int J Audiol. 2004;43:245-51.
62. Thedinger B, House WF, Edgerton BJ. Cochlear implant for tinnitus. Case reports. Ann Otol Rhinol Laryngol. 1985;94: 10-3.
63. Van de Heyning P, Vermeire K, Diebl M, et al. Incapacitating unilateral tinnitus in single-sided deafness treated by cochlear implantation. Ann Otol Rhinol Laryngol. 2008;117: 645-52.
64. Ramos A, Polo R, Masgoret E, et al. Cochlear implant in patients with sudden unilateral sensorineural hearing loss and associated tinnitus. Acta Otorrinolaringol Esp. 2012;63: 15-20.

*References with asterisks refer to critical sources.

65. Punte AK, De Ridder D, Van de Heyning P. On the necessity of full length electrical cochlear stimulation to suppress severe tinnitus in single-sided deafness. Hear Res. 2013;295:24-9.
66. Gates GA, Cobb JL, D'Agostino RB, et al. The relation of hearing in the elderly to the presence of cardiovascular disease and cardiovascular risk factors. Arch Otolaryngol Head Neck Surg. 1993;119:156-61.
67. Austin DF, Konrad-Martin D, Griest S, et al. Diabetes-related changes in hearing. Laryngoscope. 2009;119:1788-96.
68. Loprinzi PD, Lee H, Gilham B, et al. Association between accelerometer-assessed physical activity and tinnitus, NHANES 2005-2006. Res Q Exerc Sport. 2013;84:177-85.
69. Hallam RS, Jakes SC, Hinchcliffe R. Cognitive variables in tinnitus annoyance. Br J Clin Psychol. 1988;27 (Pt 3): 213-22.
70. Axelsson A, Ringdahl A. Tinnitus—a study of its prevalence and characteristics. Br J Audiol. 1989;23(1):53-62.
71. Kuk FK, Tyler RS, Russell D, Jordan H. The psychometric properties of a tinnitus handicap questionnaire. Ear Hear. 1990;11(6):434-45.
72. Wilson PH, Henry J, Bowen M, Haralambous G. Tinnitus reaction questionnaire: psychometric properties of a measure of distress associated with tinnitus. J Speech Hear Res. 1991;34(1):197-201.
73. Meikle MB, Griest SE, Stewart BJ, et al. Measuring the negativeimpact of tinnitus: a brief severity index. Abstracts of the 18th Midwinter Research Meeting. Des Moines (IA): Association for Research in Otolaryngology. 1995; p. 167.
74. Newman CW, Jacobson GP, Spitzer JB. Development of the Tinnitus Handicap Inventory. Arch Otolaryngol Head Neck Surg. 1996;122(2):143-8.
75. Meikle MB, Henry JA, Griest SE, et al. The tinnitus functional index: development of a new clinical measure for chronic, intrusive tinnitus. Ear Hear. 2012;33(2):153-76.
76. Dobie RA, Sakai CS, Sullivan MD, et al. Antidepressant treatment of tinnitus patients: report of a randomized clinical trial and clinical prediction of benefit. Am J Otol. 1993;14(1):18-23.
77. Coelho C, Figueiredo R, Frank E, et al. Reduction of tinnitus severity by the centrally acting muscle relaxant cyclobenzaprine: an open-label pilot study. Audiol Neurootol. 2012;17(3):179-88.
78. Vanneste S, Figueiredo R, De Ridder D. Treatment of tinnitus with cyclobenzaprine: an open-label study. Int J Clin Pharmacol Ther. 2012;50(5):338-44.
79. Witsell DL, Hannley MT, Stinnet S, et al. Treatment of tinnitus with gabapentin: a pilot study. Otol Neurotol. 2007; 28(1):11-5.
80. Piccirillo JF, Finnell J, Vlahiotis A, et al. Relief of idiopathic subjective tinnitus: is gabapentin effective? Arch Otolaryngol Head Neck Surg. 2007;133(4):390-7.
81. Dehkordi MA1, Abolbashari S, Taheri R, et al. Efficacy of gabapentin on subjective idiopathic tinnitus: a randomized, double-blind, placebo-controlled trial. Ear Nose Throat J. 2011;90(4):150-8.
82. Brantberg K. Paroxysmal staccato tinnitus: a carbamazepine responsive hyperactivity dysfunction symptom of the eighth cranial nerve. J Neurol Neurosurg Psychiatry. 2010; 81(4):451-5.
83. Azevedo AA, Figueiredo RR. Tinnitus treatment with acamprosate: double-blind study. Braz J Otorhinolaryngol. 2005; 71(5):618-23.
84. Sharma DK, Kaur S, Singh J, et al. Role of acamprosate in sensorineural tinnitus. Indian J Pharmacol. 2012;44(1): 93-6. doi: 10.4103/0253-7613.91876.
85. Hester TO, Theilman G, Green W, et al. Cyclandelate in the management of tinnitus: a randomized, placebo-controlled study. Otolaryngol Head Neck Surg. 1998;118(3 Pt 1): 329-32.
86. Hurtuk A, Dome C, Holloman CH, et al. Melatonin: can it stop the ringing? Ann Otol Rhinol Laryngol. 2011;120(7): 433-40.
87. Megwalu UC, Finnell JE, Piccirillo JF. The effects of melatonin on tinnitus and sleep. Otolaryngol Head Neck Surg. 2006;134(2):210-3.
88. Hilton MP, Zimmermann EF, Hunt WT. Ginkgo biloba for tinnitus. Cochrane Database Syst Rev. 2013;28;3:CD003852.

CHAPTER

21

Meniere's Disease

Daniel H Coelho, Richard A Goldman

INTRODUCTION

When Prospere Meniere presented his landmark paper to the French Imperial Academy of Medicine in January 1861, the suggestion that hearing and balance were both controlled by labyrinthine organs was considered extremely controversial and therefore poorly received. It would take 40 years before Hallpike and Portman histologically confirmed endolymphatic dilation in patients with episodic vertigo, fluctuating hearing, and low-pitched tinnitus.

The capricious nature of the disease has made it difficult to prospectively determine the efficacy of therapeutic intervention, and thus the treatment of Meniere's disease (MD) is primarily empiric. Absence of robust prospective, randomized, placebo-controlled studies has led to a variety of medical and surgical therapeutic interventions of uncertain value.[1,14] Given the therapeutic void, the aims of management of MD are limited to (1) reducing the number and severity of acute attacks of vertigo; (2) aborting or ameliorating hearing loss (HL) and tinnitus associated with such attacks; (3) alleviating any chronic symptoms (e.g. tinnitus and imbalance); and (4) preventing progression of the disease, in particular, the loss of hearing and balance that characterizes the disorder.[34] The authors prefer the term "management" in lieu of "treatment" because currently there is no known treatment option that adequately addresses all four of the above criteria.

This chapter serves to thoroughly review current understanding of MD, including pathogenesis, clinical presentation, evaluation, management, and prognosis.

PATHOGENESIS, HISTOLOGY, AND GENETICS

Even today, over 150 years since Meniere first described the now eponymous disorder, MD continues to be incompletely understood, and the true etiology and pathophysiology of this entity remain elusive. Histologically, the hallmark of MD is endolymphatic hydrops on postmortem temporal bone specimens, which was first demonstrated in simultaneous work by Hallpike and Cairns and Yamakawa in 1938.[2] This finding is characterized by dilation and distention of the membranous labyrinth and classic depictions demonstrate bulging of Reissner membrane encroaching upon the scala vestibuli in cross-sectional slides (Fig. 21.1). Dilation can be severe with membranes contacting the bony walls with near total obliteration of perilymphatic space. Similar distention of the utricle and saccule can also be seen.

Presumably aberrant fluid homeostasis causes these pathologic findings as well as the accompanying inner ear dysfunction, but the etiology of hydrops and precise mechanisms to account for the symptom complex remain unknown. An early theory was that disruption or blockage of longitudinal endolymphatic flow from the cochlea to the endolymphatic sac resulted in hydrops. This theory was supported by Kimura's guinea pig model, in which endolymphatic hydrops could be experimentally induced by surgical ablation of the endolymphatic sac.[3]

The rupture theory proposed by Schuknecht then attempted to account for how hydrops might result in the

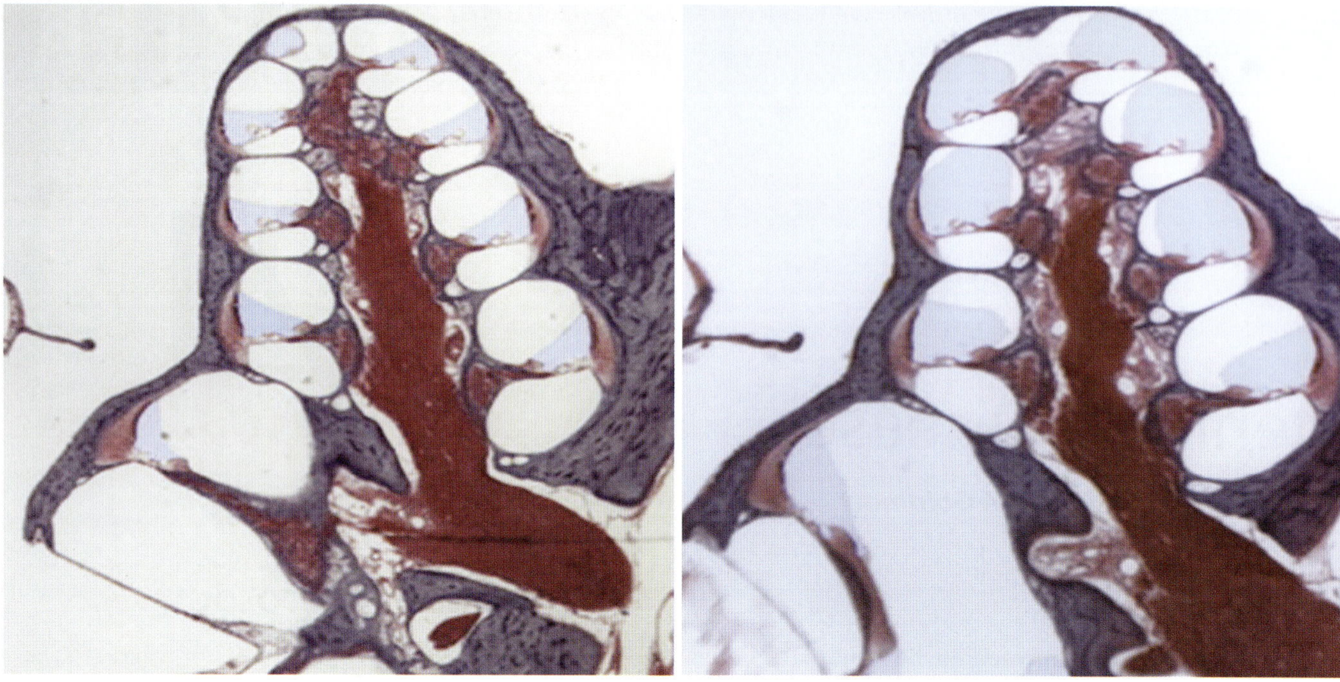

Fig. 21.1: Mid-modiolar sections through the normal guinea pig cochlea (left) and from a cochlea in which endolymphatic hydrops was induced by surgical ablation of the endolymphatic duct and sac (right). The endolymphatic space has been colored blue to highlight the endolymph enlargement into the perilymphatic space of scala vestibuli resulting from the distension of Reissner's membrane. Histology of these specimens was performed in the laboratory of Dr R Kimura as part of a collaborative study. From Salt AN, Plontke SK. Endolymphatic hydrops: pathophysiology and experimental models. Otolaryngol Clin North Am. 2010;43(5):971-83.

characteristic symptoms. In histologic studies Schuknecht demonstrated evidence of prior rupture and healing in Reissner membrane leading to the hypothesis that ruptures in the distended membrane allowed for mixing of perilymph and endolymph, thereby resulting in nerve paralysis and the characteristic episodic symptoms. Vertigo subsequently improved with healing of the rupture and restoration of the normal electrochemical gradient.[4] Other theories of endolymph or potassium leakage have also been proposed to cause symptoms in a similar fashion.

Although intuitive and appealing, the above theories are likely drastic oversimplifications and belie the complexity of inner ear physiology. Studies of endolymphatic fluid dynamics indicate that there is very little longitudinal endolymphatic flow, suggesting that radial flow in the endolymphatic space largely regulates endolymphatic volume.[5] The ionic composition is maintained by the stria vascularis with the movement of water largely following osmotic gradients.

Additional research has called into question the presumed causal relationship between endolymphatic hydrops and Meniere's symptoms. In a large series of temporal bone studies, endolymphatic hydrops was seen in all patients with MD but all cases of endolymphatic hydrops did not have MD.[6] In reviewing the above and related basic science research, Semaan et al. suggest that more subtle and yet undetermined cellular and biochemical perturbations may result in the cochleovestibular dysfunction characteristic of MD and endolymphatic hydrops could be a related epiphenomenon.[7]

Whether endolymphatic hydrops causes MD or whether it arises secondarily, the nature of the aberrant homeostatic mechanisms at work remains an area of conjecture and a variety of potentially contributing factors have been implicated including immunogenic, infectious, hormonal, and genetic. A subset of patients with a familial form of MD representing up to 15% of the patient population has been described and led to a variety of genetic studies that have yet to convincingly identify candidate gene associations.[8] Some of the genes investigated have included the COCH gene, KCNE gene family which relates to potassium channels, and AQP2, an aquaporin gene. Other interesting associations, including the high prevalence of allergy and migraine among MD patients have also been described.[9]

A common supposition is that a variety of genetic polymorphisms may predispose patients to development of the disease state when combined with a variety of environmental factors. Such a complex mechanism of disease could certainly account for the clinical heterogeneity of MD, as well as the scientific difficulty in determining a single etiology.

Research in MD has focused on what Semaan et al. described as five principal areas: genetics and autoimmunity, intralabyrinthine fluid dynamics, cellular and molecular alterations, electrophysiologic tests in diagnosis, and creating ideal animal models.[7] With recent advances in molecular biology and molecular genetics, great strides have been made in understanding MD, although no one single theory of pathogenesis has yet to become universally accepted. This inability to provide a unifying explanation for the clinical picture of MD prevents any significant translational application for more targeted and effective treatments. Lack of a unifying or single etiology likely reflects the clinically and genetically heterogeneous nature of MD and thus the lack of efficacy of any single treatment. Perhaps the most important result of ongoing research will be the earlier identification of patients with MD so that possible preventative measures can be taken.

CLINICAL FINDINGS

The prevalence of MD varies widely according to published literature, ranging from 15 to 157 per 100,000.[10] It is unlikely that these differences are the results of geographic distributions of disease, but rather due to reporting biases. Bilateral disease is found in 10% of patients with MD at initial diagnosis; with disease progression, it may be found in more than 40%.[11]

The typical onset of disease is middle age, though MD has been reported in children as young as 4 and as old as the 90s.[12] The peak incidence of MD is in the 40- to 60-year-old age group.[10] The mean age among treatment groups in some studies ranged from 49 to 67 years. These data suggest there is generally a fairly long lag-time of several years between the onset of symptoms and diagnosis/management. MD appears to be more common in women (1.3:1 to 1.8:1) and whites, though reporting biases might exist as these two populations are more likely to seek medical care.[13] For most patients, MD remains symptomatic for a limited duration of time, approximately 5 to 15 years. Once the period of "active" MD has passed, patients can still be left with significant hearing loss and disabling vestibular hypofunction that can last for the remainder of their lives.

Although the classic presentation of MD is marked by episodes of recurrent vertigo, fluctuating low-frequency sensorineural hearing loss, aural fullness, and roaring tinnitus, in reality the presentation can be highly variable and its clinical course characterized by acute exacerbation and spontaneous remission. The diagnosis is based on clinical presentation because there is no definitive objective test available. To define the certainty of diagnosis of MD, the American Academy of Otolaryngology—Head and Neck Surgery (AAO-HNS) promulgated diagnostic and reporting guidelines, published in 1972, 1985, and 1995, but these remain poorly or incorrectly used (Tables 21.1 to 21.4).[1] Although nearly 80% of the 128 papers on MD published from 1988 to 1999 used the AAO-HNS Committee on Hearing and Equilibrium (CHE) criteria, only 50% did so correctly.[14]

The vertigo attacks associated with MD are usually severe and can last from 30 min to 5 or more hours. They can be associated with nystagmus (horizontal or rotatory) and frequently involve nausea and/or vomiting. In approximately 10% of cases, vertigo attacks are accompanied by sudden drop attacks without loss of consciousness. This variant, often referred to as "Crisis of Tumarkin", can be quite dramatic. Following an attack patients generally feel unsteady and fatigued for hours to days. Many

Table 21.1: Diagnostic Scale of Meniere's Disease of American Academy of Otolaryngology—Head and Neck Surgery Committee on Hearing and Equilibrium*

- Certain Meniere's disease
  - Definitive Meniere's disease, plus histopathologic confirmation
- Definitive Meniere's disease
  - Two or more episodes of vertigo of at least 20 minutes
  - Audiometrically documented hearing loss on at least one occasion
  - Tinnitus and aural fullness
- Probable Meniere's disease
  - One definite episode of vertigo
  - Audiometrically documented hearing loss on at least one occasion
  - Tinnitus and aural fullness
- Possible Meniere's disease
  - Episodic vertigo without documented hearing loss
  - Sensorineural hearing loss, fluctuating or fixed, with disequilibrium, but without definitive episodes

*In all cases, other causes must be excluded.

From Coelho DH, Lalwani AK. Medical management of Meniere's disease. Laryngoscope. 2008;118:1100.

Originally from Committee on Hearing and Equilibrium guidelines for the diagnosis and evaluation of therapy in Meniere's disease. American Academy of Otolaryngology—Head and Neck Foundation, Inc. Otolaryngol Head Neck Surg. 1995;113:181-5.

patients are afflicted "out of the blue", whereas other patients can predict their attacks based on weather, time of year, psychosocial stressors, or menstrual cycle. Another rare variant, known as Lermoyez syndrome, is characterized by improvement in hearing during the peak of vertigo symptoms.

During attacks, patients will report hearing loss, aural fullness, and tinnitus. When documented, audiograms will display low-frequency sensorineural loss. The low-frequency loss is what accounts for complaints of nonpulsatile "roaring" or "ocean-like" tinnitus, rather than the more common high-pitched ringing. Between attacks the hearing returns to baseline and the aural fullness and tinnitus resolve. Nonetheless, the trend over time often results in progressive sensorineural hearing loss.

Of note, the terms MD, Meniere's syndrome, and endolymphatic hydrops are frequently and incorrectly used interchangeably. They are in fact separate and distinct entities. All patients have endolymphatic hydrops—when due to a known cause (allergic, auto-immune, familial, post-traumatic, etc.), the associated constellation of symptoms are referred to as Meniere's syndrome. Idiopathic endolymphatic hydrops is referred to as MD. Since definitive diagnosis requires histologic confirmation, we prefer the term MD.

Table 21.2: American Academy of Otolaryngology—Head and Neck Surgery Committee on Hearing and Equilibrium Criteria for Reporting Hearing in Meniere's Disease

Stage	*Four-tone average (dB)*
1	≤25
2	26–40
3	41–70
4	>70

From Coelho DH, Lalwani AK. Medical management of Meniere's disease. Laryngoscope. 2008;118:1100.

Originally from Committee on Hearing and Equilibrium guidelines for the diagnosis and evaluation of therapy in Meniere's disease. American Academy of Otolaryngology—Head and Neck Foundation, Inc. Otolaryngol Head Neck Surg. 1995;113:181-5.

Staging is based on four-tone average (arithmetic mean rounded to, nearest whole number) of pure-tone thresholds at 0.5, 1, 2, and 3 kHz of worst audiogram during interval 6 months before treatment. This is same audiogram that is used as baseline evaluation to determine hearing outcome from treatment. Staging should be applied only to cases of definite or certain Meniere's disease.

EVALUATION

A variety of diagnostic tests are available to help in the differentiation of MD from other, similar conditions. Although no one test is specific enough to definitively diagnose MD, laboratory, genetic, electrophysiologic, and radiographic testing can be helpful when the etiology is in question.

Blood tests are generally not used in the diagnosis of MD, but can be helpful in excluding similar conditions. Thyroid stimulating hormones (hypothyroidism), Lyme titres (Lyme disease), fluorescent treponemal antibodies (syphilis), complete blood cell counts (leukemia), and glucose levels (diabetes) can all be helpful in ruling out other causes of fluctuating hearing or imbalance. Erythrocyte sedimentation rate, anti-nuclear antibodies, and other indicators of potential autoimmune inner ear disease can

Table 21.3: American Academy of Otolaryngology—Head and Neck Surgery Committee on Hearing and Equilibrium Criteria for Reporting Function in Meniere's Disease: Functional Level Scale

	Regarding my current state of overall function, not just during attacks (check the ONE that best applies)
1	My dizziness has no effect on my activities at all
2	When I am dizzy I have to stop what I am doing for a while, but it soon passes and I can resume activities. I continue to work, drive, and engage in any activity I choose without restriction. I have not changed any plans or activities to accommodate my dizziness
3	When I am dizzy I have to stop what I am doing for a while, but it does pass and I can resume activities. I continue to work, drive, and engage in most activities I choose, but I have had to change some plans and make some allowance for my dizziness
4	I am able to work, drive, travel, take care of a family, or engage in most activities, but I must exert a great deal of effort to do so. I must constantly make adjustments in my activities and budget my energies. I am barely making it
5	I am unable to work, drive, or take care of a family. I am unable to do most of the active things that I used to. Even essential activities must be limited. I am disabled
6	I have been disabled for 1 year or longer and/or I receive compensation (money) because of my dizziness or balance problem

From Coelho DH, Lalwani AK. Medical management of Meniere's disease. Laryngoscope. 2008;118:1100.

Originally from Committee on Hearing and Equilibrium guidelines for the diagnosis and evaluation of therapy in Meniere's disease. American Academy of Otolaryngology—Head and Neck Foundation, Inc. Otolaryngol Head Neck Surg. 1995;113:181-5.

Table 21.4: American Academy of Otolaryngology—Head and Neck Surgery Committee on Hearing and Equilibrium Summary of Reporting Guidelines in Meniere's Disease

Numerical value	*Class*
0 (complete control of definitive spells)	A
1–40	B
41–80	C
81–120	D
>120	E
Secondary treatment initiated because of disability from vertigo	F

From Coelho DH, Lalwani AK. Medical management of Meniere's disease. Laryngoscope. 2008;118:1100.

Originally from Committee on Hearing and Equilibrium guidelines for the diagnosis and evaluation of therapy in Meniere's disease. American Academy of Otolaryngology - Head and Neck Foundation, Inc. Otolaryngol Head Neck Surg. 1995;113:181-5.

Numerical value = $(X/Y) \times 100$, rounded to nearest whole number, where X is average number of definitive spells per month for 6 months 18–24 months after therapy and Y is average number of definitive spells per month for 6 months before therapy.

also be helpful. Along those lines, allergy testing should be considered in patients with allergic components by history.

Audiograms are essential in the diagnosis and management of patients with MD. Although a wide range of hearing acuity can be seen, ranging from normal to profound sensorineural hearing loss, the classic pattern is that of fluctuating low-frequency sensorineural hearing loss. This is due to the fact that hydrops affects the cochlear apex more than the base. Interestingly, patients with mild low-frequency hearing loss often times do not complain of hearing impairment. Note that for some patients, use of inserts during the hearing test can give a false mild low-frequency hearing loss or exaggerate existing low-frequency hearing loss. We recommend using headphones for all patients with the potential diagnosis of MD. Ultimately, serial audiograms may play the most important diagnostic role, as fluctuation and/or progression can be seen over time.

Electrocochleography (ECoG) is another test that can be helpful in confirming suspicions of endolymphatic hydrops. ECoG measures and compares the summating potential with the action potential of the auditory nerve in response to auditory stimuli. A ratio of 40% or more may suggest elevated endolymphatic pressure, though this test has limited sensitivity and in our practice, when used, is more confirmatory than diagnostic. Generally, ECoG is most sensitive during an active episode or in advanced disease.

Electronystagmography or videonystagmography can be used to differentiate central from peripheral vestibulopathies. In MD, the caloric component can be particular helpful. Although this subtest only quantifies the function of the horizontal semicircular canals, it can be helpful in determining laterality. During the acute phase, inner ear irritation may result in ipsilateral fast-phase nystagmus, whereas chronic hypofunction typically results in diminished responses or contralateral fast-phase nystagmus. In addition to laterality, calorics can be helpful in guiding decisions to proceed with vestibular ablation (chemical or surgical) by giving information on the presumably unaffected ear.

Vestibular evoked myogenic potentials (VEMP) can be recorded when bone-conduction stimulates the saccule, causing contraction of contralateral neck muscles (cervical or cVEMP) or the extraocular muscles (ocular or oVEMP). Frequency specific VEMPs can be helpful in determining laterality in early stage, audiometrically normal MD, or may indicate the potential for the development of bilateral MD.[15] VEMPs can also be helpful in monitoring the progress of low-dose gentamicin injections.[16] The use of VEMPs in clinical practice has been well described but as of yet is not widely accepted.[17]

RADIOLOGY

Historically imaging has had no role in confirming diagnosis of MD. Traditionally, CT, and later MRI were used to rule out other causes of asymmetric hearing loss and vertigo that could mimic MD.[18] Advances in MRI resolution and sequencing, however, have allowed for improved evaluation of the microscopic anatomy of the inner ear and the possibility of visualizing endolymphatic hydrops in vivo.

This capability is made possible by the selective diffusion of gadolinium contrast agents into perilymph and not endolymph. Endolymphatic hydrops can thus be visualized as an enlarged signal void from the scala media which is bounded by the enhancing scalae vestibuli and tympani and this was first demonstrated by Niyazov et al in 2001 in the guinea pig model.[18a] A key experimental advance has been the use of intratympanic gadolinium which affords higher concentrations of contrast in perilymph and in 2007 Nakashima et al. reported successful visualization of endolymphatic hydrops in human patients with MD following intratympanic gadolinium injection.[19] While no adverse effects of dilute intratympanic gadolinium have been reported, more rigorous safety trials are required prior to wide adoption of this technique in clinical practice. Hydrops has since been demonstrated in humans using intravenous gadolinium as well, but despite advanced MRI technology, double doses of contrast were required.[20]

The potential value of imaging in MD was demonstrated by a study that showed much higher sensitivity of MRI with intratympanic contrast (95%) versus combined glycerol test and ECoG (75%) in the diagnosis of MD.[21] Further advances in technology and standardization of protocols may allow for more quantitative and objective measurement of endolymphatic hydrops. With this possibility, MRI visualization of the in vivo human ear may come to play a key role in the future diagnosis of MD, as well as provide new insights into the pathophysiology, natural history, and efficacy of therapeutic interventions.

MANAGEMENT

MD should be considered a chronic condition for which interventions do not eliminate the underlying cause of disease. Moreover, no medical treatments appear to result in long-term preservation of hearing.[22] Nonetheless, despite the relative paucity of evidence-based research, current medical regimens can control disease (as defined by vertiginous attacks) in approximately 80% of patients (Flowchart 21.1).

ACUTE MANAGEMENT

In the acute setting, vestibular suppressants and antiemetic medication have been used to control acute spells of vertigo. They can be divided into different classes, including benzodiazepines, antihistamines, anticholinergics, and antidopaminergics. Benzodiazepines act on the cerebellar GABA-ergic system that inhibits vestibular nuclei response. In the United States, benzodiazepines are favored for their vestibular suppression as well as anxiolytic properties. However, because benzodiazepines may impair vestibular compensation, their use beyond acute vertiginous episodes should be limited. Antihistamines, potent antivertiginous, and antiemetic medications, including meclizine and dimenhydrinate, have demonstrated efficacy in MD when compared with placebo.[23,24] However, care must be taken in patients with glaucoma or prostate disease because antihistamines can have excessive anticholinergic effects. Scopolamine is a naturally occurring belladonna alkaloid with anticholinergic properties that is commonly used to prevent nausea and vomiting associated with motion sickness. For the nausea associated with vertigo, a variety of anti-emetics including metoclopramide, promethazine, prochlorperazine, and ondansetron can be used. Many of these medications are available as a suppository making them especially useful for patients unable to tolerate oral intake.

In lending some credence to the immunogenic theory of MD, some authors promote the use of oral or intratympanic steroids in the acute setting to lessen the severity of attacks and possibly even promote earlier recovery of hearing, though this remains controversial.[1,25] Severe episodes can be treated with burst courses of oral steroids tapered over 5–14 days. The administration of all these and other medications, alone or in combination, have all been described and tried in the management of acute MD, although, to date, little to no strong evidence exists for any of these practices. In addition to medication, it is important to remember the role of rest and hydration (especially with emesis) as a therapeutic adjuvant in the acute setting.

CHRONIC MANAGEMENT

Lifestyle Adjustment, Avoidance of Triggers

Some patients with MD note acute exacerbations of their condition with certain triggers. Offending agents include high salt intake, caffeine, alcohol, nicotine, stress, fatigue, monosodium glutamate, and allergy. Avoidance of these triggers can play a crucial role in the prevention of Meniere's attacks. A normal hormonal milieu has also been implicated in MD; an association between MD and menstruation has been suggested, although the clinical relevance of such a correlation remains to be elucidated.[26] Emotional stress has been associated with increased frequency and severity of attacks.[27] The true relationship between stress, vertigo, and MD remains to be elucidated. Nonetheless, structured psychological support has been recommended in the management of MD.[28,29] According to Kinney et al.[28] encouragement by family support systems, social support systems, and MD support groups may significantly relieve some emotional stresses caused by MD. Thus, identification and avoidance of environmental or psychological triggers can play an important role in the management of MD. Unfortunately, for the majority of patients, no such specific trigger can be identified, and further intervention is usually necessary.

Flowchart 21.1: Algorithm for the treatment of Meniere's disease. From Coelho DH, Lalwani AK. Medical management of Meniere's disease. Laryngoscope. 2008;118:1105.

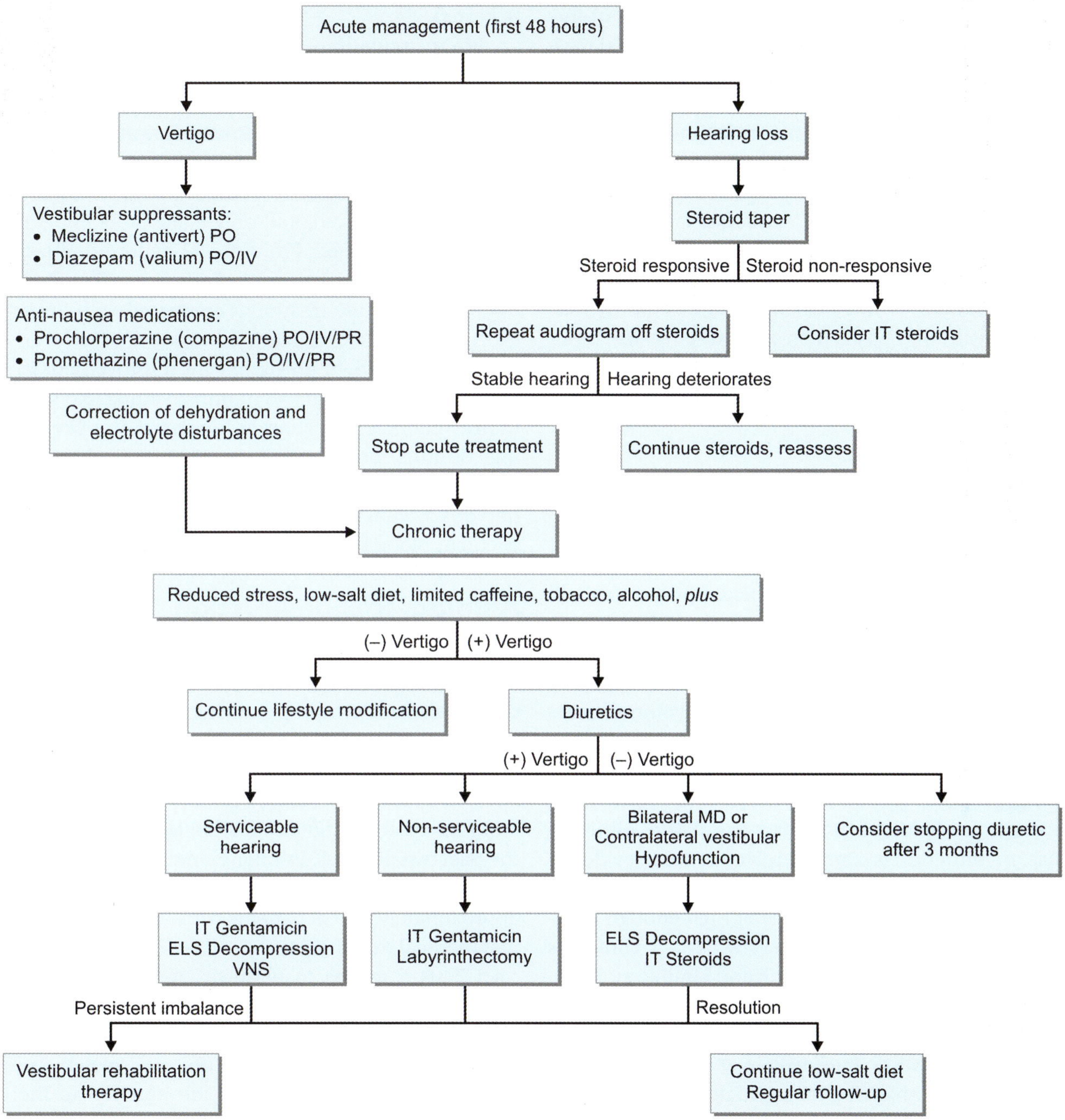

Salt Restriction

Anecdotally, some patients have described acute symptoms after high salt exposure, and treatment protocols based on sodium restriction have been a foundation of the management of MD since the 1930s.[30] Recent evidence has suggested that the effects of sodium on endolymphatic hydrops are far more complex than mere fluctuations in endolymphatic levels.[31] Despite the incomplete understanding of its role in developing hydrops, sodium restriction continues to be widely supported in both the literature and clinical practice. Claes and Van de Heyning have suggested that all patients should observe a low-salt diet with an intake of no more than 1 g of NaCl-enhanced salt per day, although no evidence for the benefit of this regimen was reviewed.[32] Various other regimens have been proposed, most restricting daily dietary sodium intake to < 2000 mg, though to date not one published study supports the efficacy of sodium restriction alone in the management of MD. Patients are advised to eliminate the use of salt at the table and limit its use in cooking and baking. Herbs and spices can be used for taste enhancement. Patients must be counseled to carefully inspect product nutritional information labels not only for sodium content but also for serving size. Many high-sodium products show low listings based on a small serving size. Input of a nutritionist should be suggested in diet modification, as other dietary factors have been implicated in MD as well.[33]

Pharmacologic Therapy

For some patients with MD, avoidance of certain triggers and dietary modification will result in adequate control of the disease. However, a significant proportion will require additional therapeutic intervention. Diuretics are frequently used along with or as an alternative to dietary salt restriction to reduce total body salt and consequently total body fluid. By decreasing the overall volume status of a patient, diuretics are believed to decrease the endolymphatic pressure and volume, or hydrops, of the inner ear. Other proposed mechanisms include the reduction in endolymph production at the stria vascularis. Although the use of diuretics is commonplace, strong evidence to support their use is limited. A recent meta-analysis of diuretics in MD found "no trials of high enough quality" to meet the standard set for review.[34] Many clinicians refer to the early studies of Klockhoff and Lindblom, which showed significant improvement in vertigo, HL, and overall quality of life when hydrochlorothiazide was compared with placebo.[35] However, Ruckenstein et al.'s re-evaluation of Klockhoff and Linblom's data found no statistical difference in measures of hearing, tinnitus, vertigo, or general condition between diuretic and placebo groups.[36] The only published randomized controlled trial (RCT) on the subject showed that after 17 weeks of Dyazide (triamterene and hydrochlorothiazide) treatment, patients had significantly improved vestibular symptoms but no change in HL or tinnitus.[37] Some clinicians have promoted the simultaneous use of diuretics together with salt restriction. With stabilization of the disease (marked by a symptom-free period of 6–12 months), patients can be slowly weaned off their particular regimen. If necessary, therapy can be restarted.

Microcirculation changes leading to ischemia of the stria vascularis has been thought to contribute to MD. Vasodilators have been used by some to relieve ischemia, with improved cochlear microcirculation leading to reduced endolymphatic pressure or possible inhibition of vestibular nuclei activity.[38] Nonetheless, not one RCT of histamine was found, and only a few RCTs of betahistine have been published. Fraysse et al. reported reduction in vertigo frequency, severity, and duration of vertigo after 60 days of betahistine treatment compared with flunarizine, a cerebrally active calcium antagonist.[39] However, other studies have shown no significant improvement in vertigo over the long-term (> 3 months) setting. No significant improvement, either short or long term, was seen in hearing, tinnitus, or aural fullness.[40] Most likely, any beneficial effects of vasodilators result from nonspecific central nervous system suppression rather than a direct effect on cochlear blood flow.

Aminoglycoside Ablation

The aminoglycosides are toxic to the inner ear; streptomycin and gentamicin are selectively vestibulotoxic and destroy the endolymph-producing dark cells in the ampullary crista.[41] These properties of aminoglycosides have been harnessed to treat vertigo associated with MD. In 1956, Schuknecht described middle ear perfusion with an aminoglycoside antibiotic for the treatment of MD. Over the past two decades, intratympanic gentamicin (ITG) has become a common weapon in the arsenal addressing the approximately 10% of patients with MD refractive to maximal medical treatment.

ITG is a means to perform chemical labyrinthectomy that essentially exploits the vestibulotoxic properties of gentamicin. It can be delivered to the middle ear via myringotomy, tympanostomy tube, microwick, or microcatheter. The exact method of introduction to the inner ear may come through the round window membrane itself, the annular ligament, or vascular channels.[42] Once in the inner ear, the mechanism of vestibulotoxicity remains incompletely understood. Only one published report of histopathologic examination of the vestibular end organs in a patient with MD exists, which showed severe atrophy of the neuroepithelium of the semicircular canal cristae ampullares with undifferentiated cells, fibrosis, and edema of the stroma.[43]

The large number of published reports on the efficacy of ITG has led to widespread adoption of its use and a relative abandonment of surgical ablation. However, a note of caution was raised by Cohen-Kerem and colleagues in their meta-analysis of published studies using ITG as a sole treatment modality and using American Academy of Otolaryngology—Head and Neck Surgery (AAO-HNS) reporting guidelines for MD: not a single acceptable double-blind or blinded prospective control trial was identified.[44] Variations in concentration, dose, frequency, and duration all limit standardization and comparison of results. Therefore, little consensus exists for the optimal protocols for delivery, even in the rare occurrence when outcomes measures are standardized. Hopefully, ongoing clinical trials will address this shortcoming.

In patients with unilateral MD, the authors prefer to use the low-dose method described by Harner et al.[45] The procedure is office-based using either lidocaine injection or topical phenol for tympanic membrane anesthesia. Unbuffered gentamicin sulfate at a concentration of 40 mg/cc is drawn into a 1-mL tuberculin syringe. A 31/2 inch, 25-gauge needle is attached, and approximately 0.5–0.75 mL are injected into the middle ear space. A second needle hole is necessary to release middle ear air to allow for adequate injection (Fig. 21.2). Patients are then left supine for 30 min and instructed to keep water out of their ear for 2 weeks. Patients return in 1 month when an audiogram is obtained. Such intervention resulted in a 76% improvement in vertigo and no change in hearing at 4 years postinjection. Approximately, 15–20% of patients require a second ITG injection usually at 1-month interval; a third injection is rarely required. This low-dose method is rarely associated with hearing loss.

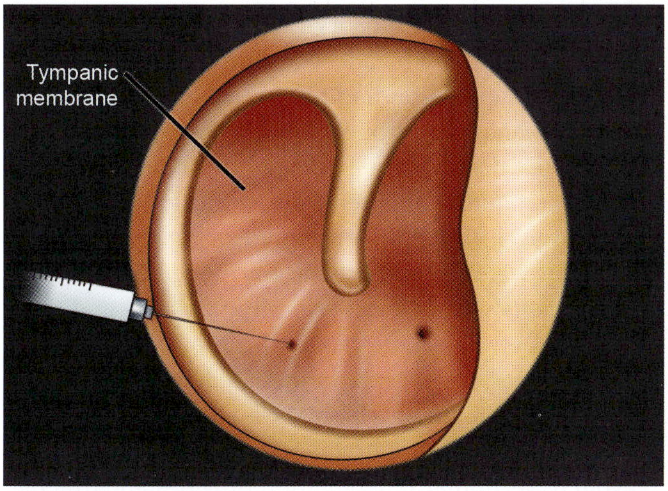

Fig. 21.2: Transtympanic perfusion technique, right ear.

While easy to use, ITG should be used with caution. Given that 20% of patients develop bilateral disease, the risk of bilateral labyrinthine hypofunction during patient's lifetime is high. The resultant disequilibrium and oscillopsia can be incapacitating and irreversible. VEMP testing may be useful in identifying patients with unilateral symptoms that actually have subclinical contralateral (bilateral) disease. In patients with bilateral MD, we favor the use of intratympanic steroids or nonablative surgery (e.g. endolymphatic sac decompression).

Steroids

The concept of MD as an inflammatory or immune-mediated disease has led to the use of corticosteroids in the management of its symptoms. In addition to immune and inflammatory regulation, corticosteroids are known to affect carbohydrate, electrolyte, protein, and lipid metabolism, making exact physiologic effects impossible to gauge. Furthermore, the discovery of glucocorticoid receptors in the inner ear suggests that steroids may also affect fluid homeostasis.[46] Nonetheless, the use of steroids in MD is largely empiric, based on successes of this technique in patients with sudden sensorineural HL, autoimmune HL, and tinnitus. More recently, despite the absence of strong evidence, intratympanic steroids have gained popularity both in the treatment of sudden sensorineural HL and in MD. Similar to ITG, the advantages are numerous, including ease of administration, avoidance of surgery, contraindications to systemic therapy (e.g. patients with hypertension and diabetes), intolerance of systemic therapy (insomnia, gastrointestinal disturbances, etc.), salvage therapy when systemic treatment fails, and selection of the active ear for treatment. Concentrations of steroids in the inner ear after intratympanic administration far exceed those seen in systemic administrations.[47,48] Complications include pain, short-lasting vertigo, otitis media, tympanic membrane perforation, vertigo (temporary or permanent), and HL. Optimal drug doses, schedule, duration, and means of delivery to the inner ear have yet to be standardized, and reporting of complications has been inconsistent. The relatively few prospective studies that have been conducted suggest that although vertigo symptoms may improve, hearing and tinnitus do not significantly change. Silverstein et al. reported a 72% rate of substantial or complete vertigo control at 18 months, although this is not significantly different from ITG or endolymphatic sac decompression.[49] Lack of effect on hearing is in contrast with the anecdotal evidence that intratympanic steroids are effective in reversing HL in sudden sensorineural HL suggest different pathophysiologies for these two disorders. In MD patients in whom hearing improvement/preservation is not of primary concern or in those who have failed other medical therapies, intratympanic steroid injection may provide substantial benefit prior to more aggressive surgical options. Clearly, more prospective and controlled studies are needed to fully understand and use this treatment option.

Complementary and Alternative Medicines

Patients with suboptimal improvement, as well as patients who have responded to allopathic treatment, are increasingly turning to complementary and alternative medicines (CAM) as both adjunct and alternative to traditional management. Anecdotal evidence abounds attesting to benefits of gingko biloba, niacin, bioflavonoids, lipoflavonoids, ginger root, and a host of other herbal supplements. Acupuncture, acupressure, yoga, and Tai Chi have long been used in the management of vertigo, nausea, and dysequilibrium. Although no evidence exists on the efficacy of these modalities or for the existence of these associations, the otolaryngologist must be aware that many patients with MD have investigated or are using these options. As early as 1998, Eisenberg et al. showed that 42% of patients have used or are using CAM, and 75% of them do not tell their physician.[50] It is therefore imperative that the clinician asks his or her patients regarding the use of CAM and attempts to integrate viable CAM strategies with proven therapeutic options to create a treatment plan that is effective, safe, and meaningful to the patient.

Devices

A common complaint of patients with MD is that symptoms can wax and wane depending on ambient pressure changes. Early investigators of this phenomenon postulated that inducement of positive pressure changes to the inner ear could lead to increased exchange of inner ear fluids via the different communication routes. In 1986, Densert et al. created a placebo controlled, randomized clinical study of 39 definitive MD patients in whom they showed electrocochleographic parameters were improved by the application of positive pressure pulses of low amplitude in the middle ear.[51] These and similar findings laid the foundation for the development of a portable low-intensity alternating pressure generator worn in the external auditory canal. The first such device was designed in Sweden and, since 2000, is now marketed in the United States as the Meniett device (Medtronic Xomed, Jacksonville, FL). In 2006, Gates et al. reported their results of a long-term follow-up clinical trial of the Meniett device for patients with classic, unilateral MD unresponsive to traditional medical treatment.[52] For the long term, the authors found a gradual improvement in vertigo for most but not all participants. The Meniett offers an attractive option to patients with MD who have failed medical treatment, although there are a few shortcomings. The device requires the insertion of a long-term tympanostomy tube, which itself has attendant complications, including middle and external ear infections. Moreover, use of the device without a patent tube can actually exacerbate symptoms because of middle ear pressure mechanics. No objective measurement of hearing has been performed, and subjective reports by patients suggest that hearing invariably does not improve in either the short or long term with the use of the Meniett device. The device is also expensive and rarely covered by insurers. In 2005, a manually operated device, the P-100 (Enttex, Hannover, Germany) debuted as a less-expensive alternative to the Meniett. However, little has been written about its efficacy.

Rehabilitation Therapy

There has been increasing interest in the use of vestibular rehabilitation in the management of vestibular dysfunction. The therapy, an exercise-based group of activities aimed at maximizing central nervous system compensation, relies on plasticity, formation of internal models, learning of limits, and sensory weighting, so that patients can "recalibrate" their balance mechanisms. Traditionally, vestibular rehabilitation had not been frequently used in the acute management of MD owing to the intermittent nature of the disease. The patients originally referred for vestibular rehabilitation therapy were those who by medical or surgical ablation were cured of their vertiginous attacks but were left with persistent dysequilibrium. Yet, many patients with MD suffer from imbalance and disequilibrium between acute vertiginous spells and therefore could benefit from vestibular rehabilitation.[53] Furthermore, for those patients with MD who have exhausted the medical (or surgical) armamentarium or for those wishing to avoid it, vestibular rehabilitation provides an attractive option.

SURGICAL MANAGEMENT

When considering surgical intervention for MD, one must realize that the goal is primarily to improve quality of life because none of the surgical options result in significantly changed long-term hearing outcome. Simply, surgery does not address the underlying disease process, and therefore a "cure" is not possible. Using questionnaires, Soderman et al. found no difference in overall quality between patients treated conservatively, surgically, or with ITG.[54] Nonetheless, surgical intervention can play a valuable role in the management of patients with MD who fail to adequately respond to initial measures. Surgery is generally only considered after an adequate trial of medical management and then additional individual patient considerations must be taken into account when selecting appropriate surgical interventions—be they nondestructive (vestibular function preserving) or destructive (vestibular and/or hearing functioned sacrificed).

Nondestructive Surgery

Endolymphatic Sac Surgery

Endolymphatic sac surgeries, both decompression and shunting procedures, can be categorized as nondestructive interventions in that they are likely to preserve hearing and vestibular function and are generally considered as first-line surgical interventions. They may be considered in patients for whom destructive procedures may be ill advised, including those who continue to have serviceable hearing and those with bilateral disease. These procedures are performed via transmastoid approach that is extended to skeletonize the posterior semicircular canal and sigmoid sinus and expose the posterior fossa dura (Fig. 21.3). The endolymphatic sac is then identified and broadly exposed (decompression) and can be opened with placement of a shunting device, such as silastic sheeting. Theoretically, the shunt would allow excess endolymph to drain to the mastoid or subarachnoid space, depending on the nature of shunt placement. The previously discussed basic science research may suggest that such a theory supporting the rationale for these procedures is flawed. Additionally, a postmortem histological study of patients who had undergone endolymphatic sac surgery showed that the sac was not exposed or the shunt did not reach the lumen in 13 of 15 cases; interestingly 8 of these experienced relief from vertigo whereas the 2 in which the surgery appeared successful histologically did not experience relief.[55]

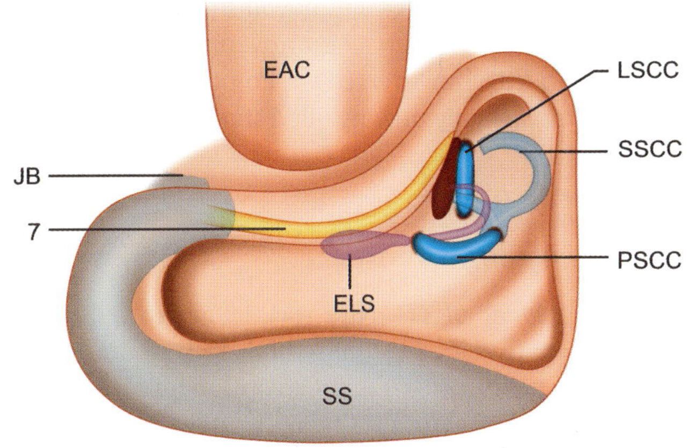

Fig. 21.3: Surgical anatomy of the endolymphatic sac, right ear. (EAC, external auditory canal; 7, facial nerve; JB, jugular bulb; ELS; endolymphatic sac; SSCC, superior semicircular canal; LSCC, lateral semicircular canal; PSCC, posterior semicircular canal; SS, sigmoid sinus).

Endolymphatic surgery remains among the more controversial topics in otology. While numerous series claim high success rates, a recent Cochrane review only identified two RCTs, both of which failed to demonstrate a benefit over control arms.[56] This review included the famous Danish sham study in which a simple mastoidectomy was performed in the control group and suggested that the significant improvement in both groups was largely due to a placebo effect. Other authors have claimed that errors in methodology and data analysis account for the failure to demonstrate benefit.

Given the paucity of evidence to suggest any long-term benefit in hearing and balance and the complexities of endolymphatic physiology, one possibility is that endolymphatic sac surgery hastens progression to a patient's natural endpoint.[57] If that is the case, then these procedures may still have a role in the management of vertigo in MD but that benefit remains unproven to modern standards of evidence-based medicine.

Novel Approaches

Additional nondestructive procedures aimed at symptomatic improvement in patients with refractory vertigo and MD have also been reported. Charpiot et al. reported a vertigo control rate of 75% and a hearing preservation rate of 82% following lateral canal plugging procedures.[58] In a retrospective review of 42 patients, Loader et al. reported statistically significant improvements in Dizziness Handicap Inventory postoperatively following stapedius and tensor tympani tenotomy.[59] It should also be noted that, while not a novel technique, tympanostomy tube placement has also been employed in the management of MD. The natural history of improvement in vertigo seen over time in MD, however, calls into question the benefit demonstrated by any uncontrolled study.

Destructive Surgery

Labyrinthectomy

With the advent of ITG, the role of ablative inner ear surgeries in the management of MD has diminished. Destructive procedures remain an option for patients with refractory vertigo who have failed gentamicin therapy or endolymphatic sac surgery. The goal of labyrinthectomy is the elimination of all vestibular function on the operated side at the expense of remaining hearing, if any. It can be performed with relatively little morbidity and is highly successful in controlling vertiginous episodes. It is generally not recommended in patients with serviceable hearing or in cases of bilateral disease due to the potential for bilateral vestibular loss. Transmastoid labyrinthectomy provides adequate access for the surgical ablation of the entirety of the bony and membranous labyrinth, while a transcanal approach requires blind probing and risks incomplete removal of all neuroepithelium and has generally fallen out of favor.

Vestibular Nerve Section

Vestibular neurectomy or nerve sectioning surgery is an additional option in the management of refractory vertigo in patients who continue to have serviceable hearing and have failed more conservative therapies (Fig. 21.4). This procedure may be performed by a middle fossa, retrolabyrinthine, or most commonly a retrosigmoid approach. While 98% vertigo control rates have been reported with 82% hearing preservation, these procedures have significantly higher morbidity when compared with labyrinthectomy. Higher rates of hearing preservation have also been reported. This procedure generally requires a craniotomy with subsequent intensive care monitoring and complications include facial nerve injury, CSF leak, and meningitis. Longer length of stay and period of disability, as well as higher cost have also been reported when compared to labyrinthectomy.[60]

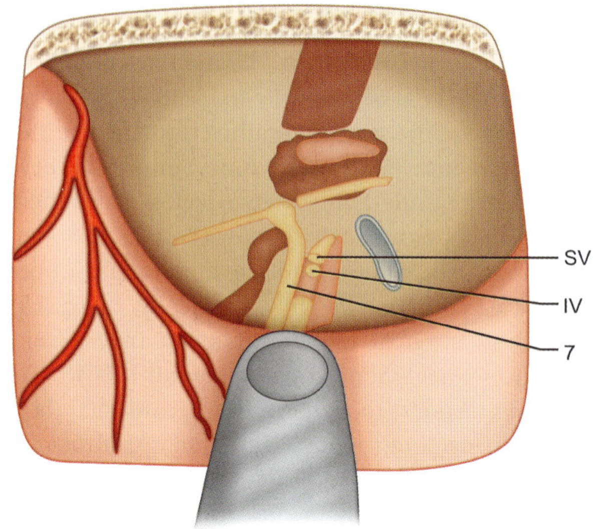

Fig. 21.4: Middle fossa approach to vestibular nerve section, right ear. (SV, superior vestibular nerve; IV, inferior vestibular nerve; 7, facial nerve).

Cochleosacculotomy

The indications for cochleosacculotomy are similar to those for labyrinthectomy and may be considered in patients deemed unfit for general anesthesia. In this procedure, a tympanomeatal flap is elevated and a right angle pick is introduced through the round window and toward the oval window. This maneuver is intended to disrupt the spiral lamina and fistulize the cochlear duct. While the procedure is simple to perform, it carries a high risk of hearing loss and its long-term efficacy is uncertain. As with transcanal labyrinthectomy, this technique has largely fallen out of favor.

PROGNOSIS

Although the management of vertigo is successful in most cases, hearing loss and tinnitus still represent a significant challenge for the patient and practitioner alike. Hearing aids are an important part of rehabilitation and should be considered for any patient with severe impairment and good compliance. However, given the fluctuating nature of HL in MD, compliance may be limited before hearing deterioration has stabilized. For patients with severe to profound loss, cochlear implants play an important role in the restoration of hearing.

Hearing aids may also prove beneficial when severe tinnitus is present, though Feenstra concluded that >95% of tinnitus in MD patients can be successfully managed with simple directive counseling.[61] Many other modalities have been proposed, none can be recommended because of lack of compelling medical evidence.

CONCLUSION

In the absence of relevant clinical studies, the management of MD remains empirical, with the use of lifestyle changes, pharmacotherapy, office-based procedures, and surgery. The development of transtympanic therapies represents a true advance in therapeutics that has largely supplanted surgical intervention. Only with increasing understanding through continued high-quality basic, translational, and clinical research can we shift our management paradigm from that of control to that of cure.

REFERENCES

1. Antonio SM, Friedman R. Meniere's disease. In: Jackler RK, Brackmann DE (eds), Neurotology. Philadelphia, PA: Elsevier; 2005. pp. 621-38.
2. Hallpike CS, Cairns H. Observations on the pathology of Meniere's syndrome: (section of otology). Proc R Soc Med. 1938;31(11):1317-36.
3. Kimura RS. Experimental blockage of the endolymphatic duct and sac and its effect on the inner ear of the guinea pig. A study on endolymphatic hydrops. Ann Otol Rhinol Laryngol. 1967;76(3):664-87.
4. Schuknecht HF. The pathophysiology of Meniere's disease. Am J Otol. 1984;5(6):526-7.
*5. Salt AN, Plontke SK. Endolymphatic hydrops: pathophysiology and experimental models. Otolaryngol Clin N Am. 2010;43(5):971-83.
*6. Merchant SN, Adams JC, Nadol JB, Jr. Pathophysiology of Meniere's syndrome: are symptoms caused by endolymphatic hydrops? Otol Neurotol. 2005;26(1):74-81.
7. Semaan MT, Alagramam KN, Megerian CA. The basic science of Meniere's disease and endolymphatic hydrops. Curr Opin Otolaryngol Head Neck Surg. 2005;13(5):301-7.
8. Hietikko E, Kotimaki J, Okuloff A, et al. A replication study on proposed candidate genes in Meniere's disease, and a review of the current status of genetic studies. Int J Audiol. 2012;51(11):841-5.
*9. Derebery MJ. Allergic and immunologic features of Meniere's disease. Otolaryngol Clin N Am. 2011;44(3):655-66, ix.
10. Minor LB, Schessel DA, Carey JP. Meniere's disease. Curr Opin Neurol. 2004;17(1):9-16.
11. Kitahara M. Bilateral aspects of Meniere's disease. Meniere's disease with bilateral fluctuant hearing loss. Acta Otolaryngol Suppl. 1991;485:74-7.
12. Paparella MM. Pathogenesis and pathophysiology of Meniere's disease. Acta Otolaryngol Suppl. 1991;485:26-35.
13. Morrison AW, Johnson KJ. Genetics (molecular biology) and Meniere's disease. Otolaryngol Clin N Am. 2002;35(3):497-516.
14. Thorp MA, Shehab ZP, Bance ML, et al. Hearing A-HCo, Equilibrium. The AAO-HNS Committee on Hearing and Equilibrium guidelines for the diagnosis and evaluation of therapy in Meniere's disease: have they been applied in the published literature of the last decade? Clin Otolaryngol Allied Sci. 2003;28(3):173-6.
15. Rauch SD, Zhou G, Kujawa SG, et al. Vestibular evoked myogenic potentials show altered tuning in patients with Meniere's disease. Otol Neurotol. 2004; 25(3):333-8.
*16. Helling K, Schonfeld U, Clarke AH. Treatment of Meniere's disease by low-dosage intratympanic gentamicin application: effect on otolith function. Laryngoscope. 2007;117(12):2244-50.
17. Young YH. Potential application of ocular and cervical vestibular-evoked myogenic potentials in Meniere's disease: a review. Laryngoscope. 2013;123(2):484-91.
18. Coelho DH, Roland JT, Jr., Golfinos JG. Posterior fossa meningiomas presenting with Meniere's-like symptoms: case report. Neurosurgery. 2008;63(5):E1001; discussion E.
18a. Niyazov DM, Andrews JC, Strelioff D, et al. Diagnosis of endolymphatic hydrops in vivo with magnetic resonance imaging. Otol Neurotol. 2001;22(6):813-7.
19. Nakashima T, Naganawa S, Sugiura M, et al. Visualization of endolymphatic hydrops in patients with Meniere's disease. Laryngoscope. 2007;117(3):415-20.
20. Nakashima T, Naganawa S, Teranishi M, et al. Endolymphatic hydrops revealed by intravenous gadolinium injection in patients with Meniere's disease. Acta Otolaryngol. 2010;130(3):338-43.
21. Fukuoka H, Takumi Y, Tsukada K, et al. Comparison of the diagnostic value of 3 T MRI after intratympanic injection of GBCA, electrocochleography, and the glycerol test in patients with Meniere's disease. Acta Otolaryngol. 2012;132(2):141-5.
*22. Coelho DH, Lalwani AK. Medical management of Meniere's disease. Laryngoscope. 2008;118(6):1099-108.
23. Babin RW, Balkany TJ, Fee WE. Transdermal scopolamine in the treatment of acute vertigo. Ann Otol Rhinol Laryngol. 1984;93(1 Pt 1):25-7.
24. Pyykko I, Magnusson M, Schalen L, et al. Pharmacological treatment of vertigo. Acta Otolaryngol Suppl. 1988; 455:77-81.
25. Fisher LM, Derebery MJ, Friedman RA. Oral steroid treatment for hearing improvement in Meniere's disease and endolymphatic hydrops. Otol Neurotol. 2012;33(9):1685-91.
26. Morse GG, House JW. Changes in Meniere's disease responses as a function of the menstrual cycle. Nurs Res. 2001;50(5):286-92.
27. Soderman AC, Moller J, Bagger-Sjoback D, et al. Stress as a trigger of attacks in Meniere's disease. A case-crossover study. Laryngoscope. 2004;114(10):1843-8.
28. Kinney SE, Sandridge SA, Newman CW. Long-term effects of Meniere's disease on hearing and quality of life. Am J Otol. 1997;18(1):67-73.
29. Coker NJ, Coker RR, Jenkins HA, et al. Psychological profile of patients with Meniere's disease. Arch Otolaryngology Head Neck Surg. 1989;115(11):1355-7.
30. Furstenberg AC, Lashmet FH, Lathrop F. Meniere's symptom complex: medical treatment. 1934. Ann Otol Rhinol Laryngol. 1992;101(1):20-31.

*References with asterisks refer to critical sources.

31. Thai-Van H, Bounaix MJ, Fraysse B. Meniere's disease: pathophysiology and treatment. Drugs. 2001;61(8):1089-102.
32. Claes J, Van de Heyning PH. Medical treatment of Meniere's disease: a review of literature. Acta Otolaryngol Suppl. 1997;526:37-42.
33. Di Berardino F, Filipponi E, Alpini D, et al. Meniere disease and gluten sensitivity: recovery after a gluten-free diet. Am J Otolaryngol. 2013;34(4):355-6.
34. Thirlwall AS, Kundu S. Diuretics for Meniere's disease or syndrome. Cochrane Database Syst Rev. 2006 (3):CD003599.
35. Klockhoff I, Lindblom U. Meniere's disease and hydrochlorothiazide (Dichlotride)—a critical analysis of symptoms and therapeutic effects. Acta Otolaryngol. 1967;63(4): 347-65.
36. Ruckenstein MJ, Rutka JA, Hawke M. The treatment of Meniere's disease: Torok revisited. Laryngoscope. 1991;101 (2):211-8.
37. van Deelen GW, Huizing EH. Use of a diuretic (Dyazide) in the treatment of Meniere's disease. A double-blind crossover placebo-controlled study. ORL J Otorhinolaryngol Rel Spec. 1986;48(5):287-92.
38. Timmerman H. Pharmacotherapy of vertigo: any news to be expected? Acta Otolaryngol Suppl. 1994;513:28-32.
39. Fraysse B, Bebear JP, Dubreuil C, Berges C, Dauman R. Betahistine dihydrochloride versus flunarizine. A double-blind study on recurrent vertigo with or without cochlear syndrome typical of Meniere's disease. Acta Otolaryngologica Suppl. 1991;490:1-10.
40. James AL, Burton MJ. Betahistine for Meniere's disease or syndrome. Cochrane Database Syst Rev. 2001;(1):CD001873.
41. Black FO, Pesznecker SC. Vestibular ototoxicity. Clinical considerations. Otolaryngol Clin N Am. 1993;26(5):713-36.
42. Hirsch BE, Kamerer DB. Role of chemical labyrinthectomy in the treatment of Meniere's disease. Otolaryngol Clin N Am. 1997;30(6):1039-49.
43. Ishiyama G, Lopez I, Baloh RW, et al. Histopathology of the vestibular end organs after intratympanic gentamicin failure for Meniere's disease. Acta Otolaryngol. 2007;127(1): 34-40.
*44. Cohen-Kerem R, Kisilevsky V, Einarson TR, et al. Intratympanic gentamicin for Meniere's disease: a meta-analysis. Laryngoscope. 2004;114(12):2085-91.
45. Harner SG, Driscoll CL, Facer GW, et al. Long-term follow-up of transtympanic gentamicin for Meniere's syndrome. Otol Neurotol. 2001;22(2):210-14.
46. Rarey KE, Gerhardt KJ, Curtis LM, et al. Effect of stress on cochlear glucocorticoid protein: acoustic stress. Hear Res. 1995;82(2):135-8.
47. Parnes LS, Sun AH, Freeman DJ. Corticosteroid pharmacokinetics in the inner ear fluids: an animal study followed by clinical application. Laryngoscope. 1999;109(7 Pt 2):1-17.
48. Chandrasekhar SS, Rubinstein RY, Kwartler JA, et al. Dexamethasone pharmacokinetics in the inner ear: comparison of route of administration and use of facilitating agents. Otolaryngol Head Neck Surg. 2000;122(4):521-8.
*49. Silverstein H, Isaacson JE, Olds MJ, et al. Dexamethasone inner ear perfusion for the treatment of Meniere's disease: a prospective, randomized, double-blind, crossover trial. Am J Otol. 1998;19(2):196-201.
50. Eisenberg DM, Davis RB, Ettner SL, et al. Trends in alternative medicine use in the United States, 1990-1997: results of a follow-up national survey. JAMA. 1998;280(18):1569-75.
51. Densert B, Densert O, Erlandsson B, et al. Transmission of square wave pressure pulses through the perilymphatic fluid in cats. Acta Otolaryngol. 1986;102(3-4):186-93.
52. Gates GA, Verrall A, Green JD, Jr, et al. Meniett clinical trial: long-term follow-up. Arch Otolaryngol Head Neck Surg. 2006;132(12):1311-6.
53. Gottshall KR, Hoffer ME, Moore RJ, Balough BJ. The role of vestibular rehabilitation in the treatment of Meniere's disease. Otolaryngol Head Neck Surg. 2005;133(3):326-8.
54. Soderman AC, Bergenius J, Bagger-Sjoback D, et al. Patients' subjective evaluations of quality of life related to disease-specific symptoms, sense of coherence, and treatment in Meniere's disease. Otol Neurotol. 2001;22(4):526-33.
55. Chung JW, Fayad J, Linthicum F, Ishiyama A, Merchant SN. Histopathology after endolymphatic sac surgery for Meniere's syndrome. Otol Neurotol. 2011;32(4):660-4.
*56. Pullens B, Verschuur HP, van Benthem PP. Surgery for Meniere's disease. Cochrane Database Syst Rev. 2013;2: CD005395.
57. Gibson WP. Hypothetical mechanism for vertigo in Meniere's disease. Otolaryngol Clin N Am. 2010 Oct;43(5):1019-27.
58. Charpiot A, Rohmer D, Gentine A. Lateral semicircular canal plugging in severe Meniere's disease: a clinical prospective study about 28 patients. Otol Neurotol. 2010;31(2): 237-40.
59. Loader B, Beicht D, Hamzavi JS, et al. Tenotomy of the middle ear muscles causes a dramatic reduction in vertigo attacks and improves audiological function in definite Meniere's disease. Acta Otolaryngol. 2012;132(5):491-7.
60. Gacek RR, Gacek MR. Comparison of labyrinthectomy and vestibular neurectomy in the control of vertigo. Laryngoscope. 1996;106(2 Pt 1):225-30.
61. Feenstra L. The management of tinnitus with or without Meniere's disease. Acta Otolaryngol Suppl. 1997;526:47-9.

*References with asterisks refer to critical sources.

CHAPTER

22

Temporal Bone Trauma

J Caleb Simmons, Alex D Sweeney, Marc-Elie Nader, Robert A Williamson

INTRODUCTION

The complex structure of the temporal bone reflects its functional importance. Occupying the majority of the lateral skull base, the temporal bone is composed of multiple bony subunits, the contents of which are crucial to our interactions with the surrounding world. It houses major arterial and venous structures, serves as a rigid boundary of the middle and posterior cranial fossae, acts as an important gateway between the intracranial contents and the head and neck, and acts as a receiver for information essential to proper hearing and balance. Undoubtedly, temporal bone injury can be catastrophic in many ways.

The development of the temporal bone is important to consider in the setting of traumatic injury. In utero, the temporal bone develops as a hybrid of intramembranous (squamous and tympanic) and intracartilaginous (petrous and mastoid) bone formation.[1] Ossification in these different locations progresses at varying rates, and the end result is bony fusion along planes that are preserved as suture lines in the adult temporal bone. As the temporal bone grows, it begins to aerate from within. Pneumatization begins as a consequence of prenatal expansion within the tympanic cavity, and it can continue for years following birth.[2,3] The developed temporal bone thus may have intrinsic weaknesses along suture lines and its more aerated portions.[4]

Anatomically, the temporal bone can be divided into four subunits: petrous, squamous, tympanic, and mastoid. These divisions are most relevant in terms of the structures contained within each portion. The petrous portion of the temporal bone is located medially and anteriorly and contains the carotid artery, cochlea, labyrinth and the labyrinthine segment of the facial nerve, which includes the geniculate ganglion. It also comprises the bony portion of the internal auditory canal. The tympanic segment of the temporal bone contains the tympanic membrane (TM), ossicles, and the horizontal segment of the facial nerve. The mastoid segment contains the vertical segment of the facial nerve, the transverse/sigmoid sinus and jugular bulb. Additionally, the inferior-most aspect of the mastoid portion—the mastoid tip—is an insertion point for neck musculature such as the posterior belly of the digastric, the sternocleidomastoid, and splenius capitus. The squamous portion of the temporal bone serves as a shield over the temporal lobe of the brain.

PATHOGENESIS

Temporal bone fractures are relatively common in the setting of closed head trauma across all age groups. Cannon and Jahrsdoerfer demonstrated in a series of 1300 consecutive head trauma patients that approximately 22% of skull fractures included a fracture of the temporal bone.[5] Additionally, upwards of 40% of patients with basilar skull fractures have been reported to have a temporal bone fracture.[6] These rates may differ based on age. Previous reports have identified temporal bone fractures following head trauma in 30-75% of adults[7,8] versus 6-14% of pediatric patients.[9] These differences may be explained by the relative elasticity of the less-pneumatized and less-fused pediatric temporal bone versus that of the adult, though evidence does suggest that even the adult skull retains the ability to deform before fracturing occurs.[10] Both populations appear to have a bimodal age distribution. Pediatric temporal bone trauma occurs more often around the ages 3 and 12,[11] while adult trauma in the adult population occurs more commonly in the 20s and 50s.[4] There is a male preponderance in both adults and children, though there appears to be less of a significant gender difference in the pediatric population (62.5% males in children versus 81.7% in adults).[4] In both age groups, fractures are unilateral in >90% of cases.[4]

The common mechanisms of temporal bone trauma depend somewhat on the patient population. In Cannon and Jarsdoerfer's series of 1300 consecutive head trauma patients, 44% occurred as a result of automobile collisions. Automobile and bicycle accidents account for a significant portion of pediatric injuries, as well.[5] Children under the age of 4 may be just as likely to have trauma due to falls.[4,11] Penetrating trauma in the form of gunshot wounds represents a smaller percentage of temporal bone injuries, though some reports suggest that there are trends toward increased penetrating temporal bone trauma due to gun violence in urban areas of the United States.[12]

Two of the most important considerations in the evaluation of temporal bone trauma are the mechanism of the trauma and the distribution of the trauma within the temporal bone. Whether penetrating or blunt, all trauma is the result of force and energy transfer from one structure to another. The degree of trauma, therefore, should be directly proportional to the mass of the object striking the temporal bone, directly proportional to the change in acceleration of that object as it strikes the temporal bone and exponentially proportional to the velocity of that object. As such, knowledge of the specific trauma mechanism can be critical in predicting the extent of injury, especially when considering the differences between traumatic forces such as a rifle round and an automobile windshield. Specifically in cases of penetrating gunshot wounds, considerations of muzzle velocity and ammunition caliber could prove helpful.

The location of temporal bone trauma may correlate with post-traumatic functional deficits. When blunt force is applied to the temporal bone, it is thought to dissipate along vectors that are predictable based on the orientation of the trauma. Blunt occipital trauma, where force is delivered perpendicular to the long access of the temporal bone, is generally associated with transverse fractures. Furthermore, longitudinal fractures are more frequently seen when the lateral aspect of the temporal bone absorbs a forceful blow.[13] Traditionally, temporal bone fractures have been characterized in terms of their orientation to the long axis of the petrous pyramid as longitudinal or transverse, the former being identified in approximately 80% of cases. However, newer studies have suggested that as many as 75% of fractures are actually oblique,[14] and characterization of fractures as oblique, longitudinal, and transverse nomenclature does not correlate well with clinical findings other than sensorineural hearing loss (SNHL).[4,15] This has led to the introduction of different classification systems that may have better clinical correlation, including otic-capsule-sparing versus otic-capsule-violating,[6,16,17-18] petrous versus nonpetrous,[15] and another system based on the four parts of the temporal bone (squama, tympanic, mastoid, and petrous)[4]. For example, describing fractures based on their involvement of the otic capsule or the petrous bone may be more predictive of facial nerve injury, cerebrospinal fluid (CSF) leak, and type of hearing loss (Table 22.1). No system has gained widespread acceptance as yet, though clinical correlation and utility seem to be highest with the otic capsule sparing/nonsparing classification. Otic violation resulted in complete ipsilateral SNHL in Figures 22.1 and 22.2, as well as facial nerve weakness that resolved in the case of Figures 22.1A to D and did not in the case of Figures 22.2A to C. A CSF leak was a sequela of the otic-violating fracture in Figures 22.3A and B; the leak resolved with conservative management. Otic-sparing fractures are demonstrated in Figures 22.4 and 22.5, resulting in conductive hearing loss (CHL) that resolved in Figures 22.4A and B and did not in Figures 22.5A and B.

CLINICAL FINDINGS: SYMPTOMS AND SIGNS

As discussed above, the findings associated with temporal bone trauma can vary widely depending on the mechanism and location of trauma. In general, an initial evaluation should begin with an in-depth history that can elicit the specific circumstances surrounding an injury (including ballistics information, when applicable) and functional deficits immediately following injury. The initial physical examination should identify associated soft tissue injury, realizing that some findings, such as an auricular hematoma, require immediate attention. Additionally, given the frequency with which temporal bone injuries can involve the carotid canal (52%) and jugular bulb (21%)[19], massive bleeding should be quickly recognized and stabilized. Ecchymosis along the skull base is commonly seen in basilar skull fractures. Battle's sign (occipital ecchymosis) and the so-called "raccoon eyes" (periorbital

Table 22.1: Three systems of classification of pattern of temporal bone fractures and their functional relevance

	Incidence	*SNHL*	*CHL*	*Facial nerve injury*	*CSF leak*	*Overall*
Longitudinal*	50%	20	46.7	20	20	
Transverse	27%	25	37.5	25%	25	
Oblique	23%	28.6	14	28.6	28.6	
p-value		Not (p=0.34)	Not (p=0.33)	Not (p>0.99)	Not (p=0.64)	p=0.48
Otic-capsule sparing*	80%	4	33.3	12	8.3	
Otic-capsule violating	20%	100	50	67	67	
p-value		p<0.001	Not (p=0.64)	p<0.05	p<0.005	p<0.001
Petrous**	11.6	70	20	22.2	33.3	
Nonpetrous	99.4	37.8	55.6	7.2	3.6	
p-value		Not (p=0.06)	p=0.0022	p=0.022	p<0.000001	

(SNHL, sensorineural hearing loss; CHL, conductive hearing loss; CSF, cerebrospinal fluid).
*Data and statistical analysis by Little et al.[18]
**Data and statistical analysis by Ishman et al.[15]
Highlighted value indicates a comparison between petrous category and nonpetrous "middle ear subgroup" that showed a significant difference in CHL.

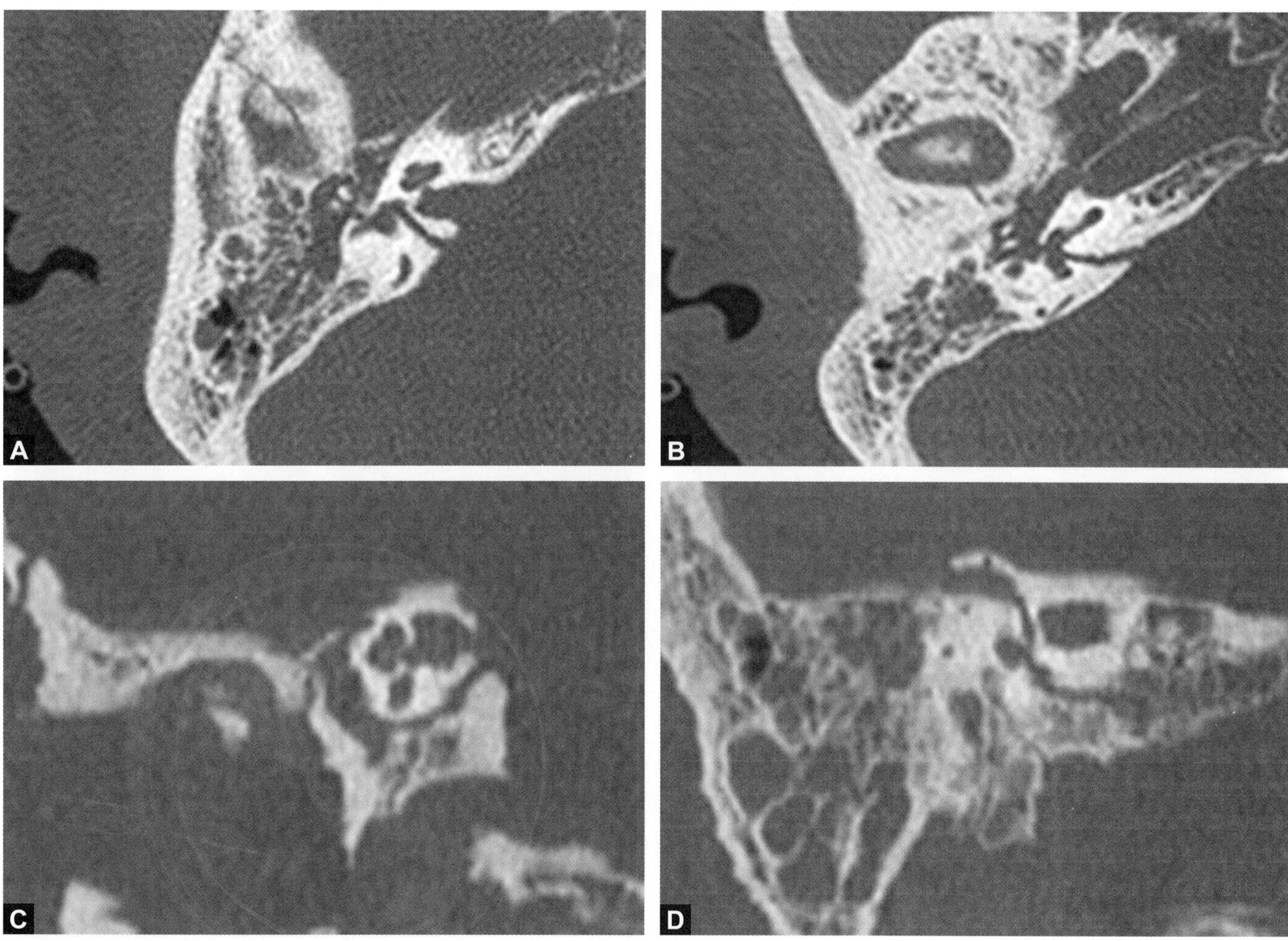

Figs. 22.1A to D: Patient with right temporal bone fracture after motor vehicle accident, resulting in traumatic brain injury. The temporal bone fracture is transverse, violating the otic capsule in the petrous bone. The patient had ipsilateral facial nerve weakness of unknown onset after his injury, likely due to injury in tympanic segment. The facial weakness resolved with conservative management. He had total ipsilateral sensorineural hearing loss on post-injury audiogram.

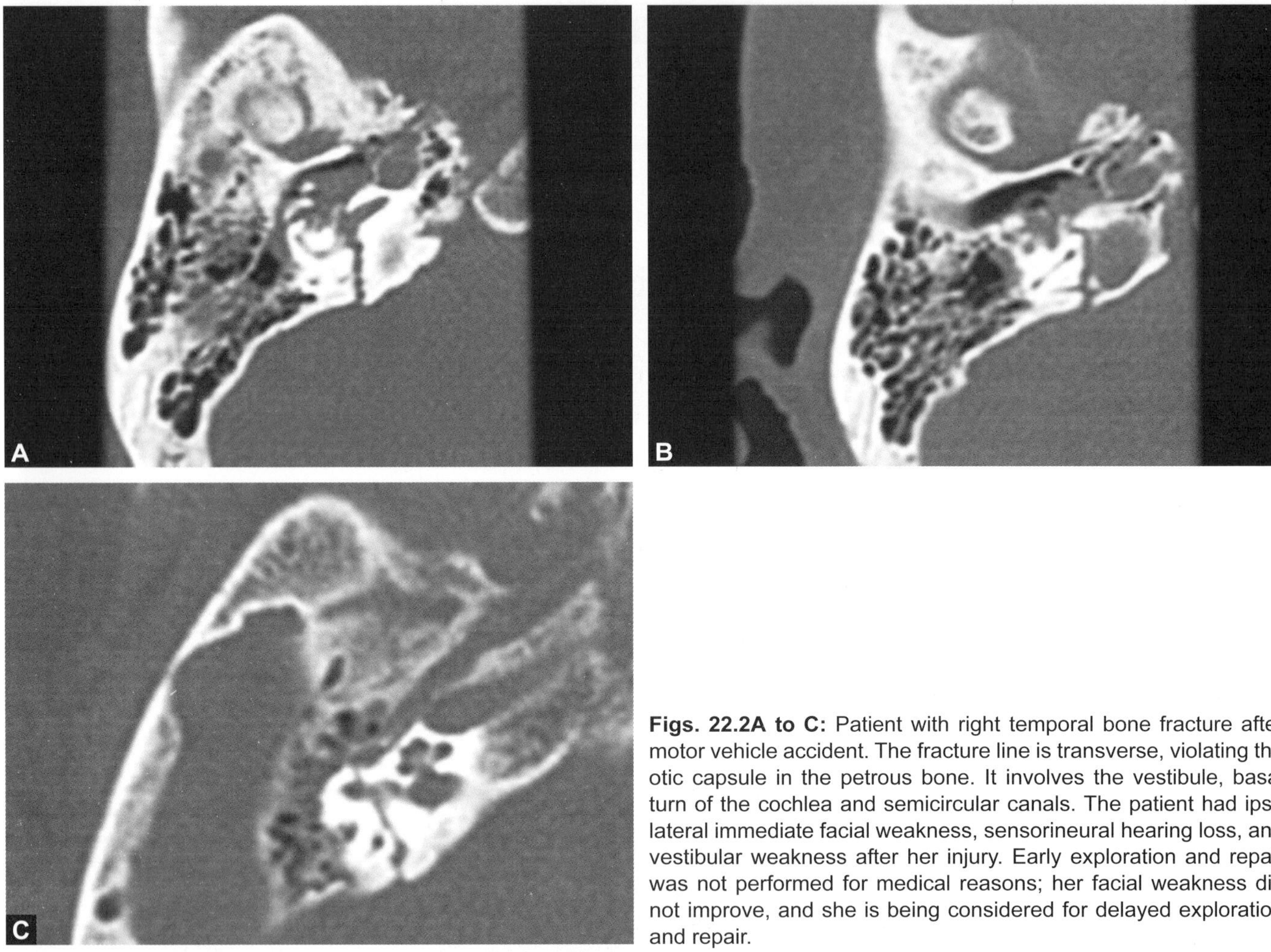

Figs. 22.2A to C: Patient with right temporal bone fracture after motor vehicle accident. The fracture line is transverse, violating the otic capsule in the petrous bone. It involves the vestibule, basal turn of the cochlea and semicircular canals. The patient had ipsilateral immediate facial weakness, sensorineural hearing loss, and vestibular weakness after her injury. Early exploration and repair was not performed for medical reasons; her facial weakness did not improve, and she is being considered for delayed exploration and repair.

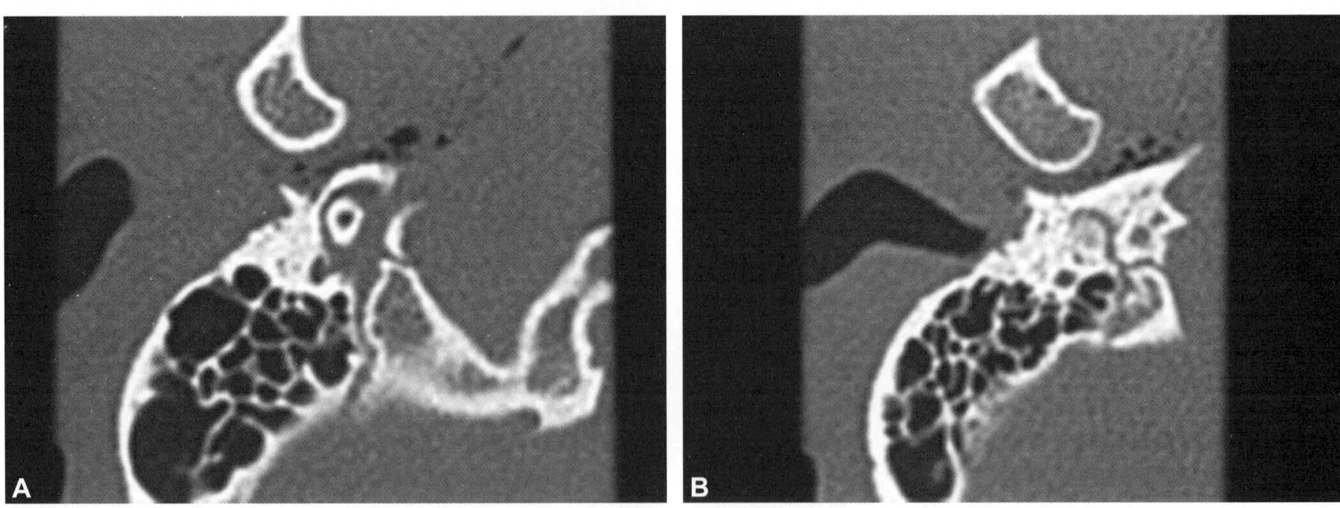

Figs. 22.3A and B: Patient with right temporal bone fracture after motor vehicle accident. The transverse fracture violates the otic capsule in the petrous bone. Patient had multiple other facial fractures and traumatic brain injury. Ipsilateral cerebrospinal fluid leak through a tegmen defect resolved with conservative treatment.

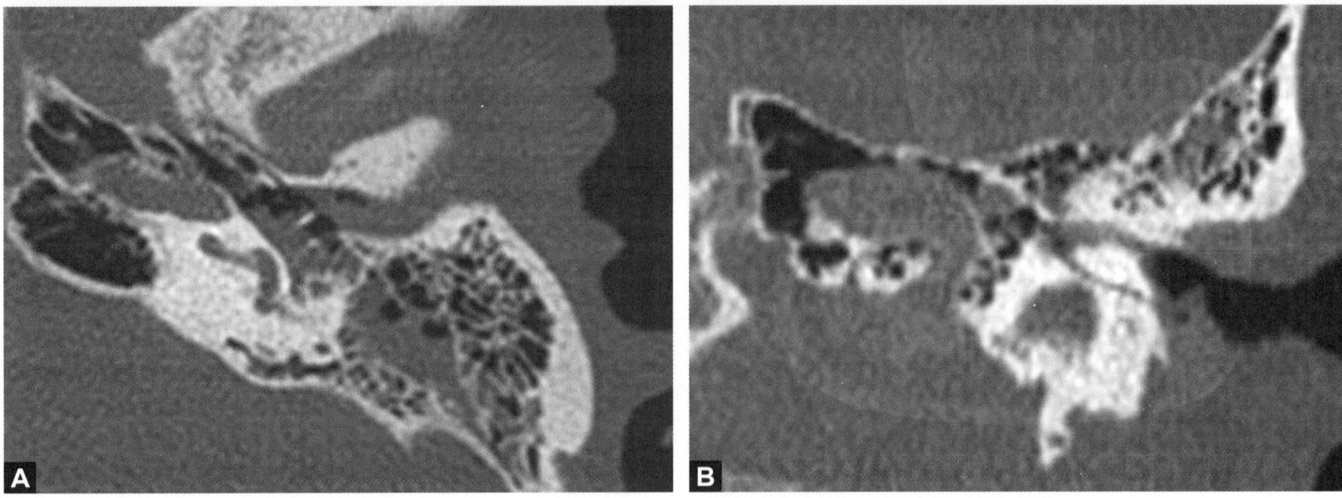

Figs. 22.4A and B: Patient with left temporal bone fracture after motorcycle accident. The longitudinal fracture spares the otic capsule and extends through the tympanic and mastoid sections of the temporal bone as well as the external auditory canal. The patient had conductive hearing loss after his injury that improved with time, indicating his ossicular chain was not involved.

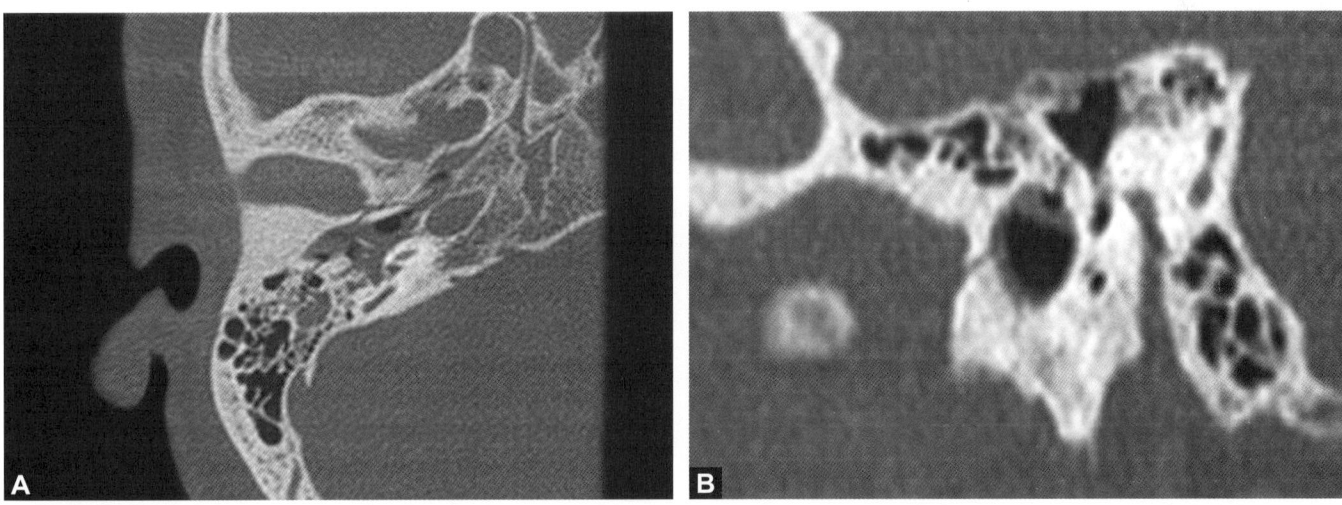

Figs. 22.5A and B: Patient with right temporal bone after motor vehicle accident. The longitudinal fracture extends through the foramina rotundum and ovale, middle ear, mastoid air cells, external auditory canal, and squamous portion of the temporal bone. There is subluxation of the malleoincudal joint on CT imaging.

ecchymosis) are two well-described examination findings. In the case of penetrating trauma, an effort should be made to identify "entry" and "exit" wounds, which allow for an assessment of trajectory and the probability of a retained foreign body. Irrigation is contraindicated as this may flush contaminated debris into the intracranial space. Packing is also avoided except in the rare case with severe hemorrhage, because if a CSF leak is present, packing will lead to stagnation of fluid and may increase the risk of meningitis.

After assessing soft tissue and potential vascular injuries, a prudent examination following temporal bone trauma should be concerned with any external auditory canal (EAC) disruption, intracranial injury with or without CSF leak, facial nerve injury, and cochleovestibular injury. Intracranial injury is frequently associated with temporal bone fractures. In a 1998 review of 43 patients with temporal bone trauma from an urban hospital, 84% of patients had one or more radiographically abnormal intracranial findings, which may be suspected based on depressed mental status (49%).[12] Cerebrospinal fluid leaks are also not uncommon. A review of complications from 820 temporal bone fractures seen at a single institution over 5 years identified an 18% incidence of CSF leak.[16] Suspicion should arise with the persistent passage of clear fluid through the external auditory meatus, the nose, or an associated soft tissue injury.

Facial nerve injuries are also commonly seen in association with temporal bone fractures. In fact, as many as 10% of fractures may have a concomitant facial nerve injury[15], though this number may be less in the more flexible pediatric temporal bone (3%).[11] Of paramount importance when facial nerve weakness is identified are efforts to distinguish between complete and incomplete paralysis and to determine the time of onset of the weakness (immediate versus delayed). The presence of an immediate, complete paralysis should arouse suspicion of injury that may require a time-sensitive repair.

Hearing loss is reported in up to 26% of temporal bone fractures, though fulminant cochleovestibular injury is relatively less common.[16] Hearing loss patterns can be conductive, sensorineural, or mixed depending on the nature of the injury. Tuning fork interrogation at 256Hz, 512Hz, and 1024Hz can be helpful to gauge the extent of the injury if the patient is alert and cooperative. Conductive losses can occur though external canal disruption, TM perforation, ossicular disruption, and the presence of fluid or blood in the middle ear. Partial SNHLs can occur as the result of concussive injury to the cochlea. Complete SNHL can be suggestive of disruption in the membranous labyrinth, which may also be associated with stimulation or deprivation of vestibulo-ocular pathways in the form of nystagmus. Horizontal nystagmus with the fast phase oriented away from the injury would be expected in vestibulocochlear injury.

EVALUATION: LABORATORY, OTOLOGIC, AND NEUROTOLOGIC TESTING

Audiogram

Bedside testing, with the use of tuning forks, may allow initial gross evaluation of the patient's hearing. A baseline audiogram is then obtained once the patient's condition is stabilized. The baseline audiogram frequently shows CHL secondary to hemotympanum, but may establish a baseline SNHL. A formal audiogram obtained 3–6 weeks after injury allows the quantitative assessment of conductive, mixed, and SNHL. A significant air-bone gap may signify ossicular chain disruption, indicating the need for ossiculoplasty. Severe SNHL or anacusis may dictate which surgical approach should be used in patients who require facial nerve decompression or CSF fistula repair. A translabyrinthine approach may be used in patients with nonserviceable hearing who need surgery. In very young patients, patients with traumatic brain injury, or those otherwise uncooperative with testing, auditory brain stem response may be used to obtain a baseline level of auditory function.[20]

Vestibular Testing

Electro- or videonystagmography (ENG or VNG), though not commonly necessary in the acute phase, may be obtained in patients who complain of vertigo following trauma to the temporal bone. VNG testing helps differentiate between central and peripheral vertigo and helps quantify the loss of vestibular function. Complete vestibular deficit may be seen with transverse or capsule-disrupting fractures. In these cases, VNG testing shows a spontaneous nystagmus with the fast phase beating toward the contralateral side and absent caloric responses on the affected side.

Benign positional vertigo may also occur following trauma to the temporal bone.[21] VNG usually shows a rotational nystagmus following the Hallpike maneuver. The nystagmus shows the classical characteristics of latency with onset, limited and short duration, and fatigability upon repeated stimulating head movements.

Electrodiagnostic Testing of Facial Nerve

Electrodiagnostic testing of the facial nerve is performed in patients with complete facial paralysis following trauma to the temporal bone. Electrical testing of the facial nerve includes the minimal nerve excitability test (NET), maximal stimulation test (MST), electroneuronography (ENoG), and standard electromyography (EMG). Of these tests, the MST and ENoG are the most commonly used ones. Electrical testing of the facial nerve helps differentiate a neuropraxic injury from neural degeneration. It allows objective measurement of the percentage of neural injury or degeneration. In turn, it helps the clinician determine the prognosis for recovery of facial function and the necessity for facial nerve surgery.

Electrical testing of the facial nerve should be performed no sooner than 3 days following the onset of paralysis to allow Wallerian degeneration to take place. The MST compares the strength of facial twitching between the paralyzed and unaffected sides in response to the strongest stimulus tolerated by the patient. The facial nerve is stimulated transcutaneously at the level of the stylomastoid foramen with a Hilger facial nerve stimulator. The strength of facial contraction is subjectively evaluated between the two sides and described as equal, mildly decreased, significantly decreased, or absent.

If electrical testing of the facial nerve is abnormal, then ENoG is performed thereafter. ENoG allows a more objective evaluation of the amplitude of the muscle compound action potential (CAP) in response to facial nerve stimulation. The facial nerve is stimulated near the stylomastoid foramen and the CAP is measured at the nasolabial fold by cutaneous electrodes. The decrease in the amplitude of the CAP is directly proportional to the percentage of degenerated nerve fibers. A degeneration of 90% of nerve fibers was determined by Fisch to be the threshold beyond which chances of spontaneous recovery are poor and, therefore, the threshold at which patients should undergo facial nerve decompression. [22]

If delayed intervention is being considered, EMG can be performed 10 days after injury and can be used to establish whether recovering axons are present. This is particularly helpful when ENoG shows absent responses. Voluntary motor units and polyphasic potentials indicate that regeneration is in progress. The lack of these and the presence of fibrillation potentials indicate a fully degenerated nerve (or a complete injury, e.g. transection) without evidence of ongoing recovery.

Laboratory

In patients with temporal bone trauma, laboratory testing may help establish the diagnosis of CSF leak. Traditionally, the appearance of a halo sign when a drop of bloody discharge is instilled on filter paper or bed linen has been associated with the presence of CSF in the sample. However, the value of this sign has been debated by some authors. Dula and Fales determined that this sign was not specific for CSF as halos would also be produced by mixtures of blood with saline, tears, or nasal secretions.[23] High glucose levels (>50 mg/100 mL) are considered to be indicative of CSF.[24]

β2-transferrin is a protein found in CSF, perilymph, and aqueous humor. It can be measured in samples of otorrhea or rhinorrhea to detect the presence of CSF. It is a noninvasive technique that requires only 50 μL of fluid. However, the prolonged time for laboratory analysis may limit the usefulness of this test. Contrast-enhanced computed tomography (CT), radioisotope dye instillation, and intrathecal dye methods may help in localizing the site of the leak if not evident. The use of intrathecal fluorescein may also be considered when laboratory testing or imaging fails to identify a suspected leak, but this is not without the potential for adverse reactions. In most cases, high-resolution CT (HRCT) imaging of the temporal bone with thin slices (1 mm or less) is adequate to visualize the likely source of leak.

Radiologic Imaging

Patients who sustain temporal bone trauma undergo a primary evaluation for life-threatening medical emergencies. Initial radiologic workup usually includes a chest X-ray, cervical spine X-rays, and brain CT.

High-resolution CT is the study of choice to evaluate temporal bone fractures. It consists of thin slices of 1.0 or 1.5 mm taken in both axial and direct coronal planes. HRCT is virtually 100% sensitive for the detection of temporal bone fractures.[25] However, brain CT with 10 mm cuts was found to miss 50% of the temporal bone fractures detected on HRCT.[26] HRCT allows for the accurate evaluation of ossicular chain integrity, fallopian canal, and tegmen tympani. Some authors argue that HRCT should not be performed in the context of isolated SNHL without any other neurologic symptoms since determining the presence a fracture through the otic capsule does not alter the treatment. Indications to obtain a HRCT include facial paralysis, CSF leak, fracture of the EAC, or suspected vascular injury. [27]

Magnetic resonance imaging (MRI) is the study of choice to evaluate intracranial complications that may otherwise be missed on CT. However, it cannot replace HRCT when evaluating the integrity of the ossicular chain or facial nerve. Air in the middle ear may mimic the appearance of the ossicles[28] and blood in the mastoid may produce a hyperintense signal that masks the facial nerve.[29] MRI is indicated when HRCT suggests a defect >2 cm, as MRI will rule out potential herniation of intracranial contents into the mastoid/middle ear space. The presence of herniation may dictate surgical approach. Temporal lobe parenchymal injury or intracranial bleeding/hematoma noted on MRI may also influence surgical decision making.

Carotid angiography is not routinely performed in patients with temporal bone trauma. It should be considered in patients who have a displaced fracture through the carotid canal, penetrating trauma involving the petrous segment, neurologic findings that are not explained by the brain CT, lateralizing neurologic deficits, Horner's syndrome, or cervical bruit.[30] CT angiography can be used in select cases to assess vascular injury, but sensitivity and the option of endovascular intervention are inferior compared to standard angiography.

TREATMENT AND PROGNOSIS

Initial treatment should be guided by general trauma principles, with special attention given to any associated intracranial and/or cervical spinal injuries. Possible carotid injury or significant hemorrhage should also be assessed and managed in the acute phase, particularly in penetrating trauma. Treatment decision making should then be guided by clinical and radiographic assessment. Audiometry should be conducted as early as possible, and facial nerve functional assessment by initial clinical evaluation and electrical testing will also guide treatment. In this section are discussed the sequelae of a temporal bone fracture that will require conservative or surgical intervention.

Facial Nerve Injury

Prevalence of facial nerve paralysis with temporal bone fractures from all etiologies has been estimated to be 7–10%.[31] Post-traumatic facial nerve injury is classically addressed in view of two factors: (1) the timing of onset of paresis or paralysis and (2) the suspected location of the lesion. The first factor has been disputed by a few authors who claim that electrophysiological testing has largely subsumed clinical onset of paralysis as the primary indication for surgical exploration and intervention.[32] The second factor is helpful in establishing an algorithm for surgical approach.

First, regarding the indications for surgical intervention, the classic dictum has been to intervene sooner in cases that demonstrated immediate facial paralysis after injury and to observe with electrophysiological testing in cases with delayed onset of paralysis. Certainly, if a patient's facial nerve is documented to be immediately paralyzed after injury, then the pretest probability of transection is high. In one study of 65 nerve explorations, 80% had immediate onset of facial paralysis.[33] The patient's best chance at recovery is then dependent on exploration and attempted anastomosis.[34-35] However, a patient who initially has intact facial function after injury but then develops significant clinical dysfunction in a delayed fashion is the most difficult to prognosticate. In Darrouzet's study, 17% of operated nerves were delayed in onset or time of onset was unknown.[33] Particularly in this category, a few authors have moved toward regarding electrophysiological testing as the most convincing indication for intervention, independent of history of clinical onset.[32] In support of this, often the patient with a temporal bone fracture has been paralyzed, intubated, and sedated as part of the primary survey. Eyewitness accounts and glancing observations obtained while stabilizing the patient can be erroneous. Thus, the time to manifesting the facial nerve injury can be difficult to ascertain. Every effort should be made to elicit facial movement by physical examination in the early hours after presentation, and if some movement is seen then often these patients can be managed conservatively. However, electrophysiological testing affords important measurable data points in the event of a nebulous history, a confounded examination, or deteriorating facial movement on clinical examination.

Second, the location of the suspected lesion largely guides the surgical approach. The suspected location may be evident to the neurotologist if the patient has an external wound in the parotid region or CT imaging demonstrating a fracture line approximating the course of the facial nerve. However, at times, the patient may have multiple injuries, significant intracranial trauma, or complex fracture pattern. At such a time, a systematic approach to the facial nerve may be helpful. The course of the nerve from the brain stem to the facial musculature is divided into three segments, including intracranial, intratemporal, and extratemporal/peripheral.[24]

The intracranial facial nerve includes that segment from the brain stem to the fundus of the internal auditory canal. This segment is rarely the site of injury except in cases of severe trauma where stretch and shock-wave type injuries occur. The segment is largely protected from penetrating trauma by the petrous bone and cranial vault, but if the area is violated by such an injury, it is often in the midst of extensive central nervous system pathology. At such a time, the patient's central nervous system pathology takes precedent and should be managed first.

The intratemporal facial nerve includes that segment extending from the internal auditory canal fundus to the stylomastoid foramen. This is often the segment of interest to the otolaryngologist/neurotologist, as it includes the areas most frequently damaged in blunt trauma to the skull, as demonstrated in Figures 22.2A to C. Regardless of fracture pattern, the facial nerve is involved at the perigeniculate region in 66–93% of cases.[33,36] Fisch et al. demonstrated that the area of the fallopian canal in the region of the meatal foramen is the point on the facial nerve's course through the temporal bone with the narrowest diameter and thus the least room for expansion in the event of neural swelling.[36] When significant edema occurs, this can prevent axoplasmic flow and thus cause neural injury, manifesting as delayed onset of facial nerve weakness. Penetrating injury such as a gunshot wound often causes more severely complex and comminuted lines of fracture and can cause lesions in the nerve in multiple locations within the bone. The rate of facial nerve injury is approximately 50% with gunshot wounds to the temporal bone with the vertical segment being the most frequently injured.[37-38] Interestingly, one series of 66 patients showed no significant difference in rate of recovery to HB 1 or 2 based on location of the nerve lesion within the temporal bone.[39]

The extratemporal facial nerve is that segment distal to the stylomastoid foramen. Injuries to this segment are often accompanied by facial injuries and lacerations. Laceration to the nerve in this area is best repaired by direct anastomosis as soon as the patient's condition permits. If segmental loss has occurred, an interpositional graft should be used. In the first 48 hours after injury, intraoperative electric nerve stimulation may be useful in order to identify the distal stump within the wound bed.[24]

In all patients, the timing of surgery is largely based on both clinical examination and electrophysiological testing. As described previously, in patients with delayed or unknown onset or incomplete paralysis, surgical intervention is indicated when >90% degeneration has been demonstrated on ENoG in order to prevent conversion of neural injury from Sunderland class II (axonotmesis) to class III (neurotmesis). Sunderland class III entails significant synkinesis in a large percentage of cases.[24] Patients in this category are typically first treated with high-dose corticosteroids during expectant management, beginning at 1mg/kg/day of prednisone for 1–3 weeks and then tapering off.[6,33] The goal of this therapy is to reduce neural edema, improve axoplasmic flow, and prevent advancement of Sunderland class. In two series, 84–93% of patients had delayed onset and met criteria for conservative management, and both series showed 100% rate of recovery to House-Brackmann (HB) grade I or II.[6,16] One of these studies demonstrated 59% of patients in this category gained spontaneous recovery by 1 month and 88% of patients showed recovery by 3 months.[16] Alternatively, one recent case series of 66 patients showed a significant difference in the rate of good recovery (HB 1 or 2) in patients who underwent surgical decompression within 2 weeks compared to those treated at 2 weeks to 2 months, suggesting there may be an optimal time period for facial nerve rescue in the event of neural swelling.[39] The question of how long is too long after the event for surgical intervention is controversial, as there have been one case series and one case study of patients recovering facial nerve function after decompression several months after the initial event. In one series of nine patients with persistent facial paralysis 3 months after injury, decompression resulted in recovery to grade I or II in seven of nine patients at 1 year follow-up.[40] Sofferman reported delayed nerve decompression in one patient that subsequently resulted in good recovery 14 months after injury, despite poor prognosis suggested by neuromuscular tests.[41] The outcomes on late decompression of the facial nerve are decidedly limited, and thus late decompression may not yield significant benefit.

Clear goals for surgery must be outlined when undertaking surgical exploration and intervention in the case of intratemporal facial nerve injury. The pathology of penetrating trauma (gunshot) appears to be primarily transection[37], found in two-thirds to three-fourths of patients. In blunt trauma, the injury is due to intraneural hemorrhage, bony fragment impingement, and/or nerve transection, in decreasing order of occurrence.[24] CT imaging is often useful in ascertaining the precise area of injury. In cases where transection is suspected, the objective is to fully expose the area of transection and to reanastamose the transected ends—either primarily or with interposition grafts—in a tension-free manner. In cases of delayed facial nerve dysfunction or degenerative ENoG testing, the objective is to relieve pressure on the nerve to allow it to expand and to decrease damage to endoneural tubules from external constriction.[24] As mentioned previously, the area where the nerve is most anatomically prone to constriction is in the fallopian canal, and this area must be exposed.

Some surgeons advocate beginning with a trans-mastoid approach with a view to convert to middle cranial fossa approach if needed.[6,16,39,42] In cases of mixed and comminuted fractures (and intact cochleovestibular function), both transmastoid and middle fossa approaches may be needed in order to fully expose the nerve for reanastamosis or decompression. In cases of comminuted gunshot wounds or fractures involving the otic capsule, a resultant dead ear on audiometry may permit a translabyrinthine approach to expose the entire facial nerve without a middle fossa approach. If the results of ENoG show < 100% degeneration, facial nerve monitoring may have some value intraoperatively and should be considered.

The approaches to the facial nerve are delineated elsewhere. Iatrogenic trauma to a vulnerable facial nerve should be minimized by leaving a thin shell of bone over the nerve throughout decompression. When drilling is finished and the exposure is finished, a dissector may be used to lift the thin roof of bone atraumatically. When the facial nerve has been unroofed, bone fragments may be seen compressing the facial nerve directly, and if so, should be removed gently. If the bone fragments are in good reduction or if fragments are removed, the facial nerve may be observed to be blood stained or diffusely enlarged; either may signify intraneural hematoma within the intact epineurium. The nerve sheath should be incised sharply with atraumatic technique until nonedematous nerve is encountered, careful to preserve the underlying nerve fascicles. The degree of nerve loss should be assessed. If the nerve loss extends out of the surgical field, the surgeon should be prepared for an additional approach in order to fully expose the injured segment of the nerve.

If complete transection is observed, then the surgeon must prepare the nerve for anastomosis. If the fibers have been partially but significantly avulsed, then the nerve can likely be classified to be within Sunderland classes III–V and experiencing neurotmesis; the surgeon must consider clean division of the remaining trunk followed by interposition graft placement. In either case, these maneuvers may require nerve rerouting through a created bony channel or interposition grafting. In select cases involving the mastoid segment, the nerve can be dissected from the stylomastoid foramen into the parotid area and mobilized proximally to anastomose primarily.[24] The goal should be to provide a tension-free end-to-end anastomosis with reliable reapproximation of nerve ends. In one case series, a nerve gap was observed in 13.8% of cases.[33] When an interposition graft is required, the great auricular nerve provides up to 7–8 cm of useable length, while the sural nerve offers greater versatility with a potential length of 30cm.[24] Previously, monofilament 9-0 or 10-0 suture has been used for anastomosis[43], but more recently there have been studies demonstrating the efficacy of fibrin glue.[44] Animal studies have demonstrated less inflammatory and fibrotic response as well as improved axonal regeneration with the use of fibrin glue on rat nerve transection models when compared to microsuture technique.[45] In one prospective human study of 11 explored nerves, 78% of patients undergoing nerve suturing recovered to at least HB III[46], while another human study showed 84% long-term recovery to grade III or better using fibrin glue for both primary reapproximation and interposition grafting.[44]

The prognosis of patients with facial paralysis undergoing indicated nerve exploration has been demonstrated to be quite hopeful. The best prognosis is obtained with early intervention during the acute phase of degeneration, and a correlation was demonstrated between longer duration of nerve interruption and worse outcome after repair.[44] One study found that 2 weeks were the optimal period for intervention for recovery to HB 1 or 2.[39] Recovery of facial function after repair averaged 7 months in one study.[44] In one series of 115 patients, 94–100% of patients showed at least a grade III recovery, 45% had grade I recovery, and no patients had worse than grade IV recovery at 2 years follow-up.[33] In another prospective series of 11 explored facial nerves, 5 showed recovery to HB I, 4 to HB II, and 2 to HB III.[46] Patients with transection or severe injuries requiring grafting should be counseled that HB grade III function represents the best outcome possible.

There are patients with delayed or unknown onset who do not meet the > 90% degeneration on ENoG who then have persistent facial paralysis or paresis even 3–4 months after injury. Reanimation or reinnervation procedures should not be offered until the patient has had 1 year to show any spontaneous recovery, for fear of disrupting a slowly but spontaneously healing nerve. Preserving eye function must be the priority during this period, and may entail gold weight lid implants, tarsorrhaphy, or other procedures to promote eye closure and prevent dryness. If at 1 year there has been no recovery, then discussion with the patient about possible interventions should proceed. Patients with HB grade I or II may be satisfied with their functional or cosmetic outcome and desire no intervention. Patients with HB grade III or IV may require various ancillary procedures or botulinum toxin injection for hyperfunction or synkinesis. Patients with grade V or VI may require various reanimation or reinnervation procedures to restore facial function, oral competence, and appearance.

CSF Leak

Incidence of CSF leak in temporal bone fracture ranges from 15% to 45%.[16,45,47] CSF otorrhea or rhinorrhea signifies an additional defect in the dural layer enveloping the brain. An injury to the skull base into the posterior or middle fossa may permit CSF to drain into the mastoid and middle ear, through the Eustachian tube, and into the nose or oropharynx. Otorrhea signifies a defect in the TM or the external ear canal. Collection of the fluid in a sterile container permits laboratory testing as outlined above.

Many imaging and radioisotope studies exist to assist in pinpointing the site of CSF egress. Often noncontrast HRCT is enough to suggest a defect in the skull base along the fracture line. However, when the site is more subtle, contrast-enhanced CT, radioisotope studies, or intrathecal dye instillation can be considered. Intrathecal dye methods are no longer in favor due to potential adverse reactions and the improvement of other methods. Radioisotope studies are useful in studies of the anterior skull base. If HRCT demonstrates a defect >2 cm, then MRI should be performed to rule out potential herniation of intracranial contents into the mastoid or middle ear, which may change surgical approach.[48]

Complications may occur in the presence of a CSF leak. The rate of meningitis in patients with temporal bone fractures and CSF leak has been demonstrated to be 7–10%[16,49]; the most significant risk factors were a leak persisting >7 days and the presence of a concurrent infection elsewhere. However, prophylactic antibiotics effective against the most common pathogen causing meningitis, *Pneumococcus spp.,* have led to a significant reduction in its incidence.[50] Routine use in trauma cases is controversial, however. Pneumocephalus may occur when air is introduced into the cranial cavity and sealed within by a ball-valve defect in the dura. The development of air within the dura is a potentially lethal complication, possibly resulting in intracranial hypertension and possible brain herniation.[51] If neurologic examination changes or if pneumocephalus is persistent, then aggressive management with the assistance of a neurosurgeon is indicated.

Initially, CSF leak can be managed with conservative measures as the majority of leaks will close spontaneously. Patients are instructed to maintain bed rest, elevate the head of the bed, and avoid straining with the use of stool softeners.[16] Spontaneous resolution with conservative management occurred in 95–100% of patients, with closure occurring in the first 7 days in 78% and between 8 and 14 days in 95%.[16,47] Placement of a lumbar drain can also be useful for persistent cases lasting 5–7 days after injury. The catheter is inserted into the subarachnoid space by aseptic lumbar puncture and left in place under sterile dressing. CSF is released through the catheter in a controlled fashion and at a defined rate to lessen the pressure differential across the dural defect and allow more expedient spontaneous closure.

CSF leaks that persist beyond the first 7 days despite these conservative methods, patients with recurrent meningitis, or patients with persistent pneumocephalus, will likely require surgical repair.[52] The proportion of patients with persistent CSF leak who require surgical repair appears to be approximately 5%.[16,47] Based on CT imaging and localization and extent of the defect, the approaches may include middle ear, mastoid, or middle fossa exposure. Depending on the size and shape of the defect, soft tissue or cartilage may be obtained for multilayer closure, usually reinforced by bone pate or free fragments or grafts taken from the mastoid in order to stabilize the repair against continuous CSF pulsation pressure and gravity. Depending on extent and persistence of the leak, temporal bone obliteration with abdominal fat grafting may be considered, possibly including removal of the TM and squamous elements of the EAC, with closure of the EAC. This latter option will result in a maximal CHL, and thus is particularly useful when sensorineural function has already been lost.

Hearing Loss

Audiometry should be performed on every patient with temporal bone fracture due to the risk of SNHL and CHL. If performed early, audiometry will likely show a component of CHL due to hemotympanum. A full audiometric workup should be obtained 3–6 weeks after injury to assess the existing level of SNHL and to examine for evidence of TM disruption or ossicular chain dislocation. At times there is total loss of one ear due to fracture, and standard otologic precautions should be taken when considering operating on the only hearing ear, including the consideration of amplification alone.

Conductive Hearing Loss

Conductive hearing loss is demonstrated more often in temporal bone fracture lines involving the attic and posterosuperior EAC wall. Associations of CHL with classifications of fracture lines may be seen in Table 22.1. Dislocation of the ossicles is frequently suggested on audiometry with a persistent air-bone gap of >20 dB, and may be seen on CT imaging as in Figures 22.5A and B. On middle ear exploration, incudostapedial dislocation is the most common finding (11–14%), followed by dislocation of the incudomallear joint, fracture of the stapes suprastructure (7%), and last malleus fracture (1%).[5,19] Children appear to have an increased incidence of stapes fracture, possibly secondary to increased deformity of the pediatric skull.[53]

Initial management is typically conservative, allowing for recovery from injury and clearance of blood products from the middle ear, TM injury and blood products in the EAC. However, if surgery is indicated for other reasons (e.g. facial nerve decompression or CSF leak repair), it may be appropriate to perform ossiculoplasty at that time.[39]

Fractures of the distal long process of the malleus near the umbo may be treated by excision of the fractured segment and tympanoplasty with temporalis fascia. More proximal malleus fractures may require removal of the malleus and either incus transposition or placement of prosthesis. Dislocation of the incus may be treated with either incus transposition, placement of prosthesis, or more conservatively with careful reduction of the dislocation and packing of the mastoid and middle ear.

Rarely, in patients with large skull base defects or after middle cranial fossa surgery, CHL can occur due to dura contacting the heads of the ossicles, resulting in a dampening of transmission. The hearing loss is generally minimal but may require skull base repair to correct, particularly with large defects or herniation.[48]

Prognosis for CHL is generally good, with closure of air-bone gap in most studies to within 10dB.[45]

Sensorineural Hearing Loss

Sensorineural hearing loss can occur after temporal bone trauma due to five proposed mechanisms: (1) direct injury to the acoustic nerve; (2) direct injury to the otic capsule with disruption of the membranous labyrinth, vascular vasospasm, thrombosis, or hemorrhage into the inner ear; (3) perilymphatic fistula; (4) occlusion of the vestibular aqueduct by the fracture line, followed by endolymphatic hydrops; and (5) pressure waves transmitted directly the cochlea, resulting in damage to the organ of Corti and concussion of the temporal bone without appreciable fracture lines.[54] Examples of otic-violating fractures resulting in complete SNHL may be seen in Figures 22.1 to 22.3.

Any sensorineural component evident on audiometry at 4–6 weeks is typically permanent and is not expected to improve with surgery. Patients with mild to moderate SNHL are treated with standard amplification. In patients with unilateral profound SNHL, bone-anchored hearing aids have traditionally been the best option for rehabilitation and to decrease the head-shadow effect. Temporal bone fracture may result in bilateral severe to profound SNHL however, and these patients may be candidates for cochlear implantation. Patients must be properly selected: there must be no significant bony discontinuity or cochlear ossification.[55-56] If a transverse temporal bone fracture occurs through the internal auditory canal, the postganglionic cochlear nerve may be injured, rendering cochlear implantation useless. If this type of injury is bilateral, an auditory brain stem implant (ABI) may be the only option for auditory rehabilitation, but these injuries are typically severe and often not survivable. Some surgeons recommend promontory testing to demonstrate an intact cochlear nerve (VIII) before implantation, though this test does not have high enough negative predictive value to preclude confidence interval (CI). High-resolution CT or heavily T2-weighted MRI sequences may be useful for establishing cochlear anatomy and patency, but shortly, the only method by which one may be sure a patient will not tolerate or benefit from CI is a CI trial.[63] Cochlear implantation in the ipsilateral ear in patients deafened by temporal bone fracture has resulted in 70-100% open-set sentence recognition. These results were found to be superior to ABI results in similar patients.[54] One study demonstrated a complication of facial nerve stimulation by CI through fracture lines in 2 of 7 patients with deafness due to temporal bone implantation. These two CIs required explantation, but the patients were able to be implanted in the contralateral ear with good hearing rehabilitation and no facial nerve stimulation.[55] Auditory brain stem implantation has been proposed as a second-line treatment for patients who fail CI.

Vestibular Injury/Dysfunction

Vertigo may be a complication of temporal bone fracture and must be fully investigated to determine etiology and help guide treatment. Short-term vestibular suppressants may be used to manage acute symptoms but chronic use prevents vestibular adaptation and rehabilitation, and should be avoided. Vestibular function testing may be helpful in analyzing the vestibular system and discerning the etiology of new-onset, postinjury vertigo.

Benign paroxysmal positional vertigo (BPPV) is certainly the most common etiology of vertigo after head trauma, usually developing days to weeks after the initial injury. BPPV symptoms are caused by traumatic displacement of otoconia into the ampulla of the semicircular canals, typically the posterior canal. Treatment is by standard repositioning maneuvers and rehabilitation. The prognosis is excellent with this therapy.

Perilymph fistula may occur at the oval or round window and may involve subluxation of the stapes footplate. This is typically treated with either repair or obliteration of niches during middle ear exploration.[5] Preservation of residual auditory and vestibular function, as well as resolution of symptoms, has been reported with surgical repair.[5,57]

When perilymph fistula has been ruled out, post-traumatic endolymphatic hydrops may be considered as an etiology for a trauma patient's vertigo. This is likely to occur in a delayed fashion after temporal bone injury, possibly secondary to occlusion of the vestibular aqueduct by the fracture line or healing process.[57] This complication is typically ongoing and chronic, with a similar prognosis to Meniere's disease. These patients usually first undergo medical management similar to Meniere's disease with low-salt diet, steroids, and diuretics. Usually the indications for intervention or surgical management follow the indications for management of Meniere's disease after failed trials of medical therapy.

Associated Lower Cranial Nerve Injury

Rarely, temporal bone fractures may present with palsies of other cranial nerves, usually V through XI. Penetrating injuries to the temporal bone may be extensive and comminuted, involving multiple foramina. Longitudinal fractures may extend to foramen ovale, while transverse may extend to foramen spinosum or lacerum.[24] The rationale for the timing of surgical intervention follows that of the facial nerve. If there was immediate onset of paralysis after injury, some authors advocate exploration. In the cases of delayed onset, expectant monitoring is usually advised and spontaneous recovery is the usual outcome.[58-59] Ongoing lower cranial nerve functional deficits, though unusual, can typically be rehabilitated according to current clinical guidelines for nontraumatic causes.

OTHER SEQUELAE

Various other rare sequelae of temporal bone trauma have been reported, and can be quite delayed. Meningocele or encephalocele may present from 1 to 21 years after the initial temporal bone trauma.[60] Presentation is generally with onset of CSF otorrhea, unilateral clear middle ear effusion, or recurrent meningitis. HRCT and MRI imaging may be required for proper diagnosis and surgical planning, and a combined mastoid and middle cranial fossa may be required for repair, similar to the previous discussion on CSF leaks.

Cholesteatoma attributable to a history of temporal bone trauma is rare with fewer than 20 reported cases.[61] Presentation may be 2–24 years after the initial injury. The development of this sequela may be due to a penetrating injury or fracture line seeding epithelial elements from the skin or EAC canal into the temporal bone. In one case series, 15% of patients surviving gunshot wounds to the temporal bone later developed secondary cholesteatoma requiring mastoidectomy.[16] Cholesteatomas from this mechanism are frequently extensive since the mastoid is typically well pneumatized and allows for uninhibited spread of the squamous elements. There have been case reports of otogenic brain abscesses due to infected cholesteatomas within fracture lines.[61] Mastoidectomy, including possible canal-wall-down or radical techniques, has been advocated as the primary treatment for penetrating gunshot wounds, as residual bullet fragments may remain lodged in the bone and become a nidus for infection as well.[24]

Patients with temporal bone fracture, particularly those violating the otic capsule, should be informed that they have an increased long-term risk for meningitis, estimated to be as high as 15%.[54] This is hypothesized to be secondary to the fibrous nature of the endochondral bone of the otic capsule, which is more porous than the native bone.[50,62] One case report illustrated the seriousness of this complication with a patient with remote history of temporal bone fracture who progressed from acute otitis media to lethal meningitis. Histopathologic analysis of the temporal bone after death showed acute purulent labyrinthitis within an old fracture line filled with fibrous tissue. The fracture line extended into the internal auditory canal and thus provided acquired access to the meningeal space.[62] In the event of such a complication, the meningitis should be treated per normal protocol. When resolved, the patient should be treated with labyrinthectomy and fat graft obliteration with closure of the EAC.

REFERENCES

1. Bailey FR, Miller AM. Text-Book of Embryology. New York, NY: William Wood and Co.

2. Nemzek WR, Brodie HA, Chong BW, et al. Imaging findings of the developing temporal bone in fetal specimens. Am J Neuroradiol. 1996;17(8):1467-77.
3. Virapongse C, Sarwar M, Bhimani S, et al. Computed tomorgraphy of temporal bone pneumatization: 1. Normal pattern and morphology. AJR. 1985;145:473-81.
4. Kang HM, Kim MG, Boo SH, et al. Comparison of the clinical relevance of traditional and new classification systems of temporal bone fractures. Eur Arch Otorhinolaryngol. 2012;269:1893-9.
5. Cannon CR, Jahrsdoerfer RA. Temporal bone fractures. Review of 90 cases. Arch Otolaryngol. 1983;109(5):285-8.
6. Dahiya R, Keller JD, Litofsky NS, et al. Temporal bone fractures: otic capsule sparing versus otic capsule violating clinical and radiographic considerations. J Trauma. 1999; 47(6):1079-83.
7. Hass AN, Ledington JA. Traumatic injuries of the temporal bone. Otolaryngol Clin North Am. 1988;21:295-316.
8. Wiet RJ, Valvassori GE, Kotsanis CA, et al. Temporal bone fractures: state of the art review. Am J Otolaryngol. 1985; 6:207-15.
9. McGuirt WF Jr., Stool SE. Temporal bone fractures in children: A review with emphasis on long-term sequelae. Clin Pediatr. 1992;31:12-8.
10. Yoganandan N, Pintar FA. Biomechanics of temporo-parietal skull fracture. Clinical Biomechanics. 2004;19:225-39.
11. Lee D, Honrado C, Har-El G, et al. Pediatric temporal bone fractures. Laryngoscope. 1998;108(6):816-21.
12. Alvi A, Bereliani A. Acute intracranial complications of temporal bone trauma. Otolaryngol Head Neck Surg. 1998;119 (6):609-13.
13. Spector GJ. Developmental temporal bone anatomy and its clinical significance: variations on themes by H.F. Schuknecht. Ann Otol Rhinol Laryngol Suppl. 1984;112:101-9.
14. Ghorayeb BY, Yeakley JW. Temporal bone fractures: longitudinal or oblique? The case for oblique temporal bone fractures. Laryngoscope. 1992;102:129-34.
15. Ishman SL, Friedland DR. Temporal bone fractures: traditional classification and clinical relevance. Laryngoscope. 2004;114(10):1734-41.
16. Brodie HA, Thompson TC. Management of complications from 820 temporal bone fractures. Am J Otol. 1997; 18(2):188-97.
17. Kelly KE, Tami TA. Temporal bone and skull base trauma. In: Jackler RK, Brackmann DE (eds), Neurotology. St Louis: Mosby; 1994. pp. 1127-47.
18. Little SC, Kesser BW. Radiographic classification of temporal bone fractures: clinical predictability using a new system. Arch Otolaryngol Head Neck Surg. 2006;132(12):1300-4.
19. Wysocki J. Cadaveric dissections based on observations of injuries to the temporal bone structures following head trauma. Skull Base. 2005;15(2):99-106.
20. Lew HL, Lee EH, Miyoshi Y. Brainstem auditory-evoked potentials as an objective tool for evaluating hearing dysfunction in traumatic brain injury. Am J Phys Med Rehabil. 2004;83(3):210-15.
21. Katsarkas A. Benign paroxysmal positional vertigo (BPPV): idiopathic versus post-traumatic. Acta Otolaryngol. 1999; 119(7):745-9.
22. Fisch U. Management of intratemporal facial nerve injuries. J Laryngol Otol. 1980;94(1):129-34.
23. Dula DJ, Fales W. The 'ring sign': is it a reliable indicator for cerebral spinal fluid? Ann Emerg Med. 1993;22(4):718-20.
24. Jenkins HA, Ator GA, Chen HH. Traumatic facial paralysis. In: Brackmann DE, Shelton C, Arriaga MA, et al. (eds), Otologic Surgery, 3rd edition. Philadelphia, PA: Saunders; 2010. pp. 347-361.
25. Johnson DW, Hasso AN, Stewart CE, et al. Temporal bone trauma: high-resolution computed tomographic evaluation. Radiology. 1984;151(2):411-5.
26. Holland BA, Brant-Zawadzki M. High-resolution CT of temporal bone trauma. AJR Am J Roentgenol. 1984;143(2):391-5.
27. Brodie HA. Management of temporal bone trauma. In: Flint PW, Haughey BH, Lund VJ, et al. (eds), Cummings Otolaryngology Head & Neck Surgery. Philadelphia: Elsevier; 2010.
28. Zimmerman RA, Bilaniuk LT, Hackney DB, Goldberg HI, Grossman RI. Magnetic resonance imaging in temporal bone fracture. Neuroradiology. 1987;29(3):246-51.
29. Haberkamp TJ, Harvey SA, Daniels DL. The use of gadolinium-enhanced magnetic resonance imaging to determine lesion site in traumatic facial paralysis. Laryngoscope. 1990;100(12):1294-300.
30. Kerwin AJ, Bynoe RP, Murray J, et al. Liberalized screening for blunt carotid and vertebral artery injuries is justified. J Trauma. 2001;51(2):308-14.
31. Chang CY, Cass SP. Management of facial nerve injury due to temporal bone trauma. Am J Otol. 1999;20:96-114.
32. Nash JJ, Friedland DR, Boorsma KJ, et al. Management and outcomes of facial paralysis from intratemporal blunt trauma: a systematic review. Laryngoscope. 2010;120 Suppl 4:S214.
33. Darrouzet V, Duclos JY, Liguoro D. Management of facial paralysis resulting from temporal bone fractures: Our experience in 115 cases. Otolaryngol Head Neck Surg. 2001; 125:77-84.
34. McKennan KX, Chole RA. Facial paralysis in temporal bone trauma. Am J Otol. 1992;13:167-72.
35. Coker NJ, Fordice JO, Moore S. Correlation of the nerve excitability test and electroneurography in acute facial paralysis. Am J Otol. 1992;13:127-33.
36. Fisch U. Facial paralysis in fractures of the petrous bone. Laryngoscope. 1974;84:2141-54.
37. Shindo ML, Fetterman BL, Shih L. Gunshot wounds of the temporal bone: A rational approach to evaluation and management. Otolaryngol Head Neck Surg. 1995;112:533-9.
38. Duncan NO 3rd, Coker NJ, Jenkins HA, et al. Gunshot injuries of the temporal bone. Otolaryngol Head Neck Surg. 1986;94:47-55.
39. Hato N, Nota J, Hakuba N, et al. Facial nerve decompression surgery in patients with temporal bone trauma: analysis of 66 cases. J Trauma. 2011;71(6):1789-93.

40. Quaranta A, Campobasso G, Piazza F. Facial nerve paralysis in temporal bone fractures: outcomes after late decompression surgery. Acta Otolaryngol. 2001;121(5):652-5.
41. Sofferman RA. Facial nerve injury and decompression. In: Nadol JB, Mckenna MJ (eds), Surgery of the Ear and Temporal Bone, 2nd edition. Philadelphia, PA: Lippincott Williams & Wilkins; 2005:435-50.
42. Coker NJ, Kendall KA, Jenkins HA, et al. Traumatic intratemporal facial nerve injury: management rationale for preservation of function. Otolaryngol Head Neck Surg. 1978;97:262-9.
43. Coker NJ. Management of traumatic injuries to the facial nerve. Otolaryngol Clin North Am. 1991;24:215-27.
44. Bozorg Grayeli A, Mosnier I, Julien N. Long-term functional outcome in facial nerve graft by fibrin glue in the temporal bone and cerebellopontine angle. Eur Arch Otorhinolaryngol. 2005;262(5):404-7
45. Nosan DK, Benecke JE Jr, Murr AH. Current perspective on temporal bone trauma. Otolaryngol Head Neck Surg. 1997; 117:67-71.
46. Ulug T, Arif Ulubil S. Management of facial paralysis in temporal bone fractures: a prospective study analyzing 11 operated fractures. Am J Otolaryngol. 2005;26(4):230-38.
47. McGuirt WF Jr., Stool SE. Cerebrospinal fluid fistula: the identification and management in pediatric temporal bone fractures. Laryngoscope. 1995;105(4 Pt 1):359-64.
48. Nishiike S, Miyao Y, Gouda S. Brain herniation into the middle ear following temporal bone fracture. Acta Otolaryngol. 2005;125(8):902-5.
49. Leech PJ, Paterson A. Conservative and operative management for cerebrospinal-fluid leakage after closed head injury. Lancet. 1973;1:1013-6.
50. Brodie HA. Prophylactic antibiotics for posttraumatic cerebrospinal fluid fistulae. A meta-analysis. Arch Otolaryngol Head Neck Surg. 1997;123(7):749-52.
51. Andrews JC, Canalis RF. Otogenic pneumocephalus. Laryngoscope. 1986;96(5):521-8.
52. Marentette LJ, Valentino J. Traumatic anterior fossa cerebrospinal fluid fistulae and craniofacial considerations. Otolaryngol Clin North Am. 1991;24:151-63.
53. Singh S, Salib RJ, Oates J. Traumatic fracture of the stapes suprastructure following minor head injury. J Laryngol Otol. 2002;116(6)457-9.
54. Medina M, Di Lella F, Di Trapani G, et al. Cochlear implantation versus auditory brainstem implantation in bilateral total deafness after head trauma: personal experience and review of the literature. Otol Neurotol. 2014;35(2):260-70.
55. Camilleri AE, Toner JG, Howarth KL, et al. Cochlear implantation following temporal bone fracture. J Laryngol Otol. 1999;113(5):454-7.
56. Simons JP, Whitaker ME, Hirsch BE. Cochlear implantation in a patient with bilateral temporal bone fractures. Otolaryngol Head Neck Surg. 2005;132(5):809-11.
57. Lyos AT, Marsh MA, Jenkins HA. Progressive hearing loss after transverse temporal bone fracture. Arch Otolaryngol Head Neck Surg. 1995;121(7):795-9.
58. Ghorayeb BY, Yeakley JW, Hall 3rd JW. Unusual complications of temporal bone fractures. Arch Otolaryngol Head Neck Surg. 1987;113(7):749-53.
59. Yildirim A, Gurelik M, Gumus C. Fracture of skull base with delayed multiple cranial nerve palsies. Pediatr Emerg Care. 2005;21(7):440-42.
60. Souliere Jr. CR, Langman AW. Combined mastoid/middle cranial fossa repair of temporal bone encephalocele. Skull Base Surg. 1998;4:185-9.
61. Majmundar K, Shaw T, Sismanis A. Traumatic cholesteatoma presenting as a brain abscess: a case report. Otol Neurotol. 2005;26(1):65-7.
62. Sudhoff H, Linthicum Jr FH. Temporal bone fracture and latent meningitis: temporal bone histopathology study of the month. Otol Neurotol. 2003;24(3)521-2.
63. Johnson F, Semaan MT, Megerian CA. Temporal bone fracture: evaluation and management in the modern era. Otolaryngol Clin North Am. 2008;41(3):597-618, x.

CHAPTER

23

Vestibular Schwannoma

Sean McMenomey, Maja Svrakic

INTRODUCTION

Historical Background

Vestibular schwannomas were described in the 18th and 19th century, but the first attempt at surgical removal was performed by Charles McBurney in 1891, followed by Sir Charles Balance and Thomas Annandale in the subsequent decade.[1,2] These early surgical efforts were largely unsafe and carried up to 78% mortality rates. The stage for modern principles of surgical removal of vestibular schwannomas was set by Harvey Cushing in the early 20th century, who with meticulous hemostasis and gentle dissection brought the mortality rate down to 20% in 1917. He utilized a bilateral suboccipital approach for removal of tumors, allowing for adequate herniation of the cerebellum, which was routinely partially resected in an effort to improve patient survival.[3] One should keep in mind that before imaging, in this era, patients presented with late, life-threatening brain stem compressing symptoms from large tumors. It was Cushing's trainee, Walter Dandy who further refined the technique with a unilateral suboccipital approach, in wide use today.[4]

The true modern era in surgical resection of vestibular schwannoma was marked by William House in the 1960s, who perfected the translabyrinthine and middle cranial fossa (MCF) approach utilizing the operating microscope and surgical drills.[5-7] By the mid-1980s, mortality rates of vestibular schwannomas were consistently under 1%.[8] Once mortality was in the background of complications of vestibular schwannoma resection, refinements in technique such as those utilized for facial nerve preservation and, more recently, hearing took precedence.

Incidence and Epidemiology

The most commonly quoted incidence rate of vestibular schwannoma in the United States is 10 per million per year, amounting to almost 3200 newly diagnosed tumors annually.[8] This incidence rate is similar to the incidence found in other countries, ranging from 10 to 20 per million people per year.[9-15] A recent review of the Denmark patient database over the last four decades reports a significant increase in incidence, from 3 per million per year in 1976, to almost 23 per million per year in 2004 and leveling off at 19 per million per year in 2008.[16] The increase in incidence is almost entirely due to improved diagnostic methods, but increased physician and patient symptom awareness certainly play a role.

Incidentally discovered vestibular schwannomas, those found in patients who had MRI scans performed for other reasons and either had no symptoms or were not pursuing the cause of their symptoms, may be as high as 2 in 10,000 adults.[17] Some older histopathologic studies have found incidental vestibular schwannomas in up to 2.7% of autopsy specimens.[18] There appears to be no gender prevalence, although men may have a higher rate of incidentally discovered schwannomas.[17]The mean age of diagnosis continues to be in the 5th decade of life for sporadic unilateral tumors.[16,19] In patients with neurofibromatosis type 2 (NF2), the initial presentation is in the 20s and 30s.[20]

Etiology and Pathology

Vestibular schwannomas arise from the vestibular division of cranial nerve VIII (CN VIII). Their common misnomer is acoustic neuromas, although the NIH consensus discourages its use. While some groups have shown an equal prevalence in origin between the superior and inferior vestibular nerve (IVN) divisions,[21] others report a strong predilection for the IVN.[22] Most vestibular nerve schwannomas originate lateral to the glial-schwannian junction.[23] The myelin sheath of CN VIII is produced proximally by the oligodendroglial cells, and distally by the Schwann cells; the switch in the type of myelin-producing cells can vary, which can account for the variable site of origin of the schwannomas along the vestibular nerve. However, most occur in the vicinity of the vestibular ganglion, where the density of Schwann cells is the highest.[24]

On gross examination, vestibular schwannomas are yellow-white or yellow-gray heterogeneous masses, with frequent cystic components covered in a smooth and regular surface. Despite the smooth surface that is distinct from the core, there is no true capsule to this tumor. Histopathologic studies have shown two morphologically distinct cells comprising vestibular schwannomas: Antoni A and Antoni B cells. Antoni A cells are small, densely packed, spindle-shaped cells, while Antoni B cells are pleomorphic, looser, and contain a vacuolated cytoplasm.[25,26]

The molecular sequence of events that leads to formation of vestibular schwannomas is still under research. The NF2 tumor suppressor gene found on chromosome 22 has been shown to be inactivated in both familial and sporadic cases. The product of the NF2 gene (merlin) regulates Schwann cell division; mutations in both copies are necessary for the phenotype of unregulated growth and resultant vestibular schwannomas.[27,28] Estrogen and progesterone hormones,[29-31] repeated radiation from diagnostic studies[32,33] and even cell phone use[34] have all been investigated as environmental factors that may contribute to the development of vestibular schwannomas, although their role is still uncertain.

Growth Characteristics

The stereotypical pattern of growth of vestibular schwannomas consists of an intracanalicular (IAC) component that later expands medially to the cisternal, followed by brain stem compressive and hydrocephalic in its late stages.[8] The symptoms of these four classically described stages are progressively more severe, starting with tinnitus or mild hearing loss and progressing to visual loss, lower CN dysfunction, and even death from tonsillar herniation. The late stages of growth are rarely encountered today owing to earlier diagnoses. The rate of growth rarely exceeds 2 mm per year, and is further discussed in the section on conservative management ("watchful waiting") of vestibular schwannomas.

Measurement of size of vestibular schwannomas is not consistent in the literature. Radiation treatment-based studies report on volumetric dimensions, while studies on surgical treatment or meta-analyses report most frequently the largest axial dimension. The morphologic feature of vestibular schwannomas is distinguished by a spherical component (the cisternal portion) and a tongue-like protrusion into the IAC portion. Thus, calculating a spherical volume from the largest axial diameter (traversing both the cisternal and IAC portion) will overestimate the true volume of tumor. As radiologic diagnostic methods become more sophisticated, a volumetric calculation will likely replace diameter-based estimates. Although there is no universally accepted terminology to describe small versus large tumors, most authors utilize the following classification:

1. *Intracanalicular*
2. *Small*: <1 cm (*see* Fig. 23.1)
3. *Medium*: <2.5 cm (*see* Figs. 23.2A and B)
4. *Large*: >2.5 cm (*see* Fig. 23.3)
5. *Giant*: >4 cm (*see* Fig. 23.4)

CLINICAL MANIFESTATIONS

The typical clinical presentation of an early (IAC) vestibular schwannoma consists of symptoms related to CNVIII—

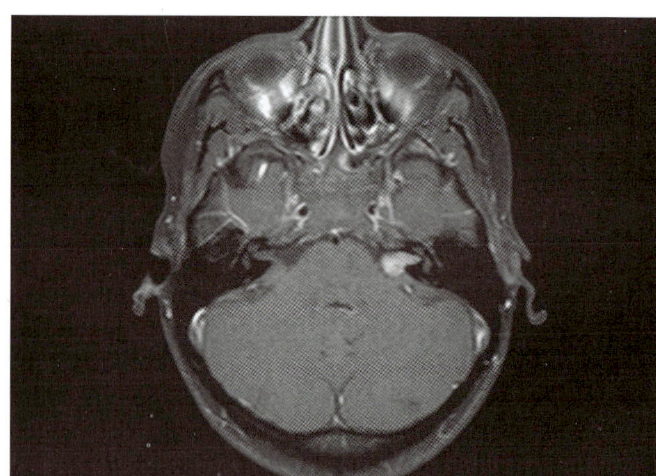

Fig. 23.1: Small vestibular schwannoma. Axial Gd-enhanced T1 MRI sequence shows a small left-sided vestibular schwannoma with both a cisternal and intracanalicular component.

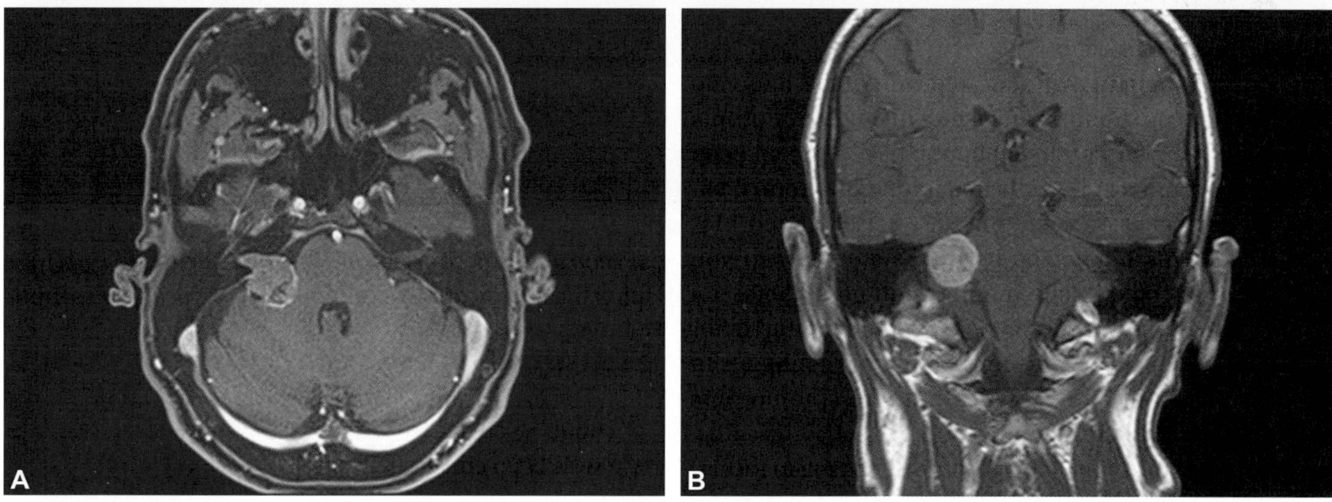

Figs. 23.2A and B: Medium-sized vestibular schwannoma. Axial and coronal Gd-enhanced T1 MRI sequence shows a medium right-sided vestibular schwannoma with both a cisternal and intracanalicular component.

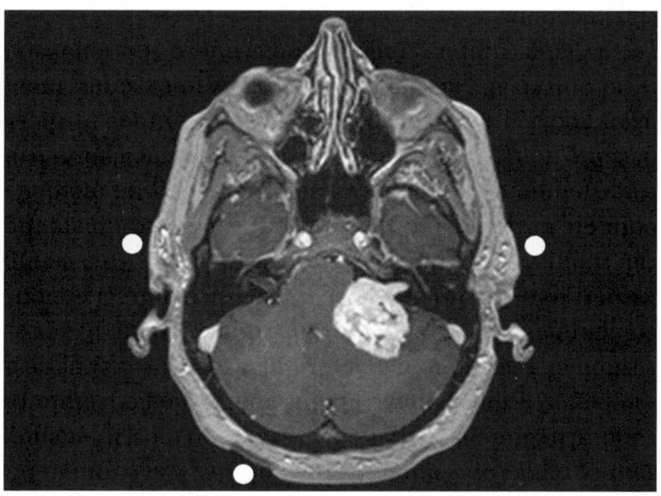

Fig. 23.3: Large vestibular schwannoma. Axial Gd-enhanced T1 MRI sequence shows a large left vestibular schwannoma with both a cisternal and intracanalicular component.

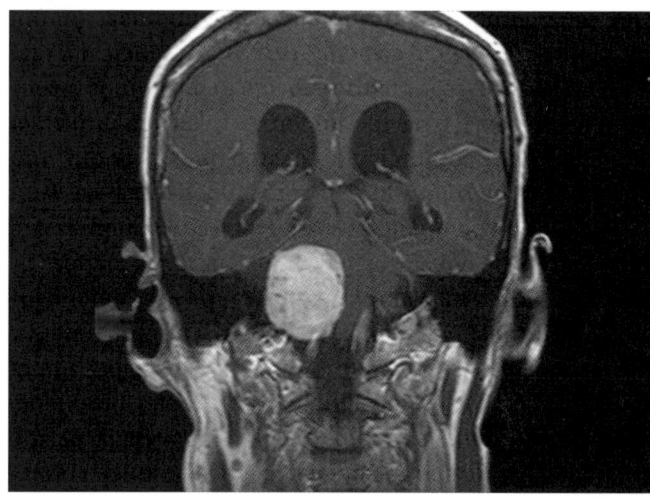

Fig. 23.4: Giant vestibular schwannoma. Coronal Gd-enhanced T1 MRI sequence shows a giant right vestibular schwannoma measuring 4.1 cm in the anteroposterior and 3.5 cm in the cranio-caudal dimension. Note the resulting hydrocephalus from brain stem and fourth ventricle compression.

hearing loss, tinnitus, and vestibular dysfunction. As the tumor grows medially, in its cisternal stage, hearing loss typically worsens and vertigo progresses to disequilibrium. Further growth with brain stem compression is accompanied with trigeminal symptoms. It is rare to encounter a patient with late brain stem compressive symptoms and hydrocephalus, although large tumors were the norm in the Cushing era, along with visual loss and headaches associated with increased intracranial pressure (ICP).

Hearing loss is a symptom found in over 95% of patients. The most likely reason is interruption of the blood supply to the inner ear and cochlear nerve by tumor compression, but also from tumor infiltration of the auditory fibers. The hearing loss is typically unilateral and asymmetric, involving preferentially high frequencies. Patients will notice a difficulty with phone use on the affected side. In up to a quarter of patients with vestibular schwannomas, a sudden decrease in hearing occurs, similar to an acute viral infection or vascular occlusion, and can be attributed to idiopathic sudden sensorineural hearing loss (SNHL) only if the presence of a vestibular schwannoma is ruled out with imaging.[19,35] The clinician should keep in mind that even in patients who have tumors the sudden loss may recover, and they should be diligent in their search for retrocochlear pathology.[36]

Normal or symmetric hearing does not rule out a vestibular schwannoma. In fact, up to 15% of patients can have subjectively normal hearing, and up to 4% can be audiometrically normal [stereotactic radiotherapy (SRT)<25dB, speech discrimination score (SDS) > 85%].[19,37] Tinnitus is seen in up to 70% of patients, vertigo in 19%, and disequilibrium is reported by up to 70% of patients with large tumors.[19,35,37] Other associated symptoms, especially with larger tumors, are a result of trigeminal nerve involvement. Altered facial sensation, most commonly hypoesthesia, can occur in up to 50% of patients with tumor >2 cm.[19] In these patients, the ipsilateral corneal reflex will likely be diminished.

Weakness of either the facial or the trigeminal nerve is a rare symptom and occurs with larger tumors. Facial twitching occurs in no >10% of patients.[19] If facial nerve function is electroneurographically impaired, the clinician should suspect an alternate diagnosis such as facial nerve neurinomas, malignant tumors of the cerebellopontine angle (CPA), or metastases.[38] Large and compressive tumors can manifest with headache and papilledema from resultant hydrocephalus, which occurs in < 4% of patients.[19] Lower CN deficits and long tract signs are very rarely seen today. Sudden neurologic deterioration can occur secondary to intratumoral hemorrhage, with acute symptoms of hearing loss, facial spasm or weakness, facial sensory disturbance, hoarseness, and altered mental status.[39,40] An emergent surgical intervention, usually with a ventriculostomy, is required. Fortunately, this potentially life-threatening event is seldom encountered. Table 23.1 demonstrates the changing trends in presentation of vestibular schwannomas over the past 100 years.

WORKUP

Auditory and Vestibular Studies

Conventional pure tone and speech audiometry is the workhorse of diagnostic studies in the initial evaluation of vestibular schwannomas. Classically, patients present with unilateral asymmetric, preferentially high frequency, gradual loss along with decreased SDS that are out of proportion to the pure tone loss. These two cost-effective audiometric tests are a screening tool used to identify those patients who should undergo an MRI imaging study. The advantage of pure tone and speech audiometry is that it is relatively inexpensive and readily available across centers and around the world.

The prevalence of vestibular schwannoma in patients with asymmetrical hearing loss has been estimated as high as 7.7%.[45-48] There is still no consensus as to what constitutes *asymmetric* hearing. Methods used include the pure-tone average (PTA) approach (average asymmetry across several specified frequencies), the single-frequency approach (hearing asymmetry is only calculated at one frequency), and multiple frequency pure-tone asymmetry approach (single frequency hearing asymmetries must be present at two or more frequencies and exceed a specified asymmetry criterion). *See* Table 23.2 for examples of these approaches.

The patient's history should always be considered, especially when hearing loss can be explained by other causes, such as significant head trauma, noise trauma, radiation therapy to the head and neck, chemotherapy, or immunosuppression. These patients may not warrant further workup for retrocochlear pathology. While trigeminal

Table 23.1: Changing trends in presentation of vestibular schwannoma

Author	*Group (year)*	*N*	*Hearing loss*	*Tinnitus*	*Disequilibrium*	*Vertigo*	*CN V*	*CN VII*	*Low CN*	*Visual symptoms*	*Acute*
Cushing[41]	Hopkins and Harvard (1917)	30	100%	77%	90% vestibular symptoms		87%	77%	70%		23% crisis
Mathew et al.[42]	Mayo Clinic (1978)	225	97%	66%	46%	5%	33%	22%		15%	
Selesnick et al.[43]	UCSF (1993)	126	85%	56%	48%	19%	20%	10%	0%	3%	
Matthies and Samii[35]	Hannover (1997)	1,000	95%	63%	61%	61%	17%	17%	3%	2%	
Harun et al.[44]	Hopkins (2012)	1,269	91%	69%	61% dizziness			4%			

(CN, cranial nerve).

Table 23.2: Auditory testing thresholds for further workup of asymmetric SNHL

Author (year) (ref)	*Frequencies (kHz)*	*Threshold criteria*	*Additional factors*
Welling et al.[49]	0.5, 1, 2, 4	≥15 dB	WRS >20% difference Vertigo Sudden SNHL Other CN
Mangham[50]	PTA (1, 2, 4, 8)	≥5 dB: ABR ≥20 dB: MRI	
Ruckenstein et al.[51] Cueva[47]	0.25, 0.5, 1, 2, 4, 8	≥15 dB at 2+ freq	WRS >15% difference
Robinette et al.[52]	PTA (0.5, 1, 2, 3)	≥15 dB	WRS <30% Vertigo Aural fullness Headache Other CN
Obholzer et al.[53]	0.25, 0.5, 1, 2, 4, 8	If PTA ≤ 30 dB 15 dB at 2 adj freq If PTA > 30 dB 20 dB at 2 adj freq	Unilateral tinnitus Sudden SNHL

(SNHL, sensorineural heart loss; CN, cranial nerve; ABR, auditory brainstem response; PTA, pure-tone average; WRS: word recognition score).

nerve dysfunction is highly suspicious for CPA lesions, fluctuant, low-frequency SNHL associated with aural fullness is rarely concerning for vestibular schwannomas. Patients who develop sudden SNHL, even if it later recovers, should undergo further testing as up to 15% of vestibular schwannomas present in this manner.[54,55] What constitutes asymmetric hearing loss that is medically significant continues to vary and is based on clinician's intuition.[56]

Asymmetric pure tone and speech audiometry can also be followed up with an auditory brainstem response (ABR). The ABR pattern most specific for presence of a vestibular schwannoma is presence of wave I only, but wave V latency is found in up to 60% of abnormal diagnostic ABRs. In the era of MRIs, the ABR test, once thought of as highly specific and sensitive, has significant false negative and false positive rates. An overall false negative rate may be as high as 15% and up to 33% in IAC tumors.[47,57] In larger tumors, however, only 4% of schwannomas had normal ABRs. The false positive rate of ABRs is also surprisingly high, and can exceed 80% in standard, nonsophisticated settings.[8] The specificity and sensitivity of ABR, especially in small tumors, can be improved upon with a stacked ABR. Stacked ABRs are composed of neural activity initiated across the whole cochlea and are able to detect by reduction in wave amplitude even IAC tumors with specificity and sensitivity in the 90% range.[58]

The role of OAEs is currently limited. OAEs can be used as a risk stratifying method in patients in whom hearing preservation is considered.[59-61] Specifically, patients with Class C or D hearing, in whom ABR is undetectable, may suffer from purely retrocochlear conduction but normal cochlear function, which would be detected with good OAEs. Unfortunately, this is not commonly the case, as vestibular schwannomas frequently disrupt cochlear hair cell function, likely by limiting the blood supply to the cochlea.[62]

Vestibular tests are infrequently used in the diagnosis for vestibular schwannomas. Most commonly this is due to high false positive rates, i.e. many patients who are found to have an abnormal vestibular test will not have a tumor when subjected to an MRI. Although up to 90% of patients with vestibular schwannoma will have an electronystagmography test battery abnormality,[63-65] the specificity rate is quite low. Caloric responses can be used to predict the origin of tumor. Since the lateral semicircular canal is sensitive to external warm or cool irrigation, the superior vestibular nerve (SVN) generates the response. Thus, if caloric response is diminished, the SVN is likely affected, and if the caloric response is normal, the IVN could be the nerve of tumor origin. In fact, 98% of SVN tumors show diminished caloric responses, compared to 60% of IVN tumors.[65]

Imaging Studies

Current diagnostic methods for radiologically detecting vestibular schwannomas almost exclusively rely on MRI. Plain films of the IAC and polytomography are of historical interest only. Computed tomography (CT) scans were utilized in the 1970s, and when contrast enhanced can detect tumors >1.5 cm. At present, a contrast-enhanced CT can be of value in patients who cannot undergo an MRI or in the elderly when detecting a small tumor would not change management and the study is done to rule out a larger, brain stem–compressing lesion.

The characteristic profile of vestibular schwannomas on gadolinium (Gd)-enhanced MRIs is a brightly enhancing lesion on T1 imaging. Lesions as small as 1 mm can be seen with thin-sectioned sequences targeted to the IAC. In gradient echo T2-weighted high-resolution images such as the constructive interference in the steady state (CISS) sequence, the individual nerves coursing through the IAC appear as hypointense linear structures surrounded by T2 hyperintense cerebrospinal fluid (CSF). Vestibular schwannoma can be seen as a hypointense mass, displacing CSF or distorting adjacent nerves. This sequence is particularly useful in detecting fluid between the lateral end of the vestibular schwannomas and the internal auditory canal fundus, absence of which can have a negative influence on hearing outcome as well as facial nerve function.[66]

Meningiomas at the CPA can have a similar MRI profile as the vestibular schwannomas. They can be distinguished by their sessile, eccentrically placed base, dural tail, solid consistency (as opposed to cystic), as well as by other morphological factors. Enhancements of the 8th nerve or within the IAC from a viral or immune-mediated neuritis have been reported as false-positive cases of vestibular schwannomas. However, Gd-enhanced MRIs remain a diagnostic gold standard, especially in the age of early detection of small tumors.[67,68]

The major downside of MRIs is their cost and relatively low yield. They can be burdensome in terms of time, expense, and inefficient utilization of health-care capacity. In screening asymmetric hearing loss, the average cost for identifying a positive patient based on MRI was $61,650.[69]

However, early detection and management of vestibular schwannomas may result in reduced morbidity, especially since hearing preservation surgery is now a realistic goal if schwannomas are diagnosed and treated before they are >2 cm. Carrier et al. have proposed one way in decreasing the cost of MRI imaging with a focused enhanced sequence.[70] Their protocol is of comparable cost to ABRs, and is able to detect small tumors with anatomical detail needed for planning surgical approach.

NF2 Testing

A definitive diagnosis of NF2 requires the presence of bilateral vestibular schwannomas or developing a unilateral vestibular schwannoma by 30 years and a first-degree blood relative with NF2, or the presence of a unilateral vestibular schwannoma and developing at least two of the following conditions known to be associated with NF2: meningioma, glioma, schwannoma, or juvenile posterior subcapsular lenticular opacity/juvenile cortical cataract[71]; *see* Figures 23.5A and B. Patients with probable NF2 should undergo further evaluation with MRI of the IAC if not already performed, as well as a complete spinal series to evaluate the spine and stage the disease.

Genetic counseling should be offered to patients with NF2. Blood screening for the specific mutation of the NF2 gene on chromosome 22 can be performed in patients who have diagnosed NF2, as the defect may be identified in up to 75% of patients, and subsequently used to screen family members. The use of blood screening for patients without a diagnosis of NF2 or with a suspected diagnosis of NF2 is not recommended.

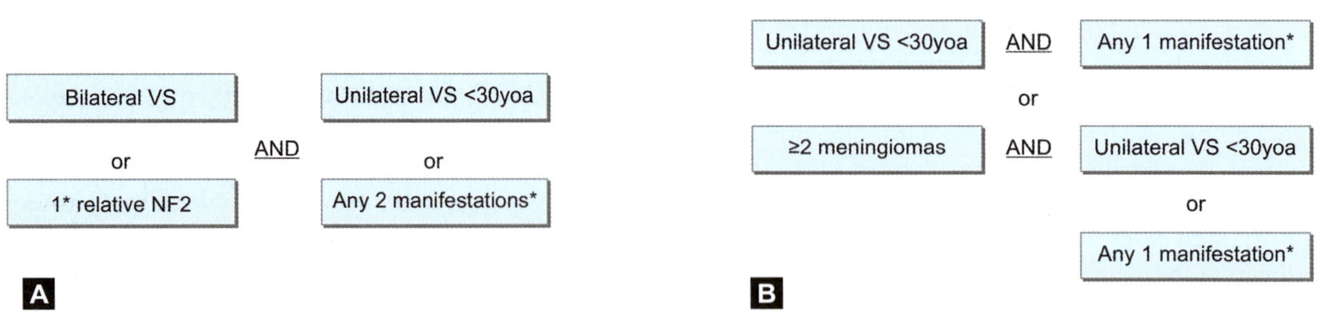

Figs. 23.5A and B: (A) Definite NF2. (B) Probable NF2 (should evaluate). *Manifestations include meningioma, glioma, schwannoma, or juvenile posterior subcapsular lenticular opacities/juvenile cortical cataract.

Delayed Diagnosis

As MRI imaging became more widespread in the use of ruling out retrocochlear pathology in those patients with asymmetric hearing loss, the delay in diagnosis from onset of symptoms to confirmation of lesion in the CPA became shorter. In 1989, Traquina et al. reported on their vestibular schwannoma patient population who experienced diminished auditory function for over 2 years in 60% of cases, and the mean duration of hearing loss prior to diagnosis was over 4 years.[72] Clear superiority of the MRI to aid in timely diagnosis was also demonstrated in a Danish study in 1990 where the use of this imaging modality was still limited at the time and a large percentage of tumors were discovered by CT scans, measuring 4 cm in size.[73] Reasons for delay may include both patient and physician factors, and are likely to diminish with increased awareness. Because there are no specific clinical findings that clearly distinguish those patients with vestibular schwannomas from other patients with sudden hearing loss,[19] an evaluation with ABR or Gd-enhanced MRI for any patient with sudden hearing loss even when hearing normalizes[74] is recommended.

MANAGEMENT STRATEGIES

Patient Counseling

Management of patients with vestibular schwannoma consists of three main strategies:

1. Observation (watchful waiting)
2. Surgical resection
3. Radiation therapy

It is especially important that the patient receives counseling with respect to all three of these strategies and that the clinician is familiar with expected outcomes, risks and benefits of observation, surgery, and radiation. This may indeed involve more than one clinician, such as a neurotologist, skull base surgeon, neurosurgeon, and radiation oncologist. Each of the management options is discussed separately below.

Choice of management strategy is based on predicted natural course of the tumor and the neurologic sequelae (such as CN deficits and brain stem compression), the ability to either surgically remove the tumor with minimal postoperative complications, or radiate the tumor with least adverse effects. Preservation of hearing, if present at diagnosis, strongly guides management. Patient-specific factors such as age, medical condition, patient's desire, their ability for follow-up, and social and economical support influence treatment options. Finally, the surgeon's operative skill and familiarity with pitfalls and their avoidance for each surgical approach may dictate the specific intervention chosen (Table 23.3).

Contemporary Treatment Trends and Expected Outcomes

A recent meta-analysis of outcomes of all three management strategies compared large studies published since 2004, with a pooled total of over 5,000 patients.[75]They summarized that observation of patients with vestibular schwannomas offers the least risk, but that growth occurs in 29–54% of the cases and about a half of those patients will require additional treatment. Risks of surgery are avoided with radiation-based treatment, but additional treatment may be required in up to 10% of cases, and radiation-induced risks are not negligible. While surgical resection offers the best control rates and most cytoreductive therapy and very rarely requires additional treatment, it poses risks such as facial nerve neuropathy in about a quarter of the cases. Hearing preservation is comparable in observation and radiation in 3 and 6 years of follow-up, respectively, and can be expected in about half of the cases. With hearing-preservation attempts in microsurgical resection, the chance of hearing preservation falls to about a third of the patients.

The most recent patient polling conducted by the Acoustic Neuroma Association in 2008 compiled data from over 2000 respondents, and compared them to the 1983 and 1998 surveys. These are the trends observed by the survey[76,77]:

1. Tumor size at diagnosis has decreased significantly
   a. Before 1998, 23.8% tumors were <1.5 cm, compared to after 1998, where 45.3% of newly diagnosed tumors are <1.5 cm
2. More patients with smaller tumors are being treated
   a. For tumors < 1.5 cm, treatment has increased from 17% in 1983 to 38% in 2008
   b. 50% of tumors treated now are >2 cm in diameter
3. Fewer patients are undergoing surgical treatment
   a. 100% of patients underwent surgical treatment in 1983; this has fallen to 85% in 1998 and 61% in 2008
4. Radiation therapy has become more common
   a. 20% of patients are treated with radiation in 2008, up from 5% in 1998 and 0% in 1983
5. Observation is playing a more significant role in management
   a. 4% of patients were followed with watchful waiting in 1998 and 20% in 2008

Table 23.3: Summary of advantages and disadvantages of management strategies

	Management strategy					
	Observation		*Radiation*		*Surgery*	
Consideration	*Advantages*	*Disadvantages*	*Advantages*	*Disadvantages*	*Advantages*	*Disadvantages*
Level of intervention	Noninvasive	Serial MRIs needed	Nonsurgical, minimally invasive (one day intervention for stereotactic)	Weekly intervention (for fractionated RT) Postintervention MRIs		Highly invasive Postoperative hospital stay Long recovery time
Hearing	Hearing-sparing (initially)	Unpredictable time to hearing loss	Can be hearing-sparing	Unpredictable time to hearing loss	Up-front hearing outcome	Higher risk of hearing loss (approach-dependent)
Balance		Unpredictable level of balance disturbance		Unpredictable level of balance disturbance	Nonaffected side compensates Predictable balance outcome	Immediate postoperative balance disturbance
Facial nerve function	Preserves facial nerve function		Mostly preserves facial nerve function			Facial nerve function at risk (approach and size-dependent)
Recurrence		Lesion persists/grows May ultimately require intervention	May involute	Lesion persists May require salvage surgery (higher risk)	Goal is eradication of disease Low recurrence rate In case of recurrence or subtotal resection, leaves radiation as option	
Sequelae	Avoids surgical and radiation risks	Unpredictable growth rate/ behavior	Avoids surgical risks	Rare malignant transformation Rare hydrocephalus Rare trigeminal nerve symptoms	Avoids radiation risks	Surgical risks: CSF leak, meningitis, wound infection
Limitations	Good for elderly Good for patients with medical comorbidities	Cystic and compressive tumors not amenable	Good for patients with medical comorbidities	Poor choice for younger patients Large tumors (> 3 cm) not amenable	Only choice for large/cystic/ compressive tumors	Poor choice for patients with significant medical comorbidities

While these trends may continue in the same direction, the pendulum may also swing in favor of one over another strategy as it becomes more refined, available technology becomes more sophisticated and more precise, and as effectiveness is maximized and risk reduced. At present, microsurgery continues to be the primary method of treatment across tumor sizes in the United States and observation remains the least common management modality.

Cost

Awareness of cost of treatment is practical for the clinician. In the United States, data from 2008 showed that the mean cost of microsurgery for patients with tumors >3 cm was $23,788 compared with $16,143 for radiation treatment. Although the upfront cost of surgery was higher, cumulative cost of radiation and follow-up remained lower only if the rate of tumor progression was <3%.[78,79] In a similar Canadian study on small (<1.5 cm) tumors, conservative management was least costly (approximately CAN$10,000) compared to microsurgical removal (CAN$22,000) and Gamma Knife radiotherapy (CAN$28,000). Thirty-five percent of patients in the conservative arm of this study progressed to surgery or radiation.[80]

Table 23.4: Reasons for management with watchful waiting

Reason for observation	*Bakkouri et al.*[94] *(n=386)*	*Tschudi et al.*[93] *(n=74)*	*Glasscock et al.*[90] *(n=34)*
Tumor size	67%	32%	68%
Risk deterioration of hearing	51%	27%	
Advanced age	42%	4%	53%
Poor general health	5%	4%	24%
Patient preference		54%	
Minimal symptoms		20%	
Only hearing ear		1%	6%

Quality of Life

Quality of life (QOL) in patients with vestibular schwannoma can be difficult to measure, and disease-specific QOL surveys rather than the generic Short Form 36 Health Survey (SF-36) may be able to provide more information in the future.[81] The few studies conducted show conflicting results. Interestingly, cochleovestibular symptoms did not correlate with the QOL score, and there was no significant difference in QOL scores between management options of observation, radiation, and surgical treatment in 2 years of prospective follow-up.[81] Another prospective study on small-to-medium size tumors found that baseline QOL was similar in all three treatment arms, and unexpectedly improved in the surgical resection group at 2 years of follow-up.[82] Overall QOL in the surgical resection group was not significantly different between age groups and different operative approaches.[83]

Watchful Waiting

When considering the most conservative management modality, the natural course of the benign vestibular schwannoma and the possible neurologic sequelae and their impact on the patient's QOL must be taken into account. Additionally, the need and length of radiologic follow-up as well as the likelihood of future treatment (failure of conservative management) must also be considered.

Watchful waiting may be appropriate in elderly patients with an estimated lifespan shorter than the estimated growth leading to symptom progression, in those patients with significant medical comorbidities, in patients who have minimal symptoms, or those whose vestibular tumor is on the side of their only hearing ear.[84-93] Table 23.4 demonstrates some changing trends in the reasons clinicians and patients have opted for conservative management over the past 25 years.

Natural History of Untreated Vestibular Schwannomas

Growth Rate

Vestibular schwannomas are by and large slow growing tumors. The most commonly reported growth rate is 1–2 mm/year.[75,85,95-97] A couple of important considerations should be taken into account when describing growth rate.

1. Growth rate is usually measured in linear dimensions, even though more recent studies advocate for volumetric and doubling growth rate analysis, as linear measurements may underestimate the three-dimensional (3D) increase in tumor size. Varughese et al. found that in their 6-year radiologic follow-up of untreated acoustic tumors in 178 patients, 77% were larger by volumetric analysis compared to only 29% by standard linear analysis.[98]
2. Most data on natural history of untreated vestibular schwannomas are retrospective in nature and usually describe those tumors that are most amenable to watchful waiting at time of diagnosis, and will thus underestimate true growth rates (Table 23.5).

From the summary table above, there is relatively wide variability of tumors that become larger over time (29–54%). Spontaneous regression may occur in 1–26% of the cases. Tumors that are large (> 2.5 cm) at presentation increase the odds of future tumor growth.[101,103] Cystic tumors are more likely to enlarge and do so at a faster rate.[104] Extracanalicular tumors grow faster than IAC ones.[105,106] A study from Johns Hopkins looking at 180 patients who were conservatively managed over 10 years found that a reported symptom of tinnitus increases the odds of future tumor growth.[101]

Radiologic Follow-Up

Growth is usually seen in the first 3 years after presentation. Most groups recommend obtaining an MRI scan at

Table 23.5: Meta-analyses and large studies of observation management: tumor growth and rate

Report (ref)	*Year*	*Number of patients*	*Mean Follow-up (years)*	*Average growth rate (mm/year)*	*Stable*	*Smaller*	*Larger*
Huet et al.[97]	1998	558	3	1.8	–	–	54%
Yamakami et al.[99]	2003	903	3	1.9	47%	4%	51%
Smouha et al.[85]	2005	1,345	3	1.9	51%	6%	43%
Yoshimoto[100]	2005	1,340	3	1.2	46%	8%	46%
Stoquart-Elsankari et al.[81]	2009	70	2	–	63%	1%	36%
Agrawal et al.[101]	2010	180	10	1.1	–	–	37%
Pennings et al.[102]	2011	47	4	–	51%	9%	40%
Varughese et al.[98]*	2012	178	6	0.6	45%	26%	29%

*By linear analysis.

6 months after presentation, followed by an annual MR for at least another 2 and up to 5 years, with lifelong MRI scans every 5 years.[104] Of the tumors that grow, 53% are detected by the initial follow-up in 6 months. More indolent tumors may take more time to manifest, but all do by the 6-year period. The yield of follow-up scans in identifying growing tumors falls considerably after the first 3 scans.[107]

Symptoms

Hearing: A not uncommon reason why patients and clinicians choose to observe and scan newly diagnosed vestibular schwannomas and why patients are reluctant to undergo treatment is the fear of hearing loss when hearing is intact at presentation (*see* Table 23.2). Both the clinician and the patient should be realistic in their expectations of the natural progression of hearing loss in cases of untreated vestibular schwannomas.

When it comes to hearing outcomes in the observation treatment arm, the initial tumor size does not impact hearing preservation rates.[79,95,102,103,108] Also, the growth pattern, i.e. IAC versus extrameatal tumors, does not appear to be correlated to the probability of hearing preservation.[79,102] Even IAC tumors and tumors that do not grow, when followed for 7 years, have caused some hearing to deteriorate in up to 89% of the cases at the conclusion of follow-up.[102] Deterioration that concludes with nonserviceable hearing usually occurs in the first 2 years of conservative management.[102] Hearing deterioration independent of size change can also be a reason for patients to ultimately undergo treatment (Table 23.5).

There is, however, a strong correlation between hearing preservation in fast versus slow growing tumors.[93,109,103,105] A recent meta-analysis of 612 patients in 34 pooled studies found that hearing preservation rate was markedly higher for patients in the group who had tumors with an average annual growth rate of ≤ 2.5 mm/year, compared with those with higher growth rates (75 vs. 32%, respectively). The follow-up range for these studies was 2–4 years, and the overall hearing preservation rate was 54% for all tumors combined. The definition of hearing preservation in this meta-analysis was having AAO-HNS class A or B hearing or Gardner-Robertson Class II or better hearing at the end of the follow-up period.[103]

Vertigo and disequilibrium: Up to three quarters of patients who are being managed by observation have complaints of either vertigo or disequilibrium.[110] In a study of 186 patients followed over 2 years, only symptoms of vertigo negatively impacted their QOL, while hearing had no effect on QOL score.[110] In another study of 241 patients over 5 years, presence of dizziness was the most significant audiovestibular predictor of low QOL scores in patients with vestibular schwannomas; similarly, hearing loss did not influence QOL.[111] For this subgroup of patients, use of intratympanic gentamicin is a viable option to control symptoms without a surgical or radiation-based intervention.[112] Disabling vertigo has been cited steadily as the sole reason for deciding to undergo active management after a period of observation in 9–14% of patients (Table 23.6).

In those cases where there is a delay in diagnosis of vestibular schwannoma, the lack of management also constitutes a "conservative" approach, albeit this was not a treating clinician or patient-driven choice. Once discovered, however, the projected time of tumor presence should be taken into account—i.e. for the patient who had symptoms for 3 years prior to the discovery of the benign lesion, they are close to their third year of

Table 23.6: Reasons for pursuing active treatment after a period of observation

Reason for treatment	*Agrawal et al.*[101] *(n=180)*[101]	*Bakkouri et al.*[94] *(n= 386)*	*Godefroy et al.*[111] *(n=70)*[111]	*Flint et al.*[113] *(n=100)*	*Tschudi et al.*[93] *(n=74)*
Tumor growth	83%	43%	89%	91%	22%
Disabling vertigo	13%	14%	11%	9%	11%
Hearing deterioration	3%	38%			
Patient choice	1%	8%			
Corneal hypoesthesia					44%
Facial weakness					22%

Table 23.7: Failure of conservative management

Report (ref)	*Year*	*Number of patients*	*Years follow-up*	*Ultimately treated*	*Radiation*	*Surgery*	*Time to treatment*
Tschudi et al.[93]	2000	74	3 (mean)	12%	0%	100%	–
Flint et al.[113]	2005	100	11	11%	0%	100%	–
Hajioff et al.[105]	2007	70	10	30%	67%	33%	3 years (mean)
Bakkouri et al.[94]	2009	386	9	24%	22%	78%	>50% in first year
Godefroy et al.[111]	2009	70	4 (mean)	39%	19%	81%	3 years (mean)
Agrawal et al.[101]	2010	180	10	35%	–	–	2.6 years (mean)
Lloyd et al.[114]	2010	481	5	50%	–	–	–
Breivik et al.[110]	2012	193	4 (mean)	38%	77%	23%	2 years (mean)

conservative "management". However, the vast majority of patients opt for active management strategies once the delay has been suspected.

Failure Rates of Conservative Management

When talking about failure of conservative management, the focus is mainly on patients who subsequently seek active treatment and not on those patients who are lost to follow-up. Tumor growth was the most important predictor of a change in strategy from conservative to either microsurgical or radiation management.[101,103] Reasons for failure of conservative management include most commonly tumor growth, worsening vertigo, progression of hearing loss, and patient decision in absence of changing clinical or radiologic status.[85,101] These are summarized in Table 23.6. Evidently, the reasons for pursuing treatment have changed over the past 30 years of follow-up, likely owing to the increase in the use of radiologic studies and the introduction of radiation-based treatments.

Table 23.7 summarizes the overall failure rate and the proportion of treatments pursued.

Most failures (75–90%) occur within the first 5 years of follow-up.[101,105] The patients who changed their treatment strategy were significantly more likely to have larger tumors at presentation, tumors located in the CPA, and they were more likely to subsequently display tumor growth at faster rates than individuals who were managed conservatively throughout the study period.[101]

Incidence of postoperative complications is not higher in patients undergoing secondary surgery than in patients undergoing primary surgery.[94,115-119] In other words, delaying the surgical decision does not seem to worsen disease treatment outcomes. Good facial nerve outcome with tumors <2 cm was found in 87% of patients operated on at diagnosis and in 84% of patients operated on after established tumor growth. In this case study, of almost 1400 patients when patients who were primarily allocated to conservative management (959 cases) were pooled, good facial function was found in 97% of them at 5 years of follow-up. This outcome was significantly better than for the 419 patients who underwent primary operation (87%), pointing to the advantage of the observation strategy for small-to-medium-sized schwannomas.[120]

Special Considerations

In certain situations, the three options for management of vestibular schwannomas do not weigh in the same—i.e.

for very small or asymptomatic tumors, the risks of surgery may initially outweigh the benefits, while for very large tumors, observation or radiation are inappropriate management strategies.

Intracanalicular Tumors

At present, treating clinicians are more often managing small and IAC schwannomas compared to prior decades, which is likely due to improved imaging and increased awareness.[121] These smaller tumors are less likely to be symptomatic and do not carry a risk of impending complications. Watchful waiting is a relatively safe approach, with the only significant risk being progression of SNHL. A more proactive approach advocates for early intervention, with the intention of preserving the hearing status at time of diagnosis for these small tumors.[122] However, hearing preservation rates for either radiation or microsurgical resection have not been consistently better than the natural history of hearing loss progression with conservatively managed IAC schwannomas. Thus, an increasing number of study groups have advocated for observation-based management.[123] In fact, quality-adjusted-life-year totals for all three management strategies in patients with small vestibular schwannomas are highest in patients who undergo a period of observation compared to those who undergo immediate surgery or radiation treatment.[124]

A recent review of over 3000 patients found that the management of small (<2 cm) vestibular schwannomas in the United States between 2004 and 2007 has seen a decrease in microsurgical resection, an increase in radiation-based treatment and a steady but low (25%) rate of observation. In light of findings that the majority of these small tumors do not grow, the authors concluded that vestibular schwannomas are overtreated in the United States.[125]

Very Large Tumors

When confronted with a patient with a large (>3 cm) vestibular schwannoma, observation rarely plays a role in management, owing mostly to the fact that these tumors are symptomatic, exhibit some brain stem compression, and risk neurologic compromise. In certain cases, however, observation may play a role:

1. When the vestibular schwannoma is in the only hearing ear; in these cases, management is usually undertaken once all hearing is compromised; a contralateral cochlear implant (CI) is an option in these patients[126]
2. When the patient has bilateral vestibular schwannomas and the one in question is smaller of the two (in cases of NF2); in a recent review of NF2 patients with bilateral brain stem compressing schwannoma, the time range between first and second surgery was 1.5–7.7 years[127]
3. When the patient refuses treatment
4. When the patient is terminally ill

Similarly, radiation rarely plays a role as there is a risk of transient increase in the size of the tumor, and in large masses even the small increase could bring upon a catastrophic outcome with hydrocephalus. Very large tumors are almost always treated with surgical resection, total or partial; this is discussed in the following section.

Microsurgical Resection

Microsurgical resection has historically had three primary goals in decreasing priority: preserve the patient's life, maintain the patient's facial nerve function, and preserve any useful hearing in the operated side. With multiple centers developing standardized resection procedures utilizing operating microscopes, electrophysiological monitoring including CN monitoring, precision instruments, and expertise of neurological and neurosurgical teams, mortality has significantly decreased. Therefore, avoidance of significant postoperative morbidity (CSF leak, meningitis, neurovascular compromise) becomes the focus over simply preserving the patient's life.[128]

There are three basic and most commonly utilized approaches in microsurgical removal: retrosigmoid (suboccipital), MCF, and translabyrinthine. The first two approaches are hearing-sparing while the last sacrifices any residual hearing. All three approaches involve bony removal via a craniotomy, craniectomy or both, and microdissection of tumor away from the brain, CNS, and adjacent vascular structures.

Decision of Surgical Approach

Choice of the approach depends on multiple factors including level of serviceable hearing, depth of tumor extension into the IAC, the size of the tumor, and the experience and familiarity of the surgeon with the various approaches.[129] In general, patients with poor hearing undergo a translabyrinthine approach; patients with good hearing and small or IAC tumors are suitable for MCF approach; and for patients with good hearing and tumors that do not extend too far lateral into the IAC the retrosigmoid approach is best (Fig. 23.6). For patients with large tumors, even in the case of good hearing, the translabyrinthine approach offers the best exposure of the entire IAC to aid in tumor removal as likelihood of preserving hearing with large tumors is low. There is debate across centers over what constitutes good and poor hearing, and even in the cases of good hearing a translabyrinthine approach is utilized when the chance of hearing preservation is low.

Table 23.8 summarizes advantages and disadvantages of all three major approaches to microsurgical vestibular schwannoma removal. Choice of approach is also largely influenced by the availability and experience of the neurosurgical and neurotologic teams. In fact, one study found that when comparing 11 different institutions, surgical team accounted for more variability in hearing and facial nerve outcome than did approach.[132] As an example, the ability to preserve hearing with the MCF approach has very high variability among institutions, and its perceived advantage in hearing outcomes may never reach statistical significance.

Theoretically, the choice of approach may change based on the most recent imaging, such as a planned retrosigmoid approach converted to a translabyrinthine with the latest MRI showing substantial lateral growth (Figs. 23.7A and B). However, a Canadian study showed that even tumors with documented growth do not extend laterally into the IAC within a year of surgery. Thus, it appears to be unnecessary to obtain imaging that is more recent than a year for concerns of lateral growth only, although it may be required for other clinical reasons.[133]

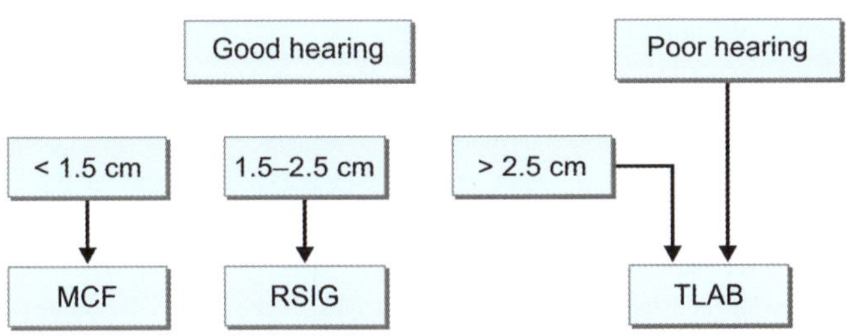

Fig. 23.6: General algorithm for surgical approach.

Hearing Status: Hearing Conservation Candidacy

Expectations of both patient and physician need to be realistic when it comes to hearing preservation in surgical treatment of vestibular schwannomas. Goals and definitions of a "successful" result should be clearly outlined; if a patient discerns little benefit from what the surgeon perceived as a successful hearing outcome, they will likely be disappointed.

Hearing classification: The American Academy of Otolaryngology—Head and Neck Surgery (AAO-HNS) has established a classification system for reporting the hearing class of patients both at presentation and after any therapeutic intervention. Figure 23.8A is a schematic for the definition of A-D hearing class. An alternative classification, frequently used in the radiation treatment literature, is the Gardner-Robertson classification,[134] which uses descriptive terms for the assigned grades: good, serviceable, nonserviceable and poor hearing and deaf for patients with profound loss (Fig. 23.8B).

Hearing conservation candidacy: For a patient to be considered a candidate for hearing conservation, they must have both good hearing at baseline and, importantly, carry a good prognosis of preserving their good hearing. Both of these factors lead to some controversy.

Table 23.8: Summary of advantages and disadvantages of surgical approaches[130,131]

	Advantages	*Disadvantages*
MCF	Hearing sparing Better hearing outcome No intradural drilling	Worse facial nerve outcome especially with tumors 10–18 mm CPA and IVN tumors Temporal lobe retraction Limited exposure of posterior fossa
RSIG	Can be hearing sparing Better facial nerve outcome Can address large tumors Placement of ABI possible	Worse hearing outcome Blind lateral dissection into IAC limit is lateral 3rd of IAC Cerebellar retraction Headaches and vertigo
TLAB	Facial nerve outcome best Early identification of facial nerve in IAC Can address large tumors Less neurological complications Extradural drill dissection Exposure of entire IAC, fundus to porus Placement of ABI possible	Destroys hearing *Limits*: high jugular bulb Longer time of dissection *Largest bony defect*: reconstruction needed More CSF leaks

(MCF, middle cranial fossa; RSIG, retrosigmoid; TLAB, translabyrinthine; IAC, intracanalicular portion; ABI, auditory brainstem implementation; CPA, cerebellopontine angle; IVN, inferior vestibular nerve).

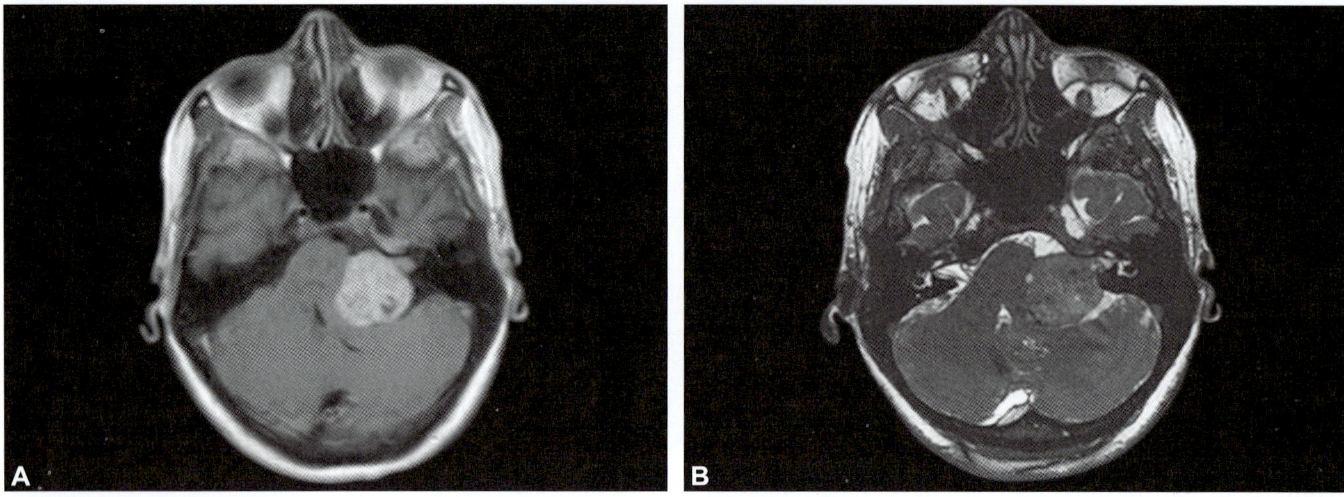

Figs. 23.7A and B: Vestibular schwannoma with primarily cisternal involvement. For this patient with large left cisternal vestibular schwannoma and limited lateral extension, retrosigmoid approach proved suitable for removal. The constructive interference in steady state gradient-echo T2 MRI sequence shows spinal fluid separating the lateral extension of the tumor from the cochlea and labyrinth.

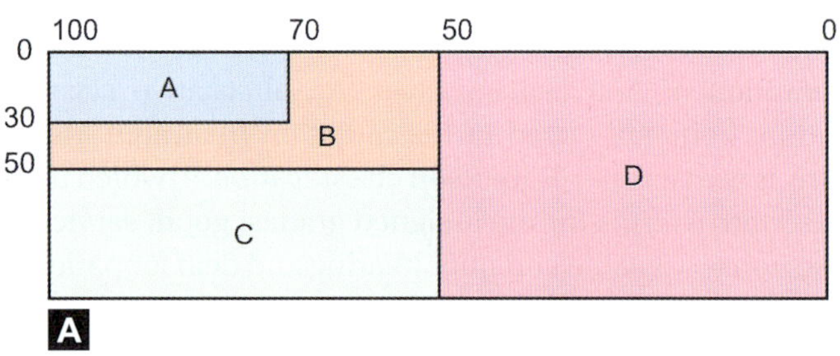

Grade	PTA (dB)	SD (%)
I Good	0–30	70–100
II Serviceable	31–50	50–69
III Non-serviceable	51–90	5–49
IV Poor	90–100	1–4
V Deaf	0	0

B

Figs. 23.8A and B: (A) The American Academy of Otolaryngology—Head and Neck Surgery classification for hearing. The horizontal axis represents the word recognition scores in percentages (%) and the vertical axis the average of pure tone dB at 500, 1000, 2000 and 3000 Hz. (B) Gardner-Robertson hearing scale.

As a general rule, the better the patient's baseline hearing, the better the chance of preserving hearing. Many authors use the "50/50" rule to define good hearing, in line with the AAO-HNS classification A and B category hearing: at least a 50% SDS AND an at least 50 dB SRT of 4 tone PTAs (500, 1k, 2k, 4k). An important distinction is that this is a good rule of thumb only if contralateral hearing is normal. Further, due to Stenger's effect, patients will gain little benefit if the postoperative side has 30 dB or greater SRT and 30% or less SDS compared to the contralateral, nonoperated side. Therefore, for a patient with normal hearing on the uninvolved side, such as 10 dB SRT and 100% SDS, even if the postoperative hearing result is 45dB SRT and 60% SDS (category B), the benefit may not be perceptible as that patient will likely be preferentially using the uninvolved side for auditory information.

The strictest criteria for useful hearing then utilize the AAO-HNS category A classification (70% SDS and 30 dB SRT) with the assumption that the contralateral ear is normal. Ultimately, few patients who opt for surgery fall into this category of good hearing, and thus few patients should expect hearing preservation. The argument can then certainly be made for early surgery before hearing deterioration sets in.[135] The specific outcomes of surgical approaches with respect to preservation of auditory function are discussed below in the surgical outcomes section. Table 23.9 outlines unfavorable prognostic factors of hearing preservation and the diagnostic method used to identify these factors.

When the surgeon is confronted with a patient who has a large tumor with minimal IAC penetration and excellent hearing with a near normal ABR, other CPA tumors (such as a meningioma) should be considered.

Size and Location

Size and location of the tumor play a significant role when choosing the surgical approach. Very large tumors are appropriately dealt with utilizing a retrosigmoid, translabyrinthine, or extended translabyrinthine approach. A review of close to 1700 vestibular schwannomas >2.5 cm

Table 23.9: Unfavorable preoperative prognostic factors for hearing preservation

Unfavorable preoperative hearing Preservation factor	*Diagnostic method*
Absent or distorted ABR Even if the hearing level by PTA is good	Auditory function test: ABR
Unaffected caloric response Suggests inferior VN origin (adjacent cochlear nerve in the inferior compartment of the IAC is at risk)[136]	Vestibular function test: calorics
Deep IAC penetration RSIG approach exposes only proximal two-thirds of IAC; complete resection of tumor in distal one-third requires partial removal of inner ear structures[129,137]	Imaging: MRI
Tumor size > 2 cm (cisternal component) With the RSIG approach useful hearing may be obtained in <25% of patients[138,139]	Imaging: MRI
Filling of IAC Less than 1 mm room between tumor and IAC fundus[140,141] Substantial IAC erosion predicts greater compression of 8th nerve[8]	Imaging: MRI

(ABR, auditory brainstem response; IAC, intracanalicular; RSIG, retrosigmoid; PTA, pure-tone average; VN, vestibular nerve).

found that 65.2% robotic surgery implementation group (RSIG) versus 62.5% TLAB resections preserved good facial nerve function (HB 1-2) and only 27.4% via the extended TLAB.[142] An earlier review of 54 tumors >3 cm in size, 84% of which were resected via a TLAB approach, good facial nerve function was preserved in 84% of cases.[143] Given that size of tumor significantly affects facial nerve outcome, consideration should be given to subtotal or planned staged resection or postoperative radiation when dealing with tumors >3.5 cm.[144]

Conversely, entirely IAC tumors (Fig. 23.9) are probably best treated with an MCF or RS approach. In a literature review comparing outcomes of surgical resection of IAC tumors with retrosigmoid versus a MCF approach, the retrosigmoid resection maintained 58% hearing preservation rates (compared to 62% via MCF) but improved facial nerve outcomes and fewer other complications.[145]

Tumors with a lateral extension into the distal IAC (Fig. 23.10) are not suitable for a retrosigmoid resection and tumors with a large cisternal component have an unfavorable location for a standard MCF resection (*see* Table 23.8). Clearly, patient priorities (facial nerve function versus hearing function) and surgeon expertise play a large role in selection. Surgical teams with expertise in one over another resection method may preferentially choose the method they have the most favorable results with, irrespective of the reported data from other centers and compiled studies.

Surgical Techniques

Much of the operative setup, equipment, surgical site preparation, and postoperative care are common to all major surgical approaches to vestibular schwannoma removal; these are summarized in Table 23.10.

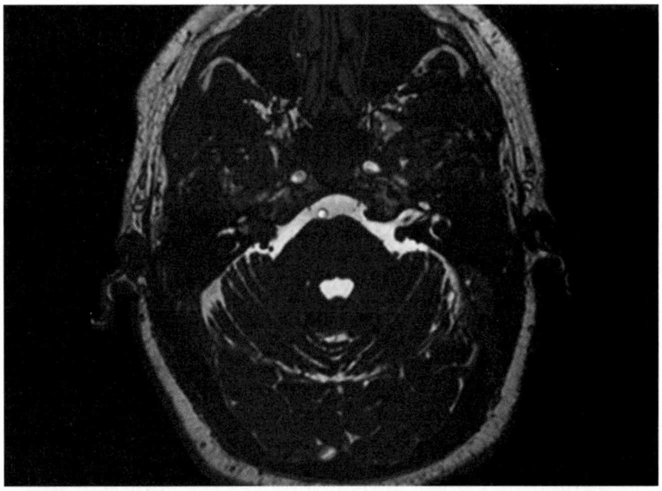

Fig. 23.9: Vestibular schwannoma with proximal intracanalicular involvement. The constructive interference in steady state gradient-echo T2 MRI sequence shows spinal fluid separating the lateral extension of the right-sided tumor from the cochlea and labyrinth. We chose a hearing-sparing middle cranial fossa approach for this patient.

Surgical removal of vestibular schwannoma carries a risk of intraoperative and postoperative complications, which is the major drawback of surgery over observation or radiation. Discussed below are some basic surgical principles that we follow for all approaches to minimize intraoperative complications and also some not uncommon postoperative complications and suggestions for their avoidance.

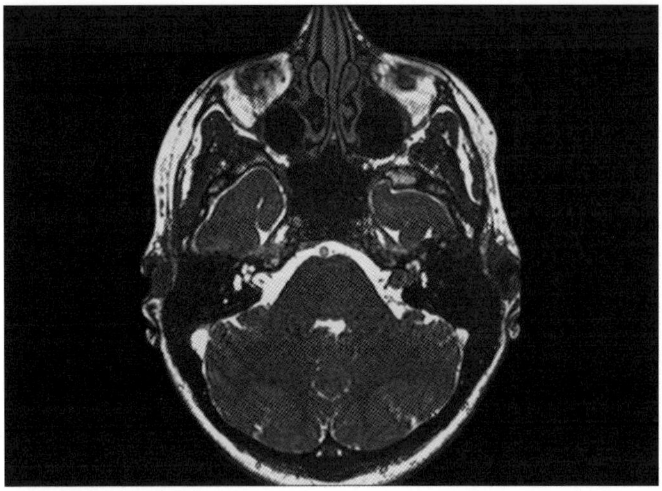

Fig. 23.10: Vestibular schwannoma involving the distal intracanalicular. The constructive interference in steady state gradient-echo T2 MRI sequence shows no spinal fluid separating the lateral extension of the left-sided tumor from the cochlea and labyrinth. We chose a TLAB approach for this patient who presented with class C hearing.

Surgical Principles

The following basic surgical principles are followed for all three approaches:

Appropriate patient selection

- Careful anatomical review of the preoperative MRI is conducted. Anatomical variants, such as a high riding jugular bulb, may limit dissection extent.
- Older patients may have thinner and more adherent dura than younger patients that is more prone to injury, increasing the chance of hematoma or CSF leak; thus approaches that necessitate more dural dissection such as the MCF route may be contraindicated.
- As hearing significantly influences the choice of surgical approach, functional hearing should be assessed with a most up-to-date preoperative test.

Maximizing exposure

For any surgery to be performed safely and effectively, good exposure of the surgical field is crucial. The tips on achieving optimum exposure for each of the three major surgical approaches are discussed under the specific approach; general principles are as follows:

- Brain retraction, crucial for RSIG and MCF approaches as well as large tumors, can be facilitated with medications (Mannitol, Lasix) and monitoring for appropriate urinary response; patient positioning with head down and also with hyperventilation in order to lower carbon dioxide to 27–28 mm Hg.
- Meticulous hemostasis allows superior visualization of the surgical field; care should be taken when using bipolar cautery; gentle pressure with Gelfoam, pledgets, utilization of thrombin to promote clotting as well as oxidized cellulose (Oxacyl or Surgicel) are safe and effective hemostatic agents.

Safe dissection and maximization of functional outcome

- Facial nerve and cochlear nerve function monitoring [ABR or cochlear nerve action potential (CNAP)] are routinely used.
- Obtain a baseline ABR once the patient is asleep.
- Resist blunt dissection and removing the tumor en bloc.
- The IAC portion is debulked with CUSA and then sharply dissected off the facial and cochlear nerves that are identified laterally; the IAC portion is removed laterally to medially toward the porus.
- The intracranial portion is debulked and the facial and audiovestibular root entry zones are identified on the pons; sharp dissection is utilized to remove the remaining capsule, medially to laterally toward the porus.
- Prass probe is used to positively identify the facial nerve and can assist in dissection off of the tumor.
- The course of the facial nerve between the brain stem, where it is just slightly inferior to the 8th nerve entry zone, and its entry into the porus where it assumes the anterosuperior location is variable as the tumor can splay the nerve and distort its fibers in almost any direction. The most difficult part of the dissection is removal of the capsule from the thinned facial nerve, just proximal to the anterior edge of the porus acusticus.
- Take care to preserve the labyrinthine artery if attempting hearing preservation surgery.
- Any maneuver that results in deterioration in the brainstem auditory-evoked responses or abnormal firing of the facial nerve requires immediate cessation to allow recovery. Irrigation with warm saline frequently quiets the facial nerve. Deterioration secondary to surgically induced vasospasm may be managed by local application of papaverine.
- Consider subtotal resection if hearing preservation is strongly desired or facial nerve function will be compromised.
- Similar principles to those outlined for 7th and 8th CNs should be followed for larger tumors that involve CNs V and IX–XI that can also be monitored intraoperatively; subtotal resection should also be considered in cases where lower CNs are involved as their

Table 23.10: Perioperative considerations

Preoperative	*Intraoperative*	*Postoperative*
Anesthesia	**Positioning**	**Postoperative care (standard protocol without any complications)**
General endotracheal anesthesia	Operating table turned to 180°	Admitted to NSICU × 24 hours, then floor care with appropriate clinical neurologic monitoring
Direct (arterial) blood pressure, heart rate, oxygen saturation, carbon dioxide concentration continuous monitoring	Supine position	DVT and PUD prophylaxis
Foley catheter for urinary output monitoring	*MCF*: ipsilateral shoulder elevated; head rotated to 45°opposite tumor; neck slightly extended	Dexamethasone × 48 hours, then taper
Short-acting neuromuscular blockade only (such as with succinylcholine)	*RSIG*: head rotated to the opposite side of tumor as far as neck mobility allows; ipsilateral shoulder taped down	Reglan, Zofran for nausea and vomiting
Medications	*TLAB*: head rotated to the opposite side of tumor	Analgesia with acetaminophen and codeine
24-hour perioperative antibiotics: Ancef or vancomycin for PCN allergy	External head fixation per team preference	Postoperative nimodipine can assist in promoting blood flow to the inner ear and maximizing hearing preservation[146]
Preoperative IV Decadron	Patient secured to bed with three straps and operating table allows inclination in all planes	Antivirals directed at the herpes virus can be used in delayed facial palsy
Mannitol (20% at 1 g/kg)	**Preparation**	**PO day 1**
RSIG and MCF	Pinna	Arterial line, Foley catheter removed
TLAB if large tumor	*MCF*: taped down over earphone with tegaderm	Patient mobilized to chair
Equipment	*RSIG*: taped anteriorly over earphone with tegaderm	Clear liquid diet, advanced as tolerated
Operating microscope with assistant head	*TLAB*: prepped into the field and retracted anteriorly	**PO day 2**
High-speed drill (cutting and diamond burs)	Shave to at least 1 cm behind incision line	JP drain removed from abdomen
Suction-irrigation system	Incision injected with subcutaneous 1% lidocaine with 1:100,000 epinephrine	Patient mobilized to ambulation with assistance
Two suction lines	Abdominal site prepared for fat graft	**PO day 3**
Monopolar and bipolar (micro and macro) cautery	Triple iodine scrub for both the craniotomy and abdominal graft site	Compressive dressing removed, wound inspected
Electrophysiologic monitoring	**Wound closure**	Discharge to home
Performed by the EP team	Bacitracin irrigation and meticulous hemostasis	PO day 10
Facial nerve: direct and transcranial	Muscle or periosteal flap and subcutaneous tissue is approximated in staggered separate layers with interrupted Vicryl stitches	Stitches removed
Earphones for far-field ABR	Skin is closed with a 3-0 nylon running interlocking stitch	
RSIG and MCF	Compressive (mastoid) dressing is applied	
Motor and somatosensory (electrodes in upper and lower extremities)	Abdominal closure with interrupted Vicryl, subcutaneous monocryl and JP drain	
Other cranial nerves (CN V, IX, X, XI)		
RSIG and TLAB if large tumors		

(RSIG, retrosigmoid; CN, cranial nerve; ABR, auditory brainstem response; TLAB, translabyrinthine; MCF, middle cranial fossa; TLAB, translabyrinthine).

compromise could significantly affect the patient's ability to swallow and expose them to a risk of aspiration pneumonia.
- Facial nerve function can be compromised by direct traction, blunt trauma, cautery, and rarely transection. Positive probe stimulation at the brainstem root exit zone portends a good prognosis. Lack of response to stimulation at elevated current levels suggests poor recovery.

Avoiding and Managing Postoperative Complications

These are some postoperative complications and tips on minimizing their occurrence as well as recommended management for all surgical approaches to vestibular schwannoma removal:

CSF leaks are a relatively common postoperative complication of vestibular schwannoma resection. CSF leak occurs either through the skin at the incision line or the fluid makes its way down the mastoid air cells, the middle ear, and the Eustachian tube manifesting as rhinorrhea or a postnasal drip. The risk of CSF leak extension through the air cells versus the skin incision is slightly higher, with approximately 60% occurring via the mastoid temporal bone air cell route.[147-149]

These general preventative measures should be undertaken:

- Use bone wax or autologous fat with TISSEEL (Fibrin Sealant) to obliterate all fat cells; apical petrous peri-IAC air cells are a common culprit.
- Pressure bandage should be applied postoperatively to minimize wound leaks.
- In patients in whom BIH is suspected, consider placing a perioperative lumbar drain.

For management of CSF leaks, we employ a graded approach.[150] Subcutaneous CSF collections ("pseudomeningoceles"), if not tense or leaking through the incision line, may be amenable to several days of pressure dressing as they typically resolve. Sterile aspiration of the wound collection can also be attempted.

Once leaking through the wound, bedside oversowing with mattress sutures, application of pressure dressing and medical measures such as bed rest, head of bed elevation, and avoidance of Valsalva maneuvers can be attempted. Indeed, conservative management has been shown to be successful in up to 53% of cases.[151] If unsuccessful, a lumbar drain can be applied for 3–5 days, clamped for 24 hours to test integrity of seal, and removed. More aggressive management with wound revision may also be indicated; in this case, additional fat, muscle, fascia can be packed and all levels of closure should be carefully inspected and revised as needed. The reported rates of success in the management of CSF leak with lumbar drain placement range from 31% to 83% in the recent literature, and reoperation rates have been reported to range from 21% to 61%.[147,149,152-155]

CSF rhinorrhea may respond to medical measures as well, acetazolamide can be added, and a lumbar drain can be applied for several days. If revision surgery is needed, a subtotal petrosectomy (in the case of no hearing) with obliteration of the extracanalicular (EAC) and ET block under direct vision with bone wax followed by muscle prevents further leaking. In the case of preserved hearing, an intact wall mastoidectomy can be performed with obstruction of the fossa incudis with fat, muscle or fascia, and TISSEEL.

In cases of refractory CSF leaks and where a disturbance in CSF production or absorption is suspected, a permanent (lumbar-peritoneal or ventriculoperitoneal) shunt should be considered.

A rare complication of CSF leak, in cases where there is a ball-valve wound effect, is a tension pneumocephalus with signs and symptoms of progressive increase ICP; these should be recognized and treated appropriately. Pneumocephalus can also occur with excessive CSF drainage via placed shunt. A more common complication of CSF leaks is meningitis, discussed below.

Postoperative meningitis can be either aseptic (chemical) from meningeal inflammation induced by blood or irritants such as bone dust or cotton wool lint entering the subarachnoid space, or it can be infectious, frequently occurring in conjunction with a CSF leak. Aseptic meningitis is usually associated with headaches, malaise, and a low-grade fever, while infectious meningitis frequently manifests with high fevers, stiff neck, excruciating headache, photophobia, and various degrees of obtundation. Head CT and lumbar puncture or analysis of CSF in cases where LD has been already been placed are diagnostic. In cases of bacterial meningitis, the most common pathogens involved are *Staphylococcus* species, *Enterobacter*, and *Propionibacterium acnes*.[156]

If the clinical presentation is highly suggestive of bacterial meningitis, intravenous antibiotics with good CSF penetration (vancomycin and ceftriaxone) are initiated immediately as disease progression may be rapid. In addition, corticosteroids and analgesics are used for both bacterial and aseptic meningitis. Because most patients presenting with meningitis present with associated CSF leak, management of CSF leak as described earlier is essential. For aseptic meningitis, not only anti-inflammatory corticosteroids but also nonsteroidal anti-inflammatory medications such as Celebrex can be tried. Of note, symptoms may recur after steroid withdrawal.

During surgery, avoidance of postoperative meningitis is achieved with the following:

- Minimize blood and debris from entering once dura is opened. This is especially important with the retrosigmoid approach as the dura is opened early in the procedure.
- Maintain a sterile field and irrigate wound with an antibiotic solution to minimize wound infections that can lead to bacterial meningitis.

Epidural hematoma can be suspected in patients with signs of increased ICP (increased BP, bradycardia, decreased level of consciousness, and/or dilation of pupils). A noncontrast CT scan is indicated in these cases if time allows, but if the onset of symptoms is rapid and the patient becomes unstable, opening the incision for removal of the cranioplasty, abdominal fat, and blood clot at the bedside may be necessary. CPA hematoma is a potentially fatal complication that leads to increased ICP and brain stem compression.

These potentially devastating intracranial complications can be minimized with:

- Careful observation for bleeding after irrigation of the operative bed after the tumor has been dissected; this is imperative to decrease the likelihood of postoperative compressive CPA hematoma. Anesthesia may be asked to apply Valsalva maneuver or temporarily elevate blood pressure to allow potential bleeders to declare themselves
- Careful elevation of the bone flap during craniotomy; some patients may have thinner or more adherent dura
- Control postoperative hypertension.

Venous infarction from injury to the sigmoid sinus or transverse sinus can occur with TLAB and RSIG approaches during the craniotomy. Some theories proposed to explain dural sinus thrombosis in vestibular schwannoma microsurgery include retraction on the sinus intraoperatively, desiccation of the sinus during tumor resection, and even propagation of bone wax used for control of emissary veins.

Venous congestion can be asymptomatic or can manifest with speech disturbance as it will usually affect the temporoparietal region. Rarely, cerebral edema or papilledema with progressive vision loss can occur, leading to headaches, visual obscuration, or blindness. The onset of symptoms may range from days to weeks after surgery; Keiper et al. found an onset range from 1 to 35 days postoperatively, with a mean onset of 15.6 days postoperatively.[157] Most importantly, signs of venous congestion should be recognized early (CT scan can be used for screening, but a magnetic resonance venography is a more definitive diagnostic tool) and treated with appropriate measures. Treatment of dural sinus thrombosis can range from supportive (steroids, volume repletion, carbonic anhydrase inhibitors) to thrombolytic, including medical anticoagulation, direct endovascular thrombolysis, and even surgical thrombectomy.

However, they are best avoided with the following:

- Review preoperative films for dominant venous outflow side
- Minimize intraoperative mechanical retraction of the sigmoid sinus
- Smaller venous tears can be controlled with layering of Gelfoam (thrombin-soaked) and neural patties for gentle pressure. An alternative method is with oxidized cellulose and gentle bipolar cautery just over the cellulose material
- Larger tears may necessitate primary repair with 6-0 Prolene suture with or without addition of muscle; larger tears increase the likelihood of ipsilateral venous outflow compromise
- Packing with Surgicel or bone wax should be avoided as this may cause sinus occlusion
- Emissary veins can usually be controlled at their root at the sinus with bipolar cautery
- Petrosal vein (Dandy's vein) is frequently ligated in larger tumors; very rarely it can lead to papilledema or cerebellar infarction, but the surgeon should be aware of this potentially devastating complication.

The cerebellum, pons, or temporal lobe is vulnerable to *traumatic parenchymal injury* either from retraction or violation of the pial lining during dissection. Temporal lobe injury from retraction during the MCF approach can be suspected in the case of postoperative seizures, aphasia, and auditory hallucinations. These should be treated medically with ICP-lowering agents and antiseizure medications. The cerebellum can be injured during a RSIG approach and this can manifest with prolonged ataxia and dysmetria. If more significant cerebellar injury has occurred and swelling occurs, surgical evacuation of any associated clots and even resection of the contused cerebellum may be necessary. Approximately one-third of the cerebellum can be resected without producing a permanent cerebellar deficit. In some cases, it may be necessary to decompress the posterior fossa including the foramen magnum.

During surgery:

- Employ all necessary medical measures to achieve appropriate "shrinking" of the temporal lobe or the cerebellum so as to avoid excessive mechanical retraction
- During the translabyrinthine approach, avoid injuring the dural covering over the temporal lobe during skeletonization of the tegmen
- Dissection should occur in the arachnoid plane as much as possible
- Larger tumors can obscure the arachnoid plane and some dissection occurs in the subpial plane, which exposes the brain to parenchymal injury
- Consider leaving a thin capsule of tumor if injury cannot be safely prevented

Intracranial vascular complications can be devastating and stem from interruption of the anterior inferior cerebellar artery (AICA) or one of its branches to the brain stem. Partial AICA syndrome in the postoperative period can not only be apparent with ataxia and dysmetria (cerebellar symptoms) but also hemiparesis or hemisensory disturbance (long tract signs). A postoperative MRI is diagnostic. Treatment is rehabilitative.

Measures to help with avoiding injury to AICA and its branches:

- These vessels are at risk even with small tumor removal as AICA can loop in the vicinity of the porus
- The surgeon should be familiar with anatomical variants
- Intraoperative motor and somatosensory EP monitoring alerts the surgeon of any impending compromise
- If bleeding occurs during tumor dissection, careful identification and isolation of vessels with mobilization away from the tumor are preferred
- Vessels are cauterized only if necessary and as to close their entrance to tumor as possible
- Bipolar cautery should be used with judiciously; only vessels that feed the tumor should be cauterized; otherwise, use topical hemostatic agent

Middle Cranial Fossa Approach

Background/Indication: The MCF approach was used as early as 1892 as a surgical method for the treatment of trigeminal neuralgia and later for infections and lesions of the petrous apex, facial nerve exposure, and grafting and repair of semicircular canal dehiscence.[158-160] It was popularized by House for microsurgical exposure of the internal auditory canal in the late 1950s.[5] Kawase elaborated on the extended MCF approach in the 1980s with the dissection of the petrous apex, which was used for exposure of aneurysms of the basilar artery and petroclival tumors.[161]

Today, the MCF approach to the IAC for the purpose of resection of vestibular schwannomas is most suitable for IAC tumors that have a minor CPA component (< 1 cm) and for patients with good hearing [(better than or near 30 dB PTA and 70% word recognition score (WRS)]. Tumors that contact the brain stem are not suitable for the standard MCF approach. Contraindications for a supratentorial craniotomy include age >69 years, ASA (American Society of Anesthesiologists) class >II, and Karnofsky performance scale score <60.[160]

In patients with an only hearing ear or with bilateral tumors in the case of NF2, there is a role for early proactive surgical management via an MCF approach in an attempt to prevent hearing deterioration.[162] Brackmann et al. have reported good hearing results in patients with NF2 in whom the MCF approach was used, maintaining hearing within 15 dB of preoperative levels in 48% of patients.[162] Decompression of the IAC (as opposed to tumor removal) can also be considered in patients with progressive hearing loss in an only hearing ear as a therapeutic option.[163]

Technical steps

Craniotomy:

- Incision is planned as a reverse question mark with the lower limb passing anterior to the pinna, the horizontal limb following the top of the EAC, and the semicircular limb following the curve of the temporalis muscle (green line in Fig. 23.11).
- Skin and subcutaneous tissue are incised down but not through the temporalis muscle fascia with a #15 blade.

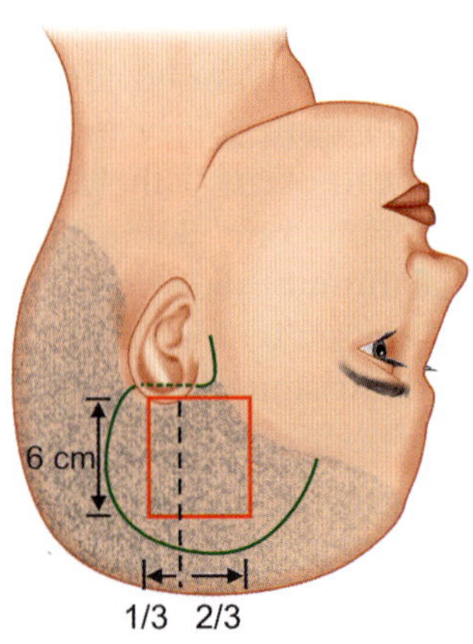

Fig. 23.11: Middle cranial fossa skin incision and craniotomy from the surgeon's view.

- Cautery is used to control bleeding of the branches of the superficial temporal artery.
- Temporalis muscle is incised with a monopolar Bovie knife leaving a cuff of muscle attached to the fascial coalescence at it inserts into the cranium.
- Muscle and soft tissue flaps are anteroinferiorly based and held out of the way with fish hooks.
- Squamous portion of the temporal bone, root of the zygoma, and temporoparietal suture line are identified as bony landmarks.
- The craniotomy is marked approximately 6 cm in height and 4.5 cm in width, centered at the one-third and two-third of the width line (1.5 cm posterior, 3 cm anterior) (red line, Fig. 23.11).
- The inferior most edge of the craniotomy should be as close to the root of the zygoma as possible to avoid an overhang limiting exposure of the MCF floor.
- The inferior aspect of the craniotomy is drilled with a 3-0 cutting diamond burr, making burr-hole type openings to the level of dura at the two inferior corners that will allow footplate attachment placement.
- The dura is identified and separated from the medial aspect of the cranium with a curved blunt periosteal elevator.
- The other three craniotomy edges are completed with a craniotome footplate.
- The bone flap is set aside wrapped in saline gauze.

Dural elevation and exposure of the floor of the middle cranial fossa:

- Operating microscope is brought into the field.
- Dura is circumferentially elevated from the bone edges with a blunt elevator, in an anterior to posterior direction.
- The middle meningeal artery is identified as it exits from the foramen spinosum (anterior most point of dissection).
- Any venous bleeding can be controlled with oxidized cellulose.
- As dura is elevated, the next landmark is the arcuate eminence, which marks the elevation of bone overlying the superior semicircular canal.
- The greater superficial petrosal nerve (GSPN) is identified; this marks the lateral margin of dissection (Fig. 23.12).
- Medially, the petrous ridge is identified and the superior petrosal sinus passing within its ridge.
- A House-Urban retractor is positioned such that the blade is caught under (just medial to) the petrous ridge and under the anticipated position of the IAC.

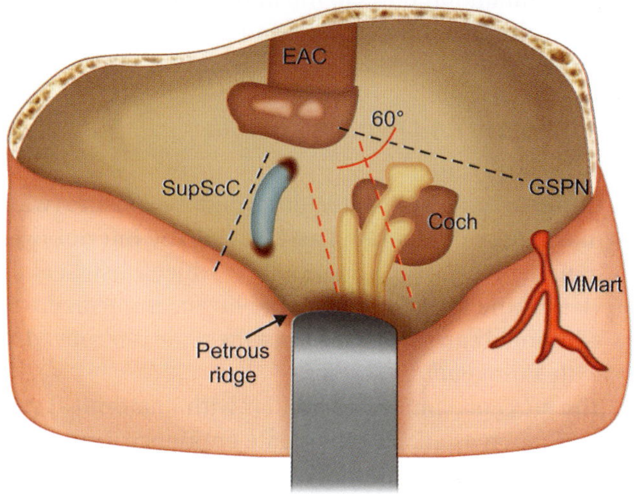

Fig. 23.12: Surgical view of middle cranial fossa floor (left side).

- The IAC is reliably found between the long axis of the arcuate eminence (squamous cell carcinoma, SCC) and the GSPN at approximately 60° posterior from the GSPN.[164,165]
- Drilling is initiated on the petrous ridge medially, where there is most bone to remove.
- The cochlea is located anteriorly, the vestibule posterolaterally, marking the limits of drill dissection.

Dissection of the IAC and tumor removal:

- The bony IAC is outlined with increasingly smaller diamond burrs until only a bony eggshell remains.
- Ideally, the IAC is circumferentially skeletonized, 270°.
- The dura of the IAC is opened with a microsurgical blade.
- The separation between the facial nerve and the SVN (Bill's bar) is identified.
- Facial nerve stimulating probe (Prass probe) is used to positively identify the facial nerve.
- The tumor is identified and separated from the facial nerve starting at the fundus to the level of the porus using sharp microdissection.
- SVN can be sectioned at the level of the fundus to allow slack for tumor mobilization.
- Extrameatal portions of tumor and larger tumors can be debulked with CUSA.

Wound closure:

- The IAC is packed with an abdominal fat graft that is harvested once tumor is removed and covered with tissue sealant such as TISSEEL.
- The craniotomy plate is secured with miniplates; two tie-down holes for dural lateralization are made with

1-mm diamond burrs in the middle of the craniotomy plate, separated by 2–3 mm and a 4-0 Neurolon stitch is used.

Specific Issues and Avoiding Pitfalls

Maximize exposure:

- Common pitfall is insufficient anterior exposure (while making the craniotomy) and leaving the inferior overhanging edge of the craniotomy, which obstructs the view of the MCF floor (this can be accomplished with additional careful drilling once the plate is removed, or with a rongeur).
- The surgeon should be familiar with anatomical variants (such as an absent arcuate eminence, prominent bony undulations of the MCF floor, dehiscent geniculate ganglion, petrous carotid artery, superior semicircular canal, and tegmen tympani) in order to avoid injury to these structures.
- The surgeon should also be familiar with alternative approaches to identifying the IAC such as those described by House,[5] Fisch,[166] and Garcia-Ibanez (outlined above).[165]
- Be able to expand approach in tumors with a larger CPA involvement.[167-169]

Maximize outcome:

- Minimize traction of GSPN that can be transmitted to facial nerve trunk via geniculate ganglion
- Decompress the meatal foramen for optimal facial nerve exposure.

Minimize complications:

- Close the IAC with fat and cover TISSEEL.
- Consider a split calvarial graft if skull base defect is large.
- Use fat with TISSEEL or bone was to occlude any peri-IAC air cells of the petrous bone.
- Total time of temporal lobe retraction should be kept at a minimum.
- Be aware and attempt to avoid bleeding into the posterior fossa with removal of the extrameatal portion as this area is poorly exposed with MCF approach.

Suboccipital Approach (Retrosigmoid)

Background/Indication: The first known attempted surgical removal of a vestibular schwannoma was performed by McBurney in 1891 who utilized a suboccipital (retrosigmoid) approach: "after opening the suboccipital plate with a mallet and gouge, the cerebellum swelled massively, so much so that it became necessary to shave off the excess". In his early attempt, no tumor was removed and the patient expired 12 days later.[170] Successful attempts were pioneered by Cushing in 1905 and later his resident trainee Dandy; while Cushing advocated for a bilateral craniotomy,[41] Dandy favored a unilateral suboccipital approach.[171] Further modifications involved placing the patient in a sitting position rather than prone, which was supplanted by the three-quarter prone (park bench) and supine positions in more recent years.[172] As with the MCF approach, introduction of the surgical microscope in the late 1950s revolutionized the surgical technique.

The retrosigmoid approach is suitable for tumors of all sizes. When hearing preservation is the goal, tumors that do not penetrate the lateral-most third of the IAC are best suited. This approach offers excellent exposure of the brainstem and CNs IV through XII. If hearing preservation is not the goal, lateral drilling into the vestibular aqueduct and posterior semicircular canal exposes the distal third of the IAC. Contraindications to the retrosigmoid approach are patients with medical conditions who cannot tolerate general endotracheal anesthesia and evidence of invasion of the labyrinth by the tumor, in which case a translabyrinthine approach would be more appropriate.[173]

Surgical centers vary in how the specific steps of the approach are allocated among neurotologists and neurosurgeons. Commonly, the neurosurgical team performs a craniotomy after skeletonization of the sigmoid sinus and exposes the surgical field. The neurosurgical team also debulks the majority of the tumor. Once this is accomplished, the otolaryngologist (neurotologist) performs the IAC drillout laterally, avoiding injury to the inner ear structures.

Technical steps: We have utilized the following modifications.[174]

Craniotomy:

- Incision is planned approximately 4–5 cm behind pinna (3 fingerbreadths) and is mostly vertical with slight curve anteriorly and posteriorly (green line in Figure 23.13).
- Anteriorly based periosteal (Palva flap) is made.
- Palva flap and skin flap incision should be staggered and approximated with interrupted Vicryl stitches.
- Soft tissue is retracted with fish hooks (anteriorly and inferiorly).
- Bony landmarks (the EAC anteriorly, mastoid tip, temporal line and the osterion) are identified and the presumed relationship to the sigmoid sinus.
- Drilling is initiated without the use of a microscope with cutting and then diamond burrs once the bony plate over the sigmoid sinus is sufficiently thinned.

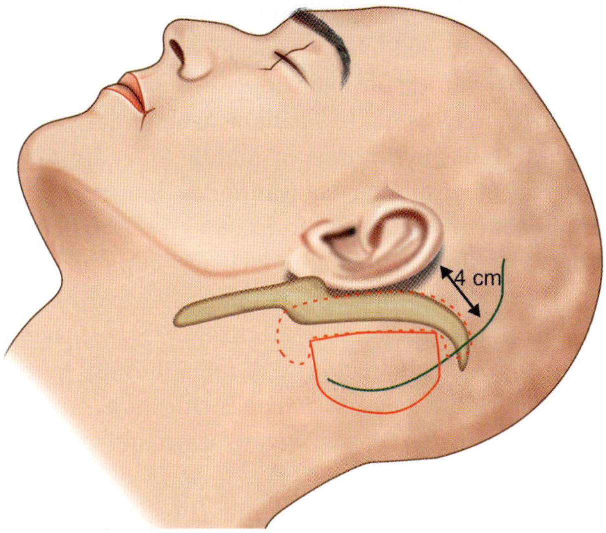

Fig. 23.13: Retrosigmoid approach incision and craniotomy.

- The sigmoid sinus is skeletonized from the lateral sinus superiorly to the horizontal curve of the occipital bone; the sinus can be completely decompressed if additional anterior exposure into the IAC is needed (red dotted line in Figure 23.13).
- Craniectomy is then made, with the superior limb parallel to the lateral sinus, and anterior edge parallel to the sigmoid sinus, making an approximately 2.5 × 2cm window.
- Bone flap is placed in saline soaked gauze.

Opening of dura and exposure of brain stem and IAC:
- The dura is opened sharply with a surgical blade and Metzenbaum scissors.
- The dural flap is anteriorly based and is secured with stitches.
- The cerebellum is gently retracted with Telfa.
- Lateral medullary cistern is rapidly identified to allow for decompression of CSF and for relaxation of the cerebellum. It is crucial to perform this step rapidly and with the use of the surgical microscope as needed since larger tumors may create significant pressure in the posterior fossa and may cause the cerebellum to herniate through the small dural opening.
- The brainstem and the CNs are identified starting from the occipital floor and moving superiorly.
- The 7th and 8th CNs are seen exiting the brain stem and penetrating into the porus acusticus with the associated tumor.
- Debulking of the cisternal portion commences.

IAC drillout and tumor removal:
- Dura over the posterior face of the temporal bone that is overlying the IAC is opened in a saloon-door fashion with a sickle beaver blade.
- The posterior aspect of the IAC is drilled to allow for lateral exposure, around 180°.
- Bony landmarks, the operculum at the entrance of the vestibular aqueduct serve as delineation of the anterior most dissection.
- Tumor is dissected laterally to medially using sharp dissection techniques.

Closure:
- Hemostasis is achieved and Telfa strips are removed under constant irrigation.
- Fat from the abdominal fat graft is placed in the drilled IAC and sealed with fibrin glue.
- Dura is closed in a watertight fashion.
- Mastoid and temporal bone air cells are plugged with fat, fibrin glue and bone wax as needed.
- Tie-down holes are made in the bone for dural lateralization.
- Craniotomy plate is secured at three ends with miniplates.
- Soft tissue closure is in two layers with an anteriorly based periosteal flap followed by cutaneous flap.

Specific Issues and Avoiding Pitfalls

Maximize exposure:
- Adequate anterior exposure can be achieved with complete sigmoid sinus decompression, allowing the anterior dural flap to decompress it.
- Superior aspect of craniotomy should be as close to the lateral sinus as possible.
- Inferior aspect of craniotomy should be as close to the horizontal curve of the occipital bone with minimal overhang (this can be modified with a rongeur).
- Passive retraction of cerebellum should be optimized.
- Rapid identification of the lateral medullary cistern space and decompression of CSF is key.

Maximize outcome:
- Preserve AICA loop and labyrinthine artery; the surgeon should be aware of the anatomical variants of the AICA and its branches.
- In the event that a semicircular canal is entered, it should be immediately closed with bone wax in hopes of preserving hearing.

- Superior aspect of the IAC should be drilled with caution to avoid injury to the facial nerve as it runs in the anterosuperior quadrant of the IAC.
- The most difficult part of the tumor to dissect is the transitional or junction zone. This is a 1 cm long area along the ventrolateral portion of the tumor just proximal to the porus acusticus. In this region the tumor capsule and nerves are extremely adherent as a result of tumor invasion of the arachnoid. Facial nerve stimulation is vital as it facilitates identification of the facial nerve fibers that may be difficult, despite high magnification, to distinguish from arachnoidal adhesions or filaments of the eighth CN.

Minimize complications:

- Prevention of bone dust contamination of the CSF space may be accomplished with materials commonly used for hemostasis or neural protection.
- Obliteration of IAC with fat and TISSEEL, held in position by a "saloon-door" dural flap.
- Use bone wax to block perimeatal cells in all cases.
- Meticulous obliteration of the mastoid and temporal bone air cells with bone wax, fat and TISSEEL.
- Dura should be tested for watertight closure and allograft can be used if the edges cannot approximate.
- Replacement of the bone flap or placement of adipose graft within the craniotomy defect has been associated with decreased rates of long-term postoperative headache (from 12% down to 1%).[175,176]
- Bone flap should be elevated carefully.
- Before dura is open all measures to promote brain retraction should be employed (hyperventilation, Mannitol, Lasix, corticosteroids, head elevation).
- Cisternal drainage of the CSF should occur promptly after the dura is opened.
- In large tumors, consider placing EMG ET tubes to monitor 9/10; also 5 and 11.
- Cerebellum should only be retracted with Telfa (no retractors).
- Excessive head turning or flexion can compromise venous sinus drainage and should be avoided.
- Sigmoid sinus should be carefully skeletonized to avoid injury.

Postoperative and Long-Term Headache

Headaches are a common postoperative complaint; up to 65% patients report headache beyond the immediate postoperative period after vestibular schwannoma resection.[175,177,178] Patients undergoing the retrosigmoid approach to resection of vestibular schwannoma may be particularly vulnerable to postoperative headaches.[175,177,178] In a meta-analysis of 1653 patients who underwent retrosigmoid, translabyrinthine, or middle fossa approach for resection of vestibular schwannoma, long-term significant headache was reported in 36% of the patients who underwent retrosigmoid approach as compared with 16% and 1% of those who underwent translabyrinthine and middle fossa approaches, respectively.[178] Specifically, with a retrosigmoid craniectomy, dural adhesion to nuchal musculature has been associated with dural stretch and headache; for this reason we advocate utilizing a craniotomy plate instead.[131,150,174]

Headache within the immediate postoperative period may be caused by incisional pain, slight reduction in CSF pressure, dural irritation, dural stretch, spasm of nuchal musculature and irritating substances within the subarachnoid space.[131,178] Immediate postoperative headache may be reduced by minimizing retraction, decreasing tension of dural closure, and the use of lactated ringers for irrigation.[131] Prevention of desiccation of dural flaps may facilitate dural closure minimizing dural stretch and irritation.[178] In addition, placement of absorbable gelatin sponge (Gelfoam), Telfa, or cottonoids during IAC drillout helps to prevent the collection of bone dust in the posterior fossa, which has been associated with postoperative headache and chemical meningitis.[131,178] Most often, headaches within the immediate postoperative period may be managed with acetaminophen and opioid analgesia.

Translabyrinthine Approach

Background/Indication: The translabyrinthine craniotomy as an approach to the CPA was first described by and performed by otologists at the beginning of the 20th century. However, due to the difficulty of dissection and poor hemostatic control the approach was deemed "a wholly impractical suggestion" by Dandy in 1925; in 1928 Cushing said of the translabyrinthine approach: "If the otologist has ambitions to treat these lesions there is no possible route more dangerous or difficult than this one... a proposal of this sort I am sure would never occur to an otologist who has general surgical training before he engaged in the particular surgery of his specialty".[179]

William F. House reintroduced this approach in the 1960s, and it has since been routinely used in every surgical center worldwide for removal of vestibular schwannomas. Although hearing is sacrificed, the translabyrinthine craniotomy allows the most direct access to the CPA, as well as exposure of the facial nerve from brainstem to stylomastoid foramen. All drilling is extradural, and this minimizes intracranial complications and bone dust entering the cranial cavity. The entire length of the internal auditory canal (IAC) from fundus to porus, as well as the CPA, is routinely exposed.[180]

The translabyrinthine approach is suitable for patients with preoperative loss of functional hearing with either small IAC tumors or large tumors. For any tumor >2–2.5 cm this approach should be utilized, as chance of hearing preservation is low. For patients who can tolerate general endotracheal anesthesia, special consideration should be given for patients who have active chronic ear disease, for patients who have the tumor in an only hearing ear and for whom a subtotal resection via a retrosigmoid approach is considered, and for patients who have a high-riding jugular bulb.[173]

Technical steps

Craniotomy:

- Incision is planned approximately 3 cm behind pinna (2 fingerbreadths) and is C-shaped.
- Anteriorly based periosteal (Palva flap) is made.
- Palva flap and skin flap incision should be staggered and approximated with interrupted Vicryl stitches.
- Soft tissue is retracted with fish hooks (anteriorly).
- Bony landmarks (the EAC anteriorly, spine of Henle, mastoid tip, temporal line) are identified.
- Drilling is initiated without the use of a microscope with cutting and then diamond burrs.
- Standard landmarks are identified: tegmen plate, sigmoid sinus and sinodural angle, antrum, incus, lateral SCC.
- Facial nerve is identified with thinning the bone over it with a 4 diamond burr from its 2nd genu and inferior toward the stylomastoid foramen.
- Bony plates over the middle fossa, sigmoid sinus, and posterior fossa are thinned, egg-shelled, and removed.
- The larger the tumor, the more the retrosigmoid dura needs to be exposed to allow access, and the further posterior an incision is needed.
- Bipolar cautery is used to shrink the dura and facilitate further dural separation from bone and further bone removal.
- Labyrinthectomy with preserving the inferior half of the lateral SCC in order to protect the facial nerve.
- Inferior extent of dissection: jugular bulb.
- Cochlear aqueduct is encountered in this location, parallel and inferior to the IAC, which may lead to CSF leakage.

IAC:

- Ampullae of lateral SCC and superior SCC followed into the vestibule and this marks the entrance of the SVN and the superior and most lateral edge of the IAC.
- Troughs are made superiorly and inferiorly around the IAC allowing for 180–270° of removed bone.
- Dura over the IAC is incised with a sickle knife.
- Tumor is debulked; resection is in lateral to medial direction.

Closure:

- Remove incus; scar mucosa and place fat followed by TISSEEL into antrum.
- Dura over IAC approximated in a "girdle" fashion.
- Fat "corks" placed in between the girdle stitches and covered with TISSEEL.
- Fat strips packed into the remainder of cavity with TISSEEL.

Specific Issues and Avoiding Pitfalls

Maximize exposure:

- In cases of anteriorly based sigmoid sinus or a contracted mastoid, full bony removal and decompression of the sigmoid sinus and the temporal lobe may be necessary before further dissection commences.
- Inferior dissection should be carried down all the way to the jugular bulb, especially in larger tumors.

Maximize outcome:

- Counsel patients appropriately with respect to expected facial nerve outcome: with larger tumors (>3.5cm) about 50% of patients will have a HB1 or 2 1 year postoperatively.[144]
- Facial nerve should be quickly identified in its descending portion in the mastoid.
- The inferior bony half of the lateral semicircular canal should be left up as long as possible to protect the nerve at its 2nd genu.
- If making a trough at the superior aspect of the IAC, avoid drilling in the anterior direction as the labyrinthine portion of the facial nerve.

Minimize complications:

- Avoid drilling the facial recess; if any facial recess cells are opened, they should be sealed to prevent CSF leak.
- The antrum should always be packed off as described above to prevent CSF rhinorrhea.

- Avoid injury to the sigmoid sinus, especially if dominant.
- More medial drilling along the sinodural angle raises the risk of tearing the superior petrosal sinus. This angle of intersection of the posterior fossa dura and tentorium makes the sinodural intersection a difficult area to achieve full bony decompression and places the superior petrosal sinus at greater risk.
- Bleeding from the superior petrosal sinus also can be controlled with topical hemostatic agents, but one must be aware of the anatomic variant where the vein of Labbé drains into this sinus.
- Drilling along the inferior trough of the IAC can place the dome of the jugular bulb at risk, particularly when the bulb is elevated. Jugular bulb tears can be controlled similarly to those of sigmoid sinus tears, although in rare instances ligation of the jugular vein in the neck with extraluminal packing of the sigmoid sinus may be required.

CSF Leaks and Cranioplasty after a Translabyrinthine Approach

Translabyrinthine resection, compared to the other two approaches, leaves the largest cranial defect. The highest rates of reoperation for CSF leak repair have been reported with the translabyrinthine approach.[153] Special attention should be given to wound closure and also reconstruction of the bony defect. The rates of CSF leak after translabyrinthine craniotomy have dropped over the past few decades.

Some centers perform a cranioplasty with hydroxyapatite cement recontouring with or without titanium mesh, which secures the autologous fat packing; this type of reconstruction has dropped the incidence of postoperative CSF leak to <4%.[181] However, while hydroxyapatite and titanium mesh reconstruction is associated with improved outcome, they increase the cost of surgery; for this reason some advocate a vascularized cranioplasty bone flap instead.[182] Wu et al. reported a decrease in CSF leak rates from 28 to 7% with the use of musculoperiosteal flap closure, although the soft tissue may complicate follow-up imaging.[149] There are also reports of <1% leak rates without the use of cranioplasty and relying on meticulous closure techniques.[183,184] Leaks through the wound are very rare with carefully layered, watertight closures.

We favor closure with autologous adipose tissue grafts (*see* Figs. 23.14A to C). Fat grafting assists in the imaging follow-up of patients with vestibular schwannoma. In addition, fat grafting has been found to decrease the rate of CSF leak from 5.7% to 2.2% when compared with muscle flap reconstruction.[185] With limited facial recess dissection, minimal dissection of the incus buttress, and packing of temporalis fascia around the incus to obstruct the mastoid antrum in addition to fat obliteration of the mastoid cavity, no CSF leaks were encountered in 61 patients after translabyrinthine approach vestibular schwannoma resection.[183]

Extended and Modified Approaches

The three standard approaches described above may need to be extended in cases of large tumors or unfavorable anatomy. For the translabyrinthine approach, when the vestibular schwannoma extends anteriorly or when the jugular bulb is high (especially in the case of a dominant sinus) a transotic/transcochlear approach may be necessary. Usually, the surgeon plans the extended approach based on preoperative imaging, but sometimes the decision to expand the surgical field happens intraoperatively. With this extension, the content of the middle ear is removed, the wall of the EAC is taken down, and the EAC and the Eustachian tube are obliterated. The facial nerve can either be left in its bony canal between the geniculate ganglion and the stylomastoid foramen[186,187] or it can be rerouted. Facial nerve rerouting can interrupt the deep petrosal artery supply of the perigeniculate segment and lead to ischemia. This technique requires additional surgical time and expertise and carries a more significant risk of paresis, in some cases of up to 74%.[188] Posterior rerouting of the facial nerve can be indicated in cases of residual tumor and preoperative facial nerve deficit.[187]

Apart from the transcochlear extension, the translabyrinthine approach can be extended via a transapical approach. The main principle of this extension is an increase of bone removal around the IAC from 270° to up to 320°, in addition to a broad mastoidectomy in which bone anterior and posterior to the sigmoid sinus and around the middle fossa is completely removed and inferior dissection and decompression of the jugular bulb is achieved. In a review of 100 tumors that were >4 cm and an enlarged translabyrinthine transapical approach was used, total removal was achieved in 92% of cases; facial nerve function was a HB1-3 in 75% of cases and CSF leaks occurred 1.8% of the time.[189]

The retrosigmoid approach can be extended anterolaterally for large tumors with a significant IAC component by drilling through the posterior aspect of the petrous bone and sacrificing vestibular organs and hearing. The MCF approach can be extended posteriorly by dividing

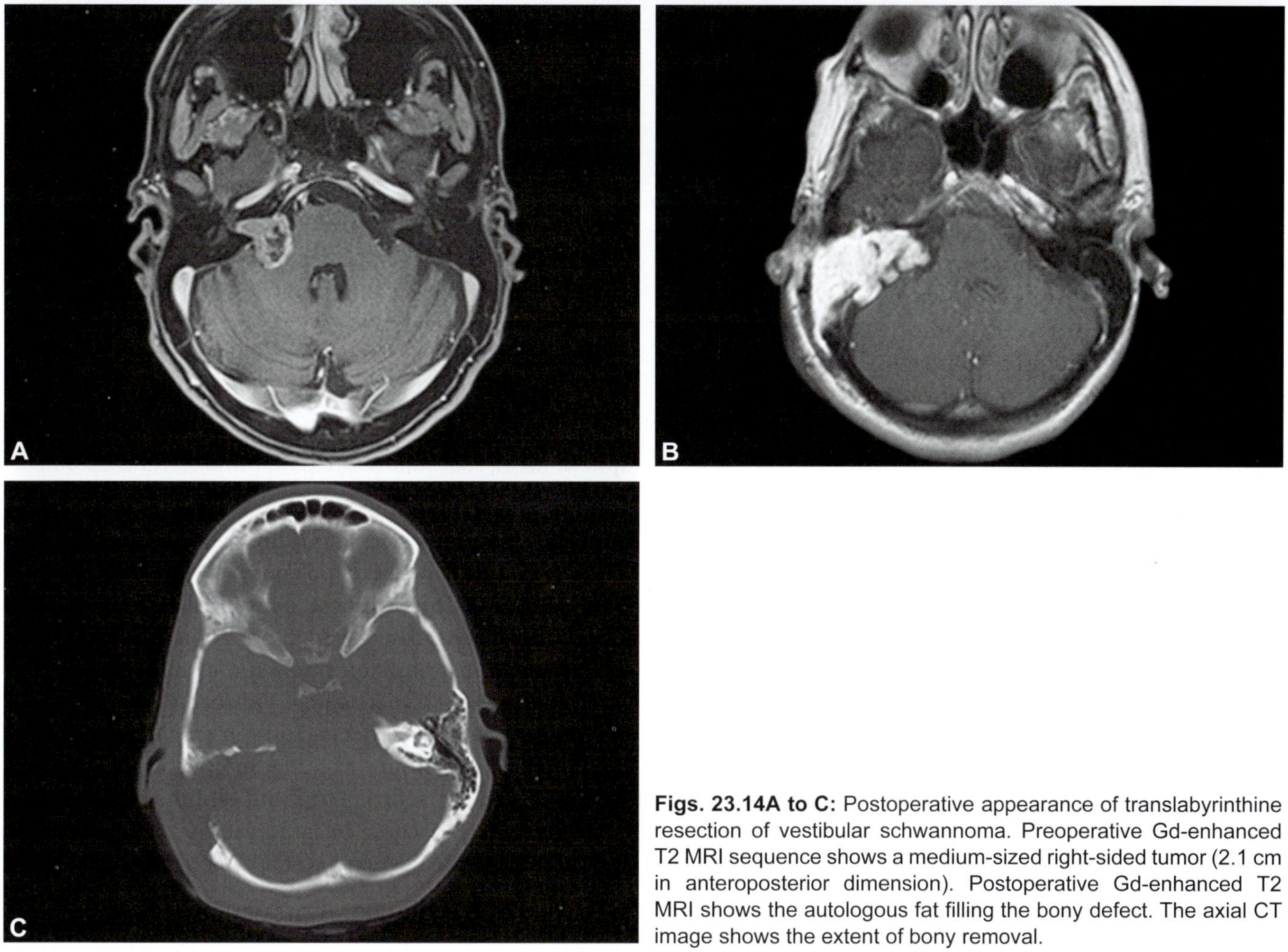

Figs. 23.14A to C: Postoperative appearance of translabyrinthine resection of vestibular schwannoma. Preoperative Gd-enhanced T2 MRI sequence shows a medium-sized right-sided tumor (2.1 cm in anteroposterior dimension). Postoperative Gd-enhanced T2 MRI shows the autologous fat filling the bony defect. The axial CT image shows the extent of bony removal.

the superior petrosal sinus to reach tumors in the CPA. This maneuver, however, does increase the risk of injury to the facial nerve applying more traction via the GSPN to the geniculate area.

In an attempt to preserve hearing with medium to large tumors with a significant lateral IAC component, a presigmoid retrolabyrinthine approach has been described. The patient's anatomy needs to be favorable such that the space between the sigmoid sinus and the posterior semicircular canal, once the sinus has been decompressed, allows for adequate exposure and dissection. In more recent years, the addition of surgical endoscopes can assist in total tumor resection with this technique.[190] In a review of 10 patients who underwent a presigmoid retrolabyrinthine endoscopy assisted dissection, 8 patients had complete removal of tumor, the facial nerve was postoperatively impaired in two patients, and one patient experience a deterioration in hearing.[191]

Another strategy for hearing preservation and maximized exposure is the transcrusal approach. After a wide mastoidectomy and skeletonization of the sigmoid sinus, the superior and inferior canals from the ampullae to the common crus are sacrificed by drilling and then are occluded with bone wax and bone dust. In the six patients presented, who almost all had tumors >3 cm in size, hearing preservation was achieved 100% of the time.[192]

The terminology and extent of the approaches discussed above were been defined previously (Table 23.11).[192]

Surgical Outcomes

When discussing the surgical options with a patient, expected outcomes with respect to preservation of hearing, preservation of facial function, extent of tumor removal and any possible complications as well as options for rehabilitation, need for adjunctive treatment and follow-up must be thoroughly discussed. This section compares

Table 23.11: Transpetrosal approaches

Approach	*Resection*
Retrolabyrinthine	Semicircular canals remain intact
Transcrusal	Superior and posterior SCCs are removed from the ampullae to the common crus
Translabyrin-thine	Horizontal canal and vestibule are entered; the IAC is opened laterally
Transotic	Complete removal of SCCs and skeletonization of the facial nerve; EAC obliteration
Transcochlear	Includes transotic, with posterior mobilization of the facial nerve, removal of cochlea, and exposure of the petrous carotid artery

(SCC, squamous cell carcinoma; IAC, intracanalicular; EAC, extracanalicular).

the outcomes and complications of the three major surgical approaches with respect to VII and VIII CNs and those related to other factors.

VII and VIII Cranial Nerves

Hearing preservation: As described above, not all patients are candidates for hearing preservation approaches. Once their adequate candidacy has been determined, they usually undergo either the MCF or the retrosigmoid resection. The success of hearing preservation varies significantly among centers. Also, definition of "success" is not always consistent; the clinician should keep these reporting inconsistencies in mind when reviewing studies. Tables 23.12 A to C outline hearing preservation outcomes in studies published in the past decade.

A recent meta-analysis of 49 articles and 998 patients with 6 months to 7 years of follow-up revealed an overall hearing preservation rate of 52% for the RSIG and MCF approach combined.[193] Hearing preservation was defined as the percentage of patients who postoperatively had class A or B hearing out of the total number of patients with preoperative class A or B hearing. When separated by approach, 63% out of the total 286 MCF cases and 47% out of the total 702 RSIG cases achieved successful hearing preservation. The advantage that the MCF approach has over the RSIG approach was shown to be significant even when controlling for the size of tumors addressed by the RSIG route. This meta-analysis also confirmed that hearing preservation declines with increasing tumor size. A literature review of only IAC vestibular schwannomas found similar results with an overall hearing preservation rate for the RSIG and MCF approach of 58% and 62%, respectively.[145]

There are a few centers that perform comparable number of both MCF and RSIG approaches. More typically, one surgical team prefers one approach over the other and achieves better results with the preferred method. There is large variability between centers in hearing preservation rates for both the RSIG and MCF approach (Tables 23.12A and 23.12B). Interestingly, within one center, when tumors are controlled for size, data show similar hearing outcomes (Table 23.12C). This is probably due to reporting bias.[132]

With MCF resections, the long-term results of hearing preservation are good even after 5 years. One study showed that the initial postoperative class A hearing was preserved in class A or B in 95% of the cases at the conclusion of the 5-year follow-up; in another, WRS class I hearing (SDS>70%) was maintained in 23 (88%) of 26 patients with >5 years of follow-up.[194,195]

Intraoperative monitoring of hearing function with ABR or CNAP during vestibular schwannoma surgery is routinely performed by many surgeons. A review from Stanford found that monitoring by CNAP is significantly associated with a higher chance of hearing preservation,[196] while monitoring by ABR did not have a positive influence on hearing preservation results. Superiority of direct (CNAP) 8th nerve monitoring was also demonstrated by Danner et al. hearing was preserved in 71% of patients with tumors 1 cm or less and in 32% of patients with tumors between 1 and 2.5 cm, compared to 41% and 10% when ABR was used for the same size matched tumors.[197] Another intraoperative predictor of hearing outcome may be severity of adhesion of the tumor to the 8th nerve; tumors with severe adhesions may be associated with a hearing preservation rate of <20%.[198]

Facial nerve function: Facial nerve function is one of the most important outcomes with vestibular schwannoma surgery. Facial nerve deficits are a cause of significant morbidity for the patient—not just for cosmetic reasons, which can be devastating and socially isolating, but also for the functional reasons of impaired eye closure, oral competence and nasal valve function. Patients who present with a benign tumor that is affecting their hearing will more likely consent to a surgical procedure that may cause further hearing deterioration, but will be harder pressed to undergo a procedure that may cause a facial palsy or paralysis when they did not present with one to begin with. Preservation of facial nerve function is the most important concern of patients undergoing surgery of the CPA.[119,211,212]

All of the surgical approaches can impair facial nerve function. Function can be compromised by direct traction,

Table 23.12A: Hearing preservation outcomes in recent studies: MCF

Author (ref)	*Group (year)*	*No patients*	*Hearing outcome (tumor size)*
Jackson et al.[196]	Stanford (2000)	21	76% A/B
Thomsen et al.[199]	Denmark (2000)	21	44% A/B
Arts et al.[200]	U of Michigan (2006)	63	73% A/ B (<1 cm) 58% A/B (>1 cm)
Gjuric et al.[201]	Zagreb (2007)	29	55% A/B
Woodson et al.[195]	Iowa (2010)	49	96% WRS >50%

Table 23.12B: Hearing preservation outcomes in recent studies: RSIG

Author (ref)	*Group (year)*	*No patients*	*Hearing outcome (tumor size)*
Mazzoni et al.[202]	Ospedali Riuniti (2000)	64	48% A/B
Kaylie et al.[203]	Oregon (2001)	44	29% A/B (<2 cm)
Somers et al.[204]	Belgium (2001)	26	46% A/B
Lee et al.[205]	Jefferson (2002)	51	25% GR 1/2 (<1.5 cm) 19% GR 1/2 (1.5–3 cm)
Maw et al.[206]	Bristol (2003)	40	38% A/B
Mangham[132]	Seattle (2004)	22	72% A/B
Yamakami et al.[207]	Japan (2009)	22	78% A/B
Nonaka et al.[208]	Duke (2013)	170	74% A/B

Table 23.12C: Hearing preservation outcomes in recent studies: MCF versus RSIG (intrainstitutional)

Author (center, year) (ref)	*Group (year)*	*No patients/approach*	*Hearing outcome*
Rabelo et al.[209]	Gruppo Otologico (2012)	90 MCF 82 RSIG	18.9% A/B 10.6% A/B
Moriyama et al.[198]	N Carolina (2002)	10 MCF 20 RSIG	70% A/B 70% A/B
Staecker et al.[210]	Harvard (2000)	15 MCF 15 RSIG	46% A/B 40% A/B

(RSIG, retrosigmoid; MCF, middle cranial fossa).

blunt trauma, cautery and even transection. All factors taken into consideration, the major predictor of postoperative facial nerve deficit is tumor size. For small tumors, < 1.5 cm in diameter, facial nerve outcomes are excellent (HB class 1 or 2) in 95–100% cases.[203,213] The outcomes for larger tumors are more variable, but generally for tumors >3 cm at 1 year of follow-up >85% of patients will have a HB class 1 or 2 function, and in some centers as low as 30%.[143,203,213,214] A meta-analysis of 79 studies and 11,873 patients found the cutoff size to be 2 cm; for tumors <2 cm 90% patients preserved excellent facial nerve function while for those 2 cm or larger, the average preservation rate was 67%.[215]

Since size of tumor affects approach, comparison of facial nerve outcome between approaches should be conducted for size-matched tumors. For larger tumors, the surgeon is often faced with the decision between the RSIG and TLAB approach (Table 23.13A). Similarly, for smaller tumors where hearing preservation is attempted, the choice is between the MCF and RSIG approach (Table 23.13B). Regarding the hearing preservation approaches, while the hearing outcomes favor the MCF approach, the facial nerve outcomes have been thought to favor the RSIG approach. However, in a large meta-analysis of studies conducted over the past two decades and controlling for tumor size, the MCF approach has led to excellent outcomes in 85%

Table 23.13A: Facial nerve outcomes: RSIG versus TLAB

Author (ref)	*Group (year)*	*Approach (n)*	*HB 1+2 outcome (size of tumor)*
Samii et al.[217]	Hannover, Germany (2006)	RSIG (*n*=22)	95% (intracanalicular)
Tonn et al.[218]	Wuerzburg, Germany (2000)	RSIG (*n*=396)	89% (<30 mm)
Maw et al.[206]	Bristol, UK (2003)	RSIG (*n*=40)	90% (<30 mm)
Mazzoni et al.[202]	Ospedali Rinuiti, Italy (2000)	RSIG (*n*=150)	85% (<20 mm)
Danner et al.[197]	UCSD (2004)	RSIG (*n*=242)	95% (<10 mm) 100% (10–15 mm) 89% (15–20 mm) 77% (20–25 mm) 66% (>25 mm)
Darwish et al.[219]	New Zealand (2005)	RSIG (*n*=97)	80% (<15 mm) 81% (15–30 mm) 22% (>30 mm)
Mamikoglu et al.[220]	Northwestern, IL (2003)	TLAB (*n*=81) RSIG (*n*=17)	68% (20–30 mm) 59% (20–30 mm)
Anderson et al.[221]	Loyola, IL (2005)	TLAB (*n*=25) RSIG (*n*=22)	72% (>30 mm) 81% (>30 mm)
Wu and Sterkers[222]	Paris, France (2000)	TLAB (*n*=40)	65% (>30 mm)
Zhang et al.[223]	Xijing Hospital, China (2005)	RSIG (*n*=105)	57% (>40 mm)

(RSIG, retrosigmoid; TLAB, transylabyrinthine).

Table 23.13B: Facial nerve outcomes: smaller tumors

Author (ref)	*Group (year)*	*Approach (n)*	*HB 1+2 outcome (Size of tumor)*
Staecker et al.[210]	Harvard (2000)	MCF (*n*=15) RSIG (*n*=15)	93% (intracanalicular) 93% (intracanalicular)
Moriyama et al.[198]	Raleigh, NC (2002)	MCF (*n*=10) RSIG (*n*=20)	100% (intracanalicular) 95% (intracanalicular)
Sanna et al.[224]	Piacenza, Italy (2004)	MCF (*n*=56) RSIG (*n*=41)	52% (<15 mm) 95% (<15 mm)
Satar et al.[225]	Meta-analysis (2003)	MCF (*n*=797)	99% (<1 mm) 94% (1–10 mm) 86% (10–19 mm)
Arts et al.[200]	Ann Arbor, MI (2006)	MCF (*n*=73)	96% (3–18 mm)
Isaacson et al.[226]	Ann Arbor, MI (2005)	TLAB (*n*=63) MCF (*n*=61)	100% (<10 mm) 93% (10–18 mm) 94% (<10 mm) 92% (10–18 mm)
Mann et al.[38]	Mainz, Germany (2002)	MCF (*n*=129) TLAB (*n*=136) RSIG (*n*=111)	85% (intracanalicular) 79% (<15 mm) 79% (15–25 mm) 100% (intracanalicular) 93% (<15 mm) 81% (15–25 mm) 77% (<15 mm) 49% (15–25 mm)

(RSIG, retrosigmoid; MCF, middle cranial fossa; TLAB, translabyrinthine).

of cases and was significantly higher than the RSIG resection with excellent outcomes in 78%. The TLAB approach in the same analysis led to an average 81% of patients with a HB class 1 or 2 outcome.[215] A multivariate analysis of 624 patients found no significant difference in facial nerve outcomes between approaches when controlling for tumor size.[216]

One consideration with large tumors, which are known to carry a greater risk of facial nerve palsy after resection, is to perform a near-total resection, leaving a piece of tumor capsule on the facial nerve part that is most splayed out and at most risk. While this strategy implies a better prognosis theoretically, the studies conducted so far have not shown significant difference in long-term facial function outcomes between gross total and near-total resection.[216,227,228] The risk of recurrence between near-total resection and gross total resection is comparable, and thus many authors advocate for leaving a capsule behind, especially with unfavorable facial nerve anatomy or significant tumor adhesion to the nerve. The role of near-total and subtotal resection in microsurgical treatment of vestibular schwannoma is discussed in a separate section below.

Other factors that have been investigated with respect to their influence on facial nerve functional outcomes include age of patient, experience of the surgeon, presence of a cystic component and intraoperative monitoring of facial nerve activity. While the large meta-analysis found that age of the patient significantly influenced outcome, with patients younger than 65 having unexpectedly worse outcomes than those older than 65 (71% vs. 84% with HB class 1 or 2 function, respectively), other studies have not found a significant association.[215,216] Experience of the surgeon may play a role in the first 2 years of practice.[216,228] In a Danish study of 773 patients with vestibular schwannomas, solid versus cystic large tumors were compared with respect to facial nerve outcomes. Even though the solid tumors were more adherent to the surrounding structures, 27% of patients with the solid tumors had a significant (HB 6) facial nerve function deficit compared to 41% of patients with cystic tumors.[229]

Most of today's major vestibular schwannoma treatment centers monitor facial nerve activity during microsurgical resection. Electrophysiologic monitoring is indeed associated with significantly better functional outcomes, with one study showing a 70% good or excellent function (HB 3 or better) without monitoring compared to 89% when monitoring is utilized; similar results have been demonstrated in larger meta-analyses.[215,218,230,231] Intraoperative electrophysiologic studies have reduced the rate of complete facial nerve palsy from 14% to 1.5%.[218]

Vestibular disturbance: Apart from hearing preservation and facial nerve function outcomes, the possibility of vestibular disturbance should also be discussed with the patient. Both the inferior and superior division of the vestibular nerves can be affected by the tumor. Further, disequilibrium can be caused by cerebellar damage, brain stem injury, residual vestibular nerve dysfunction, and compromise of AICA vessels as well as direct damage to the vestibule while drilling the posterior aspect of the petrous bone during the retrosigmoid approach.

In one study, balance disturbance was the most frequently reported symptom after vestibular schwannoma surgery in up to 10.2% of patients immediately following surgery and remained in 6.3% of patients in long-term follow-up.[208] This same group examined the incidence of vestibular function according to surgical approach and found that it occurred in 12% of patients with the retrosigmoid approach, 11.7% of patients with the MCF, and 5% of patients undergoing the translabyrinthine approach. In a large meta-analysis, the TLAB approach and smaller tumors were associated with significantly less postoperative disequilibrium.[232] When it comes to the retrosigmoid approach, most commonly associated with postoperative symptom of dizziness, a review of 104 patients found that up to 77.2% complained of postoperative imbalance.[233] Young age, large tumors, and female gender as well as preoperative vestibular complaints can all increase this surgical risk.

Incidence of Other Complications

A recent, statistically powerful meta-analysis of 100 articles including close to 33,000 patients who underwent vestibular schwannoma surgery found that in 22% of patients at least one complication was not related to the VII and VIII CNs.[232] CSF leaks were found in 8.5% cases, followed by 3.8% total infections rate (of which 78% were meningitis and the remaining were wound infections and fat graft site infections), 1.3% complications consisted of other CN deficits (trochlear, abducens, glossopharyngeal, vagus and accessory nerves), ischemic injury or hemorrhage was found in 1% and mortality in 0.2% of cases.

CSF leak: Cerebrospinal fluid (CSF) leak is the most commonly reported complication of microsurgical resection of vestibular schwannoma. The TLAB approach appears to carry the highest risk of CSF leaks, ranging from 0% to 31%,[148,149,152,183,184,234,235] followed by the MCF approach with 4-20% incidence.[236,237] The lowest rate of CSF leaks may be associated with the RSIG approach, reported to be in the 3% to 12% incidence range.[147,152,238,239] The difference among approaches, however, was not found to be significant in two large meta-analyses.[148,153]

Other variables that can influence the incidence of postoperative CSF leak may be the patient's age (carrying a 5% increase in risk in those patients older than 50),[153] as well as increase in tumor size.[151,152,240] .The notion that larger tumors carry a higher risk of CSF leak, however, has been challenged by other reports.[153,241-243] Also, incidence of CSF leakage was found to be higher in patients with tumor recurrence needing additional surgery (11%) than in patients undergoing surgery for the first time (4%).[244] Management and tips on prevention of postsurgical CSF leaks are discussed above.

Meningitis: Meningitis is the second most common complication of vestibular schwannoma microsurgery. Reported incidence of meningitis ranges from 0.14% to 9.9%.[148,151,153,183,184,205,208,234,245,246] Large review studies have found a significant increase in the risk of meningitis in patients who also developed a CSF leak after surgical resection of vestibular schwannoma.[148,153] In an analysis of patients with meningitis after vestibular schwannoma resection, 82% of patients had a history of postoperative CSF leak.[240] A large majority of patients (56–72%) with postoperative meningitis have aseptic (chemical) meningitis compared to culture-confirmed bacterial meningitis, found in 22% of patients.[245,247]

Wound infections: Of the 3.8% total infection rate found in the meta-analysis of close to 33,000 vestibular schwannoma resections, wound infection accounted for 16%, and fat graft site infection for 3.4% of cases.[232] Other studies have found wound infection rates in the range of 2–3%.[205,208] There was no significant correlation between approach for tumor resection or tumor size and wound infections.[232]

Cranial nerve deficits not related to nerves in the IAC (CN VII and VIII): In addition to the cochlear nerve and facial nerve, deficiency in other CNs may be encountered after vestibular schwannomas microsurgical resection. Deficits in CNs outside of the IAC are typically associated with larger vestibular schwannomas or extended approaches.[243,246] From these reports, trochlear nerve deficits can be seen in up to 4.2% of cases; the abducens nerve may be transiently or permanently affected in 1.7% and up to 5.8% of cases; the trigeminal nerve was affected in 0.9% of cases; and vagus nerve deficits were seen in 0.3% of patients undergoing microsurgery for removal of vestibular schwannomas.

Vascular injury, thrombosis, intracranial hemorrhage, seizures, and death: With the advent of microsurgical technique and advances in perioperative care, rates of vascular injury, intracranial hemorrhage, parenchymal injury, and associated mortality have declined precipitously. Rates of postoperative intracranial hemorrhage range from approximately 0.8% to 1.7%.[151,243,246] Rates of dural sinus thrombosis reported in the literature range from 0.1% to 4.6%.[151,157,248,249]

Recently reported mortality rates in association with vestibular schwannoma microsurgery are <2%.[151,243,246] Although the reported incidence is low, mortality seems to be associated with larger tumors.[250] Vascular fatalities are commonly associated with injury to the AICA.[250]

Seizures can be associated with vascular or parenchymal injury. In a review of 120 patients after vestibular schwannoma microsurgical resection, a 6.6% rate of seizure was reported; 3.3% of patients experienced 1 seizure, and 3.3% of patients experienced multiple seizures requiring medication.[157] Slattery et al. reported a 1.2% rate of seizure in their review of 162 patients.[251]

Recurrence and Postoperative Surveillance

A distinction should be made between recurrence rates of those tumors where the goal of treatment was complete resection and recurrence rates of tumors where fragments or parts were purposefully left behind by the surgical team. The success rate of GTR declines in parallel with tumor size; in a recent report, GTR was achieved in 100% of intrameatal tumors, 98.2% of small tumors, 77.7% of medium tumors, 67.5% of moderately large tumors, 45.4% of large tumors, and 44.8% of giant tumors.[208] However, even with intended complete tumor resection, residual cell rests may remain adherent to intact or remnant nerves. Recurrence typically represents regrowth of these residual tumor rests.

Mamikoglu et al. reported a tumor recurrence rate of 1% after complete resection of large vestibular schwannomas at 5-year follow-up.[234] In a review of >1,500 translabyrinthine approach microsurgical resections of vestibular schwannoma, a 0.3% rate of recurrence was described.[252] Similarly, a review of 735 cases of complete tumor resection via the middle fossa approach revealed a 0.3% rate of tumor recurrence.[253] Carlson et al. compared recurrence rates of tumors after gross total resection at 3.5 years of follow-up among all approaches; the overall recurrence rate was 3.5%; the TLAB and RSIG approaches carried a risk of recurrence of 2.2% and 2.4% respectively, while

2 out of the 15 patients who underwent the MC approach (12.3%) had tumor recurrence.[254] Residual and recurrent tumors typically remain asymptomatic until tumor regrowth is sizable.

Tumor regrowth is most commonly assessed with postoperative MRIs. Based on their follow-up of 350 patients over 3.5 years, Carlson et al. have recently proposed an algorithm for the timing and optimal schedule of postsurgical surveillance.[254] The initial MRI should be obtained 6 months postoperatively to serve as a baseline for further comparison of subsequent imaging. The average linear diameter growth rate for recurrent tumors is similar to untreated tumors, ranging from 0 to 5 mm per year.[95,252,255,256]

Postoperative enhancement along the surgical bed is almost ubiquitous (occurring in 98.5% patients).[254] Linear-type enhancements are not predictive of regrowth, and a repeat MRI may be obtained years later. For patients who underwent gross total resection and have a nodular-type enhancement on a baseline 6-month postoperative MRI, more frequent MRI scans are suggested (the authors advocate a follow-up scan at year 3, 7, and 15). Subtotal resection and nodular enhancement increase the risk of recurrence rates by up to 9- and 16-times fold, respectively. Accordingly, these individuals should have imaging performed more aggressively at 2, 5, 10, and 15 years. An increased risk of recurrence based on completeness of resection[257,258] and nodular-type enhancement on MRIs[259] has been confirmed by other studies. Fat suppression protocol MRI facilitates postoperative surveillance in patients who underwent reconstruction of operative defects with adipose tissue grafting.[252]

Role for Incomplete/Subtotal Resection

The definition of difference between NTR and STR is not consistent; typically a cutoff between 2 mm and 5 mm of linear capsule remnant is used. Decision to perform a gross total resection (GTR) versus near-total (NTR) or subtotal (STR) resection can be made intraoperatively in an effort to preserve CN function or may be mandatory in the case of adverse patient response during surgery. Less than complete removal can also be elected preoperatively, despite the possible risk of regrowth, with intention to subsequently treat or observe the tumor.[255,257,260]

Cranial nerve preservation: The hearing status of the contralateral ear is also relevant. If it is impaired from a second vestibular schwannoma (as in cases of NF2) or other otologic disease, incomplete removal may increase the chance of hearing conservation.[261] Nonaka et al. analyzed their series of 170 patients in whom hearing preservation was attempted and correlated to the extent of approach; out of 150 GTR, 75.3% patients achieved an A or B class hearing, compared to 82.4% of 14 total NTR and 66.7% of 3 total STR.

The benefit of more conservative resection appears to favor facial nerve outcomes, although this has not been consistently demonstrated (Table 23.14).

Recurrence rates: The location of tumor remnant can influence tumor recurrence rates, with those tumors left at the fundus of the IAC are more capable of regrowth, presumably due to a richer blood supply.[8,258,260] Cystic tumors may also be more likely to recur if merely debulked.[8,257] While some studies show a significantly increased risk of recurrence with subtotal resection, others have not found a difference in the extent of resection and recurrence rates (*see* Table 23.14).

Subsequent treatment: Within most patients, tumor regrowth does not occur. However, in the selected cohort of patients in whom regrowth is encountered, subsequent treatment is frequently necessary in 59–100% of cases.[257,258] The patient's age, functionality, medical comorbidities, and rate of tumor growth must be factored into the clinical decision making about the management of recurrence and regrowth. Because of higher chance of regrowth over time with incomplete resections, total resections are favored in younger patients.

Treatment options with recurrent or incompletely resected tumors include repeating microsurgical resection or administering postoperative radiation. Multimodality treatment with adjunctive or delayed use of radiation is discussed in the subsequent section. Surgical resection of a recurrent tumor (revision surgery) should be distinguished from planned staged surgical resection, as the former is used as a salvage technique and the latter is performed in a controlled, predetermined matter. Revision surgery has been associated with elevated rates of facial nerve injury,[263,264] while planned staged tumor removal appears to carry improved facial nerve outcomes.[144,265,266]

Planned staged microsurgical resection of vestibular schwannomas has been described for large tumors (>3 cm) by using a RSIG approach for initial debulking, followed by a second staged TLAB approach for completion of tumor removal 4–6 months later.[265] In their series of 34 patients, Patni and Kartush have described up to 94% HB

Table 23.14: Extent of tumor resection: recurrence and cranial nerve outcomes

Report (ref)	*Center (year)*	*Extent of resection (n)*	*Recurrence (years follow-up)*		*Cranial nerve preservation*	
Bloch et al.[257]	UCSF (2004)	GTR (*n*=455)	—		Intact FN function (HB1)	
		NTR (*n*= 76)	3% (3 years)		61%†	
		STR (*n*= 93)	32%		51%†	
					55†	
Nonaka et al.[208]	Duke (2002)	GTR (*n*=306)	0.1%† (3 years)		Good FN function	HP success rate
		NTR (*n*=73)	3%†		89%	75%
		STR(*n*= 31)	10%†		77%	82%
					77%	67%
Carlson et al.[254]	Mayo clinic (2012)	GTR (*n*=144)	4% (3.5 years)		—	
		NTR (*n*=32)	3%			
		STR (*n*=27)	22%			
Sughrue et al.[262]	UCSF (2011)	GTR (*n*=571)	10†(5 years)	9%† (10 years)	—	
		NTR (*n*=89)	22%†	8%†		
		STR (*n*=112)	16%†	8%†		
Gurgle et al.[142]	Stanford (2012)*	GTR (*n*=336)	—		Good FN function	
		NTR (*n*=55)			47%	
		STR (*n*=80)			75%	
					93%	
Seol et al.[227]	Kangwon National University, ROK (2006)	GTR (*n*=26)	4%		Good FN function (immediate postoperative)	
		NTR (*n*=32)	9%†		15%	
		STR (*n*=58)	28%		41%	
					47%	

*Literature review.
†No stat sig.

grade I facial nerve function in staged resection of large tumors. Raslan et al. have also proposed a similar staged resection as a strategy to improve facial nerve outcomes and morbidity in large tumors.[266] In the first stage, a RSIG approach is utilized to debulk the CPA portion of tumor without meatal drilling. The decision for staging was made based on presence of cerebellar or brain stem edema, tumor adherence to the facial nerve or brain stem, poor facial nerve stimulation or a thin or splayed facial nerve. Twenty-eight patients underwent such staged resections. Compared to size-matched tumors removed with the traditional single staged approach, gross or near-total resection was achieved for 96% of patients (compared to 79% of single stage); good facial nerve function was achieved in 82% versus 53% of staged vs. nonstaged resections, respectively. However, CSF leak was more common in two-stage microsurgical removal of vestibular schwannoma. The patient's age should also factor into deciding on a staged approach, as younger patients may tolerate a two-stage tumor resection, and older patients may not tolerate a second craniotomy.

Salvage Surgery after Radiation

For those patients in whom vestibular schwannoma was primarily treated with radiation, salvage microsurgical treatment carries higher morbidity then for patients undergoing primary microsurgical resection, including relatively poor facial nerve outcomes and nearly impossible hearing preservation.[267-269] Poor facial nerve outcomes are thought to occur because an irradiated facial nerve's regeneration potential is diminished, and the recovery from microsurgical trauma is not as robust. It may take anywhere between 1 and 10 years for salvage surgery, with the most common reason to undergo secondary treatment being tumor growth.[268,269] The tumor may quadruple in volume before salvage surgery is considered.[269]

An alternative strategy is to perform a more conservative resection compared to nonirradiated cases.[270] Friedman et al. found a significant difference in facial nerve outcomes with partial (near-total or subtotal) resection following radiation in their series of 73 recurrent tumors.[271] At 1 year of follow-up, good facial nerve function (H-B I/II) was found in 85.7% of patients with partial removal and 50% of those with gross total removal. They found no evidence of treatment success compromise.

Radiation

Introduction and Definition of Terms

In addition to watchful waiting and microsurgical resection, radiation-based treatment forms the third broad category of management strategies of vestibular schwannomas. This option is appealing to both patients and clinicians as its intent is to minimize treatment-related morbidity, yet still provide an active management strategy.

Conventional radiotherapy (as opposed to modern stereotactic radiation) is seldom used, and few studies have published outcomes, which are poor with respect to significant recurrence, treatment-related morbidity and even mortality.[272,273] Stereotactic radiation-based treatments are varied, and the definition of the type of treatment should be precise as there are significant differences in protocols (one- versus multi-day) and outcomes as they relate to hearing preservation, preventing recurrence, and minimization of other complications. A distinct difference exists between radiosurgery and radiation therapy. Radiosurgery is so named as it can essentially be utilized as a one-time treatment, akin to a surgical intervention, but also as a staged course of two to five sessions (referred to as hypofractionated). Radiation therapy implies fractionating or dividing the radiation dose over multiple treatments, usually longer than 5 days and up to 30 treatments.

Minimizing radiation of uninvolved tissues is achieved with differential distribution of energy in radiosurgery, relying on a specified radiation dose to the target surrounded by an area of a steep dose falloff in its vicinity. In radiation therapy or hypofractionated therapy, minimization of injury to healthy adjacent tissue is in addition achieved by dose fractionation. *Dose conformality* is defined as the ratio of the total volume of all tissue receiving the prescribed radiation dose over the planned target volume, an important concept in treatment optimization. High dose conformality implies a very favorable ratio of tissues that are intended for radiation (tumor) versus the surrounding and likely vulnerable neurovascular structures (CNs, cochlea, etc.). The point in space through which the central rays of the radiation beam pass is the treatment *isocenter*, while the lines around the tumor confines, in centrifugal order, mark *isodose lines*. The same dose is delivered to the area between the two adjacent isodose lines.

Delivery of radiation for either radiosurgery or radiation therapy is achieved with various technology and software. Some systems require the utilization of a stereotactic frame, while others are frameless. *Stereotactic* refers to a method in which a precise 3D coordinate in space is defined (either with a Cartesian or polar system) and then used to describe the exact location of the intended treatment delivery, as well as the exact location of tissues to be excluded from treatment. Stereotactic method can be achieved with a mounted frame with reference fiducials or with a real-time imaging that is frameless.

Historical Background

Lars Leksell, a Swedish neurosurgeon, is credited for pioneering a radiation-based method of destroying discrete anatomical regions within the brain while minimizing the effect on the surrounding tissues. Leksell and Borje Larsso, a physicist and radiobiologist, were the first to utilize gamma rays from multiple directions to treat small and specific areas within the cranium in 1951 at the Uppsala University in Stockholm, Sweden.[274] Leksell used the polar coordinate system (relying on a fixed point, with a specified distance, angle and direction from it) for his original Gamma Knife device. The first treatment of a vestibular schwannoma in a human was performed by Leksell in 1969 with the help of his Gamma Knife, a stereotactic device that contained multiple radioactive cobalt (cobalt-60) sources.[275]

Almost 20 years later, first linear accelerator (LINAC) systems were developed. Stereotactic radiosurgery (SRS) and SRT can both be achieved with the (Leksell)Gamma Knife or a linear accelerator (LINAC) system (X-knife, Novalis and Cyberknife).While the original Gamma Knife relied on a stereotactic headframe with reference fiducials, newer technology (Cyberknife)does not require a stereotactic headframe but relies on orthogonal radiographs and an optical tracking system.

Current Delivery Systems

Leksell Gamma Knife: The Leksell Gamma Knife (Elekta Instruments, Norcross, GA, USA) uses either 201 (models U, B, C, 4-C) or 192 (model Perfexion) fixed Co 60 radiation sources that can be collimated to radiation beams of 4–18 mm (16 mm with Perfexion). Dose plans generally consist of several weighted isocenters to create a conformal 3D volume to cover the desired target. A stereotactic headframe is used to provide reference fiducials for stereotactic accuracy and fixation in the device.

Linear accelerator systems: Multiple linear accelerator (LINAC) systems have been developed during the second half of the last century, with the first system described by Betti and Derechinsky in 1984,[276] and first patient trials published in 1985 by Colombo et al. from Vicenza, Italy.[277] The LINAC technology has subsequently been modified to achieve improved precision and accuracy. The LINAC systems commercially available today include the X-knife (Radionics Inc, Burlington, MA, USA), Novalis (BrainLAB, Heimstetten, Germany), and Cyberknife (AccurayInc, Sunnyvale, CA, USA).

Rather than relying on multiple fixed radiation sources collimated to a set point, in a LINAC system the radiation source moves around the patient in multiple arcs with the radiation entering the cranium through many different points. Various techniques have been developed to improve dose conformality, including dynamic techniques, in which both the patient seat and arc radiation delivery system move to shape target volume. These systems are also used in conjunction with a stereotactic headframe or mask.

Cyberknife: In the 1990s, John Adler created the CyberKnife, a robotic frameless radiotherapy system that uses real-time acquisition of the patient's bony anatomy for image-guidance.[278] The Cyberknife is a frameless, image-guided, robotic radiotherapy system that uses a LINAC mounted on a 6-axis robotic arm and a real-time optical tracking system. The arm is programmed to move the linear accelerator sequentially through a predetermined series of locations. At each location, radiation is delivered to the target volume. The trajectory and dose delivered at each location are calculated so that their cumulative effect optimizes the coverage of the target volume while minimizing the exposure of adjacent tissues. The Cyberknife can generate beams from >1200 directions. This allows for nonisocentric radiation planning that can optimize dose conformality and homogeneity. The use of Cyberknife, for its frameless image-guided technology, has made the delivery of staged radiation therapy more practical in the treatment of vestibular schwannoma.

Candidacy

Radiation therapy-based treatment is generally used in the following settings:

1. Patients with unilateral or bilateral vestibular schwannomas that are <3 cm in diameter within the CPA.
2. Patients who have residual tumor after a planned subtotal microsurgical resection or those that recur despite apparent gross total removal.
3. Patients who demonstrate tumor growth following radiotherapy or radiosurgical treatment can also be considered for retreatment; retreatment is considered no sooner than 1 year after initial radiotherapy.
4. Patients who are not microsurgical candidates because of advanced age or other risk factors or patients who do not wish to undergo microsurgical treatment.
5. Patients who have neurofibromatosis type II (NF2) can also be candidates for radiotherapy, although as a group this population does not seem to respond as well to treatment as do patients who have sporadic unilateral tumors.[279]
6. Patients who prefer radiation therapy over other management options.

Delivery Techniques

Single treatment delivery: The following protocol is utilized by the Mayo Clinic in conjunction with the Leksell Gamma Knife and the associated software Gamma Plan for 3D dose planning[280]:

- At an outpatient center, the patient is given a low-dose oral benzodiazepine; younger patients may require general anesthesia; however, treatment is generally well tolerated.
- Patient's head is cleaned with alcohol and infiltrated with a local anesthetic at the points where headframe will be applied.
- Stereotactic headframe (Leksell Model G) is applied with a 4-point fixation.
- MRI followed by CT imaging (1 mm slices for both modalities) is utilized to define the exact 3D volumetric locations of the vestibular schwannoma and critical temporal bone structures surrounding the tumor.
- The MRI and CT scan images are fused with the Gamma Plan software.

- A conformal radiation dose plan is then developed, utilizing a combination of isocenters with various-sized collimators and differential weighting. The Perfexion model divides 192 Co 60 radiation sources into 8 sectors of 24 sources each. Each sector can be completely blocked from contributing to the isocenter or collimated to sizes of 4, 8, or 16 mm; these manipulations allow for more complex-shaped isocenters.
- Patients are typically discharged from outpatient observation within several hours of completing treatment and can resume all daily activities with no restrictions.

Single treatment radiation dose: With any type of radiation-based treatment, a higher dose is more successful at preventing recurrence of tumor, but comes at a cost of increased treatment induced toxicity. In the 1990s, with mean tumor margin doses of 18 Gy (range 16–20 Gy) the tumor control rate was excellent, yet the rate of new onset facial weakness after radiation treatment was as high as 21%, loss of serviceable hearing occurred in up to 75% of cases and 36% patients developed trigeminal sensory disturbance. As the mean tumor margin dose was decreased to 13 Gy (range 12–16 Gy) in 1997, the toxicity of treatment declined. With the new lowered margin dose, no patients developed new facial weakness, trigeminal symptoms occurred in < 4% of cases, and serviceable hearing loss was reduced to 23%. In addition, dose conformality improved by simultaneously increasing the number of isocenters from a mean number of 5 in the early 90s and increasing to 8 toward the end of the century.[280]

Presently, most protocols utilize a dose of 12–13 Gy for patients with serviceable hearing and 13–14 Gy for patients with poor hearing. Most cases are treated using the 50% to 60% isodose line, which maintains a high intratumoral dose with a steep radiation falloff.[280]

Single-fraction SRS using LINAC-based units is very similar, except that the tumor margin dose of 12 to 14 Gray (Gy) is usually prescribed to the 80% or 90% isodose line.[281] This results in a more homogeneous radiation distribution, but the maximum dose is less than typically used in Gamma Knife procedures.

Hypofractionated treatment delivery: Injury to adjacent uninvolved CNs may be mitigated in part by fractionating or staging a course of treatment into a series of smaller doses of radiation.[282-284] The Cyberknife, obviating the need for a fixed headframe, has been utilized to deliver hypofractionated therapy in three consecutive daily treatments.

Below is the protocol used by Stanford University School of Medicine.[285]

Pretreatment evaluation:
- Gadolinium-enhanced MRI is obtained in all patients within the 3 months before treatment and the tumor is measured in three orthogonal dimensions.
- Pretreatment audiograms (including WRS and PTAs) are obtained within 3 months before treatment.
- Cranial nerve status is evaluated, with special attention given to the fifth, seventh, and eighth CN examination.

Treatment planning and delivery:
- The patient is fitted with a custom made Aquaplast mask and thin foam headrest (ensures consistent positioning).
- High-resolution CT scan (1.25 mm slice) with IV contrast is obtained.
- The acquired images are transferred to the Cyberknife treatment planning workstation.
- If the tumor morphology and dimensions are consistent in the acquired CT and the pretreatment MRI, target planning can be done using CT imaging alone (nearly all cases); in the case of contrast intolerance, 2 mm Gd-enhanced T1-weighted MRI is used for planning, and a noncontrast CT is used for real-time patient tracking during treatment.
- The treating surgeon manually defines/outlines the tumor volumes and critical structures on axial images; the window levels may need to be adjusted to soft tissue versus bone when delineating tumor versus outlining the cochlea, respectively.
- The Cyberknife treatment planning software performs nonisocentric, inverse planning to achieve a highly conformal radiotherapy dose that minimizes dose to the adjacent critical structures.
- The treatment plan is evaluated by the treating surgeon and the radiation oncologist. The number of paths and beams used for each patient varies and is determined by the selected individual treatment plan.
- The patient is placed supine on the treatment couch and the Aquaplast mask is put on the patient and affixed to the treatment couch; alignment is confirmed.
- Each treatment fraction lasts between 30 and 45 minutes.
- Following each radiotherapy fraction, patients are treated with an oral dose of 4 mg of dexamethasone for prophylaxis of acute radiation toxicity.

Hypofractionated treatment radiation dose: Hypofractionated (multisession) SRS procedures for patients with vestibular schwannoma generally use 18 to 21 Gy in 3 daily fractions and up to 20 to 25 Gy in 5 daily fractions.[282,286] In the above protocol from Stanford University, a total of 21 Gy over 3 days (7 Gy per treatment) are delivered, which is equivalent to a 14-Gy single dose session. In patients in whom hearing preservation is attempted and who are at low risk of recurrence, the dose is lowered to 6 Gy fractions, for a total of 18 Gy (equivalent to 11.5-Gy single dose).The treatment dose is prescribed to the 70% to 80% isodose contour line at the periphery of the tumor.[285]

Conventional fractionated stereotactic radiotherapy delivery: Conventional fractionated radiotherapy has been used to treat vestibular schwannomas. The relative reduction in accuracy and conformality compared with radiosurgery methods is the main drawback to this approach. Even with the most precise techniques for external beam radiation therapy setup, such as relocatable headframes (e.g. the Gill-Thomas-Cosman system), the targeting of radiation is less accurate than that which can be achieved with frame-based radiosurgical methods. Radiation can be delivered with photon or proton beams.

Proton-based therapy has the advantage of delivering most of its energy at a fixed point, with minimal entry and exit radiation compared with photon-based radiation delivery systems. This property is advantageous if trying to avoid critical structures in way of treatment beans, such as the cochlea or brainstem. However, the technology is significantly higher in cost, and thus there has been limited use in treatment of vestibular schwannoma.

The following is a typical treatment protocol administered over 6 weeks, 5 days a week (total of 30 treatments):

- To allow repeatable radiation delivery over several weeks, a molded mask and bite block is created for each patient.
- Alternatively, an individual mask system can be immobilized to the patient's skull with two titanium screws under local anesthesia.[287,288]
- Stereotactic localization system is attached to the base frame.
- Patient is placed in treatment position and thin section CT and MRI imaging is performed for treatment planning.
- CT and MRI images are fused, and the target volume and surrounding critical organs at risk are delineated in a 3D manner.
- The planning target volume encompasses the contrast enhancing tumor and a safety margin of 2 mm, accounting for motion and repositioning uncertainty.
- Treatment plan consists of 4 static isocentric, irregularly shaped, noncoplanar fields that are collimated by a multileaf collimator.
- The total dose is prescribed to the reference point; the 90% isodose encompassed the planned target volume.
- Patient is positioned with the stereotactic mask system. Target isocenter coordinates as defined by 3D planning are adjusted with a stereotactic positioning device.
- Radiotherapy is delivered using 6- and 15-MV photons generated by a linear accelerator.
- All fields are irradiated daily, and the total treatment time does not exceed 25 min.

Conventional fractionated stereotactic radiotherapy dose: Typical fractionation schemes in radiation oncology involve delivering 1.8 to 2.0 Gy per fraction with a maximum dose of 45.0 to 57.6 Gy of photon beams. This dose has historically been proven to be safe for adjacent normal tissues and allows for total doses in excess of 50 Gy to be delivered over a course of approximately 6 weeks.[287,289-293]

For proton beam SRT, similar fractionation schemes have been developed with the radiation dose being expressed as cobalt Gray equivalents (CGE). These doses have ranged from 1.8 to 2.0 CGE per fraction delivered in 30 to 33 fractions with a maximum dose of 54 to 60 CGE for patients with useful hearing before treatment.[294-296]

Follow-Up

For SRS, follow-up audiograms and MRI scans are performed at 6-month intervals for the first year, then yearly for the next several years, eventually moving to MRI imaging every 3–4 years if no evidence of tumor growth is detected. The chance for tumor growth is extremely low for stable tumors 4 years post-GKRS (Gamma Knife radiosurgery).[297-299]

Outcomes

Gamma knife stereotactic radiosurgery (single treatment)

Tumor control rates: When discussing tumor control rate after radiosurgery, a distinction should be made between radiologic control (post-treatment imaging demonstrating either no growth or regression of tumor) and clinical control, indicating that no further treatment was needed. Another important concept to keep in mind is that transient tumor swelling (growth) occurs in as many as 80% of cases after GKRS, which peaks around the 6th month after treatment, but may continue for up to 3 years later.[298,300-304] Serial MRI scans aid in differentiating true tumor growth versus associated edema.

Factors that have been associated with subsequent tumor growth of sporadic unilateral vestibular schwannoma include imaging/targeting error, tumor biology, tumor volume and presence of cystic components. Tumor control rates with current lower tumor margin treatment doses of 12–13 Gy have remained the same when compared to earlier treatments with margin doses higher than 13 Gy.[297,305-307]

Table 23.15 summarizes tumor control rates in some representative large retrospective studies conducted over the past 15 years. Currently, for unilateral vestibular schwannomas treated with GKRS, radiologic control ranges from 89% to 96%, whereas clinical control ranges from 91% to 98% (*see* Table 23.15).

Hearing preservation: For most radiation-based treatment outcomes, hearing results are reported on a Gardner-Robertson scale, with serviceable hearing including Gardner-Robertson class 1 and 2 hearing (PTA 50 dB or less, SDS 50% or greater). A recent review of 74 articles and 5825 patients found that overall hearing preservation rate of about 57% can be expected after radiosurgical treatment, and patients treated with 12.5 Gy were more likely to have preserved hearing (59% vs. 53% for >12.5 Gy).[313] Age of the patient was not a significant prognostic factor for hearing preservation rates.

In those patients whose hearing worsens, hearing loss typically develops 3–12 months after radiation treatment, but may continue to deteriorate for up to 10 years post treatment.[309] In a recent study, Carlson et al. found that durable hearing preservation a decade after low-dose SRS for vestibular schwannomas occurs in less than one-fourth of patients.[314]

In general, hearing preservation rates worsen as tumor size increases.[315] Better pretreatment hearing predicts improved hearing outcomes as well.[314,316] One of the most significant factors in hearing preservation after SRS appears to be radiation dose to the cochlea.[316-319] For single session SRS, a maximum cochlear dose <4.0 to 4.2 Gy has been shown to correlate with better hearing preservation (Table 23.16).

Complications

Acute complications: Acute side effects after GKRS are usually mild and self-limited.[323,324] In the immediate period, patients may complain of headaches, nausea, vomiting

Table 23.15: GKRS: tumor control rates

Author (ref)	*Group (year)*	*N (previous microsurgery)*	*Mean tumor volume (range)*	*Marginal dose (range)*	*Mean follow-up (range)*	*Post treatment size*	*Further treatment needed*
Kondziolka et al.[308]	U of Pittsburgh (1998)	162 (55)	2.2 cm (0.8–3.9 cm)	16.6 Gy (12–20 Gy)	(5–10 years)	62% smaller 33% same 6% larger	2%
Prasad et al.[309]	U of Virginia (2000)	153 (56)	2.8 cm^3 (0.02–18.3 cm^3)	13 Gy (9–20 Gy)	4 years (1–10 years)	81% smaller 12% same 6% larger	0.7%
Chung et al.[310]	Taipei (2005)	195 (76)	4.1 cm^3 (0.04–23.1 cm^3)	13 Gy (11–18 Gy)	3 years	58% smaller 35% same 7% larger	3%
Hasegawa et al.[298]	Komaki City (2005)	317 (73)	5.6 cm^3 (0.2–36.7 cm^3)	13.2 Gy (10–18 Gy)	7 years (5–10 years)	61% smaller 31% same 7% larger	9%
Myrseth et al.[311]	Bergen, Norway (2005)	102 (5)	0–0.1 cm 17.5% 1.1–2.0 cm 66% 2.1–3.0 cm 16.5%	12 Gy (10–20 Gy)	6 years (1–14 years)	49% smaller 40% same 11% larger	5%
Chopra et al.[312]	U of Pittsburgh (2007)	216 (0)	1.3 cm^3 (0.08–37.5 cm^3)	13 Gy (12–13 Gy)	6 years	9% larger	1.4%

(GKRS, Gamma Knife radiosurgery).

Table 23.16: GKRS: Hearing preservation

Author (ref)	Group (year)	Patients with pretreatment hearing (N)	Mean follow-up (range)	Hearing preservation
Kondziolka et al.[308]	U of Pittsburgh (1998)	32	>5 years (5–10 years)	47%
Prasad et al.[309]	U of Virginia (2000)	36	4 years (1–10 years)	58%
Andrews et al.[320]	T Jefferson (2001)	69	3 years	33%
Rowe et al.[321]	Sheffield, UK (2003)	49	3 years	76%
Lunsford et al.[297]	U of Pittsburgh (2005)	267	>3 years (3–15 years)	79%
Hasegawa et al.[298]	Komaki City (2005)	74	7 years (5–10 years)	68%
Myrseth et al.[311]	Bergen, Norway (2005)	31	6 years (1–14 years)	43%
Baschnagel et al.[322]	William Beaumont, MI (2013)	40	3 years (1–5 years)	74%
Carlson et al.[314]	Mayo Clinic (2013)	44	3 years 5 years 10 years	55% 48% 23%

(GKRS, Gamma Knife radiosurgery).

and fatigue. Acute facial paralysis (occurring within the first week after treatment) has also been reported.[325-328] Acute paralysis resolved in almost all cases to HB grade1 or 2 within 6 months to 2 years after onset. Oral or intravenous steroids were given in each case. A case of permanent profound SNHL secondary to acute intracochlear hemorrhage has also been reported.[325]

Facial paralysis and hemifacial spasm: Development of a new facial nerve neuropathy is rare after GKRS with current 12–13-Gy marginal doses. Facial weakness typically occurs within the first year of treatment. Even for those patients who develop a temporary facial paralysis, the symptom usually resolves after 6 months to a year (Table 23.17). Similarly, hemifacial spasm occurs in rare cases and typically develops between 1 and 2 years after treatment.[300,304] Pollock et al. have postulated that hemifacial spasm is the result of tumor expansion with irritation of the facial nerve or a delayed vascular insult; it improves with carbamazepine.[304,329]

Trigeminal neuralgia/neuropathy: In a recent meta-analysis, Sughrue et al. have found that 2.4% of patients develop a non CN7 or CN8 CN neuropathy after GKRS, the overwhelming majority of which is involvement of the trigeminal nerve (paresthesia or facial tingling).[332] They also found that patients receiving >13 Gy marginal dose radiation were significantly more likely to develop trigeminal nerve neuropathy than those receiving a dose <13 Gy. Flickinger et al. have found that the risk of trigeminal neuropathy increases with increasing tumor volume.[305] Similar to facial nerve dysfunction, trigeminal symptoms have been reported to develop between 5 and 48 months post-treatment.[305,309]

Vestibular symptoms: An increase in pretreatment vestibular symptoms after Gamma Knife surgery varies widely in the current literature, and where reported, occurs from 13% to 37% (Table 23.17). Pollock et al. investigated the progression of the symptom of vertigo after treatment and found a steady decline from 13% at the 3-month mark to 3% at last follow-up.[304] In the meta-analysis conducted by Sughrue et al., out of 2,383 patients who received marginal radiation doses >13 Gy, 1.1% reported new vertigo or balance disturbance, which was significantly less for 3,248 patients who received radiation doses of <13 Gy (1.8%).[332]

Hydrocephalus: After GKRS, hydrocephalus is believed the result of tumor necrosis, with proteinaceous debris blocking CSF flow. The development of hydrocephalus is more common after treatment of larger (>25 mm diameter) tumors, and the median time to development of hydrocephalus is 1 year.[333] The rates of post-treatment hydrocephalus are relatively low, and occur in <4% of cases (*see* Table 23.17). In the meta-analysis by Sughrue et al., the mean rate of post-GKRS hydrocephalus was 0.85%,

Table 23.17: Adverse effects of GKRS

Author (ref)	*Group (year)*	*Dose (N)*	*CN 7 symptoms*	*Vestibular symptoms*	*CN 5 symptoms*	*Hydrocephalus*
Regis et al.[300]	Marseille, France (2002)	12–14 Gy (104)	2% temp 0% perm 3% spasm	37% vertigo 26% imbalance	4%	3%
Flickinger et al.[305]	U of Pittsburgh (2004)	12–13 Gy (313)	0%	NR	2.5%	NR
Myrseth et al.[311]	Bergen, Norway (2005)	10–12 Gy (103)	5%	NR	NR	4%
Rowe et al.[321]	Sheffield, UK (2003)	13–15 Gy (232)	4.5% temp 1% perm 1.3% spasm	13% nonspec	8%	1.2%
Chung et al.[310]	Taipei, Taiwan (2005)	11–18 Gy (195)	1% temp	NR	1%	2%
Hempel et al.[330]	Munich, Germany (2006)	10–14.5 Gy (123)	0%	13.3% dizziness	5.8%	2.4%
Pollock[304]	Mayo Clinic (2006)	12.2 Gy, mean (82)	0%	16% (3 months) 7% (1 year) 3% (>1 year)	1.2%	4%
Murphy et al.[331]	Cleveland Clinic (2011)	12–13 Gy, (117)	6% temp 3% perm	4% vertigo 18% imbalance	1%	1%

(GKRS, Gamma Knife radiosurgery).

three-quarters of which necessitated intervention with a VP shunt.[332] The development of hydrocephalus was not reduced with lower radiation doses.

Special Considerations: Large and Cystic Tumors

For tumors >3 cm in diameter, GKRS is not a recommended treatment modality. Significant tumor-associated edema occurs almost invariably for tumors that are >3 cm, which can cause immediate and severe headaches, vomiting and dizziness.[334] Brainstem compression may develop, leading to ataxia and obstructive hydrocephalus. Another reason why large tumors should not be irradiated primarily is that tumor control rates are decreased even with higher doses.

Studies of SRS of large tumors have had variable outcomes and have consequently recommended varied cutoff values to define "large" vestibular schwannomas. Hasegawa et al. have found that for tumors >15 cm^3 (equivalent to >3 cm in diameter) 10-year progression free survival was 57%, compared to 95% for tumors <15 cm^3.[298] Link et al. have found in their 34 patient series with tumors >2.7 cm an 18% failure rate at 5 years, and an incidence of 14% of facial nerve impairment, both significantly higher than for smaller tumors.[280] Yang et al. studied 65 patients with tumors between 3 and 4 cm in size.[335] They report remarkably good results, with a 3% failure rate (necessitating surgery), 82% patients retaining good hearing at 2 years of follow-up, 2% of patients developing new facial nerve symptoms, 6% of patients with trigeminal complaints and 5% patients with hydrocephalus necessitating shunt placement. Their conclusion is that most vestibular schwannomas with a maximum diameter <4 cm and without significant mass effect can be managed satisfactorily with GKRS.

Cystic vestibular schwannomas may represent a unique subtype of tumor. Relative to solid vestibular schwannoma, vestibular schwannoma with intratumoral cysts is associated more commonly with sudden expansion and associated morbidity.[336,337] In a study by Pendl et al. six out of 74 patients with cystic tumors demonstrated post-treatment enlargement (8%), and half of those required a subsequent microsurgical intervention.[338] Delsanti et al. have also shown a 6.4% treatment failure rate in their series of 54 cystic vestibular schwannomas, 3 times higher than for solid tumors.[339] However, Hasegawa et al. have not found such correlations.[303] While presence of cystic components is not an absolute contraindication to GKRS, patients should be advised about potentially increased risk of failed primary treatment and acute worsening of symptoms.

Radiation Treatment after Surgery

Radiation treatment after primary microsurgical removal of vestibular schwannomas can be considered as adjunctive, planned treatment in cases of STGR or NTGR, or in cases

Table 23.18: Outcomes after microsurgical treatment followed by radiation

Author (ref)	*Group (year)*	*Residual/recurrent (N)*	*Median time after surgery*	*New CN symptoms*	*Revision surgery needed*
Pollock et al.[342]	Mayo Clinic (1998)	78 52/26	4.8 years	23% CN7 10% CN5	8%
Unger et al.[343]	Graz, Austria (2002)	50 34/16	3.3 years	10% CN7 8% CN5	4%
Yang et al.[334]	Goyang, ROK (2008)	61 61/0	0.5 years	0% CN7 0% CN5	2%
Pollock and Link[341]	Mayo Clinic (2008)	55 22/33	5 years	10% CN7 4% CN5	6%
van de Langenberg et al.[344]	Maastricht, the Netherlands (2011)	50 50/0	0.7 years	6% CN7 2% CN5	8%

(CN, cranial nerve).

where there is unplanned recurrence or regrowth of tumor. In fact, documented tumor growth after surgical treatment is the indication for undergoing GKRS in up to 86% of patients.[340,341] Table 23.18 summarizes the outcomes of radiosurgery after initial microsurgical treatment for both residual (planned) and recurrent (unplanned) tumors; in newer studies, CN, and treatment failures are comparable to those encountered when radiosurgery is the primary treatment modality.

Repeated Radiation Therapy

A percentage of patients with vestibular schwannoma who undergo radiation-based vestibular schwannoma treatment will experience tumor enlargement requiring further therapy. To date, the experience with repeating vestibular schwannoma SRS is limited, with each center only reporting a small number of cases and short follow-up after repeated SRS. Using tumor margin doses similar to the initial treatment (11–13 Gy), control rates have ranged from 90% to 100%. The morbidity of repeating SRS has been low, with most patients already deaf before a second SRS and new facial weakness occurring in <10%.[345,346]

Cyberknife Radiosurgery

With the arrival of the Cyberknife in 1996, fractionating radiation treatments has become more practical. Distributing radiation over several rather than one treatment allows for a reduction of treatment-related morbidity without a decrease in tumor control. In a study from Stanford, 61 patients underwent 3 consecutive daily treatments of 7 Gy (equivalent of a one-time 14 Gy dose).[285] In this study, no patients developed facial palsy or trigeminal symptoms, and two patients (3%) developed transient facial twitching. Of the 35 patients who had GR hearing 1–2, 74% maintained hearing in the same class at last follow-up. One patient (2%) required subsequent microsurgical treatment for tumor enlargement.

Fractionated Stereotactic Radiotherapy

Fractionated Stereotactic Radiotherapy (FSRT) is defined as radiation treatment that is longer than 3 days (3 treatments). Advocates of dose fractionation have posited that SRT may provide better hearing outcomes than single-fraction SRS. However, some of the reports of SRT have relied on patients' subjective hearing function rather than audiometric data.[290,292] A recent review of SRT outcomes found that hearing preservation rates for conventional and hypofractionated schemes are no better than what has been reported for single-session SRS.[291,313] In studies on SRT administered over 25–30 fractions over 5–6 weeks, new facial nerve weakness varied from 0% to 2%; useful hearing was maintained in 56–84% cases and tumor failure rate occurred in 2–4% cases in long-term (>5 years) follow-up.[290-293] Proton beam radiotherapy seems to have similar tumor control and facial nerve outcomes, with hearing preservation rates reported from 31% to 42%.[294-296]

Malignant Transformation

Radiation therapy is being utilized with increasing frequency in treatment of vestibular schwannomas. As the experience with SRS grows, long-term serious complications such as malignant transformation of these benign tumors have only begun to emerge. The number of reports of radiation-induced malignant transformation is nearing 20 cases, albeit not all have been biopsy-proven benign before treatment.[347,348] The most common malignant pathology is GBM and malignant peripheral nerve sheath tumors, although sarcomas have also been diagnosed.[349] There appears to be a predilection for radiation-induced malignant transformation in NF2 patients.[347,350]

In all cases, the malignancies carry a grave prognosis; they are frequently discovered >5 years after radiation treatment, and even a case of 19-year latency has been reported.[351] It is generally advocated that this therapeutic modality should be used with caution in NF2 cases and young patients. The clinician should monitor irradiated patients for life, as the secondary malignancy may appear many years after treatment.

Radiation Treatment Compared to Microsurgical Treatment

With advancements in radiation treatment technology and availability of long-term follow-up, the direct outcome comparison between two active management strategies, microsurgery and radiation, is finally possible. The debate between the superiority of one treatment over another is most relevant for small- and medium-sized tumors, as large tumors (>3 cm) are still reserved for surgical management. Planned combined treatment, especially of larger tumors, with partial resection followed by definitive radiation has also entered the stage as a viable and even preferred management option for vestibular schwannomas.

When comparing treatment outcomes, the clinician should be cautious to take note of the specific radiation dose and administration schedule utilized, as older studies that reported higher radiation-related morbidity were based on high radiation doses.[352] In a recent review of developments over the past decade in management of vestibular schwannoma, Theodosopoulos et al. have redefined the treatment algorithm.[76] In their review, at present, the best tumor control rates are achieved with stereotactic radiosurgery, the best hearing preservation rates with limited dose fractionated radiation therapy and the best cytoreductive therapy with microsurgery. Although microsurgery, even in the best hands, has worse facial nerve and hearing outcomes than current radiation-based treatments, it remains the preferred treatment for lesions causing mass effect.

At present, the best quality of evidence (prospective cohort studies and case-control series) show superior outcomes for vestibular schwannoma patients having stereotactic radiosurgery compared to surgical resection, allowing a grade B recommendation for this approach.[353] Pollock et al. have thus concluded that unless long-term follow-up shows frequent tumor progression at currently used radiation doses, radiosurgery should be considered the best management strategy for the majority of vestibular schwannoma patients.

REHABILITATION

Facial Nerve Deficit Management and Rehabilitation

Facial nerve deficits affect the QOL of the patient, and much has been written on the rehabilitative options. These include immediate repair in cases where the nerve was transected (either deliberately when inseparable from tumor or inadvertently) with either end-to-end anastomosis, cable graft from sural or greater auricular nerves, or even a jump graft from the hypoglossal nerve to the distal unaffected facial nerve. Most vestibular schwannomas do not require facial nerve resection, and thus most injuries are from mechanical stretch or vascular compromise to the nerve, but can also occur secondary to heat injury from either drilling or the microscope light.[354] The best strategies in avoiding these intraoperative injuries were discussed in the previous section. The speed of recovery after facial nerve injury generally falls under two categories—return of function within 2 months for less severe injuries or 8–15 months for more severe injuries (those where remyelination needs to occur). The sooner recovery is seen, the better the overall prognosis. In more severe injuries with delayed recovery, some degree of synkinesis is expected.

After tumor resection, the surgeon is sometimes faced with a dilemma when presented with an anatomically intact but electrically silent nerve (nerve that does not stimulate at brainstem level). Carlson et al. have found that in this specific population, the most likely outcome was a HB3 facial nerve functioning that recovers at around 9 months postoperatively.[355] They have concluded that current electroprognostic testing is not reliable in predicting poor facial function outcomes and thus advocate that facial nerve repair should not be pursued at time of surgery.

Delayed facial nerve paralysis is not uncommon after microsurgical resection of vestibular schwannomas. Even in the case when no facial nerve deficits were noted initially, the ipsilateral facial muscle function may deteriorate within the next 72 hours and even up to 2 weeks after surgery. Etiologies proposed for delayed facial palsy include ischemic injury from postoperative edema within the labyrinthine segment of the nerve or from herpes virus reactivation.[356,357] Prophylactic or postoperative antiviral acyclovir treatment has been used for delayed facial palsy as well as nimodipine in cases where ischemia is suspected. Strauss et al. have found a significantly higher rate of complete facial function recovery in patients treated with nimodipine postoperatively.[358] Perioperative and postoperative corticosteroids are almost routinely used, and theoretically assist with decreasing inflammatory injury to the facial nerve, although no studies have been done to support or dismiss their efficacy.

In cases of anatomically intact nerve but compromised function, great care must be taken, as always, to prevent ipsilateral corneal injury from exposure. When the expected recovery time is long (>6 mos) or likely to not be complete, and the patient is at risk of corneal injury, a gold weight or lid tightening procedures should be considered. If recovery is not full, but the patient has some mimetic function, facial nerve exercises are a part of the rehabilitative program. Electrodiagnostic tests can aid with prognosis.

In most cases of questionable or incomplete recovery, patients should be referred to facial plastic surgeons who specialize in facial nerve and facial reanimation. Botox injections to the contralateral side may aid in relaxing the contralateral face and improving symmetry. Hypoglossal to facial nerve grafts may be considered after 18 months to 2 years of loss of activity, as well as static procedures or microvascular grafts in cases of severe asymmetry or disability.

Auditory Rehabilitation

Hearing loss is the most frequent presenting symptom of vestibular schwannomas. It is also a risk of all three management approaches: watchful waiting, microsurgery and radiation treatment. It is likely that the patient will at some point in time be faced with considering rehabilitative options of single-sided deafness.

Hearing Aids and Options for Single-Sided Deafness

Options are as with any other cause of single-sided deafness, including a CROS aid, bone-anchored hearing device (BAHA or SoundBite), preferential positioning, and raised awareness for noise and toxin protection for the uninvolved ear. While cochlear implants (CIs) are now playing a role in other patients with SSD, in the context of vestibular schwannomas, they are considered only for NF2 patients with bilateral tumors and intact nerves (such as after radiation). A CI, however, may play a role in patients who have a vestibular schwannoma in the only hearing ear, and should be considered in the nontumor ear side, and placed prior to vestibular schwannoma intervention. This should be carefully planned, as current CIs require removal of the magnet to be compatible with MRI scans.

ABIs

While the cochlear nerve is usually affected with vestibular schwannoma, the 8th nerve root entry zone and the cochlear ganglia are not. This leaves an option for an auditory brainstem implant (ABI), which processes an auditory signal received from the environment with a microphone and converts it to an electric stimulus directly on the brainstem. The ABI has been used and approved in cases of NF2 where patients have bilateral tumors and are at risk of bilateral deafness; it is further discussed in the NF2 section below. ABI has not been used in cases of patients with tumors in the only hearing ear, as CIs are still an option in the contralateral ear, and currently patients with CIs continue to outperform patients with ABIs.

Vestibular Rehabilitation

Dizziness can have a significant impact on the patient's QOL. Vestibular symptoms may occur as a part of the natural progression of tumor growth, and patients should be appropriately counseled when opting for the wait and scan strategy. They are also common in patients who undergo radiation treatment. With respect to surgical resection, patients usually experience acute vertigo after a TLAB approach, which subsides with time as compensation with the contralateral vestibular system occurs. Most advocate for a complete transection of the vestibular nerves during tumor removal in RSIG and MCF approaches. However, Mann et al. have found that preserving the uninvolved division of the vestibular nerve accelerates vestibular compensation in the early postoperative period; this effect was not significant 6 months after surgery.[38] In a study by Feigl et al., 43.5% of patients complained of dizziness prior to tumor removal and 77.2% experienced dizziness after RSIG approach to tumor resection.[233] Their study shows that dizziness has a negative effect on the course of recovery, and they advocate for administration of antiemetics preoperatively in addition to widely utilized postoperative therapies.

Preoperative status of the contralateral vestibular system affects the time and extent of compensation after surgical resection of tumor as well as after radiation treatment. Presence of contralateral Meniere disease, labyrinthitis, or vestibular neuritis will likely result in poorer outcomes and longer recovery time. For symptomatic management, vestibular rehabilitative therapy plays an important role in patients with vestibular schwannomas, either as a part of postoperative, postradiation or wait-and-scan management strategy. Another option in patients with severe symptoms is ablation of the ipsilateral vestibular system with intratympanic gentamicin, even at the expense of hearing. In postradiation cases, or cases where the transection of vestibular nerves was not complete and even in patients who opt to not undergo tumor removal, an ipsilateral labyrinthectomy can be considered.

NF2-ASSOCIATED VESTIBULAR SCHWANNOMAS

Background

Approximately 5% of patients who have a vestibular schwannoma have Neurofibromatosis 2 (NF2). NF2 vestibular schwannomas are histologically distinct from sporadic vestibular schwannomas.[359]

NF2 is a rare autosomal dominant syndrome characterized by bilateral vestibular schwannomas, multiple meningiomas, CN and spinal tumors, and eye abnormalities. The incidence is estimated to be 1 in 33,000 to 1 in 87,000 live births.[360,361] NF2 is distinctly genetically and clinically separate from NF1; NF1 has been localized to chromosome 17 and NF2 to chromosome 22. NF1 is a multisystem disorder in which some features may be present at birth and others are age-related manifestations (among them café au lait spots, optic gliomas, neurofibromas, iris hamartomas, etc.). NF1 and NF2 can be distinguished by a careful examination and detailed history of the patient's symptoms.

The most common presenting symptom of a patient with NF2 is a neurologic complaint (found in 17.5% patients), followed by an appearance of a skin tumor (11.7% patients) and vision loss (10.7%); up to 10.7% of patients are asymptomatic at time of diagnosis.[362] Despite these trends, there is significant heterogeneity in presentation. While some patients may have a very mild form with small vestibular schwannomas manifesting later in life, in others the disease can be aggressive, disseminated and locally invasive, and may require a multispecialist team approach.

Management

The treatment options for NF2 patients who have bilateral vestibular schwannomas depend on the patient's clinical presentation and tumor size. Loss of useful hearing, the status of other intracranial tumors, presence of brainstem compression, or hydrocephalus must all be considered when discussing the management options.

Watchful Waiting

Watchful waiting with serial imaging is the most common management option utilized in patients with NF2, be it in the setting of a small tumor in the only-hearing ear or of bilateral tumors too large for hearing preservation attempts. As with sporadic vestibular schwannomas, an MRI is performed 6 months after the diagnosis and then annually. Microsurgical removal should be considered if there is a change in clinical status (brainstem compression, progression to unserviceable hearing) or if the tumor significantly enlarges. There have even been reports of patients in whom the contralateral tumor decreased in size after surgical removal of the opposite-side schwannoma.[363]

Medical Management

Medical management of NF2-associated vestibular schwannoma is still early in development. Therapy in the form of antibodies targeted against VEGF (bevacizumab) may hold some promise not only in the reduction in size of vestibular schwannomas but also in improvement in hearing.[364,365] Other clinical trials are investigating lapatinib and rapamycin to stop the growth of NF2 vestibular schwannomas.[366] Erlotinib held initial promise in a case report but failed to show benefit in a larger study, and in fact many patients suffered side effects.[367,368] Although early results of drug therapies have been promising, long-term studies are still needed to demonstrate benefit.

Surgical Management

Hearing preservation: Hearing preservation in patients with NF2-associated vestibular schwannoma is a reasonable option for those patients who have bilateral tumors smaller than 2 cm and good hearing (class A or B). The tumor that should be resected first is on the side of the worse hearing ear or if it is the larger of the two. If hearing preservation is successful, then the contralateral tumor may be addressed 6 months later. Hearing preservation results in patients with NF2 seem to be worse compared to patients who have unilateral sporadic tumors.[251] In one series, 67% of patients qualified for hearing preservation.[369] The MCF approach offers the best results in hearing preservation for patients with NF2-associated vestibular schwannomas, with the highest preservation rates reaching 50%.[370,371] Therefore, microsurgical removal via the MCF approach should be offered to patients who qualify, including children, and potentially preserve hearing in both ears.

In patients with NF2, the retrosigmoid approach to vestibular schwannoma removal is particularly risky for hearing preservation, as the cochlear fibers are dispersed throughout the tumor, unlike what is typically seen in unilateral vestibular schwannomas. This anatomical relationship is likely the reason why even partial tumor removal of NF2-associated schwannomas risks hearing.[366]

Prophylactic MCF and IAC decompression: In patients whose tumors are observed and suffer some progression of hearing loss, a decompression of the IAC via the MCF approach can be considered as a prophylactic measure against complete hearing deficit. Not only can stabilization of current level of hearing occur, but improvement in hearing has been documented as well.[372] For this specific indication, the tumor itself is not removed as this may increase the risk of hearing loss. In a review of 49 patients who underwent IAC decompression via a MCF craniotomy, hearing preservation was successful in 90% in the immediate postoperative period and approximately 75% 1 year later. While the advantage may be only an average of an extra 2 years of hearing, some patients continue to have auditory function up to 10 years later.[372]

Nonhearing preservation: Most patients with NF2 vestibular schwannoma present with tumors that are too large to be considered for hearing preservation. Therefore, the most common microsurgical removal is achieved with the TLAB or RSIG approach. If there is brainstem compression, even in cases where patients still have some hearing, the TLAB or RSIG craniotomy should be performed as they allow safest and complete tumor removal. Of the two, the TLAB approach is preferred as the RSIG may not allow for dissection of the most lateral aspect of the IAC, and thus carries a slightly higher risk of recurrence.

Radiation treatment: From the reported results on GKRS for NF2-associated vestibular schwannoma, it appears that GKRS is less effective in treating tumors secondary to NF2 compared to sporadic cases.[279,280, 373-375] In the largest study of 122 tumors, the average marginal dose was 15 Gy, higher than what is used for unilateral cases, and clinical tumor control rate was 79% at 4 years of follow-up.[375] Twenty percent of the tumors were treated with one or more prior microsurgical resections. The majority of patients were treated for documented tumor growth; other indications for GKRS in this population included a rapid deterioration in hearing, tumor near 3 cm in size, or planned adjuvant therapy for significant residual tumor after microsurgery. The serviceable hearing preservation rate in those patients who qualified was 22% at 4 years of follow-up, lower than the results seen with sporadic tumors. Mathieu et al. found in their series hearing preservation rates of 73%, 59% and 48% at 1-, 2- and 5-year follow-up, respectively, indicating that the radiation effects continue long after radiation treatment.[279] Patients and their families should be counseled appropriately with respect to their expectations.

An important and concerning consideration in this population is that radiation of NF2-associated vestibular schwannoma may lead to malignant tumor transformation, especially because of an already defective tumor suppressor gene.[376] Of the 14 cases reported with histologically verified intracranial malignancy arising in a stereotactically irradiated field, four were patients with NF2.[377] At least 5 of 106 patients with NF2 who underwent radiotherapy developed radiation-induced malignancies, and nearly 50% of reports of malignant degeneration occur in the context of NF2.[376,378]

Auditory rehabilitation: Auditory rehabilitation in patients with NF2 leaves two basic options: (1) for patients with smaller tumors (<2 cm) who can undergo SRS and preserve an anatomically intact cochlear nerve, an ipsilateral CI may be subsequently implanted; (2) for patients with larger tumors (>2.5 cm), an ABI can be placed at the time of microsurgical resection (TLAB or RSIG approach).[280,379,380]

Prior to placing a CI, electrical promontory stimulation can help determine the presence and functionality of the cochlear nerve. In the group of 10 patients with NF2-associated tumors who underwent SRS, hearing outcomes after CIs were favorable.[381]

In the United States, the ABI, a device intended to stimulate the dorsal cochlear nucleus at the brainstem, is FDA-approved for use in individuals with NF2 older than 2 years of age. The ABI can be placed with the first tumor removal as a "sleeper" even when useful hearing may still be present on the contralateral ear, and then be activated at a later date. With progression of contralateral disease, a second ABI can be placed at removal of the second tumor, offering the advantage of bilateral ABIs. Most patients with NF2-associated tumors have achieved enhanced communication skills with ABIs.

An important consideration in patients with NF2 is the need for frequent surveillance MRIs, and thus the magnet should be removed from the receiver stimulator when implanting either CI or ABI.

REFERENCES

1. Ramsden RT. The bloody angle: 100 years of acoustic neuroma surgery. J R Soc Med. 1995;88(8):464-8.
2. Ramsden RT. A brilliant surgical result, the first recorded: Annandale's case, 3 May 1895. J Laryngol Otol. 1995;109(5): 369-73.
3. Cushing H. Intracranial Tumours: Notes Upon a Series of Two Thousand Verified Cases with Surgical-Mortality Percentages Pertaining Thereto. Balliere: Tindall & Cox n.d. ix, 150 p.
4. Pearce JM. Walter Edward Dandy (1886-1946). J Med Biogr. 2006;14(3):127-8.
5. House WF. Surgical exposure of the internal auditory canal and its contents through the middle, cranial fossa. Laryngoscope. 1961;71:1363-85.
6. House WF. Transtemporal bone microsurgical removal of acoustic neuromas. Evolution of transtemporal bone removal of acoustic tumors. Arch Otolaryngol. 1964;80: 731-42.
7. House WF. The acoustic neuroma saga. J Laryngol Otol. 1995;109(5):367-8.
8. Jackler RK, Brackmann DE. Neurotology, 2nd edition. Philadelphia, PA: Mosby; 2005. xxiii, 1411p.
9. Tos M, et al. What is the real incidence of vestibular schwannoma? Arch Otolaryngol Head Neck Surg. 2004;130(2): 216-20.
10. Howitz MF, et al. Incidence of vestibular schwannoma in Denmark, 1977-1995. Am J Otol. 2000;21(5):690-4.
11. Gudmundsson TH, Petersen H. Acoustic neuroma in Iceland for 30 years (1979-2009). Laeknabladid. 2013;99(6): 289-92.
12. Frohlich AM, Sutherland GR. Epidemiology and clinical features of vestibular schwannoma in Manitoba, Canada. Can J Neurol Sci. 1993;20(2):126-30.
13. Barker DJ, Weller RO, Garfield JS. Epidemiology of primary tumours of the brain and spinal cord: a regional survey in southern England. J Neurol Neurosurg Psychiatry. 1976; 39(3):290-6.
14. Nestor JJ, et al. The incidence of acoustic neuromas. Arch Otolaryngol Head Neck Surg. 1988;114(6):680.
15. Evans DG, et al. Incidence of vestibular schwannoma and neurofibromatosis 2 in the North West of England over a 10-year period: higher incidence than previously thought. Otol Neurotol. 2005;26(1):93-7.
16. Stangerup SE, et al. True incidence of vestibular schwannoma? Neurosurgery. 2010;67(5):1335-40; discussion 1340.
17. Lin D, et al. The prevalence of "incidental" acoustic neuroma. Arch Otolaryngol Head Neck Surg. 2005;131(3): 241-4.
18. Thomsen J, Jorgensen MB. Undiagnosed acoustic neurinomas. A presentation of 4 cases. Arch Klin Exp Ohren Nasen Kehlkopfheilkd. 1973;204(3):175-82.
19. Selesnick SH, Jackler RK. Atypical hearing loss in acoustic neuroma patients. Laryngoscope. 1993;103(4 Pt 1):437-41.
20. Glasscock ME, 3rd, Hart MJ, Vrabec JT. Management of bilateral acoustic neuroma. Otolaryngol Clin North Am. 1992;25(2):449-69.
21. Clemis JD, et al. Relative frequency of inferior vestibular schwannoma. Arch Otolaryngol Head Neck Surg. 1986;112 (2):190-4.
22. Komatsuzaki A, Tsunoda A. Nerve origin of the acoustic neuroma. J Laryngol Otol. 2001;115(5):376-9.
23. Xenellis JE, Linthicum Jr. FH. On the myth of the glial/ schwann junction (Obersteiner-Redlich zone): origin of vestibular nerve schwannomas. Otol Neurotol. 2003;24(1):1.
24. Tallan EM, et al. Does the distribution of Schwann cells correlate with the observed occurrence of acoustic neuromas? Am J Otol. 1993;14(2):131-4.
25. Kitamura K, Sugimoto M. Histological structures of bilateral acoustic tumors. Adv Otorhinolaryngol. 1988;42:172-6.
26. Nager GT. Acoustic neurinomas. Pathology and differential diagnosis. Arch Otolaryngol. 1969;89(2):252-79.
27. Lanser MJ, Sussman SA, Frazer K. Epidemiology, pathogenesis, and genetics of acoustic tumors. Otolaryngol Clin North Am. 1992;25(3):499-520.
28. Wolff RK, et al. Analysis of chromosome 22 deletions in neurofibromatosis type 2-related tumors. Am J Hum Genet. 1992;51(3):478-85.
29. Carroll RS, Zhang JP, Black PM. Hormone receptors in vestibular schwannomas. Acta Neurochir (Wien). 1997;139 (3):188-92; discussion 193.
30. Beatty CW, et al. Acoustic schwannoma and pregnancy: a DNA flow cytometric, steroid hormone receptor, and proliferation marker study. Laryngoscope. 1995;105(7 Pt 1): 693-700.
31. Filipo R, et al. Expression of steroid receptors in acoustic neuroma. Clin Otolaryngol Allied Sci. 1995;20(5):413-7.
32. Han YY, et al. Are frequent dental x-ray examinations associated with increased risk of vestibular schwannoma? J Neurosurg. 2012;117 Suppl:78-83.
33. Corona AP, et al. Risk factors associated with vestibular nerve schwannomas. Otol Neurotol. 2012;33(3):459-65.
34. Muscat JE, et al. Handheld cellular telephones and risk of acoustic neuroma. Neurology. 2002;58(8):1304-6.
35. Matthies C, Samii M. Management of 1000 vestibular schwannomas (acoustic neuromas): clinical presentation. Neurosurgery. 1997;40(1):1-9; discussion 9-10.
36. Berg HM, et al. Acoustic neuroma presenting as sudden hearing loss with recovery. Otolaryngol Head Neck Surg. 1986;94(1):15-22.
37. Fahy C, Nikolopoulos TP, O'Donoghue GM. Acoustic neuroma surgery and tinnitus. Eur Arch Otorhinolaryngol. 2002;259(6):299-301.
38. Mann WJ, Maurer J Marangos N. Neural conservation in skull base surgery. Otolaryngol Clin North Am. 2002;35(2): 411-24, ix.
39. Odabasi AO, Buchman CA, Morcos JJ. Tumor-associated hemorrhage in patients with acoustic neuroma. Am J Otol. 2000;21(5):706-11.
40. Tos M, Thomsen J. Acoustic Neuroma: Proceedings of the First International Conference on Acoustic Neuroma, Copenhagen, Denmark , August 25-29, 1991: Kugler Publications; 1992.
41. Cushing H. Tumors of the nervus acusticus and the syndrome of the cerebellopontile angle. Philadelphia: Saunders; 1917. viii, 296p.

42. Mathew GD, et al. Symptoms, findings, and methods of diagnosis in patients with acoustic neuroma. Laryngoscope. 1978;88(12):1893-903, 1921.
43. Selesnick SH, Jackler RK, Pitts LW. The changing clinical presentation of acoustic tumors in the MRI era. Laryngoscope. 1993;103(4 Pt 1):431-6.
44. Harun A, et al. Sex and age associations with vestibular schwannoma size and presenting symptoms. Otol Neurotol. 2012;33(9):1604-10.
45. Daniels RL, et al. Causes of unilateral sensorineural hearing loss screened by high-resolution fast spin echo magnetic resonance imaging: review of 1,070 consecutive cases. Am J Otol. 2000;21(2):173-80.
46. Baker R, et al. Should patients with asymmetrical noise-induced hearing loss be screened for vestibular schwannomas? Clin Otolaryngol Allied Sci. 2003;28(4):346-51.
47. Cueva RA. Auditory brainstem response versus magnetic resonance imaging for the evaluation of asymmetric sensorineural hearing loss. Laryngoscope. 2004;114(10):1686-92.
48. Suzuki M, et al. Prevalence of acoustic neuroma associated with each configuration of pure tone audiogram in patients with asymmetric sensorineural hearing loss. Ann Otol Rhinol Laryngol. 2010;119(9):615-8.
49. Welling DB, et al. Acoustic neuroma: a cost-effective approach. Otolaryngol Head Neck Surg. 1990;103(3):364-70.
50. Mangham CA. Hearing threshold difference between ears and risk of acoustic tumor. Otolaryngol Head Neck Surg. 1991;105(6):814-7.
51. Ruckenstein MJ. et al. A prospective study of ABR and MRI in the screening for vestibular schwannomas. Am J Otol. 1996;17(2):317-20.
52. Robinette MS, et al. Auditory brainstem response and magnetic resonance imaging for acoustic neuromas: costs by prevalence. Arch Otolaryngol Head Neck Surg. 2000;126(8):963-6.
53. Obholzer RJ, Rea PA, Harcourt JP. Magnetic resonance imaging screening for vestibular schwannoma: analysis of published protocols. J Laryngol Otol. 2004;118(5):329-32.
54. Pensak ML, et al. Sudden hearing loss and cerebellopontine angle tumors. Laryngoscope. 1985;95(10):1188-93.
55. Yanagihara N, Asai M. Sudden hearing loss induced by acoustic neuroma: significance of small tumors. Laryngoscope. 1993;103(3):308-11.
56. Margolis RH, Saly GL. Asymmetric hearing loss: definition, validation, and prevalence. Otol Neurotol. 2008;29(4):422-31.
57. Wilson DF, et al. The sensitivity of auditory brainstem response testing in small acoustic neuromas. Laryngoscope. 1992;102(9):961-4.
58. Don M, Kwong B, Tanaka C. Interaural stacked auditory brainstem response measures for detecting small unilateral acoustic tumors. Audiol Neurootol. 2012;17(1):54-68.
59. Filipo R, et al. Role of transient-evoked otoacoustic emissions for hearing preservation in acoustic neuroma surgery. Am J Otol. 1997;18(6):746-9.
60. Telischi F. An objective method of analyzing cochlear versus noncochlear patterns of distortion-product otoacoustic emissions in patients with acoustic neuromas. Laryngoscope. 2000;110(4):553-62.
61. Brackmann DE, et al. Prognostic factors for hearing preservation in vestibular schwannoma surgery. Am J Otol. 2000;21(3):417-24.
62. Odabasi AO, et al. Effect of acoustic tumor extension into the internal auditory canal on distortion-product otoacoustic emissions. Ann Otol Rhinol Laryngol. 2002;111(10):912-5.
63. Benitez JT, Arsenault MD. Brainstem auditory evoked response sensitivity: comparison with other neurologic tests in the detection of retrocochlear lesions. ORL J Otorhinolaryngol Relat Spec. 1989;51(6):332-8.
64. Haapaniemi JJ, et al. Audiovestibular findings and location of an acoustic neuroma. Eur Arch Otorhinolaryngol. 2000;257(5):237-41.
65. Linthicum FH, Jr, et al. Infrared/video ENG recording of eye movements to evaluate the inferior vestibular nerve using the minimal caloric test. Otolaryngol Head Neck Surg. 1988;98(3):207-10.
66. Rompaey VV, et al. Fundus obliteration and facial nerve outcome in vestibular schwannoma surgery. Skull Base. 2011;21(2):99-102.
67. Zealley IA, et al. MRI screening for acoustic neuroma: a comparison of fast spin echo and contrast enhanced imaging in 1233 patients. Br J Radiol. 2000;73(867):242-7.
68. Annesley-Williams DJ, et al. Magnetic resonance imaging in the investigation of sensorineural hearing loss: is contrast enhancement still necessary? J Laryngol Otol. 2001;115(1):14-21.
69. Wilson YL, et al. Cost analysis of asymmetric sensorineural hearing loss investigations. Laryngoscope. 2010;120(9):1832-6.
70. Carrier DA, Arriaga MA. Cost-effective evaluation of asymmetric sensorineural hearing loss with focused magnetic resonance imaging. Otolaryngol Head Neck Surg. 1997;116(6 Pt 1):567-74.
71. Gutmann DH, et al. The diagnostic evaluation and multidisciplinary management of neurofibromatosis 1 and neurofibromatosis 2. JAMA. 1997;278(1):51-7.
72. Traquina DN, Guttenberg I, Sasaki CT. Delayed diagnosis and treatment of acoustic neuroma. Laryngoscope. 1989;99(8 Pt 1):814-8.
73. Thomsen J, Tos M. Acoustic neuroma: clinical aspects, audiovestibular assessment, diagnostic delay, and growth rate. Am J Otol. 1990;11(1):12-9.
74. Saunders JE, et al. Sudden hearing loss in acoustic neuroma patients. Otolaryngol Head Neck Surg. 1995;113(1):23-31.
75. de Beer BA, et al. Hearing deficits in young adults who had a history of otitis media in childhood: use of personal stereos had no effect on hearing. Pediatrics. 2003;111(4 Pt 1):e304-8.
76. Theodosopoulos PV, Pensak ML. Contemporary management of acoustic neuromas. Laryngoscope; 2011;121(6):1133-7.

77. Patel J, Vasan R, van Loveren H, et al. The changing face of acoustic neuroma management in the USA: Analysis of the 1998 and 2008 patient surveys from the acoustic neuroma association. Br J Neurosurg. 2014;28(1):20-4.
78. Banerjee R, et al. Comparison of the surgical and follow-up costs associated with microsurgical resection and stereotactic radiosurgery for vestibular schwannoma. J Neurosurg. 2008;108(6):1220-4.
79. Graamans K, Van Dijk JE, Janssen LW. Hearing deterioration in patients with a non-growing vestibular schwannoma. Acta Otolaryngol. 2003;123(1):51-4.
80. Verma S, et al. Evaluation of cost effectiveness for conservative and active management strategies for acoustic neuroma. Clin Otolaryngol. 2009;34(5):438-46.
81. Stoquart-Elsankari S, et al. Motor and cognitive slowing in multiple sclerosis: an attentional deficit? Clin Neurol Neurosurg. 2010;112(3):226-32.
82. Di Maio S, Akagami R. Prospective comparison of quality of life before and after observation, radiation, or surgery for vestibular schwannomas. J Neurosurg. 2009;111(4):855-62.
83. Schwartz MS, Riddle SA, Delashaw JB Jr, et al. Quality of life following acoustic neuroma surgery. Neurosurg Focus. 1998;5(3):e3.
84. Strasnick B, et al. The natural history of untreated acoustic neuromas. Laryngoscope. 1994;104(9):1115-9.
85. Smouha EE, et al. Conservative management of acoustic neuroma: a meta-analysis and proposed treatment algorithm. Laryngoscope. 2005;115(3):450-4.
86. Anand VT, et al. Non-surgical management of acoustic neuromas. Clin Otolaryngol Allied Sci. 1992;17(5):406-10.
87. Bederson JB, et al. Conservative treatment of patients with acoustic tumors. Neurosurgery. 1991;28(5):646-50; discussion 650-1.
88. Charabi S, et al. Vestibular schwannoma growth—long-term results. Acta Otolaryngol Suppl. 2000;543:7-10.
89. Fucci MJ, et al. Acoustic tumor growth: implications for treatment choices. Am J Otol. 1999;20(4):495-9.
90. Glasscock ME, 3rd, et al. Management of acoustic neuroma in the elderly population. Am J Otol. 1997;18(2):236-41; discussion 241-2.
91. Hoistad DL, et al. Update on conservative management of acoustic neuroma. Otol Neurotol. 2001;22(5):682-5.
92. Perry BP, Gantz BJ, Rubinstein JT. Acoustic neuromas in the elderly. Otol Neurotol. 2001;22(3):389-91.
93. Tschudi DC, Linder TE, Fisch U. Conservative management of unilateral acoustic neuromas. Am J Otol. 2000;21(5): 722-8.
94. Bakkouri WE, et al. Conservative management of 386 cases of unilateral vestibular schwannoma: tumor growth and consequences for treatment. J Neurosurg. 2009;110(4): 662-9.
95. Rosenberg SI. Natural history of acoustic neuromas. Laryngoscope. 2000;110(4):497-508.
96. Valvassori GE, Guzman M. Growth rate of acoustic neuromas. Am J Otol. 1989;10(3):174-6.
97. Huet AC, et al. Validation of an optical surface plasmon resonance biosensor assay for screening (fluoro)quinolones in egg, fish and poultry. Food Addit Contam Part A Chem Anal Control Expo Risk Assess. 2009;26(10):1341-7.
98. Varughese JK, et al. Growth of untreated vestibular schwannoma: a prospective study. J Neurosurg. 2012;116(4): 706-12.
99. Yamakami I, et al. Conservative management, gamma-knife radiosurgery, and microsurgery for acoustic neurinomas: a systematic review of outcome and risk of three therapeutic options. Neurol Res. 2003;25(7):682-90.
100. Yoshimoto Y. Systematic review of the natural history of vestibular schwannoma. J Neurosurg. 2005;103(1):59-63.
101. Agrawal Y, et al. Predictors of vestibular schwannoma growth and clinical implications. Otol Neurotol. 2010;31(5):807-12.
102. Pennings RJ, et al. Natural history of hearing deterioration in intracanalicular vestibular schwannoma. Neurosurgery. 2011;68(1):68-77.
103. Sughrue ME, et al. The natural history of untreated sporadic vestibular schwannomas: a comprehensive review of hearing outcomes. J Neurosurg. 2010;112(1):163-7.
104. Martin TP, et al. A protocol for the conservative management of vestibular schwannomas. Otol Neurotol. 2009;30 (3):381-5.
105. Hajioff D, et al. Conservative management of vestibular schwannomas: third review of a 10-year prospective study. Clin Otolaryngol. 2008;33(3):255-9. doi: 10.1111/j.1749-4486.2008.01705.x.
106. Battaglia A, Mastrodimos B, Cueva R. Comparison of growth patterns of acoustic neuromas with and without radiosurgery. Otol Neurotol. 2006;27(5):705-12.
107. Kondziolka D, et al. The newly diagnosed vestibular schwannoma: radiosurgery, resection, or observation? Neurosurg Focus. 2012;33(3):E8.
108. van Leeuwen JP, et al. Acoustic neuroma: correlation among tumor size, symptoms, and patient age. Laryngoscope. 1995;105(7 Pt 1):701-7.
109. Massick DD, et al. Tumor growth and audiometric change in vestibular schwannomas managed conservatively. Laryngoscope. 2000;110(11):1843-9.
110. Breivik CN, et al. Conservative management of vestibular schwannoma—a prospective cohort study: treatment, symptoms, and quality of life. Neurosurgery. 2012;70(5): 1072-80; discussion 1080.
111. Godefroy WP, et al. Conservative treatment of vestibular schwannoma: a follow-up study on clinical and quality-of-life outcome. Otol Neurotol. 2009;30(7):968-74.
112. Giannuzzi AL, Merkus P, Falcioni M. The use of intratympanic gentamicin in patients with vestibular schwannoma and disabling vertigo. Otol Neurotol, 2013. 30: p. 30.
113. Flint, D., P. Fagan, and A. Panarese, Conservative management of sporadic unilateral acoustic neuromas. J Laryngol Otol, 2005. 119(6): p. 424-8.
114. Lloyd SK, et al. Audiovestibular factors influencing quality of life in patients with conservatively managed sporadic vestibular schwannoma. Otol Neurotol. 2010;31(6): 968-76.
115. Dhanachai M, et al. Fractionated stereotactic radiotherapy for bilateral vestibular schwannomas associated with neurofibromatosis type 2: early experiences in Ramathibodi Hospital. J Med Assoc Thai. 2004;87(9):1076-81.

116. Martin HC, et al. Patient-assessed outcomes after excision of acoustic neuroma: postoperative symptoms and quality of life. J Neurosurg. 2001;94(2):211-6.
117. Nicoucar K, et al. Surgery for large vestibular schwannomas: how patients and surgeons perceive quality of life. J Neurosurg. 2006;105(2):205-12.
118. Walsh RM, et al. The role of conservative management of vestibular schwannomas. Clin Otolaryngol Allied Sci. 2000;25(1):28-39.
119. Wiegand DA, Fickel V. Acoustic neuroma—the patient's perspective: subjective assessment of symptoms, diagnosis, therapy, and outcome in 541 patients. Laryngoscope. 1989;99(2):179-87.
120. Kaltoft M, Stangerup SE, Caye-Thomasen P. Facial nerve function after vestibular schwannoma surgery following failed conservative management. Neurosurgery. 2012;70(2):278-82.
121. Stangerup SE, et al. True incidence of vestibular schwannoma? Neurosurgery. 2010;67(5):1335-40.
122. Regis J, et al. Wait-and-see strategy compared with proactive Gamma Knife surgery in patients with intracanalicular vestibular schwannomas. J Neurosurg. 2010;113:105-11.
123. Quesnel AM, McKenna MJ. Current strategies in management of intracanalicular vestibular schwannoma. Curr Opin Otolaryngol Head Neck Surg. 2011;19(5):335-40.
124. Morrison D. Management of patients with acoustic neuromas: a Markov decision analysis. Laryngoscope. 2010;120(4):783-90.
125. Lau T, et al. Paradoxical trends in the management of vestibular schwannoma in the United States. J Neurosurg. 2012; 117(3):514-9.
126. Thedinger BA, Cueva RA, Glasscock ME, 3rd. Treatment of an acoustic neuroma in an only-hearing ear: case reports and considerations for the future. Laryngoscope. 1993;103(9):976-80.
127. Peyre M, et al. Increased growth rate of vestibular schwannoma after resection of contralateral tumor in neurofibromatosis type 2. Neuro Oncol. 2011;13(10):1125-32.
128. Koerbel A, Gharabaghi A, Safavi-Abbasi S, et al. Evolution of vestibular schwannoma surgery: the long journey to current success. Neurosurg Focus. 2005;18(4):e10.
129. Jackler RK, Pitts LH. Selection of surgical approach to acoustic neuroma. Otolaryngol Clin North Am. 1992;25(2): 361-87.
130. Chamoun R, MacDonald J, Shelton C, Couldwell WT. Surgical approaches for resection of vestibular schwannomas: translabyrinthine, retrosigmoid, and middle fossa approaches. Neurosurg Focus. 2012;33(3):e9.
131. Bennett M, Haynes DS. Surgical approaches and complications in the removal of vestibular schwannomas. Otolaryngol Clin North Am. 2007;40(3):589-609.
132. Mangham CA, Jr. Retrosigmoid versus middle fossa surgery for small vestibular schwannomas. Laryngoscope. 2004; 114(8):1455-61.
133. Clark M, et al. Lateral Intracanalicular growth of vestibular schwannomas and surgical planning. Otol Neurotol. 2010;31(2):267-70.
134. Gardner G, Robertson JH. Hearing preservation in unilateral acoustic neuroma surgery. Ann Otol Rhinol Laryngol. 1988;97(1):55-66.
135. Noudel R, Ribeiro T, Roche PH. Microsurgical treatment of intracanalicular vestibular schwannomas. Prog Neurol Surg. 2008;21:183-91.
136. Shelton C, et al. Acoustic tumor surgery. Prognostic factors in hearing conversation. Arch Otolaryngol Head Neck Surg. 1989;115(10):1213-6.
137. Kartush JM, et al. Anatomic basis for labyrinthine preservation during posterior fossa acoustic tumor surgery. Laryngoscope. 1986;96(9 Pt 1):1024-8.
138. Cohen NL, Lewis WS, Ransohoff J. Hearing preservation in cerebellopontine angle tumor surgery: the NYU experience 1974-1991. Am J Otol. 1993;14(5):423-33.
139. Irving RM, Jackler RK, Pitts LH. Hearing preservation in patients undergoing vestibular schwannoma surgery: comparison of middle fossa and retrosigmoid approaches. J Neurosurg. 1998;88(5):840-5.
140. Mohr G, et al. Preservation of hearing in patients undergoing microsurgery for vestibular schwannoma: degree of meatal filling. J Neurosurg. 2005;102(1):1-5.
141. Kocaoglu M, et al. Comparison of contrast-enhanced T1-weighted and 3D constructive interference in steady state images for predicting outcome after hearing-preservation surgery for vestibular schwannoma. Neuroradiology. 2003;45(7):476-81.
142. Gurgel RK, Dogru S, Amdur RL, Monfared A. Facial nerve outcomes after surgery for large vestibular schwannomas: do surgical approach and extent of resection matter? Neurosurg Focus. 2012;33(3):e16.
143. Roland JT, Jr. et al. Cranial nerve preservation in surgery for large acoustic neuromas. Skull Base. 2004;14(2):85-90.
144. Brackmann DE, Cullen RD, Fisher LM. Facial nerve function after translabyrinthine vestibular schwannoma surgery. Otolaryngol Head Neck Surg. 2007;136(5);773-7.
145. Noudel R, et al. Hearing preservation and facial nerve function after microsurgery for intracanalicular vestibular schwannomas: comparison of middle fossa and retrosigmoid approaches. Acta Neurochir. 2009;151(8):935-44.
146. Scheller C, et al. The influence of prophylactic vasoactive treatment on cochlear and facial nerve functions after vestibular schwannoma surgery: a prospective and open-label randomized pilot study. Neurosurgery. 2007;61(1):92-7; discussion 97-8.
147. Bayazit YA, et al. Management of cerebrospinal fluid leak following retrosigmoid posterior cranial fossa surgery. ORL J Otorhinolaryngol Relat Spec. 2009;71(6):329-33.
148. Selesnick SH, et al. The incidence of cerebrospinal fluid leak after vestibular schwannoma surgery. Otol Neurotol. 2004;25(3):387-93.
149. Wu H, et al. Comparison of different wound closure techniques in translabyrinthine acoustic neuroma surgery. Skull Base Surg.1999;9(4):239-42.
150. Heman-Ackah SE, Golfinos JG, Roland, Jr JT. Management of surgical complications and failures in acoustic neuroma surgery. Otolaryngol Clin North Am. 2012;45(2):455-70.

151. Slattery WH, 3rd, Francis S, House KC. Perioperative morbidity of acoustic neuroma surgery. Otol Neurotol. 2001; 22(6):895-902.
152. Brennan JW, et al. Cerebrospinal fluid leak after acoustic neuroma surgery: influence of tumor size and surgical approach on incidence and response to treatment. J Neurosurg. 2001;94(2):217-23.
153. Becker SS, Jackler RK, Pitts LH. Cerebrospinal fluid leak after acoustic neuroma surgery: a comparison of the translabyrinthine, middle fossa, and retrosigmoid approaches. Otol Neurotol. 2003;24(1):107-12.
154. Fishman AJ, et al. Prevention and management of cerebrospinal fluid leak following vestibular schwannoma surgery. Laryngoscope. 2004;114(3):501-5.
155. Fishman AJ, et al. Cerebrospinal fluid drainage in the management of CSF leak following acoustic neuroma surgery. Laryngoscope. 1996;106(8):1002-4.
156. O'Malley MR, Haynes DS. Assessment and management of meningitis following cerebellopontine angle surgery. Curr Opin Otolaryngol Head Neck Surg. 2008;16(5):427-33.
157. Keiper GL, Jr., et al. Dural sinus thrombosis and pseudotumor cerebri: unexpected complications of suboccipital craniotomy and translabyrinthine craniectomy. J Neurosurg. 1999;91(2):192-7.
158. Hartley F. I. Intracranial neurectomy of the fifth nerve. Ann Surg. 1893;17(5):511-26:1.
159. Monfared A, Mudry A, Jackler R. The history of middle cranial fossa approach to the cerebellopontine angle. Otol Neurotol. 2010;31(4):691-6.
160. Angeli S. Middle fossa approach: indications, technique, and results. Otolaryngol Clin North Am. 2012;45(2): 417-38.
161. Kawase T, et al. Transpetrosal approach for aneurysms of the lower basilar artery. J Neurosurg. 1985;63(6):857-61.
162. Brackmann DE, et al. Early proactive management of vestibular schwannomas in neurofibromatosis type 2. Neurosurgery. 2001;49(2):274-80; discussion 280-3.
163. Gadre AK, et al. Middle fossa decompression of the internal auditory canal in acoustic neuroma surgery: a therapeutic alternative. Laryngoscope. 1990;100(9):948-52.
164. Tanriover N, et al. Middle fossa approach: microsurgical anatomy and surgical technique from the neurosurgical perspective. Surg Neurol. 2009;71(5):586-96.
165. Garcia-Ibanez, E, Garcia-Ibanez JL. Middle fossa vestibular neurectomy: a report of 373 cases. Otolaryngol Head Neck Surg. 1980;88(4):486-90.
166. Fisch U. Transtemporal surgery of the internal auditory canal. Report of 92 cases, technique, indications and results. Adv Otorhinolaryngol. 1970;17:203-40.
167. Wigand ME, Haid T, Berg M. The enlarged middle cranial fossa approach for surgery of the temporal bone and of the cerebellopontine angle. Arch Otorhinolaryngol. 1989;246 (5):299-302.
168. Wigand ME, et al. Extended middle cranial fossa approach for acoustic neuroma surgery. Skull Base Surg. 1991;1(3): 183-7.
169. Haid CT, Wigand ME. Advantages of the enlarged middle cranial fossa approach in acoustic neurinoma surgery. A review. Acta Otolaryngol. 1992;112(3):387-407.
170. Greenblatt SH, Dagi TF, Epstein MH. A history of neurosurgery: in its scientific and professional contexts. 1997, Park Ridge, Ill.: American Association of Neurological Surgeons. xiv, 625 p.
171. Fox WL. The Cushing—Dandy controversy. Surg Neurol. 1975;3(2):61-6.
172. Elhammady MS, Telischi FF, Morcos JJ. Retrosigmoid approach: indications, techniques, and results. Otolaryngol Clin North Am. 2012;45(2):375-97.
173. Bailey BJ. Head and neck surgery—otolaryngology, 3rd edition. Philadelphia: Lippincott Williams & Wilkins; 2001.
174. Heman-Ackah SE, et al. Retrosigmoid approach to cerebellopontine angle tumor resection: surgical modifications. Laryngoscope. 2012;122(11):2519-23.
175. Rameh C, Magnan J. Quality of life of patients following stages III-IV vestibular schwannoma surgery using the retrosigmoid and translabyrinthine approaches. Auris Nasus Larynx. 2010;37(5):546-52.
176. Teo MK, Eljamel MS. Role of craniotomy repair in reducing postoperative headaches after a retrosigmoid approach. Neurosurgery. 2010;67(5):1286-91; discussion 1291-2.
177. Ruckenstein MJ, et al. Pain subsequent to resection of acoustic neuromas via suboccipital and translabyrinthine approaches. Am J Otol. 1996;17(4):620-4.
178. Schaller B, Baumann A. Headache after removal of vestibular schwannoma via the retrosigmoid approach: a long-term follow-up-study. Otolaryngol Head Neck Surg. 2003; 128(3):387-95.
179. Nguyen-Huynh AT, et al. The aborted early history of the translabyrinthine approach: a victim of suppression or technical prematurity? Otol Neurotol. 2007;28(2):269-79.
180. Arriaga MA, Lin J. Translabyrinthine approach: indications, techniques, and results. Otolaryngol Clin North Am. 2012;45(2):399-415.
181. Arriaga MA, Chen DA, Burke EL. Hydroxyapatite cement cranioplasty in translabyrinthine acoustic neuroma surgery-update. Otol Neurotol. 2007;28(4):538-40.
182. Yuen HW, Chen JM. Reconstructive options for skull defects following translabyrinthine surgery for vestibular schwannomas. Curr Opin Otolaryngol Head Neck Surg. 2008;16(4):318-24.
183. Goddard JC, Oliver ER, Lambert PR. Prevention of cerebrospinal fluid leak after translabyrinthine resection of vestibular schwannoma. Otol Neurotol. 2010;31(3):473-7.
184. Merkus P, et al. Less than 1% cerebrospinal fluid leakage in 1,803 translabyrinthine vestibular schwannoma surgery cases. Otol Neurotol. 2010;31(2):276-83.
185. Ludemann WO, et al. Fat implant is superior to muscle implant in vestibular schwannoma surgery for the prevention of cerebrospinal fluid fistulae. Neurosurgery. 2008;63 (1 Suppl 1):42-3.
186. Gantz BJ, Fisch U. Modified transotic approach to the cerebellopontile angle. Arch Otolaryngol. 1983;109(4): 252-6.

187. Fisch U, Mattox D. Microsurgery of the skull base. New York: Thieme; 1988. xxxii, 669 p.
188. Parhizkar N, Hiltzik DH, Selesnick SH. Facial nerve rerouting in skull base surgery. Otolaryngol Clin North Am. 2005; 38(4):685-710.
189. Angeli RD, et al. Enlarged translabyrinthine approach with transapical extension in the management of giant vestibular schwannomas: personal experience and review of literature. Otol Neurotol. 2011;32(1):125-31.
190. Pieper DR. The endoscopic approach to vestibular schwannomas and posterolateral skull base pathology. Otolaryngol Clin North Am. 2012;45(2):439-54.
191. Iacoangeli M, et al. Microsurgical endoscopy-assisted presigmoid retrolabyrinthine approach as a minimally invasive surgical option for the treatment of medium to large vestibular schwannomas. Acta Neurochir. 2013;155(4): 663-70.
192. Horgan MA, et al. Transcrusal approach to the petroclival region with hearing preservation. Technical note and illustrative cases. J Neurosurg. 2001;94(4):660-6.
193. Sughrue ME, et al. Hearing preservation rates after microsurgical resection of vestibular schwannoma. J Clin Neurosci. 2010;17(9):1126-9.
194. Wang AC, et al. Durability of hearing preservation after microsurgical treatment of vestibular schwannoma using the middle cranial fossa approach. J Neurosurg. 2013;15:15.
195. Woodson EA, et al. Long-term hearing preservation after microsurgical excision of vestibular schwannoma. Otol Neurotol. 2010;31(7):1144-52.
196. Jackson LE,Roberson, Jr. JB, Acoustic neuroma surgery: use of cochlear nerve action potential monitoring for hearing preservation. Am J Otol. 2000;21(2):249-59.
197. Danner C, Mastrodimos B, Cueva RA. A comparison of direct eighth nerve monitoring and auditory brainstem response in hearing preservation surgery for vestibular schwannoma. Otol Neurotol. 2004;25(5):826-32.
198. Moriyama T, et al. Hearing preservation in acoustic neuroma surgery: importance of adhesion between the cochlear nerve and the tumor. J Neurosurg. 2002;97(2):337-40.
199. Thomsen J, et al. Middle fossa approach in vestibular schwannoma surgery. Postoperative hearing preservation and EEG changes. Acta Otolaryngol. 2000;120(4):517-22.
200. Arts HA, et al. Hearing preservation and facial nerve outcomes in vestibular schwannoma surgery: results using the middle cranial fossa approach. Otol Neurotol. 2006;27(2): 234-41.
201. Gjuric M, et al. Vestibular schwannoma volume as a predictor of hearing outcome after surgery. Otol Neurotol. 2007;28(6):822-7.
202. Mazzoni A, Calabrese V, Danesi G. A modified retrosigmoid approach for direct exposure of the fundus of the internal auditory canal for hearing preservation in acoustic neuroma surgery. Am J Otol. 2000;21(1):98-109.
203. Kaylie DM, et al. Acoustic neuroma surgery outcomes. Otol Neurotol. 2001;22(5):686-9.
204. Somers T, et al. Prognostic value of magnetic resonance imaging findings in hearing preservation surgery for vestibular schwannoma. Otol Neurotol. 2001;22(1):87-94.
205. Lee SH, Willcox TO, Buchheit WA. Current results of the surgical management of acoustic neuroma. Skull Base. 2002;12(4):189-95.
206. Maw AR, et al. Hearing preservation and facial nerve function in vestibular schwannoma surgery. Clin Otolaryngol Allied Sci. 2003;28(3):252-6.
207. Yamakami I, et al. Hearing preservation and intraoperative auditory brainstem response and cochlear nerve compound action potential monitoring in the removal of small acoustic neurinoma via the retrosigmoid approach. J Neurol Neurosurg Psychiatry. 2009;80(2):218-27.
208. Nonaka Y, Fukushima T, Watanabe K. Contemporary surgical management of vestibular schwannomas: analysis of complications and lessons learned over the past decade. Neurosurgery. 2013;72(2 Suppl Operative):103-15.
209. Rabelo de Freitas M, et al. Analysis of hearing preservation and facial nerve function for patients undergoing vestibular schwannoma surgery: the middle cranial fossa approach versus the retrosigmoid approach--personal experience and literature review. Audiol Neurootol. 2012;17(2):71-81.
210. Staecker H, et al. Hearing preservation in acoustic neuroma surgery: middle fossa versus retrosigmoid approach. Am J Otol. 2000;21(3):399-404.
211. Cross T, et al. Impact of facial paralysis on patients with acoustic neuroma. Laryngoscope. 2000;110(9):1539-42.
212. Parving A, et al. Some aspects of life quality after surgery for acoustic neuroma. Arch Otolaryngol Head Neck Surg. 1992;118(10):1061-4.
213. Briggs RJ, Fabinyi G, Kaye AH. Current management of acoustic neuromas: review of surgical approaches and outcomes. J Clin Neurosci. 2000;7(6):521-6.
214. Wiet RJ, et al. Long-term results of the first 500 cases of acoustic neuroma surgery. Otolaryngol Head Neck Surg. 2001;124(6):645-51.
215. Sughrue ME, et al. Preservation of facial nerve function after resection of vestibular schwannoma. Br J Neurosurg. 2010;24(6):666-71.
216. Bloch O, et al. Factors associated with preservation of facial nerve function after surgical resection of vestibular schwannoma. J Neurooncol. 2011;102(2):281-6.
217. Samii M, Gerganov V, Samii A. Improved preservation of hearing and facial nerve function in vestibular schwannoma surgery via the retrosigmoid approach in a series of 200 patients. J Neurosurg. 2006;105(4):527-35.
218. Tonn JC, et al. Acoustic neuroma surgery as an interdisciplinary approach: a neurosurgical series of 508 patients. J Neurol Neurosurg Psychiatry. 2000;69(2):161-6.
219. Darwish BS, et al. Facial nerve function and hearing preservation after retrosigmoid excision of vestibular schwannoma: Christchurch Hospital experience with 97 patients. ANZ J Surg. 2005;75(10):893-6.
220. Mamikoglu B, Esquivel CR, Wiet RJ. Comparison of facial nerve function results after translabyrinthine and retrosigmoid approach in medium-sized tumors. Arch Otolaryngol Head Neck Surg. 2003;129(4):429-31.
221. Anderson DE, et al. Resection of large vestibular schwannomas: facial nerve preservation in the context of surgical approach and patient-assessed outcome. J Neurosurg. 2005;102(4):643-9.

222. Wu H, Sterkers J. Translabyrinthine removal of large acoustic neuromas in young adults. Auris Nasus Larynx. 2000;27 (3):201-5.
223. Zhang, X., et al. Facial nerve function after excision of large acoustic neuromas via the suboccipital retrosigmoid approach. J Clin Neurosci. 2005;12(4):405-8.
224. Sanna, M, et al. Hearing preservation surgery in vestibular schwannoma: the hidden truth. Ann Otol Rhinol Laryngol. 2004;113(2):156-63.
225. Satar B, Yetiser S, Ozkaptan Y. Impact of tumor size on hearing outcome and facial function with the middle fossa approach for acoustic neuroma: a meta-analytic study. Acta Otolaryngol. 2003;123(4):499-505.
226. Isaacson B, Telian SA, El-Kashlan HK. Facial nerve outcomes in middle cranial fossa vs translabyrinthine approaches. Otolaryngol Head Neck Surg. 2005;133(6):906-10.
227. Seol HJ, et al. Optimal extent of resection in vestibular schwannoma surgery: relationship to recurrence and facial nerve preservation. Neurol Med Chir (Tokyo). 2006;46(4): 176-80; discussion 180-1.
228. Marouf R, Noudel R, Roche PH. Facial nerve outcome after microsurgical resection of vestibular schwannoma. Prog Neurol Surg. 2008;21:103-7.
229. Fundova P, et al. Cystic vestibular schwannoma: surgical outcome. J Laryngol Otol. 2000;114(12):935-9.
230. Morikawa M, et al. Long-term results of facial nerve function after acoustic neuroma surgery--clinical benefit of intraoperative facial nerve monitoring. Kobe J Med Sci. 2000;46(3):113-24.
231. Youssef AS, Downes AE. Intraoperative neurophysiological monitoring in vestibular schwannoma surgery: advances and clinical implications. Neurosurg Focus. 2009;27(4):e9.
232. Sughrue ME, et al. Beyond audiofacial morbidity after vestibular schwannoma surgery. J Neurosurg. 2011;114(2): 367-74.
233. Feigl GC, et al. Analysis of risk factors influencing the development of severe dizziness in patients with vestibular schwannomas in the immediate postoperative phase. Clin Neurol Neurosurg. 2011;113(1):52-6.
234. Mamikoglu B, Wiet RJ, Esquivel CR. Translabyrinthine approach for the management of large and giant vestibular schwannomas. Otol Neurotol. 2002;23(2):224-7.
235. Godefroy WP, et al. Surgery for large vestibular schwannoma: residual tumor and outcome. Otol Neurotol. 2009; 30(5):629-34.
236. Shelton C, et al. Middle fossa acoustic tumor surgery: results in 106 cases. Laryngoscope. 1989;99(4):405-8.
237. Kanzaki J, et al. Postoperative complications in acoustic neuroma surgery by the extended middle cranial fossa approach. Acta Otolaryngol Suppl. 1991;487:75-9.
238. Harner SG, Beatty CW, Ebersold MJ. Retrosigmoid removal of acoustic neuroma: experience 1978-1988. Otolaryngol Head Neck Surg. 1990;103(1):40-5.
239. Dutton JE, et al. Acoustic neuroma (schwannoma) surgery 1978-1990. J Laryngol Otol. 1991;105(3):165-73.
240. Bryce GE, et al. Cerebrospinal fluid leaks and meningitis in acoustic neuroma surgery. Otolaryngol Head Neck Surg. 1991;104(1):81-7.
241. Celikkanat SM, et al. Cerebrospinal fluid leak after translabyrinthine acoustic neuroma surgery. Otolaryngol Head Neck Surg. 1995;112(6):654-8.
242. Gillman GS, Parnes LS. Acoustic neuroma management: a six-year review. J Otolaryngol. 1995;24(3):191-7.
243. Tos M, Thomsen J, Harmsen A. Results of translabyrinthine removal of 300 acoustic neuromas related to tumour size. Acta Otolaryngol Suppl. 1988;452:38-51.
244. Stieglitz LH, et al. Factors affecting postoperative cerebrospinal fluid leaks after retrosigmoidal craniotomy for vestibular schwannomas. J Neurosurg. 2009;111(4):874-83.
245. Sanchez GB, et al. Chemical meningitis following cerebellopontine angle tumor surgery. Otolaryngol Head Neck Surg. 2008;138(3):368-73.
246. Sluyter S, et al. Analysis of the results obtained in 120 patients with large acoustic neuromas surgically treated via the translabyrinthine-transtentorial approach. J Neurosurg. 2001;94(1):61-6.
247. Zarrouk V, et al. Evaluation of the management of postoperative aseptic meningitis. Clin Infect Dis. 2007;44(12): 1555-9.
248. Hadeishi H, Yasui N, Suzuki A. Mastoid canal and migrated bone wax in the sigmoid sinus: technical report. Neurosurgery. 1995;36(6):1220-3; discussion 1223-4.
249. Crocker M, et al. Symptomatic venous sinus thrombosis following bone wax application to emissary veins. Br J Neurosurg. 2008;22(6):798-800.
250. Wiet RJ, Teixido M, Liang JG. Complications in acoustic neuroma surgery. Otolaryngol Clin North Am. 1992;25(2): 389-412.
251. Slattery WH, 3rd, Brackmann DE, Hitselberger W. Middle fossa approach for hearing preservation with acoustic neuromas. Am J Otol. 1997;18(5):596-601.
252. Shelton C. Unilateral acoustic tumors: how often do they recur after translabyrinthine removal? Laryngoscope. 1995; 105(9 Pt 1):958-66.
253. Gjuric M, Wigand ME, Wolf SR. Enlarged middle fossa vestibular schwannoma surgery: experience with 735 cases. Otol Neurotol. 2001;22(2):223-30; discussion 230-1.
254. Carlson ML, et al. Magnetic resonance imaging surveillance following vestibular schwannoma resection. Laryngoscope. 2012;122(2):378-88.
255. Kemink JL, et al. Operative management of acoustic neuromas: the priority of neurologic function over complete resection. Otolaryngol Head Neck Surg. 1991;104(1):96-9.
256. Nikolopoulos TP, et al. Acoustic neuroma growth: a systematic review of the evidence. Otol Neurotol, 2010. 31(3): p. 478-85.
257. Bloch DC, et al. The fate of the tumor remnant after less-than-complete acoustic neuroma resection. Otolaryngol Head Neck Surg. 2004;130(1):104-12.
258. El-Kashlan HK, et al. Recurrence of acoustic neuroma after incomplete resection. Am J Otol. 2000;21(3):389-92.
259. Bennett ML, et al. Postoperative imaging of vestibular schwannomas. Otolaryngol Head Neck Surg. 2008;138(5): 667-71.
260. Thedinger BS, Whittaker CK, Luetje CM. Recurrent acoustic tumor after a suboccipital removal. Neurosurgery. 1991;29 (5):681-7.

261. Wigand ME, et al. Preservation of hearing in bilateral acoustic neurinomas by deliberate partial resection. Acta Otolaryngol. 1992;112(2):237-41.
262. Sughrue ME, et al. Extent of resection and the long-term durability of vestibular schwannoma surgery. J Neurosurg. 2011;114(5):1218-23.
263. Roche PH, Khalil, Thomassin JM. Microsurgical removal of vestibular schwannomas after failed previous microsurgery. Prog Neurol Surg. 2008;21:158-62.
264. Freeman SR, et al. Revision surgery for residual or recurrent vestibular schwannoma. Otol Neurotol. 2007;28(8): 1076-82.
265. Patni AH, Kartush JM. Staged resection of large acoustic neuromas. Otolaryngol Head Neck Surg. 2005;132(1):11-9.
266. Raslan AM, et al. Staged resection of large vestibular schwannomas. J Neurosurg. 2012;116(5):1126-33.
267. Battista RA, Wiet RJ. Stereotactic radiosurgery for acoustic neuromas: a survey of the American Neurotology Society. Am J Otol. 2000;21(3):371-81.
268. Husseini ST, et al. Salvage surgery of vestibular schwannoma after failed radiotherapy: the Gruppo Otologico experience and review of the literature. Am J Otolaryngol. 2013;34(2):107-14.
269. Roche PH, et al. Surgical removal of vestibular schwannoma after failed gamma knife radiosurgery. Prog Neurol Surg. 2008;21:152-7.
270. Slattery WH, 3rd. Microsurgery after radiosurgery or radiotherapy for vestibular schwannomas. Otolaryngol Clin North Am. 2009;42(4):707-15.
271. Friedman RA, et al. A paradigm shift in salvage surgery for radiated vestibular schwannoma. Otol Neurotol. 2011;32(8):1322-8.
272. Wallner KE, et al. Efficacy of irradiation for incompletely excised acoustic neurilemomas. J Neurosurg. 1987;67(6): 858-63.
273. Maire JP, et al. Fractionated radiation therapy in the treatment of stage III and IV cerebello-pontine angle neurinomas: preliminary results in 20 cases. Int J Radiat Oncol Biol Phys. 1992;23(1):147-52.
274. Leksell L. The stereotaxic method and radiosurgery of the brain. Acta Chir Scand. 1951;102(4):316-9.
275. Leksell L. Stereotactic radiosurgery. J Neurol Neurosurg Psychiatry. 1983;46(9):797-803.
276. Betti O, Derechinsky V. Multiple-beam stereotaxic irradiation. Neurochirurgie. 1983;29(4):295-8.
277. Colombo F, et al. Stereotactic radiosurgery utilizing a linear accelerator. Appl Neurophysiol. 1985;48(1-6):133-45.
278. Adler JR, Jr, et al. The Cyberknife: a frameless robotic system for radiosurgery. Stereotact Funct Neurosurg. 1997;69 (1-4 Pt 2):124-8.
279. Mathieu D, et al. Stereotactic radiosurgery for vestibular schwannomas in patients with neurofibromatosis type 2: an analysis of tumor control, complications, and hearing preservation rates. Neurosurgery. 2007; 60(3):460-8; discussion 468-70.
280. Link MJ, et al. Radiation therapy and radiosurgery for vestibular schwannomas: indications, techniques, and results. Otolaryngol Clin North Am. 2012;45(2):353-66.
281. Friedman WA, et al. Linear accelerator radiosurgery for vestibular schwannomas. J Neurosurg. 2006;105(5):657-61.
282. Lederman G, et al. Acoustic neuroma: potential benefits of fractionated stereotactic radiosurgery. Stereotact Funct Neurosurg. 1997;69(1-4 Pt 2):175-82.
283. Lo YC, Ling CC, Larson DA. The effect of setup uncertainties on the radiobiological advantage of fractionation in stereotaxic radiotherapy. Int J Radiat Oncol Biol Phys. 1996;34(5):1113-9.
284. Williams JA. Fractionated stereotactic radiotherapy for acoustic neuromas. Int J Radiat Oncol Biol Phys. 2002;54(2): 500-4.
285. Sakamoto GT, Blevins N, Gibbs IC. Cyberknife radiotherapy for vestibular schwannoma. Otolaryngol Clin North Am. 2009;42(4):665-75.
286. Chang SD, et al. Staged stereotactic irradiation for acoustic neuroma. Neurosurgery. 2005;56(6):1254-61;discussion 1261-3.
287. Fuss M, et al. Conventionally fractionated stereotactic radiotherapy (FSRT) for acoustic neuromas. Int J Radiat Oncol Biol Phys. 2000;48(5):1381-7.
288. Fuss M, et al. Fractionated stereotactic intensity-modulated radiotherapy (FS-IMRT) for small acoustic neuromas. Med Dosim. 2002;27(2):147-54.
289. Andrews DW, et al. Toward dose optimization for fractionated stereotactic radiotherapy for acoustic neuromas: comparison of two dose cohorts. Int J Radiat Oncol Biol Phys. 2009;74(2):419-26.
290. Chan AW, et al. Stereotactic radiotherapy for vestibular schwannomas: favorable outcome with minimal toxicity. Neurosurgery. 2005;57(1):60-70; discussion 60-70.
291. Combs SE, et al. Differences in clinical results after LINAC-based single-dose radiosurgery versus fractionated stereotactic radiotherapy for patients with vestibular schwannomas. Int J Radiat Oncol Biol Phys. 2010;76(1):193-200.
292. Koh ES, et al. Fractionated stereotactic radiotherapy for acoustic neuroma: single-institution experience at The Princess Margaret Hospital. Cancer. 2007;109(6):1203-10.
293. Thomas C, et al. Hearing preservation following fractionated stereotactic radiotherapy for vestibular schwannomas: prognostic implications of cochlear dose. J Neurosurg. 2007;107(5):917-26.
294. Bush DA, et al. Fractionated proton beam radiotherapy for acoustic neuroma. Neurosurgery. 2002;50(2):270-3; discussion 273-5.
295. Vernimmen FJ, et al. Long-term results of stereotactic proton beam radiotherapy for acoustic neuromas. Radiother Oncol. 2009;90(2):208-12.
296. Weber DC, et al. Proton beam radiosurgery for vestibular schwannoma: tumor control and cranial nerve toxicity. Neurosurgery. 2003;53(3):577-86; discussion 586-8.
297. Lunsford LD, et al. Radiosurgery of vestibular schwannomas: summary of experience in 829 cases. J Neurosurg. 2005;102 Suppl:195-9.
298. Hasegawa T, et al. Stereotactic radiosurgery for vestibular schwannomas: analysis of 317 patients followed more than 5 years. Neurosurgery. 2005;57(2):257-65; discussion 257-65.

299. Inoue HK. Low-dose radiosurgery for large vestibular schwannomas: long-term results of functional preservation. J Neurosurg. 2005;102 Suppl:111-3.
300. Regis J, et al. Functional outcome after gamma knife surgery or microsurgery for vestibular schwannomas. J Neurosurg. 2002;97(5):1091-100.
301. Nakamura H, et al. Serial follow-up MR imaging after gamma knife radiosurgery for vestibular schwannoma. AJNR Am J Neuroradiol. 2000;21(8):1540-6.
302. Yu CP, et al. Sequential volume mapping for confirmation of negative growth in vestibular schwannomas treated by gamma knife radiosurgery. J Neurosurg. 2000;93 Suppl 3:82-9.
303. Hasegawa T, et al. Evaluation of tumor expansion after stereotactic radiosurgery in patients harboring vestibular schwannomas. Neurosurgery. 2006;58(6):1119-28; discussion 1119-28.
304. Pollock BE. Management of vestibular schwannomas that enlarge after stereotactic radiosurgery: treatment recommendations based on a 15 year experience. Neurosurgery. 2006;58(2):241-8; discussion 241-8.
305. Flickinger JC, et al. Acoustic neuroma radiosurgery with marginal tumor doses of 12 to 13 Gy. Int J Radiat Oncol Biol Phys. 2004;60(1):225-30.
306. Wowra B, et al. Outpatient gamma knife surgery for vestibular schwannoma: definition of the therapeutic profile based on a 10-year experience. J Neurosurg. 2005;102 Suppl:114-8.
307. Pellet W, et al. Relative indications for radiosurgery and microsurgery for acoustic schwannoma. Adv Tech Stand Neurosurg. 2003;28:227-82; discussion 282-4.
308. Kondziolka D, et al. Long-term outcomes after radiosurgery for acoustic neuromas. N Engl J Med. 1998;339(20):1426-33.
309. Prasad D, Steiner M, Steiner L. Gamma surgery for vestibular schwannoma. J Neurosurg. 2000;92(5):745-59.
310. Chung WY, et al. Gamma knife surgery for vestibular schwannoma: 10-year experience of 195 cases. J Neurosurg. 2005;102:87-96.
311. Myrseth E, et al. Vestibular schwannomas: clinical results and quality of life after microsurgery or gamma knife radiosurgery. Neurosurgery. 2005;56(5):927-35; discussion 927-35.
312. Chopra R, et al. Long-term follow-up of acoustic schwannoma radiosurgery with marginal tumor doses of 12 to 13 Gy. Int J Radiat Oncol Biol Phys. 2007;68(3):845-51.
313. Yang I, et al. Hearing preservation after stereotactic radiosurgery for vestibular schwannoma: a systematic review. J Clin Neurosci. 2009;16(6):742-7.
314. Carlson ML, et al. Long-term hearing outcomes following stereotactic radiosurgery for vestibular schwannoma: patterns of hearing loss and variables influencing audiometric decline. J Neurosurg. 2013;118(3):579-87.
315. Litvack ZN, et al. Preservation of functional hearing after gamma knife surgery for vestibular schwannoma. Neurosurg Focus. 2003;14(5):e3.
316. Hasegawa T, et al. Factors associated with hearing preservation after Gamma Knife surgery for vestibular schwannomas in patients who retain serviceable hearing. J Neurosurg. 2011;115(6):1078-86.
317. Kano H, et al. Predictors of hearing preservation after stereotactic radiosurgery for acoustic neuroma. J Neurosurg. 2009;111(4):863-73.
318. Massager N, et al. Irradiation of cochlear structures during vestibular schwannoma radiosurgery and associated hearing outcome. J Neurosurg. 2007;107(4):733-9.
319. Timmer FC, et al. Gamma knife radiosurgery for vestibular schwannomas: results of hearing preservation in relation to the cochlear radiation dose. Laryngoscope. 2009;119(6):1076-81.
320. Andrews DW, et al. Stereotactic radiosurgery and fractionated stereotactic radiotherapy for the treatment of acoustic schwannomas: comparative observations of 125 patients treated at one institution. Int J Radiat Oncol Biol Phys. 2001;50(5):1265-78.
321. Rowe JG, et al. Gamma knife stereotactic radiosurgery for unilateral acoustic neuromas. J Neurol Neurosurg Psychiatry. 2003;74(11):1536-42.
322. Baschnagel AM, et al. Hearing preservation in patients with vestibular schwannoma treated with Gamma Knife surgery. J Neurosurg. 2013;118(3):571-8.
323. St George EJ, et al. Acute symptoms after gamma knife radiosurgery. J Neurosurg. 2002;97(5 Suppl):631-4.
324. Werner-Wasik M, et al. Immediate side effects of stereotactic radiotherapy and radiosurgery. Int J Radiat Oncol Biol Phys. 1999;43(2):299-304.
325. Franco-Vidal V, et al. Intracochlear hemorrhage after gamma knife radiosurgery. Otol Neurotol. 2007;28(2):240-4.
326. Ogunrinde OK, et al. Cranial nerve preservation after stereotactic radiosurgery for small acoustic tumors. Arch Neurol. 1995;52(1):73-9.
327. Pollack AG, et al. Acute neurological complications following gamma knife surgery for vestibular schwannoma. Case report. J Neurosurg. 2005;103(3):546-51.
328. Tago M, et al. Immediate neurological deterioration after gamma knife radiosurgery for acoustic neuroma. Case report. J Neurosurg. 2000;93 Suppl 3:78-81.
329. Noren G. Long-term complications following gamma knife radiosurgery of vestibular schwannomas. Stereotact Funct Neurosurg. 1998;70 Suppl 1:65-73.
330. Hempel JM, et al. Functional outcome after gamma knife treatment in vestibular schwannoma. Eur Arch Otorhinolaryngol. 2006;263(8):714-8.
331. Murphy ES, et al. Long-term outcomes of Gamma Knife radiosurgery in patients with vestibular schwannomas. J Neurosurg. 2011;114(2):432-40.
332. Sughrue ME, et al. Non-audiofacial morbidity after Gamma Knife surgery for vestibular schwannoma. Neurosurg Focus. 2009;27(6):E4.
333. Battista RA. Gamma knife radiosurgery for vestibular schwannoma. Otolaryngol Clin North Am. 2009;42(4):635-54.
334. Yang SY, et al. Evaluation of tumour response after gamma knife radiosurgery for residual vestibular schwannomas based on MRI morphological features. J Neurol Neurosurg Psychiatry. 2008;79(4):431-6.
335. Yang HC, et al. Gamma Knife radiosurgery for larger-volume vestibular schwannomas. Clinical article. J Neurosurg. 2011;114(3):801-7.

336. Charabi S, et al. Cystic vestibular schwannoma—clinical and experimental studies. Acta Otolaryngol Suppl. 2000; 543:11-3.
337. Benech F, et al. Cystic versus solid vestibular schwannomas: a series of 80 grade III-IV patients. Neurosurg Rev. 2005;28(3):209-13.
338. Pendl G, et al. Acoustic neurinomas with macrocysts treated with Gamma Knife radiosurgery. Stereotact Funct Neurosurg. 1996;66 Suppl 1:103-11.
339. Delsanti C, Regis J. Cystic vestibular schwannomas. Neurochirurgie. 2004;50(2-3 Pt 2):401-6.
340. Pollock BE, et al. Vestibular schwannoma management. Part II. Failed radiosurgery and the role of delayed microsurgery. J Neurosurg. 1998;89(6):949-55.
341. Pollock BE, Link MJ. Vestibular schwannoma radiosurgery after previous surgical resection or stereotactic radiosurgery. Prog Neurol Surg. 2008;21:163-8.
342. Pollock BE, et al. Vestibular schwannoma management. Part I. Failed microsurgery and the role of delayed stereotactic radiosurgery. J Neurosurg. 1998;89(6):944-8.
343. Unger F, et al. Radiosurgery of residual and recurrent vestibular schwannomas. Acta Neurochir (Wien). 2002;144(7):671-6; discussion 676-7.
344. van de Langenberg R, et al. Management of large vestibular schwannoma. Part I. Planned subtotal resection followed by Gamma Knife surgery: radiological and clinical aspects. J Neurosurg. 2011;115(5):875-84.
345. Yomo S, et al. Repeat gamma knife surgery for regrowth of vestibular schwannomas. Neurosurgery. 2009;64(1):48-54; discussion 54-5.
346. Dewan S, Noren G. Retreatment of vestibular schwannomas with Gamma Knife surgery. J Neurosurg. 2008;109 Suppl:144-8.
347. Husseini ST, Piccirillo E, Sanna M. On "malignant transformation of acoustic neuroma/vestibular schwannoma 10 years after gamma knife stereotactic radiosurgery" (skull base 2010;20:381-388). Skull Base. 2011;21(2):135-8.
348. Demetriades AK, et al. Malignant transformation of acoustic neuroma/vestibular schwannoma 10 years after gamma knife stereotactic radiosurgery. Skull Base. 2010;20(5): 381-7.
349. Schmitt WR, et al. Radiation-induced sarcoma in a large vestibular schwannoma following stereotactic radiosurgery: case report. Neurosurgery. 2011;68(3):E840-6; discussion E846.
350. Yang T, et al. A case of high-grade undifferentiated sarcoma after surgical resection and stereotactic radiosurgery of a vestibular schwannoma. Skull Base. 2010;20(3):179-83.
351. Markou K, et al. Unique case of malignant transformation of a vestibular schwannoma after fractionated radiotherapy. Am J Otolaryngol. 2012;33(1):168-73.
352. Kaylie DM, McMenomey SO. Microsurgery vs gamma knife radiosurgery for the treatment of vestibular schwannomas. Arch Otolaryngol Head Neck Surg. 2003;129(8):903-6.
353. Pollock BE. Vestibular schwannoma management: an evidence-based comparison of stereotactic radiosurgery and microsurgical resection. Prog Neurol Surg. 2008;21:222-7.
354. Tos M, et al. Causes of facial nerve paresis after translabyrinthine surgery for acoustic neuroma. Ann Otol Rhinol Laryngol. 1992;101(10):821-6.
355. Carlson ML, et al. The anatomically intact but electrically unresponsive facial nerve in vestibular schwannoma surgery. Neurosurgery. 2012;71(6):1125-30.
356. Franco-Vidal V, et al. Delayed facial paralysis after vestibular schwannoma surgery: role of herpes viruses reactivation—our experience in eight cases. Otol Neurotol. 2004; 25(5):805-10.
357. Sampath P, et al. Late-onset facial nerve degeneration after vestibular schwannoma surgery: incidence, putative mechanisms, and prevention. Neurosurg Focus. 1998;5(3):e6.
358. Strauss C, et al. Preservation of facial nerve function after postoperative vasoactive treatment in vestibular schwannoma surgery. Neurosurgery. 2006;59(3):577-84; discussion 577-84.
359. Sobel RA. Vestibular (acoustic) schwannomas: histologic features in neurofibromatosis 2 and in unilateral cases. J Neuropathol Exp Neurol. 1993;52(2):106-13.
360. Evans DG, et al. Birth incidence and prevalence of tumorprone syndromes: estimates from a UK family genetic register service. Am J Med Genet A. 2010;152A(2):327-32.
361. Antinheimo J, et al. Population-based analysis of sporadic and type 2 neurofibromatosis-associated meningiomas and schwannomas. Neurology. 2000;54(1):71-6.
362. Brackmann DE, Shelton C, Arriaga MA. Otologic surgery, 3rd edition. Philadelphia, PA: Saunders/Elsevier; 2010. xxi, 831p.
363. von Eckardstein KL, et al. Spontaneous regression of vestibular schwannomas after resection of contralateral tumor in neurofibromatosis Type 2. J Neurosurg. 2010;112(1): 158-62.
364. Plotkin SR, et al. Hearing improvement after bevacizumab in patients with neurofibromatosis type 2. N Engl J Med. 2009;361(4):358-67.
365. Wong HK, et al. Anti-vascular endothelial growth factor therapies as a novel therapeutic approach to treating neurofibromatosis-related tumors. Cancer Res. 2010;70(9): 3483-93.
366. Hoa M, Slattery WH, 3rd. Neurofibromatosis 2. Otolaryngol Clin North Am. 2012;45(2):315-32, viii.
367. Plotkin SR, et al. Erlotinib for progressive vestibular schwannoma in neurofibromatosis 2 patients. Otol Neurotol. 2010; 31(7):1135-43.
368. Plotkin SR, et al. Audiologic and radiographic response of NF2-related vestibular schwannoma to erlotinib therapy. Nat Clin Pract Oncol. 2008;5(8):487-91.
369. Doyle KJ, Shelton C. Hearing preservation in bilateral acoustic neuroma surgery. Am J Otol. 1993;14(6):562-5.
370. Slattery WH, 3rd, Brackmann DE, Hitselberger W. Hearing preservation in neurofibromatosis type 2. Am J Otol. 1998; 19(5):638-43.
371. Slattery WH, 3rd, et al. Hearing preservation surgery for neurofibromatosis Type 2-related vestibular schwannoma in pediatric patients. J Neurosurg. 2007;106(4 Suppl): 255-60.

372. Slattery WH, et al. Middle fossa decompression for hearing preservation: a review of institutional results and indications. Otol Neurotol. 2011;32(6):1017-24.
373. Kida Y, et al. Radiosurgery for bilateral neurinomas associated with neurofibromatosis type 2. Surg Neurol. 2000; 53(4):383-89; discussion 389-90.
374. Roche PH, et al. Neurofibromatosis type 2. Preliminary results of gamma knife radiosurgery of vestibular schwannomas. Neurochirurgie. 2000;46(4):339-53; discussion 354.
375. Rowe JG, et al. Clinical experience with gamma knife stereotactic radiosurgery in the management of vestibular schwannomas secondary to type 2 neurofibromatosis. J Neurol Neurosurg Psychiatry. 2003;74(9):1288-93.
376. Baser ME, et al. Neurofibromatosis 2, radiosurgery and malignant nervous system tumours. Br J Cancer. 2000; 82(4):998.
377. Carlson ML, et al. Radiation-induced rhabdomyosarcoma of the brainstem in a patient with neurofibromatosis type 2. J Neurosurg.2010;112(1):81-7.
378. Evans DG, et al. Malignant transformation and new primary tumours after therapeutic radiation for benign disease: substantial risks in certain tumour prone syndromes. J Med Genet. 2006;43(4):289-94.
379. Lustig LR, et al. Cochlear implantation in patients with neurofibromatosis type 2 and bilateral vestibular schwannoma. Otol Neurotol. 2006;27(4):512-8.
380. Ahsan S, et al. Cochlear implantation concurrent with translabyrinthine acoustic neuroma resection. Laryngoscope. 2003;113(3):472-4.
381. Trotter MI, Briggs RJ. Cochlear implantation in neurofibromatosis type 2 after radiation therapy. Otol Neurotol. 2010;31(2):216-9.

CHAPTER

24

Meningioma and Other Non-vestibular Schwannoma Tumors of the CPA

Adam A Master, Maura K Cosetti

INTRODUCTION

The term cerebellopontine angle (CPA) refers to the intracranial space bounded by the cerebellum, pons, and the petrous portion of the temporal bone. Traversed by a large number of neurovascular structures, tumors in this region can be diverse in clinical presentation and subject to a variety of available treatment options. Although the most common CPA tumor is a vestibular schwannoma (VS), a benign growth of the vestibular portion of the eighth cranial nerve (CN VIII), a long list of potential pathologies may be found in this region. VSs account for approximately 90% of pathology in the CPA, while meningiomas, epidermoids, facial schwannomas, and other more rare lesions comprise the remaining 10% of tumors (Table 24.1). This chapter will discuss the clinical findings and audiovestibular evaluation of non-VS pathology of the CPA, as well as the pathogenesis, imaging, and treatment specific to CPA meningiomas, epidermoids, arachnoid cysts, facial schwannomas, hemangiomas, metastatic disease, and intra-axial lesions.

Table 24.1: Differential diagnosis of cerebellopontine angle pathology

Common lesions (in order of decreasing frequency)
Vestibular schwannoma
Meningioma
Epidermoid
Facial nerve schwannoma
Arachnoid cyst
Uncommon lesions
Hemangioma
Lipoma
Dermoid
Teratoma
Metastatic disease
Intra-axial lesions
Glioma
Medulloblastoma
Choroid plexus papillomas
Ependymomas
Hemangioblastoma

CPA ANATOMY

A thorough understanding of CPA anatomy provides the foundation on which to base a discussion of the diverse pathology of this intracranial area. Situated in the posterior fossa, the CPA is bounded anteriorly by the petrous portion of the temporal bone and the lateral clivus and posteriorly by the flocculus and the petrosal surface of the cerebellum (Fig. 24.1). The lateral aspect of the tentorium marks the superior border, while the inferior extent approaches the lateral surface of the medulla. Laterally, the space is bounded by the internal auditory meatus (or porus acusticus) along with the entirety of the posterior petrous temporal bone. The pons, as well as the beginning of the contralateral CPA cistern, represents the medial extent. The apex of the CPA abuts the lateral recess of the fourth ventricle and approximates the region of the pontomedullary junction where the cochlear and vestibular divisions of CN VIII enter the brain stem. The choroid plexus of the fourth ventricle may occasionally protrude through the foramen of Luschka into this area.

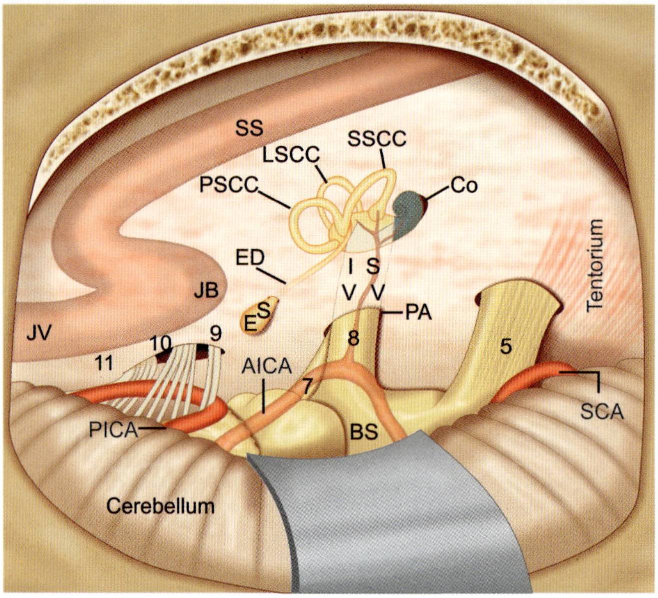

Fig. 24.1: Anatomy of the cerebellopontine angle. (5, cranial nerve 5 (trigeminal); 7, cranial nerve 7 (facial); 8, cranial nerve 8 (vestibulocochlear); 9, cranial nerve 9 (glossopharyngeal); 10, cranial nerve 10 (vagus); 11, cranial nerve 11 (spinal accessory); AICA, anterior inferior cerebellar artery; BS, brainstem; Co, cochlea; ES, endolymphatic sac; ED, endolymphatic duct (also known as the vestibular acqueduct); IV, inferior vestibular nerve; JB, jugular bulb; JV, jugular vein; LSCC, lateral semicircular canal; PICA, posterior inferior cerebellar artery; PSCC, posterior semicircular canal; SCA, superior cerebellar artery; SSCC, superior semicircular canal; SS, sigmoid sinus; SV, superior vestibular nerve).

The CPA is lined by meninges, filled with cerebrospinal fluid (CSF), and traversed by a number of neurovascular structures entering and exiting the skull base. The vestibulocochlear (CN VIII) and facial (CN VII) nerves are the core neural structures within the CPA. With respect to vascular structures, the CPA includes the anterior and posterior inferior cerebellar arteries (AICA and PICA, respectively) and their branches (including the important internal auditory artery), as well as the venous drainage of the cerebellum, pons, and medulla.

CLINICAL FINDINGS

Symptoms and signs of CPA tumors are directly related to the neurovascular anatomy of the skull base region they involve. As mentioned above, the primary CN VII and VIII course through the CPA cistern as they travel from their origin in the brain stem to the fundus of the internal auditory canal (IAC). Tumors extending medially can involve the trigeminal nerve, CN V, while those extending inferiorly can abut the lower CNs (glossopharyngeal, vagus, accessory and hypoglossal, CN IX–XII, respectively). Although the list of symptoms caused by CPA pathology can be diverse, it is not surprising that the most common are hearing loss, imbalance/disequilibrium, and tinnitus. Symptoms related to the facial and trigeminal nerves, specifically facial paresis, paralysis, spasm, pain and paresthesias, as well as cerebellar symptoms, such as ataxia, are also frequent.[1,2] Unsurprisingly, complaints of papilledema, diplopia, abducens palsy, which are related to structures anatomically distant from the CPA (i.e. the optic and oculomotor nerves), are less common. Similarly, symptoms related to lower CN dysfunction, such as dysarthria, hoarseness, and dysphagia, are less also frequent. CPA tumors can induce symptoms indicative of increased intracranial pressure or mass effect, including headache, hemiparesis, and dementia. Often, due to the nonspecific nature of some complaints and the complexity of the anatomic structures in this region, many of the above symptoms (i.e. imbalance) may have a multifactorial etiology.

Overall, CPA tumors may present with a variety of complaints and they may also remain asymptomatic. For this reason, it is not possible to diagnosis CPA pathology using symptomatology alone. Following identification of a CPA mass, it is similarly impossible to differentiate between tumor pathology on the basis of presenting symptoms. Clinical findings unique to various pathologies will be discussed in more detail below.

AUDIOVESTIBULAR AND FACIAL NERVE TESTING

Audiometry

Prior to the advent of sophisticated imaging technology such as magnetic resonance imaging (MRI; discussed at length in an upcoming section), audiovestibular testing played a larger role in the diagnosis of CPA pathology. Unsurprisingly, the vast majority of studies on audiometric evaluation of CPA tumors included patients with VS. There are significantly less data available on the audiometric presentation of non-VS tumors. Available evidence suggests that meningiomas and other non-VS CPA pathology do not have unique audiometric features distinguishing them from VS. Importantly, however, while audiometry currently functions as a useful (not mandatory) adjunct in the diagnosis of CPA pathology, it is a crucial and required element in treatment decision making and should be performed in all non-VS tumors.

Mechanisms of damage to the audiovestibular system from a non-VS CPA tumor mimic those from a VS, including direct compression on CN VIII or the brain stem nuclei, neural, or cochlear ischemia from disrupted arterial supply or impaired venous drainage, biochemical alteration of the inner ear, hair cell degeneration secondary to neuronal loss within CN VIII (i.e. deafferentation), as well as direct or indirect effects from primary cortical or cerebellar pathology.[3]

Although not independently diagnostic of a CPA lesion, auditory brain stem response testing (ABR) is the most useful audiometric test for diagnosis of CPA pathology.[4] For VS, it has been shown to have a sensitivity of 100% and a specificity of 61.9%.[5] This surpasses that of behavioral audiometry, including various "site of lesions" tests indicative of retrocochlear pathology such as reduced word discrimination, abnormal acoustic reflex thresholds, and presence of acoustic reflex decay. Data suggest that sensitivity and specificity of ABR in diagnosis of non-VS tumors of the CPA is less than for VS; as many as 15% of non-VS tumors may have normal ABRs. [6]

At present, use of electrophysiologic studies such as ABR, stacked ABR, auditory steady-state response testing (ASSR), and otoacoustic emissions in the diagnosis and management of non-VS lesions is variable and physician or institution dependent. As the sensitivity and specificity of MRI has surpassed that of available audiometric testing, routine use of these tests for diagnosis is not advocated.[7,8]

Following diagnosis, the presence or degree of hearing loss is an important factor in CPA tumor management and may specifically impact the timing, candidacy, or success of various treatment options (additional discussion in the treatment section, below). Behavioral audiometry (including pure tone air and bone levels and speech discrimination testing) remains the gold standard for functional hearing assessment and should be performed in all patients with known or suspected CPA tumors.

Vestibular Testing

Vestibular testing, including video- and electronystagmography, is used inconsistently in the diagnosis and management of CPA tumors. A reduction in caloric responses has been documented in two-third of patients with CPA meningiomas; however, the findings are nonspecific.[9] In VS management, vestibular testing may be useful in distinguishing between tumors arising from the inferior or superior vestibular nerve. These data may occasionally be useful in counseling patients on tumor management, such as the opportunity for hearing preservation surgery. It is not widely applied to non-VS tumors of the CPA.

Electroneuronograhpy

Electroneuronography (ENoG) assesses facial muscle response to maximal bipolar stimulation at the stylomastoid foramen and has also been inconsistently applied in diagnosis of these tumors. Measurements obtained give indirect information about the quantity of synchronous functional motor units of the facial nerve (FN), including the motor axon, end plate, and muscle fibers. These measurements may suggest reduced function even when not clinically evident. Overall, ENoG testing is of limited value in slow-growing, progressive lesions in which the motor units may experience partial degeneration and regeneration. [10] For these reasons, it is not commonly employed in the diagnosis or management of CPA lesions, including facial schwannomas.

MENINGIOMAS

Pathogenesis

Meningiomas are the most common extra-axial, intracranial tumor pathology; however, they account for only 3–12% of CPA tumors. Overall, the CPA ranks 8th in intracranial location, although it represents the most common location in the posterior fossa. Meningiomas arise from meningothelial cells, specifically the arachnoid cap cells located in the tips of arachnoid villi that are responsible for CSF absorption. Within the cranial vault, meningiomas are found along skull base foramina, dural sinuses, and large tributary veins. Other locations for meningioma growth in the posterior fossa include the clival and petroclival region, Meckel's cave, the jugular foramen, IAC, and foramen magnum.

Epidemiologically, meningiomas have an overall annual incidence of approximately 6 per 100,000 individuals. In symptomatic patients, however, the overall incidence is less, estimated at 2–3 per 100,000. Due to their benign pathology and overall slow growth, meningiomas represent >30% of incidental brain tumors found postmortem.

Meningioma incidence increases with age, peaking in the 6th and 7th decades, and is rare in children (accounting for <2% of childhood intracranial neoplasms). A long-recognized gender predominance in females has been supported with molecular studies demonstrating estrogen and progesterone receptors on meningioma cells. Hormonal effects may also underlie the well-known association between breast cancer and meningiomas, as well as the data demonstrating meningioma growth during pregnancy. Epidemiologic studies in both the United States and Africa have suggested a slight increased incidence of meningiomas in African Americans (3.1 vs. 2.3 per 100,000). Trauma has also been proposed as an important risk factor for meningioma development; however, data on this topic are conflicting.

Overall, the most well-recognized and significant risk factor for meningioma development is a prior history of radiation. In the central nervous system (CNS), meningiomas are the most common neoplasm resulting from prior radiation therapy. Radiation-induced meningiomas have been classified into three types based on amount of radiation exposure: low (< 10 Gy), medium (10–20 Gy), and high (> 20 Gy). Although there appears to be a long latency period (ranging from 19 to 35 years) between radiation exposure and meningioma diagnosis, studies suggest tumors in the high-dose category present earlier.[11] Many patients in these studies received radiation in childhood for a variety of noncancerous conditions, such as tinea capitis, and their data suggest an inverse relationship between radiation dose and age with high-dose recipients presenting at a younger age. In addition, radiogenic meningiomas are more likely to be histologically aggressive or "atypical" and have a higher recurrence rate after surgical removal.[11,12]

The identification and understanding of the molecular pathogenesis of meningiomas have been closely linked to that of neurofibromatosis type 2 (NF2). Although >95% of meningiomas are sporadic, the remainder are associated with a variety of hereditary syndromes, including NF2 as well as Werner's, Gorlin's, and Cowden's syndromes. NF2 is an autosomal dominant disease characterized by the development of multiple intracranial and spinal tumors, specifically bilateral VS, meningiomas, and ependymomas. Between 30% and 50% of NF2 patients develop meningiomas. It was the initial cytogenetic analysis of meningiomas samples that led to the identification of the NF2 gene, Merlin. Located on the long arm of chromosome 22, Merlin is thought to be a tumor suppressor gene involved in cytoskeletal transport and cell architecture. Mutations in this gene have been documented in up to 80% of all meningiomas.[13] Additional mutations in other chromosomes such as 1p, 6q, 10q, 14q, 17p, 18q have been associated with an increase in tumor histoplasmic atypia and even malignancy.[14,15]

Due to their generally benign pathology and slow rate of growth, however, the average time from symptom onset to diagnosis of meningiomas is approximately 4–6 years. As mentioned above, meningiomas most commonly present with symptoms related to CN VIII, specifically hearing loss, vertigo, and imbalance. Tumors that extend medially to the petroclival junction can present with pain or facial paresthesia due to involvement of CNV.[1,2]

Imaging

As discussed above, symptomatology, physical examination, and audiovestibular evaluation cannot diagnose a CPA tumor with a specificity and sensitivity that surpasses MRI. Therefore, MRI is well recognized as both the gold standard and the most efficient examination of suspected CPA pathology[5,16] (Table 24.2). MRI sequences should be performed with and without intravenous gadolinium diethylene triamine pentaacetic acid (Gd-DTPA) and include thin slice (2 mm) pre- and postcontrast T1-weighted sequences in the axial and coronal planes. Comprehensive

Table 24.2: Magnetic resonance imaging (MRI) characteristics of nonvestibular schwannoma cerebellopontine angle tumors

Pathology	*T1-weighted*	*T2-weighted*	*Gadolinium enhancement*	*Notes*
Meningioma	↓	↑→	Yes	Dural tail
Epidermoid	↓	↑	No	*
Arachnoid cyst	↓	↑	No	*
Lipoma	↑	↑→	Yes	May use fat suppression sequences
FNS	↓	↑	Yes	May be multifocal; enlargement of the FN canal on CT
Hemangioma	↓	↑	Yes	Ca^{++}, bony speculation on CT
Metastasis	↓	↑	Yes	Brain edema, leptomeningeal carcinomatosis
Intra-axial lesions	↓	↑	Yes	Lack of CSF between tumor and brainstem; narrowing of CPA cistern

↑, hyperintense; ↓, hypointense; → isointense; FNS, facial nerve schwannoma; CT, computed tomography; CPA, cerebellopontine angle; CSF, cerebrospinal fluid.

*Epidermoids and arachnoid cysts may be differentiated on fluid-attenuated inversion recovery sequences (FLAIR) and diffusion weighted imaging (DWI) sequences: only arachnoid cysts will suppress completely on FLAIR and have no restriction on DWI.

imaging should also include postcontrast fat saturation as well as heavily T2-weighted three-dimensional sequences, such as fast imaging using steady-state acquisition or constructive interference in the steady state.[16] Diffusion-weighted imaging (DWI) and magnetic resonance spectroscopy (MRS) can also be performed depending on institutional preferences. Tumor characteristics on MRI, occasionally in combination with computed tomography (CT) and other radiologic modalities, often allow differentiation between various CPA tumor pathologies (Fig. 24.1).

On MRI, meningiomas are hypo- to isointense to cerebral cortex on T1- and iso- to hyperintense on T2-weighted images. Gd-DPTA transverses the abnormal blood–brain barrier associated with meningioma growth and accumulates in the interstitial tumoral spaces. Therefore, there is avid enhancement with gadolinium in >95% of meningiomas. Although heterogeneous intensity on T1-weighted images can be seen in both VS and meningiomas, the T2 signal profile can allow differentiation between these pathologies. Specifically, heterogeneity due to intratumoral cysts demonstrates hyperintensity on T2 images and is suggestive of VS. In contrast, regions of lower intensity caused by calcification will remain low intensity on T2-weighted images and are therefore more consistent with a meningioma.

Like VS, meningiomas are typically well-circumscribed, sessile masses causing "cortical buckling", a phenomenon in which compression of the adjacent grey matter and distortion of the underlying white matter can be visualized.[17] One of the primary features distinguishing it from VS on MRI is the presence of a dural tail, a layer of enhancement extending a few millimeters from the lesion (Fig. 24.2). Histopathologic correlation studies suggest this enhancement could represent either tumor invasion or nontumoral reactive changes, such as hypervascularity, vasodilation, or tissue proliferation or increased permeability to contrast. [18] Presence of tumor cells within the peritumoral dura advocates for wide surgical resection of this region to prevent recurrence (discussed in more depth below). Occasionally, a dural tail is observed with an otherwise appearing VS – this pseudomeningeal sign is not a true dural tail and is related to bone marrow signal in the temporal bone near the porus acusticus. It can be seen on T1 images before and after Gd-DPTA contrast, thereby distinguishing it from a true dural tail seen only after contrast.

Controversy currently exists over meningioma characteristics on DWI or MRS imaging, with some data suggesting lower apparent diffusion coefficient values may be indicative of malignant or atypical histological subtypes.

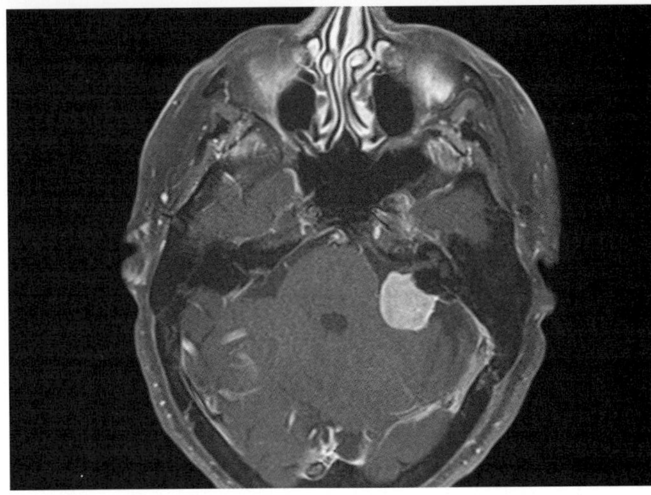

Fig. 24.2: Cerebellopontine angle (CPA) meningioma. Axial T1-weighted gadolinium-enhanced magnetic resonance image (MRI) demonstrating a left cerebellopontine angle meningioma. Note its broad sessile base and dural tail.

As these parameters have proven unreliable, DWI and MRS imaging are inconsistently used in MRI algorithms.[16,17] Unusual imaging features, such as intratumoral cysts, dense calcification, vasogenic white matter edema in adjunct parenchyma and metaplastic changes, are rare, occurring in <4% of meningiomas and may also lead to heterogeneous or minimal tumoral enhancement with gadolinium.[17] En-plaque meningiomas (discussed in more detail below) are rare pathological subtypes, which present as diffuse enhancement along the skull base, often with significant hyperostosis.

CT is a complementary modality best for identifying unique bony changes associated with meningiomas, specifically calcification and hyperostosis of adjacent bone, seen in 20–25% of tumors.[17] Following administration of iodinated intravenous contrast, meningiomas are typically hyperdense with homogenous enhancement and have a broad dural attachment.[17] Changes in the surrounding bone may represent hyperostosis, erosion secondary to direct pressure or direct tumor invasion with bony destruction. Although best visualized with CT, tumor infiltration can be seen on T1-weighted MRI images in which the normally hyperintense bone marrow fat has a lowered signal intensity. [19]

While both CPA meningiomas and VS can invade the IAC, bone erosion and widening of the porus acusticus (the opening of the IAC along the posterior petrous pyramid) are more common with VS compared to meningiomas. However, meningiomas have a greater tendency to invade other neural foramina, such as Meckel's cave, compared with VS.

Gross Pathology

Meningiomas are firm, rubbery, well-circumscribed tumors with either a smooth or nodular surface. Pinkish gray or yellow prior to formalin fixation, tumor color is indicative of lipid accumulation within cells or hemosiderin deposition following variably aged hemorrhages. Intratumoral consistency is associated with tumor contents, with calcifications and psammoma bodies endowing a gritty texture and cysts or necrosis leading to softness or fluctuance. Macroscopically, exophytic tumors (most common) have a broad, firm dural attachment, while the rare, en-plaque meningiomas are wide, sheetlike meningeal expansions most commonly seen at the sphenoid ridge and skull base.

Microscopic Histopathology

Although controversy exists in histopathological classification of meningiomas, the World Health Organization (WHO) meningioma classification scheme is the best cited and recognized of its kind. Expanding on a pioneering histologic study of approximately 1800 meningiomas, the WHO defines meningioma subtypes by grade and likelihood of recurrence.[20] Overall, tumor grade is inversely related to prognosis. Grade I tumors comprise 90% of meningioma histology and are benign with a very low risk of recurrence or aggressive growth (Figs. 24.3 and 24.4). Grade II represents 7% of meningiomas and is composed of atypical pathologic subtypes with an intermediate risk of recurrence. On histological analysis, they demonstrate ≥4 mitosis per high-power field in combination with three of the following five characteristics: increased cellularity, increased nuclear to cytoplasmic ratio, prominent nucleoli, sheetlike growth, and necrosis or brain invasion. Anaplastic, aggressive tumors with a >20 mitosis per high-power field and features of malignancy are characterized as grade III. They comprise 3% of meningiomas and have a high risk of recurrence and an overall poor prognosis (median 2 year survival of < 2 years after diagnosis).

Treatment

As with VS, there are three overarching treatment options for CPA meningiomas, including microsurgical resection, observation with serial imaging, and fractionated and stereotactic radiosurgery. Treatment choice should be guided by tumor pathology, size, location, signs, and symptoms as well as patient age, health, comorbidities, and preference.

Selection of surgical approach must be also be individualized, and skull base surgical teams should ideally be skilled in multiple techniques. A variety of hearing preservation [retrosigmoid (RS) and middle fossa] and non-hearing preservation approaches [translabyrinthine (TL) and transcochlear] have been applied to CPA meningiomas with success (Fig. 24.5).

The RS approach is an efficient and flexible hearing preservation approach commonly employed in CPA meningioma resection. A RS craniotomy allows access to a large portion of the posterior fossa extending from the tentorium cerebelli to the foramen magnum and is ideal

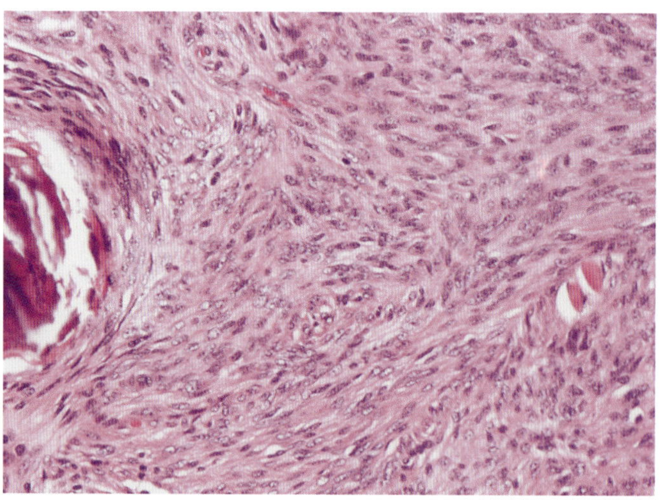

Fig. 24.3: Histologic image of a WHO grade I cerebellopontine angle (CPA) meningioma demonstrating both myxoid and microcystic morphology. Note the predominately spindle-shaped, fibroblast-like cells that form parallel and interlacing bundles (H&E, x 40).

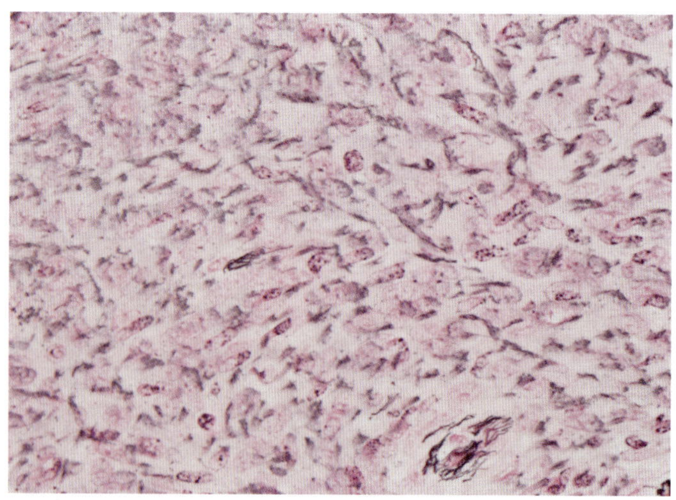

Fig. 24.4: Reticulin staining of a WHO grade I cerebellopontine angle (CPA) meningioma. Reticulin highlights the fibrous collagen deposition common in this histopathologic type of meningioma.

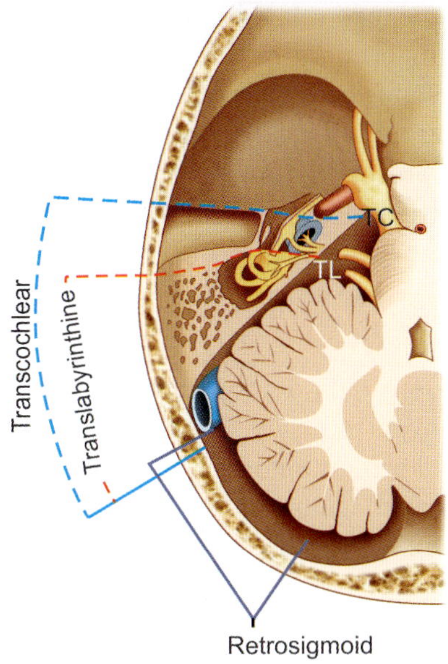

Fig. 24.5: Diagram of various surgical approaches to the cerebellopontine angle.

for meningiomas that extend outside the CPA, but not to the fundus of the IAC. Unlike VS, site of dural origin of CPA meningioma dictates its relationship to the CN VIII nerve bundle and, therefore, influences rates of both hearing preservation and FN injury.[21] For example, meningiomas arising anterior to the IAC displace the vestibulocochlear nerve posteriorly and place them at greater risk of injury from an RS approach.

Although the RS approach offers the opportunity for hearing preservation, success depends on tumor size and location but may be better than similarly sized schwannomas. Overall, rates of hearing preservation in meningioma resection are greater than that with VS surgery and approach 100% in some series.[22,23] Involvement of the lateral one-third of the IAC, the increased incidence of postoperative headache, and the need for cerebellar retraction are considerations in the RS approach.

Extended middle fossa surgery employs a temporal craniotomy to provide wide and direct exposure to the entire IAC and CPA. Bone removal within Kawase's triangle bordered by the internal carotid artery and the cochlea posteriorly allows access to CPA tumors with IAC and petroclival extension. Limited to tumors with <1 cm extension into the CPA, this hearing preservation surgery has been successfully applied to a small group of CPA meningiomas.[24] Specific disadvantages of this approach include the potential for morbidity associated with temporal lobe retraction.

The standard non-hearing preservation approach to the CPA is unarguably the TL approach. Virtually any size tumor of the CPA angle can be resected from this approach, with better FN outcomes and overall less morbidity as retraction of the cerebellum or temporal lobe is not required.[22] This approach requires complete sacrifice of labyrinth, and therefore patients selected for this approach typically lack serviceable hearing preoperatively.

The transcochlear and transotic approaches offer the widest conceivable exposure to the CPA angle with extension of dissection to the petrous tip.[25] The two methods differ in their risk of injury to the FN: in the transcochlear approach, the FN is transposed, while in the transotic approach, it is left in its anatomic position within the fallopian canal. These approaches have been successfully employed for large posterior fossa meningiomas involving the petrous apex and clivus, but also may be used as an alternative to TL approach when additional exposure is desired.[25,26] Compared to the TL approach, there is increased risk of damage to the FN. In a retrospective review at the House Ear Clinic of 24 patients who underwent transcochlear resection of CPA meningioma, 95% had postoperative facial paralysis, with 12 of 20 patients improving to House–Brackmann (HB) grade III or better.[27] Despite its drawbacks, there are few rival approaches that can provide unobstructed access to the petroclivus, basilar artery, and ventral pons.

Gamma knife radiosurgery (GKR) has been employed for the treatment of skull base meningiomas for over 25 years. Recently published long-term data show radiographic progression-free survival to be 98%, 96%, and 78% at 3, 5, and 10 years post-treatment.[28] A majority of patients (91%) had no deterioration in the neurological condition since treatment. Overall, tumor progression was associated with age >65 and limited dose to the tumor margin.[29]

In selected cases, expectant management of CPA meningiomas may be viable treatment option. In general, observation is recommended for tumors that are unresectable due to their location, slow-growing small asymptomatic tumors, as well patients who are poor surgical candidates. In a review of 252 patients with asymptomatic incidentally found meningiomas, one third demonstrated no growth with a mean follow-up of 67 months.[30]

EPIDERMOIDS

Pathogenesis

Epidermoids are the third most common CPA lesion, following VS and meningiomas. They are congenital rest lesions postulated to originate from ectodermal squamous epithelium trapped during neural tube closure between weeks 3 and 5 of intrauterine development.[31] Like primary cholesteatoma found within the middle ear and mastoid, the stratified squamous epithelial lining encases desquamated keratin and slowly enlarges. Grossly, epidermoid tumors have both a smooth or lobulated surface and a pearly, white capsule consistent with the tumor's pathogenesis as squamous epithelium. Calcium may be present in 10% of these tumors and epidermoid fluid is typically thick, brown, and viscous resulting from cholesterol and hemosiderin by-product of cell membrane decomposition.[31] Like many CPA lesions, epidermoids are slow growing with enlargement seemingly parallel to desquamation rates of normal epithelial cells.[32] They typically expand toward areas of least resistance, including cisterns, fissures, and ventricles and often occupy multiple intracranial compartments. Although most commonly found intradurally in the CPA or parasellar region, intraparenchymal and fourth ventricle lesions have also been reported.[33-35] Unlike other tumors in the CPA, epidermoids tend to surround or encase neurovascular structures instead of compressing or pushing them to the periphery. This feature is of great importance for surgical management as the neurovascular structures often course within the tumor instead of on the external surface. Rarely, epidermoids may degenerate into malignant squamous cell carcinoma.[36-38] Due to their slow and insidious growth pattern, epidermoids often reach considerable size before causing symptoms (typically hearing and balance related complaints). Although large at presentation, epidermoids rarely present with obstructive hydrocephalus as the fissured, cystic wall allows CSF spread around the tumor. Patients with epidermoids may occasionally present with chemical or aseptic meningitis from extrusion of cyst fluid into the subarachnoid space.[34]

Imaging

On MRI, epidermoids demonstrate hypointensity on T1 images and hyperintensity on T2 (Figs. 24.6 and 24.7). However, unlike meningiomas and VS, epidermoids do not enhance with gadolinium. (Minimal enhancement of the epidermoid capsule has been documented in approximately 25% of tumors.[31]) Epidermoids share similar CT characteristics with arachnoid cysts; both present as well-circumscribed, homogenous, lobulated masses without surrounding edema of adjacent parenchyma. For this reason, CT alone is not sufficient for diagnosis.[39] On MRI and CT, epidermoid and arachnoid cyst contents match the density and intensity of CSF. However, specific MRI sequences allow distinction between these two pathologies: epidermoids are differentiated from arachnoid cysts by their relative hyperintensity to CSF on FLAIR (fluid-attenuated inversion recovery sequences) and DWI sequences. Other lesions with FLAIR and DWI hyperintensity include abscesses and cholesteatoma. These can be differentiated from epidermoids by thick rim enhancement and temporal bone destruction, respectively.[31]

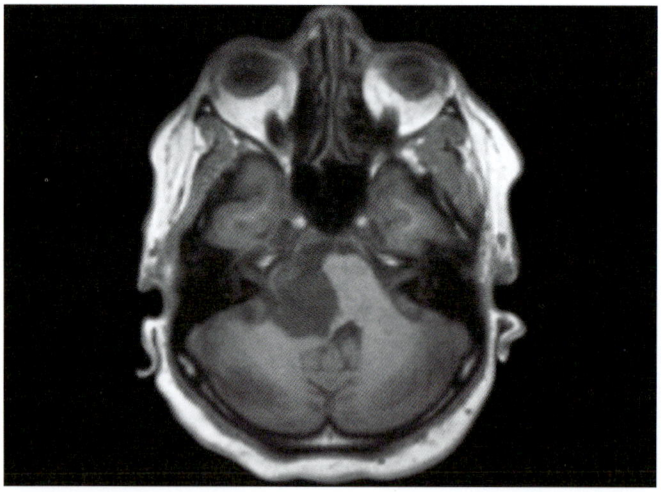

Fig. 24.6: Cerebellopontine angle (CPA) epidermoid. Axial T1-weighted magnetic resonance imaging (MRI) of a CPA epidermoid demonstrating low signal intensity. Note the compression of brainstem and fourth ventricle.

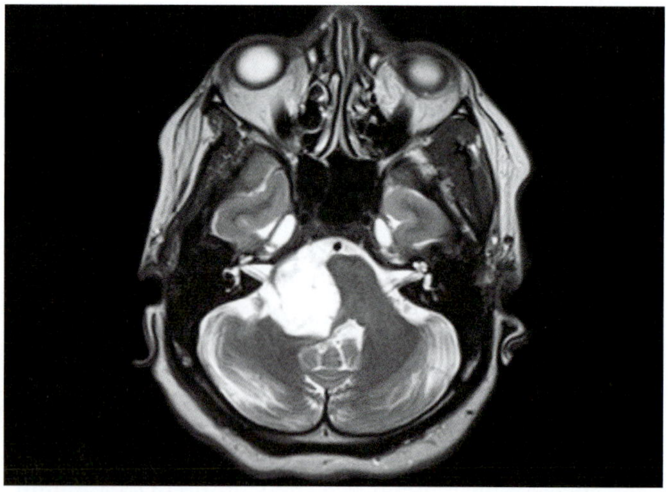

Fig. 24.7: Cerebellopontine angle (CPA) epidermoid. Axial T2-weighted magnetic resonance imaging (MRI) of a CPA epidermoid demonstrating hyperintensity. Note cranial nerves VII and VIII visible in the internal auditory canal.

Areas of contrast enhancement within epidermoids have been reported in the literature and have been shown to correlate with malignant transformation to squamous cell carcinoma, an extremely rare event.[36-38,40,41] Also rare are "white epidermoids"—tumors whose high proteinaceous content leads to reverse signal intensity with hyperintensity on T1 and hypointensity on T2.[31,42]

Treatment

Treatment of epidermoids is gross total resection, often via an RS craniotomy.[31] As discussed previously, these tumors are typically avascular and friable, but may encase or even adhere to neurovascular structures within the CPA. To avoid permanent nerve or vascular injury, subtotal resection with preservation of vital structures has been strongly advocated. Although subtotal resection would intuitively suggest a higher risk of recurrence, there are studies supporting similar recurrence rates following total and sub-/near-total resections. [43] Overall, published data suggest a high rate of hearing preservation for subtotal resection, even if performed for the second time.[44,45] At present, data on GKS of epidermoid tumors are scarce. For tumors with malignant transformation, the addition of adjuvant radiotherapy to surgical resection appears to confer a survival benefit.[46]

FACIAL NERVE SCHWANNOMAS

Pathogenesis

Schwannomas of the FN can occur anywhere along the FN course and intratemporal lesions are often multifocal. Although most commonly located in the perigeniculate region, facial nerve schwannomas (FNS) may also occur in the CPA.[10,47] Isolated CPA FNS represent <2% of all FNS lesions and can be challenging, if not impossible, to differentiate from VS preoperatively.[48] Like VS, FNS are slow growing, predominately benign neoplasms of Schwann cells. Documented growth rates are slightly higher than that of VS with an average of <1 cm^3/year and malignancy is extremely rare, with few reported cases in the literature.[47,49] FNS are uncommon in children and rarely bilateral.[10] Unlike meningiomas and VS, there are no known genetic loci involved in the development of FNS.

Not surprisingly, signs and symptoms of these lesions relate to the location(s) of the FN they involve. Extratemporal involvement may present as a parotid mass; middle ear FNS can cause conductive hearing loss and sensorineural hearing loss; and FNS of the CPA may present with a range of clinical findings common to all CPA tumors. Of note, FNS located intratemporally (within the bony FN canal) can lead to neural entrapment and FN symptoms even at very small sizes; therefore, they often present earlier than FNS confined to the CPA. Facial paresis, often subtle, is more common in the initial presentation of facial schwannomas compared with other CPA lesions.[48]

Imaging

On MRI, nonvestibular nerve schwannomas, such as FNS or schwannomas of the lower CNs, are identical to both meningiomas and VS in signal intensity and enhancement, but may be identified by their location and appearance. FNS may cause abnormal enhancement along the length of the intratemporal FN on postcontrast T1-weighted images, occasionally presenting as "beads on a string" with multifocal enhancement.[16,48] Enlargement of the FN canal on CT may also be diagnostic of a FNS. Of note, lower CN schwannomas (such as tumors of CN IX, X, XI and XII) are suspected by their intimate relationship to the corresponding skull base foramina. Unlike the FN, these nerves do not course through the CPA cistern, and therefore rarely involve the CPA unless quite large.

Treatment

Although management of FNS has evolved in recent years, timing of intervention remains controversial. Surgery is the mainstay of treatment options and traditional teaching supported tumor observation until symptoms of FN paresis reached or surpassed HB grade III–IV. Surgical excision nearly always leads to complete disruption of the continuity of the FN, and therefore expectedly necessitates nerve reconstruction or adjunctive reanimation procedures. (Isolated instances of complete tumor removal with preservation of FN continuity have been reported.[10]) FN reconstruction techniques may restore facial function to a HB grade III, thus the timing of surgical excision must balance these two outcomes. Consensus supports surgical intervention when tumor effects reach a HB III–IV. Maintaining an expectant approach until HB V or complete paralysis occurs confers a distinct disadvantage in outcome—published data supports better functional outcomes with less preoperative deficit. [47,50] Conservative surgical approaches, specifically decompression and debulking, may also be employed to prolong native facial function as

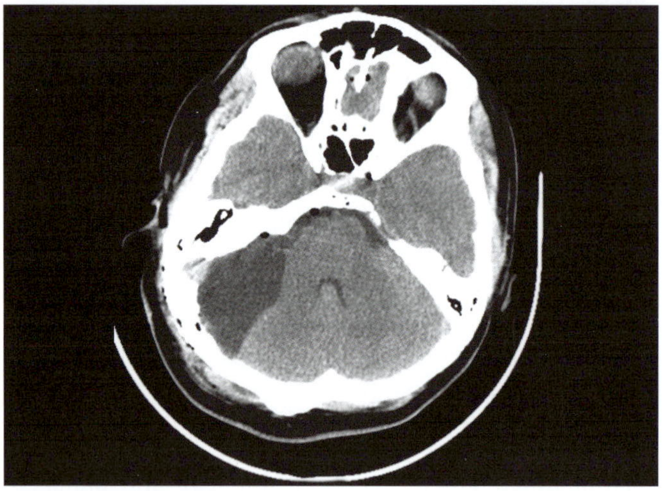

Fig. 24.8: Computed tomography (CT) image of an arachnoid cyst.

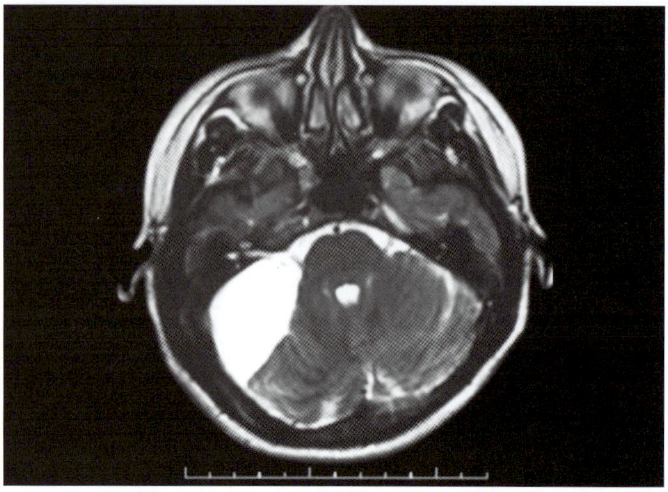

Fig. 24.9: Arachnoid cyst. Axial T1-weighted magnetic resonance imaging (MRI) of a large cerebellopontine angle (CPA) arachnoid cyst with characteristic hyperintensity matching the signal intensity of cerebrospinal fluid (CSF).

long as possible. These methods may also be utilized when a FNS is encountered unexpectedly during surgical excision for presumed VS. As described above, preoperative determination of FNS pathology in patients without FN paresis or radiographic involvement of the intratemporal FN may be extremely challenging or impossible. When faced with an unexpected FNS intraoperatively, surgical management choices include complete resection, subtotal resection of debulking, or decompression. A recent study described excellent FN function (HB < III) in a group of 16 patients where tumor debulking and/or FN decompression were performed.[48]

GKS has also been advocated as a modality allowing long-term preservation of FN function. In small published series, GKS allowed long-term preservation of innate FN function leading authors to promote GKS as a first-line treatment option for FNS.[51,52]

ARACHNOID CYSTS

Pathogenesis

Arachnoid cysts are believed to be a congenital developmental abnormality in which a thin-walled sac is created by aberrant or increased pulsatile CSF flow. The lesion consists of arachnoid membrane lined with collagen and arachnoid cells and slowly enlarges with trapped CSF.[53] Acquired arachnoid cysts that are comparatively rare appear to occur after trauma or intracranial surgery. [54] As with other CPA lesions, these are slow growing and cause symptoms from mass effect on surrounding neurovascular structures. Without free communication with the subarachnoid space, enlarging cysts may initially present with symptoms of increased intracranial pressure. Representing < 1% of all intracranial neoplasms, they are most commonly found in the middle cranial fossa and are rare lesions of the CPA.[55] Less than 10% of all intracranial arachnoid cysts are found in the posterior fossa. [56,57] In their study of approximately 300 tumors, Helland et al. suggest a possible relationship between gender and location with temporal cysts occurring more commonly in males and CPA location predominating in females.[55]

Imaging

As stated above, epidermoids and arachnoid cysts may have similar imaging characteristics on both MR and CT (Figs. 24.8 and 24.9). MRI allows differentiation between these tumors: only arachnoid cysts will suppress completely on FLAIR and have no restriction on DWI. Other rare pathologies that may be confused with arachnoid cysts include mega cisterna magna, which has identical MRI characteristics on T1-, T2-weighted images, FLAIR and DWI but has no mass effect on the cerebellum or vermis.[53]

Treatment

In the case of incidentally discovered, asymptomatic arachnoid cysts, observation is strongly encouraged.[58-61] For symptomatic cysts, a range of surgical options has been proposed ranging from craniotomy with complete removal to stereotactic cyst needle drainage. Endoscopic cyst fenestration, subtotal removal, cystoperitoneal shunting, drainage, and fistulization with the subarachnoid space have also been advocated. [53,61] Rarity of pathology and overall lack of published data make a comparison of various interventions challenging; however, multiple groups have reported recovery of SNHL as well as return of FN function following fenestration of CPA arachnoid cysts.[62,63] Overall, surgical drainage is preferred in most centers, typically via an RS approach. Diuretics have been reported to reduce symptoms in some patients; however, they are not widely used. GKS is no employed in the treatment of arachnoid cysts.

LIPOMAS

Pathogenesis

Like arachnoid cysts, lipomas are more commonly found in the supratentorial brain and are rare in the posterior fossa and CPA. Composed of mature adipose tissue, they are benign, slow-growing masses that can often become large before inducing symptoms. They are congenital malformations resulting from malabsorption of the meninx primitive, a mesenchymal derivative of neural crest cells. Lipomas are predominately asymptomatic and found incidentally on imaging or at autopsy. Symptomatic lipomas usually present with hearing and balance complaints and may be limited to the IAC or involve both the IAC and CPA. As with epidermoid tumors, lipoma growth progressively encases surrounding neurovascular structures and can often be inseparable from arachnoid and neural tissue. Although symptoms results from mass effect, the trabeculated, fibrovascular consistency of lipomas has been shown to cause demyelination and may be histopathologically indistinguishable from neural fibers.[64-66] This microscopic anatomy is an important consideration in timing and approach of surgical management.

Imaging

Because they are composed of fat, lipomas demonstrate a distinct MRI appearance, allowing them to be distinguished from other CPA pathology: they are hyperintense on pregadolinium T1 images and hypointense on T2 images (Fig. 24.10). Although lipomas typically enhance with gadolinium, the signal may be difficult to distinguish from bone marrow enhancement on postcontrast T1 images. MRI may also allow visualization of the neurovascular structures traversing the body (versus the periphery) of the tumor and can be a distinguishing feature. In challenging cases, chemically selective fat-suppression sequences can allow differentiation from other CPA pathology.

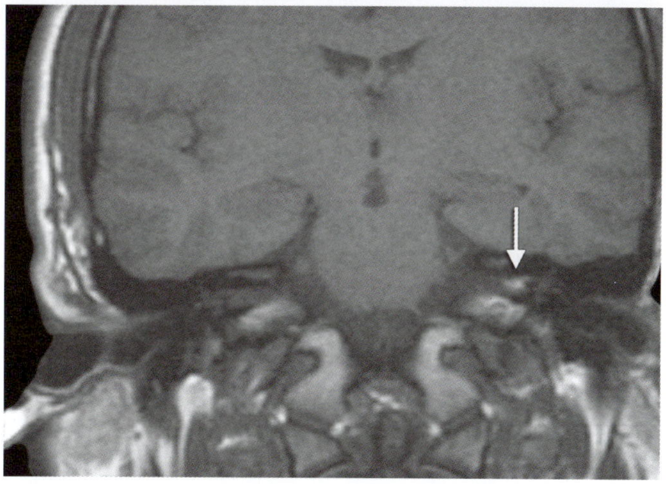

Fig. 24.10: Lipoma of the internal auditory canal. Axial T1-weighted precontrast magnetic resonance imaging (MRI) image with white arrow indicating lesion. Note that unlike most other cerebellopontine angle (CPA) pathology, this lesion is hyperintense on pregadolinium T1 images.

Treatment

Pathogenic features described above make observation the primary treatment modality for CPA lipomas. Their dense adherence to neurovascular structures of the CPA make hearing loss and FN injury common sequelae of surgical excision. Published reports demonstrate hearing loss and FN paresis/paralysis in most patients subjected to surgical removal.[67] Supported by very low growth rates and lack of malignant transformation, expectant management with serial imaging is now a well-documented, low-morbidity treatment of CPA lipomas.[68] In rare cases of significant growth or progressive CN/neurologic dysfunction, subtotal surgical resection may be considered. Approach for surgical excision is often guided by preoperative audiologic baseline and may proceed via hearing or nonhearing preservation approaches. At present, GKS does not have a role in treatment of CPA lipomas.

HEMANGIOMAS

Pathogenesis

Benign hamartomatous lesions arising from blood vessels, hemangiomas are characterized as capillary or cavernous.

They are extremely rare, accounting for < 0.01% of CPA tumors. Capillary hemangiomas have a predilection for the perigeniculate capillary plexus, while cavernous are more common in the IAC/CPA. For reasons that are not fully understood, they often cause symptoms of hearing loss and facial paresis more rapidly than other CPA lesions and at a comparatively smaller size. Data suggest that most, if not all, untreated patients with hemangiomas of the CPA will progress to complete CN dysfunction of VII and VIII.[69]

Imaging

Capillary hemangiomas can be suspected when CT demonstrates bone erosion, calcium deposits or spiculated bone surrounding the geniculate ganglion. Cavernous hemangiomas of the CPA are rarely calcified. MRI features are similar to that of VS and meningiomas with hypo- or intermediate intensity on T1 images, hyperintensity on T2 and enhancement with gadolinium (Fig. 24.11) Facial paresis/paralysis in the presence of a small IAC or perigeniculate tumor should raise suspicion for a hemangioma.

Treatment

Overall, published data advocates surgical excision with complete or gross total resection.[69,70] This can be accomplished via a hearing preservation (MCF, RS) or non-hearing preservation approach (TL) depending on level of residual hearing at the time of intervention. Intraoperatively, meticulous sharp dissection of CN is advocated to carefully separate the dense tumor attachments and many authors report preservation of neural continuity. Due to the rarity of these extra-axial lesions, scant published data exist on observation or stereotactic radiosurgery for hemangiomas of the CPA. Radiosurgery has been used to successfully treat hemangiomas of the cavernous sinus as well as brain stem and other intra-axial cavernomas; however, this experience has not yet been extrapolated to hemangiomas of the temporal bone.

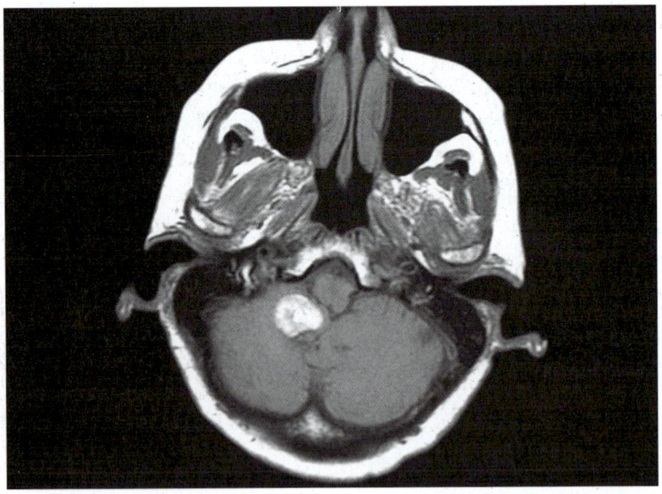

Fig. 24.11: Cerebellopontine angle (CPA) cavernoma. Axial T1-weighted gadolinium-enhanced magnetic resonance imaging (MRI) demonstrating a cavernous hemangioma of the posterior fossa and CPA.

METASTATIC LESIONS

Pathogenesis

Primary malignant neoplasms from other sites may uncommonly metastasize to the CPA via hematogenous spread. Overall, the most common CNS metastases arise from cancer of the breast, lung, melanoma and lymphoma, in decreasing frequency, although all are rare in the CPA.[71] In fact, data suggests that the coexistence of a known extracranial malignancy and an isolated CPA mass should not presume metastatic disease. In particular, a unifocal CPA tumor in a woman with breast cancer is more likely to be a meningioma than metastatic disease.[72]

Malignant melanoma has a predilection for metastasis to the CNS, likely due to the melanin producing cells within the leptomeninges (pia and arachnoid). Metastatic CNS melanoma can be multifocal with lesions in both the brain and spine as well as diffuse with widespread meningeal involvement. Isolated metastatic disease to the CPA is exceedingly rare with an incidence of <1%.[73] Brackmann and Doherty reviewed the House Ear clinic experience and found 8/6500 CPA lesions to be melanoma (incidence of 0.12%).[73] Of these, many were bilateral and occurred many years after primary melanoma diagnosis. Diagnosis can be challenging, but may be caught with CSF analysis for malignant cells and unique imaging characteristics.

For these rare CPA lesions, the symptom constellation or onset may occasionally be suggestive (although not diagnostic) of pathology. For example, patients with malignant or metastatic disease often present with more rapid and severe symptom progression compared with other CPA lesions.[36,73]

Imaging

Metastases may present as a CPA mass or with leptomeningeal carcinomatosis, typically characterized as a "seeding" or a multiple enhancing lesion pattern on postcontrast MRI images. The MRI appearance of CPA metastasis is variable and can mimic more common CPA lesions such as VS or meningioma (i.e. hypointensity on T1, hypo- or hyperintensity on T2 and enhancement with gadolinium) (Fig. 24.12). Unique features signaling malignancy include indistinct brain–tumor interface (signifying tumor invasion) and/or significant peritumoral edema of the surrounding brain, best seen as increased intensity on T2 images. Suspected malignancy warrants a thorough total body evaluation, with specific attention to areas of common primaries (i.e. breast, lung, and liver) as well as a CSF analysis for malignant cells.

Treatment

Unlike the previously discussed non-VS tumors of the CPA, treatment of metastatic lesions is multimodality, including surgical extirpation, radiation therapy or stereotactic radiosurgery, and/or chemo- or immunotherapy. Surgical intervention may be indicated for tissue diagnosis or, in cases of isolated intracranial metastasis (i.e. CSF negative for malignant cells), complete tumor excision. As with other CPA masses, surgical approach may be influenced by multiple factors, including hearing status and tumor location. Both resection and radiosurgery of isolated CPA metastasis have been shown to improve survival.[73]

INTRA-AXIAL LESIONS

Intra-axial lesions may extend into the CPA from their primary site of origin, including the brain stem (gliomas), cerebellum (hemangioblastomas, medulloblastoma from the vermis or astrocytoma from the peduncles), or the fourth ventricle [choroid plexus papillomas (CPPs) and ependymomas]. In general, intra-axial lesions may be identified by the lack of CSF between the tumor and adjacent brain parenchyma. Unlike extra-axial lesions, which cause mass effect on the cerebellum and brain stem, these lesions narrow the CPA cistern.[16] Like metastatic lesions, treatment of intra-axial pathology is multidisciplinary and commonly involves multiple modalities. Stereotactic biopsy may be employed to gain tissue diagnosis prior to initiation of definitive treatment. Depending on pathology, a variable combination of surgical excision, stereotactic radiosurgery, or chemo- or immunotherapy is employed.[74] For intra-axial lesions, survival rates depend largely on pathology with medulloblastoma greatly exceeding that of brain stem gliomas.[74] Imaging characteristics and treatment considerations unique to each pathology are briefly described below.

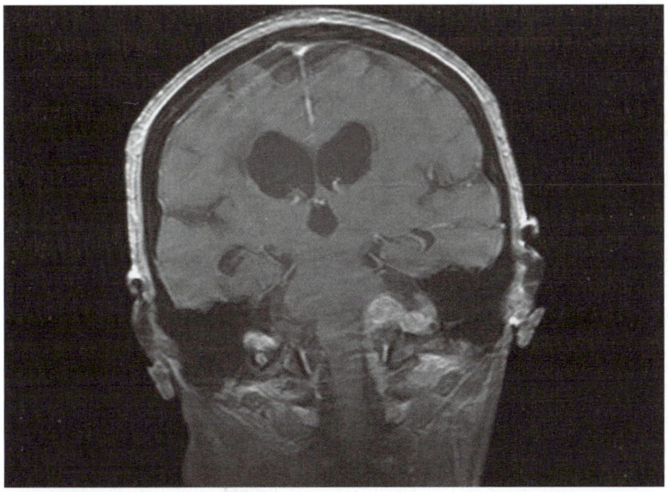

Fig. 24.12: Cerebellopontine angle (CPA) metastasis. Coronal T1-weighted gadolinium enhanced magnetic resonance imaging (MRI) demonstrating renal cell carcinoma metastasis to the cerebellopontine angle.

Gliomas

Brainstem gliomas are the most common CPA lesion in children and represent a diverse group of astrocytic tumors with variable outcome. Exophytic gliomas may extend into the CPA from their origin on the surface of the pons, while intrinsic, diffuse gliomas may enlarge within the brain stem itself. Unlike other CPA lesions, intra-axial brain stem gliomas are more likely to present with cerebellar and long tract signs instead of the typical CPA symptoms of hearing loss or imbalance. On T2-weighted MRI images, diffuse signal intensity may extending up and down the brain stem with inconsistent enhancement onT1 postcontrast images. Overall, surgical goals are diagnosis and re-establishment of CSF pathways and, depending on tumor location, may not always include significant tumor resection. Diffuse gliomas are generally treated with external beam radiotherapy; hyperfractionated radiation dosing and addition of chemotherapy have not shown a survival advantage. Prognosis is variable, but generally poor with median survival of 1 year.[75]

Medulloblastomas

Medulloblastomas are intrinsic cerebellar lesions arising from the superficial granular layer of the cerebellar folia. The most prevalent malignant CNS tumor in children, they are highly aggressive with frequent metastasis and early local invasion.[76] They are most commonly diagnosed between 5 and 10 years of age and appear to have a slight male predominance. In general, hearing loss is uncommon with primary cerebellar lesions such as medulloblastoma. These patients commonly present with imbalance (versus vertigo) and often have shorter symptom duration of days or months (versus years with VS or meningiomas).[77] Many children present with symptoms of increased intracranial pressure due to tumor growth into the subarachnoid space and fourth ventricle causing obstructive hydrocephalus.[77] Histopathologically, their features typify primitive neuroectodermal tumors and consist of densely packed, poorly differentiated, small, blue cells. On MRI, heterogenous enhancement with cystic changes on postcontrast T1 images is more common than with VS or meningiomas. Leptomeningeal spread may also be seen. Treatment involves surgical extirpation with the goal of removing > 75% of tumor mass and re-establishing CSF drainage pathways followed by chemoradiation. Treatment decision making is complex and coordinated, multidisciplinary neuro-oncoloigc management is credited with improved survival, up to 70% at 5 years.[78]

Choroid Plexus Papillomas and Ependymomas

CPPs and ependymomas arise from similar regions within the fourth ventricle and may represent variants of a common papillary tumor. Like other posterior fossa intra-axial tumors, they are more common in children than adults; CPP is most common in newborns and those under 2 years of age. Both reach the CPA by extension through the foramen of Luschka, leading to early intracranial hypertension in nearly all cases. Because they affect the apex of the CPA first, they can also produce early audiovestibular symptoms. On CT, calcification is common while cystic changes are rare. MRI characteristics are similar to more common CPA pathology with hypo- or isointensity on T1 images and homogenous enhancement with gadolinium. Treatment of these tumors differs with gross total resection rarely possible in ependymomas and curative in CPP. Ependymomas are commonly treated with adjuvant radiation, while the role for chemoradiation in CPP is unclear. Survival rates following multidisciplinary treatment may reach 80% at 10 years.[79]

Hemangioblastomas

Intracranially, hemangioblastomas originate in the blood vessels of the cerebellum, but they can also be multifocal, often with a concurrent retinal tumor. Although they may be associated with von Hippel–Lindau (VHL) disease, most are sporadic. Genetic testing to confirm loss of the tumor suppressor VHL gene on chromosome 3 is available and encouraged in diagnosis.[80] As with other intra-axial lesions, ataxia and increased ICP are more common than hearing loss or vertigo. On CT and MRI, hemangioblastomas are vascular, cystic, and enhance with contrast. Flow voids related to their increased vascularity may be a distinguishing feature on MRI. Angiographic embolization followed by surgical resection is the mainstay of treatment with an adjuvant chemotherapy and stereotactic radiation playing a role in recurrent disease and VHL-associated tumors.

CONCLUSION

There is a variety of non-VS lesions of the CPA, including meningioma, epidermoid, arachnoid cyst, facial and other CN schwannomas, metastatic disease, and primary intra-axial lesions. If symptomatic, complaints related to the structures of the CPA, namely the nerves of hearing and balance, are most common, although patients may manifest a variety of intracranial symptoms. Differentiation between tumor pathology using presentation, physical examination, or audiovestibular testing is challenging. Current practice recognizes MRI as the most efficient and effective method to diagnose CPA pathology. Once diagnosed, a variety of treatment options may be employed, including observation, surgery, or stereotactic radiosurgery.

REFERENCES

1. Shulev Y, Trashin A, Gordienko K. Secondary trigeminal neuralgia in cerebellopontine angle tumors. Skull Base. 2011;21(5):287-94.
2. Son DW, Choi CH, Cha SH. Epidermoid tumors in the cerebellopontine angle presenting with trigeminal neuralgia. J Korean Neurosurg Soc. 2010;47(4):271-7.
3. Prasher DK, Tun T, Brookes GB, et al. Mechanisms of hearing loss in acoustic neuroma: an otoacoustic emission study. Acta Otolaryngol. 1995;115(3):375-81.
4. Turner RG, Shepard NT, Frazer GJ. Clinical performance of audiological and related diagnostic tests. Ear Hear. 1984;5(4):187-94.
5. Rupa V, Job A, George M, et al. Cost-effective initial screening for vestibular schwannoma: auditory brainstem response or magnetic resonance imaging? Otolaryngol Head Neck Surg. 2003;128(6):823-8.
6. Bozorg Grayeli A, Refass A, Smail M, et al. Diagnostic value of auditory brainstem responses in cerebellopontine angle tumours. Acta Otolaryngol. 2008;128(10):1096-100.

7. Fortnum H, O'Neill C, Taylor R, et al. The role of magnetic resonance imaging in the identification of suspected acoustic neuroma: a systematic review of clinical and cost effectiveness and natural history. Health Technol Assess. 2009;13(18):iii-iv, ix-xi, 1-154.
8. Mobley SR, Odabasi O, Ahsan S, et al. Distortion-product otoacoustic emissions in nonacoustic tumors of the cerebellopontine angle. Otolaryngol Head Neck Surg. 2002;126 (2):115-20.
9. Baguley DM, Beynon GJ, Grey PL, et al. Audio-vestibular findings in meningioma of the cerebello-pontine angle: a retrospective review. J Laryngol Otol. 1997; 111(11):1022-6.
10. McMonagle B, Al-Sanosi A, Croxson G, et al. Facial schwannoma: results of a large case series and review. J Laryngol Otol. 2008;122(11):1139-50.
11. Soffer D, Pittaluga S, Feiner M, et al. Intracranial meningiomas following low-dose irradiation to the head. J Neurosurg. 1983;59(6):1048-53.
12. Harrison MJ, Wolfe DE, Lau TS, et al. Radiation-induced meningiomas: experience at the Mount Sinai Hospital and review of the literature. J Neurosurg. 1991;75(4):564-74.
13. Seizinger BR, de la Monte S, Atkins L, et al. Molecular genetic approach to human meningioma: loss of genes on chromosome 22. Proc Natl Acad Sci U S A. 1987;84(15):5419-23.
14. Perry A, Cai DX, Scheithauer BW, et al. Merlin, DAL-1, and progesterone receptor expression in clinicopathologic subsets of meningioma: a correlative immunohistochemical study of 175 cases. J Neuropathol Exp Neurol. 2000;59(10):872-9.
15. Patel NP, Mhatre AN, Lalwani AK. Molecular pathogenesis of skull base tumors. Otol Neurotol. 2004;25(4):636-43.
16. Lakshmi M, Glastonbury CM. Imaging of the cerebellopontine angle. Neuroimaging Clin N Am. 2009;19(3):393-406.
17. Hallinan JT, Hegde AN, Lim WE. Dilemmas and diagnostic difficulties in meningioma. Clin Radiol. 2013;68(8):837-44.
18. Engelhard HH. Progress in the diagnosis and treatment of patients with meningiomas. Part I: diagnostic imaging, preoperative embolization. Surg Neurol. 2001;55(2):89-101.
19. Ginsberg LE. Radiology of meningiomas. J Neurooncol. 1996;29(3):229-38.
20. Maier H, Ofner D, Hittmair A, et al. Classic, atypical, and anaplastic meningioma: three histopathological subtypes of clinical relevance. J Neurosurg. 1992;77(4): 616-23.
21. Voss NF, Vrionis FD, Heilman CB, et al. Meningiomas of the cerebellopontine angle. Surg Neurol. 2000;53(5):439-46; discussion 46-7.
22. Batra PS, Dutra JC, Wiet RJ. Auditory and facial nerve function following surgery for cerebellopontine angle meningiomas. Arch Otolaryngol Head Neck Surg. 2002;128(4): 369-74.
23. Schaller B, Heilbronner R, Pfaltz CR, et al. Preoperative and postoperative auditory and facial nerve function in cerebellopontine angle meningiomas. Otolaryngol Head Neck Surg. 1995;112(2):228-34.
24. Danner C, Cueva RA. Extended middle fossa approach to the petroclival junction and anterior cerebellopontine angle. Otol Neurotol. 2004;25(5):762-8.
25. Siwanuwatn R, Deshmukh P, Figueiredo EG, et al. Quantitative analysis of the working area and angle of attack for the retrosigmoid, combined petrosal, and transcochlear approaches to the petroclival region. J Neurosurg. 2006;104 (1):137-42.
26. Thedinger BA, Glasscock ME, 3rd, Cueva RA. Transcochlear transtentorial approach for removal of large cerebellopontine angle meningiomas. Am J Otol. 1992;13(5):408-15.
27. Angeli SI, De la Cruz A, Hitselberger W. The transcochlear approach revisited. Otol Neurotol. 2001;22(5):690-5.
28. Starke RM, Nguyen JH, Rainey J, et al. Gamma Knife surgery of meningiomas located in the posterior fossa: factors predictive of outcome and remission. J Neurosurg. 2011; 114(5):1399-409.
29. Sheehan JP, Starke RM, Mathieu D, et al. Gamma Knife radiosurgery for the management of nonfunctioning pituitary adenomas: a multicenter study. J Neurosurg. 2013.
30. Herscovici Z, Rappaport Z, Sulkes J, et al. Natural history of conservatively treated meningiomas. Neurology. 2004;63 (6):1133-4.
31. Nagasawa D, Yew A, Safaee M, et al. Clinical characteristics and diagnostic imaging of epidermoid tumors. J Clin Neurosci. 2011;18(9):1158-62.
32. Niikawa S, Hara A, Zhang W, et al. Proliferative assessment of craniopharyngioma and epidermoid by nucleolar organizer region staining. Childs Nerv Syst. 1992;8(8):453-6.
33. Berhouma M, Bahri K, Jemel H, et al. Intracerebral epidermoid tumor: pathogenesis of intraparenchymal location and magnetic resonance imaging findings. J Neuroradiol. 2006;33(4):269-70.
34. Forghani R, Farb RI, Kiehl TR, et al. Fourth ventricle epidermoid tumor: radiologic, intraoperative, and pathologic findings. Radiographics. 2007;27(5):1489-94.
35. Sener RN, Mechl M, Prokes B, et al. Epidermoid tumor of the pons. J Neuroradiol. 2004;31(3):225-6.
36. Chon KH, Lee JM, Koh EJ, et al. Malignant transformation of an epidermoid cyst in the cerebellopontine angle. J Korean Neurosurg Soc. 2012;52(2):148-51.
37. Raghunathan A, Barber SM, Takei H, et al. Primary intracranial sarcomatoid carcinoma arising from a recurrent/ residual epidermoid cyst of the cerebellopontine angle: a case report. Am J Surg Pathol. 2011;35(8):1238-43.
38. Hao S, Tang J, Wu Z, et al. Natural malignant transformation of an intracranial epidermoid cyst. J Formos Med Assoc. 2010;109(5):390-6.
39. Dutt SN, Mirza S, Chavda SV, et al. Radiologic differentiation of intracranial epidermoids from arachnoid cysts. Otol Neurotol. 2002;23(1):84-92.
40. Michael LM, 2nd, Moss T, Madhu T, et al. Malignant transformation of posterior fossa epidermoid cyst. Br J Neurosurg. 2005;19(6):505-10.
41. Hamlat A, Hua ZF, Saikali S, et al. Malignant transformation of intra-cranial epithelial cysts: systematic article review. J Neurooncol. 2005;74(2):187-94.
42. Timmer FA, Sluzewski M, Treskes M, et al. Chemical analysis of an epidermoid cyst with unusual CT and MR characteristics. AJNR Am J Neuroradiol. 1998;19(6):1111-2.

43. Schiefer TK, Link MJ. Epidermoids of the cerebellopontine angle: a 20-year experience. Surg Neurol. 2008;70(6):584-90; discussion 90.
44. Miller ME, Mastrodimos B, Cueva RA. Hearing preservation in management of epidermoids of the cerebellopontine angle: CPA epidermoids and hearing preservation. Otol Neurotol. 2012;33(9):1599-603.
45. Tuchman A, Platt A, Winer J, et al. Endoscopic-assisted resection of intracranial epidermoid tumors. World Neurosurg. 2013.
46. Nagasawa D, Yew A, Spasic M, et al. Survival outcomes for radiotherapy treatment of epidermoid tumors with malignant transformation. J Clin Neurosci. 2012;19(1):21-6.
47. Falcioni M, Russo A, Taibah A, et al. Facial nerve tumors. Otol Neurotol. 2003;24(6):942-7.
48. Mowry S, Hansen M, Gantz B. Surgical management of internal auditory canal and cerebellopontine angle facial nerve schwannoma. Otol Neurotol. 2012;33(6):1071-6.
49. O'Reilly BF, Mehanna H, Kishore A, et al. Growth rate of non-vestibular intracranial schwannomas. Clin Otolaryngol Allied Sci. 2004;29(1):94-7.
50. Kim CS, Chang SO, Oh SH, et al. Management of intratemporal facial nerve schwannoma. Otol Neurotol. 2003;24(2):312-6.
51. Kida Y, Yoshimoto M, Hasegawa T. Radiosurgery for facial schwannoma. J Neurosurg. 2007;106(1):24-9. Epub 2007/01/24.
52. Madhok R, Kondziolka D, Flickinger JC, et al. Gamma knife radiosurgery for facial schwannomas. Neurosurgery. 2009;64(6):1102-5; discussion 5.
53. Atmakuri M, Garritano FG, Kanekar SG, et al. Radiology quiz case 1: suspected arachnoid cyst of the right cerebellopontineangle. JAMA Otolaryngol Head Neck Surg. 2013;139(5):519-21.
54. Krisht AF, O'Brien MS. Acquired mirror-image cerebellopontine angle arachnoid cysts: case report. Neurosurgery. 1992;30(5):798-800.
55. Helland CA, Lund-Johansen M, Wester K. Location, sidedness, and sex distribution of intracranial arachnoid cysts in a population-based sample. J Neurosurg. 2010;113(5):934-9.
56. Pappas DG, Brackmann DE. Arachnoid cysts of the posterior fossa. Otolaryngol Head Neck Surg. 1981;89(2):328-32.
57. Erdincler P, Kaynar MY, Bozkus H, et al. Posterior fossa arachnoid cysts. Br J Neurosurg. 1999;13(1):10-7.
58. Olaya JE, Ghostine M, Rowe M, et al. Endoscopic fenestration of a cerebellopontine angle arachnoid cyst resulting in complete recovery from sensorineural hearing loss and facial nerve palsy. J Neurosurg Pediatr. 2011;7(2):157-60.
59. Pradilla G, Jallo G. Arachnoid cysts: case series and review of the literature. Neurosurg Focus. 2007;22(2):E7.
60. Samii M, Carvalho GA, Schuhmann MU, et al. Arachnoid cysts of the posterior fossa. Surg Neurol. 1999;51(4):376-82.
61. Ottaviani F, Neglia CB, Scotti A, et al. Arachnoid cyst of the cranial posterior fossa causing sensorineural hearing loss and tinnitus: a case report. Eur Arch Otorhinolaryngol. 2002;259(6):306-8.
62. Jayarao M, Devaiah AK, Chin LS. Recovery of sensorineural hearing loss following operative management of a posterior fossa arachnoid cyst. Case report. J Neurosurg Pediatr. 2009;4(2):121-4.
63. Lanzino G, diPierro CG, Ruth RA, et al. Recovery of useful hearing after posterior fossa surgery: the role of otoacoustic emissions: case report. Neurosurgery. 1997;41(2):469-72; discussion 72-3.
64. Ashkenasi A, Royal SA, Cuffe MJ, et al. Cerebellopontine angle lipoma in a teenager. Pediatr Neurol. 1990;6(4):272-4.
65. Christensen WN, Long DM, Epstein JI. Cerebellopontine angle lipoma. Hum Pathol. 1986;17(7):739-43.
66. Dahlen RT, Johnson CE, Harnsberger HR, et al. CT and MR imaging characteristics of intravestibular lipoma. AJNR Am J Neuroradiol. 2002;23(8):1413-7.
67. Kitamura K, Futaki T, Miyoshi S. Fluctuating hearing loss in lipoma of the cerebellopontine angle. ORL J Otorhinolaryngol Relat Spec. 1990;52(5):335-9.
68. White JR, Carlson ML, Van Gompel JJ, et al. Lipomas of the cerebellopontine angle and internal auditory canal: Primum Non Nocere. Laryngoscope. 2013;123(6):1531-6.
69. Deshmukh VR, Albuquerque FC, Zabramski JM, Spetzler RF. Surgical management of cavernous malformations involving the cranial nerves. Neurosurgery. 2003;53(2):352-7; discussion 7.
70. Albanese A, Sturiale CL, D'Alessandris QG, et al. Calcified extra-axial cavernoma involving lower cranial nerves: technical case report. Neurosurgery. 2009;64 (3 Suppl):onsE135-6; discussion onsE6.
71. Warren FM, Shelton C, Wiggins RH, 3rd, et al. Imaging characteristics of metastatic lesions to the cerebellopontine angle. Otol Neurotol. 2008;29(6):835-8.
72. Swensen R, Kirsch W. Brain neoplasms in women: a review. Clin Obstet Gynecol. 2002;45(3):904-27.
73. Brackmann DE, Doherty JK. CPA melanoma: diagnosis and management. Otol Neurotol. 2007;28(4):529-37.
74. Spina A, Boari N, Gagliardi F, et al. Review of cerebellopontine angle medulloblastoma. Br J Neurosurg. 2013;27(3):316-20.
75. Grimm SA, Chamberlain MC. Brainstem glioma: a review. Curr Neurol Neurosci Rep. 2013;13(5):346.
76. Polkinghorn WR, Tarbell NJ. Medulloblastoma: tumorigenesis, current clinical paradigm, and efforts to improve risk stratification. Nat Clin Pract Oncol. 2007;4(5):295-304.
77. Crawford JR, MacDonald TJ, Packer RJ. Medulloblastoma in childhood: new biological advances. Lancet Neurol. 2007;6(12):1073-85.
78. Muzumdar D, Deshpande A, Kumar R, et al. Medulloblastoma in childhood-King Edward Memorial hospital surgical experience and review: Comparative analysis of the case series of 365 patients. J Pediatr Neurosci. 2011;6(Suppl 1):S78-85.
79. Wolff JE, Sajedi M, Brant R, Coppes MJ, Egeler RM. Choroid plexus tumours. Br J Cancer. 2002;87(10):1086-91.
80. Conway JE, Chou D, Clatterbuck RE, et al. Hemangioblastomas of the central nervous system in von Hippel-Lindau syndrome and sporadic disease. Neurosurgery. 2001;48(1):55-62; discussion -3.

CHAPTER

25

Jugular Bulb and Jugular Foramen in Ear Diseases

C Eduardo Corrales, John S Oghalai

INTRODUCTION/BACKGROUND

The jugular foramen is formed at the junction between the temporal and occipital bones, with the anterolateral wall arising from the petrous portion of the temporal bone and the posteromedial wall from the occipital bone. The jugular foramen courses anteriorly and laterally as it exits the skull base. Vital neural and vascular structures are contained within the jugular foramen including the sigmoid sinus, jugular bulb, inferior petrosal sinus (IPS), meningeal branches of the ascending pharyngeal and occipital arteries, and cranial nerves IX (glossopharyngeal nerve), X (vagus nerve), and XI (spinal accessory nerve). Classically, the jugular foramen has been described as containing an anteromedial portion (pars nervosa) and a larger posterolateral portion (pars vascularis).[1] However, the jugular foramen has recently been divided into three anatomic compartments[2]: a posterior division known as the *sigmoid compartment* receiving the sigmoid sinus; an anterior division known as the *petrous compartment* receiving the IPS; and the intermediate division known as the *neural intrajugular compartment* receiving cranial nerves IX, X, XI, and meningeal branches from the ascending pharyngeal and occipital arteries. After exiting the brainstem, CN IX, X, and XI ascend in a fan ventral to foramen of Luschka, choroid plexus, and flocculus, then complete a 90° turn inferiorly upon entering the jugular foramen. The lower cranial nerves IX, X, XI are located medial to the jugular vein. There is a fibrous septum separating CN IX from CN X and CN XI in over 86% of patients, and a complete bony septum in the remaining.[3] Within the jugular foramen, cranial nerve IX forms the inferior ganglion that gives rise to the auricular branch (Jacobsen's nerve), which ascends across the cochlear promontory to form a sensory plexus and the lesser superficial petrosal nerve. Likewise, cranial nerve X also forms a ganglion as it leaves the cranial vault and forms the auricular branch of the vagus nerve (Arnold's nerve), which provides sensory innervation to the posterior wall of the external auditory canal. The IPS, which commonly consists of multiple branches, is the main drainage site for the cavernous sinus and empties into the medial aspect of the jugular bulb (JB). The relationship between IPS and the lower cranial nerves is highly variable but often the IPS courses between CN IX anteriorly and CNs X and XI posteriorly.[4]

The jugular foramen is separated from the hypotympanum by a bony plate and is medial to the descending facial canal and inferomedial to the posterior semicircular canal. The jugular foramen is separated from the anteromedial carotid canal by the caroticojugular spine and from the inferomedial hypoglossal canal by the jugular tubercle. The size of the jugular foramen varies greatly, but averages 1.5 cm in length and 1.0 cm in width.[1] In two thirds of temporal bones analyzed, the right jugular foramen is larger than the left.[3] These anatomic landmarks will be important in understanding jugular foramen disorders (Figs. 25.1A and B).

The confluence of the lateral dural venous sinuses at the jugular fossa and the connecting conduit between the sigmoid sinus and the internal jugular vein is termed the jugular bulb (JB). The JB receives the venous outflow from the IPS that opens at its petrous compartment. The upper region of the bulb is rounded and frequently termed the "dome" of the JB. The development of the JB is highly variable

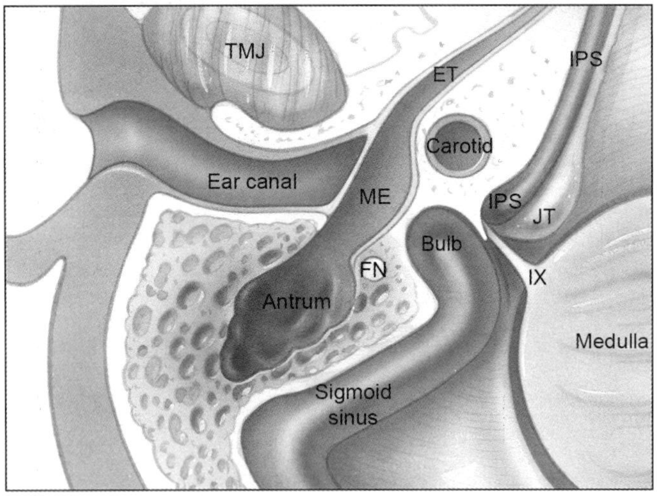

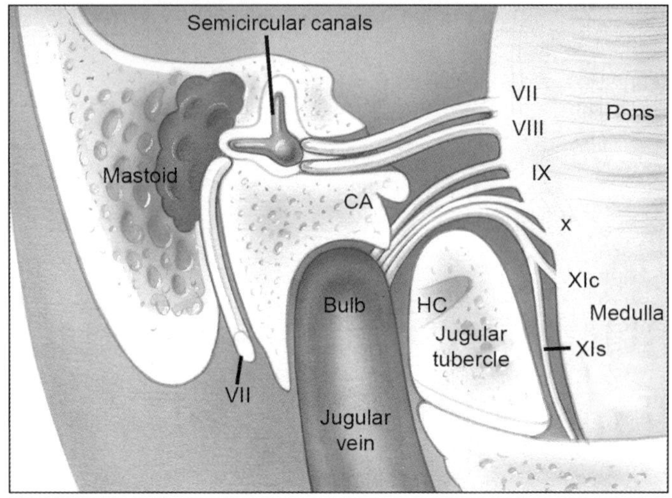

Figs. 25.1A and B: (A) Schematic drawing of the jugular foramen in axial view. (B) Schematic drawing of the jugular foramen in coronal view. Copyright RK Jackler and C Gralapp, Stanford University.

and is directly related to both embryology and postnatal development of the brain coupled with hemodynamic changes in intracranial circulation. The JB varies greatly with regard to its size, location, and shape. At birth, the JB is absent, followed by bulbous enlargement starting at around 2 years of age with continued enlargement into adulthood, and remaining stable in the elderly.[5] This observation suggests that abnormalities of the JB are acquired rather than congenital in origin, and may insinuated that venous blood flow dynamics determine the ultimate size and position of the JB with its potential for abnormal development.[5] The JB is right-sided venous dominant in over 70% of cases studied.[5,6] Similar to other venous structures, anatomical variations and developmental abnormalities are seen with the JB and mainly consist of JB dehiscence, high-riding JB, and JB diverticulum. Tissue types found in the territory of the jugular foramen include nerve, vessel, bone, fibrocartilage, mucosa, and paraganglia. Disorders can arise from any of these structures. Additionally, the relationship and significance of the jugular foramen to the deep fascial planes of the neck are extremely important. Both infections and tumors in these spaces can track cephalad along these potential spaces. The middle layer of the deep cervical fascia (buccopharyngeal fascia) lies anteromedially, the deep layer of the deep cervical fascia (prevertebral fascia) lies posterolaterally, and the superficial layer of the deep cervical fascia lies laterally.[7]

DEVELOPMENTAL AND STRUCTURAL ABNORMALITIES OF THE JUGULAR BULB

Jugular bulb abnormalities consist mainly of high-riding jugular bulb (HRJB) and jugular bulb diverticulum (JBD). Jugular bulb abnormalities are not uncommon, with a reported incidence ranging from 6% to 34% for HRJB, and 1% to 8% for JBD.[8,9] A HRJB has been defined if it rises to the level of the basal turn of the cochlea,[10] if the dome of the bulb encroaches within 2 mm of the floor of the internal auditory canal,[11] or if the bulb extends above the inferior border of the tympanic annulus.[12] A JBD is an irregular vessel outpouching or bulge that may project into the middle ear cavity, mastoid cavity, or medially toward the petrous apex.[13] The prevalence of JB abnormalities increases during the first 4 decades of life and plateaus thereafter. Both HRJB and JBD can erode into neighboring structures of the middle ear, inner ear, and mastoid. In a recent study of over 1,500 temporal bone specimens, the incidence of HRJB and JBD involving the tympanic cavity was 1% occurring with similar frequency among men and women.[9] Erosion of the inner ear by HRJB and JBD is rare and likely under-reported, but an incidence of 1–3% has been reported for HRJB eroding into the inner ear.[14,15] Jugular bulb abnormalities most commonly erode into the vestibular aqueduct, followed by vertical segment of the facial nerve and posterior semicircular canal.[14] Interestingly, two-thirds of the dehiscence was on right venous dominant side, suggesting that blood flow dynamics may be critical in the etiology of JB abnormalities.

Clinical Manifestations

Jugular bulb abnormalities including HRJB and JBD may present with a multitude clinical symptoms including hearing loss, pulsatile tinnitus, and vertigo.[14] In most patients, jugular bulb-mediated inner ear dehiscence was clinically and radiologically silent.[15] In a published series of 30 patients, jugular bulb-mediated inner ear dehiscence was associated with multiple clinical symptoms including hearing loss, pulsatile tinnitus, and vertigo.[14] Equally important, almost half of these patients with radiologically demonstrated inner ear dehiscence were asymptomatic. Common clinical findings of jugular foramen pathology are described in Table 25.1.

Diagnostic Studies

Patients presenting with hearing loss (conductive or sensorineural), vertigo or pulsatile tinnitus or tonal tinnitus could undertake imaging studies. High-resolution computer tomography (HRCT) and or magnetic resonance imaging (MRI) are critical to assess external, middle, and inner ear anatomy. High-resolution computer tomography can delineate bony abnormalities and MRI is useful to evaluate asymmetric hearing loss. High-resolution computer tomography is often sufficient for the diagnosis of JBA and imaging should focus on bony integrity of the jugular bulb, vestibular aqueduct, and vertical segment of the facial nerve. Contrast-enhanced MRI supplements the HRCT, as it provides critical information regarding course, caliber, and patency of the transverse-sigmoid-jugular bulb-internal jugular venous system (Fig. 25.2)

Vestibular evoked myogenic potentials (VEMP) responses can be obtained should the imaging demonstrate

Table 25.1: Common clinical findings in jugular foramen tumors

Region	*Test*	*Findings*
Ear	Otoscopy-Paragangliomas	Red, pulsatile retrotympanic mass
		Bruit audible with a stethoscope
		Brown's sign: a decrease in apparent size and redness of the middle ear mass upon application of positive pressure with a pneumatic otoscope; in our experience, positive pressure increases the apparent tumor size as the tympanic membrane drapes over the tumor
	Otoscopy-Schwannoma and meningioma	Usually normal
		Pale, nonpulsatile retrotympanic mass
	Audiologic testing	Conductive, sensorineural, or mixed hearing loss
		Pulse-synchronous excursions of tympanic membrane on impedance testing
Eye	Eye movement	Nystagmus
	Lid	Ptosis-Horner's syndrome
	Visual acuity	Decrease color vision, visual acuity, and papilledema from increase intracranial pressure
Throat	Oral cavity	Unilateral failure to elevate palate
		Pharyngeal anesthesia or unilateral decrease gag reflex
		Tongue weakness or atrophy
		Bulging tonsillar fossa suggestive of parapharyngeal space component
	Laryngoscopy	True vocal cord paresis or palsy
Face	Facial tone	Facial weakness or spasm
	Facial sensation	Sensory disturbance
	Masticatory muscle tone	Loss of masticatory muscle tone
Neck	Neck palpation	Parotid or carotid triangle fullness
	Muscle tone	Trapezius or SCM muscle weakness or atrophy

Source: Adapted from Rigby PL, Jackler RK. Clinicopathologic presentation and diagnostic imaging of jugular foramen tumors. Oper Tech Head Neck Surg. 1996;7:99-105.

JB-related inner ear dehiscence. In these patients, the VEMP test shows decrease in thresholds similar to superior canal dehiscence syndrome consistent with third window effect.[16]

Treatment

Most patients should be managed conservatively with serial imaging, but treatment options include decompression, embolization, resurfacing, and ligation.[9,17]

JUGULAR FORAMEN PARAGANGLIOMAS

Paragangliomas or glomus tumors are uncommon neoplasms of the temporal bone that comprise small lesions limited to the middle ear to extensive lesions involving the skull base. Over 90% of the paragangliomas are detected in the adrenal gland and are termed pheochromocytomas. The remaining 10% of paragangliomas are found in extra-adrenal sites including abdomen, thorax, and the head and neck region. Approximately 3% of paragangliomas are found in the head and neck region.[18] Of all head and neck tumors, 1 in 30,000, is a paraganglioma.[19] The most common paraganglioma in the head and neck region is the carotid body tumor, followed by paraganglioma of the JB (jugulare) and middle ear (tympanicum) and finally vagal paragangliomas.[20] Tympanic paragangliomas are the most common primary neoplasms of the middle ear[21] and jugular paragangliomas are the most common tumors of the jugular foramen.[22] This chapter focuses on paragangliomas of the JB (jugulare).

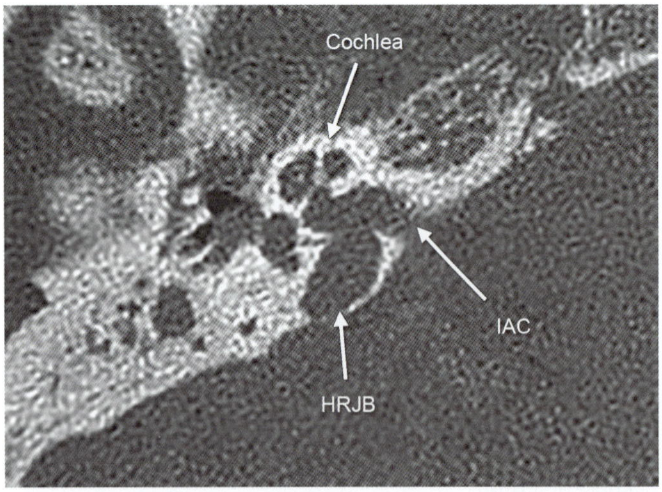

Fig. 25.2: High-resolution computed tomography (HRCT) of the right ear showing a high-riding jugular bulb (HRJB) at the level of the internal auditory canal (IAC).

History

It was Valentin in 1840 who first described the tympanic ganglion to Jacobsen's nerve in the middle ear.[23] The histological characterization of a glomus tumor was done by Stacy Guild in 1941 where he described the glomus jugulare as small formations in the adventitia of the dome of the JB along the tympanic branch (Jacobsen's nerve) of the glossopharyngeal nerve and the auricular branch (Arnold's nerve) of the vagus nerve.[24] Further descriptions and reports culminated with Alford and Guilford's publication in 1960 classifying glomus tumors into *glomus tympanicum* (tumors located in the middle ear) and *glomus jugulare* (tumors involving the JB and jugular foramen with extension into the middle ear). Since these initial descriptions, rapid advancements in genetics have augmented our understanding of paragangliomas in terms of responsible genes and risks assessment for tumors located outside the temporal bone.

Terminology

Many terms have been used to describe glomus tumors in the literature including paraganglioma, chemodectoma, glomus tumors, and nonchromaffin paraganglioma.[25] Originally, paragangliomas were termed "glomus" tumors because of the belief that the chief cells were derived from specialized pericytes as seen in true cutaneous arteriovenous (glomus) anastomosis tumors (glomangiomas). But these cutaneous tumors are unrelated to paragangliomas developmentally and functionally.[26,27] The term "nonchromaffin" paraganglioma derives from histologic examination of adrenal autonomic paraganglia that is intensely positive for chromium salts (staining used to determine the presence or absence of catecholamines), whereas extra-adrenal paraganglia does not stain with chromium salts, hence the term "nonchromaffin" paragangliomas.[25] A "chemodectoma" is an incorrect term since it inaccurately describes all paragangliomas of the head and neck region, but the only known paraganglia in the head and neck region to act as a chemoreceptor is the carotid body.[25]

Pathology

The paraganglion system constitutes chromaffin positive neural crest-derived cells that are located in extra-adrenal sites. The paraganglia in the human temporal bone are distributed along the auricular branch of the vagus nerve (Arnold's nerve) and the tympanic branch of the glossopharyngeal nerve (Jacobson's nerve). Approximately 70%

of paraganglia related to the vagus nerve occur on the jugular bulb. Paraganglia along the glossopharyngeal nerve occur anywhere from the origin of the nerve at the petrosal ganglion (10%) to the JB (28%), tympanic canaliculus (40%), promontory of the middle ear (20%), and beyond (2%). Paragangliomas of the JB may consequently be related with either the vagus or glossopharyngeal nerve, although the former is most likely. Paraganglioma tympanicums are almost always associated with the glossopharyngeal nerve (Jacobson's nerve) or rarely, the auricular branch of the vagus nerve (Arnold's nerve). Histologically, all sympathetic and parasympathetic paragangliomas are identical regardless of their site of origin. They display two types of cells that are arranged in a typical nest-like or alveolar architectural pattern: type I cells or chief cells are polygonal-shaped epithelioid cells often with enlarged hyperchromatic nuclei, abundant granular eosinophilic cytoplasm and arranged in solid groups called "Zellballen"[26] (Fig. 25.3A). Chief cells are derived from the neural crest and migrate closely with the autonomic ganglia of the sympathetic nervous system.[28] The chief cells are surrounded by a spindle-shaped basophilic type II cells or sustentacular cells, which are positive for staining with the S-100 protein and are homologous to satellite cells in the autonomic ganglia (Fig. 25.3B). Both type I and type II cells lie within a dense network of capillaries.[29] Chief cells may show nuclear pleomorphism and cellular hyperchromatism but should not be considered evidence of malignancy. Importantly, there are no histologic or immunohistochemical markers for the diagnosis of a malignant paraganglioma, and the only current criteria of malignancy is the presence of metastasis to nonneuroendocrine tissue.[30,31]

Pathogenesis

Baysal et al.[32] was the first to identify germ-line mutations of the succinate dehydrogenase subunit D gene (SDHD gene) as the underlying cause of paraganglioma syndrome 1 (PGL1) in the year 2000. Since then other mutations in the SDH complex have been discovered: Niemann et al.[33] described mutation in SDHC gene causing PGL3, and Astuti et al.[34] describing PGL4 as a mutation in the SDHB gene (Table 25.2). Mutations of SDHA do not predispose to the formation of paragangliomas but instead cause Leigh's disease, a form of encephalopathy.[35] Research has clearly demonstrated that mutations in SDHB, SDHD, and SDHC causes a loss of function of SDH resulting in a pseudohypoxic state and activation of hypoxic-inducible factors (HIFs) pathways that leads to accumulation of succinate and resulting inhibition of prolyl hydroxylase enzymes that are essential for proteosomal degradation of HIF-a subunits.[36] Currently, most of the head and neck paragangliomas are sporadic in nature, but up to 30% of these seemingly sporadic paragangliomas are due to genetic mutations.[37-40] The majority of these hereditary paragangliomas are due to PGL1, 3, and 4. Important for molecular screening, a study by Neumann et al. demonstrated a single mutation in a cohort of 598 patients with sporadic head and neck paragangliomas who were screened for all three mutations (SDHB, SDHC, and SDHD).[38] Compared to patients with sporadic paragangliomas of the head and neck, patients with PGL syndromes develop paragangliomas earlier in life as described by Burnichon et al.[41] They showed that in patients with PGL syndromes the average age at tumor diagnosis was 36 years compared to 50.2 years in patients with sporadic tumors. Furthermore,

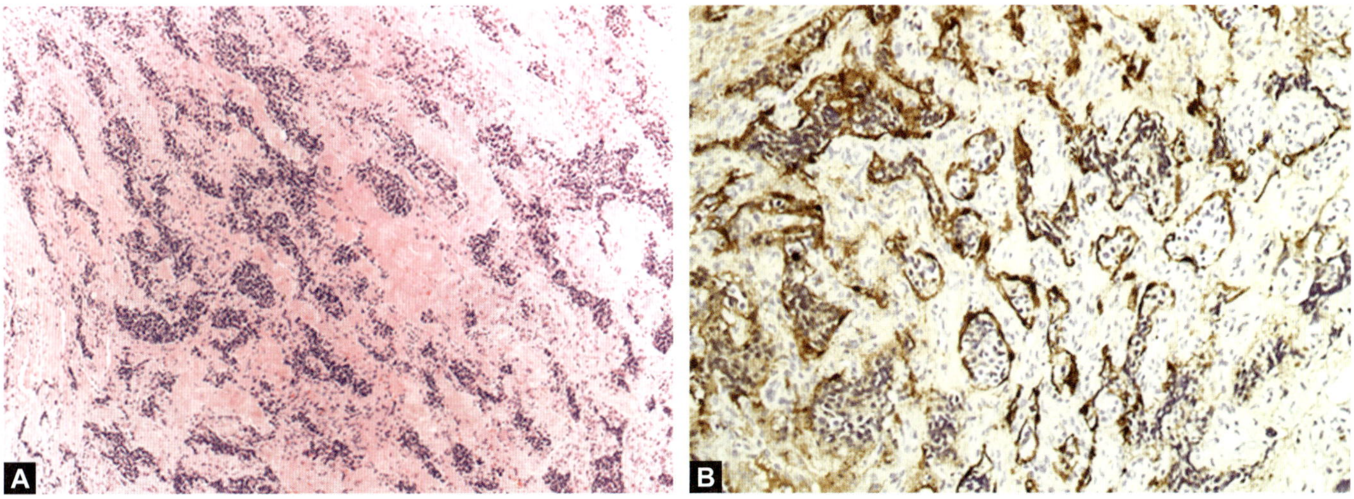

Figs. 25.3A and B: (A) Hematoxylin and eosin stain of a paraganglioma, 100x. (B) S-100 staining of a paraganglioma, 20x.

Table 25.2: Paraganglioma syndromes with their associated gene mutations. Syndrome characteristics are also shown

Syndrome	*Gene mutation*	*Characteristics*
PGL1	SDHD	Most common gene mutation, head and neck paraganglio-mas > pheochromocytomas, malignant potential
PGL2	SDHAF2 (SDH5)	Paraganglioma development
PGL3	SDHC	Develop benign single head and neck paraganglioma but 20% may have 2 PGs. Rare malignant potential
PGL4	SDHB	Develop pheochromocytomas > head and neck paraganglio-mas, high risk of malignancy

patients with PGL syndromes tend to have a higher risk of presenting with a malignant paragangliomas compared to patients with sporadic paragangliomas, but this is likely due to patients with the SDHB (PGL4) mutation who have a higher propensity to develop malignant paragangliomas compared to patients with sporadic or other PGL syndromes.[31,41]

Paraganglioma Syndrome 1 (PGL1)

Gene mutation: Baysal et al. first described the SDHD gene mutation causing PGL1.[32] PGL1 represents the most common PGL syndrome.

Mode of inheritance and penetrance: Autosomal dominant with a "parent-of-origin-dependent inheritance" since the syndrome is observed exclusively when the mutation is transmitted from the father.[42] However, SDHD mutation carriers who inherit the mutation through the maternal line will still pass the mutation to their offspring in 50% of the cases. Tumor penetrance in PGL1 is high as described by Neumann et al.[39] They reported that SDHD mutations conferred 50% penetrance by age 31 increasing to 86% by age 50. Hensen et al.[43] reported 54% penetrance at 40 years of age and increasing to 87% by age 70.

Multifocality and malignancy: In a literature review performed by Pasini and Stratakis,[44] they pooled 395 patients with the SDHD mutation. Out of the 395 patients with SDHD mutation, 91% had at least one head and neck paraganglioma and 79% had multiple head and neck paragangliomas. In a multicenter study performed by Neumann et al.,[38] 598 patients with apparently sporadic head and neck paragangliomas were screened for mutations of the genes SDHD, SDHB, and SDHC. Sixty percent of patients with the SDHD gene mutation presented with multiple head and neck paragangliomas. Malignant paragangliomas are frequently seen and can be as high as 10% of patients with SDHD mutation.[38]

Paraganglioma Syndrome 2 (PGL2)

Gene mutation: Hao et al. first described the SDH5 (also known as SDHAF2).[45]

Mode of inheritance and penetrance: similar to PGL1, PGL2 has an autosomal dominant inheritance pattern with a "parent-of-origin-dependent inheritance". There are only two reports in two families with this mutation. Tumor penetrance is high in both of these families.[35,45]

Patients with an isolated head and neck paraganglioma who do not have gene mutations in SDHD, SDHC, or SDHB should be analyzed for SDH5 gene mutation.[35]

Paraganglioma Syndrome 3 (PGL3)

Gene mutation: PGL3 is caused by a mutation in the SDHC gene.[33] These mutations are not as common as SDHD or SDHB. In the multicenter study by Neumann,[38] of a total of 598-pooled patients, 26 (4%) had a mutation in the SDHC gene.

Mode of inheritance and penetrance: autosomal dominant.[40,46] Tumor penetrance is low as reported by Neumann,[38] where the group described a positive pertinent family history in only 11.5% of the SDHC-positive patients.

Multifocality and malignancy: The majority of patients with SDHC gene mutation develop exclusively a single head and neck paraganglioma.[38,40] Malignant paragangliomas have been described but are very rare and no report has been described in either jugular or tympanic paragangliomas.[46]

Paraganglioma Syndrome 4 (PGL4)

Gene mutation: Astuti et al. first described that PGL4 is caused by a mutation in the SDHB gene.[34]

Mode of inheritance and penetrance: autosomal dominant.[34,38,39] Age-related tumor penetrance in patients with the SDHB mutation is 29% at 30 years and 45% at 40 years.[31,47]

Multifocality and malignancy: Patients with SDHB mutation develop head and neck paragangliomas and pheochromocytomas but compared to patients with SDHD mutation (PGL1), SDHB mutation carriers develop more pheochromocytomas than head and neck paragangliomas. In addition, patients with SDHB mutation develop less frequently multiple head and neck paragangliomas compared to PGL1 patients.[36,38,44,48]

Patients with PGL4 have a higher rate of malignancy in both head and neck paragangliomas and pheochromocytomas compared to all other PGL syndromes.[36,38,39,44,49] Pasini and Stratakis et al. performed a literature review on SDHB mutation carriers and showed a malignancy rate of 41% in both head and neck paragangliomas and pheochromocytomas.[44] Neumann et al.[38] showed malignant paraganglioma tumors in 13 out of 63 (20.6%) SDHB mutation carriers. Boedeker et al.[49] analyzed 195 head and neck paragangliomas for mutations of the genes *SDHC, SDCD,* and *SDHB*. He found 53.8% of the patients with SDHB mutation presented with a malignant head and neck paraganglioma, but only one patient had a jugular paraganglioma, while all others presented with a carotid body tumor. Additionally, patients with PGL4 have a high risk of developing renal carcinomas.[36,50]

Age at Presentation, Multifocality and Catecholamine Secretion

Paragangliomas may occur at any age, and most patients become symptomatic in adulthood between fourth and fifth decades of life. There is a clear earlier presentation in patients with PGL syndromes as described above. Female-to-male ratio of 3:1 to 4:1 has been reported.[21,31]

The majority of paragangliomas are solitary, but multiple or synchronous tumors occur in 3–10% of patients with the most common tumor combination being a carotid body tumor with an ipsilateral paraganglioma tympanicum.

Functional catecholamine secretion from paragangliomas of the head and neck region is reported to be 1–3%.[25,51] All paragangliomas have neurosecretory granules that contain catecholamines, though few tumors actually manifest with symptoms. Norepinephrine is the most common secreted catecholamine, but dopamine secretion has also been reported. Patients should specifically be asked about signs and symptoms of catecholamine secretion including excessive perspiration, hypertension, tachycardia, nervousness, weight loss, headaches, nausea, pallor, and flushing. Patients with above signs and symptoms should be evaluated with a plasma metanephrine level or a 24-hour urine collection measuring levels of norepinephrine and its metabolites including metanephrine and vanillylmandelic acid (VMA). Importantly, paragangliomas of the temporal bone are unable to convert norepinephrine to epinephrine due to lack of the enzyme phenylethanolamine-*N*-methyltransferase. Thus, if high levels of epinephrine or metanephrine are found, this should prompt suspicion for a concomitant adrenal pheochromocytoma and evaluated with an abdominal computer axial tomography scan. Preoperative screening for urinary metanephrines and VMA and serum catecholamines is indicated for glomus jugulare, carotid body tumors, multiple glomus tumors, and familial paragangliomas.

Malignancy and Occult Paragangliomas

Overall, <10% of all paragangliomas in the head and neck region are malignant. Of these, malignant jugulotympanic paragangliomas constitute 2–4%[49]; however, in our experience it is <1%. The presence of regional or distant metastasis to nonneuroendocrine tissues is the sole criteria to define a malignant paraganglioma. There are no histologic or immunohistochemical methods or markers yet available to determine paraganglioma malignancy. As mentioned above, patients with mutations in the SDHB gene have a higher likelihood of developing malignant paragangliomas.[49]

There is a high prevalence of occult paragangliomas in asymptomatic carriers of *SDHD* and *SDHB* gene mutations. As radiation therapy is increasingly being used for multiple benign tumors of the temporal bone including jugular paragangliomas, radiation-induced malignancies are being reported.[52] Though rare, these tumors have poor prognosis.

Clinical Manifestations and Growth Patterns

Jugular paragangliomas demonstrate a slow and insidious growth pattern. The time of onset of symptoms largely depends on site of origin of the paraganglioma. Otologic symptoms are the most common presenting complaints for both jugular and tympanic paraganglioma.

The three most common symptoms for both jugular and tympanic paragangliomas are pulsatile tinnitus, hearing loss, and otalgia.[21,53-56]

Tympanic paragangliomas have a tendency to present earlier than jugular paragangliomas due to close proximity and earlier involvement of the tympanic membrane with resultant pulsation transmission and subsequent conductive hearing loss.

Jugular paragangliomas are the most common lesions of the jugular foramen and tend to invade and migrate through vascular channels, fissures, and foramina of the temporal bone along paths of least resistance (Figs. 25.4A to C). Jugular paragangliomas have the potential to grow through the Eustachian tube to the nasopharynx, invade the petrous apex through the peritubal air cells or track through the petrous portion of the carotid artery and reach the middle cranial fossa and cavernous sinus. Superior extension into the hypotympanum is typical and the tumor can extend proximally within the lumen of the sigmoid sinus and distally into the upper portion of the jugular vein. Similar to tympanic paragangliomas, they can also erode out laterally through the tympanic membrane and into the external auditory canal. Patients with jugular paragangliomas may present with neurologic deficits and usually represents substantial tumor growth. Spector et al.[57] described the incidence of cranial nerve involvement by paraganglioma to be 37% and of intracranial extension of 15%. The facial nerve is usually involved by tumor at its mastoid segments as tumor growth proceeds laterally into the descending segment. As jugular paragangliomas extend into the jugular foramen, compression of cranial nerves IX, X, XI, and XII is possible. Patients may present with Horner's syndrome as the sympathetic plexus is compressed at the internal carotid artery. Common clinical findings of jugular foramen pathology are described in Table 25.1.

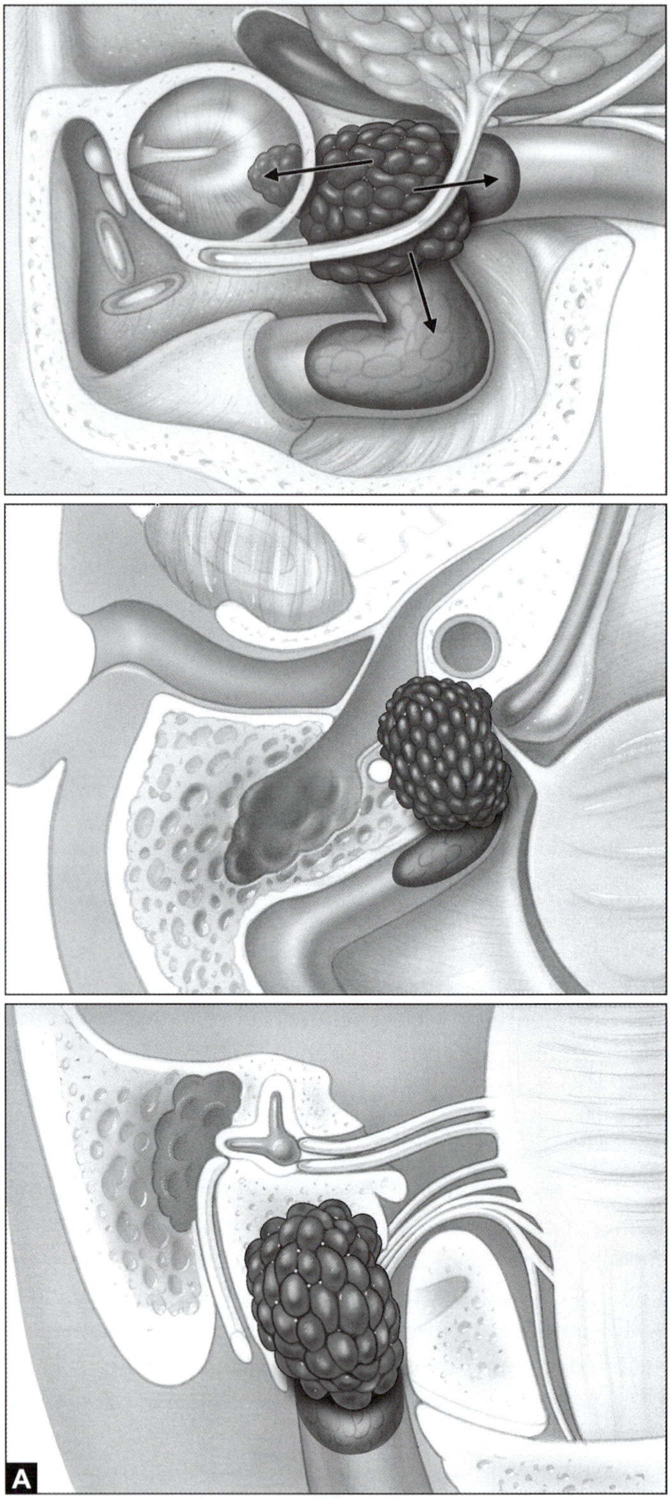

Fig. 25.4A: Jugular paraganglioma with typical extension into the hypotympanum. The tumor extends proximally within the lumen of the sigmoid sinus (coronal view), and distally into the upper portion of the jugular vein (sagittal view). Copyright RK Jackler and C Gralapp, Stanford University.

Diagnostic Studies

Patients presenting with unexplained pulsatile tinnitus, CN deficits, balance disorders, and evidence of increased intracranial pressure are all indications for imaging the jugular foramen.

Audiologic and vestibular testing: Full audiologic examination including air bone and speech audiometry should be performed to assess the degree of conductive and sensorineural hearing loss. Should the patient present with symptoms of disequilibrium or vertigo, formal videonystagmography should be performed.

Imaging: Computed tomography (CT) and MRI allow accurate preoperative assessment of tumor involvement of the temporal bone, skull base, and evaluate for intracranial involvement.

High-resolution computed tomography: Thin-section HRCT scan (<1 mm) in both axial and coronal planes is the

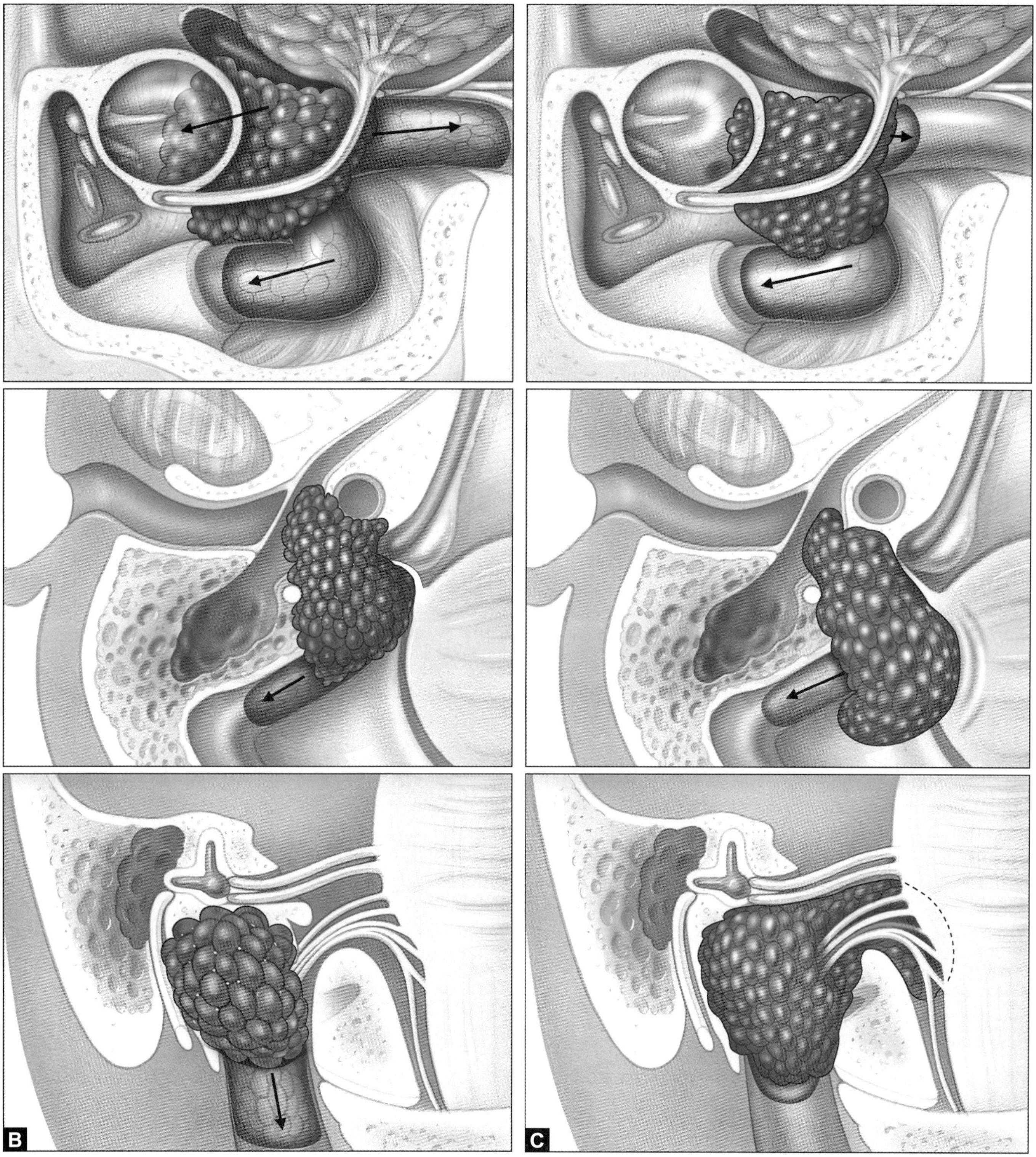

Figs. 25.4B and C: (B) Jugular paraganglioma with further extension into the sigmoid sinus proximally and into the upper portion of the jugular vein distally. Note the erosion of the carotid and fallopian canals in the axial view. (C) Jugular paraganglioma with extension into the posterior cranial fossa, with superior erosion of the internal auditory canal and medial into jugular foramen. Copyright RK Jackler and C Gralapp, Stanford University.

imaging modality to assess for temporal bone involvement, visualize bony structures and tumor extension. High-resolution CT scan is very useful to classify between paragangliomas that arise from the middle ear (tympanic) and paragangliomas arising from the JB (jugular). It provides information regarding tumor extension beyond the tympanic annulus and allows for defining bone erosion in the temporal bone. On CT scans, paragangliomas enhance intensely postcontrast. Contrasted HRCT may differentiate paragangliomas from most but not all benign and malignant tumors of the skull base. Arteriovenous fistulas (AVF) can appear similar to paragangliomas on HRCT. More specifically, HRCT helps with the differentiation of a middle ear vascular mass such as paraganglioma, aberrant internal carotid artery, and dehiscent jugular bulb. This is the main reason why a biopsy of a vascular mass in the middle ear is not recommended prior to imaging. Lastly, it identifies synchronous tumors of the temporal bone and upper neck.

Tympanic paragangliomas appear as well-circumscribed soft tissue masses in the middle ear (usually at the cochlear promontory) without bone erosion.

Jugular paragangliomas involve the hypotympanum and demonstrate an irregular or "moth-eaten" appearance at the jugulocarotid spine, jugular foramen, or hypoglossal canal (Fig. 25.5A). Careful attention must be given to the relationship between the tumor and the bony covering of the jugular bulb, the jugular plate. Erosion of the jugular plate suggests a jugular paraganglioma.

Magnetic resonance imaging: Gadolinium enhanced-MRI provides exquisite soft tissue details of tumor involvement and is superior to HRCT in its ability to characterize the vascular nature of the tumors involving the JB and skull base since it lacks bone artifact that is seen on CT scans. T1-weighted images, with and without contrast, highlight the enormous vascularity of these tumors (Fig. 25.5B), while T2-weighted images provide exceptional soft tissue contrast. In larger tumors over 2 cm, the characteristic "salt and pepper" appearance of paragangliomas corresponds to macroscopic flow voids and displays intense enhancement on MRI. Additionally, MRI is useful to identify tumor extension intracranially. Magnetic resonance angiography (MRA), magnetic resonance venography (MRV), and angiography provide information on the involvement of the great vessels and allow for preoperative embolization. Compression of the internal carotid artery can be evaluated with MRA, while MRV is useful to evaluate for collateral circulation within the dural sinuses of the skull, which can indicate occlusion of the JB and sigmoid sinus by tumor.

Angiography and embolization: Angiography serves multiple purposes. First, it allows the complement diagnosis of paragangliomas by visualizing the characteristic vascular nature. Formal intravascular angiography should not be performed prematurely for mere diagnostic purposes, but rather combined with embolization in the preoperative period. Second, paraganglioma tumor size can be determined. Third, it allows identification of dominant feeding vessels that can then be embolized to reduce blood loss during surgical removal (Fig. 25.6). Fourth, it helps identify collateral vessels associated with the carotid and vertebral arteries that must be spared during surgery. Fifth, it determines contralateral venous system patency. Sixth, it shows the presence of major venous sinus occlusion by tumor. Seventh, it identifies multifocal tumors.

Studies have demonstrated decreased operative time and intraoperative blood loss with preoperative embolization of jugular paragangliomas. Thus, preoperative embolization facilitates complete resection of jugular paragangliomas. Angiography with embolization for jugular paragangliomas is usually performed 1 or 2 days before surgical excision because a longer interval between embolization and surgery may result in revascularization of the tumor, which may paradoxically, increase intraoperative blood loss.

Nuclear medicine imaging: Multiple nuclear modalities have been applied for detection of head and neck paragangliomas. Octreotide is a somatostatin analog that when coupled to a tracer produces a scintigraphy image of neuroendocrine tumors that express somatostatin type 2 receptors.[58] Octreotide scintigraphy imaging has been applied for the diagnosis of head and neck paragangliomas with a sensitivity of 97% and specificity of 82%.[59,60] The 123I-Metaiodobenzylguanidin-scintigraphy (123I-MIBG scintigraphy) is paraganglioma specific but has disadvantages including two patient visits since the images are captured 2 and 24 hours after tracer injection, the tracer accumulates at salivary glands hindering clear diagnosis and the tracer affects many common cardiac medications and antidepressants.[61] More recently, PET/CT fusions have increased specificity and sensitivity in the diagnosis of head and neck paragangliomas.

Our recommended imaging is noncontrast HRCT of the skull base, MRI of the skull base and neck, and angiography and embolization in the preoperative period.

Differential Diagnosis

The differential diagnosis of jugulotympanic paragangliomas consists of differentiating middle ear vascular masses and tumors of the jugular foramen causing cranial nerve

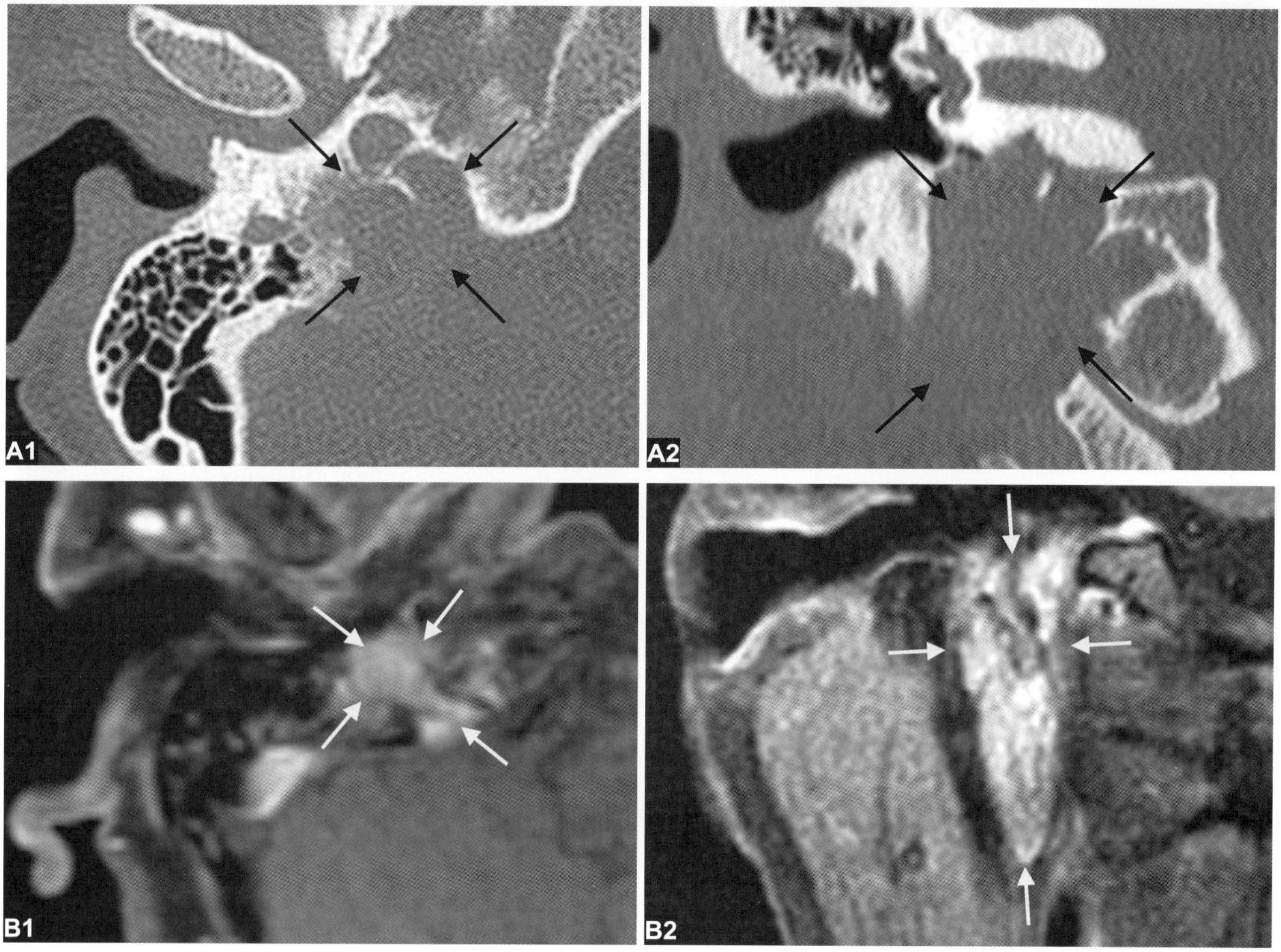

Figs. 25.5A and B: (A) High-resolution CT scan of a right jugular paraganglioma (arrows) showing bony erosion on axial view A1. Coronal view A2. (B) Gadolinium-enhanced T1-weighted axial MRI with fat suppression showing tumor (arrows) involvement of the right jugular foramen B1. Coronal view in B2 with arrow showing tumor.

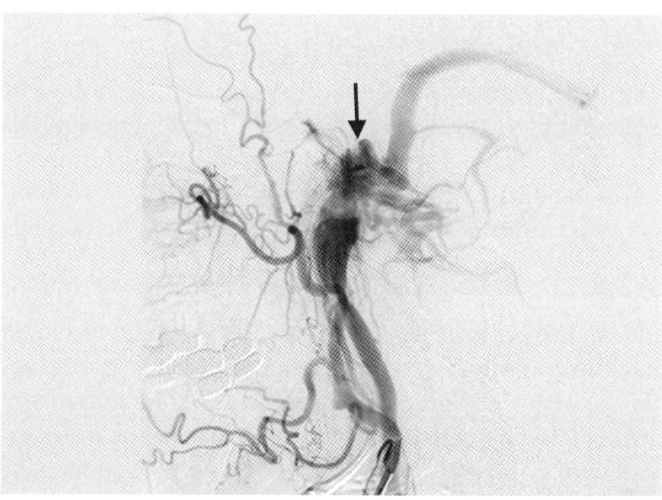

Fig. 25.6: Angiography demonstrating vascularization of a jugular foramen tumor (arrow) before embolization.

deficits (Table 25.3). The importance of radiographic imaging of paragangliomas at the skull base cannot be underestimated, with HRCT the preferred imaging choice for middle ear vascular masses and MRI for tumors located at the jugular foramen.

The differential diagnosis of middle ear vascular masses include the aberrant or laterally displaced internal carotid artery, the dehiscent or HRJB, AVF, and the congenital or acquired intratympanic carotid artery aneurysms. Aberrant internal carotid arteries are more frequently diagnosed in female patients (90%) and in the right ears (75%).[25,62,63]

The differential diagnosis of jugular foramen masses includes benign and malignant neoplasms. Schwannomas of cranial nerves IX, X, XI, and XII, meningiomas, or metastatic lesions can present with lower cranial nerve neuropathies.

Table 25.3: Differential diagnosis of jugular paragangliomas

Differential diagnosis of jugular paraganglioma
Schwannomas of the IXth, Xth, XIth, and XIIth cranial nerves
Meningiomas
Aberrant or laterally displaced internal carotid artery
Congenital or acquired internal carotid artery aneurysm
Dehiscent or high-riding jugular bulb
Arteriovenous fistula (AVF)
Thrombosis of the jugular bulb, sigmoid sinus, internal jugular vein
Chondrosarcoma, invasive squamous cell carcinoma, or metastatic disease

Tumor Classification and Selection of Surgical Approach

The fact that there are multiple classification schemes indicates that none are universally accepted. Paragangliomas of the temporal bone have been organized into three classification schemes:

1. *Fisch-Mattox classification*[64]: Includes four main categories:
   a. *Type A (glomus tympanicum)*: Tumors limited to the middle ear cleft.
   b. *Type B (glomus hypotympanicum)*: These tumors originate in the canalis tympanicus of the hypotympanum and invade the middle ear and mastoid. Jugular bulb plate is intact.
   c. *Type C*: These tumors originate at the dome of the JB and erode the overlying plate. Further classification denotes degree of carotid canal erosion (C1–C4). C1 tumors erode the carotid foramen but do not invade the carotid artery. C2 tumors erode the vertical carotid canal between the carotid foramen to the carotid bend. C3 tumors grow along the horizontal portion of the carotid artery but do not reach the foramen lacerum. C4 tumors grow to the foramen lacerum and along the carotid artery to the cavernous sinus.
   d. *Type De (extradural)*: Intracranial extension of glomus tumors displacing the posterior fossa dura. De1: <1 cm and De2: >2 cm.
   e. *Type Di (intracranial)*: Tumors with intracranial extension. Di1: <2 cm and Di2: >2 cm.
2. *Glasscock-Jackson classification*[65]: This classification has completely separate categories for tympanic and jugular paragangliomas:
   a. *Tympanic paragangliomas*:
      i. *Type I*: Small mass limited to the promontory.
      ii. *Type II*: Tumor completely filling the middle ear space.
      iii. *Type III*: Tumor filling the middle ear and extending into the mastoid.
      iv. *Type IV*: Tumor filling the middle ear, extending into the mastoid or through the tympanic membrane to fill the external auditory canal; may also extend anterior to the internal carotid artery.
   b. *Jugular paragangliomas*:
      i. *Type I*: Small tumor involving the jugular bulb, middle ear and mastoid.
      ii. *Type II*: Tumor extending under the internal auditory canal; may have intracranial extension.
      iii. *Type III*: Tumor extending into the petrous apex; may have intracranial extension.
      iv. *Type IV*: Tumor extending beyond the petrous apex into the clivus or infratemporal fossa; may have intracranial extension.
3. *De la Cruz classification*[25]: This classification consists of a tumor category paired with a surgical approach:
   a. *Tympanic*: Transcanal
   b. *Tympanomastoid*: Mastoid-extended facial recess
   c. *Jugular bulb*: Mastoid-neck (possible limited FN rerouting)
   d. *Carotid artery*: Infratemporal fossa ± subtemporal
   e. *Transdural*: Infratemporal fossa/intracranial
   f. *Craniocervical*: Transcondylar
   g. *Vagal*: Cervical

Molecular Genetic Screening

The first proposed screening protocol was described by Young et al. in 2002 who recommended genetic analysis for head and neck paraganglioma and pheochromocytoma patients with a positive family history.[66] Advantageous to molecular screening is the fact that no patients have presented with more than one mutation when tested for SDHB, SDHC, or SDHD mutations.[38] Since then multiple studies have clearly demonstrated the need to screen patients presenting with a head and neck paraganglioma.[37,39,40,44,47,67] Because of these studies, the majority of authors regard molecular genetic screening as an international standard[31] and tests are usually commercially available in large academic centers. Multiple molecular genetic screening algorithms have been proposed, and

Table 25.4: Algorithm for molecular screening of patients with head and neck paragangliomas

Clinical parameters	*Test sequence*	*Test*
Patient with multiple head and neck paragangliomas	1	SDHD
	2	SDHB
	3	SDHC
Solitary head and neck paraganglioma, and positive family history	1	SDHD
	2	SDHB
	3	SDHC
Head and neck paraganglioma with pheochromocytomas(s)	1	SDHD
	2	SDHB
	3	SDHC
Solitary head and neck paraganglioma, negative family history	1	SDHB
	2	SDHD
	3	SDHC
Malignant head and neck paraganglioma	1	SDHB
	2	SDHD
	3	SDHC

Source: Adapted from Boedeker.[31]

Boedeker et al.[31] has proposed a cost-effective screening algorithm without the risk of missing a mutation. Recommended approach depends on certain clinical parameters summarized in Table 25.4.

In patients who are carriers of PGL syndrome mutations, screening recommendations include an annual complete history and thorough physical examination that should include blood pressure measurement, annual levels of urinary catecholamines and metanephrines, and an annual MRI with contrast of the head and neck, the thorax, and the abdomen.[31,68]

Treatment

Nonsurgical Treatment

Observation-"watchful waiting"-"wait and scan": Considering the slow growth and the benign histopathology of paragangliomas, patients presenting with no or minimal symptoms can be safely observed with serial MRI scans. Additionally, elderly patients, patients with small tumors, or patients with multiple comorbidities, a wait and scan protocol should be discussed. Timing of repeat imaging is usually performed 6 months after initial diagnosis and 12 months thereafter. Surgical resection or radiation therapy can be then considered should the paraganglioma prove growth. Furthermore, observation should not be considered as first-line treatment in healthy young patients since tumor growth is likely to occur during their life span.

Radiation therapy (conventional and stereotactic): It can be recommended to patients as a primary treatment option, as a complement treatment for patients in whom total tumor removal was not achieved or as salvage treatment after surgical failure. Multiple variables should be considered for radiation therapy as a primary treatment option including the patient's age and general health status, number of cranial nerve deficits and size and location of the tumor. Multiple serious complications have been reported in patients with jugulotympanic paragangliomas treated with primary radiation including skull base osteomyelitis, temporal bone osteoradionecrosis, brain abscess, pituitary gland insufficiency, and radiation-induced malignancies.[52,69] Less serious complications include chronic otitis media, temporomandibular joint disorder, and stenosis of the external auditory canal.[70,71]

Conventional radiation: Doses range between 40 and 50 Gy scheduled over 4–5 weeks. Several studies have demonstrated local tumor control rates of 90–100% of jugulotympanic paragangliomas treated with conventional radiation with follow-up periods ranging from 1 to 12 years.[72–74]

Stereotactic radiotherapy (SRT) (Cyberknife, Gamma Knife, or LINAC): It has also been introduced for the primary treatment of jugulotympanic paragangliomas. Stereotactic radiation is thought to deliver a high dose of radiation to a limited area with sharp dose decrease at the margin causing cellular and vascular damage and eventually tumor necrosis. The usual doses recommended for paragangliomas using SR range between 14 and 20 Gy and can be given in a single day.

Surgery

Patients should be counseled of the inherent risks involved with removing paraganglioma tumors. The surgical approach for resection of paragangliomas of the temporal bone is determined by the location and extent of the tumor. For jugular paragangliomas, a larger surgical approach is required with inherently more risks involved including facial nerve palsy, lower cranial nerve deficits, vascular injury, and hearing loss. Additionally, if the clinical examination or preoperative imaging suggests metastasis, adjacent lymph node resection should be performed.[30,31]

Continuous cranial nerve monitoring for CN VII, IX, X, and XI is routinely used for resection of jugular paragangliomas:

- *Mastoid-neck approach*: Small jugular paragangliomas that do not involve the carotid artery or posterior cranial fossa are removed via mastoid-neck approach. The neck portion of the procedure in small jugular paragangliomas is necessary for jugular vein ligation. This approach begins similarly to a mastoidectomy with extended facial recess approach, and the skin incision is carried inferiorly to the neck on a natural skin crease. This approach requires preservation of a thin covering of bone surrounding the facial nerve circumferentially and drilling of the air cells medial to the nerve (Fallopian bridge technique).[75,76] The sternocleidomastoid and digastric muscles are amputated from the mastoid tip, and the mastoid tip is then removed. The internal jugular vein and internal carotid artery are identified and dissected superiorly to skull base. Sigmoid sinus and JB are exposed using diamond burrs. The proximal sigmoid sinus is occluded with extraluminal packing. Ligation of the internal jugular vein in the upper neck is then performed immediately before tumor resection to prevent tumor emboli, air emboli, and to reduce back-bleeding. The sigmoid sinus and JB are opened for tumor removal. Brisk bleeding may occur from the IPS and condylar vein, and can be controlled with gently application of Surgicel (Johnson and Johnson, USA). Cautery of the medial wall of the bulb should not be used due to the lower cranial nerves located medially risking nerve injury.
- *Infratemporal approach*: Larger jugular paragangliomas with extensive carotid artery involvement may require a larger infratemporal fossa approach. This exposure permits dissection of the tumor from the internal carotid artery into the petrous apex. This approach rarely requires transposition of the facial nerve. Resection of intracranial tumor should be performed after tumor at the JB has been removed and hemostasis achieved to reduce intracranial hemorrhage. Packing of the Eustachian tube and closure of the external auditory canal is often required.

Outcomes

Recurrence Rates

Jugular paragangliomas tend to have higher rates of recurrence compared to tympanic paragangliomas of approximately 5–10% in the setting of subtotal resections (necessary for cavernous sinus tumor extension, remnant left in the inferior neural compartment, marrow of the lower clivus or involvement of the central nervous system). In our experience, we have seen a pattern of recurrence due to residual tumor localized within infracochlear cell tracts between the cochlea and the carotid artery.

Cranial Nerve Deficits

Utilization of cranial nerve monitoring conducted via needle electrodes placed in the pharyngeal plexus (IX), larynx (X), trapezius muscle (XI), and tongue (XII), permits earlier identification of the lower cranial nerves in a distorted operative field and facilitates surgical removal via microdissection. Preoperative cranial nerve deficits are usually associated with jugular paragangliomas and very seldom from tympanic paragangliomas. Published series have reported preoperative cranial nerve deficits between 39% and 46% in jugular paragangliomas. The relative incidence of lower cranial nerve deficit due to tumor growth is X>IX>XI>XII. In our experience, however, most patients after surgery have intact external auditory canal walls and hearing is preserved. Overall, 59–72% of patients have one or more new cranial nerve deficits detected after surgery.

Complications

The most common postoperative complications are cerebrospinal fluid (CSF) leak, aspiration/pneumonia, wound infection, meningitis, and stroke. Indications for ear canal closure include extensive erosion of the ear canal, deaf ear, and tumor extension anterior to cochlea and encasing carotid.

JUGULAR FORAMEN SCHWANNOMAS

Jugular foramen schwannomas are rare, benign, noninfiltrative tumors of the lower cranial nerves. They represent the second most common tumor in the jugular foramen after paraganglioma jugulare.[25] These tumors arise from the sheaths of cranial nerves IX, X, and XI, and in over 90% of patients the nerve of origin is either the vagus (predominantly) and glossopharyngeus but clear identification of tumor origin is difficult.[77] Jugular foramen schwannomas usually arise from the posterior fossa and tend to expand the jugular foramen as they extend inferiorly. Notably more common in females, most patients with jugular foramen schwannomas present between the fourth and sixth decades of life.

Clinical Manifestations and Growth Patterns

The early signs and symptoms of jugular foramen abnormalities are often subtle and frequently overlooked until progressive multiple CN deficits become apparent. Presenting clinical features tend to reflect intracranial versus extracranial extension of tumor. Most recent large series report auditory symptoms to have the highest frequency, regardless of tumor histology (paraganglioma, meningioma, or schwannomas). Pulsatile tinnitus, hearing loss, and hoarseness are the most common presenting symptoms in patients with jugular foramen tumors including schwannomas. On otoscopy, a retrotympanic mass can be found in 11% patients with a jugular foramen schwannomas.[78] Patients with schwannomas of the jugular foramen tend to present more commonly with shoulder weakness and absent gag reflex compared to patients with paragangliomas.

Jugular foramen schwannomas are well-circumscribed tumors that tend to expand rather than invade surrounding structures. These tumors extend in paths of least resistance whether this may be into the infratemporal fossa, perijugular skull base or posterior fossa (Figs. 25.7A to F). Three types of jugular foramen schwannomas have been described: type A, predominantly intracranial; type B, predominantly in the skull base; and type C, predominantly extracranial. Type A schwannomas tend to present with VIIIth nerve and cerebellar signs and symptoms, while type B and C schwannomas tend to present with lower cranial nerve palsies. Common clinical findings of jugular foramen pathology are described in Table 25.1.

Pathology

Schwannomas are typically unilateral, well circumscribed, range in color from tan-white to yellow and have varying amounts of surface vascularity. Microscopic analysis demonstrates tumor cells that are spindle-shaped and are arranged in both Antoni type A (dense pattern) and Antoni type B (hypocellular pattern). Antoni type A tissue consists of densely packed long bipolar spindle cells with a palisading nuclei pattern known as Verocay bodies. In contrast, Antoni type B tissue is characterized by loose, disordered cells associated with a myxoid stroma (Fig. 25.8). Cystic degeneration, intratumoral hemorrhage, and necrosis is a common feature of large tumors, but even small lesions may contain these changes.

Diagnostic Studies

Similar to paragangliomas, full audiologic testing including air bone and speech audiometry should be performed to assess the degree of conductive and sensorineural hearing loss. Should the patient present with symptoms of disequilibrium or vertigo, formal videonystagmography should be performed.

Imaging: Radiologic evaluation consists of MRI and HRCT. On HRCT scans, schwannomas tend to show smooth and expanded erosion of the jugular foramen, in contrast to jugular paragangliomas that demonstrate an irregular or "moth-eaten" appearance at the jugulocarotid spine, jugular foramen, or hypoglossal canal as described above (Fig. 25.9). Magnetic resonance imaging features of jugular foramen schwannomas show a smooth, contoured mass that is isodense on T1-weighted images, high-signal intensity on T2-weighted images and intense enhancement on postgadolinium scans similar to paragangliomas but the flow voids are absent (Figs. 25.10A and B). Gadolinium-enhanced MRI provides superior visualization of any intracranial component, including tumor–brain interface (including edema), and the relationship to the vertebrobasilar system. It also shows the inferior-most extension of tumor into the neck (infratemporal fossa). We prefer to use both MRI and HRCT, in both axial and coronal planes for preoperative assessment.

Angiography with preoperative embolization can be performed before surgical resection of a schwannoma, but this is not typical. However, if there is a question about the patency of the contralateral sigmoid sinus-jugular bulb-jugular vein system, it can be helpful. This is important to assess preoperatively because if the ipsilateral venous system is dominant and needs to be resected as part of the surgery, there must be sufficient collateral circulation. Otherwise, disastrous cerebral venous infarction may occur.

Treatment Options

Observation-"watchful waiting"-"wait and scan": Considering the slow growth and the benign histopathology of jugular foramen schwannomas, patients presenting with no or minimal symptoms can be safely observed with serial MRI scans. Additionally, elderly patients, patients with small tumors, or patients with multiple comorbidities, a wait and scan protocol should be discussed. Timing of repeat imaging is usually performed 6 months after initial diagnosis and 12 months thereafter.

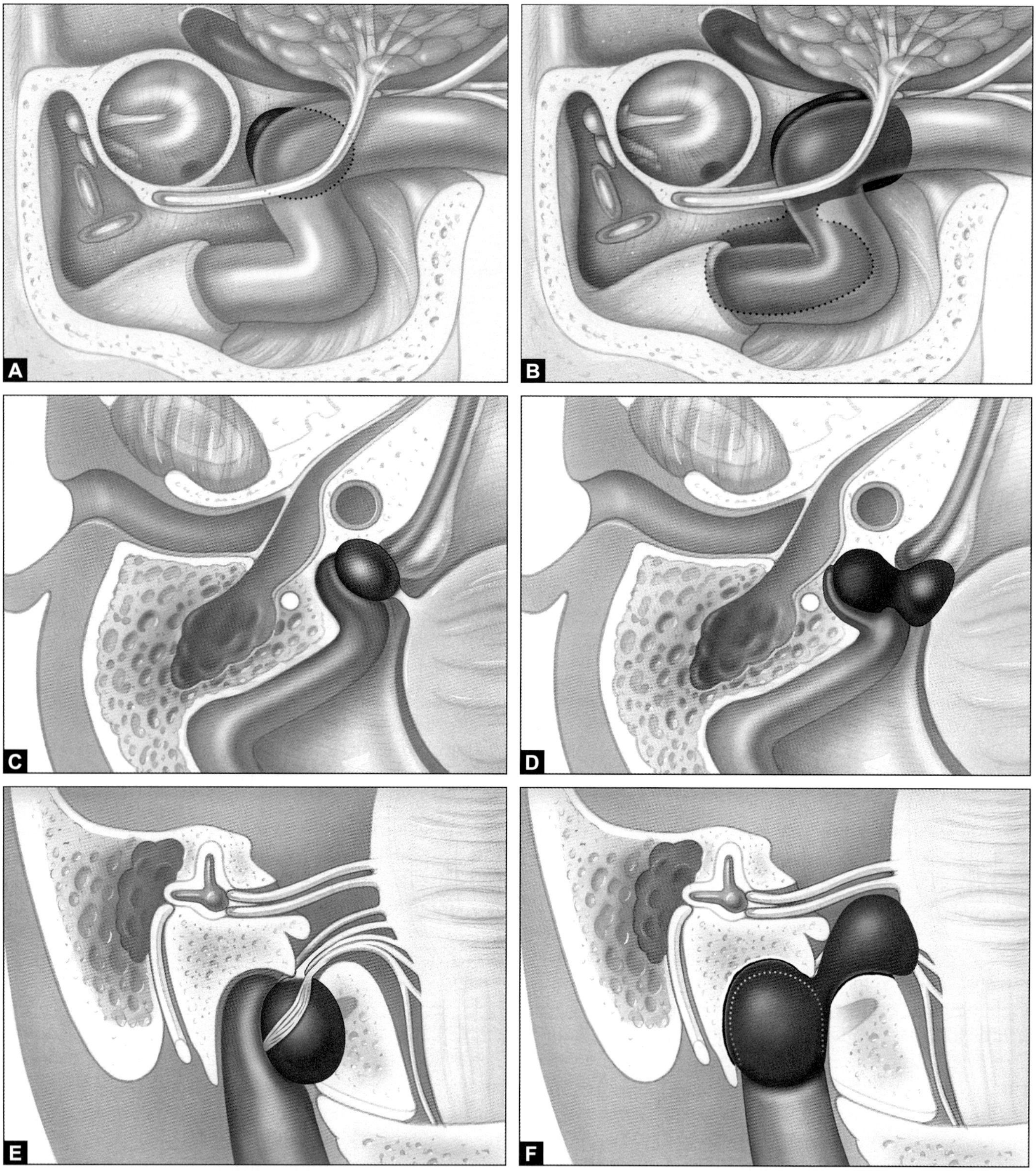

Figs. 25.7A to F: Growth patterns of jugular foramen schwannomas. Copyright RK Jackler and C Gralapp, Stanford University.

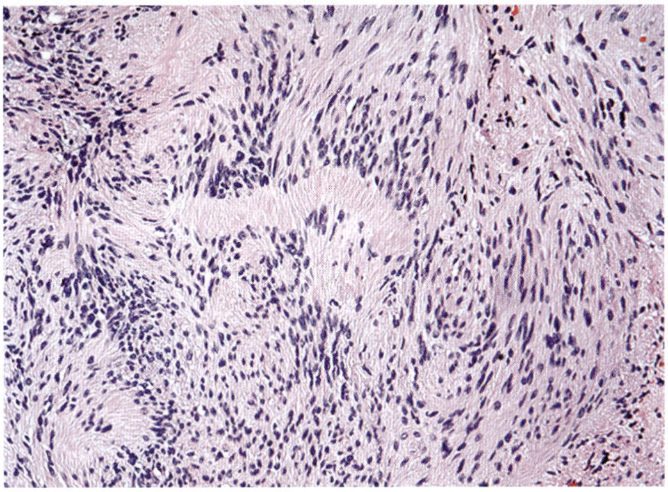

Fig. 25.8: Histology of schwannoma Antoni A and Antoni B—Verocay bodies.

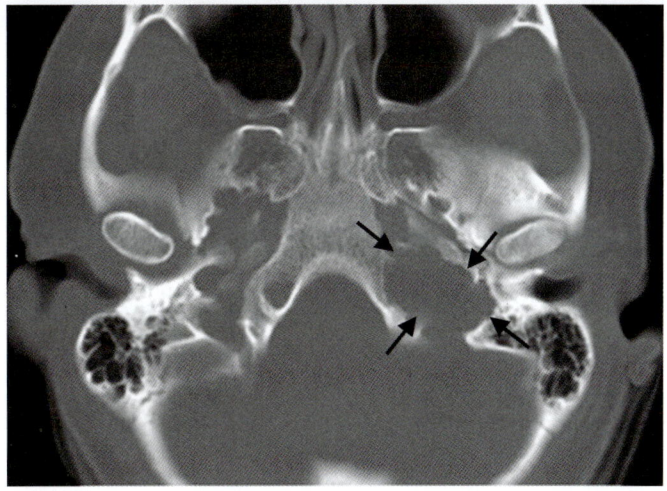

Fig. 25.9: High-resolution computer tomography (HRCT). Axial HRCT showing a schwannoma with smooth and expanded erosion of the jugular foramen (arrows).

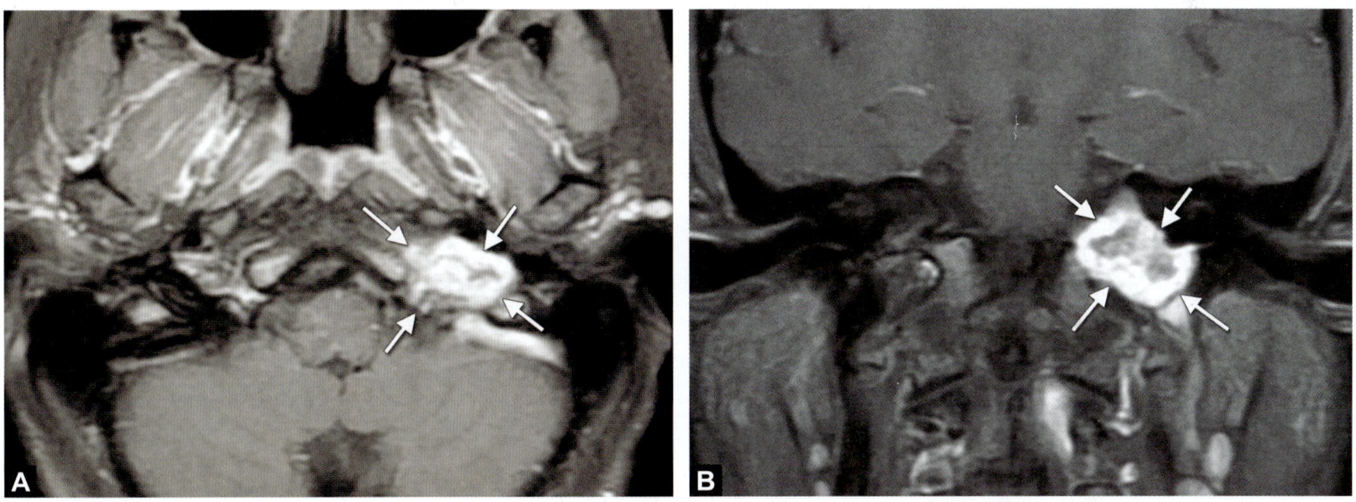

Figs. 25.10A and B: MRI of JF schwannomas. Axial gadolinium-enhanced MRI showing schwannoma centered at the jugular foramen with intense enhancement (arrows) (A). Note widened jugular foramen compared to contralateral foramen. Coronal contrast-enhanced MRI showing schwannoma centered at the jugular foramen (arrows) (B).

Surgery

The surgical approach for resection of jugular foramen schwannomas is determined by the location and extent of the tumor. For large jugular foramen schwannomas, a large surgical approach is required with inherently surgical risks including facial nerve palsy, lower cranial nerve deficits, vascular injury, and hearing loss. Depending on the extent of tumor, both the mastoid-neck and infratemporal approaches are used as described above. Tumors that are mainly intracranial with minimal extension into the jugular foramen can be resected with either a retrosigmoid approach or via a retrolabyrinthine approach. Tumors arising within the jugular foramen and extending into the infratemporal fossa can be managed via an infratemporal fossa approach combined with a transjugular approach with adequate visualization of the jugular foramen and upper neck.

Stereotactic Radiotherapy (Cyberknife, Gamma Knife, or LINAC)

Complete tumor resection is the desirable curable approach for benign jugular foramen schwannomas. However, it is not always feasible to achieve complete resection without risking injury to the lower cranial nerves. Multiple studies have shown not only long-term tumor control but also neurofunctional preservation with SRT.[79-82] Similar to paragangliomas, patients with large tumors and symptomatic mass effect are generally considered poor SRS candidates and surgical resection is often recommended. Nevertheless, complete resection is not necessarily required as residual tumor can be safely treated with SRS with neural preservation.

MENINGIOMAS

Meningiomas are the third most common tumors arising in the jugular foramen. These tumors are extra-axial neoplasms that presumably arise from arachnoidal cap cells that are located along dura, neurovascular foramina, or venous sinuses (Fig. 25.11).

Most jugular foramen meningiomas are sporadic but may occur in familial syndromes such as NF2 and Gorlin syndrome. Meningiomas are commonly encountered in middle-aged patients with a female predominance ratio of 2:1 to males.

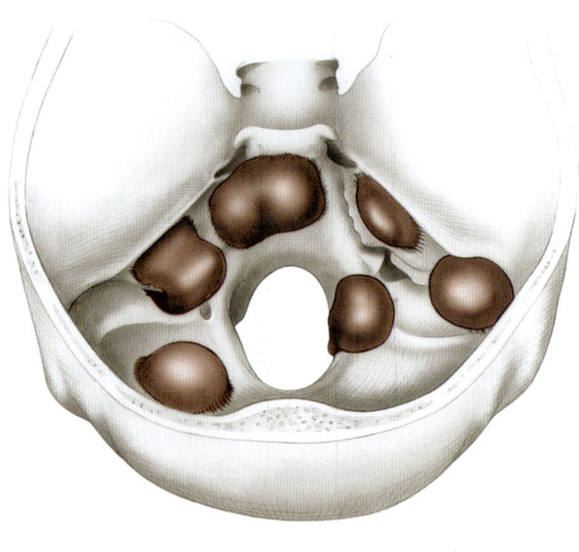

Fig. 25.11: Meningiomas at different sites in the posterior cranial base. Copyright RK Jackler and C Gralapp, Stanford University.

Clinical Manifestations and Growth Patterns

Meningiomas are benign, slow growing tumors that may arise either within the jugular foramen or penetrate it secondarily after having taken origin from an adjacent dural surface. The latter route is more common, with tumor invading the foramen via en plaque growth from either the posterior petrous surface or the lower clivus (Figs. 25.12A to F). Meningiomas are described as either being primary or secondary. Primary meningioma refers to tumor centered at the jugular foramen with possible extension into the infralabyrinthine cells or the middle ear. Additionally, primary meningiomas can extend intracranially into the cerebellopontine angle and extracranially into the infratemporal fossa. Secondary meningiomas refer to primary intracranial meningiomas that have extended into the jugular foramen, and examples include petroclival and cerebellopontine angle meningiomas. Because meningiomas, either primary or secondary, are in close proximity to cranial nerves IX–XII, VII/VIII nerve complex, and middle ear, patients present with hearing loss (sensorineural, conductive, and mixed), pulsatile tinnitus, disequilibrium, hoarseness, and dysphagia. A visible middle ear mass may be visible in over half of the patients diagnosed with a jugular foramen meningioma. Common clinical findings of jugular foramen pathology are described in Table 25.1.

Pathology

Meningiomas originate from the arachnoidal cap cells from the outer layer of the arachnoid sheath. On gross pathology, meningiomas are firm, rubbery, and well circumscribed. Microscopic analysis reveals round, polygonal, ovoid or spindle-shaped cells that are organized in nests of concentric whorls with small, rounded laminated calcific bodies termed psammoma bodies (Fig. 25.13).

Diagnostic Studies

Full audiologic testing including air bone and speech audiometry should be performed to assess the degree of

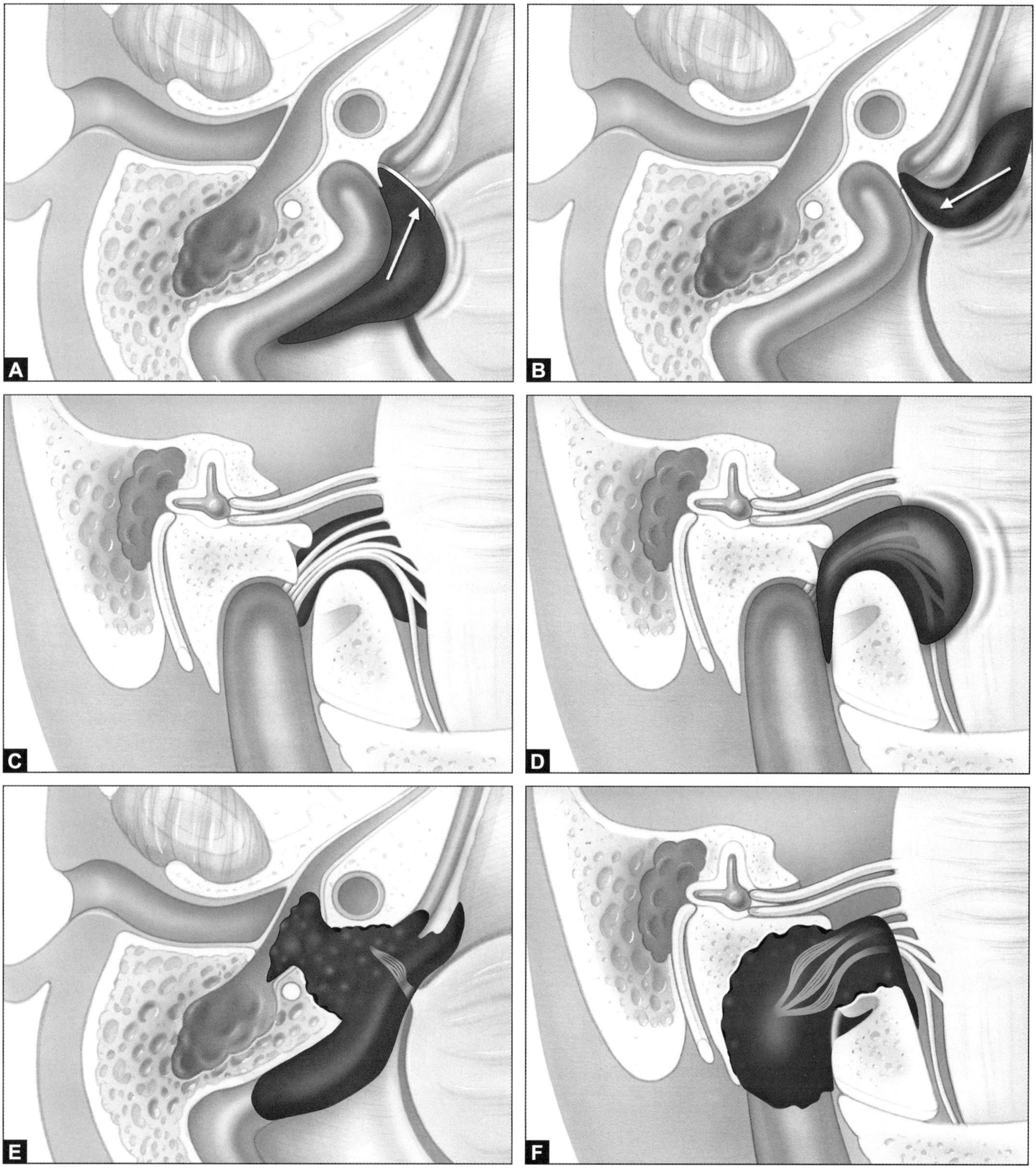

Figs. 25.12A to F: Jugular foramen meningioma growth patterns. Copyright RK Jackler and C Gralapp, Stanford University.

conductive and sensorineural hearing loss. Should the patient present with symptoms of disequilibrium or vertigo, formal videonystagmography should be performed.

Imaging: High-resolution computed tomography and gadolinium-contrasted MRI allow accurate preoperative assessment of jugular foramen meningiomas in terms of elucidating the diagnosis, tumor extension and surgical planning. On noncontrast HRCT, meningiomas appear as iso- or hyperdense tumors with areas of calcification in the internal matrix. High-resolution computer tomography also demonstrates smooth expansile bony changes with subjacent hyperostosis (Fig. 25.14A). On contrast-enhanced HRCT, meningiomas show intense and homogenous enhancement (Fig. 25.14B). Gadolinium-enhanced MRI is the imaging modality of choice for the diagnosis of meningiomas. Magnetic resonance imaging provides better delineation of intracranial and extracranial components of meningiomas originating at the jugular foramen. Characteristic MRI features of meningiomas include hypo- or isointensity on T1-weighted images, with heterogenous intensity on T2-weighted images, and homogenous and intense enhancement with gadolinium (Figs. 25.15A and B). Internal tumor matrix calcifications appear dark on T1- and T2-weighted images. Meningiomas, in contrast to schwannomas, are sessile, i.e. broad-based leading to an obtuse angle at the petrous face, demonstrate meningeal enhancement ("dural tail sign"), and show subjacent hyperostosis. Angiography with preoperative embolization is a complement imaging modality for highly vascular meningiomas of the jugular foramen.

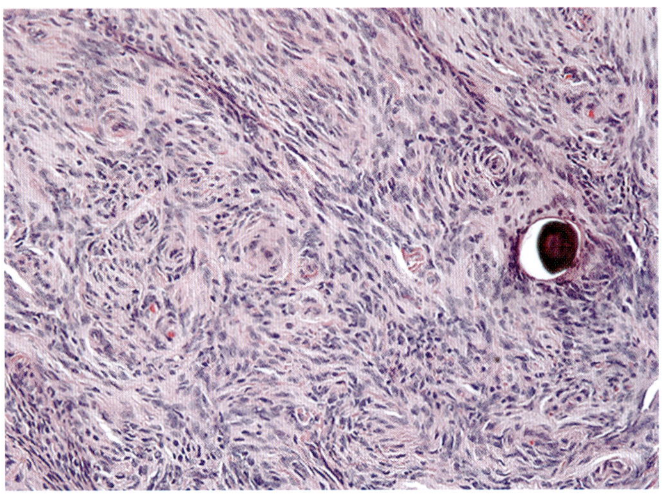

Fig. 25.13: Pathology of meningioma.

Treatment Options

Treatment options for jugular foramen meningiomas include observation with serial imaging, SRT, and microsurgery. Patients presenting with small tumors and minimal or absent symptoms are great candidates for watchful waiting with serial imaging between 6 and 12 months. Likewise, observation should not be considered as first-line treatment in healthy young patients since tumor growth is likely to occur during their life span. Patients diagnosed with large jugular foramen meningiomas and symptomatic mass effects are candidates for microsurgery. Primary treatment with SRT should be contemplated in older patients and patients in poor general health who have documented worsening symptoms and proven tumor growth.

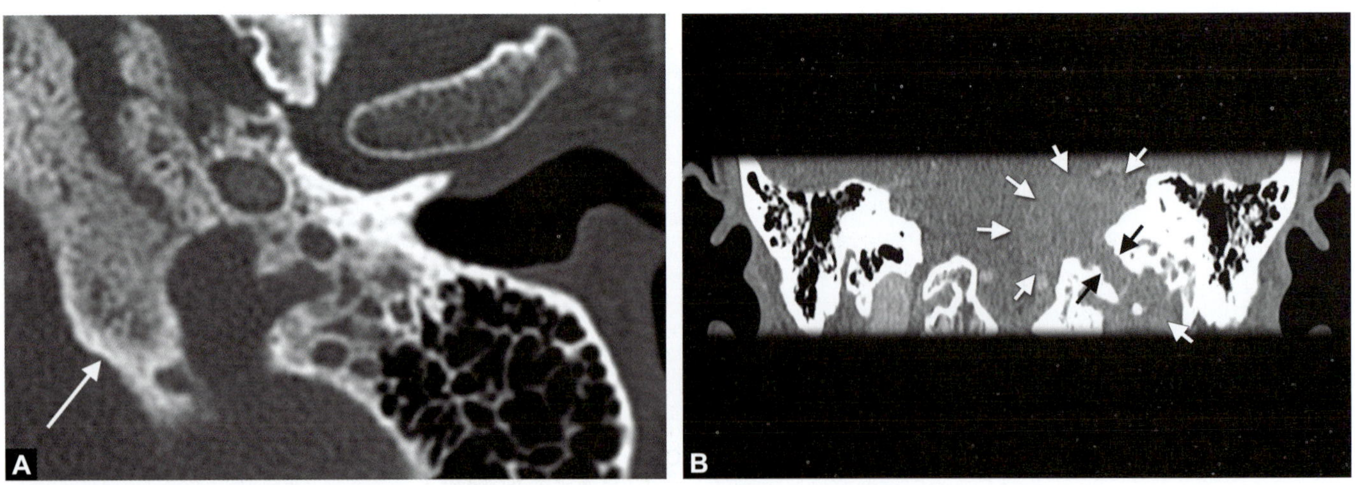

Figs. 25.14A and B: (A) High-resolution computer tomography (HRCT) axial meningioma. HRCT in the axial plane at the level of the jugular foramen showing hyperostosis (arrow). (B) HRCT coronal meningioma. Contrasted HRCT in the coronal plane at the level of the jugular foramen. White arrows depicts intracranial and extracranial extension of meningioma. Black arrows show a widened jugular foramen compared to the contralateral foramen.

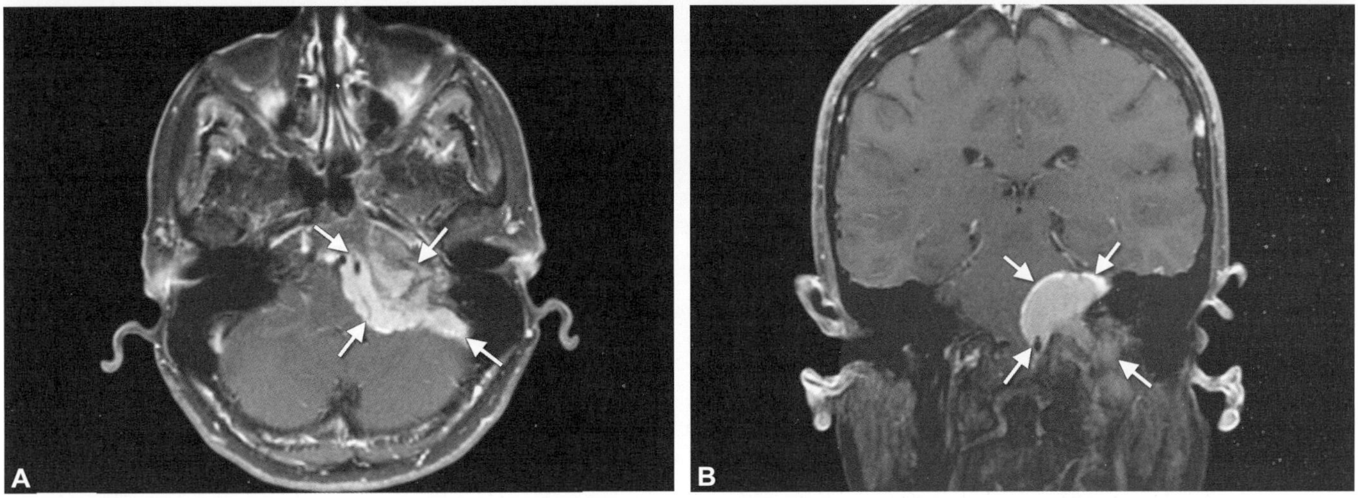

Figs. 25.15A and B: MRI meningioma. Axial gadolinium-enhanced MRI showing a large meningioma centered at the jugular foramen with extension into the infratemporal fossa (A). Coronal gadolinium-enhanced MRI showing meningioma centered at the jugular foramen. Note the meningeal enhancement and the broad dural base with an obtuse angle (B).

The premise of surgery is to prolong life and preserve neurovascular function. The surgical approach is largely determined by the size, location, vascularity, and tumor extension. The decision to operate is forthright when the patient presents with cranial nerve dysfunction prior to surgery. Yet, many patients have absent or varying degrees of lower cranial nerve dysfunction, making the decision to operate difficult. Briefly, a retrosigmoid approach may be used for meningiomas located at the cerebellopontine angle and jugular foramen. For patients diagnosed with a large jugular foramen meningioma and ipsilateral anacusis, the tumor may be resected with a translabyrinthine approach. Jugular foramen meningiomas with anterior extension may be addressed with a combined infratemporal/subtemporal approach and transjugular approach.

REFERENCES

1. Caldemeyer KS, Mathews VP, Azzarelli B, et al. The jugular foramen: a review of anatomy, masses, and imaging characteristics. Radiographics. 1997;17:1123-39.
2. Katsuta T, Rhoton AL Jr, Matsushima T. The jugular foramen: microsurgical anatomy and operative approaches. Neurosurgery. 1997;41:149-201; discussion 201-2.
3. Keles B, Semaan MT, Fayad JN. The medial wall of the jugular foramen: a temporal bone anatomic study. Otolaryngol Head Neck Surg. 2009;141:401-7.
4. Rhoton AL, Jr. Jugular foramen. Neurosurgery. 2000;47: S267-85.
5. Friedmann DR, Eubig J, McGill M, et al. Development of the jugular bulb: a radiologic study. Otol Neurotol. 2011; 32:1389-95.
6. Durgun B, Ilglt ET, Cizmeli MO, et al. Evaluation by angiography of the lateral dominance of the drainage of the dural venous sinuses. Surg Radiol Anat. 1993;15:125-30.
7. Vogl TJ, Bisdas S. Differential diagnosis of jugular foramen lesions. Skull Base. 2009;19:3-16.
8. Okudera T, Huang YP, Ohta T, et al. Development of posterior fossa dural sinuses, emissary veins, and jugular bulb: morphological and radiologic study. AJNR Am J Neuroradiol. 1994;15:1871-83.
9. Kuhn MA, Friedmann DR, Winata LS, et al. Large jugular bulb abnormalities involving the middle ear. Otol Neurotol. 2012;33:1201-6.
10. Wadin K, Thomander L, Wilbrand H. Effects of a high jugular fossa and jugular bulb diverticulum on the inner ear: a clinical and radiologic investigation. Acta Radiol Diagn. 1986;27:629-36.
11. Rauch SD, Xu WZ, Nadol JB Jr. High jugular bulb: implications for posterior fossa neurotologic and cranial base surgery. Ann Otol Rhinol Laryngol. 1993;102:100-107.
12. Hourani R, Carey J, Yousem DM. Dehiscence of the jugular bulb and vestibular aqueduct: findings on 200 consecutive temporal bone computed tomography scans. J Comp Assist Tomogr. 2005;29:657-62.
13. Pappas DG, Jr, Hoffman RA, Cohen NL, et al. Petrous jugular malposition (diverticulum). Otolaryngol Head Neck Surg. 1993;109:847-52.
14. Friedmann DR, Eubig J, Winata LS, et al. A clinical and histopathologic study of jugular bulb abnormalities. Arch Otolaryngol Head Neck Surg. 2012;138:66-71.
15. Friedmann DR, Eubig J, Winata LS, et al. Prevalence of jugular bulb abnormalities and resultant inner ear dehiscence: a histopathologic and radiologic study. Otolaryngol Head Neck Surg. 2012;147:750-56.
16. Friedmann DR, Le BT, Pramanik BK, et al. Clinical spectrum of patients with erosion of the inner ear by jugular bulb abnormalities. Laryngoscope. 2010;120:365-72.

17. Kobanawa S, Atsuchi M, Tanaka J, et al. Jugular bulb diverticulum associated with lower cranial nerve palsy and multiple aneurysms. Surgical Neurol. 2000;53:559-62.
18. Sykes JM, Ossoff RH. Paragangliomas of the head and neck. Otolaryngol Clin North Am. 1986;19:755-67.
19. Wasserman PG, Savargaonkar P. Paragangliomas: classification, pathology, and differential diagnosis. Otolaryngol Clin North Am. 2001;34:845-62, v-vi.
20. Wenig BM. Atlas of head and neck pathology. Philadelphia, PA: Saunders/Elsevier; 2008.
21. O'Leary MJ, Shelton C, Giddings NA, et al. Glomus tympanicum tumors: a clinical perspective. Laryngoscope. 1991; 101:1038-43.
22. Jackler RK, Brackmann DE. Neurotology. Philadelphia, PA: Elsevier Mosby; 2005.
23. Valentin G. Über eine gangliose Anschwellung in der Jacobsonchen Anastomose des Menschen. Arch Anat Physiolog Lpz. 1840;16:287-90.
24. Guild S. A hitherto unrecognized structure, the Glomus Jugularis, in man. Anat Rec. 1941;79:28.
25. Jackler RK, Driscoll CLW. Tumors of the ear and temporal bone. Philadelphia: Lippincott Williams & Wilkins; 2000.
26. Mills SE. Histology for pathologists. Philadelphia: Wolters Kluwer/Lippincott Williams & Wilkins Health; 2012.
27. Winship T, Klopp CT, Jenkins WH. Giomus-jugularis tumors. Cancer. 1948;1:441-8.
28. Le Douarin N. The neural crest. New York: Cambridge University Press; 1982.
29. Offergeld C, Brase C, Yaremchuk S, et al. Head and neck paragangliomas: clinical and molecular genetic classification. Clinics (Sao Paulo). 2012; 67(Suppl 1):19-28.
30. Lee JH, Barich F, Karnell LH, et al. National cancer data base report on malignant paragangliomas of the head and neck. Cancer. 2002; 94:730-37.
31. Boedeker CC. Paragangliomas and paraganglioma syndromes. GMS Curr Top Otorhinolaryngol Head Neck Surg. 2011;10:Doc03.
32. Baysal BE, Ferrell RE, Willett-Brozick JE, et al. Mutations in SDHD, a mitochondrial complex II gene, in hereditary paraganglioma. Science. 2000;287:848-51.
33. Niemann S, Muller U. Mutations in SDHC cause autosomal dominant paraganglioma, type 3. Nat Genet. 2000;26: 268-70.
34. Astuti D, Latif F, Dallol A, et al. Gene mutations in the succinate dehydrogenase subunit SDHB cause susceptibility to familial pheochromocytoma and to familial paraganglioma. Am J Hum Gen. 2001;69:49-54.
35. Bayley JP, Kunst HP, Cascon A, et al. SDHAF2 mutations in familial and sporadic paraganglioma and phaeochromocytoma. Lancet Oncol. 2010;11:366-72.
36. Ricketts CJ, Forman JR, Rattenberry E, et al. Tumor risks and genotype-phenotype-proteotype analysis in 358 patients with germline mutations in SDHB and SDHD. Hum Mutat. 2010;31:41-51.
37. Neumann HP, Bausch B, McWhinney SR, et al. Germ-line mutations in nonsyndromic pheochromocytoma. New Engl J Med. 2002;346:1459-66.
38. Neumann HP, Erlic Z, Boedeker CC, et al. Clinical predictors for germline mutations in head and neck paraganglioma patients: cost reduction strategy in genetic diagnostic process as fall-out. Cancer Res. 2009;69:3650-56.
39. Neumann HP, Pawlu C, Peczkowska M, et al. Distinct clinical features of paraganglioma syndromes associated with SDHB and SDHD gene mutations. JAMA. 2004;292:943-51.
40. Schiavi F, Boedeker CC, Bausch B, et al. Predictors and prevalence of paraganglioma syndrome associated with mutations of the SDHC gene. JAMA. 2005;294:2057-63.
41. Burnichon N, Rohmer V, Amar L, et al. The succinate dehydrogenase genetic testing in a large prospective series of patients with paragangliomas. J Clin Endocrinol Metabol. 2009;94:2817-27.
42. Mariman EC, van Beersum SE, Cremers CW, et al. Fine mapping of a putatively imprinted gene for familial nonchromaffin paragangliomas to chromosome 11q13.1: evidence for genetic heterogeneity. Hum Genet. 1995;95:56-62.
43. Hensen EF, Jansen JC, Siemers MD, et al. The Dutch founder mutation SDHD.D92Y shows a reduced penetrance for the development of paragangliomas in a large multigenerational family. Eur J Hum Genet.2010;18:62-6.
44. Pasini B, Stratakis CA. SDH mutations in tumorigenesis and inherited endocrine tumours: lesson from the phaeochromocytoma-paraganglioma syndromes. J Int Med. 2009;266:19-42.
45. Hao HX, Khalimonchuk O, Schraders M, et al. SDH5, a gene required for flavination of succinate dehydrogenase, is mutated in paraganglioma. Science. 2009;325:1139-42.
46. Niemann S, Muller U, Engelhardt D, et al. Autosomal dominant malignant and catecholamine-producing paraganglioma caused by a splice donor site mutation in SDHC. Hum Genet. 2003;113:92-4.
47. Benn DE, Gimenez-Roqueplo AP, Reilly JR, et al. Clinical presentation and penetrance of pheochromocytoma/paraganglioma syndromes. J Clin Endocrinol Metabol. 2006;91: 827-36.
48. Erlic Z, Rybicki L, Peczkowska M, et al. Clinical predictors and algorithm for the genetic diagnosis of pheochromocytoma patients. Clin Cancer Res. 2009;15:6378-85.
49. Boedeker CC, Neumann HP, Maier W, et al. Malignant head and neck paragangliomas in SDHB mutation carriers. Otolaryngol Head Neck Surg. 2007;137:126-9.
50. Vanharanta S, Buchta M, McWhinney SR, et al. Early-onset renal cell carcinoma as a novel extraparaganglial component of SDHB-associated heritable paraganglioma. Am J Hum Genet. 2004;74:153-9.
51. Schwaber MK, Glasscock ME, Nissen AJ, et al. Diagnosis and management of catecholamine secreting glomus tumors. Laryngoscope. 1984;94:1008-15.
52. Lustig LR, Jackler RK, Lanser MJ. Radiation-induced tumors of the temporal bone. Am J Otol. 1997;18:230-35.
53. Green JD Jr, Brackmann DE, Nguyen CD, et al. Surgical management of previously untreated glomus jugulare tumors. Laryngoscope. 1994;104:917-21.
54. House WF, Glasscock ME, 3rd. Glomus tympanicum tumors. Arch Otolaryngol. 1968;87:550-54.

55. Jackson CG, Welling DB, Chironis P, et al. Glomus tympanicum tumors: contemporary concepts in conservation surgery. Laryngoscope. 1989;99:875-84.
56. Larson TC 3rd, Reese DF, Baker HL Jr, et al. Glomus tympanicum chemodectomas: radiographic and clinical characteristics. Radiology. 1987;163:801-6.
57. Spector GJ, Gado M, Ciralsky R, et al. Neurologic implications of glomus tumors in the head and neck. Laryngoscope. 1975;85:1387-95.
58. Telischi FF, Bustillo A, Whiteman ML, et al. Octreotide scintigraphy for the detection of paragangliomas. Otolaryngol Head Neck Surg. 2000;122:358-62.
59. Bustillo A, Telischi F, Weed D, et al. Octreotide scintigraphy in the head and neck. Laryngoscope. 2004;114:434-40.
60. Bustillo A, Telischi FF. Octreotide scintigraphy in the detection of recurrent paragangliomas. Otolaryngol Head Neck Surg. 2004;130:479-82.
61. Hoegerle S, Ghanem N, Altehoefer C, et al. 18F-DOPA positron emission tomography for the detection of glomus tumours. Eur J Nucl Med Mol Imaging. 2003;30:689-94.
62. Lo WW, Solti-Bohman LG, McElveen JT Jr. Aberrant carotid artery: radiologic diagnosis with emphasis on high-resolution computed tomography. Radiographics. 1985;5:985-93.
63. McElveen JT, Jr., Lo WW, el Gabri TH, et al. Aberrant internal carotid artery: classic findings on computed tomography. Otolaryngology Head Neck Surg. 1986;94:616-21.
64. Brackmann DE, Ear Research Foundation of Florida, House Ear Institute. Neurological surgery of the ear and skull base. New York: Raven Press; 1982.
65. Jackson CG, Glasscock ME 3rd, Harris PF. Glomus tumors: diagnosis, classification, and management of large lesions. Arch Otolaryngol. 1982;108:401-10.
66. Young AL, Baysal BE, Deb A, et al. Familial malignant catecholamine-secreting paraganglioma with prolonged survival associated with mutation in the succinate dehydrogenase B gene. J Clin Endocrinol Metabol. 2002;87:4101-5.
67. Bayley JP, van Minderhout I, Weiss MM, et al. Mutation analysis of SDHB and SDHC: novel germline mutations in sporadic head and neck paraganglioma and familial paraganglioma and/or pheochromocytoma. BMC Medical Genet. 2006;7:1.
68. Drucker AM, Houlden RL. A case of familial paraganglioma syndrome type 4 caused by a mutation in the SDHB gene. Nat Clin Pract Endocrinol Metabol. 2006;2:702-6; quiz following 706.
69. Lalwani AK, Jackler RK, Gutin PH. Lethal fibrosarcoma complicating radiation therapy for benign glomus jugulare tumor. Am J Otol. 1993;14:398-402.
70. Hinerman RW, Mendenhall WM, Amdur RJ, et al. Definitive radiotherapy in the management of chemodectomas arising in the temporal bone, carotid body, and glomus vagale. Head Neck. 2001;23:363-71.
71. Gabriel EM, Sampson JH, Dodd LG, et al. Glomus jugulare tumor metastatic to the sacrum after high-dose radiation therapy: case report. Neurosurgery. 1995;37:1001-5.
72. Powell S, Peters N, Harmer C. Chemodectoma of the head and neck: results of treatment in 84 patients. Int J Radiat Oncol Biol Phys. 1992;22:919-24.
73. Chino JP, Sampson JH, Tucci DL, et al. Paraganglioma of the head and neck: long-term local control with radiotherapy. Am J Clin Oncol. 2009;32:304-7.
74. Boyle JO, Shimm DS, Coulthard SW. Radiation therapy for paragangliomas of the temporal bone. Laryngoscope. 1990; 100:896-901.
75. Oghalai JS, Leung MK, Jackler RK, et al. Transjugular craniotomy for the management of jugular foramen tumors with intracranial extension. Otology Neurotol. 2004;25:570-79; discussion 579.
76. Pensak ML, Jackler RK. Removal of jugular foramen tumors: the fallopian bridge technique. Otolaryngol Head Neck Surg. 1997;117:586-91.
77. Samii M, Babu RP, Tatagiba M, et al. Surgical treatment of jugular foramen schwannomas. J Neurosurg. 1995;82: 924-32.
78. Fayad JN, Keles B, Brackmann DE. Jugular foramen tumors: clinical characteristics and treatment outcomes. Otol Neurotol. 2010;31:299-305.
79. Hasegawa T. Stereotactic radiosurgery for nonvestibular schwannomas. Neurosurg Clin North Am. 2013;24:531-42.
80. Elsharkawy M, Xu Z, Schlesinger D, et al. Gamma Knife surgery for nonvestibular schwannomas: radiological and clinical outcomes. J Neurosurg. 2012;116:66-72.
81. Choi CY, Soltys SG, Gibbs IC, et al. Stereotactic radiosurgery of cranial nonvestibular schwannomas: results of single- and multisession radiosurgery. Neurosurg. 2011;68: 1200-1208; discussion 1208.
82. Nishioka K, Abo D, Aoyama H, et al. Stereotactic radiotherapy for intracranial nonacoustic schwannomas including facial nerve schwannoma. Int J Radiat Oncol Biol Phys. 2009;75:1415-19.

CHAPTER

26

Encephalocele and CSF Leak

Shawn M Stevens, Habib Rizk, Ryan A Crane, Ted A Meyer

INTRODUCTION/BACKGROUND

Caboche was the first to describe the herniation of brain content into the temporal bone in the French literature as early as 1902.[1] Since that time, authors have used a variety of terms to describe the same pathology, including brain hernia, brain prolapse, brain fungus, fungus cerebri, cerebral hernia, meningoencephalocele, and encephalocele. The modern nomenclature has come to rest on "encephalocele", but all are a pathologic process defined by the presence of cranial contents beyond the normal confines of the skull. Two types of encephalocele have been described: cranial and basal. Cranial encephaloceles are the most common type, followed by the basal type. The latter is further subdivided into midline and lateral encephaloceles. Temporal lobe or middle cranial fossa (MCF) encephaloceles are considered to be basal–lateral and represent the most common type of basal encephalocele reported.[2]

For an encephalocele to develop, by definition a gap in the bone of the skull base must be present or created. Causes for this are varied. In and of itself, an encephalocele is not necessarily a cause for concern. However, the unsupported weight of the overlying brain tissue and intracranial pressure (ICP) gradients as well as exposure to the nonsterile compartments of the temporal bone can lead to a rupture of the dural sac of the encephalocele and cerebrospinal fluid (CSF) leakage.[3] A variety of sites exist for leakage of CSF along the lateral skull base. The most common are the tegmen tympani and tegmen mastoideum. Less common locations include perilabyrinthine, translabyrinthine, or elsewhere along the posterior fossa plate. In one series by Semaan et al, defects involving the middle fossa floor were reported in 90% of all patients presenting with encephalocele. The tegmen tympani and mastoideum had equal representation, comprising approximately 40% of patients each. Multiple dehiscences in the tegmen were seen in 22% and in 55% exceeded 1 cm in diameter.[2] The perilabyrinthine route most often results from operations involving the petrous apex such as posterior fossa or retrosigmoid removal of acoustic tumors. Translabyrinthine leaks are typically associated with congenital inner ear malformations. Posterior fossa encephaloceles are rare.

Violation of the leptomeninges in conjunction with a skull base dehiscence may lead to leakage of CSF from the subarachnoid space into the lateral ear compartments. The potential routes for CSF leakage into the tympanic cavity and/or mastoid cavity are varied and usually related to an underlying pathologic process (Figs. 26.1A and B). A CSF leak can represent a life-threatening clinical entity secondary to the risk of contamination of the normally sterile subarachnoid space. Studies have suggested the overall prevalence of meningitis secondary to CSF leak to range between 4% and 50%, depending on the cause and circumstances of the leak.[4,5] Furthermore, patients may succumb to otogenic cerebral abscesses, epidural abscesses, seizure activity secondary to irritation of the herniated cerebral tissue, and rarely even death. Consequently, CSF otorrhea and otorhinorrhea should prompt an expeditious referral to a neurotologist for consideration of surgical repair. The advent of directed antibiotic regimens, together with the implementation of advanced microsurgical procedures and imaging techniques, has greatly decreased the morbidity and mortality of this process.[6]

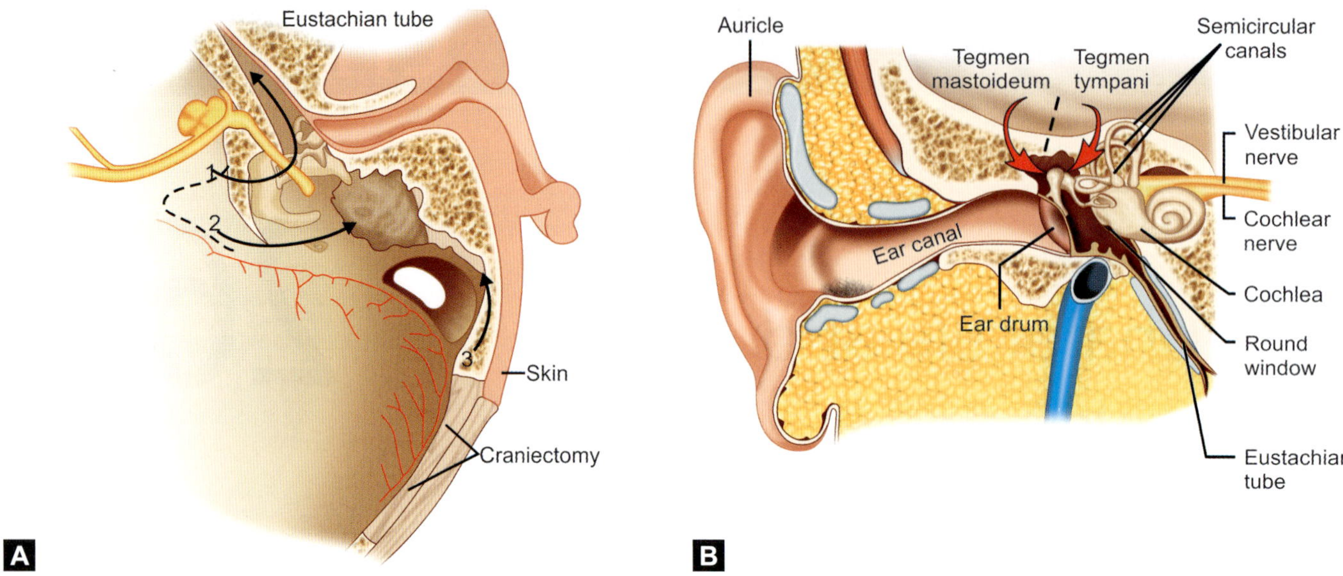

Figs. 26.1A and B: Potential routes of ingress and egress of cerebrospinal fluid (CSF) with respect to the tympanic cavity and mastoid air cells. (A) 1. Leak via the internal auditory canal exiting through the Eustachian tube; 2. Leak via the retrolabyrinthine air cells; 3. Leak via the retrosigmoid air cells. (B) Leaks via defects in the tegmen tympani.
Source: Adapted from Savva et al.[26]

PATHOGENESIS

The pathogenesis of encephalocele formation and/or temporal bone CSF leak may be varied and difficult to accurately discern at the time of presentation. Authors have described a host of etiologies including iatrogenic, infectious, traumatic, neoplastic, congenital, and spontaneous. Each of these processes is described in further detail later in this section. A summation of selected literature regarding etiologies of lateral skull base dehiscence with or without CSF leak is shown in Table 26.1.

Iatrogenic

Breach of the lateral skull base and leptomeninges during temporal bone surgery likely constitutes the most common cause for encephalocele formation and/or CSF leak. Leaks may be noted intraoperatively, during the early postoperative period, or late in the perioperative course. Intraoperative leaks generally are associated with drilling upon the dura leading to tissue maceration and immediate release of CSF. Later leaks may be associated with progressive encephalocele prolapse through iatrogenic skull base dehiscences secondary to the weight of the overlying brain tissue and ICP gradients. Indeed, the evolution of modern neurotologic surgical techniques has been geared toward the avoidance/prevention of future CSF leaks. In this regard, it is well established that the various surgical approaches to the lateral skull base each carry an inherent risk of CSF leak. In their 2004 meta-analysis, Selesnick et al. described CSF leak rates of 10.6%, 9.5%, and 10.6% of retrosigmoid, translabyrinthine, and middle fossa surgeries, respectively.[7] Thanks to evolving surgical technique, a steady improvement in these rates has been reported. The House group notes that rates in the 1980s and 1990s were as high as 20–30%.[8]

Infectious/Cholesteatoma

The mechanism here is thought to be combination of the inflammation associated with chronic otitis media (COM), negative pressures generated within the aerated temporal bone by Eustachian tube dysfunction, and infection/inflation/enzymatic reactions especially in the presence of cholesteatoma. However, iatrogenic effects cannot be overlooked as this patient population is also likely to have undergone prior surgical intervention for their disease. In one series by Jackson et al., as many as 86% of all encephaloceles reported were in patients with a history of COM with or without cholesteatoma.[3] Of these, 77% had undergone one or more prior mastoid operations and the skull base dehiscence was almost exclusively found in the postsurgical cavity.

Neoplastic

A variety of neoplasms, both benign and malignant, may arise from the tissues of the outer, middle, and inner ear,

Table 26.1: Etiologies of lateral skull base encephalocele with or without CSF leak

	Iatrogenic	*Infectious/cholesteatoma*	*Traumatic*	*Spontaneous*	*Congenital*	*Total*
Semaan et al. 2011[2]	0	2	1	25	3	31
Sanna et al. 2010[6]	61	29	10	33	0	133
Savva et al. 2003[26]	53	2	29	8	0	92
Kveton and Coelho 2004[28]	73	10	4	7	2	96
Total	187/352 (53.1%)	43/352 (12.2%)	44/352 (12.5%)	73/352 (20.7%)	5/352 (1.4%)	352

Various etiologies of dehiscence in the lateral skull base with encephalocele formation. The presented numbers are not associated with cerebrospinal fluid (CSF) leak in all cases. Selection of the studies demonstrated here was contingent upon reporting of at least four out of five etiologic categories. The most commonly reported etiology across studies was Iatrogenic followed by infectious/cholesteatoma, traumatic, spontaneous, and congenital. Neoplasm was not directly reported as an etiology in the above studies but was grouped in combination with iatrogenic dehiscence.

the cerebellopontine angle, the temporal bone, the leptomeninges, and neural structures. Encephalocele formation and/or CSF leak may occur secondary to bony erosion, secondary infection/cholesteatoma formation, or direct invasion of the skull base. Resection of neoplastic disease also carries the risk of iatrogenic CSF leak as mentioned previously. An in-depth discussion of neoplastic processes of the temporal bone and lateral skull base is beyond the scope of this chapter and is covered elsewhere in this text (*see* Chapters 9, 15, 23, and 24).

Congenital

Congenital CSF leaks are a rare clinical entity and usually result from a disturbance in the normal ossification of the temporal bone, mainly at the junction between the petrosquamous junction. Fusion of the petrosquamous suture is usually complete by 1 year of age, but delays in this process may arise secondary to growth abnormalities, chemotherapy, and/or radiation. The resulting defect serves as a route for transmission of CSF.[2] CSF leaks may also be produced by an abnormally patent cochlear aqueduct, a persistent Hyrtl fissure, or a patent petromastoid canal.[9] Some of these abnormalities, such as patent cochlear aqueduct, may also be associated with a dehiscent stapes footplate or oval window niche.[10,11] Another rare entity is CSF leak via a congenitally patent fallopian canal. The facial nerve is normally sealed from the subarachnoid space by a tight sheath of dura extending laterally from the fundus along the fallopian canal. The seal is buttressed by the tight enclosure of the labyrinthine segment of the canal around the facial nerve. If this normally tight section is abnormally large, it is possible that the subarachnoid space could extend out to fill such an enlargement. CSF pressure may cause a progressive stretching of facial nerve fibers without necessarily causing paralysis. The CSF pulsations may also cause erosion of surrounding bone, eventually leading to fistulization.[10] Congenital CSF leak by any mechanism is quite rare. When detected, it may be in association with repeated bouts of meningitis and/or sensorineural hearing loss. Case reports also note the rare finding of CSF egress after tympanostomy tube placement for presumed COM with effusion.[10]

Traumatic

Temporal bone trauma or fracture may be associated with dural tear, possible infection, short-term elevation of ICP, and bony healing defects. All of these may account for encephalocele and/or CSF leak. Further discussion on the presentation, workup, and treatment of temporal bone trauma may be found in another chapter in this book (*see* Chapter 22).

Spontaneous

Spontaneous CSF otorrhea is defined as the presence of CSF within the confines of the temporal bone not secondary to traumatic, iatrogenic, neoplastic, and/or infectious causes. It typically occurs in middle-aged adults, females more often than males, and has been significantly associated with benign intracranial hypertension (BIH), radiographically empty sella, and obese habitus.[12-14] Single or multiple dehiscences within a broadly attenuated tegmen coupled with normal inner ear anatomy are typical findings (Figs. 26.2 and 26.3). Significant uncertainty remains regarding the pathophysiology of spontaneous CSF otorrhea. The two predominant theories are as follows: (1) increased CSF pressure causes gradual attenuation of the tegmen and/or enlargement of congenital tegmen dehiscences with eventual dural herniation and CSF otorrhea; and (2) abnormally located arachnoid granulations within the tegmen act as minor CSF reservoirs that are unable to properly return CSF to the venous system and cause subsequent erosion of bone via persistent pressure at the bony sites underlying these granulations. Of the two theories, recent evidence seems to point to the former as the most likely/common mechanism. Treatment of spontaneous CSF leak is challenging and associated with a high rate of recurrence.[15]

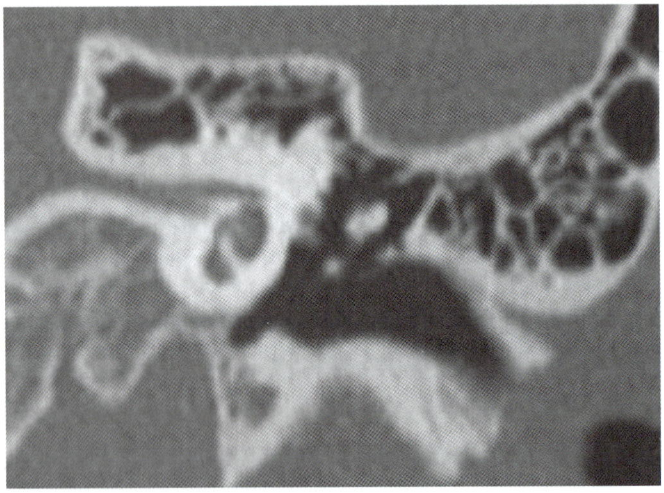

Fig. 26.2: Coronal computed tomography (CT) image, left ear, depicting a normal tegmen tympani overlying the ossicular heads.

CLINICAL FINDINGS: SYMPTOMS AND SIGNS

Diagnosis of encephalocele and CSF leak begins in the clinic with a thorough history and physical examination. As the early signs and symptoms are often vague and nonspecific, a high index of suspicion must be maintained. A prior history of ear surgery, trauma, or chronic otitis should be sought. Table 26.2 provides a listing of the most commonly reported symptoms as described in selected literature. Overall, the most frequent symptom is hearing loss, present in up to 87% of cases.[6] Pulsatile tinnitus, surprisingly, is not a commonly reported complaint. In the majority of cases, presenting symptoms may be related to the concomitant disease (e.g. otorrhoea in COM), and thus more difficult to decipher. Symptoms more specific for encephalocele such as CSF rhinorrhea (clear rhinorrhea, salty post-nasal drip), meningismus, cephalalgia, and/or seizure activity tend to occur more often in cases of spontaneous leak. Active CSF leak is often absent at the time of initial presentation and diagnosis (as few as 10% of cases in one series) except in cases of trauma or spontaneous leaks.[6] Meningitis may be the initial manifestation of encephalocele and/or leak in congenital and spontaneous cases. Repeated episodes of bacterial meningitis without other clear causation should draw attention to the temporal bone and anterior skull base.

On examination, findings vary based on etiology, comorbid conditions, and patient-specific factors. The

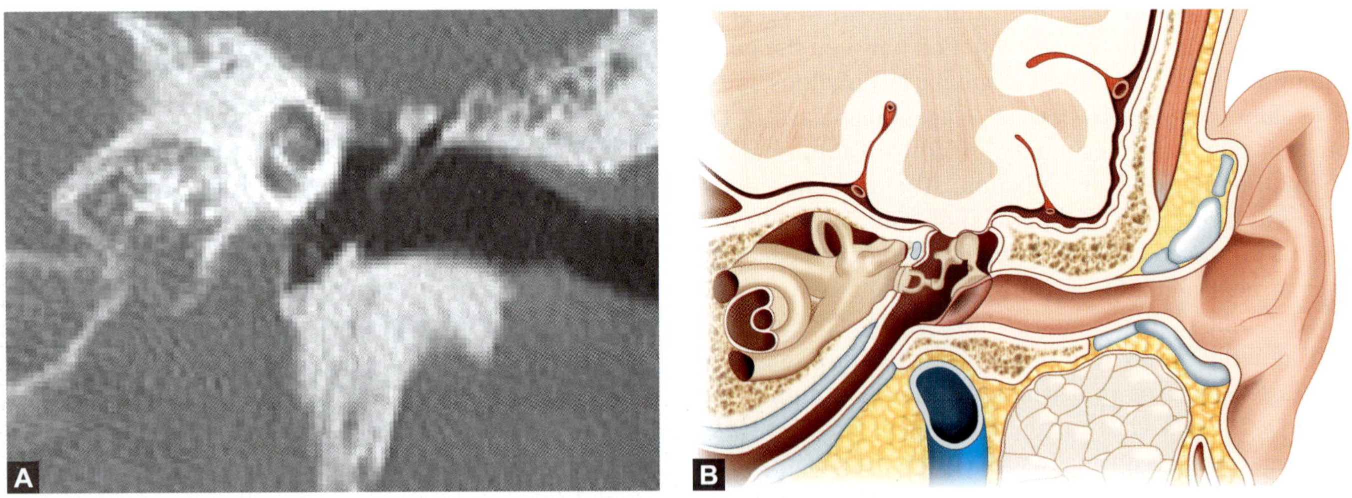

Figs. 26.3A and B: (A) Coronal computed tomography (CT) image, left ear, depicting an attenuated tegmen with a large dehiscence overlying the ossicles. The soft tissue density encroaching into the epitympanum is an encephalocele. This patient presented with spontaneous cerebrospinal fluid (CSF) otorrhea. In such cases, broad attenuation of the tegmen is common. (B) Illustration depicting dehiscence of the tegmen tympani with an encephalocele abutting the ossicular chain. The illustration is identical in orientation to the image shown on the left and is included for enhanced presentation of the soft tissues and two-dimensional special anatomy.
Source: B adapted from Gubbels et al.[31]

Table 26.2: Presenting symptoms of lateral skull base encephalocele and/or CSF leak

Symptom	Semaan et al. 2001[2] (n=31)	Jackson et al. 1997[3] (n=35)	Sanna et al. 2010[6] (n=133)	Kutz et al. 2008[30] (n=17)	Total (Percentage)
Otorrhea or middle ear effusion	21	24	14	15	74/216 (34.2%)
Hearing loss	25	18	116	8	167/216 (77.3%)
Tinnitus	4	14	—	—	18/66 (27.2%)
Vertigo	0	7	30	—	37/199 (18.5%)
Otalgia	0	3	—	—	3/66 (4.5%)
Aural fullness	0	3	—	15	18/83 (21.6%)
Meningismus/Meningitis	—	—	14	4	18/150 (12.0%)
Facial weakness	0	1	—	—	1/66 (1.5%)
Rhinorrhea	1	0	—	5	6/83 (7.2%)
Seizures/epilepsy	0	1	4	—	5/199 (2.5%)

Presenting symptoms of lateral skull base encephalocele and/or cerebrospinal fluid (CSF) leaks described as derived from selected literature. The most common presenting symptoms were hearing loss followed by otorrhea/middle ear effusion and vertigo. Aural fullness and meningitis were also reported relatively frequently. The above symptoms were not stratified according to causation of the encephalocele/leak. Not all symptoms were reported in each study while some were reported with no occurrences (0); omissions are depicted above with a dash. Relative percentage (in parentheses) of patients presenting with a particular symptom is derived from the number of patients with that symptom as a factor of all patients asked about that symptom. Patients in studies where a symptom was omitted were not included in the overall total for calculation of percentage.

encephalocele sac may be seen protruding into the middle ear, mastoid (in canal wall down cavities), or external auditory canal (EAC) through various tegmen defects. Classically, this mass is pulsatile, smooth, and may be surrounded by a watery discharge (CSF). Pulsation may be elicited or enhanced by Valsalva maneuver, which may also reproduce the leak. In postoperated ears, especially after acoustic neuroma resection, the surgical wound should be assessed for leak and/or a fluctuant collection of CSF directly deep to the surgical wound (CSFoma). In cases of a persistent, clear middle ear effusion in an otherwise healthy and nonoperated ear, a spontaneous leak should be suspected. In such cases, performance of a mryingotomy with immediate return of clear fluid may be confirmatory of the suspected diagnosis. Findings during exploratory surgery may include an avascular mass in the mesotympanum, EAC, or mastoid cavity. Other potential intraoperative findings are inflammation, moisture, mucosal thickening, granulation tissue, and/or cholesteatoma. This is especially true in chronic ears and may make identification of the encephalocele sac more difficult.[3,16] In cases associated with trauma, one may detect Battle sign, raccoon eyes, hemotympanum, canal laceration/hematoma, mandible fracture, closed head injury, and/or c-spine injury.

EVALUATION: LABORATORY, OTOLOGIC, AND NEUROTOLOGIC TESTING

Beta-2 Transferrin

Considered the gold standard test to confirm presence of CSF, beta-2 transferrin has greater sensitivity and specificity than in-office glucose testing using multireagent strip.[17] Transferrin is converted in the central nervous system to beta-2 transferrin by the enzyme neuraminidase, which is located only in the CSF, the vitreous humor, and the perilymph, making this assay a highly reliable method for detecting the presence of CSF. It is undetectable in blood and nasal secretions as well as tears and mucosal effusions except in chronic liver disease and inborn errors of glycoprotein metabolism. These rare causes of false positive are, however, easily circumvented by a protocol that includes testing the patient's serum for beta-2 transferrin as well as the suspicious fluid.[18] Beta-2 transferrin assays carry a sensitivity of 84–100% and specificity of 95–100%.[19,20] The protein is very stable, which allows for the patient with intermittent otorrhea or rhinorrhea to collect the fluid at home and send it to the lab for analysis.

Minimal amounts of fluid are needed; as little as 0.5 mL of fluid has been advocated by some authors.[17] The time for the assay is between 2 and 6 hours.

Glucose

Glucose testing can be performed in office with a multi-reagent strip. These are often overly sensitive and have been shown to give false-positive results in 45–75% of cases.[4] CSF has lower glucose levels than blood but higher than either nasal or lacrimal secretions (when testing nasal drainage). Interpretation may be difficult, but collected fluid with a concentration of 30 mg/dL glucose combined with normal blood glucose levels suggests CSF. If the patient has no active meningitis (which may lower the glucose levels) and one is able to collect the fluid without contamination by blood or wound secretions, the test may be more reliable.[21] However, due to its overall lack of specificity and the inherent difficulty in obtaining a pure specimen, glucose testing has been relatively abandoned as a primary diagnostic tool.[22]

Beta-Trace Protein

A newer, more rapid assay called beta-trace assay has been recently introduced. The beta-trace protein is actually prostaglandin D synthase. Although found in CSF, minimal concentrations are also detectable in blood, urine, aqueous humor, and vitreous humor. It is, however, one of the most abundant proteins in CSF with a high CSF:serum ratio. Current quantitative assays allow for a quick result on the order of 20 minutes. Like beta-2 transferrin, the protein is very stable, which allows for the patient with intermittent otorrhea or rhinorrhea to collect the fluid at home and send it to the lab for analysis. While some studies cite a high precision and reproducibility, diagnostic cut-off values for the various assays have yet to be definitively determined.[23] Interpretation of the results must take into account the renal function of the patient because the serum levels may be increased in renal failure. Overall, it is less specific to CSF than beta-2 transferrin such that relatively high concentrations of beta-trace protein must be present for a diagnosis of CSF. For this reason, dilution and specimen contamination are as much a problem as they are in glucose measurements. Conditions such as normal pressure hydrocephalus, and meningitis, where the levels of beta-trace proteins in the CSF might be diminished for these reasons, often yield high false negative rates.[24] Overall, beta-trace protein assays may be considered a quick screening test but confirmation of results may require an assay for beta-2 transferrin.

Otologic, Audiometric, and Immittance Testing

Otoscopic examination findings were discussed earlier in this chapter. Pneumatic otoscopy may note immobility of the drum correlating with a type B tympanogram and normal canal volumes on immittance testing. Rarely, positive or negative pressure applied across the tympanic membrane may elicit nystagmus and transient vertigo (Hennebert sign), which may indicate a fistulous exposure of the perilymph-containing labyrinth (neoplasm, trauma). Vestibular testing is typically of little diagnostic benefit. In cases of CSF otorrhea behind an intact tympanic membrane, audiograms will typically show a conductive or mixed hearing loss, although severe to profound sensorineural hearing losses may be detected in association with meningitis, congenital encephalocele/leak, neoplasm, and in some trauma cases.

Evaluation: Radiologic Imaging

Imaging may greatly assist in the diagnosis of encephalocele and CSF leak, but the importance of thorough clinical examination and good history taking cannot be understated. Employment of imaging techniques should be considered as an adjunct to a sound clinical workup and may help demonstrate the location of the encephalocele and/or leak, determine if multiple dehiscences exist, and help guide surgical planning. The diagnostic accuracy of these studies is not perfect, however, and the surgeon should be prepared to deal with the unexpected at the time of surgery.

Computed Tomography (CT)

Some advocate that high-resolution CT (HRCT) might be the only radiologic investigation necessary. This imaging modality is excellent for depicting size and location of bony defect(s) but is not truly suited to detect the site of dural tear, which is important in cases of multiple defects. A search for bilateral dehiscences should be conducted in cases of suspected spontaneous leak and in chronic ears. Sensitivity is reported around 90%, specificity up to 100%, and positive predictive value at 100%.[17,19] It should be noted that encephalocele may be difficult to distinguish from cholesteatoma, granulation tissue, cholesterol granuloma, or other soft-tissue masses within the middle ear and mastoid on HRCT. A combination of CT with MRI may boost sensitivity and aid in distinguishing these entities and in the location of a dural tear.[6,19] False positive results have also been described related to volume averaging and vascular grooves.[20] A bony algorithm with dedicated temporal bone protocol and fine cuts of 1 mm should be employed to maximize diagnostic capabilities. Coronal and sagittal reconstructions are well suited to detect tegmen defects (Figs. 26.2 to 26.4). Rare posterior cranial fossa herniations are better defined with axial sections. Other findings found to be associated with leak/encephalocele include a broadly attenuated bony skull base (Figs. 26.3 and 26.4) and arachnoid pits (secondary to the bony impressions from the arachnoid villi and present in 63% of patients with spontaneous CSF rhinorrhea in one study).[25]

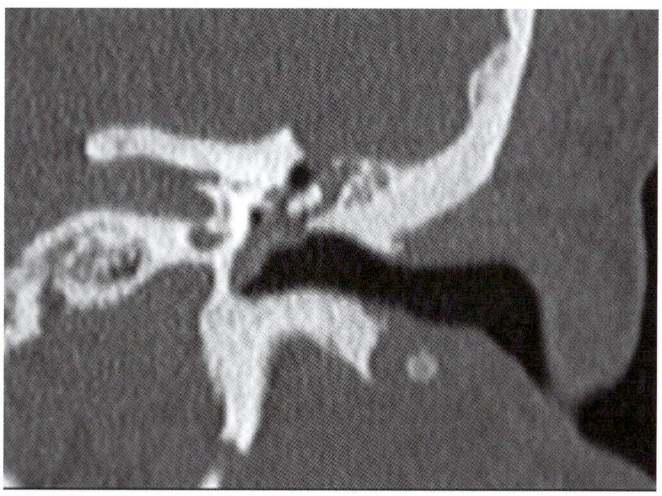

Fig. 26.4: Coronal computed tomography (CT) image, left ear, depicting a tegmen tympani dehiscence with encephalocele and cerebrospinal fluid (CSF) filling the tympanic cavity.

Magnetic Resonance Imaging (MRI)

MRI typically serves as an adjunct to CT in cases of encephalocele. Possible exceptions to this might be in chronic ear cases where cholesteatoma is expected and in the workup of erosive skull base neoplasms. In general, herniated meningoencephalic tissue is seen as a nonenhancing contiguous mass, isointense to brain in all sequences. Cholesteatoma, on the other hand, appears hyperintense in T2-weighted images, and a cholesterol granuloma appears hyperintense both in T1- and in T2-weighted images.[6] Non-echo-planar diffusion-weighted MRI also is useful for differentiating cholesteatoma in patients with chronic ear disease. Pre- and postgadolinium-enhanced, T1-weighted, thin-section images may be of great help in differentiating mucosal thickening (enhancing) from encephalocele (isointense) and neoplasms (generally enhancing). T2-weighted images are typically the most valuable in visualizing CSF leaks (Fig. 26.5) as well as herniation of the CSF-filled dura mater and neural tissue into the temporal bone (Figs. 26.6 and 26.7). In contrast to CT imaging, it does not show bony detail or any discontinuity of the underlying temporal bone cortex and is usually of limited direct diagnostic value. Recently, several authors have used MRI as an adjunctive modality to identify anatomic features often associated with CSF leak. Prichard et al. in 2006 examined radiographic studies in patients with spontaneous CSF otorrhea, finding 71% of cases to have a radiographically empty sella (known to be strongly correlated with BIH and obesity) (Figs. 26.8A and B).[13]

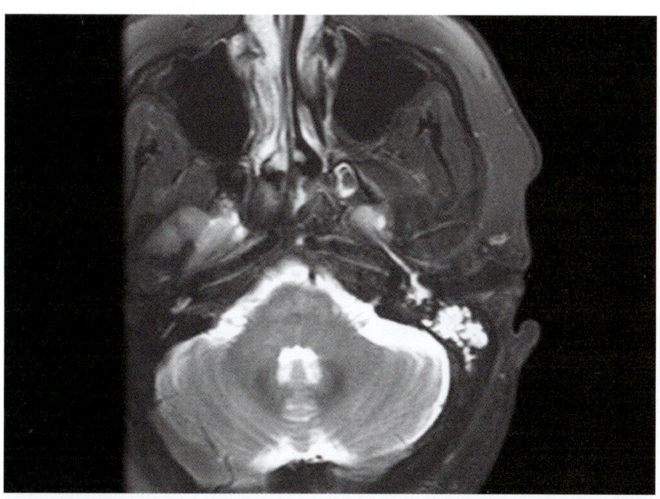

Fig. 26.5: Axial, T2-weighted magnetic resonance imaging (MRI) depicting a left ear cerebrospinal fluid (CSF) leak into the mastoid and tympanic cavities. The image also captures CSF draining into the nasopharynx via the Eustachian tube.

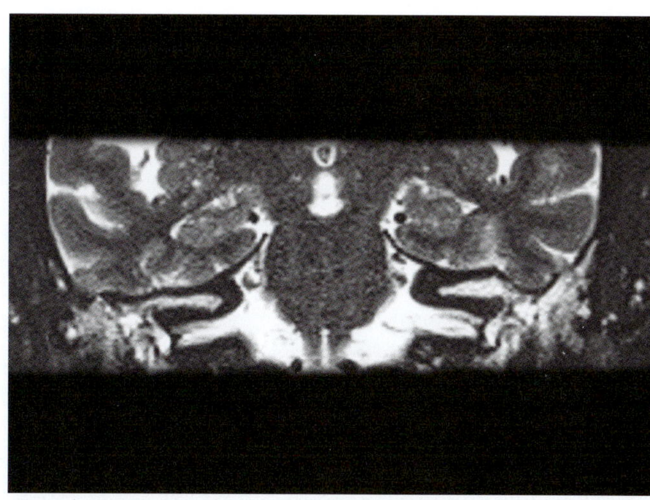

Fig. 26.6: Coronal, T2-weighted magnetic resonance imaging (MRI) depicting bilateral mastoid cavity cerebrospinal fluid (CSF) leaks via tegmen dehiscences. An encephalocele may be seen protruding through the left lateral aspect of the tegmen plate.

Goddard et al. furthered this work in 2010 through a retrospective review of individuals presenting with spontaneous CSF otorrhea and found an empty or partially empty sella in 80%. Mean BMI of these patients was 38.0 kg/m^2 compared with 28.5 kg/m^2 for those without an empty sella.[14] The quoted rate of empty sella in the general population is between 5% and 6%.[14,15]

CT Cisternography

Radionuclide cisternography may serve as an adjunct in cases where an active leak is suspected but the diagnosis unconfirmed. The most widely used radiotracer is technetium 99m-labeled diethylene-triamine-penta-acetic acid. Other tracers such as Indium 111 may also be selected for their longer half-life, especially in the setting of intermittent CSF leaks.[17] Between 3 and 10 cc of the contrast agent of choice is administered intrathecally via lumbar drain. Agents are typically diluted in saline or the patient's own CSF. The patient is then placed in Trendelenburg position to opacify the basal cisterns. In an effort to improve sensitivity, some authors have described the placement of ear wicks that may absorb the colored tracer dye. Other techniques to boost yield include use of Valsalva, and laying the patient prone or in a head-hanging position. Even with these methods, the sensitivity of the technique ranges between 40% and 85% depending on whether the leak is inactive or active, respectively.[26] For this reason, CT cisternography likely should be reserved for complex cases with a diagnosis that is in question. Cisternography is contraindicated in patients with meningitis and elevated ICP secondary to the risk of herniation.

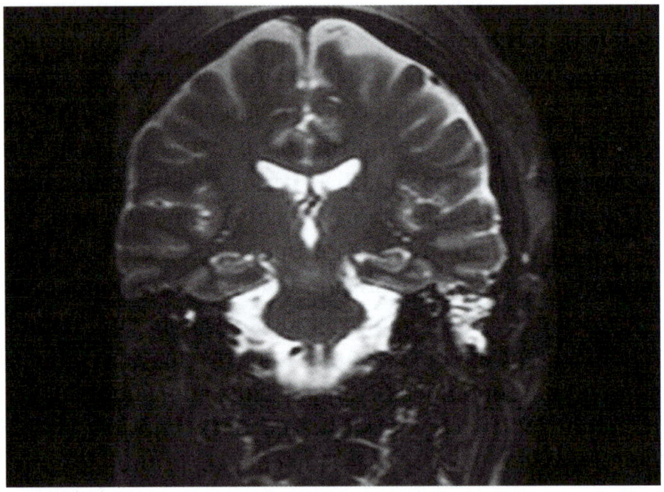

Fig. 26.7: Coronal, T2-weighted magnetic resonance imaging (MRI) of a left ear encephalocele within the mastoid cavity and associated cerebrospinal fluid (CSF) leak. The posterior semicircular canal may be appreciated medial to the CSF-filled mastoid cavity.

MRI/MR Cisternography

This newer imaging modality involves heavily T2-weighted, fast spin echo sequences with fat suppression to enhance visualization of a CSF leak via the deletion of surrounding tissues. The advantage of this technique over CT cisternography is that it is a fully noninvasive method. When an active leak is present, sensitivity of the modality may approach 90%.[27] The addition of intrathecal gadolinium-enhanced cisternography has also been associated with promising results. However, both the inability of MR to

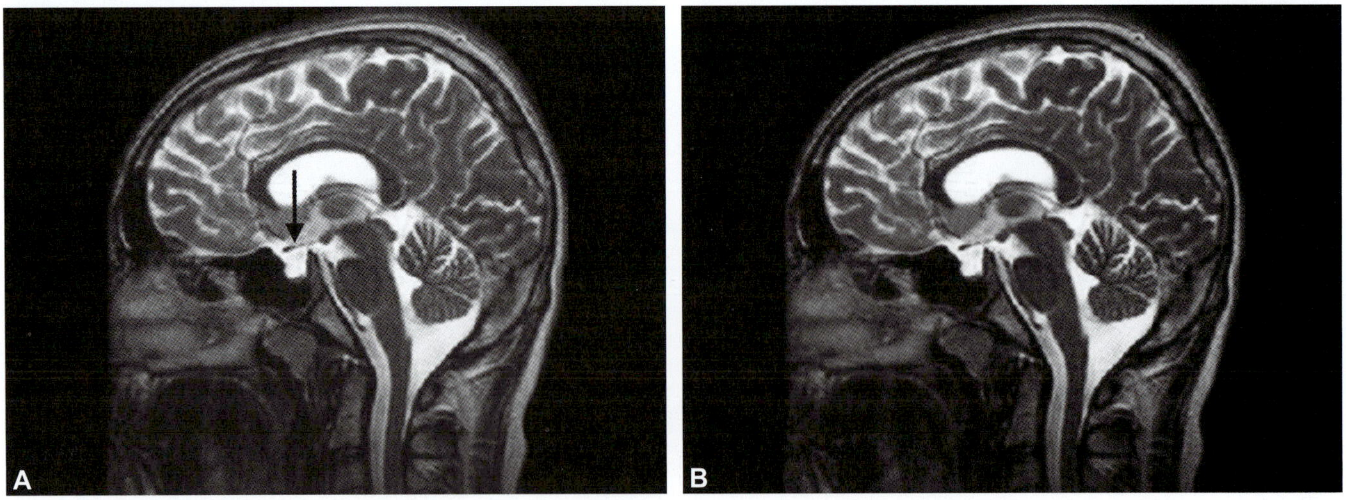

Figs. 26.8A and B: Sagittal, T2-weighted magnetic resonance imaging (MRI) image of an empty sella (black arrow).

visualize an osseous defect and the excellent sensitivity and specificity of HRCT have marginalized this modality to use in only the most complex or confusing cases. The safety of intrathecal gadolinium also has not been established and its use for this purpose has not been approved.[27]

HISTOLOGY

A detailed discussion of histopathology is beyond the scope of this text, but it is important to understand that a herniated encephalocele will be pedicled to intracranial contents via a tegmen defect of variable size. With the exception of very large dehiscences with gross protrusion of brain and leptomeninges, a typical encephalocele sac will contain extensively gliotic, degraded, and inflamed neural tissue. The herniated tissue is considered devitalized and functionless. This becomes important during surgical intervention and reconstructive planning as described below.[3]

TREATMENT/PROGNOSIS: MEDICAL AND SURGICAL

Management of temporal bone CSF leaks and encephalocele is dictated by the cause and location. A few overarching treatment concepts require discussion prior to detailed explanation of surgical approaches and materials, however. First, understanding that the various etiologies of encephalocele and CSF leak follow different natural histories is of vital importance in safe and appropriate treatment planning. For instance, traumatic CSF leaks will often cease spontaneously with only conservative measures while iatrogenic and spontaneous leaks nearly always require surgical closure and carry a high risk of developing meningitis. Second, surgical approaches are not highly varied and basically include transmastoid, MCF and hybrid procedures. However, proper selection of technique and approach is important to avoid excessive morbidity, and the operating surgeon should be prepared to alter his/her approach when indicated. Middle ear obliteration (MEO) with closure of the EAC and plugging of the Eustachian tube remains a viable option for refractory, recurrent, and overly difficult cases.

When an encephalocele is identified, it is important to know that the neural contents are usually devitalized and nonfunctional and that this tissue is exposed to a contaminated and in some cases infected environment. Thus, reduction of encephalocele tissue back into the sterile cranial vault should be avoided, and convention holds that this tissue should be amputated (usually with bipolar electrocautery and sharp scissors).[3] When amputation is complete and/or a disruption of the leptomeninges is identified, primary dural closure alone is not adequate and will lead to high failure rates. Closures using two or more supporting materials appear to lead to the best outcomes, with some authors reporting use of up to five.[3,7] Overall, the principles of skull base reconstruction should include (1) formation of a watertight seal to stop CSF leak, (2) restoration of intracranial vault integrity, and (3) avoidance of leak recurrence with strong enough reconstruction to resist ICP. In achieving these basic principles, one should be aware that no literature consensus exists on any single material or combination thereof. Thus, surgeons base strategy more on personal experience and technical comfort level to achieve success. The following discussion will provide a detailed but nonexhaustive account of the various interventions, approaches, and materials currently in use with the hope that they may be employed dynamically on a case-specific basis to achieve the greatest outcomes possible. Table 26.3 provides a listing of the various interventions described later in this text.

Table 26.3: Interventions for the treatment of lateral skull base encephalocele and CSF leak

Noninvasive interventions	*CSF diversion*	*Surgical approaches*
Head of bed elevation (30–45°)	Lumbar drain	Transmastoid approach
Bed rest	Ventriculoperitoneal shunt	Middle cranial fossa approach
Anti-emetics	External ventricular drain	Mini-middle cranial fossa approach
Antitussives	Other ventricular shunt	Transmastoid extradural, intracranial approach
Stool softeners		Middle ear obliteration

Various interventions in the surgeon's armamentarium for treating cerebrospinal fluid (CSF) leak and/or encephalocele. Noninvasive methods should be considered in most cases unless directly contraindicated. CSF diversion may be useful in select cases but is not commonly reported by most neurotologists. A nonexhaustive listing of surgical approaches is depicted in the far right column.

Conservative Measures

The basic tenets of care in patients presenting with suspected or known CSF leak mimic those of postoperative prevention protocols. Restrictions are geared primarily toward prevention of acute ICP spikes. Such restrictions may include avoidance of straining and/or lifting, bed rest, head of bed elevation (30–45°), and the use of antiemetics, antitussives, and stool softeners. As mentioned previously, conservative measures alone may be sufficient for the treatment of traumatic CSF leaks. Savva et al. noted success in 82% of traumatic leaks using this approach. The period required for cessation of the leak ranged from 1 to 18 days (median period, 3 days).[26]

In suspected or known iatrogenic leaks, the use of the above measures for a 3-and 4-day trial period has been advocated.[3] When CSF is seen to be leaking directly from the wound, the wound may be oversewn using a silk or other permanent suture in mattress fashion with a goal of sealing the skin and the underlying soft tissues. A pressure dressing is then applied. In cases of postoperative CSF rhinorrhea, the addition of a lumbar drain for a few days may lead to successful resolution of the leak.[8] However, if a leak can still be demonstrated after a few days, the patient is offered a surgical procedure to explore the wound and repair the leak, typically with a combination of autologous materials.

CSF Diversion

Lumbar Drain

In cases of spontaneous CSF otorrhea, authors within the neurosurgical community have advised the use of lumbar drain for CSF diversion and tout its utility as both a diagnostic and therapeutic tool. Kenning et al. describe placement of the drain immediately after induction of general anesthesia. At this time, an opening pressure (OP) can be obtained (helpful in diagnosis of spontaneous leaks and BIH), followed by maintenance of the drain intraoperatively. OP also may play a role in the decision to perform ventriculoperitoneal (VP) shunting as discussed in the next section. Use of the drain was typically continued for 48–72 hours postoperatively to aid with decompression of the dural repair. The authors also describe a benefit derived from temporal lobe relaxation during evaluation for sites of dehiscence.[15] As placement and maintenance of a lumbar drain typically require cross-service collaboration with neurosurgery, and since the procedure adds some inherent risk, lumbar drainage has not gained popularity among otolaryngologists, with little reporting in the literature.

Ventriculoperitoneal Shunt

Similar to the use of lumbar drains, VP shunts are not routinely employed within the otolaryngology and neurotology literature. One author does pose an interesting algorithm in which VP shunt placement is considered for patients and clinical factors found to be associated with the highest risk of recurrence. Factors include spontaneous CSF leak, high-volume leaks, OP >20 cm H_2O, BMI >30 kg/m^2, preoperative imaging demonstrating additional cranial base cortical defects (i.e. contralateral tegmen or anterior cranial base), and/or an empty sella turcica.[15] Additionally, these authors felt VP shunting warranted consideration in the presence of any event leading to inflammation of the arachnoid granulations and impairment of CSF absorption, such as meningitis, intracranial hemorrhage, and significant closed-head injury.

Surgical Approaches

Selection of the most appropriate surgical approach for the treatment of an encephalocele and/or leak must be based on the location, size, and number of skull base defect(s). Consideration should also be given to preoperative auditory function, the presence of active infection, patient capacity for healing, and comorbid conditions. When choosing an approach, the surgeon is tasked with fully understanding the benefits and risks of the various techniques with an emphasis on sound preoperative planning to avoid unnecessary morbidity. This concept especially holds in cases of single, small, and easily reached skull base defects. In cases of large encephalocele, multiple defects, poor preoperative hearing, or a broadly attenuated skull base, a more aggressive surgical approach may be appropriate.

Transmastoid Approach

For small and laterally based defects, a transmastoid repair is chosen by many otologic surgeons. This approach allows extracranial visualization and assessment of the middle and posterior fossa plates, while avoiding retraction of intracranial tissues (Figs. 26.9A and B).[2] Herniated tissues should be cauterized with bipolar cautery and truncated under microscopic visualization. For more anterior defects located in the tegmen tympani, the transmastoid

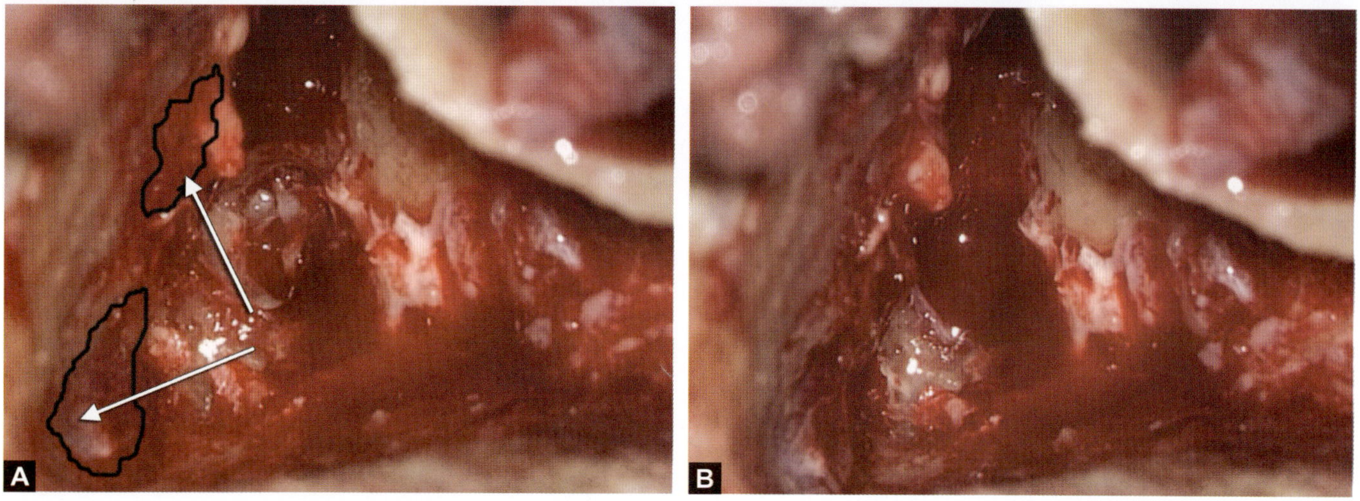

Figs. 26.9A and B: Transmastoid approach on a right ear with identification of multiple tegmen dehiscences (outlines) with visible encephaloceles (arrows).

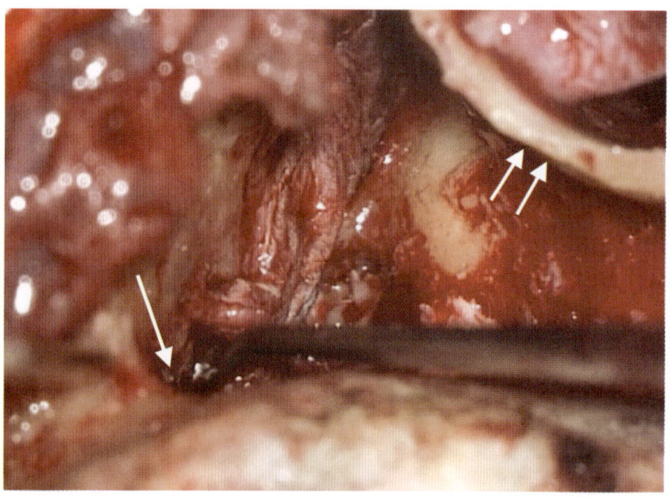

Fig. 26.10: Transmastoid approach on a right ear. Image depicts the surgeon repairing a tegmen mastoideum dehiscence with a temporalis fascia graft (long single arrow). Short double arrows point to the bony external auditory canal.

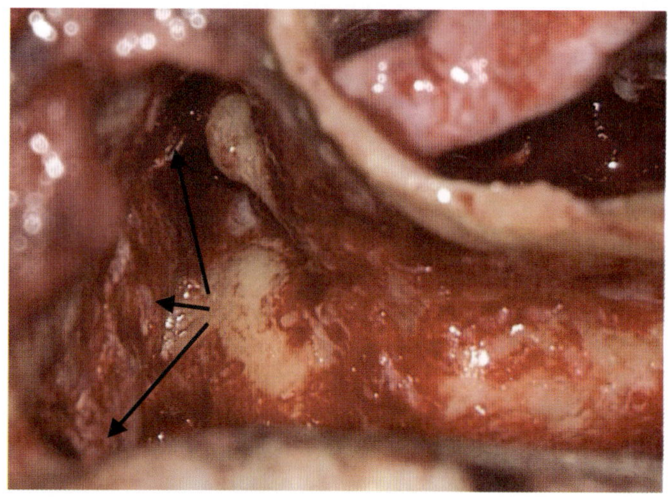

Fig. 26.11: Transmastoid approach on a right ear. Image depicts completed repair with temporalis fascia (arrows). Note that this dehiscence extended partially into the tegmen tympani overlying a well-visualized incus body and short process.

approach may provide inadequate exposure for the purposes of repair. If the ossicular chain is removed for reasons related to the encephalocele and/or concomitant COM, a transmastoid approach may work well in combination with a facial recess, extended facial recess, or posterior tympanotomy.[6] Dural defects can be packed with free autologous soft tissue plugs and covered with a layer of fascia between the dura mater and tegmen plate (Figs. 26.10 and 26.11). Second-layer closure with calvarial bone or conchal/tragal cartilage may be employed for bony defects larger than 1 cm (Fig. 26.12). Bone wax, bone dust, and free temporalis muscle plugs have also been used to good effect.[6,26] After closure of the leak and skull base defect, the surgeon may also decide to obliterate the mastoid cavity with a free abdominal fat graft or pedicled temporalis muscle flap, although this is not usually necessary. Other biomaterials have also been utilized as adjuncts to skull base reconstruction and are discussed in further detail later in this chapter.

Middle Cranial Fossa (MCF) Approach

The MCF approach provides the surgeon with potential access to the entire MCF floor. The concept underlying a MCF approach is to employ the weight of the overlying temporal lobe to bolster the repair and better resist postoperative ICP spikes.[3] The advantages of this approach are

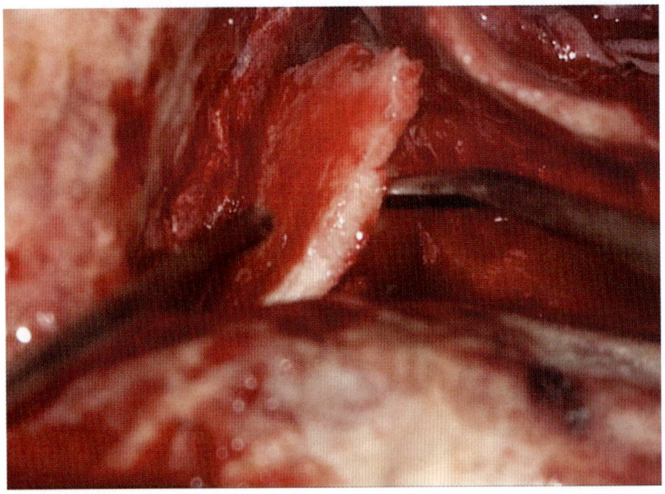

Fig. 26.12: Transmastoid approach on a right ear. The image depicts the surgeon reinforcing the temporalis fascia graft with tragal cartilage graft. The mastoid cavity was later filled with hydroxyapatite cement to fully secure this dual-layered reconstruction (not shown).

access to an anterior dehiscence, better exposure of large defects (compared with transmastoid alone), and avoidance of ossicular chain disruption. Regarding the latter, some have employed this approach to truncate tegmen tympani encephaloceles from above and then leave the herniation contents in the middle ear with little negative effect on hearing or recurrence rates.[6] Additional uses of the MCF approach include cases involving acutely infected ears (the operation remains primarily within the sterile intracranial vault) and in cases of multifocal tegmen defects. Other authors also advocate use of the MCF approach for defects larger than 2 cm and those defects extending toward the petrous apex.[2,26] Disadvantages include increased risk of iatrogenic CSF leak, increased retraction on the temporal lobe (seizure risk), and violation of the intracranial vault. Significant postsurgical bleeding, while rare, is a known clinical entity and should be kept under consideration during surgical planning.

To perform a MCF approach, a variety of skin incisions can be made in a cranial direction from the pinna (Fig. 26.13). This may extend as a straight cephalad, bow in a curvilinear fashion, or wrap around to form an anterior or posteriorly based skin flap. Elevation of the underlying temporalis muscle in a subperiosteal plane exposes the squamous temporal bone. An appropriately sized craniotomy is then performed (Fig. 26.14), with the lower edge of the craniotomy at the level of the temporal line/zygomatic process. The dura of the temporal lobe is carefully elevated until the neck of the hernia is identified, coagulated, and

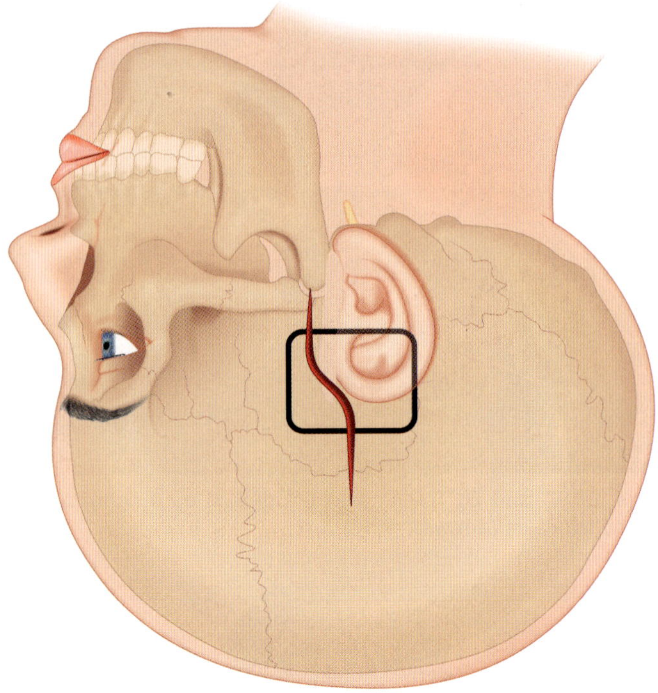

Fig. 26.13: Illustration demonstrating a preauricular incision overlying the planned craniotomy site (faint box) for a middle cranial fossa approach as would be seen by the surgeon. The incision shown above is one of many available.
Source: Adapted from Gubbels et al.[31]

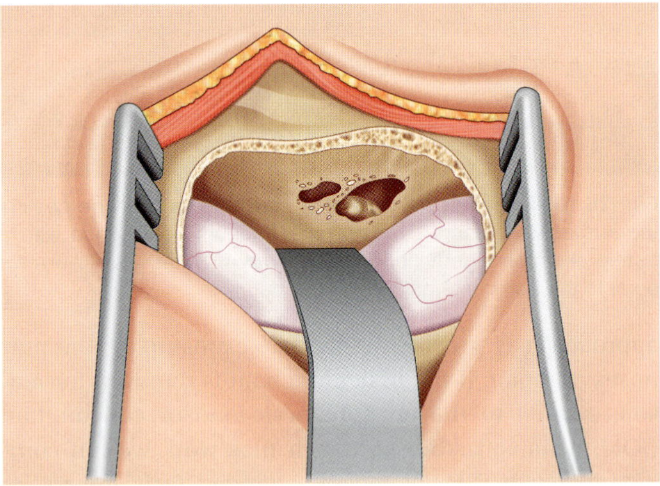

Fig. 26.14: Illustration demonstrating the surgeon's view following craniotomy and retraction of the temporal lobe. Multiple tegmen dehiscences are demonstrated allowing visualization of the ossicles. The bottom of the image correlates to the top of the patient's head.
Source: Adapted from Gubbels et al.[31]

cut (Figs. 26.14 and 26.15). The herniated tissue may be left in the middle ear or mastoid or removed at this time. A piece of cartilage is placed between the bony defect and

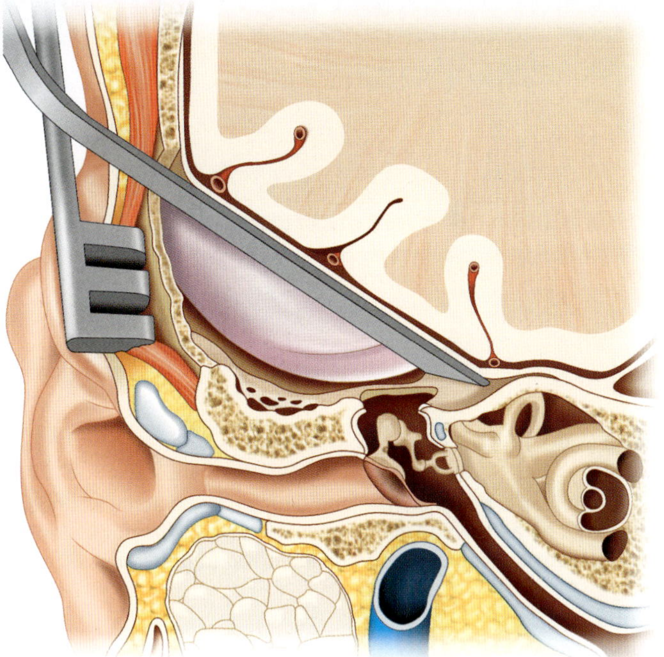

Fig. 26.15: Illustration depicting coronally oriented cross-section of middle fossa approach. The temporal lobe is retracted via the craniotomy. The encephalocele has been elevated out of the tegmen tympani dehiscence.
Source: Adapted from Gubbels et al.[31]

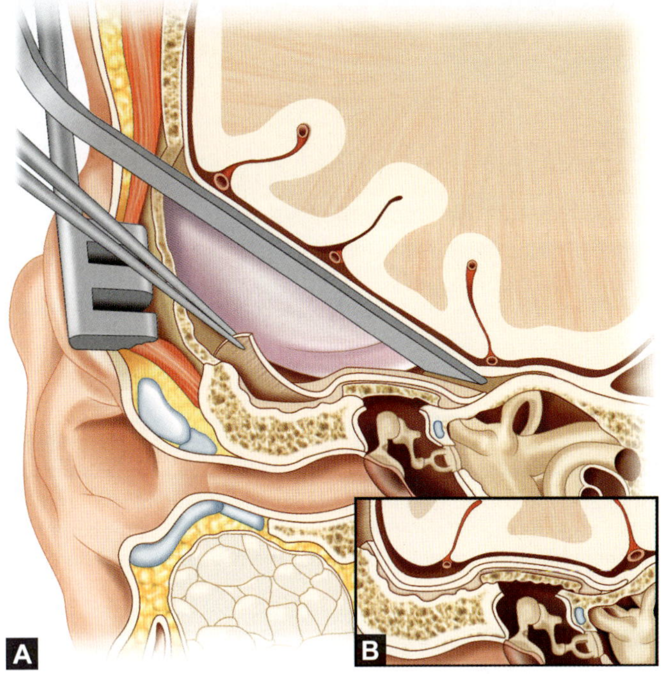

Figs. 26.16A and B: Illustration depicting coronally oriented-cross section of middle fossa approach. The temporal lobe is retracted via the craniotomy. (A) The tegmen tympani dehiscence has been repaired with a piece of autologous cartilage in an overlay fashion. An additional piece of fascia has been draped over this for multilayered closure of the defect. (B) The downward weight of the overlying temporal lobe secures the grafts and facilitates watertight closure.
Source: Adapted from Gubbels et al.[31]

the dura. The defect is then further reinforced with temporalis fascia placed between the dura and the cartilage (Figs. 26.16A and B).

Hybrid Approaches

The above approaches are often combined to maximize the benefits of each while limiting anticipated morbidity. In some cases, the surgeon may decide intraoperatively to extend an initially conservative transmastoid approach with a small craniotomy or to expand an existing defect for the same purpose of exposure. Preplanned hybrid approaches similar to this have also been described in the literature with a central concept of maximizing exposure via the least invasive route possible. Kenning et al. described a combined mastoid/mini-middle fossa approach and reported success rates of leak repair approaching 96%.[15] Groups such as Ramalingam et al. describe the use of transmastoid, minicraniotomy approaches for select defects to avoid the increased risk of full MCF approach. In both series, surgery began with a standard transmastoid approach followed by the creation of a smaller rectangular window in the temporal bone squama and/or tegmen to give access to the middle fossa. The bone from this window was typically banked and used later to repair the encephalocele defect. Skull base repair was typically facilitated by a three-layer (fascia–bone–fascia) closure in both series and both met with good success rates. Figures 26.17 and 26.18 depict the excellent visualization allowed by the mastoid/mini-middle fossa approach with regard to a large skull base dehiscence.

Semaan et al. provide an excellent description of a widely used variation of the technique described above.[2] A mastoidectomy is performed and any granulation tissue/reactive bone removed around the encephalocele (if present). The encephalocele sac is then cauterized and truncated and the tegmen defect widened using a small diamond burr. The dura is then elevated off the floor of the MCF via this enlarged bone defect with a small elevator for at least 5 mm circumferentially (Fig. 26.19). The elevation is extradural and intracranial and purposed to create a tight pocket for eventual placement of an intracranial cartilage graft. Cartilage utilized for repair is shaped to fit the defect and inserted in such a way that it "locks" into place under the dura of the temporal lobe (Fig. 26.20). This locking

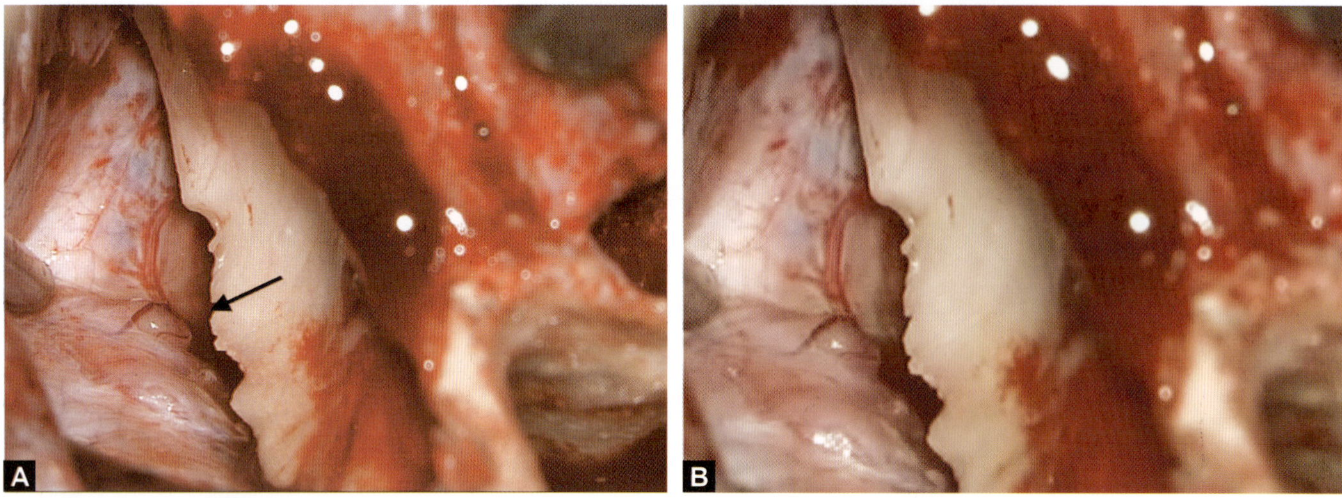

Figs. 26.17A and B: Combined transmastoid and middle cranial fossa approach on a right ear. The combination approach was chosen in this case as the full extent of the encephalocele/tegmen dehiscence could not be addressed via the mastoid alone. The image depicts an encephalocele retracted back into the middle fossa. The bony ridge (black arrow) would later be drilled down to better visualize the dehiscence.

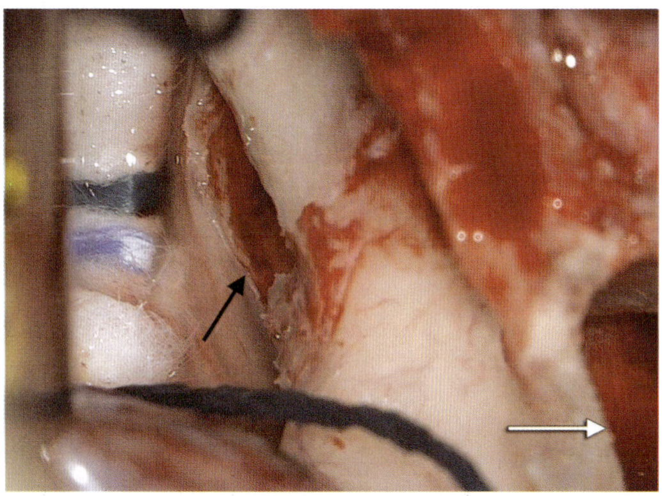

Fig. 26.18: Combined transmastoid and middle cranial fossa approach on a right ear. The combination approach was chosen in this case as the full extent of the encephalocele/tegmen dehiscence could not be addressed via the mastoid alone. The image depicts retracted temporal lobe/encephalocele and the middle fossa floor with a large dehiscence (black arrow) overlying both the tympanic and mastoid cavities. The bony ridge shown in Figure 26.17 has been drilled down. The white arrow points inferiorly toward the mastoidectomy cavity.

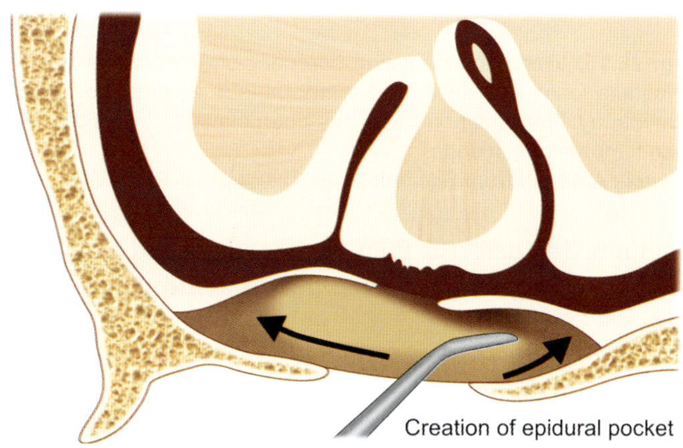

Fig. 26.19: Illustration depicting a surgeon working through an existing tegmen dehiscence to form an epidural pocket on the middle fossa floor. This pocket will be utilized for multilayered repair of the defect and capitalize on the downward force of the overlying temporal lobe to hold the reconstructive elements in place.
Source: Adapted from Semaan et al.[2]

maneuver stabilizes the graft, whose relative surface area is greater than that of the bony defect allowing for stable, secure coverage. Following this, temporalis fascia is inserted for multilayer closure followed by optional obliteration of the mastoid cavity. In defects involving the tegmen tympani, the authors performed disarticulation of the incus followed by ossicular chain reconstruction using autologous incus or a partial ossicular replacement prosthesis. In these cases, an additional posterior tympanotomy was performed to gain access to the mesotympanum without elevating a tympanomeatal flap and to adequately visualize the position of the prosthesis. In this series, all 31 patients had resolution of their CSF leakage and middle ear effusion with no clinical recurrences seen.

Middle Ear Obliteration (MEO)

Obliteration is not typically employed by most authors for the primary treatment of encephalocele and/or CSF leak except, perhaps, in difficult/refractory cases and some

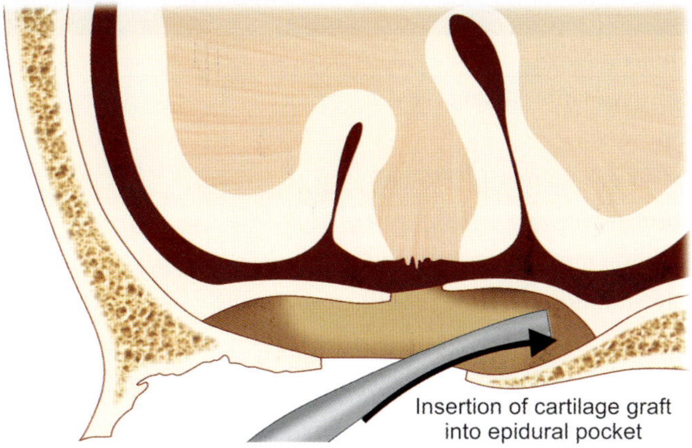

Fig. 26.20: Illustration depicting placement of a cartilage graft through the tegmen dehiscence into the epidural pocket. A secondary option that we often perform is to start with a temporalis fascia or perichondrial graft as this better contours to the irregular tegmen plate and overlying dural defect. The cartilage graft is then inserted and acts as a bolster.
Source: Adapted from Semaan et al.[2]

translabyrinthine approaches.[3,6] The technique entails performing a blind sac closure of the EAC, removing the ossicular chain, obliterating the eustachian tube, stripping the middle ear mucosa, and filling middle ear and/or surgical cavity with fat. The eustachian tube may be occluded with bone wax, muscle, ossicular remnants, and/or fascia.[8,26] The EAC should be oversewn in layers to prevent leakage via this route. In sum, MEO maximizes isolation of the middle ear from the external environment, which in turn minimizes the risks of recurrence and other complications. MEO is, however, associated with a significant loss of hearing function and will result in a maximal conductive hearing loss (generally around 60 dB). Because of the closure of the EAC, postoperative management of patients undergoing MEO necessitates radiologic follow-up in surveillance for cholesteatoma.

Repair of Congenital CSF Leak

Repair of a CSF leak due to congenital inner-ear or tegmen malformation is usually done by either repairing the defect with temporalis fascia or packing the vestibule with muscle or fascia. These entities are rare and may be difficult to fully identify and isolate intraoperatively. Thus, traditional repair methods have been associated with a surgical failure rate of 30–60%.[10] As such, multilayer closure of defects with fibrin glue, muscle, and fascia should be employed whenever possible.

Materials for Skull Base Reconstruction

Whether performed at the time of primary surgery, during a take-back procedure, or for a de novo approach to a newly diagnosed encephalocele and/or leak, the surgeon has a variety of options when it comes to reconstruction of lateral skull base defects. A great deal of literature has analyzed various techniques for the repair of translabyrinthine and retrosigmoid defects to prevent CSF leak, and it is from this body of work that the principles and tools of encephalocele repair are derived. As stated earlier in this text, no definitive reconstructive material or combination of materials has been associated with a 100% success rate. This has led authors to develop and investigate a wide variety of substances for reconstructive purposes, both autologous and synthetic.[7]

Autologous materials include, but are not limited to, abdominal free fat, temporalis muscle (pedicled flaps and free grafts), temporalis fascia, tragal or conchal cartilage free grafts, calvarial bone grafts, and bone dust (acquired from drilling). Synthetic materials include bone wax, hydroxyapatite cement (HAC), bovine-derived gelatin matrix (Floseal), and fibrin glue products. Biologically inert implants made of titanium have also been described.[8] Overall, the most commonly employed reconstruction materials tend to be autologous secondary to low infection rates, elimination of graft rejection risk, and good overall success rates. Autologous materials are also readily accessible, usually through existing surgical incisions, have a low harvest-related morbidity profile, and are very familiar to surgeons. As mentioned above, the use of multilayered closure is generally thought to lead to better outcomes although randomized controlled studies do not currently exist to back this assertion. The following discussion will focus primarily on synthetic materials as the use and harvest of autologous grafts has been well established. Table 26.4 provides a list of various reconstructive materials utilized in lateral skull base reconstruction.

Hydroxyapatite Cement (HAC)

Use of HAC has been described for the closure of a variety of postcraniotomy defects, including translab, middle fossa, transcochlear, and retrosigmoid approaches.[7,28,29] It has also been successfully employed for reconstructing posterior canal wall defects caused by trauma or cholesteatoma. HAC is a calcium-phosphate cement that sets to HA, the major component of human skeletal bone. This is accomplished through a chemical reaction in which tetracalcium phosphate and dicalcium phosphate dihydrate dissolve in

Table 26.4: Materials for surgical reconstruction of bony defects

Autologous	*Synthetic*
Temporalis fascia	Hydroxyapatite cement (HAC)
Temporalis muscle (rotational flap or free graft)	Bone wax
Abdominal free fat graft	Bovine gelatin matrix (Floseal)
Tragal free cartilage graft	Fibrin glue
Conchal free cartilage graft	Titanium mesh plate
Calvarial free bone graft	Polytetrafluoroethylene (PTFE) mesh
Bone dust	
Bone paste/Pâté	

Various materials, both autologous and synthetic used in the reconstruction/repair of the lateral skull base.

water and reprecipitate as microporous HAC. Where HAC differs from other available HA preparations is that it is a cement and not a ceramic, which can become quite brittle. Success rates, defined as successful cessation of a CSF leak, have been reported as high as 97%.[28] HAC has also proven effective when compared with autologous materials. In one retrospective comparison of abdominal fat graft versus HAC (for the closure of translabyrinthine craniotomies) Arriaga and Chen reported lower leak rates in the cement group (3.7%) compared to the fat group (12.9%).[29] These studies suggest that the use of HAC may be a promising surgical adjunct, especially for prophylaxis against CSF leakage in translabyrinthine acoustic surgery. It may also be employed in revision cases where autologous materials may not be as readily available to backfill a widely attenuated skull base or one with multiple defects. Overall, it is associated with low infection (2.8%) and resorption rates. The disadvantages of HAC are its costliness, potential disruption of future surgical revisions, and unintentional conductive hearing loss if it is allowed to enter the middle ear cleft and fuse the ossicles. Overall complication rates have ranged from 0% to 11%, with the vast majority of these complications occurring early in the postoperative period.[28] Figures 26.21 and 26.22 depict application of HA cement to obliterate a mastoid cavity following dual layer closure of a large tegmen dehiscence.

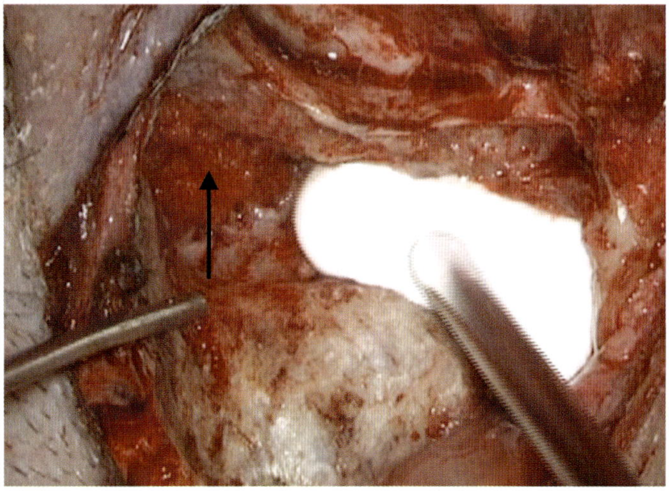

Fig. 26.21: Transmastoid approach on a right ear. The surgeon is filling the mastoid cavity with hydroxyapatite cement. The aditus ad antrum has been packed off with Gelfoam (black arrow) to prevent extravasation of the cement into the tympanic cavity, which may cause a conductive hearing loss.

Fibrin Glue

The properties of fibrin glue with regard to its use in the closure of CSF leaks and reconstruction of craniotomy defects are still being explored. Based on fibrinogen and thrombin and sometimes mixed with the adhesive N-butyl cyanoacrylate, the glue solidifies as it comes into contact with thrombin (converts fibrinogen to fibrin) in the presence of moisture. Thus, depending on the thrombin concentration, the solidification may take anywhere from 5 to 15 seconds. This is of special interest considering the environment inherent to CSF leaks. While the marketed glues are associated with minimal tissue toxicity, low infection rates, and remain radiopaque, neuropathological side effects have been reported when cyanoacrylate comes in contact with brain tissue. Thus, craniotomy defects should first be packed with muscle or fascia before injecting the product.[11] Fibrin glues are typically not used alone.

Titanium Mesh Closure

The House group has published a large series of 389 patients who underwent titanium mesh closure over free

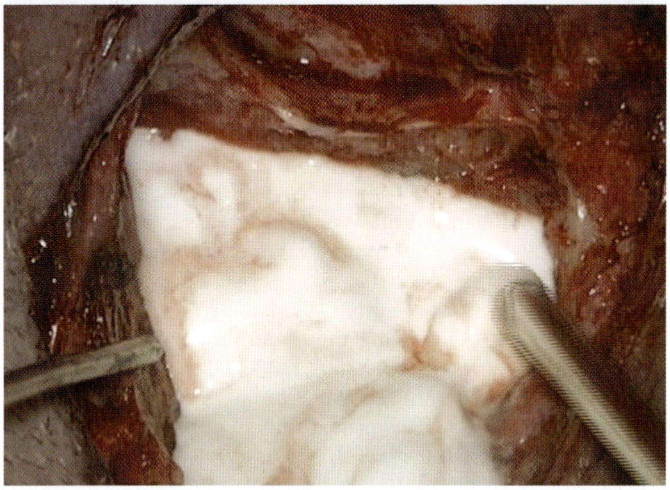

Fig. 26.22: Transmastoid approach on a right ear. The surgeon is filling the mastoid cavity with hydroxyapatite cement. The bony external auditory canal may be appreciated as the lateral-most extent to which the mastoid cavity is filled with cement.

abdominal fat graft following translabyrinthine craniotomy for the resection of acoustic neuromas. They noted that the use of titanium materials to repair various craniotomy defects had already been well established in the neurosurgical literature. Nonferrous and relatively radiolucent, the biologically inert titanium allows for postoperative use of MRI and CT. In addition to creating an anatomic reconstruction of the cranial surface, this cranioplasty technique is thought to provide additional support for the underlying abdominal fat grafting. Out of their cohort of 389, Fayad and Brackmann noted only thirteen patients (3.3%) to have postoperative CSF leaks, which compared favorably to their prior rates using fat graft alone (8.7%; p=0.003).[8]

PROGNOSIS

Outcomes following surgery for reconstruction of encephaloceles and CSF leaks will vary depending on the location, cause, and surgical planning as mentioned above. Complications rates following surgery are generally low when patients are managed thoroughly and appropriately. Of greatest concern is the development of recurrent CSF leak that may portend the development of postoperative meningitis. Leak recurrence typically mandates revision surgery and in some cases MEO. Among all etiologies for CSF leaks, those occurring spontaneously are known to have the highest rate of recurrence.[15] Other postoperative complications described include seizure activity, transient ischemic event/stroke, sepsis, graft extrusion, conductive hearing loss, and sensorineural hearing loss. In summary, encephalocele and CSF leaks represent challenging clinical entities that require extensive diagnostic and technical prowess on the part of the surgeon. A solid understanding of critical treatment concepts and the wide armamentarium at one's disposal should lead to successful outcomes.

REFERENCES

1. Caboche H. De la hernie cerebrale dans les interventions intracraniennes dirigees contre les otitis moyennes suppurees. Annales des maladies de l'oreille, de larynx, du nex et du pharynx. 1902;28:278-94.

*2. Semaan MT, Gilpin DA, Hsu DP, et al. Transmastoid extradural-intracranial approach for repair of transtemporal meningoencephalocele: a review of 31 consecutive cases. Laryngoscope. 2011;121(8):1765-72.

*3. Jackson CG, Pappas DG Jr, Manolidis S, et al. Brain herniation into the middle ear and mastoid: concepts in diagnosis and surgical management. Am J Otol. 1997;18(2):198-205.

4. Nuss DW, Costantino PD. Diagnosis and management of cerebrospinal fluid leaks: highlights of the instructional courses of the American Academy of Otolaryngology—Head Neck Surgery. Otolaryngol Head Neck Surg. 1995;8:79-95.

*5. Sonig A, Thakur JD, Chittiboina P, et al. Is posttraumatic cerebrospinal fluid fistula a predictor of posttraumatic meningitis? A US Nationwide Inpatient Sample database study. Neurosurg Focus. 2012;32(6):E4.

*6. Sanna M, Fois P, Russo A, et al. Management of meningoencephalic herniation of the temporal bone: personal experience and literature review. Laryngoscope. 2009;119(8):1579-85.

*7. Selesnick SH, Liu JC, Jen A, et al. The incidence of cerebrospinal fluid leak after vestibular schwannoma surgery. Otol Neurotol. 2004;25(3):387-93.

*8. Fayad JN, Schwartz MS, Slattery WH, et al. Prevention and treatment of cerebrospinal fluid leak after translabyrinthine acoustic tumor removal. Otol Neurotol. 2007;28(3):387-90.

9. Rich PM, Graham J, Phelps PD. Hyrtl's fissure. Otol Neurotol. 2002;23(4):476-82.

10. Foyt D, Brackmann DE. Cerebrospinal fluid otorrhea through a congenitally patent fallopian canal. Arch Otolaryngol Head Neck Surg. 2000;126(4):540-2.

11. Tyagi I, Syal R and Goyal A. Cerebrospinal fluid otorhinorrhea due to inner ear malformations: clinical presentation and new perspectives in management. J Laryngol Otol. 2005;119:714-8.

12. Schlosser RJ, Woodworth BA, Wilensky EM, et al. Spontaneous cerebrospinal fluid leaks: a variant of benign intracranial hypertension. Ann Otol Rhinol Laryngol. 2006;115(7):495-500.

13. Prichard CN, Isaacson B, Oghalai JS, et al. Adult spontaneous CSF otorrhea: correlation with radiographic empty sella. Otolaryngol Head Neck Surg. 2006;134(5):767-71.

*References with asterisks refer to critical sources.

14. Goddard JC, Meyer T, Nguyen S, et al. New considerations in the cause of spontaneous cerebrospinal fluid otorrhea. Otol Neurotol. 2010;31(6):940-5.
*15. Kenning TJ, Willcox TO, Artz GJ, et al. Surgical management of temporal meningoencephaloceles, cerebrospinal fluid leaks, and intracranial hypertension: treatment paradigm and outcomes. Neurosurg Focus. 2012;32(6):E6.
16. Ramalingam KK, Ramalingam R, Sreenivasa Murthy TM, et al. Management of temporal bone meningo-encephalocoele. J Laryngol Otol. 2008;122(11):1168-74.
*17. Lloyd K, DelGaudio JM, Hudgins PA, Imaging of skull base cerebrospinal fluid leaks in adults. Radiology. 2008;248: 725-36.
18. Tabaouti K, Kraoul L, Alyousef L, et al. The role of biology in the diagnosis of cerebrospinal fluid leaks. Ann Biol Clin. 2009;67:141-51.
19. Chan D, Poon WS, Ip CP, et al. How useful is glucose detection in diagnosing cerebrospinal fluid leak? The rational use of CT and Beta-2 Transferrin assay in detection of cerebrospinal fluid fistula. Asian J Surg. 2004;27:39-42.
20. Bullock R, Soares D. Current imaging of cerebrospinal fluid leaks. West Indian Med J. 2009;58:362-6.
21. Brown NE, Grundfast M, Jabre A, et al. Diagnosis and management of spontaneous cerebrospinal fluid-middle ear effusion and otorrhea. Laryngoscope. 2004;114:800-805.
22. Gorog T, Rudolph P, Meyer JE, et al. Separation of β2 transferrin by denaturing gel electrophoresis to detect cerebrospinal fluid in ear and nasal fluids. Clin Chem. 2005; 51:1704-10.
23. Reiber H, Walther K, Althaus H. Beta-trace protein as sensitive marker for CSF rhinorrhea and CSF otorrhea. Acta Neurol Scand. 2003;108:359-62.
24. Warnecke A, Averbeck T, Wurster U, et al. Diagnostic relevance of β2-transferrin for detection of cerebrospinal fluid fistulas. Arch Otolaryngol Head Neck Surg. 2004;130: 1178-84.
25. Wang EW, Vandergrift WA 3rd, Schlosser RJ. Spontaneous CSF leaks. Otolaryngol Clin North Am. 2011;44(4): 845-56.
*26. Savva A, Taylor MJ, Beatty CW. Management of cerebrospinal fluid leaks involving the temporal bone: report on 92 patients. Laryngoscope. 2003;113(1):50-6.
27. Selcuk H, Albayram S, Ozer H, et al. Intrathecal gadolinium-enhanced MR cisternography in the evaluation of CSF leakage. Am J Neuroradiol. 2010;31:71-5.
*28. Kveton JF, Coelho DH. Hydroxyapatite cement in temporal bone surgery: a 10 year experience. Laryngoscope. 2004; 114(1):33-7.
29. Arriaga MA, Chen DA. Hydroxyapatite cement cranioplasty in translabyrinthine acoustic neuroma surgery. Otolaryngol Head Neck Surg. 2002;126:512-7.
30. Kutz JW, Husain IA, Isaacson B, et al. Management of spontaneous cerebrospinal fluid otorrhea. Laryngoscope. 2008;118:2195-9.
*31. Gubbels S, Selden NR, Delashaw Jr JB, et al. Spontaneous middle fossa encephalocele and cerebrospinal fluid leakage: diagnosis and management. Otol Neurotol. 2007;28: 1131-9.

CHAPTER

27

Presbystasis and Balance in the Elderly

David A Schessel

INTRODUCTION

For the purpose of this discussion, presbystasis is defined as the deterioration in balance function associated with aging. This is neither a specific disease nor does it originate from a singular organ system or part of the body. Rather, it represents the symptoms caused by changes in the balance system that occur with aging. The "balance system", in this case, is subtended by a complex of interacting afferent, central processing, and efferent elements.

Presbystasis is ideally a diagnosis of exclusion. Thus, it is "ruled out" by the identification of specific diseases as cause for the balance problem. These diseases are more the topic of other sections of this text. However, it has to be recognized that the common endpoint of both specific diseases of specific end-organs as well as presbystasis, all cause the common symptom of imbalance and dizziness.

Thus, while this chapter deals with presbystasis, the contents are generalizable to virtually all diseases and factors that affect balance. This is invariably the case when it comes to treatment options. Thus, while studies conclude that with our improved ability to identify specific diagnoses causing problems with balance in elderly individuals, and therefore exclude the diagnosis of presbystasis, we still have to consider how the disease affects the individual through assessment of the balance system as a whole. Lastly, as will be discussed in this chapter, there is an age-related "deterioration" in most of the components of the equilibrium system. Presbystasis may therefore be a consequence of this "natural" process. Whether we then consider these age-related changes that underlie presbystasis a disease versus a consequence of getting older, will have to be left for more philosophical discussions.

To get an idea of the importance of this symptom, the clinical presentation of presbystasis includes symptoms such as dizziness and imbalance and perhaps its most extreme manifestation, falling. The symptom of dizziness represents one of the commonest complaints of elderly individuals. Dizziness is the reason for 8% of patient visits to their primary care provider in individuals over 65 years of age. This number increases to 18% for the oldest individuals. It is a quality of life influence in 20% of people over age 60. Imbalance is reported in 51% of women and 29% of men over age 70. This increases to 50% in everyone between 80 and 90 years of age.

One of the most significant manifestations of dysfunction of the balance system is that of falling. Falls will occur in one third of community-dwelling individuals[3] 65 years of age and 60% of nursing home residents annually. In 2010, 2.3 million nonfatal falls were treated in emergency departments, requiring over 600,000 admissions to hospitals and accounting for 40% of nursing home admissions. This alone cost about $30 billion dollars in direct medical expenses that year. Falls are responsible for up to 70% of accident-related deaths in people > 75 years of age. It is the commonest cause of traumatic brain injury, which in turn is the cause of death in almost half of fatal falls. In 2009, 20,400 older adults died from unintentional fall injuries. Just considering hip fractures alone, >90% of hip fractures, particularly in those over 70, are the consequence of falls. One quarter of those suffering a hip fracture will die within 6 months of the injury. Overall life expectancy is reduced by 10–15%, along with a reduction in quality of life, when hip fracture occurs. Even when falls do not produce injury, they do produce a fear of future falls. This in turn results in a reduction in activity with a consequent loss of physical fitness. Loss of physical fitness and anxiety are each factors increasing the risk of falling. Dizziness and balance problems represent a tremendous impact of quality of life and morbidity and mortality in the elderly individual and a tremendous cost to society.

This discussion begins with an overview of the components of the balance system and an understanding of their contribution in maintaining equilibrium. We will discuss what happens to these separate elements of the balance system as we age and how age-related dysfunction contributes to the global complaint of loss of balance and its consequences. As will be seen, this includes both specific age-related changes to end-organ function as well as dysfunction related to additive small changes in multiple systems underlying balance control. It not only includes intrinsic changes in the components of the balance system, but also extrinsic influences, such as medications, illness, and features of the environment. This chapter will discuss some of the more specialized components in the evaluation of the elderly dizzy patient who may be experiencing presbystasis. Lastly, we will discuss some of the therapeutic options aimed at improving balance and reducing its most serious consequence, that of falling.

THE BALANCE SYSTEM

The balance system is composed of those afferent, central processing, and efferent elements responsible for helping us maintain body orientation and visual acuity as we navigate our environment. Simply, afferent elements include vestibular, visual, and proprioceptive systems. Central processing, of course, occurs in the central nervous system. Efferent elements include primarily muscle groups and skeletal components responsible for moving the eyes and maintaining balance.

The anatomy and physiology of these systems are discussed in depth elsewhere in this text. Briefly, the contribution of vestibular system is through its detection of both angular and linear acceleration, including gravity, associated with head/body movement. Included here are the five receptors in the inner ears and the afferent eighth cranial nerves responsible for passing this information to central processing areas. Vestibular information is utilized in several ways. One is to help stabilize vision while our head moves. This is the vestibulo-ocular reflex (VOR). Head movement information is used to rapidly generate eye movements exactly opposite the direction and speed of the head. This allows the eyes to stay focused on the world despite motion of the head. Vestibular information is also used, via the vestibulo-spinal system to help us orient our body and center of gravity while we move or the support surface moves, such as standing on a boat.

The afferent visual system consists of the eyes. Vision serves a number of processes. With reference to balance, it provides information related to head orientation through spatial awareness of the horizon, detection of body position relative to fixed objects including their position and size, and details of the support surface. It also provides necessary information about movement both of the environment and self. This is used not only to gather information about the environment, but also, like the vestibulo-ocular system, to enable the visual system itself to function by image stabilization. This later aspect is accomplished by the detection of retinal slip, the movement of visual images across the retina. Retinal slip information is processed through two different pathways, the optokinetic and smooth pursuit systems. The optokinetic is particularly sensitive to movement of the entire visual field across the nonfoveate retina, for example, the motion of the environment as we move our head. It is responsible for the sensation of movement, or vection, that occurs when the visual field moves, as in a large screen movie theater. The smooth pursuit system is to enable tracking of more discrete objects in the visual field. These can be objects that are moving, such as the bird as it flies; it also allows us to focus on the fixed object as we move.

Both the visual and vestibular systems are critical in enabling us to use our visual system. In this regard, they serve overlapping and complementary functions. The visually driven smooth pursuit and optokinetic system detects low-frequency and low-velocity movements while the vestibular receptors process higher speed motion. This frequency difference can be demonstrated by trying to read a written passage while shaking the page in front of our eyes. It is very difficult to focus on the words. However, one can easily fix on words if the page is held still and the head is shaken. The former utilizes the visual tracking system and the latter the high-frequency-detecting VOR.

The somatosensory system includes proprioceptors for the sensation of the position of the body and cutaneous somatosensation, which conveys information relative to the body's interface with the environment. In the case of proprioception, muscle tension is conveyed by muscle spindles. Position and weight distribution is detected by joint and tendon-based receptors, including Golgi tendon organs, Ruffini's endings, and other articular receptors. The system provides sensory feedback about the nature of the environment also. Information such as the consistency and position of the support surface and weight distribution and changes in support interface is detected by cutaneous pressure receptors, including cutaneous Merkel's disk, Pacinian corpuscles, and hair follicle receptors, which are distributed throughout the body surface. The plantar surface of the foot is particularly rich in fast-adapting receptors. These make the sole of the foot particularly sensitive to slight changes in weight distribution and quality of the contact surface.

Central connections of these systems and processing areas are diffuse. It is said that the vestibular system itself is one of the most disseminated systems in the brain. The vestibular system relays via the eighth cranial nerve primarily with the brainstem-located vestibular nuclei as well as by direct connections with the deep cerebellar nuclei. There is a strong connection with the cerebellum, particularly to the vermis and the flocculonodular areas. The vestibular nuclei and brainstem connections with oculomotor nuclei and spinal motor pathways are responsible for the vestibulo-ocular and vestibulospinal reflexes. Together the vestibulocerebellum, vestibular nuclei, and other brainstem areas are responsible for modulation of the reflexes such as the VOR gain during natural behaviors such as accommodation for the distance, of viewed objects and changes in gain necessitated by changes in eyeglass prescription. They also are capable of reflex inhibition when reflex movements are not desirable during tasks such as tracking environmental motion and perhaps during sleep where stimulation of reflexive vestibular responses would be disruptive. These centers are also involved in the process of vestibular adaptation to injury of the peripheral vestibular receptors or adjustment to a new eyeglass prescription. Cortical connections are in the region of the posterior insular cortex. There does not appear to be a singular vestibular cortex. Rather, this area receives input from all three sensory modalities, vestibular, visual, and somatosensory. There are also connections to the stress centers in the hippocampus. This connection is documented in animals. The connection does appear present in humans where stress appears to act as both promoter and interference to vestibular compensation. Control of autonomic reflexes, such as orthostatic blood pressure changes, may also be influenced by the vestibular system. Vestibular connections to autonomic centers for vomiting are certainly well known.

Visual information is also processed centrally through a number of pathways. In the case of smooth pursuit, retinal slip information goes to the primary visual cortex and the medial temporal visual area. From the cortex it goes to the cerebellum, which then feeds the brainstem oculomotor nuclei. The optokinetic reflex alternatively receives information via subcortical pathways including the accessory optic nuclei. In this case information is processed through the vestibular system and distributed to the appropriate oculomotor nuclei.

Somatosensory information is used reflexively at the level of the spinal cord. Information is also passed to subcortical and cortical centers for more refined voluntary movements.

A discussion of the central nervous system processes responsible for the integration of sensory information and volitional demands and ultimately with motor behavior is complicated and beyond the needs of this chapter. In addition, many of the ways the balance system functions to maintain balance and orientation to the environment are seemingly reflexive. Yet, the sensory information used and motor responses generated to accomplish the task of maintaining balance are open to modification centrally. Selective use of one sensory modality or another is one example. For instance, quiet stance prioritizes proprioception and somatosensory inputs, particularly from the lower extremities and soles of the feet to keep us upright and balanced. While walking and running, there is a greater prioritization of the visual system. Navigating in a dark environment with an irregular surface, such as outdoors on open ground, will rely on the vestibular system. The motor responses themselves are learned processes with sequences of activations of various muscle groups ultimately committed to memory. There are differences in pathway if this is a new motor sequence versus a modification of a previously used learned movement, such as in response to muscle fatigue or injury. Interestingly, sleep appears to be an important factor in the consolidation of such behaviors.

Efferent connections include oculomotor connections to move the eyes and motor neurons responsible for controlling the muscles responsible for maintaining desired body position relative to gravity. The balance system relies heavily on the musculoskeletal system to regulate body position and the movement and positioning of the eyes, including not only the muscles that enact the motion but also their partnered skeletal elements.

EFFECTS OF AGING ON THE BALANCE SYSTEM

Age affects the balance system in a number of ways. While there are a multitude of diseases and other factors that can produce deterioration in function, when it comes to presbystasis, we are dealing with extrinsic and "nonpathologic" intrinsic changes that seem to be specifically associated with age and influence our ability to maintain balance. As expected, the effect of age is apparent throughout the balance system.

General Changes in Balance Associated with Aging

Changes in gait are common as we age. Overall, the elderly walk slower and take shorter steps with a wider step width. They spend more time in the double support position, both feet on the ground simultaneously. These changes may be to enhance safety but may be a response to physical limitations of the balance system. Responses to obstacles also change. They reduce speed and take smaller steps with a narrower step width. They will misstep and often hit the object they are trying to avoid. This is particularly true if the obstacle is unexpected or attention is divided. They are less able to incorporate changes in gait pattern, such as sidestepping, turning, or stopping, in their normal gait patterns. There is always a slight sway to our bodies as we stand quietly in one position. Older individuals will typically have increased amplitude of sway. The degree of sway correlates linearly with age and greater risk of falling.

An extension of sway is tripping. In this case, the center of mass moves beyond the limits of support and has to be countered with a step. Elderly individuals tend to make smaller steps in response, which are more often inadequate at stopping horizontal and vertical motion. Potential causes include inability to move the stepping limb, actual muscle weakness and differences in amplitude, and latency of muscle activation. Studies have suggested that the reduction in muscle recruitment is often responsible for the problem. Slowing of reflex reaction time is well known to occur with aging, the source of which may also be multifactorial. On the afferent side, there may be a reduction in afferent sensitivity, processing may be delayed. Alternatively, on the efferent side there may be inadequate recruitment of efferent corticospinal motorneurons or problems in the muscle itself.[8] Also important in the ability to respond to a sudden unexpected perturbation is the activation of muscles in an orderly fashion. Elderly individuals demonstrate a loss of this organization and will tend to respond with coactivation of agonist/antagonist muscle groups. This serves to stiffen the joints, such as the ankle, but is less effective at re-establishing balance if the center of balance has gone too far off center. Interestingly, this is a response also seen in infants. Cocontraction of lower extremity muscles is used generically regardless of sensory input.[4] Similarly, when the perturbation is to the side and a cross step is elicited, the crossing leg will hit the weight bearing leg in 55% of cases in the elderly as opposed to 8% in the young. This is a common cause of lateral falls, which are particularly problematic due to the increased risk of hip fracture compared to falls forward or back.

These observations of the functional consequences of aging on balance function and functional ability represent the collective effect of age-related changes on the individual components of the balance system.

Effect of Age on the Vestibular System

Dysfunction of the vestibular system is very common in elderly individuals. Population studies in which the contribution of the vestibular system is evaluated in isolation, with minimization of the roles of visual and somatosensory input, suggest that vestibular function is reduced in 50% of individuals in their 70th decade and 85% in individuals 90 and over. Studies on specific end organs have demonstrated similar effect. Deterioration in utricular function has been demonstrated to occur linearly over our lifetimes. This was measured as the gain of the ocular counter-rolling reflex between 20 and 80 years of age. It affected women more than men. This was correlated with balance behaviors felt indicative of the health of the balance system—specifically, how much an individual sways under conditions that isolate the vestibular system. When vision was removed and proprioception was reduced by standing on soft foam, there was a linear increase in sway in advancing age groups. Putting these together, it was determined that reductions in otolith function are correlated to sway measures. As noted above, increased sway is strongly correlated to the risk of falling. This effect of age on the utricle is mirrored in the saccule. It is manifested by age-related reductions in vestibular-evoked myogenic potential (VEMP) thresholds.[22] Similar findings have been observed looking at the semicircular canal system via the VOR. In a large study by Baloh et al.[3] in 1993, age-related changes included decreases in VOR gain, a reduction in VOR time constant, reduced peak optokinetic slow phase velocity and a reduction in the visual–vestibular interaction causing reduced VOR suppression by vision and a reduced VOR gain enhancement with vision. These were all felt to reflect changes in the vestibular–visual and oculomotor pathways. Similar results were obtained by Agrawal et al.[12] In this case canal, utricular and saccular function were evaluated with the head impulse test, the ocular VEMP (o-VEMP), and the cervical VEMP (c-VEMP), respectively. All receptors demonstrated age-related deterioration. However, the semicircular canals appeared to be affected to a greater degree and earlier than the otolith receptors. Decreases in saccular function have also been noted to mirror age-related high-frequency hearing loss. This was further exacerbated if history included increased noise exposure. This was identified by decreases in the amplitude of the c-VEMP as opposed to measurements of utricular function via o-VEMP and canal-specific gains, using the canal-specific head impulse test.[32] Age-related high-frequency hearing loss, especially with concomitant history of noise exposure, might serve as an indicator for risk of balance-related disability.

Anatomic studies of the vestibular system in humans and animals have demonstrated age-related changes also. Hair cell number has been recognized to decrease with age. When this occurs is variable, with some reports suggesting loss beginning in the fourth decade and others in the seventh. Rauch et al[20] studied the inner ear of normal humans ranging from birth to their 90s. He used Nomarski optics to enable differentiation of cell type as well as number. Results demonstrated a continuous reduction in total hair cell number throughout life. Type I hair cells were lost from the crista of the semicircular canals, sooner than the otolithic receptor maculae. Type II hair cells were lost at the same rate in all five receptors.

Age-related reduction and deterioration of the otolithic membrane has been observed. This may be associated with a reduction in production of otoconia. Decrease in the globular substance masses that serve as precursors to the otoconia are reduced in animal studies. There is a general demineralization and deformity of otoconia. Studies have suggested that such degeneration might also correlate with body calcium metabolism. This is postulated to contribute to the increased incidence of benign paroxysmal positional vertigo in the elderly and individuals with conditions such as osteopenia.

Other changes to the vestibular end-organs have also been noted in the aging vestibular system. These include accumulation of lipofuscin as well as reduction in blood supply to the receptors.

Morphologic changes also occur in the central vestibular pathways. At the level of the vestibular nuclei, the primary relay nucleus and processing area for vestibular input, changes include a loss of cells particularly of the inferior and lateral nuclei. There is relative sparing of the superior nucleus, which is a principal component of the VOR. In line with this, the VOR tends to be less affected over our lifetime while vestibulospinal reflexes and vestibular adaptive functions may be more age sensitive.[2]

Effect of Age on the Somatosensory System

Aging affects virtually all receptors of the afferent proprioceptor and cutaneous sensory system. Some changes are likely due to age and wear-and-tear alone, but there is also the influence of decrease in weight bearing and activity feeding back on the system. Proprioceptive muscle spindles show changes reflective of loss of innervation, peripheral neuropathy, and reduction in diameter and constituents and sensitivity of the receptors.[23] There are changes in the myosin expression in receptor spindles as well as skeletal muscles. This alters the speed of muscle contraction within the receptors as well as the efferent side of the system, skeletal muscles. Joint and tendon receptors (Golgi tendon organs, Pacinian corpuscles, Ruffini's endings, and free nerve endings) all decrease in number in tendons and joint capsules. Nerve atrophy and slowing of conduction velocity of afferent nerves has also been demonstrated. Loss of proprioception has been demonstrated by a reduction in the ability of the elderly to detect changes and set joint position as well as younger individuals. This is more significant for the distal lower extremities—ankles—than for more proximal joints such as the hip. Osteoarthritic joints demonstrate greater loss of joint position sense than non-arthritic. Animal studies have demonstrated that loss of mechanoreceptors and nerve atrophy may precede development of osteoarthritis of the joint. These studies have suggested that such loss might be a causative factor in the development of osteoarthritis.

Cutaneous sensory reception is also reduced with age. This reduction tends to be worse in the lower body. The ability to detect vibration as well as a reduction in the sensitivity of vibration receptors is notably reduced above age 70. A 92% reduction in two-point sensation has been noted in the foot over age 65. The plantar surface of the foot is also affected more than the dorsal surface. This is suggested to reflect the greater degree of wear-and-tear on the sole of the foot. Anatomically, this is reflected in a global reduction in the number of all cutaneous receptors throughout the body in older individuals. As stated above, the detection of weight distribution is critical in maintaining stance. This is again reflected in the greater proportion of fast-adapting receptors particularly sensitive to changes in weight distribution and quality of the contact surface. The consequence of the reduction in tactile sensitivity, in this case two-point discrimination, has been found to correlate with increased mediolateral sway and incidence of multiple falls when compared with nonfalling age-matched elderly individuals.

Extrinsic causes of loss of peripheral sensation are very common, for example, diabetes. Peripheral nerve damage occurs in up to 25% of diabetics after 10 years of disease and in 50% of individuals after 20 years. Peripheral vascular disease will have similar consequences as well as spinal degenerative problems and arthritis, as mentioned above. Diseases of the foot have been shown to be associated with an increased risk of falling, particularly multiple falls, as well as reduced mobility overall.[18] This included foot pain as well as deformities, in particular corns. Deficits are especially notable when active tasks, such as walking up or down stairs, are evaluated. This is reasonable given that the problem is manifested more as the weight is shifted to various positions on the foot. Deformities of the toes were also associated with greater problems shifting balance forward. Other extrinsic causes include factors such as excessive alcohol use, vitamin b-12 deficiency and chemotherapy, all known causes of peripheral numbness.

Effect of Age on the Visual System

Alterations to the lens and cornea and retina affecting visual acuity, contrast sensitivity, glare sensitivity, dark adaptation, and depth perception are well known to occur with aging. Occurrence of cataracts is 16%, macular degeneration 9%, and glaucoma 3% of individuals over 65. Certainly, more common are refractive errors. There is also a reduction in the speed of central visual processing with a loss in fast motion detection manifested as a reduction in flicker frequency. Other changes include reduction in ocular motility and slowing of visual pursuit and rapid eye movements. These latter occurrences are common findings on videonystagmogram (VNG) records from elderly individuals.

Central Nervous System Changes Associated with Age

Some of these changes were mentioned in the context of the specific sensory motor systems above, but there are more general changes in the way the brain functions when it comes to dealing with balance function. In some cases these would seem to be adaptive in response to deterioration of the afferent input and efferent capabilities. However, they are also a byproduct of a general deterioration in brain function and capacity. It is generally recognized that the brain reaches its full volume at age 13. It then begins a slow decrease in size that accelerates to a rate of 0.5% after age 60.[12] General reductions in motor learning and adaptation, while generally resistant to an age effect, do show negative changes as tasks become more complex and there is extraneous interference. This is manifested in reductions in the ability to perform balance-related tasks when there are distractions or multiple tasks to be performed. One thought is that this reflects an age-related decrease in working memory and cognitive processing speed. Physiologic changes felt to reflect this change include reductions in volume of the frontal cortex and striatum and specific reduction in dopamine, a transmitter shown to facilitate sequence learning and formation of motor memory. The loss of integrity of the white matter tracts responsible for motor learning and integration is also implicated.[15]

Mild cognitive impairment has been associated with the risk of falling in the elderly. It has been found that the change is most significant when the deficit is in executive functions as opposed to amnestic.[9] Loss of visuospatial processing has been additionally identified as playing a role in the incidence of falls in a prospective study.[17]

Studies have also suggested that as opposed to utilization of "automatic" and specified areas of the brain for balance as well as shutting off inputs when not needed, as in the prioritization of sensory inputs discussed previously, elderly individuals will use generic processing resources or cognitive areas of the brain to integrate, process, and control balance. This use of a more fixed and limited resource means that balance may be more easily compromised by more complex balance tasks and by unrelated simultaneous tasks.[7] Furthermore, elderly individuals are less able to shift from one balance strategy to another based on need, for instance, responding to changing levels of illumination or changing qualities of the support surface. This is supported by dual-task behavioral studies as well as imaging studies. This change in the brain areas used for processing is supported by functional magnetic resonance imaging studies of mentally imaged balance tasks. Again seen are differences in the areas of the brain activated based on age. Specifically, in young individuals, sensory inputs were inactivated based on need. In the elderly there was activation of the cortical multisensory vestibular areas of the cortex for most activities. This can be interpreted as a way of adapting to a decreased input from the aging sensory systems, but it has the potential to be detrimental when sensory input is contradictory or distorted. It also would make it more susceptible to interference by extraneous input and activity, such as moving about in a crowd.[33]

Efferent Changes Associated with Aging

Efferent changes associated with aging are numerous. This includes all the age-related changes that occur in muscles and skeleton. Muscle changes have been discussed above. It is important to recognize the role of disuse in this regard. The lack of muscle strength and joint flexibility creates a self-perpetuating cycle of deterioration that limits activity and increases imbalance and its consequences, including falling. Pain in muscles and joints is well known to cause maladaptive changes in gait and balance that contribute to limitation in activity, and by default, falls. Thus disorders such as arthritis, as discussed above, have a significant impact. Foot problems have been associated with individuals who fall repeatedly.[18] As noted above, lesions such as bunions, corns, and overgrown toenails are included in this. Problems of particular note are those causing pain. While quiet standing is not affected, dynamic tasks including alternate stepping tasks, walking and stair ascent–descent tasks are affected. Given that many of these problems can be remediated, such podiatric problems should be considered.

Extrinsic Factors Influencing Dizziness and Falls

Extrinsic factors include all those factors that influence the functioning of the components of the balance system directly, such as medications and medical conditions. Also included are those things that interact with the balance system, such as ambient lighting, shoes, obstacles, complexity of the visual environment, and support surface as well as those that interfere with concentration on the balance task such as mental interferences and extraneous tasks.

The number of medical conditions that can influence balance is quite large. To give an idea of what we are speaking of, issues like diabetes are well known in this regard. This can directly influence sensory inputs like vision and proprioception. Cardiovascular disease with circulatory problems affects global function. However, issues such as arrhythmia or hypotension can produce more direct and sudden changes. Disorders that alter mental status, such as thyroid disease, vascular disease, and neurodegenerative diseases, can all affect balance. Disease causing changes in muscle strength and joint mobility are influential. Diverse infections carry much more potential to alter the level of alertness and cognitive ability in the elderly and thus influence balance. The effect of stress/anxiety, perhaps due to its involvement of areas of the brain shared with the processing of balance information, especially in the elderly as noted above, can interfere with balance performance. Multitasking while walking has been shown to be problematic in the elderly. The effect of anxiety and fear of falling alone causes problems with gait and a spiraling deterioration when it causes the individual to become more limited in their activity and therefore less fit. This in turn further restricts activity and general physical health. Suffice it to say, the list is monumental.

Medications

Given what we know about issues that affect balance function and cause dizziness in the elderly, any medication that has the potential to cause dizziness, sedation, loss or distortion of sensory input, or loss of cognitive function has the potential to worsen balance. Anecdotally, there are very few medications that do not list dizziness or fatigue or sensory changes somewhere in their adverse reaction or drug interaction profiles. When looking at the consequence of this effect, there are a number of drug classes that have been specifically associated with increased incidence of falling in numerous studies.[29] Medication classes found to be causative include sedatives and hypnotics, neuroleptics and antipsychotics, antidepressants, benzodiazepines, cardiac, analgesics including nonsteroidal medications, and antihypertensive medications including diuretics. The odds ratio for falling is as high as 3.6 for antipsychotic medications. There is further support for these findings in that removal of psychotropic medications has been associated with a decrease in falls. It appears that any sedating medications, including nonbenzodiazepine-containing sedatives such as diphenhydramine, have the potential to compromise balance function.

Special mention is also made of medications used in the treatment of vertigo or dizziness. Drowsiness, dizziness, and impaired coordination lead the list in common side effects of these medications. Given this, it is not surprising that these have the capacity to exacerbate presbystasis. It is important that such medications be used where indicated for active vertigo, but the dose needs to be tapered and the drug discontinued when the acute phase of the disease is over. They should not be used indiscriminately for all complaints of dizziness and imbalance.

Polypharmacy has been associated with a propensity to cause falls in elderly individuals. Studies have shown that the number of drugs is an independent variable in fall risk. However, many of these evaluations have found the effect of polypharmacy was realized only when medications known to increase the risk of falls, such as sedative-hypnotics, were included.

Vitamin D deficiency has been associated with the risk of falls and consequent fractures.[5,14] This is not only due to its association with bone strength but muscle strength as well. Histopathologically, it is reflected in atrophy of muscle fibers, particularly type II fibers. Elderly individuals are especially subject to deficits in vitamin D due to factors such as decreased dietary intake, decreased skin thickness, reduced sunlight exposure, impaired intestinal absorption, and reduced hydroxylation in the liver and kidneys. Vitamin D deficiency, defined as serum vitamin D3 levels < 30 nmol/L, was identified in 36% of men and 47% of women in a wintertime study in the Northern Hemisphere. The effect is most prominent in proximal muscle groups and presents as a sensation of heaviness in the legs, fatiguing easily, and problems with activities such as climbing stairs and getting up from a chair. It has been associated with increased falls also. Studies have demonstrated that the risk of falls was increased in individuals with serum levels < 60 nmol/L and those receiving low-dose supplementation (< 600 IU/day) when compared with individuals with levels > 60 nmol/L and high-dose supplementation (700–1000 IU/day). Meta-analysis studies of randomized controlled trials suggest the effect can be as much as a 19–23% reduction in falls in the higher dose/serum level studies. There is no apparent difference in efficacy of active versus supplemental forms of vitamin D when assessed for fall-risk reduction.

DIAGNOSIS OF PRESBYSTASIS

Presbystasis represents disequilibrium associated with no identifiable pathologic cause. It seems to be the consequence of the accumulated age-related extrinsic and intrinsic changes resulting in balance problems. The diagnosis of presbystasis is one of exclusion, but its diagnosis follows the same outline as in the assessment of any individual complaining of dizziness or balance problems. Thus, the differential that has to be excluded is large, including any problem of the afferent, processing, and efferent systems underlying equilibrium. Studies suggest that presbystasis can be ruled out in over 80% of cases of individuals presenting with imbalance or falling. Readers are referred to appropriate sections of this text for detailed review of the evaluation of the dizzy patient and diseases of the inner ear. Diseases that are particularly common in the elderly population include benign paroxysmal positional vertigo. As opposed to the typically described isolated spells associated with change in position, in the elderly, subtle abnormal stimulation of the vestibular system associated with moving about can cause much more chronic symptoms that impact global balance function. Surprisingly, bed associated spells are often unreported. Hallpike testing must be performed. Other causes of injury to the vestibular system, such as vestibular neuronitis or Meniere's disease or perhaps age-related deterioration in function, can manifest as imbalance in a number of ways. Permanent loss of vestibular function resulting from any cause can result in inadequate vestibular input to support the vestibular driven reflexes. The same injury can also produce symptoms due to inadequate adaptation to a vestibular injury. Adaptation to vestibular injury is often slower or compromised as we age. This is presumably associated with changes in central mechanisms responsible for such adaptation. This would include the brainstem vestibular nuclei as well as areas of the vestibular cerebellum. Difficulties in vestibular adaptation associated with age are well known and need to be considered before performing vestibular ablative procedures. Alternatively, after vestibular injury, elderly individuals have to be encouraged to begin vestibular adaptive activities to encourage recovery.

Migraines as well as headaches in general are less common in elderly individuals. In the elderly, 50% of migraines will be unassociated with pain with a greater incidence of symptoms such as hearing loss, tinnitus and vertigo, and dizziness. Typical migraines occurring in younger years will occasionally change to the more atypical forms noted above.

There are a number of central neurologic diseases that can present to the otolaryngologist due to their associated gait problems as part of their presentation. Examples of these include normal pressure hydrocephalus. This condition is most often idiopathic. It is commonest in elderly individuals. It can be the consequence of prior head trauma and intracranial bleeding, infections such as meningitis, stroke, and brain tumors. Hydrocephalus, in this case, is felt to be a form of communicating hydrocephalus with a slow or fluctuating obstruction causing gradual dilatation of the ventricles and pressure on the brain. Cerebrospinal fluid (CSF) pressure is characteristically within the normal range. Symptoms differ from acute hydrocephalus, e.g. headaches, nausea and vomiting, and instead include gait disturbance, urinary incontinence, and dementia-like cognitive dysfunction. It consequently is often misdiagnosed as Alzheimer's disease, dementia or Parkinson's disease. It is particularly important to diagnose normal pressure hydrocephalus due to its reversibility with CSF diversion.

These represent a very few examples of the differential that have to be considered when approaching the individual with balance problems, including presbystasis.

HISTORY

As always, the history is perhaps the most critical factor in sorting through the extensive differential. This begins with a thorough understanding of the complaint. It is important to have the individual explain their symptoms without words like dizziness or even vertigo.

It is useful to know how the problem arose. Was it a gradual onset or sudden? If spells, what is the duration of the attacks? This is useful to differentiate states such as central degenerative conditions and presbystasis from diseases such as Meniere's disease or a stroke.

What are the circumstances that produce the symptoms? This would include the place and environmental characteristics, such as in the dark, in crowds, or on irregular surfaces. This includes determination of the type of activity associated with symptoms. Presbystasis is largely symptomatic when walking or standing. There is likely to be no abnormal sensation when sitting or lying. True vertigo is typically going to be absent. The individual will often express trepidation about getting about and often significant reduction in ability to get around, loss of independence, and fear of falling. The occurrence of and causes of falls are of special importance. A detailed history of falls and their circumstance is important.

Associated features need to be determined. Aside from those associated with the usual dizziness history, bodily weakness, numbness, incoordination, stiffness and pain of body, incontinence, shortness of breath, and cognitive and behavioral changes are important examples.

Medical history is critical, given the number of medical conditions that can influence the balance system. Diseases such as diabetes or cerebral and cardiovascular disease and associated problems such as neuropathy and retinopathy must be defined. History should include information about vision and corrective lenses. Progressive lenses have been associated with an increased incidence of imbalance. Bodily cutaneous sensation and strength is important. This should include the presence of pain or limitation of motion and diseases such as arthritis, osteoporosis, orthopedic procedures, and podiatric conditions. A list of medications with prescription timing relative to the onset of symptoms is critical. Social history has to include living situation, the type of shoes worn, or the use of a cane or other assistive device. Specific activities and limitations caused by the problem should be defined along with characteristics of the environment.

EXAMINATION

In addition to the typical components of the neuro-otologic examination of all patients presenting with dizziness, the examination has to include evaluation of those systems responsible for maintenance of upright posture. Thus, measures of strength and coordination are important. Observation of gait and quiet standing is useful. Normal gait is characterized by an alignment of the medial side of the foot or medial malleolus along a straight line. Standing is done with the feet together with patient's eyes open as well as closed. Standing on an unstable support surface, such as foam block, can also be performed. Degree of body sway is assessed. Marked increase in sway with eye closure is often a sign of proprioceptive or vestibular deficit. Specific testing of proprioception includes vibration sensation and joint position sense of the lower extremities, i.e. the big toe. Cerebellar/central disease is characterized by a wide-based, drunken gait. There is often significant sway when standing with feet together (Rhomberg sign). Unlike proprioceptive and vestibular system deficits, removing vision with eye closure will not worsen function significantly in central disease. Strength and flexibility have to be assessed. Hyperactive reflexes and spasticity suggest upper motor neuron damage. Reduced reflexes, muscle atrophy, and fasciculations occur with lower motor neuron problems. Generalized weakness can also be from myopathic and neuropathic problems as well as chronic disuse. Specific muscle deficits cause variations in abnormal gait. If there is unilateral hip girdle weakness, the hips will shift to the side of weakness. Bilateral weakness results in a waddling gait. Quadriceps weakness causes the individual to swing the leg forward and lock the knee to take a step, and foot drop causes an over-elevation of the affected leg to take a step. Central disorders such as Parkinson's disease are associated with a festinating gait, sudden stops, and falls. The progress of movement is slow but the gait is made of rapid, short, narrow steps with the heel and toe striking the ground simultaneously as opposed to normal, heel first.

A number of clinical tests have been developed in an attempt to assess balance and risk of falling in particular. The timed up-and-go test is one example that has been suggested as predictive of falls. Test instructions and one example of interpretation are shown in Table 27.1. Various interpretations have been suggested. For example, <10 seconds is normal, 11–20 seconds is normal for frail

Table 27.1: Timed up and go test

The person may wear their usual footwear and can use any assistive device they normally use
1. Have the person sit in the chair with their back to the chair and their arms resting on the arm rests
2. Ask the person to stand up from a standard chair and walk a distance of 10 ft. (3 m)
3. Have the person turn around, walk back to the chair, and sit down again
Timing begins when the person starts to rise from the chair and ends when he or she returns to the chair and sits down
The person should be given one practice trial and then three actual trial. The times from the three actual trials are averaged
Predictive results
Seconds Rating
<10 Freely mobile
<20 Mostly independent
20–29 Variable mobility
>20 Impaired mobility

and disabled individuals, >20 seconds suggests the need for assistive devices or intervention (i.e. balance training/therapy), and >30 seconds suggesting possible fall risk. Other studies have suggested a normal cutoff of 12 seconds. Meta-analysis of clinical trials has questioned the validity of this test for healthy, independent-living elderly. A moderate correlation has been found for lower-functioning older people. No time cutoff point has been suggested.[21] Other tests used similarly include the alternate-step test, stair ascent and decent, sit to stand test, and the 6-m walk test. Studies suggest that these together are 69% sensitive and 56% specific in predicting multiple falls.[25] Other clinical test protocols have been developed that similarly use combinations of several tests of balance, functional reach, strength and flexibility. These include the Tinetti Balance Assessment Tool and the Berg Balance Test (Table 27.2). Higher scores on these tests indicate better balance function. Studies have suggested that, for example, a high score on the Berg Balance Test suggests a lesser likelihood of falling. Low scores did not predict future falls, though.[6] Some clinical assessment tools have included combinations of tests of physical ability with social and medical factors.[26] These also have limited utility. It has been suggested that these tests can be considered screens for identifying individuals who may require remediation and increased surveillance.

Typical quantitative tests of vestibular function, such as VNG and rotory chair, are by definition going to be normal in individuals with presbystasis. However, an effort

Table 27.2: Berg balance scale

Equipment needed: ruler, two standard chairs (one with arm rests, one without), footstool or step, stopwatch or wristwatch, 15 ft walkway
Scoring: a five-point scale, ranging from 0–4. "0" indicates the lowest level of function and "4" the highest level of function. Total score = 56
Interpretation: 41–56 = low fall risk
21–40 = medium fall risk
0 –20 = high fall risk
A change of eight points is required to reveal a genuine change in function between two assessments
Sitting to standing—instructions: Please stand up. Try not to use your hand for support
Standing unsupported—instructions: Please stand for two minutes without holding on
Sitting with back unsupported but feet supported on floor or on a stool—instructions: Please sit with arms folded for 2 minutes
Standing to sitting—instructions: Please sit down
Transfers—instructions: Arrange chair(s) for pivot transfer Ask subject to transfer one way toward a seat with armrests and one way toward a seat without armrests. You may use two chairs (one with and one without armrests) or a bed and a chair
Standing unsupported with eyes closed—instructions: Please close your eyes and stand still for 10 seconds
Standing unsupported with feet together—instructions: Place your feet together and stand without holding on
Reaching forward with outstretched arm while standing—instructions: Lift arm to 90°. Stretch out your fingers and reach forward as far as you can
Pick up object from the floor from a standing position—instructions: Pick up the shoe/slipper, which is in front of your feet
Turning to look behind over left and right shoulders while standing—instructions: Turn to look directly behind you over the left shoulder. Repeat to the right
Turn 360°—instructions: Turn completely around in a full circle. Pause. Then turn a full circle in the other direction
Place alternate foot on step or stool while standing unsupported—instructions: Place each foot alternately on the step/stool. Continue until each foot has touched the step/stool four times
Standing unsupported one foot in front—instructions: Place one foot directly in front of the other
Standing on one leg—instructions: Stand on one leg as long as you can without holding on

Readers are referred to the full description of the test for scoring details.

has been made toward defining tests that can predict the symptoms and consequence of presbystasis. Laboratory tests utilizing electromyographic and quantitative balance information such as measures of sway and reaction times for perturbations in weight distribution have improved prediction slightly. They are better at identifying nonfallers than those at risk. Comparative studies of computerized dynamic posturography (CDP) and electronystagmography (ENG) identify both tests as having some predictive value. Within the ENG protocol (60% sensitive), oculomotor testing (saccades, visual pursuit, optokinetic testing) was most sensitive (40%). CDP was 79% sensitive. The limits of stability component of the CDP test was the only test that seemed predictive of those who had experienced multiple falls.[11] Similar results were identified in a study utilizing a "Physiological Profile Assessment", which included measures of visual contrast, knee proprioception, leg extension, reaction time for hand, and sway on foam block. This was compared with a quantitated measurement of sway during tasks of maximum leaning ability and sway, the latter including ability to change direction of sway and reaction time.[27] Results showed a correlation with age and strong correlations between individuals having single and no falls versus multifallers (two or more falls in 12 months). Reaction time, the time to terminate or change sway direction, was 20–60% slower in multifallers. This is felt to be reflective of the fact that most falls are caused by an inability to react rapidly enough to recover from a loss of balance during daily activity. It was concluded that reaction time was more sensitive than measures of static sway.

TREATMENT

As noted above, presbystasis is the consequence of dysfunction of the balance system. It is likely that it represents subtle age-related changes and extrinsic influences that add up to difficulties with balance and orientation. The most extreme manifestation of presbystasis is falling, the cause of which is also multifactorial. Studies have identified over 400 risk factors that may be associated with falls.[27] Because of this, the approach to helping improve function and balance and prevent occurrences like falling must also reflect a varied approach that removes or modifies those extrinsic factors and optimizes conditions to maximize the use of intrinsic sensory, processing and efferent capacities. Many different modalities of therapy have been used in this regard. These can be categorized as adaptation, habituation, optimization, and substitution (Table 27.3).

Adaptation refers to activities that force the use of deficient areas of the balance system to improve their function. This is one of the goals of vestibular rehabilitation therapy. In this case, exercises are aimed at improving vestibular function itself by forcing the individual to create the situation where the vestibular system fails, either vestibuleocular or vestibulespinal. Therapy forces correction of any asymmetry in performance in the compromised vestibular system. In the case of presbystasis, it can also help encourage use of the vestibular system, as well as other sensory modalities to optimize balance function. While discussion of the specific exercises used is not the topic of this chapter, the sort of activities will invariably be tasks that require visual fixation while the head and body are moving, or tasks where other inputs are compromised, such as with eyes closed or while looking in a different direction. There are many activities of daily life that can be used to serve to enhance function, for instance, sending the individual to the grocery store and having them walk aisles looking for items or riding a stationary bike or treadmill while trying to read or watch a nearby television.

Table 27.3: Balance rehabilitation

Adaptation—activities highlight the disability to force compensation
Habituation—repetition of difficult activity improves performance
Optimization—adjustments to self or environment to enhance balance system needs
Substitution—ensure optimal utilization of all available systems, i.e. cervico-ocular reflex, reduce dependence on visual system

Habituation is the process of repetition of activities or patterns of activity to make them more automatic. This is used in rehabilitation of individuals with bilateral vestibular loss. In this case, the repetition of a desired activity eventually becomes learned. Thus instead of using automatic reflexes to control activities, motor preprogramming of the activity enables one to function without the reflexive sensory input. This will work for complex motor activities too.

Optimization is a very large component in improving balance and preventing falls. This includes those modifications that improve the performance of all components of the balance system and the demands placed on it, for example, optimizing vision by treating cataracts, getting corrective lenses, and putting a light on when walking about. At the same time, problems with visual orientation have arisen due to progressive lenses in glasses. Possible use of single-lens glasses when walking outside is recommended. Even the use of a hat to reduce glare is helpful.

Proprioception can be improved by managing neuropathic problems, wearing low and tie shoes that couple the individual to the ground and enhance sensory input as well as the ability to react to perturbations more quickly, as opposed to higher heels or floppy slippers. In this regard, work is ongoing to produce inserts for shoes to enhance proprioception.[19] The use of a cane or walking stick has been shown to be of marked assistance in such individuals, not for leaning on but to give information about the support surface. Elderly individuals with presbystasis will frequently report that simply putting a finger on a support surface takes away all disability. It is suggested that the input gained from the use of such a device is equivalent to a set of eyes. Sound cues have also been shown to be used to orient in space in elderly individuals. Body sway during quiet standing was reduced when there was a fixed noise source present.[31] It suggests that balanced and serviceable hearing might be important for physical balance in the elderly.

Given the recognized effect of medications in causing changes in alertness and balance, consideration needs to be given to prescribed medications. As noted previously, sedative hypnotic medications are particularly problematic. This would also include medications for the treatment of dizziness/vertigo. Treatment of medical conditions, such as diabetes, cardiac arrhythmia, and blood pressure, is understandably important.

The characteristics of the environment are also of importance. Reduction in clutter and optimal illumination become critical in creating a safe environment. Care must be taken when walking on irregular surfaces or thick carpets. Assistive supports on stairs, in corridors, and in bathing facilities have to be considered.

Behavioral modification is also important. Elderly individuals have to recognize unsafe behaviors such as like climbing ladders, walking about in the dark, and carrying bundles up and down stairs. Counseling is often helpful to indicate areas of risk, the importance of assistive devices and optimizing use of devices and lifestyle and exercise programs in improving balance and safety.

Substitution refers to the enhanced utilization of inputs that are working to replace those that are not. One interesting example is that of the cervico-ocular reflex. There are sensors for head rotation in the neck muscles. These can actually drive the eyes like the vestibular system. Nonhuman primates use this reflex routinely. Normal humans do not normally, but these inputs can be recruited. The same goes for overuse of the eyes to balance. The vestibular system might be fine, but the brain has decided not to use it. This too can be adjusted with exercises that force the individual to rely on the ears as opposed to the eyes. This happens to be a common problem for elderly individuals.

A formal program of vestibular rehabilitation addresses the above issues. Formal programs have been shown to be effective at improving balance, confidence, and lessening fear of falling, flexibility strength, and reaction time. Pure strength training has been shown to be less effective at reducing falls, but clearly is important in improving global function of other systems.[24] A systematic review of various exercise programs, including balance training, strength training, Tai Chi, dance and qi gong as well as enhanced daily activity, showed that they were only weakly beneficial at improving balance.[13] These studies used the timed up and go test, Berg balance, and walking speed to assess efficacy. Although they are excellent clinical measuring tools, there are questions as to their usefulness. Programs that require the individual to go to the therapist's office in addition to home exercises have been suggested to be better than home therapy alone. However, many exercise programs are effective, including Yoga and Tai Chi. However, studies are contradictory, with some identifying an 18% reduction in fall risk following group sessions combined with home exercises. Other studies have not found this benefit. The failure of these programs has been ascribed to factors including inability to perform the exercises in more frail individuals, as well as lack of adherence to the program. One study of perturbation training using unpredictable translation of the support surface and cable pulls of the torso did reduce the occurrence of multiple small steps in recovery, foot collisions, and grasp time. It did not correlate to reduction in falls, though. Other studies comparing intensive, individualized therapy with counseling sessions, medical interventions and exercise, counseling alone, and no intervention, did not identify efficacy in reducing falls.[16]

In a recent review aimed at identifying measures that would be effective at fall reduction and fall-risk reduction, multicomponent group therapy and home therapy and to a lesser degree, Tai Chi, all reduced fall rate and risk.[10] They also reduced the risk of a fall-related fracture. The same was found for home assessments and modification of the environment. This was especially true for more frail and visually impaired clients. Oddly, improving vision was variable in efficacy. It helped to give active multifocal lens wearers single-lens distance glasses. However, perhaps because of the increase in activity, more frail clients given better vision had an increased fall risk. This may have been due to their doing more activity as a consequence of the better vision and thus having more opportunity to fall.

Other findings included the benefits of vitamin D, having a cataract removed, pacemaker placement where indicated, podiatric treatment, and improved shoes.

As discussed, presbystasis falls into the category of problems that cause imbalance. While it is unique in being a diagnosis of exclusion, its symptoms are those of imbalance and dizziness, the same as many diagnosed conditions. The consequences are severe, in many cases including loss of independence and psychological stress and even morbidity and mortality. The causes of presbystasis are by definition multiple and diverse and represent the sum of subtle influences that in themselves do not constitute disease, but in sum do. It is because of this that the evaluation of such individuals has to be inclusive and treatment multifaceted to correct as many of the component problems that result in presbystasis.

REFERENCES

1. AgrawalY, et al. Decline in semicircular canal and otolith function with age. Otol Neurotol. 2012;33:832-9.
2. Alvarez JC, et al. Aging and the human vestibular nuclei: morphometric analysis. Mech Aging Dev. 2000;114(3): 149-72.
3. Baloh RW, et al. The effect of aging on the visual-vestibuloocular responses. Exp Brain Res. 1993;95(3):509-16.
4. Benjuya N, et al. Age-induced shifts from a reliance on sensory input to muscle contraction during balanced standing. J Gerontology. 2004;59A(2):166-71.
5. Bischoff-Ferrari HA, et al. Fall prevention with supplemental and active dorms of vitamin D: a meta-analysis of randomized controlled trials. BMJ. 2009; 339:b3692.
6. BogleThorbahn LD, Newton RA. Use of the Berg balance test to predict falls in elderly persons. Physical Therapy. 1996;76(6):576-83.
7. Boisgontier MP, et al. Age-related differences in attentional cost associated with postural dual tasks: increased recruitment of generic cognitive resources in older adults. Neurosci Biobehavioral Rev. 2013;37(8):1824-37.
8. Cronin NJ, et al. Decreased lower limb muscle recruitment contributes to the inability of older adults to recover with single step following a forward loss of balance. J Electromyograph Kinesiol. 2013:23(5):1139-44.
9. Delbaere K, et al. Mild cognitive impairment as a predictor of falls in community-dwelling older people. Am J Geriatric Psychiatry. 2012;20(10):845-53.
10. Gillespie LD, et al. Interventions for preventing falls in older people living in the community (review). Cochrane Rev. 2012;11.
11. Girardi M, et al. Predicting fall risk in an elderly population: computer dynamic posturography versus electronystagmography test results. Laryngoscope. 2001;111(9):1528-32.
12. Hedman AM, et al. Human brain changes across the life span: a review of 56 longitudinal magnetic resonance imaging studies. Human Brain Mapping. 2012;33:1987-2002.
13. Howe TE, et al. Exercise for improving balance in older people. Cochrane Database Syst Rev. 2007(4):CD004963.
14. Janssen H, et al. Vitamin D deficiency, muscle function, and falls in elderly people. Am J Clin Nutr. 2002;75:611-15.
15. King BR. et al. Neural correlates of the age-related changes in motor sequence learning and motor adaptation in older adults. Front Hum Neurosci. 2013;7(142):1-13.
16. Lord SR, et al. The effect of an individualized fall prevention program on fall risk and falls in older people: a randomized, controlled trial. J Am Geriatr Soc. 2005;53:1296-304.
17. Martin KL, et al. Cognitive function modifies the effect of physiological function on the risk of multiple falls-A population-based study. J Gerontology A BiolSci Med Sci. 2013;68(9):1091-7.
18. Menz HB, et al. The contribution of foot problems to mobility impairment and falls in community-dwelling older people. J Am Geriatrics Soc. 2001;49:1651-6.
19. Perry SD, et al. Efficacy and effectiveness of a balance enhancing insole. J Gerontol A Biol Med Sci. 2008;63(6):595-602.
20. Rauch SD, et al. Decreasing hair cell counts in aging humans. Ann N York Acad Sci. 2001;942:220-7.
21. Schoene D, et al. Discriminative ability and predictive validity of the timed up and go test in identifying older people who fall: systematic review and meta-analysis. J Am Geriatrics Soc. 2013;61(2):202-8.
22. Serrador JM, et al. Loss of otolith function with age is associated with increased postural sway measures. Neurosci Lett. 2009:465(1):10-5.
23. Shaffer SW, Harrison AL. Aging of the somatosensory system: a translational perspective. Phys Ther. 2007;87(2):193-207.
24. Sturnieks DL, et al. Balance disorders in the elderly. Clin Neurophysiol. 2008;38:467-78.
25. Tiedemann A, et al. The comparative ability of eight functional mobility tests for predicting falls in community dwelling older people. Age Aging. 2008;37:430-5.
26. Tiedemann A, et al. The development and validation of a brief performance-based fall risk assessment tool for use in primary care. J Gerontology. 2010;65(8):896-903.
27. Tucker MG, et al. What are the relations between voluntary postural sway measures and falls-history status in community-dwelling older adults? Arch Phys Med Rehabl. 2010;91:750-8.
28. Woo J, et al. Development of a simple scoring tool in the primary care setting for prediction of recurrent falls in men and women aged 65 years and over living in the community. J Clin Nursing. 2009;18:1038-48.
29. Woolcott JC, et al. Meta-analysis of the impact of 9 medication classes on falls in the elderly. Arch Intern Med. 2009; 169(21):1952-60.
30. Woollacott MH, Shumway-Cook A. Changes in posture control across the lifespan—a systems approach. Phys Ther. 1990;70:799-807.
31. Zhong X, Yost WA. Relationship between postural stability and spatial hearing. J Am Acad Audiol. 2013;24(9):782-8.
32. Zuniga MG, et al. Association between hearing loss and saccular dysfunction in older individuals. Otol Neurotol. 2012;33(9):1586-92.
33. Zwergal A, et al. Aging of human supraspinal locomotor and postural control in fMRI. Neurobiol Aging. 2012;33:1073-84.

CHAPTER

28

Inner Ear Dehiscence

Jason A Beyea, Lorne S Parnes, Sumit K Agrawal

INTRODUCTION/BACKGROUND

The normal functioning of the inner ear relies on the mechanical isolation of the perilymph and endolymph from surrounding structures by the thick bone of the otic capsule. The round and oval windows permit controlled access by outside sound and pressure changes to the inner ear fluids. In disease states that have other bony openings in the otic capsule, specific signs and symptoms will be observed, with their distinct characteristics based on the location of the bony dehiscence. Historically, this was recognized in the context of a horizontal semicircular canal (SCC) fistula in patients with an advanced cholesteatoma. More recently, primary dehiscences of the superior SCC, posterior SCC, and cochlea have been described.

SUPERIOR SEMICIRCULAR CANAL DEHISCENCE

Pathogenesis

Superior semicircular canal dehiscence (SSCD) is the most studied type of otic capsule dehiscence, and will serve as the archetype for a discussion of inner ear dehiscence. Lessons learned from the study of superior SCC dehiscence can be applied to the evaluation and management of other types of inner ear dehiscence. The SSCD syndrome was first described by Minor et al.[37] Studies on cadaveric temporal bones have found a dehiscence of the overlying bone of the superior SSC in 0.5% of specimens.[11] In an additional 1.4% of specimens, the bone coverage was <0.1mm, such that it might appear dehiscent even on ultra-high-resolution computed tomography (CT) of the temporal bone. Despite the high radiographic and histological prevalence, the clinical prevalence is much lower.

The underlying pathophysiology is related to an opening in the bone that overlies the superior SCC. This creates a third mobile window (the first and second being the oval and round windows) into the inner ear. As a result, the vestibular labyrinth responds to sound and pressure changes.

Excitation of the superior canal occurs with application of positive pressure in the external auditory canal (EAC), Valsalva maneuver against pinched nostrils, and presentation of loud sound to the ear.[11] Positive pressure to the EAC and Valsalva against pinched nostrils creates a positive pressure gradient from the middle to the inner ear, the pressure is released through the dehiscence over the superior canal, and resultant utriculofugal flow in the superior canal is excitatory. The mechanism of loud sound-induced excitation has been postulated to occur through a different mechanism, which may be due to rectified stapes motion, excitation/inhibition asymmetry, and/or vestibular nerve afferent phase-locking.[11]

Inhibition of the superior canal occurs with creation of negative pressure in the EAC, Valsalva maneuver against a closed glottis, and jugular venous compression. These stimuli create a positive pressure gradient from the middle cranial fossa to the inner ear at the dehiscence, the pressure is released at the round or oval windows, and the resultant utriculopetal flow in the superior canal is inhibitory.

The resultant eye movements (Figs. 28.1A and B) typically align themselves with the plane of the affected superior SCC. With eyes in center gaze, excitation of the right superior SCC (tone presentation to right ear) results in slow phase-induced eye movements directed upward with a torsional rotation of the superior pole of the eyes toward the patient's left side.[13] Fast phase nystagmus (if present) is directed downward with a torsional rotation of the superior pole of the eyes toward the patient's right side. Conversely, excitation of the left superior SCC (tone presentation to the left ear) results in slow phase induced eye movements directed upward with a torsional rotation of the superior pole of the eyes toward the patient's right side. Fast phase nystagmus (if present) is directed downward with a torsional rotation of the superior pole of the eyes toward the patient's left side. The presence of the torsional and vertical components of the induced eye movements is dependent on direction of gaze (neutral, right, and left gaze—*see* Figs. 28.1A and B).

Dehiscence of the bone overlying the superior SCC is presumed to arise from a reduction of the normal thickening of bone over the superior canal that occurs during

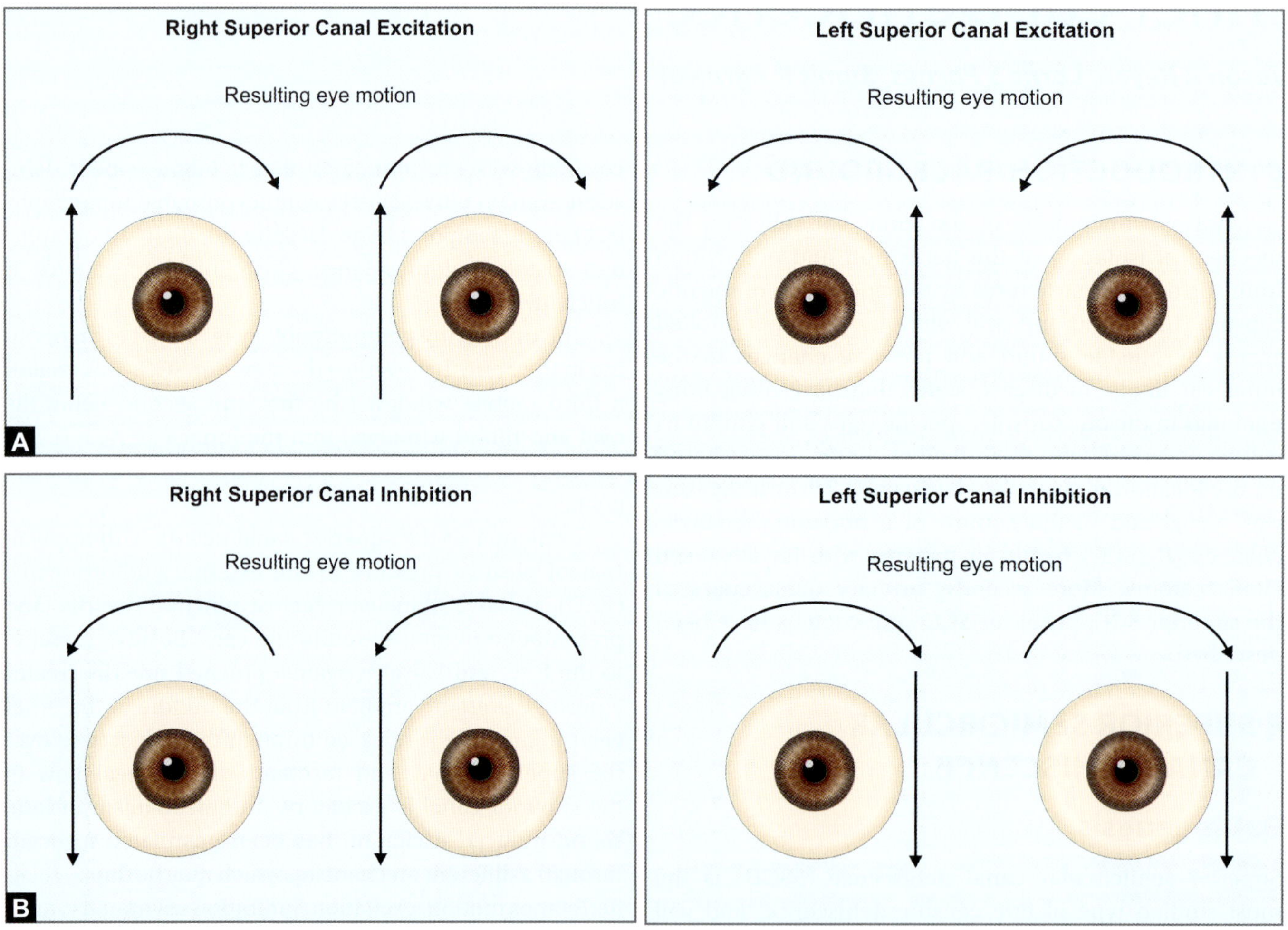

Figs. 28.1A and B: Slow phase resulting eye motion upon excitation (A) and inhibition (B) of the superior semicircular canal in neutral gaze position. Excitation of the superior canal is caused by application of positive pressure in the external auditory canal, Valsalva maneuver against pinched nostrils, and presentation of loud sound to the ear. Conversely, inhibition of the superior canal is caused by creation of negative pressure in the external auditory canal, Valsalva maneuver against a closed glottis, and jugular venous compression. This figure demonstrates slow phase resulting eye motion only in neutral gaze. For excitation of a given superior semicircular canal with gaze toward that ipsilateral side, resulting eye motion is purely upward. For excitation of a given superior semicircular canal with gaze toward the contralateral side, resulting eye motion is purely torsional with the superior pole of the eyes beating toward the contralateral side. For inhibition of a given superior semicircular canal with gaze toward that ipsilateral side, resulting eye motion is purely downward. For inhibition of a given superior semicircular canal with gaze toward the contralateral side, resulting eye motion is purely torsional with the superior pole of the eyes beating toward the ipsilateral side.
Source: Adapted with permission from Beyea et al.[5]

the first 3 postnatal years,[11] although this postnatal developmental cause of SSCD remains controversial. Tsunoda and Terasaki[51] used a computer simulation model to propose that SSCD arises during the fetal developmental period. Wang and Parnes[54] described a case of bilateral SSCD in a patient with external, middle, and inner ear abnormalities, providing support to a congenital etiology. In contrast, a recent retrospective radiological series of temporal bone CT scans demonstrated a statistically significant increase in superior canal dehiscence with increasing age,[40] lending support to an acquired cause. Precipitating events of the SSCD syndrome remain speculative. These include direct trauma, activities that produced changes in middle ear or intracranial pressure,[3] and systemic bony demineralization that occurred with increasing age.[40]

Clinical Findings: Symptoms and Signs

This syndrome can include vestibular and audiologic symptoms (Table 28.1). Vestibular symptoms manifest as vertigo, oscillopsia, chronic disequilibrium, and motion intolerance.[37] Minor[34] reported that 60 (92%) of 65 patients with superior canal dehiscence had vestibular symptoms that were attributed to the dehiscence of the superior canal. In this same series, 54 (83%) had Tullio phenomenon, and 44 (68%) had pressure-induced (induced by coughing, sneezing, and straining) vertigo.[34] The Tullio phenomenon, which is a sense of brief transient motion or vertigo induced by loud sounds, is one of the key characteristics of this syndrome. This phenomenon can also be seen with Meniere's disease, other causes of perilymph fistula and vestibulofibrosis, so these should remain in the differential diagnosis. A complete focused history includes a search for other causes of vestibular symptoms.

Associated auditory symptoms include hearing loss, autophony, pulsatile tinnitus, and hyperacusis of bone-conducted sounds such as the sound of the patient's own footsteps and their eyes moving in their orbits.[36,34] In the series of Minor,[34] 39 patients (60%) had autophony and 34 patients (52%) had hyperacusis of bone-conducted sounds. Chi et al.[12] found that 27% of their patients reported tinnitus, often described by the patients as pulsatile. Although the mechanism of pulsatile tinnitus is unknown, the proposed pathophysiology involves transmission of normal intracranial pulse-related pressure changes through the superior canal dehiscence to the cochlea.[8]

Interestingly, SSCD can present purely as a conductive hearing loss, without associated vestibular symptoms.[30] In this manner, SSCD can mimic otosclerosis. Patients may undergo failed middle ear surgery for a presumed otosclerosis.[25] A key distinguishing factor is the presence of the acoustic reflex in patients with SSCD,[30] whereas this will typically be absent in patients with otosclerosis.[47] Furthermore, Röösli et al.[46] highlight the role of obtaining a CT scan prior to revision stapes surgery to identify abnormalities such as SSCD, and to avoid performance of unnecessary surgeries. These findings emphasize the importance of screening patients with suspected otosclerosis for vestibular symptoms. SSCD should be on the clinician's differential diagnosis of conductive hearing loss.

Table 28.1: Findings in superior semicircular canal dehiscence syndrome

	Patients affected
Symptoms	
Tullio phenomenon	83% (54/65)[34]
Hearing loss	82% (9/11)[12]
Aural fullness	80% (4/5)[50]
Pressure-induced vertigo	68% (44/65)[34]
Autophony	60% (39/65)[34]
Hyperacusis of bone conducted sounds	52% (34/65)[34]
Pulsatile tinnitus	27% (3/11)[12]
Signs	
Sound-evoked eye movements	77% (46/60)[34]
256 Hz tuning fork heard at lateral malleolus	75% (3/4)[55]
Valsalva-evoked eye movements	70% (42/60)[34]
External auditory canal applied pressure evoked eye movements	43% (26/60)[34]
Sound-evoked head tilt in plane of SSC	18% (11/60)[34]
Investigations	
Audiogram—air-bone gap ≥10 dB at 250 Hz	72% (38/53)[34]
Audiogram—depressed bone conduction <0 dB	67% (2/3)[49]
Audiogram—acoustic reflexes absent	11% (2/18)[58]
VEMP—lowered threshold	91% (32/35)[58]

Source: Adapted with permission from Beyea et al.[5]
(SSC, superior semicircular canal; VEMP, vestibular-evoked myogenic potential).

An explanation for the variability in symptomatology experienced by different patients has been proposed by Pfammatter et al.[44] These investigators found patients with both vestibular and cochlear symptoms had significantly larger dehiscences of the superior canal (mean of 4.1mm) on high-resolution CT scan than those with only vestibular or cochlear symptoms (mean of 1.9mm) ($p < 0.001$).

Sound or pressure-evoked eye movements should be observed in the absence of visual fixation,[13] as visual fixation can suppress the nystagmus of labyrinthine origin. However, the torsional nystagmus component is poorly inhibited by visual fixation,[28] as point fixation can only suppress the vertical and horizontal components of the nystagmus. Avoidance of visual fixation suppression can be achieved with the use of infrared video equipment or Frenzel's glasses.[13] Cremer et al.[13] recommend assessment of evoked eye movements during presentation of tones (125 Hz to 6 kHz, intensity of 110 dB HL), Valsalva maneuvers, and tragal compression. Direction of the evoked nystagmus will be as previously described (*see* Figs. 28.1A and B). Minor[34] found that of patients with vestibular signs associated with SSCD, 82% had sound-evoked eye movements, 75% had Valsalva-evoked eye movements, and 45% had EAC pressure-evoked eye movements. Furthermore, a tilt of the head in the plane of the superior canal evoked by sound was detected in 20% of these patients. In dehiscences ≥5mm, nystagmus evoked by tone presentation aligns between the plane of the superior and horizontal canals.[36] Weber 512 Hz tuning fork will lateralize to the affected ear, and a low-frequency tuning fork (128 and 256 Hz) placed on the lateral malleolus of the ankle may rarely be heard by the patient.[20,55] The evaluation should include a complete head and neck examination, Dix–Hallpike, and a focused neurological exam.

Evaluation: Otologic and Neurotologic Testing

Audiometry often reveals a low-frequency conductive hearing loss on the affected side, with normal word recognition and intact acoustic reflexes.[37,8,35] Bone conduction thresholds may be <0 dB HL.[49] Tympanometry demonstrates normal pressures and the testing may induce vertigo and eye movement from the pressure change in the middle ear.[3] As noted, the intact acoustic reflexes may be the significant clue that differentiates SSCD from otosclerotic conductive hearing loss.[1]

Routine electronystagmography fails to identify objective abnormal findings, but the patient may report vertigo with the application of pressure to the EAC.[39] Caloric testing will typically be normal.[9]

Vestibular-evoked myogenic potentials (VEMPs) are enhanced in SSCD, displaying a reduced response threshold on the affected side [49,34] (Fig. 28.2). Crane et al.[14] found 13 of their 18 SSCD patients tested with cervical VEMP had decreased thresholds on the affected side. Pfammatter et al.[44] demonstrated that with a bone dehiscence on high-resolution CT scan of ≥2.5mm, the VEMP threshold was more often lowered (≤80dB SPL) than if the dehiscence was <2.5mm (p=0.009). The VEMP responses typically reported for SSCD syndrome are cervical VEMPs,

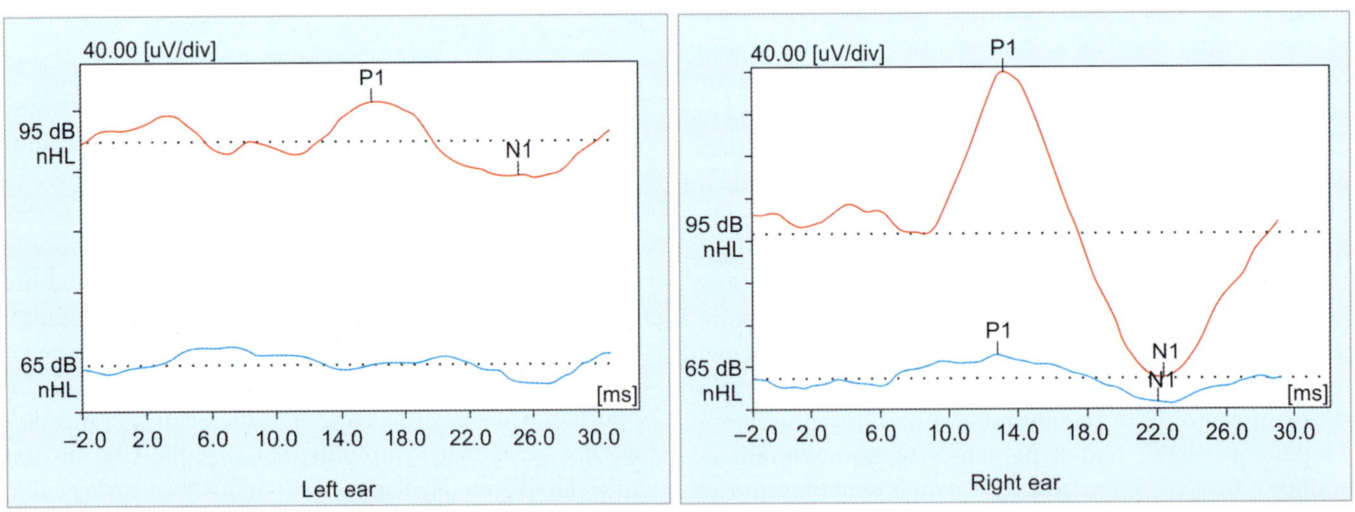

Fig. 28.2: Cervical vestibular-evoked myogenic potential (VEMP) responses (click-evoked, measured from the ipsilateral sternocleidomastoid muscle) in a patient with right superior semicircular canal dehiscence syndrome and a normal left ear. The right superior canal dehiscence was confirmed with high-resolution computed tomography (CT) and intraoperatively via a transmastoid approach. Left panel demonstrates left ear response at 95 dB nHL stimulation (50 microV amplitude response), and an absence of response at 65 dB nHL stimulation. Right panel demonstrates right ear response at 95 dB nHL stimulation (289 microV amplitude response) and at 65 dB nHL stimulation (43 microV amplitude response). This clinical example highlights both the reduced threshold on the right side (response is present at 65 dB nHL stimulation) and >2:1 ratio of amplitude on the affected side (right: 289 microV response at 95dB nHL stimulation) compared with the normal side (left: 50 microV response at 95dB nHL stimulation).

as electromyography is recorded from the sternocleidomastoid muscle. Ocular VEMPs, measured from electrodes placed on the cheek below the eye, have been shown to be equally useful in diagnosis and follow-up of SSCD syndrome,[56] but demonstrate better test-retest reliability than cervical VEMP.[42] Our center currently uses cervical VEMPs.

Evaluation: Radiologic Imaging

High-resolution CT scanning is necessary to accurately diagnose the bony dehiscence. The use of 0.5mm collimation and oblique reformats in the plane of the superior SCC has been demonstrated to improve specificity and positive predictive value of a finding of dehiscence.[6] Belden et al.[6] found that the positive predictive value (PPV) of an apparent dehiscence in SSCD was 50% with 1.0mm collimation using coronal and transverse images, which improved to 93% with 0.5mm collimation and CT reformatting in the plane of the superior SCC. An example of a patient with surgically confirmed right superior SCC dehiscence with 0.625-mm collimation is shown in Figures 28.3A and B. New technology using Cone-Beam Volumetric Tomography holds promise for improved diagnostic accuracy related to its ability to provide greater information content and spatial resolution compared to multi-slice CT.[43]

SSCD syndrome is diagnosed by the presence of vestibular and/or audiologic symptoms characteristic of the syndrome, evoked eye movements in the plane of the affected superior SCC, and radiological confirmation of bony dehiscence over the superior SCC.[34] A low-frequency conductive hearing loss and normal word recognition on audiometry, the presence of intact acoustic reflexes, and lowered thresholds on VEMP testing aid in the diagnosis.

Differential Diagnosis

Careful consideration of the presenting symptoms of SSCD syndrome permits formulation of a broad differential diagnosis. Although SSCD is the most commonly reported of the primary inner ear dehiscences, other types of inner ear dehiscence (including posterior SCC dehiscence and cochlear dehiscence, as discussed later) should be actively sought and excluded with the observation of the direction of evoked eye movements (if present) and the use of high-resolution CT. Furthermore, a labyrinthine fistula can be caused by post-traumatic leakage of perilymph from the inner to the middle ear and from disruption of the labyrinthine bone caused by cholesteatoma or chronic otitis media.[33] Clinical history, the direction of evoked eye movements, and CT scan findings will distinguish these pathologies from SSCD.[33]

A history of transient vertigo raises the possibility of benign paroxysmal positional vertigo (BPPV). This can be distinguished from SSCD syndrome by the absence of audiologic symptoms, the absence of sound/pressure-evoked nystagmus, a positive Dix–Hallpike, and the presence of bony coverage of the superior canal on CT scan. Otosclerosis also presents with a conductive hearing loss, but can be distinguished based on the absence of vestibular symptoms on history, the absence of acoustic reflexes, and the presence of bony coverage of the superior canal on CT scan. Patulous Eustachian tube shares with SSCD the symptom of autophony. Poe[45] noted in his series that the patients with patulous Eustachian tube had autophony of their breathing, whereas those with SSCD syndrome did not. Clinical evaluation of respiratory excursion of the tympanic membrane and a high-resolution CT scan will further clarify the diagnosis. Finally,

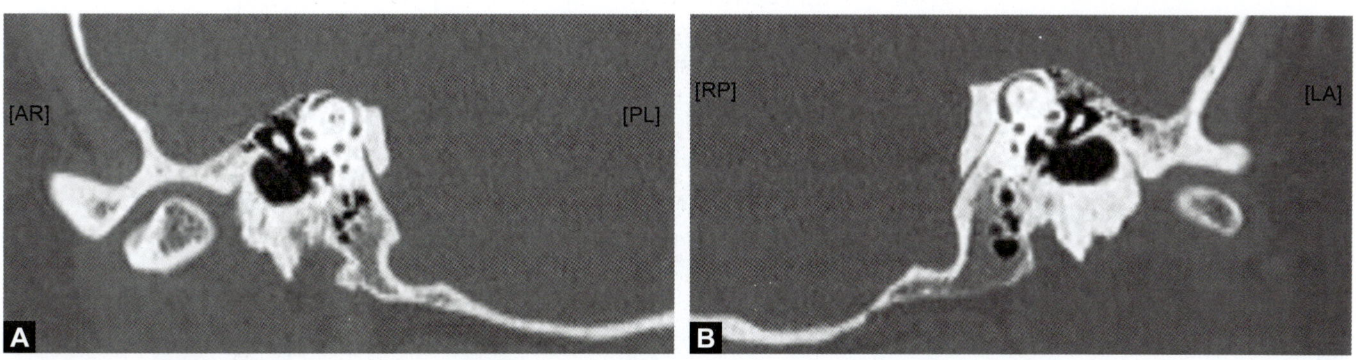

Figs. 28.3A and B: 0.625 mm collimated computed tomography (CT) scan of the temporal bones in a patient with surgically confirmed right superior semicircular canal dehiscence syndrome. Multiplanar reformation in oblique sagittal orientation demonstrates (A) dehiscence of bone over the right superior semicircular canal and (B) bony covering over the normal left superior semicircular canal. (AR, anterior right; PL, posterior left; RP, right posterior; LA, left anterior).

migraine-associated vertigo should be considered. Migraine-related vertigo (MV) is the most common cause of spontaneous nonpositional episodic vertigo.[16] Brief migraine-related vertigo attacks lasting seconds with possible migraine-associated symptoms of hearing loss, tinnitus, and aural fullness can be difficult to distinguish from SSCD on clinical history. Typically, noise or Valsalva-precipitated vertigo is not present in MV.[16] The absence of sound and pressure-evoked eye movements and the presence of bony coverage of the superior canal on CT scan will distinguish MV from SSCD.

TREATMENT

In most patients, control of symptoms is achieved by avoidance of symptom-evoking sound and pressure stimuli.[32] A conscientious patient can often avoid their distinct triggers. Only after attempted trigger avoidance and in the presence of debilitating vestibular or auditory symptoms should surgical management be pursued. The Dizziness Handicap Inventory (DHI) can be used to quantify the disability that SSCD syndrome is causing for the patient and to evaluate postoperative response to surgery.[15]

Surgical management of SSCD syndrome is through resurfacing or plugging of the superior SCC. Resurfacing is typically performed through a middle fossa approach[34] although recently successful transmastoid resurfacing has been described.[2,50] Plugging is performed through a middle fossa[37] (as shown in Figures 28.4A and B) or transmastoid[8,1,17] approach. A recent meta-analysis[52] has demonstrated the superiority of canal plugging or capping (with hydroxyapatite cement) over resurfacing for resolution of symptoms.

The transmastoid approach to superior SCC plugging has become our surgical approach of choice (📹 28.1). This approach has the advantages of obviating a craniotomy, avoidance of temporal lobe retraction, familiarity of the approach for experienced otologists, and the ability to occlude the canal without manipulating the defect.[1] In the minority of patients with a very low-lying tegmen, the middle fossa approach would be considered. The authors do not have personal experience with the middle fossa approach for SSCD, and we refer the reader to Minor[32] for a review of this technique. We use bone dust for canal plugging, as opposed to bone wax, as bone dust has been shown to promote less inflammation and to demonstrate improved osteogenesis.[23] Briefly, a 5–6 cm postauricular incision is made, a standard mastoidectomy is performed, and the horizontal canal is visualized (Figs. 28.5A to D). Bone between the horizontal canal and tegmen is carefully drilled layer by layer with a small diamond burr to blue-line the superior canal on both sides of the dehiscence. A 1 × 3 mm endosteal island is made on both the ampulated and nonampulated sides of the canal, and gently elevated with a fine 90° hook to visualize the membranous labyrinth. To enable better and easier insertion of the bone dust, we create a type of bone putty by mixing the bone dust from the drilled off mastoid cortex with fibrinogen sealant (Tisseel). A "plug", fashioned to be just a bit larger than the fenestration is gently packed into both fenestrations. The intent is to completely occlude

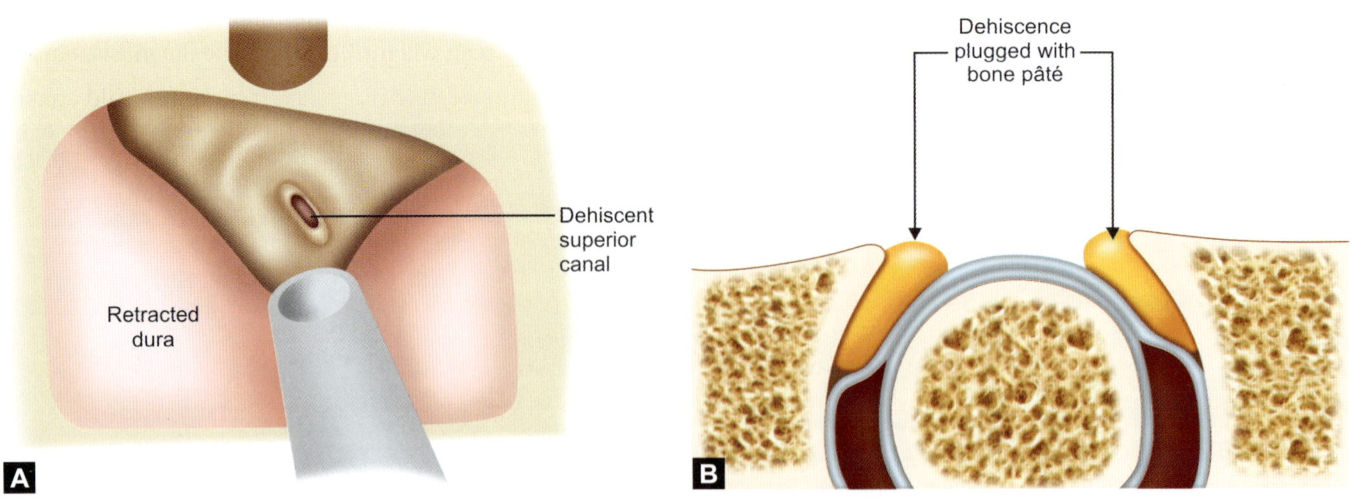

Figs. 28.4A and B: Right ear. Middle fossa approach to superior semicircular canal plugging. A standard middle fossa craniotomy is performed, and the dura is gently retracted (A) to reveal the dehiscent superior semicircular canal. (B) Tissue sealant and bone dust are mixed to form a bone pâté, which is used to plug the superior canal, ensuring that both ends of the dehiscence are plugged.

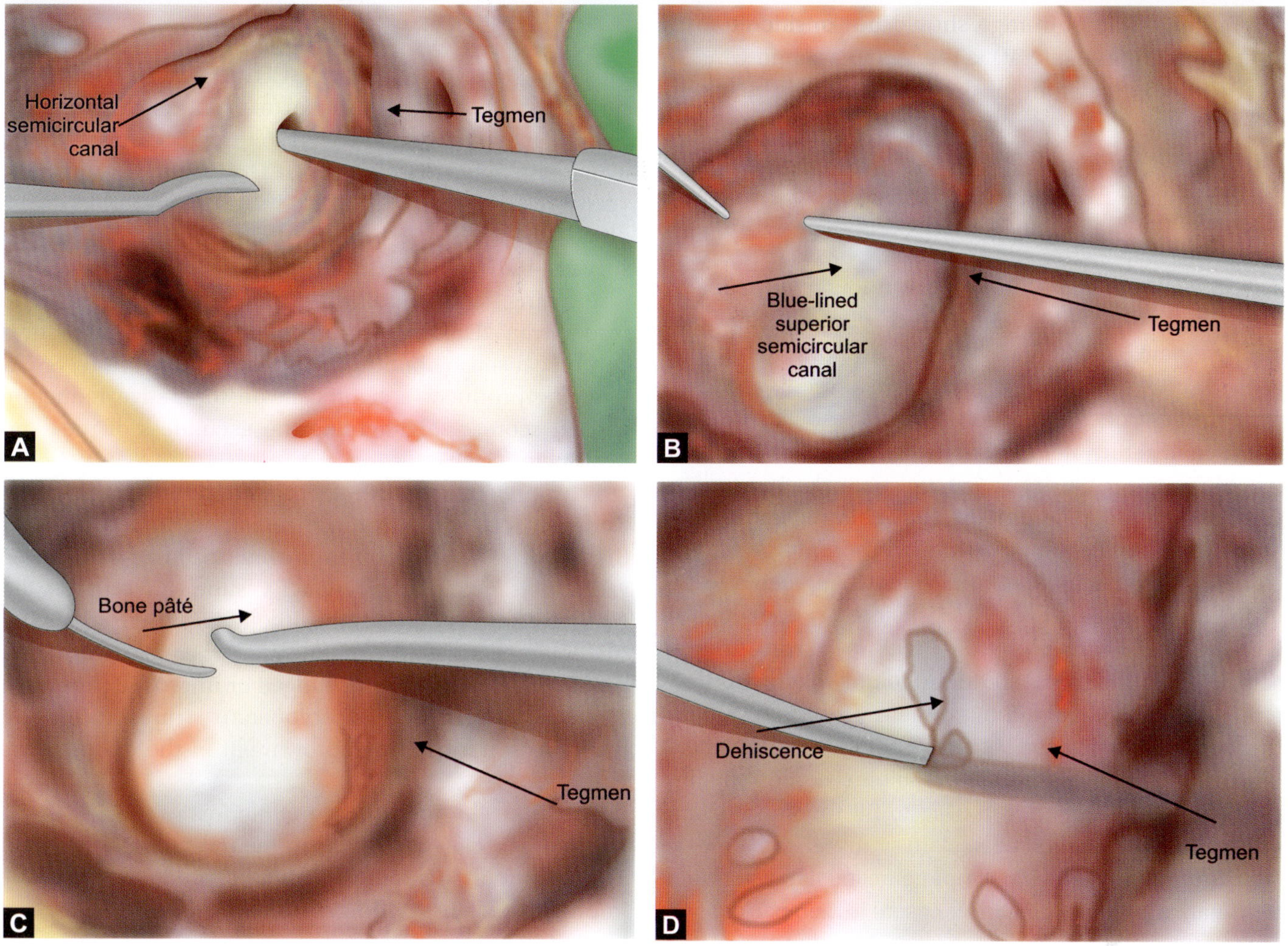

Figs. 28.5A to D: Left ear. Transmastoid approach to superior semicircular canal plugging. (A) A standard mastoidectomy is performed, and the horizontal semicircular canal visualized. (B) The superior semicircular canal is blue lined on both the ampulated and nonampulated sides of the dehiscence. (C) Bone pate is gently packed into the two fenestrations. This occludes the canal and functionally isolates the region of dehiscence. (D) Following insertion of both plugs, the dura is gently mobilized to verify the dehiscence.
Source: Adapted with permission from Beyea et al.[5]

the bony and membranous canal on either side of the dehiscence, and thereby completely and permanently partitioning the dehiscent region from the remainder of the inner ear. We are careful in our attempts to not overfill the canal lumen so as to not occlude the common crus or the ampulla, though we admit that this is a potential pitfall of our technique. The bone putty will ossify in time thus creating a permanent solid occlusion of the canal. In our opinion, the "plug" needs to be solid. We have treated a patient who remained symptomatic after middle fossa canal occlusion with fascia. During the transmastoid procedure, we noted that although the fascia was filling the lumen of the superior canal at the dehiscence, it was still mobile and attached to the undersurface of the dura, so in essence, the patient still had the third window effect.

Only after the plugs are firmly inserted should consideration be given towards drilling out the superior canal bone between the plugs to directly examine the dehiscence. With good imaging that clearly shows the dehiscence, this part is purely elective and slightly increases the risk of dural damage. We have felt comfortable exploring the dehiscences in all of our cases, and have found them as small as the tip of a Rosen needle and as large as 5 mm in length. In our experience of more than 30 cases, we have never seen the dura herniating down into the lumen of the canal. At this point, the fenestrations and exposed dehiscence are covered with temporalis fascia and fibrinogen sealant to further protect against perilymph leakage.

In patients whose SSCD ear is their only hearing ear and/or their only ear with vestibular function, or who are elderly/medically unfit for transmastoid or middle fossa SCC occlusion, consideration is given to a round window reinforcement. Patching of the round window theoretically dampens its hypercompliance and makes the inner ear less sensitive to sound and pressure.[48] This approach is minimally invasive and does not preclude future transmastoid/middle fossa procedures if round window reinforcement is unsuccessful. To date, we have treated nine ears in eight patients with round window reinforcement. These patients have demonstrated relief or significant improvement in pulsatile tinnitus, autophony, and hyperacusis of bone conducted sounds. At present, the long-term success of this procedure is not known. A recent multi-center study demonstrates the efficacy and safety of this technique.[59] We are aware that several other tertiary care otology groups are performing this procedure with overall positive results (personal communication). Our technical approach to round window augmentation is as follows (Figs. 28.6A and B). A standard tympanomeatal flap is elevated through a transcanal approach. If necessary, overhanging bone above the round window niche is removed with a diamond burr. The mucosa from around the window is freshened with a 90° pick. A small piece of areolar tissue harvested from a small incision just behind the pinna is fashioned as a plug to fill the entire round window niche. Fibrinogen sealant is dispensed over the fascia/round window. The tympanomeatal flap is returned to its native position, and the ear canal is then packed with absorbable gelatin sponge in the usual fashion.

PROGNOSIS

Most outcome literature on SSCD surgical repair is from series that used a middle cranial fossa approach. Complete vestibular symptom and sign resolution occur more often in patients who underwent SSCD plugging (8 out of 9) versus resurfacing (7 out of 11).[34] This is supported by the meta-analysis of Vlastarakos et al.[52] who demonstrated success rates of 32/33, 8/16, and 14/15 for plugging, resurfacing, and capping with hydroxyapatite-cement, respectively. Delayed failures of resurfacing procedures can be caused by bone graft resorption.[18] Of note, SSCD plugging produces a significant postoperative reduction in DHI scores,[15] highlighting the usefulness of pre- and postoperative DHI testing.

Our previous report[1] of 3 cases of transmastoid superior SCC occlusion has now been substantiated by a further 13 cases.[4] Symptoms improved or abated in 15 of the 16 patients. One of our patient's vestibular symptoms did not improve postoperatively although she refused further treatment of her contralateral superior canal dehiscence. All patients had either unchanged or improved pure-tone thresholds compared to preoperative thresholds. Two patients demonstrated improvement in their conductive hearing loss.

Limb et al.[26] found that middle fossa repair of SSCD was not associated with sensorineural hearing loss, and a small group of patients demonstrated postoperative improvement in conductive hearing loss. The risk of sensorineural hearing loss is higher in patients who have

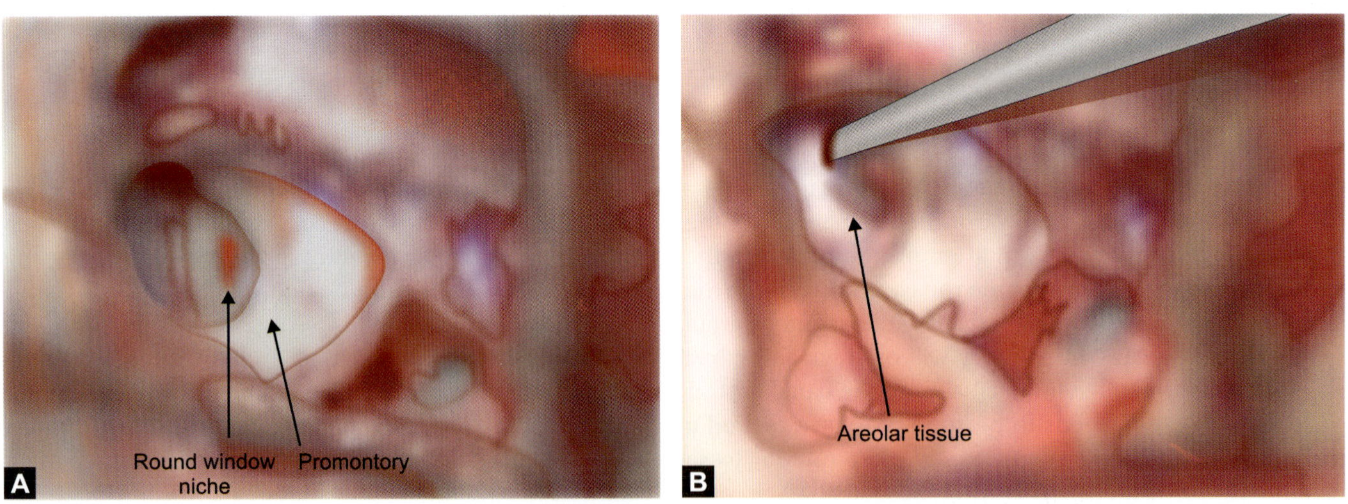

Figs. 28.6A and B: Left ear. Transcanal approach to round window reinforcement. (A) A standard tympanomeatal flap is elevated, and the round window niche visualized. If necessary, overhanging bone above the round window niche is removed with a small diamond burr. The mucosa around the round window is freshened with a 90° pick. A small piece of areolar tissue is harvested from a small post-auricular incision. (B) The areolar tissue is used to augment the entire round window niche, and fibrinogen sealant is dispensed over the areolar tissue/round window.

previously undergone inner ear surgery.[26] Superior SCC dehiscence plugging results in reduced function in the surgically repaired canal, but typically does not impair the function of the other two ipsilateral SCCs.[10] Interestingly, VEMP thresholds have been found to normalize after corrective surgical plugging of the superior SSCD.[56]

POSTERIOR SEMICIRCULAR CANAL DEHISCENCE

Pathogenesis

Posterior semicircular canal dehiscence (PSCD) was first radiologically described by Wadin et al.[53] in a study of patients with a high jugular bulb. PSCD has since been described in temporal bone fibrous dysplasia,[29] enlarged vestibular aqueduct with Mondini malformation, Apert syndrome, microtia/aural atresia, and as a result of iatrogenic injury.[19]

Clinical Findings: Symptoms and Signs

Symptoms include aural fullness, autophony, pulsatile tinnitus, disequilibrium, vertigo, and Tullio phenomenon.[19] Krombach et al.[24] found in their series of 23 patients with PSCD that 86% presented with vertigo, 9% with hearing loss or tinnitus, and 5% with symptoms unrelated to the inner ear.

Evaluation: Otologic and Neurotologic Testing

Hearing loss can be mixed, purely conductive, or purely sensorineural.[19] Gopen et al.[19] found reduced VEMP thresholds in all 10 (of 12) patients tested.

Evaluation: Radiologic Imaging

Diagnosis is confirmed with high-resolution CT scan of the temporal bones (Fig. 28.7), with standard axial and coronal views. Interestingly, there may be a right-sided predilection for PSCD, theorized to be related to the more common right dominant jugular venous drainage.[19]

Treatment

Treatment is similar to that for SSCD. Trigger avoidance should be attempted first. For those patients with poor symptomatic control, surgical management is pursued with transmastoid posterior SCC occlusion,[31] as is performed for intractable BPPV. The authors note that since most commonly the dehiscence is from the jugular bulb near the ampulla, partitioning of that area may be very difficult with transmastoid posterior canal occlusion, although Mikulec and Poe[31] did obtain successful results with this approach.

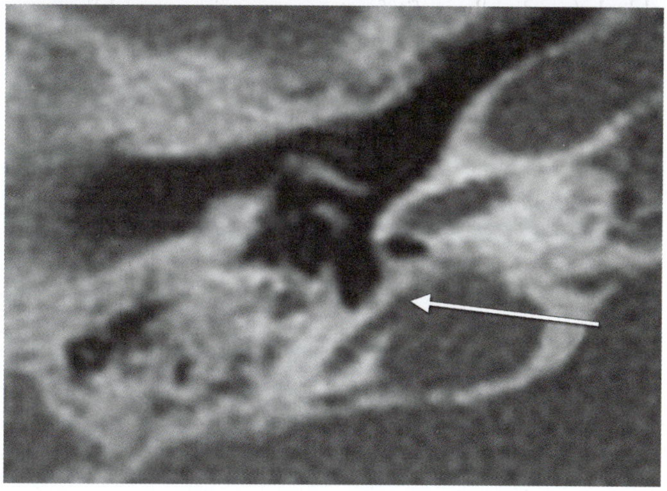

Fig. 28.7: Computed tomography (CT) scan (axial section) of a right ear. The posterior semicircular canal is dehiscent into the jugular fossa (arrow).
Source: Adapted with permission from Gopen et al.[19]

Prognosis

Given the paucity of reports of PSCD in the literature, the details of long-term prognosis are not yet reported. Conservative management with trigger avoidance is the mainstay of management for most patients.

COCHLEAR DEHISCENCE

Pathogenesis

Three types of cochlear dehiscences have been described: cochlear-carotid, cochlear-internal auditory canal (IAC), and cochlear-facial nerve.

Cochlear-carotid dehiscence was first described in 2004 by Modugno,[38] and subsequently described by four other groups.[22, 27,41,57] In a CT temporal bone study of 30 normal patients, Young et al.[57] defined the normal range of the distance between the cochlea and carotid artery (which they termed the Cochlear-Carotid Interval) as 0.2 to 3.8 mm on the right side and 0.2 to 5.0 mm on the left side. These groups explain the symptoms of cochlear-carotid dehiscence through the concept of a mobile pathologic third window, as has been proposed in the pathophysiology of superior and posterior SCC dehiscence syndromes. Cochlear-IAC dehiscence has been described in a patient who presented with short episodes of vertigo and a mixed hearing loss.[21] This patient was found to have a Mondini-like dysplasia with a shortened cochlea, a deficient modiolus, and a communication between the IAC and the basal turn of the cochlea (a third window). Most recently, the cochlear-facial nerve dehiscence has been described by Blake et al.[7] They concluded that the cochlear-facial nerve dehiscence contributed to their patients' symptoms through the mechanism of a third mobile window. They hypothesized a genetic or systemic predisposition to this condition, as both of their patients had bilateral involvement. They also raise the interesting possibility that the frequency of the hearing loss notch on the audiogram may correspond to the region of the cochlea that has a bony dehiscence, as this region may demonstrate increased dissipation of acoustic energy due to the absence of bony coverage.

Clinical Findings: Symptoms and Signs

Presenting symptoms include hearing loss, pulsatile tinnitus, and autophony, with the cochlear-IAC dehiscence patient also experiencing short episodes of vertigo.[21] Ipsilateral carotid pressure may decrease the severity of pulsatile tinnitus in patients with cochlear-carotid dehiscences.[27] Facial nerve function is typically normal in patients with cochlear-facial nerve dehiscence.[7]

Evaluation: Otologic and Neurotologic Testing

Audiometric testing can reveal conductive, mixed, or sensorineural hearing losses. Of particular interest is the finding of notching of the air conduction thresholds at a particular frequency and the possible association with the region of the cochlea that has a bony dehiscence.[7] VEMP testing typically does not reveal lowered thresholds as in SSCD; however, one group did report lowered VEMP thresholds.[38]

Evaluation: Radiographic Imaging

High-resolution CT with axial and coronal views is the standard for diagnosis of cochlear dehiscences. This reveals a dehiscence of the bony septum between the cochlea and carotid artery in cochlear-carotid dehiscences[22,27,38,41] (Fig. 28.8). Cochlear-IAC dehiscence may demonstrate

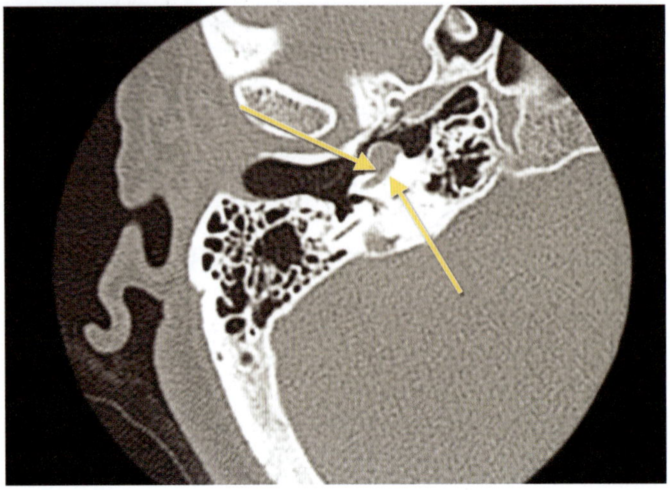

Fig. 28.8: Computed tomography (CT) scan (axial section) of the right ear. The vertical segment of the petrous internal carotid artery is dehiscent (arrows) into the basilar turn of the cochlea. *Source*: Adapted with permission from Lund and Palacios.[27]

a deficient modiolus and a communication between the IAC and the basal turn of the cochlea[21] (Fig. 28.9). In patients with a cochlear-facial nerve dehiscence, imaging reveals a bone dehiscence between the basal turn of the cochlea and labyrinthine segment of the facial nerve, with both patients demonstrating bilateral cochlea-facial nerve dehiscences[7] (Fig. 28.10).

Treatment

Hearing amplification should be considered in appropriately selected candidates. In cases of cochlear-carotid dehiscence, observation is initially implemented for all patients. In only the most severely symptomatic patients, Lund and Palacios[27] suggest considering a chemical or surgical labyrinthectomy to deafen the ear. Certainly, this would never be performed in any only-hearing and/or only-vestibular ear, and the operative risk of damage to the carotid would be significant. Another theoretical option would be carotid balloon occlusion,[27] but this entails even graver risks. For cochlear-IAC and cochlear-facial nerve dehiscences, observation is the management of choice.

Prognosis

Patient education regarding the presence of the bony dehiscence and the cause of their symptomatology can be reassuring for many patients. As more of these patients are identified and followed clinically, the long-term prognosis will be characterized.

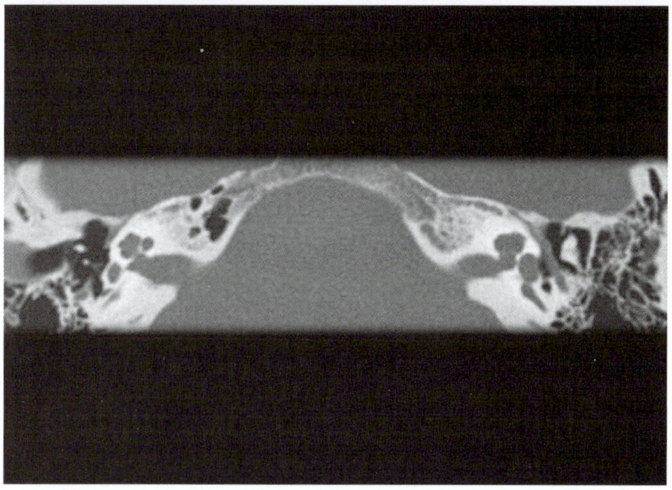

Fig. 28.9: Computed tomography (CT) scan (axial section) of the temporal bones. The left cochlea is shorter and has a deficient modiolus. The normal right cochlea is shown for comparison.
Source: Adapted with permission from Karlberg et al.[21]

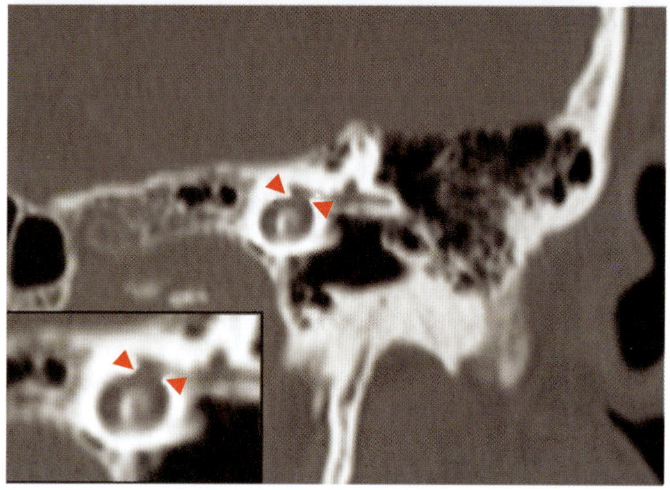

Fig. 28.10: Computed tomography (CT) scan (coronal section) of the left ear. There is merging of the facial canal and cochlea (arrowheads).
Source: Adapted with permission from Blake et al.[7]

SUMMARY

SSCD is the most widely known form of primary inner ear dehiscence. However, there are multiple other types that have been reviewed in this chapter. Careful history and physical examination, in conjunction with audiometric and vestibular testing, can suggest a diagnosis. High-resolution CT scan is mandatory in all patients suspected of inner ear dehiscence and is the gold standard for diagnosis. Management is typically conservative with education and trigger avoidance. In patients with severe and/or poorly controlled symptoms and a surgically amenable dehiscence, surgical intervention is entertained.

SSCD represents the first described of a broad spectrum of inner ear dehiscences that exist. Further thoughtful identification, evaluation, and documentation of these patients will aid in the characterization and management of the gamut of inner ear dehiscence disorders.

VIDEO LEGEND

Video 28.1: Transmastoid superior semicircular canal occlusion.

REFERENCES

1. Agrawal SK, Parnes LS. Transmastoid superior semicircular canal occlusion. Otol Neurotol. 2008;29:363-7.
2. Amoodi HA, Makki FM, McNeil M, et al. Transmastoid resurfacing of superior semicircular canal dehiscence. Laryngoscope. 2011;121:1117-23.
3. Banerjee A, Whyte A, Atlas MD. Superior canal dehiscence: review of a new condition. Clin Otolaryngol. 2005;30:9-15.
4. Beyea JA, Agrawal SK, Parnes LS. Transmastoid semicircular canal occlusion: a safe and highly effective treatment for benign paroxysmal positional vertigo and superior canal dehiscence. Laryngoscope. 2012;122:1862-6.
5. Beyea JA, Parnes LS, Agrawal SK. Superior semicircular canal dehiscence syndrome: evaluation and management. In: Lalwani AK and Pfister MHF (eds), Recent Advances in Otolaryngology: Head and Neck Surgery. New Delhi, India: Jaypee Brothers; 2012.
6. Belden CJ, Weg N, Minor LB, et al. CT evaluation of bone dehiscence of the superior semicircular canal as a cause of sound- and/or pressure-induced vertigo. Radiology. 2003;226:337-43.
7. Blake DM, Tomovic S, Vazquez A, et al. Cochlear-facial dehiscence—a newly described entity. Laryngoscope. 2014;124:283-9.
8. Brantberg K, Bergenius J, Mendel L, et al. Symptoms, findings and treatment in patients with dehiscence of the superior semicircular canal. Acta Otolaryngol. 2001;121:68-75.
9. Brantberg K, Bergenius J, Tribukait A. Vestibular-evoked myogenic potentials in patients with dehiscence of the superior semicircular canal. Acta Otolaryngol. 1999;119:633-40.
10. Carey JP, Migliaccio AA, Minor LB. Semicircular canal function before and after surgery for superior canal dehiscence. Otol Neurotol. 2007;28:356-64.
11. Carey JP, Minor LB, Nager GT. Dehiscence or thinning of bone overlying the superior semicircular canal in a temporal bone survey. Arch Otolaryngol Head Neck Surg. 2000;126:137-47.
12. Chi FL, Ren DD, Dai CF. Variety of audiologic manifestations in patients with superior semicircular canal dehiscence. Otol Neurotol. 2010;31:2-10.
13. Cremer PD, Minor LB, Carey JP, et al. Eye movements in patients with superior canal dehiscence syndrome align with the abnormal canal. Neurology. 2000;55:1833-41.

14. Crane BT, Lin FR, Minor LB, et al. Improvement in autophony symptoms after superior canal dehiscence repair. Otol Neurotol. 2010;31:140-6.
15. Crane BT, Minor LB, Carey JP. Superior canal dehiscence plugging reduces dizziness handicap. Laryngoscope. 2008; 118:1809-13.
16. Eggers SD. Migraine-related vertigo: diagnosis and treatment. Curr Pain Headache Rep. 2007;11:217-26.
17. Fiorino F, Barbieri F, Pizzini FB, et al. A dehiscent superior semicircular canal may be plugged and resurfaced via the transmastoid route. Otol Neurotol. 2010;31:136-9.
18. Friedland DR, Michel MA. Cranial thickness in superior canal dehiscence syndrome: implications for canal resurfacing surgery. Otol Neurotol. 2006;27:346-54.
19. Gopen Q, Zhou G, Poe D, et al. Posterior semicircular canal dehiscence: first reported case series. Otol Neurotol. 2010; 31:339-44.
20. Halmagyi GM, Aw ST, McGarvie LA, et al. Superior semicircular canal dehiscence simulating otosclerosis. J Laryngol Otol. 2003;117:553-7.
21. Karlberg M, Annertz M, Magnusson M. Mondini-like malformation mimicking otosclerosis and superior semicircular canal dehiscence. J Laryngol Otol. 2006;120:419-22.
22. Kim HH, Wilson DF. A third mobile window at the cochlear apex. Otolaryngol Head Neck Surg. 2006;135:965-6.
23. Kim TH, Nam BH, Park CI. Histologic changes of lateral semicircular canal after transection and occlusion with various materials in chinchillas. Korean J Otolaryngol-Head Neck Surg. 2002;45:318-21.
24. Krombach GA, DiMartino E, Schmitz-Rode T, et al. Posterior semicircular canal dehiscence: a morphologic cause of vertigo similar to superior semicircular canal dehiscence. Eur Radiol. 2003;13:1444-50.
25. Li PM, Bergeron C, Monfared A, et al. Superior semicircular canal dehiscence diagnosed after failed stapedotomy for conductive hearing loss. Am J Otolaryngol. 2011;32:441-4.
26. Limb CJ, Carey JP, Srireddy S, et al. Auditory function in patients with surgically treated superior semicircular canal dehiscence. Otol Neurotol. 2006;27:969-80.
27. Lund AD, Palacios SD. Carotid artery-cochlear dehiscence: a review. Laryngoscope. 2011;121:2658-60.
28. Maire R, Duvoisin B. Localization of static positional nystagmus with the ocular fixation test. Laryngoscope. 1999; 109:606-12.
29. McCall AA, Curtin HD, McKenna MJ. Posterior semicircular canal dehiscence arising from temporal bone fibrous dysplasia. Otol Neurotol. 2010;31:1516-7.
30. Mikulec AA, McKenna MJ, Ramsey MJ, et al. Superior semicircular canal dehiscence presenting as conductive hearing loss without vertigo. Otol Neurotol 2004;25:121-9.
31. Mikulec AA, Poe DS. Operative management of a posterior semicircular canal dehiscence. Laryngoscope. 2006; 116:375-8.
32. Minor L.B. Superior canal dehiscence syndrome. Am J Otol 2000;21:9-19.
33. Minor LB. Labyrinthine fistulae: pathobiology and management. Curr Opin Otolaryngol Head Neck Surg. 2003;11:340-6.
34. Minor LB. Clinical manifestations of superior semicircular canal dehiscence. Laryngoscope. 2005;115:1717-27.
35. Minor LB, Carey JP, Cremer PD, et al. Dehiscence of bone overlying the superior canal as a cause of apparent conductive hearing loss. Otol Neurotol. 2003;24:270-8.
36. Minor LB, Cremer PD, Carey JP, et al. Symptoms and signs in superior canal dehiscence syndrome. Ann N Y Acad Sci. 2001;942:259-73.
37. Minor LB, Solomon D, Zinreich JS, Zee DS. Sound- and/or pressure-induced vertigo due to bone dehiscence of the superior semicircular canal. Arch Otolaryngol Head Neck Surg. 1998;124:249-58.
38. Modugno GC, Brandolini C, Cappello I, et al. Bilateral dehiscence of the bony cochlear basal turn. Arch Otolaryngol Head Neck Surg. 2004;130:1427-9.
39. Mong A, Loevner LA, Solomon D, et al. Sound- and pressure-induced vertigo associated with dehiscence of the roof of the superior semicircular canal. AJNR Am J Neuroradiol. 1999;20:1973-5.
40. Nadgir RN, Ozonoff A, Devaiah AK, et al. Superior semicircular canal dehiscence: congenital or acquired condition? AJNR Am J Neuroradiol. 2011;32:947-9.
41. Neyt P, Govaere F, Forton GE. Simultaneous true stapes fixation and bilateral bony dehiscence between the internal carotid artery and the apex of the cochlea: the ultimate pitfall. Otol Neurotol. 2011;32:909-13.
42. Nguyen KD, Welgampola MS, Carey JP. Test-retest reliability and age-related characteristics of the ocular and cervical vestibular evoked myogenic potential tests. Otol Neurotol. 2010;31:793-802.
43. Penninger RT, Tavassolie TS, Carey JP. Cone-beam volumetric tomography for applications in the temporal bone. Otol Neurotol. 2011;32:453-60.
44. Pfammatter A, Darrouzet V, Gartner M, et al. A superior semicircular canal dehiscence syndrome multicenter study: is there an association between size and symptoms? Otol Neurotol. 2010;31:447-54.
45. Poe DS. Diagnosis and management of the patulous eustachian tube. Otol Neurotol. 2007;28:668-77.
46. Röösli C, Hoffmann A, Treumann T, et al. Significance of computed tomography evaluation before revision stapes surgery. HNO. 2008;56:895-900.
47. Shahnaz N, Bork K, Polka L, et al. Energy reflectance and tympanometry in normal and otosclerotic ears. Ear Hear. 2009;30:219-33.
48. Silverstein H, Van Ess MJ. Complete round window niche occlusion for superior semicircular canal dehiscence syndrome: a minimally invasive approach. Ear Nose Throat J. 2009;88:1042-56.

49. Streubel SO, Cremer PD, Carey JP, et al. Vestibular-evoked myogenic potentials in the diagnosis of superior canal dehiscence syndrome. Acta Otolaryngol Suppl. 2001;545:41-9.
50. Teixido M, Seymour PE, Kung B, et al. Transmastoid middle fossa craniotomy repair of superior semicircular canal dehiscence using a soft tissue graft. Otol Neurotol. 2011;32:877-81.
51. Tsunoda A, Terasaki O. Dehiscence of the bony roof of the superior semicircular canal in the middle cranial fossa. J Laryngol Otol. 2002;116:514-8.
52. Vlastarakos PV, Proikas K, Tavoulari E, et al. Efficacy assessment and complications of surgical management for superior semicircular canal dehiscence: a meta-analysis of published interventional studies. Eur Arch Otorhinolaryngol. 2009;266:177-86.
53. Wadin K, Thomander L, Wilbrand H. Effects of a high jugular fossa and jugular bulb diverticulum on the inner ear. A clinical and radiologic investigation. Acta Radiol Diagn (Stockh). 1986;27:629-36.
54. Wang JR, Parnes LS. Superior semicircular canal dehiscence associated with external, middle, and inner ear abnormalities. Laryngoscope. 2010;120:390-3.
55. Watson SRD, Halmagyi GM, Colebatch JG. Vestibular hypersensitivity to sound (Tullio phenomenon): structural and functional assessment. Neurology. 2000;54:722-8.
56. Welgampola MS, Myrie OA, Minor LB, et al. Vestibular-evoked myogenic potential thresholds normalize on plugging superior canal dehiscence. Neurology. 2008;70:464-72.
57. Young RJ, Shatzkes DR, Babb JS, et al. The cochlear-carotid interval: anatomic variation and potential clinical implications. Am J Neuroradiol. 2006;27:1486-90.
58. Zhou G, Gopen Q, Poe DS. Clinical and diagnostic characterization of canal dehiscence syndrome: a great otologic mimicker. Otol Neurotol. 2007;28:920-6.
59. Silverstein H, Kartush JM, Parnes LS, et al. Round window reinforcement for superior semicircular canal dehiscence: a retrospective multi-center case series. Am J Otolaryngol. 2014;35:286-93.

CHAPTER

29

Peripheral Vertigo

Jeffrey T Vrabec, Marc-Elie Nader

INTRODUCTION

Dizziness is a very common complaint in the general population, significantly increasing with advancing age.[1,2] While dizziness is a broad term that encompasses nonvestibular dizziness and disequilibrium, this chapter is concerned with vertigo. Vertigo is defined as the illusion of motion when none is occurring. Patients usually describe a sensation that either they or the environment is spinning. Vertigo has traditionally been classified as being of central or peripheral origin. The clinical history and physical examination findings usually help the clinician differentiate a peripheral vertigo from a central one. Peripheral vertigo can be associated with hearing loss, mild-to-moderate imbalance, unidirectional nystagmus that decreases with fixation, rapid recovery, and rarely other neurologic symptoms. Central vertigo is usually associated with other neurologic symptoms, more severe imbalance, a nystagmus that can change direction, and that does not decrease with fixation and an overall slower recovery.

The lifetime prevalence of peripheral vertigo (assessed by questionnaire) is estimated to be 7.4%.[2] It is associated with significant burden on quality of life, with 70% of patients seeking medical help, 41% being on sick leave, 40% interrupting their daily activities, and 19% avoiding leaving the house.[2] Agrawal et al. examined data from the NHANES survey, in which participants were asked to perform the Romberg test on a compliant foam surface. In this study, 35% of adults over 40 failed the test, implying some vestibular dysfunction.[3] Nonambulatory, obese subjects, and those requiring assistance to stand were excluded, yet the 4-year prevalence was substantial. Age and diabetes were associated with increased prevalence, while gender and race were not statistically significant variables.

Obtaining an adequate clinical history is essential when trying to determine the exact cause of peripheral vertigo. The key elements of the questionnaire include (1) onset and duration of each episode, (2) frequency, (3) associated otologic symptoms (e.g. hearing loss, aural fullness, and tinnitus), (4) precipitating factors (e.g. specific head positions or movements, loud sounds), and (5) previous or concomitant otologic diseases. The differential diagnosis of peripheral vertigo can be categorized according to the duration of the vertigo and the associated otologic symptoms (Table 29.1). The most common causes of peripheral vertigo among those listed are benign paroxysmal positional vertigo (BPPV), vestibular neuritis (VN)/labyrinthitis, Meniere's disease, and third window disorders including superior canal dehiscence syndrome. Disorders covered in other chapters are not reiterated here.

BENIGN PAROXYSMAL POSITIONAL VERTIGO

Background

Though undoubtedly recognized by many earlier physicians, BPPV was initially characterized by Dix and Hallpike in 1952.[4] They outlined the clinical course and diagnostic method using a specific positioning technique. It is considered to be the most common disorder of the peripheral vestibular system, accounting for 40% or more of patients

Table 29.1: Frequent causes of peripheral vertigo

Duration	*Diagnosis*	*Hearing loss*	*Tinnitus*	*Aural fullness*
Seconds	Benign positional paroxysmal vertigo	No	No	No
	Third window disorders	Possible conductive loss	Pulsatile	Yes
Minutes to hours	Meniere's disease	Yes	Yes	Yes
	Vestibulopathy	No	No	No
Hours to days	Vestibular neuronitis	No	No	No
	Labyrinthitis	Yes	Yes	No
	Labyrinthine trauma	Yes	Yes	
	Ototoxicity	Possible, (drug dependent)	Possible	No

with peripheral vertigo.[5] The true prevalence of this disease is difficult to measure accurately because of its self-limiting nature. Because of this, patient series from referral practices will undoubtedly underestimate the true prevalence among all patients with vestibular disorders. BPPV is seen in all age groups, increasing in prevalence with advancing age.[6] It seems to be more common in women, stroke patients, and in association with other vestibular disorders and migraines.[7-10] BPPV is most commonly idiopathic with no specific etiology identified in 50–70% of cases. The two most common causes of secondary BPPVs are head injuries and VN.[11,12] BPPV has also been observed following some surgical procedures such as stapedectomy[11] and cochlear implantation.[13]

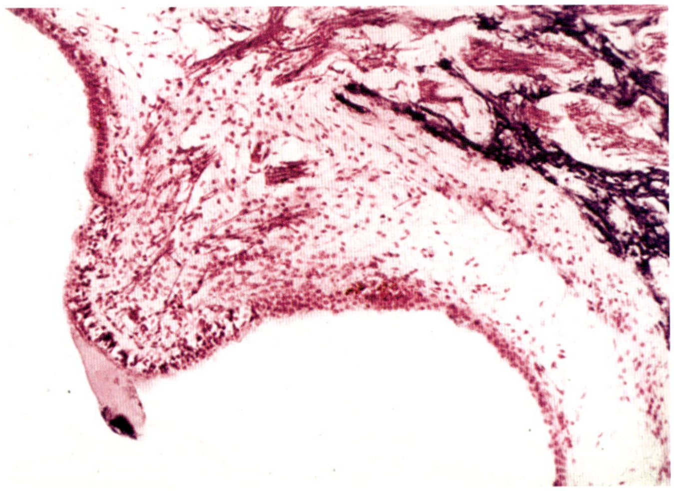

Fig. 29.1: Histopathology slide depicting cupulolithiasis.

Pathogenesis

BPPV involves the posterior semicircular canal in the majority of cases. The most commonly accepted pathophysiologic theory is canalolithiasis, with particles originating from the otolith organs being trapped in the posterior canal. This notion is supported by the characteristics of the nystagmus elicited during an episode of BPPV and by findings of free-floating particles in the endolymph of patients undergoing posterior canal surgery for recalcitrant BPPV.[14] Another mechanism of BPPV that was previously proposed by Schuknecht and termed cupulolithiasis involves loose otoconia that get deposited on the cupula causing its deflection (Fig. 29.1).[15]

Clinical Findings

The typical features of the nystagmus observed in posterior canal BPPVs are best explained by canalolithiasis: (1) the latency of the nystagmus is consistent with the time required for gravity to initiate the movement of the particles in the endolymph, (2) the short duration of the nystagmus represents the time required for the debris to reach the lowest portion of the canal, (3) the reversal of the nystagmus observed when the patient sits up can be explained by movement of the endolymph flow in the opposite direction, (4) fatigability of the nystagmus upon repeated stimulating head movements may be due to dispersion of the debris within the canal, and (5) the direction and torsional features of the nystagmus can be explained physiologically.

In the head-hanging position with the head hyperextended and turned 45° toward the side of the lesion, the canaloliths trapped in the posterior canal move away from the cupula causing an ampullofugal flow of endolymph. The resulting deflection of the cupula produces an excitatory stimulation of the posterior canal. The ipsilateral superior oblique muscle is activated causing depression and intorsion of the ocular globe, which corresponds to the slow phase of the nystagmus. The clinician then observes the fast component of the nystagmus in the opposite direction with elevation and extortion of the globe. In other terms, the nystagmus is seen to be upbeating and geotropic (toward the ground).

The horizontal semicircular canal is less commonly involved, and studies report that horizontal canal BPPV accounts for 5–10% of cases.[16-18] In horizontal canal canalolithiasis, the particles are more often found in the long arm of the canal away from the cupula. When the patient turns his head toward the side of the lesion, an ampulopetal flow of endolymph occurs, producing an excitatory stimulation of the lateral canal. The ipsilateral medial rectus muscle is activated and produces adduction of the ocular globe. The clinician observes the fast component of the horizontal nystagmus in the opposite direction toward the affected ear and the nystagmus is viewed as geotropic. When the patient turns his head to the contralateral side, inhibition of the involved horizontal canal occurs and the nystagmus is in the opposite direction. This nystagmus is still geotropic. However, it is weaker compared to the one caused by movement of the head toward the side of the lesion, helping the physician determine which side is affected.

In horizontal canal cupulolithiasis, with the head turned toward the affected side, cupular deflection produces inhibition of the lateral canal and a corresponding ageotropic nystagmus is observed. When the head is turned to the opposite direction, activation of the canal results in a stronger ageotropic nystagmus.

Evaluation

Diagnosis of BPPV is based on the suggestive clinical history and characteristic findings on physical examination. The history usually recounts episodes of vertigo elicited by specific head movements. These include rolling over in bed, lying down, extending the neck, and bending over. The side of the lesion can often be identified by the patient. The duration of the vertigo is typically less than a minute, although many patients experience dizziness, disequilibrium, and nausea lasting several minutes or hours after an attack. The episodes tend to occur in clusters over several weeks and can recur frequently.

Idiopathic BPPV is not associated with other otologic or neurologic symptoms. However, the clinician should include in his questionnaire the pertinent symptoms associated with pathologies that may predispose to BPPV, such as VN, head trauma, Meniere's disease, and migraine.

The physical examination should include the Dix–Hallpike maneuver. This diagnostic procedure is performed by having the patient first seated with the head turned 45° toward the side to be tested. The clinician then quickly brings down the head of the patient ideally 30° below the level of the table. After a variable latency period of several seconds, nystagmus can be observed that lasts less than a minute. The patient is brought back up and the eyes are examined for reversal of the nystagmus. These steps allow evaluation of the ipsilateral posterior semicircular canal, and the nystagmus observed will be upbeating and geotropic as described previously. Superior canal BPPV is a much rarer pathology occurring only in 1–3% of patients with BPPV.[17,19] Since the superior canal lies in the same plane as the posterior canal of the contralateral side, the Dix–Hallpike maneuver can also be used to test for superior canal BPPV. However, the maneuver done on one side evaluates the contralateral superior canal and the nystagmus is downbeating and ageotropic.

A modification of the Dix–Hallpike procedure can be used to test for horizontal canal BPPV. The patient lies in the supine position with the neck flexed 30°. The head is turned toward one side and the eyes are observed for a horizontal nystagmus. The head is then turned toward the contralateral side. The direction of the nystagmus (geotropic or ageotropic) and its intensity allow the clinician determine which horizontal canal is affected and the probable underlying pathophysiology as discussed previously.

Evaluation: Additional Studies

BPPV is not associated with hearing loss or other otologic or neurologic symptoms. Clinical practice guidelines published by the AAO-HNS emphasize the diagnostic utility of the physical examination and discourage the use of imaging and ENG, while offering no recommendation on routine audiometry for routine cases.[20] If the history and neurotological examination detect atypical features or clinical findings, then additional testing is pursued as appropriate.

Treatment: Medical

The primary treatment of BPPV consists of noninvasive physical maneuvers. They rely on gravity to displace particles trapped in the semicircular canal back into the utricle. Medication can be given prior to initiating these therapies to minimize nausea and dizziness in patients who are particularly susceptible to these symptoms. However, medication by itself was not found to be a successful treatment option for BPPV and routine use is discouraged. [20,21]

The particle repositioning technique was developed by Epley in 1992 for posterior canal canalolithiasis (Fig. 29.2).[22] This maneuver is started in the Dix–Hallpike position with the head turned toward the affected canal. After the nystagmus stops, the head is turned 90° and the eyes are observed for a secondary nystagmus that reflects movement of the particles within the canal away from the cupula. Once the nystagmus subsides, the head is turned another 90°. The patient rolls onto his side until he is facing down. Afterwards, the patient sits back in the upright position.

The Semont liberatory maneuver is an alternative therapeutic option to treat posterior canal cupulolithiasis (Fig. 29.3).[23] The patient starts in the sitting position

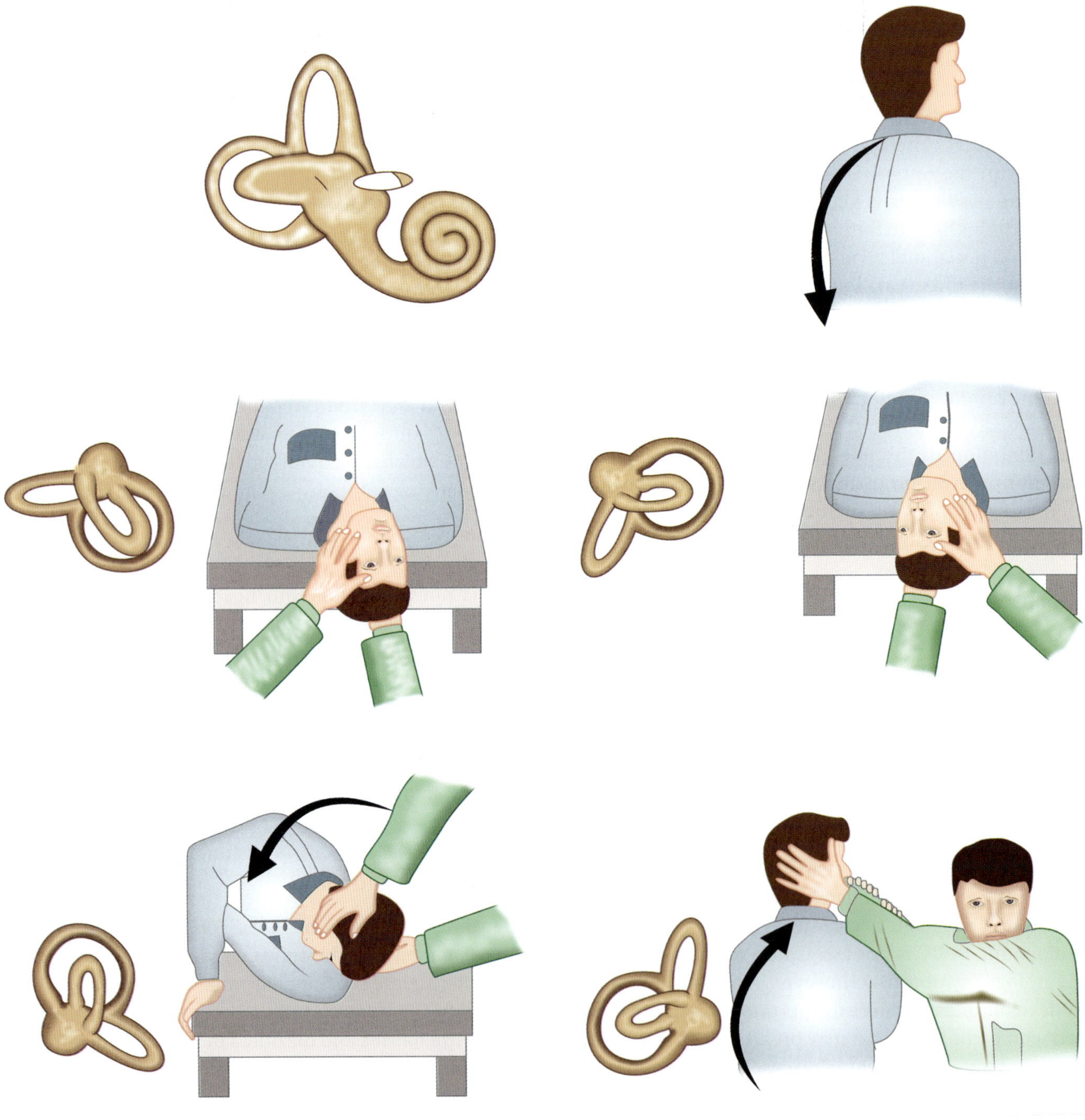

Fig. 29.2: Epley maneuver.

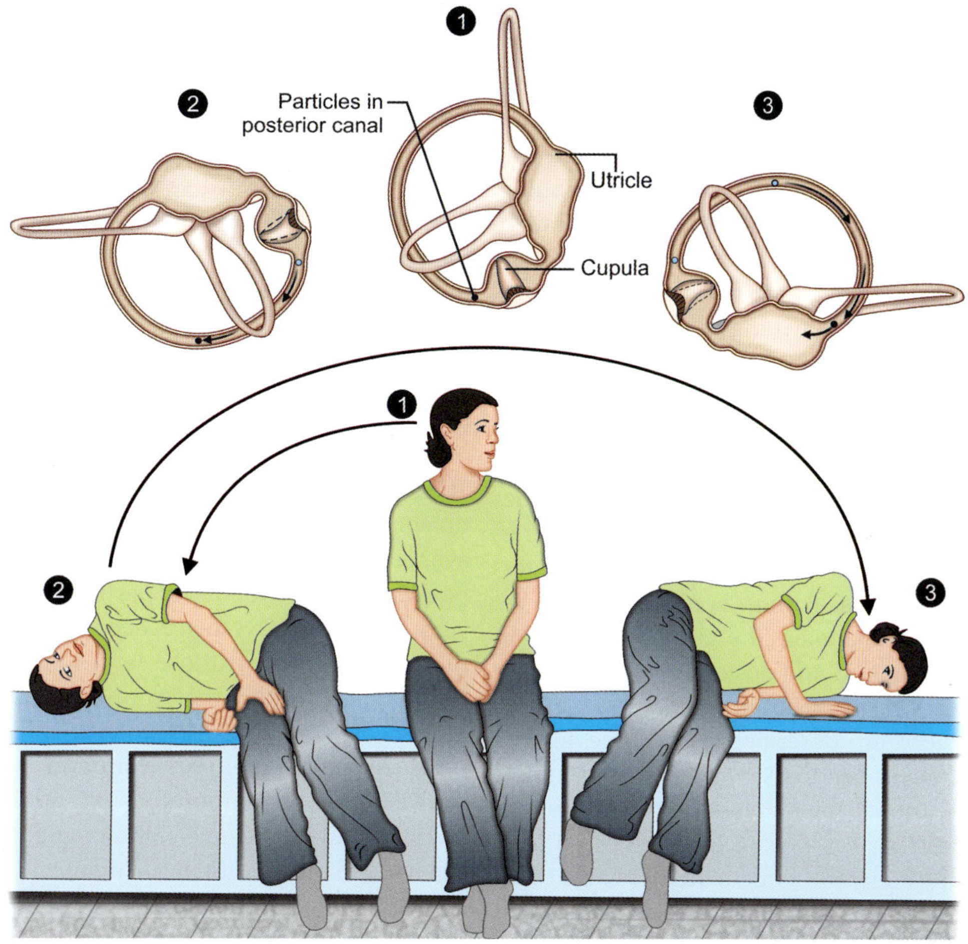

Fig. 29.3: Semont maneuver.

with the head turned away from the affected canal. The patient is rapidly brought backward to the lying position on the affected side and remains in that position for several minutes. Without turning the head, the patient is then rapidly moved to the opposite side lying face down. After several minutes, the patient sits up slowly. Patients can be easily taught this technique and can perform it at home as needed for recurrence. However, this maneuver is less easily employed in obese or elderly patients with limited mobility.

Particle repositioning maneuvers have also been developed for lateral canal BPPV. The barrel roll initially described by Epley[24] consists in having the patient roll 360° starting with the head turned toward the affected canal. The patient turns the whole body 90° at a time away from the affected side until a full turn is achieved and the patient is back in the supine position.

Studies comparing particle repositioning techniques find both are highly effective, with no significant difference in outcomes.[16] Success rates of >80% are seen with single treatment approaches.[25] Further improvement in outcomes is seen with repetition of maneuvers. While most studies have been conducted by physicians or therapists providing supervised performance of the maneuvers, it is likely that high rates of success can be achieved by self-taught techniques. In the digital age, it is easy to locate instructional videos demonstrating the Dix-Hallpike test and the particle repositioning techniques.

Treatment: Surgical

Given the ease of particle repositioning, it is difficult to define a surgical candidate. Our practice emphasizes repetitive particle repositioning that continues until resolution is documented. The risk of repetitive particle repositioning is extremely low; the technique is noninvasive and economical. While recurrences are expected intermittently, the burden of disease must be great and the response to particle repositioning very poor to consider offering surgical intervention. Using this algorithm, surgical candidates in the authors' practice represent less than 1:1000 BPPV cases.

Surgical intervention for BPPV initially focused on deafferentation. This can be accomplished by vestibular neurectomy, though complete loss of ipsilateral vestibular function is an extreme approach for isolated dysfunction of the posterior canal. The need for selective neurectomy necessitated a technique for dividing the singular nerve. A transcanal approach was described by Gacek in the early 1970s, while others approached the nerve via middle or posterior fossa craniotomy with medial sectioning in the IAC.[26]

Singular neurectomy is technically challenging as the nerve must be divided on its lateral aspect, medial to the round window, and anterior to the ampulla of the posterior canal. In this anatomically narrow region, the nerve measures <0.5 mm in diameter. The close proximity of the basal turn of the cochlea and posterior canal ampulla place these structures at risk of surgical injury.[27]

Results of surgery are described as positive in the majority of cases. Gacek reports 97% success in a series of 252 procedures, though documentation of resolution with Dix-Hallpike testing was inconsistently reported. The length of follow-up (if any for some patients) is also not stated, and it is uncertain if the results are as durable as claimed. Questions arise due to the difficulty in performing and confirming sectioning of the nerve intraoperatively. Other series are not as successful as Gacek, though postoperative assessment is also more critical.[28] The rate of sensorineural hearing loss is at least 4%, though again, documentation is poor. It is interesting that Gacek reports significant hearing loss in 4 of the last 55 cases, yet claimed this occurred in only 5 of the first 197 cases.

A more practical and reproducible surgical solution for intractable BPPV is posterior semicircular canal occlusion. First described by Parnes and McClure, the goal of surgery is to occlude the canal preventing fluid movement.[29] The occluded canal is rendered insensitive to angular movement or gravity, while other labyrinthine structures are preserved. Canal occlusion has been used as an adjunct to central skull base approaches and for the treatment of superior canal dehiscence syndrome, therefore it is familiar to neurotologists. A transmastoid approach is used to skeletonize the posterior semicircular canal. Controlled fenestration of the canal is performed and the canal is occluded with bone pate (Figs. 29.4A to D). Long-term sustained elimination of BPPV is reported in over 90% of patients.[30-32] Transient hearing loss and dizziness is seen in the early postoperative period. Persistent disequilibrium is rare. The hearing loss is more severe at higher frequencies but typically recovers within 6 weeks. Permanent high frequency hearing loss can occur. Severe sensorineural hearing loss occurs in < 5% of cases. Postoperative reduction in caloric response in the operated ear is not uncommon suggesting that a mild labyrinthitis may develop in these cases. Since the technique is similar to that described in superior canal dehiscence, the complication profile is expected to be similar.

Prognosis

The natural history of BPPV includes a high rate of spontaneous resolution. The mean duration of symptoms averages <2 weeks.[2] Those seeking medical attention can be successfully treated with particle-repositioning maneuvers with success rates exceeding 95% if repeated up to three times, even those with long-standing BPPV.[16,23] Additional treatment may continue until full resolution is documented.

Recurrences are very common with an incidence of 16% in the first 6 months. With additional duration of follow-up, the incidence will increase. Recurrent BPPV is expected to respond to particle repositioning with similar success rates as described for primary episodes.

VESTIBULAR NEURITIS

Background

Vestibular neuritis is probably the third most common cause of peripheral vertigo, after BPPV and Meniere's disease. Among patients presenting to an outpatient clinic for vertigo and dizziness, VN accounted for 8.1% of the diagnoses.[33] VN is an acute inflammatory disorder of the vestibular nerve characterized by vertigo, nausea, and vomiting. The onset is very rapid and the vertigo is not associated with other otologic or neurologic symptoms. Other terms have been used interchangeably with VN that may have rendered the older medical literature more confusing, including vestibular neuronitis, epidemic vertigo, and vestibular paralysis.

Pathogenesis

The exact etiology and underlying pathophysiology of VN have not been completely elucidated. Clinical symptoms and histopathology implicate isolated involvement of the

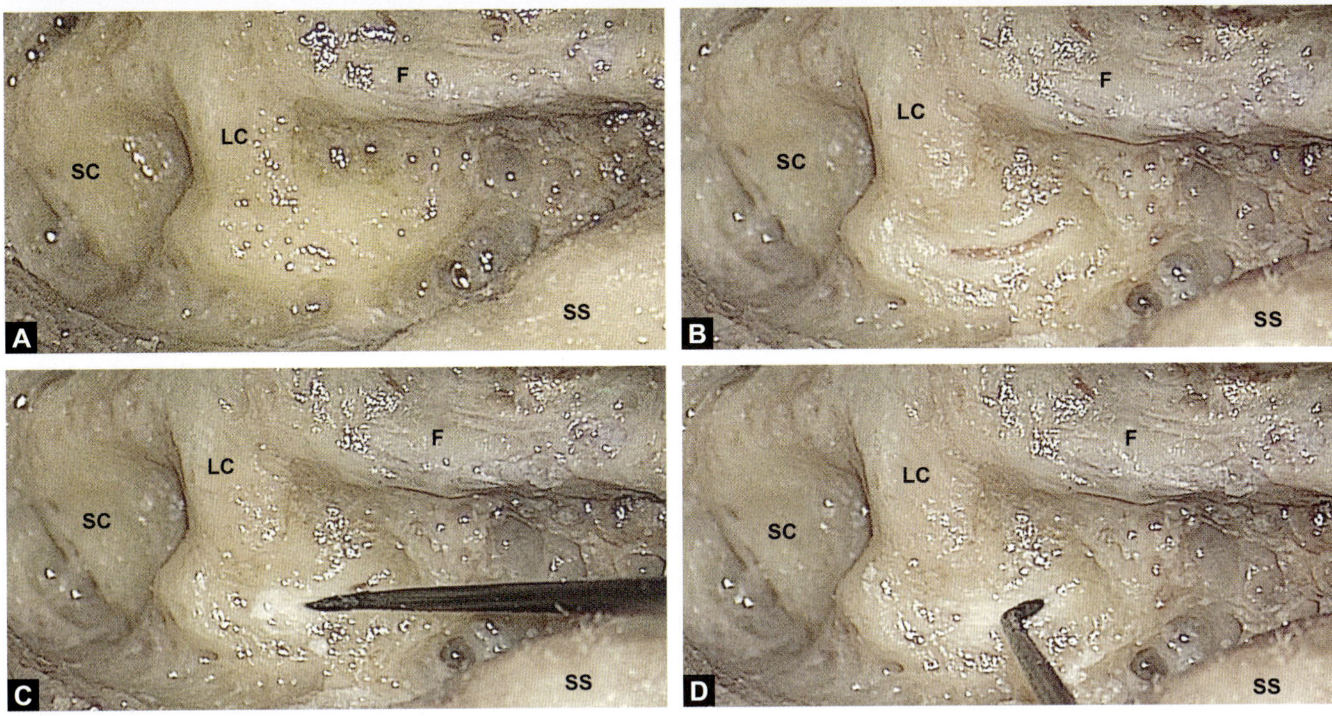

Figs. 29.4A to D: Posterior semicircular canal occlusion for intractable benign paroxysmal positional vertigo (BPPV) through a transmastoid approach. (F, facial nerve; LC, lateral semicircular canal; SC, superior semicircular canal, SS, sigmoid sinus).

vestibular nerve. Temporal bone specimens show atrophy within the vestibular ganglion and preservation of the end organs and sensory epithelium. There is no vascular pathology to implicate an ischemic phenomenon. Histopathological findings are similar to that seen in herpes zoster oticus, suggesting a viral etiology.[34] Supporting evidence includes the frequent isolation of viral DNA from the vestibular ganglion in autopsy series.[35-37] Both herpes simplex virus type 1 (HSV-1) and varicella zoster virus are observed, though the quantity of virus is highly variable.[38] In addition, an animal model of acute, reversible vestibular dysfunction after inoculation of HSV in the middle ear has been described.[39] VN most commonly affects the superior vestibular nerve with or without involvement of the inferior vestibular nerve. Three-dimensional recordings of the spontaneous nystagmus and vestibulo-ocular reflex (VOR) showed sparing of the posterior semicircular canal in 21 of 29 patients with VN.[40] The utricular and saccular function may be impaired in patients with VN, and recording ocular and cervical vestibular evoked myogenic potentials (VEMP) has been proposed as a mean to determine which division(s) of the vestibular nerve is/are affected.[41] The reason for preferential involvement of the superior division of the vestibular nerve is unclear. Among the possible explanations are greater susceptibility to viral invasion of the ganglion via vestibulofacial anastomoses and anatomic differences of the cribrose region leaving it more susceptible to injury due to entrapment and ischemia.[42]

Clinical Findings

The patient affected by VN usually suffers an initial acute episode of sudden rotational vertigo associated with nausea and vomiting. The vertigo is independent of the head position and usually lasts several hours to days. The symptoms are exacerbated by head movements, and their intensity is such that the patient usually prefers to stay still in the supine position. The vertigo subsides in a predictable manner, though associated disequilibrium is more variable. It may last for several months depending on amount of vestibular function impairment, activity, and associated deficits including vision, proprioception, and extremity strength.

Evaluation: Physical Examination

If the patient is seen during an acute episode of VN, the clinician can observe a horizontal rotary nystagmus toward the unaffected side that may be suppressed with fixation. The intensity of the nystagmus correlates with the degree of vestibular dysfunction and decreases over time due to recovery of vestibular function, central compensation, or both. Within a few days, spontaneous nystagmus may not be observed, though gaze nystagmus in the direction of the fast phase may persist. Late findings include nystagmus after head shaking or a pathologic head thrust test, with corrective saccades observed when the head is briskly turned toward the affected side. Some patients also may develop a positive Dix–Hallpike test due to secondary BPPV.

Evaluation: Physiologic Tests

Electronystagmography can document reduced caloric responses on the affected side in the acute phase. However, this finding may be absent in cases involving only the inferior division of the vestibular nerve. Thus, combining caloric testing with VEMP testing may better determine which division of the vestibular nerve is affected. The superior vestibular nerve innervates the utricle and anterosuperior part of the saccule while the inferior division innervates the posteroinferior part of the saccule. Ocular VEMPs (oVEMPs) reflect the function of the utricle and cervical VEMPs (cVEMPs) the function of the saccule. Therefore, the pattern of changes in oVEMPs and cVEMPs can help classify VN as involving the superior division only (reduced oVEMPs, intact cVEMPs), the inferior division only (reduced cVEMPs, intact oVEMPs) or both divisions (both cVEMPs and oVEMPs reduced). However, some clinicians argue that this distinction is not clinically relevant, especially since a small percentage of cases involve only the inferior vestibular nerve.

Evaluation: Radiographic Tests

Magnetic resonance imaging (MRI) with gadolinium rarely shows enhancement of the eighth nerve in VN.[43] If hearing loss or atypical neurologic findings are present, MRI should be ordered to exclude intracranial lesions.

Treatment: Medical

The medical treatment of VN involves (1) symptomatic relief during the initial acute episode of vertigo, (2) vestibular exercises to promote central compensation, (3) particle-repositioning maneuvers to treat secondary BPPV, and (4) possible treatment of the underlying pathophysiologic cause. Initially, vestibular suppressants, benzodiazepines, and antiemetics can help control the symptoms of vertigo, nausea, and vomiting. Vestibular suppressants should be tapered as soon as possible to avoid compromising central compensation. Inpatient admission should be considered for patients presenting with severe vomiting and dehydration. Patients should start vestibular exercises that reinforce the VOR as soon as possible to promote central compensation. Secondary BPPV is successfully managed with particle-repositioning maneuvers as noted earlier. Untreated BPPV may be an impediment to performing adequately the vestibular exercises, and its resolution is essential to allow maximal central compensation.

The hypothesis of latent viral reactivation as the etiology of VN opens the door to therapies aimed at the underlying causes of vestibular dysfunction, namely viral replication and neural edema. To date, only one study evaluated the role of antiviral agents in the management of VN. Strupp et al. determined that valacyclovir did not result in improved outcomes when used alone compared to placebo and did not act synergistically with methylprednisolone when used in combination.[44] Several studies have investigated the role of corticosteroids in the management of VN.[44-49] Some of these papers showed faster improvement in symptoms at short-term[46,47] and long-term follow-up,[47] and improved recovery of peripheral vestibular function at long-term follow-up.[44,49] However, Shupak et al. recently reported no differences in occurrence of symptoms or Dizziness Handicap Inventory scores in patients treated with prednisone compared to placebo despite an earlier recovery of the peripheral vestibular function on ENG.[45] Overall, these studies present important limitations in their design, including a small sample size and high risk of bias. Because of these studies' limitations and their conflicting results, recommendations for the use of corticosteroids in VN cannot be firmly supported by the current literature.

Surgical management of persistent symptoms is described. The indications for surgery are not clear and presume that persisting labyrinthine asymmetry as a result of neural degeneration is responsible for ongoing symptoms of vertigo or disequilibrium. There is not a reliable method for determining what symptoms are due to labyrinthine dysfunction and which are due to incomplete central compensation. Results of vestibular neurectomy for VN are less favorable than in Meniere's disease, and persisting labyrinthine dysfunction is more likely.[50]

Prognosis

Vestibutar neuritis is a benign, self-limited disease that has a good prognosis. The general rule is complete recovery of balance with resolution of disequilibrium after a variable amount of time. Patients may show persisting sensitivity to rapid head movements toward the affected side if vestibular function does not recover. Recurrence of vertigo may occur in 2–11% of patients, although it is usually less intense than during the initial attack.[51,52] Secondary BPPV may develop in up to 15% of patients with VN, and it is treated with particle repositioning maneuvers.[52]

LABYRINTHITIS

Pathogenesis

The term labyrinthitis is defined as an inflammation or infection of the cochlea and vestibular organs. All types of infectious organisms entering the inner ear can induce a significant inflammatory response, as there are case reports of labyrinthitis due to many different viruses, bacteria, and fungi. Theoretical routes of entry to the labyrinth include the round and oval windows, cochlear aqueduct, internal auditory canal and defects in the bony labyrinth secondary to cholesteatoma, trauma, or surgery as well as via hematogenous spread. Infectious spread from the middle ear is termed otogenic, while spread from intracranial infections is deemed meningogenic.

The degree of labyrinthine injury is determined by the complex interaction of the infecting organism, treatment rendered, and host defenses. In general, it is not possible to identify the pathogen based on degree of hearing loss or severity of vertigo. Other clinical findings (rash, middle ear effusion, meningeal signs) are suggestive, though definitive identification rests with specific culture or genetic data. Bilateral labyrinthine involvement usually suggests a meningogenic etiology, while a unilateral dysfunction suggests an otogenic origin.

Histologically, labyrinthitis has been classified as serous or suppurative. This cannot be defined clinically or radiographically, making it more of an academic distinction. In a series of temporal bones from individuals succumbing to bacterial meningitis, both types of changes are seen.[53] In cases of suppurative labyrinthitis, inflammatory cells are seen exclusively in the perilymph, are always seen in the cochlea, but are seen in the vestibular system in only 50% of cases. In contrast, cases of eosinophilic staining (traditionally referred to as serous labyrinthitis) display an inflammatory response predominantly within the superior and posterior canals, show equal involvement of endolymph and perilymph spaces, and have cochlear involvement in only 40% of cases. Seventeen percent of the temporal bones from individuals with bacterial meningitis did not show any inflammatory response.[53] Within this series, the inflammatory response observed was not uniform for a given infecting organism, and can even differ in temporal bones from the same individual. The likely route of entry to the labyrinth was the cochlear modiolus, as inflammatory changes in this area strongly correlated with the presence of suppurative infection, while patency of the cochlear aqueduct was not as specific.[53]

Histological findings in viral labyrinthitis are less commonly described.[54-57] The paucity of specimens is attributable to the rarity of fatal infections, difficulty in establishing a definitive diagnosis, and reduction in disease prevalence due to widespread immunization for measles, mumps, and rubella. Some features of the histopathology in viral disease include both distension and collapse of endolymph spaces and involvement of the stria vascularis, neither of which was observed by Merchant and Gopen in cases of bacterial infection.[53]

A late feature of labyrinthitis is fibrosis, termed labyrinthitis ossificans (LO). A severe inflammatory response, usually due to bacterial infection, is necessary to induce the fibrosis. LO occurs in up to 60% of cases of deafness due to meningitis and any of the common meningogenic bacteria are capable of inducing labyrinthine fibrosis.[58] The basal turn of the scala tympani is most commonly involved, independent of the source of the infection.[59] Scala vestibuli involvement is less common allowing an alternative route for cochlear implant placement when the scala tympani is blocked.[16] The onset of fibrosis in the inner ear was seen as early as 3 days after intrathecal infection in an animal model for meningogeniclabyrinthitis.[60] This finding emphasizes the importance of early cochlear implantation in patients with profound hearing loss secondary to meningitis.

Clinical Findings

Labyrinthitis is characterized by vestibular symptoms similar to those seen in VN, but including a variable degree of hearing loss. The vertigo and disequilibrium also follow a similar pattern of gradual improvement over days to weeks. Persisting disequilibrium would be expected in some cases, though the incidence is not well defined, and is probably organism specific. The hearing loss may be limited and transient in mild cases of labyrinthitis. More virulent infections, treatment delay, and altered host immune response may contribute to a profound hearing loss.

Evaluation

Clinical vestibular findings will be similar to those described for VN. The physical examination may provide significant information regarding the etiology of the infection specifically, examination of the middle ear and assessment for signs of meningismus. Myringotomy with culture of a middle ear effusion or assay of the cerebrospinal fluid is important for identification of the responsible pathogen. Audiometric evaluation is necessary to document severity of hearing loss and planning of auditory rehabilitation including the potential need for cochlear implantation.

Evaluation: Radiographic Tests

High-resolution computed tomography (HRCT) and MRI can be useful in the radiographic evaluation of labyrinthitis. Acutely, labyrinthitis is often hemorrhagic and a high-intensity signal can be seen on unenhanced T1-weighted images. Enhancement with contrast may occur, though this resolves with time. If fibrosis develops, the T2 signal will diminish. Dense ossification within the labyrinth is well seen on CT, though areas of fibrosis are indistinct. The observation of ossification increases with time following the onset of deafness due to meningitis.[61]

Treatment: Medical

As with VN, vestibular suppressants and antiemetics can provide symptomatic relief during the acute attack of vertigo. After the initial episode subsides, vestibular rehabilitation promotes central compensation and allows faster recovery of balance. Parenteral antibiotics are indicated in patients with bacterial labyrinthitis. Steroids seem to have a role independent of the actual pathogen due to a nonspecific anti-inflammatory effect. Recent studies have shown protective effects of systemic steroids on auditory function in animal models of pneumococcal meningitis.[62,63] Steroids also seem to prevent the development of LO in patients with meningogeniclabyrinthitis.[64]

Prognosis

Recovery of hearing is dependent on the severity of the hearing loss, infecting organism, and treatment given. Vestibular hypofunction is more likely to be permanent than in VN. Central compensation will ameliorate the disequilibrium.

*References with asterisks refer to critical sources.

REFERENCES

1. Furman JM, Raz Y, Whitney SL. Geriatric vestibulopathy assessment and management. Curr Opin Otolaryngol Head Neck Surg. 2010;18(5):386-91.
2. Neuhauser HK, Radtke A, von Brevern M, et al. Burden of dizziness and vertigo in the community. Arch Intern Med. 2008;168(19):2118-24.
3. Agrawal Y, Carey JP, Della Santina CC, et al. Disorders of balance and vestibular function in US adults: data from the National Health and Nutrition Examination Survey, 2001-2004. Arch Intern Med. 2009;169 (10):938-44. (*)
4. Dix MR, Hallpike CS. The pathology, symptomatology and diagnosis of certain common disorders of the vestibular system. Ann Otol Rhinol Laryngol. 1952;61(4):987-1016.
5. Nedzelski JM, Barber HO, McIlmoyl L. Diagnoses in a dizziness unit. J Otolaryngol. 1986;15(2):101-4.
6. von Brevern M, Radtke A, Lezius F, et al. Epidemiology of benign paroxysmal positional vertigo: a population based study. J Neurol Neurosurg Psychiatry. 2007;78(7):710-5.
7. Lee NH, Ban JH, Lee KC, et al. Benign paroxysmal positional vertigo secondary to inner ear disease. Otolaryngol Head Neck Surg. 2010;143(3):413-7.
8. Lempert T, Leopold M, von Brevern M, et al. Migraine and benign positional vertigo. Ann Otol Rhinol Laryngol. 2000;109(12 Pt 1):1176.
9. Gross EM, Ress BD, Viirre ES, et al. Intractable benign paroxysmal positional vertigo in patients with Meniere's disease. Laryngoscope. 2000;110(4):655-9.
10. Ishiyama A, Jacobson KM, Baloh RW. Migraine and benign positional vertigo. Ann Otol Rhinol Laryngol. 2000;109(4):377-80.
11. Baloh RW, Honrubia V, Jacobson K. Benign positional vertigo: clinical and oculographic features in 240 cases. Neurology. 1987;37(3):371-8. (*)
12. Katsarkas A. Benign paroxysmal positional vertigo (BPPV): idiopathic versus post-traumatic. Acta Otolaryngol. 1999; 119(7):745-9.
13. Viccaro M, Mancini P, La Gamma R, et al. Positional vertigo and cochlear implantation. Otol Neurotol. 2007;28(6): 764-7.
14. Agrawal SK, Parnes LS. Human experience with canal plugging. Ann N Y Acad Sci. 2001;942:300-5.
15. Schuknecht HF. Cupulolithiasis. Arch Otolaryngol. 1969;90 (6):765-78.
16. Steenerson RL, Cronin GW, Marbach PM. Effectiveness of treatment techniques in 923 cases of benign paroxysmal positional vertigo. Laryngoscope. 2005;115(2):226-31.
17. Fife TD. Recognition and management of horizontal canal benign positional vertigo. Am J Otol. 1998;19(3):345-51.
18. Korres S, Balatsouras DG, Kaberos A, et al. Occurrence of semicircular canal involvement in benign paroxysmal positional vertigo. Otol Neurotol. 2002;23(6):926-32.
19. Honrubia V, Baloh RW, Harris MR, et al. Paroxysmal positional vertigo syndrome. Am J Otol. 1999;20(4):465-70.

20. Bhattacharyya N, Baugh RF, Orvidas L, et al. Clinical practice guideline: benign paroxysmal positional vertigo. Otolaryngol Head Neck Surg. 2008;139(5 Suppl 4):S47-81.
21. McClure JA, Willett JM. Lorazepam and diazepam in the treatment of benign paroxysmal vertigo. J Otolaryngol. 1980;9(6):472-7.
22. Epley JM. The canalith repositioning procedure: for treatment of benign paroxysmal positional vertigo. Otolaryngol Head Neck Surg. 1992;107(3):399-404.
23. Semont A, Freyss G, Vitte E. Curing the BPPV with a liberatory maneuver. Adv Otorhinolaryngol. 1988;42:290-3.
24. Epley JM. Positional vertigo related to semicircular canalithiasis. Otolaryngol Head Neck Surg. 1995;112(1):154-61.
25. Herdman SJ, Tusa RJ, Zee DS, et al. Single treatment approaches to benign paroxysmal positional vertigo. Arch Otolaryngol Head Neck Surg. 1993;119(4):450-4. (*)
26. Gacek RR. Transection of the posterior ampullary nerve for the relief of benign paroxysmal positional vertigo. Ann Otol Rhinol Laryngol. 1974;83(5):596-605.
27. Ohmichi T, Rutka J, Hawke M. Histopathologic consequences of surgical approaches to the singular nerve. Laryngoscope. 1989;99(9):963-70.
28. Silverstein H, Wanamaker H, Flanzer J, et al. Vestibular neurectomy in the United States--1990. Am J Otol. 1992;13(1):23-30.
29. Parnes LS, McClure JA. Posterior semicircular canal occlusion for intractable benign paroxysmal positional vertigo. Ann Otol Rhinol Laryngol. 1990;99(5 Pt 1):330-4.
30. Shaia WT, Zappia JJ, Bojrab DI, et al. Success of posterior semicircular canal occlusion and application of the dizziness handicap inventory. Otolaryngol Head Neck Surg. 2006;134(3):424-30.
31. Beyea JA, Agrawal SK, Parnes LS. Transmastoid semicircular canal occlusion: a safe and highly effective treatment for benign paroxysmal positional vertigo and superior canal dehiscence. Laryngoscope. 2012;122(8):1862-6. (*)
32. Kisilevsky V, Bailie NA, Dutt SN, et al. Lessons learned from the surgical management of benign paroxysmal positional vertigo: the University Health Network experience with posterior semicircular canal occlusion surgery (1988-2006). J Otolaryngol Head Neck Surg. 2009;38(2):212-21.
33. Strupp M, Brandt T. Vestibular neuritis. Semin Neurol. 2009;29(5):509-19. (*)
34. Schuknecht HF, Kitamura K. Second Louis H. Clerf Lecture. Vestibular neuritis. Ann Otol Rhinol Laryngol Suppl. 1981;90(1 Pt 2):1-19.
35. Furuta Y, Takasu T, Fukuda S, et al. Latent herpes simplex virus type 1 in human vestibular ganglia. Acta Otolaryngol Suppl. 1993;503:85-9.
36. Arbusow V, Schulz P, Strupp M, et al. Distribution of herpes simplex virus type 1 in human geniculate and vestibular ganglia: implications for vestibular neuritis. Ann Neurol. 1999;46(3):416-9.
37. Vrabec JT, Payne DA. Prevalence of herpes viruses in cranial nerve ganglia. Acta Otolaryngol. 2001;121(7):831-5.
38. Vrabec JT, Alford RL. Quantitative analysis of herpes simplex virus in cranial nerve ganglia. J Neurovirol. 2004;10(4):216-22. (*)
39. Esaki S, Goshima F, Kimura H, et al. Auditory and vestibular defects induced by experimental labyrinthitis following herpes simplex virus in mice. Acta Otolaryngol. 2011;131(7):684-91.
40. Aw ST, Fetter M, Cremer PD, et al. Individual semicircular canal function in superior and inferior vestibular neuritis. Neurology. 2001;57(5):768-74.
41. Govender S, Colebatch JG. Ocular vestibular evoked myogenic potential (oVEMP) responses in acute vestibular neuritis. Clin Neurophysiol. 2012;123(5):1054-5; author reply 5-6; discussion 6-7.
42. Gianoli G, Goebel J, Mowry S, et al. Anatomic differences in the lateral vestibular nerve channels and their implications in vestibular neuritis. Otol Neurotol. 2005;26(3):489-94.
43. Karlberg M, Annertz M, Magnusson M. Acute vestibular neuritis visualized by 3-T magnetic resonance imaging with high-dose gadolinium. Arch Otolaryngol Head Neck Surg. 2004;130(2):229-32.
44. Strupp M, Zingler VC, Arbusow V, et al. Methylprednisolone, valacyclovir, or the combination for vestibular neuritis. N Engl J Med. 2004;351(4):354-61.
45. Shupak A, Issa A, Golz A, et al. Prednisone treatment for vestibular neuritis. Otol Neurotol. 2008;29(3):368-74.
46. Ariyasu L, Byl FM, Sprague MS, et al. The beneficial effect of methylprednisolone in acute vestibular vertigo. Arch Otolaryngol Head Neck Surg. 1990;116(6):700-3.
47. Kitahara T, Kondoh K, Morihana T, et al. Steroid effects on vestibular compensation in human. Neurol Res. 2003;25(3):287-91.
48. Ohbayashi S, Oda M, Yamamoto M, et al. Recovery of the vestibular function after vestibular neuronitis. Acta Otolaryngol Suppl. 1993;503:31-4.
49. Karlberg ML, Magnusson M. Treatment of acute vestibular neuronitis with glucocorticoids. Otol Neurotol. 2011;32(7):1140-3.
50. Silverstein H, White DW. Wide surgical exposure for singular neurectomy in the treatment of benign positional vertigo. Laryngoscope. 1990;100(7):701-6.
51. Huppert D, Strupp M, Theil D, et al. Low recurrence rate of vestibular neuritis: a long-term follow-up. Neurology. 2006;67(10):1870-1.
52. Kim YH, Kim KS, Kim KJ, et al. Recurrence of vertigo in patients with vestibular neuritis. Acta Otolaryngol. 2011;131(11):1172-7.
53. Merchant SN, Gopen Q. A human temporal bone study of acute bacterial meningogenic labyrinthitis. Am J Otol. 1996;17(3):375-85. (*)
54. Strauss M. A clinical pathologic study of hearing loss in congenital cytomegalovirus infection. Laryngoscope. 1985;95(8):951-62.
55. Lindsay JR. Histopathology of deafness due to postnatal viral disease. Arch Otolaryngol. 1973;98(4):258-64.
56. Mizushima N, Murakami Y. Deafness following mumps: the possible pathogenesis and incidence of deafness. Auris Nasus Larynx. 1986;13 (Suppl 1):S55-7.

*References with asterisks refer to critical sources.

57. Karmody CS. Viral labyrinthitis: early pathology in the human. Laryngoscope. 1983;93(12):1527-33.
58. Douglas SA, Sanli H, Gibson WP. Meningitis resulting in hearing loss and labyrinthitis ossificans - does the causative organism matter? Cochlear Implants Int. 2008;9(2):90-6.
59. Green JD, Jr., Marion MS, Hinojosa R. Labyrinthitis ossificans: histopathologic consideration for cochlear implantation. Otolaryngol Head Neck Surg. 1991;104(3):320-6.
60. Tinling SP, Colton J, Brodie HA. Location and timing of initial osteoid deposition in postmeningitic labyrinthitis ossificans determined by multiple fluorescent labels. Laryngoscope. 2004;114(4):675-80.
61. Durisin M, Bartling S, Arnoldner C, et al. Cochlear osteoneogenesis after meningitis in cochlear implant patients: a retrospective analysis. Otol Neurotol. 2010;31(7):1072-8.
62. Kim HH, Addison J, Suh E, et al. Otoprotective effects of dexamethasone in the management of pneumococcal meningitis: an animal study. Laryngoscope. 2007;117(7):1209-15.
63. Worsoe L, Brandt CT, Lund SP, et al. Systemic steroid reduces long-term hearing loss in experimental pneumococcal meningitis. Laryngoscope. 2010;120(9):1872-9.
64. Hartnick CJ, Kim HH, Chute PM, Parisier SC. Preventing labyrinthitis ossificans: the role of steroids. Arch Otolaryngol Head Neck Surg. 2001;127(2):180-3.

CHAPTER

30

Central Vertigo

Robert W Eppsteiner, Deema Fattal, Marlan R Hansen

INTRODUCTION

Vertigo is the false sense of motion. Central vertigo results from cerebellar or brainstem pathology. In contrast, peripheral vertigo is caused by pathology of the balance end organ or the eighth cranial nerve. The dizzy patient is often referred to the otolaryngologist before the distinction between central or peripheral vertigo has been established. It is important for the otolaryngologist to be able to distinguish central from peripheral vertigo, as neurologists primarily manage central vertigo whereas otolaryngologists manage peripheral vertigo. In patients with central causes of dizziness, it is not as important to differentiate if dizziness is spinning versus lightheadedness versus presyncopal because often patients are vague about the type; e.g., in a survey, when patients were asked to describe their dizziness, more than half of patients picked a different response on retest approximately 6 minutes later[1]; secondly, when diagnosing stroke, patients with vertigo do not have a higher odds of stroke/TIA (transient ischemic attack) than those with dizziness, while patients with imbalance have higher odds of having stroke than patients with either type of dizziness.[2] For the remainder of the chapter, the term central vertigo is used, but keep in mind that patients who describe their dizziness as nonvertiginous or imbalance can still have central causes.

There are many causes of central vertigo, some of which are acute medical conditions that require prompt diagnosis and treatment. The diagnosis of central vertigo can usually be made in the office without advanced otoneurologic testing, although such testing is often helpful. This chapter will highlight the most common causes of central vertigo including vestibular migraine, vascular causes, cerebellar ataxia, cervical vertigo, and vertigo caused by mass lesions; and this chapter will also discuss the clinical diagnosis and workup of these various conditions (Table 30.1). Each disorder will be considered in turn.

CLINICAL EVALUATION OF THE DIZZY PATIENT

The clinical evaluation of the dizzy patient should be standardized and broad so as to allow for the diagnosis of any pathological process, be it peripheral or central in origin. This begins with a thorough history, which is often the most important diagnostic tool. It is important to characterize the dizzy spells by asking whether the patient is experiencing true rotatory vertigo or simply general dizziness or imbalance. In addition, the duration of the spells should be characterized, e.g. benign paroxysmal positional vertigo (BPPV) spells last seconds, TIAs last minutes, Meniere's disease episodes last hours, stroke or labyrinthine disease lasts days, and the duration of migraine dizziness is variable but typically less than a day.

Patients presenting with new onset constant vertigo for more than 24 hours are termed to have acute vestibular syndrome, which can be again peripheral (such as viral labyrinthitis) or central due to stroke. Such patients may present with isolated vertigo, or with associated otologic and/or neurologic symptoms. Note that isolated vertigo may have associated nausea, vomiting, sense of unsteadiness, sweating, or blurry vision. Any other associated symptoms such as hearing loss, tinnitus, weakness, numbness, diplopia, dysarthria, dysphagia, neck pain, or headache

Table 30.1: Common causes of central vertigo

	Diagnosis	*Vestibular testing*	*Workup*	*Treatment*	*Prognosis*
Migraine	Meet IHS migraine criteria, exclude peripheral causes, Migraine occurs during episodes of vertigo	Variable nystagmus with fixation suppression, decreased VEMP response	Clinical diagnosis	Diet modification TCA, beta-blocker, calcium channel blocker	Responds well to diet modification, refractory cases require medical therapy, spontaneous remission is common
Vascular	Acute onset of vertigo with neurologic symptoms	ENG may show caloric paresis	Acute vertigo with other neurologic symptoms	TPA, vestibular therapy, risk factor modification	Often recurrent and irreversible
Ataxia syndromes	Associated ataxia with other neurologic symptoms, family history	Vestibulo-ocular reflex testing with decreased gain, saccades with increased latency and square wave jerks	Genetic testing	Vestibular therapy, acetazolamide (episodic ataxia)	Often progressive, irreversible
Multiple sclerosis	Usually diagnosis is established prior to vertigo onset	Increased latency on VEMP	Imaging, lumbar puncture	Steroids	Varied
Cervical	Diagnosis relies on history, if underlying anatomic abnormality other associated neurologic sequelae usually present	Generally not pursued	Clinical history, imaging (Chiari malformation)	Avoid triggers Surgical intervention	Depends on etiology
Tumors	Isolated vertigo or disequilibrium, vertigo with hearing loss and/or tinnitus, concomitant cerebellar or other neurologic signs	Depends on tumor type and location, may have absent calorics	Imaging, auditory brainstem response	Observation, excision, targeted radiation	Varied depending on clinical behavior of tumor

(VEMP, vestibular-evoked myogenic potential; TPA, tissue plasminogen activator).

should be explored. It is important to note whether the episodes are triggered by change in head position such as rolling over in bed or extension of the neck or getting out of bed in the morning. It should also be noted whether the episodes have been progressive.

Physical examination findings characteristic of central vertigo include nystagmus that changes direction with changes in gaze, vertical nystagmus, nystagmus that fails to exhibit fixation suppression, and spontaneous nystagmus that is chronic (since peripheral nystagmus lasts days). It is important to complete a thorough neurologic assessment in an attempt to elicit concomitant neurologic deficits that point to a central cause of vertigo. Ataxia is a symptom characteristic of central vertigo of cerebellar origin and is not typical with peripheral causes of vertigo.

MIGRAINE-ASSOCIATED VERTIGO

Migraine headache is a common medical condition with defined diagnostic criteria established by the International Headache Society (Table 30.2). Migraine headache is commonly associated with dizziness and vertigo. Migraine-associated vertigo, also termed vestibular migraine, has diagnostic criteria distinct from those for migraine headache. Migraine-associated vertigo is a common central cause of vertigo. It has been estimated to have a lifetime prevalence of about 1% of the population, and 25–50% of migraineurs have dizziness.[3]

The pathophysiological basis of migraine headache is poorly understood and that of migraine-associated vertigo is even less well recognized. There are several theories that attempt to explain the pathogenesis of migraine-associated vertigo. The review by Furman and Marcus[4] provides a detailed description of this condition. Patients with migraine-associated vertigo demonstrate both central and peripheral signs of vestibular dysfunction. As such, current theories about the pathophysiology of migraine-associated vertigo suggest a complex interplay between classical migraine pathways (thalamus, trigeminal nucleus, pterygopalatine ganglion, trigeminal nucleus) and vestibular centers (vestibular nucleus) with resultant vasodilation of cerebral and labyrinthine vessels, which triggers neurotransmitter release, activation of pain pathways, and stimulation of vestibular end organs. This neurologic pathway has been suggested but not validated.

The International Headache Society established strict criteria for migraine headache both with and without aura (Table 30.2). Migraine without aura is more common. Diagnosis of migraine without aura requires (1) at least five headaches lasting 4–72 hours; (2) headaches with at least two of the following characteristics: unilateral throbbing, pulsating quality, moderate-to-severe pain intensity, headache resulting in avoidance of normal physical activity; and (3) during headaches at least one of the following must occur: nausea or vomiting, photophobia, and phonophobia (hyperacusis) (International Headache Society website http://www.ihs-classification.org/en). Migraine with aura has similar criteria; however, only two headache episodes are required in addition to aura (reversible visual symptoms, sensory symptoms such as numbness or paresthesias, or dysphasic speech disturbance). A diagnosis of migraine-associated vertigo requires that the patient meet International Headache Society criteria for migraine and in addition have a central balance disorder (peripheral causes of dizziness/vertigo must be ruled out) and in addition migrainous symptoms (e.g. headache) must occur during episodes of dizziness/vertigo or the dizziness has migraine features such as if light or sound exacerbates the dizziness.[4]

It has been demonstrated that dizziness/vertigo occurs in over half of patients with migraine; however, the symptoms of vertigo generally lag the onset of migraine headaches by several years.[5] Most patients with migraine-associated vertigo who present for evaluation are not actively dizzy but rather are between episodes. As such, vestibular testing is typically not fruitful. When vestibular testing has been completed on patients with migraine-associated vertigo with active symptoms, results point to both central and peripheral perturbations in the balance system. Patients tested during an acute attack of vestibular migraine most commonly demonstrate nystagmus on positional testing when fixation is suppressed (100%); less commonly nystagmus can be seen with headshake (35%) or be spontaneous (19%). Nystagmus may be only elicited with fixation suppression. The direction of nystagmus is most often horizontal, but it can be vertical or torsional.[6] Patients with vestibular migraine may have increased vestibular-evoked myogenic potential (VEMP) thresholds and decreased amplitudes.

Table 30.2: Diagnostic criteria of migraine

Diagnostic criteria for migraine without aura:
1. At least five attacks that meet criteria 2-4
2. Attacks last 4–72 hours
3. Headache involves at least two characteristics: a. Unilateral b. Pulsatile quality c. Pain is moderate to severe d. Exacerbated by physical activity
4. At least one associated symptom during headache: a. Nausea or vomiting b. Photophobia and phonophobia
5. Headache not attributed to another disorder
Diagnostic criteria for migraine with aura:
1. At least two attacks that meet criteria 2-4
2. Aura consisting of one of the following characteristics (no motor weakness): a. Reversible visual symptoms b. Reversible sensory symptoms c. Reversible dysphasic speech
3. Aura with at least two of the following characteristics: a. Homonymous visual symptoms or unilateral sensory symptoms b. Aura develops gradually over >5 minutes, or multiple symptoms occur in succession over >5 minutes c. Each symptom lasts between 5 and 60 minutes
4. Headache fulfills migraine without aura criteria 2-4. Migraine without aura begins during aura or within 60 minutes of aura ending
5. Headache not attributed to another disorder

The treatment of migraine-associated vertigo is essentially the same as treating migraine headache. Pharmacologic treatment of migraine can be divided into treatments that abort attacks and those which are preventative (Tables 30.3 and 30.4, respectively).[7] Lifestyle modification, including diet modification such as decreasing stimulants

Table 30.3: Abortive medications for migraine

Class	*Medication*	*Dose*	*Adverse effects*
NSAID	Ibuprofen	400–800 mg	Gastroesophageal reflux disease (GERD), gastric ulcer, renal dysfunction, cardiovascular (especially if previous myocardial infarction or heart failure)
	Naproxen	500–1000 mg	GERD, gastric ulcer, renal dysfunction, less cardiovascular adverse effects
Triptan	Sumatriptan	50–100 mg	Coronary spasm, serotonin syndrome if used concurrently with SSRI
	Zolmitriptan	2.5 mg	
	Naratriptan	2.5 mg	
	Rizatriptan	10 mg	
	Eletriptan	40 mg	
	Almotriptan	12.5 mg	
Ergot derivative	Ergotamine	2 mg	Nausea, vasoconstriction (including coronary), xerostomia, drowsiness

Source: Adapted from Goadsby and Sprenger.[7]
Ergot derivatives are generally not first-line treatment.

Table 30.4: Preventative first-line medications for migraine

Class	*Medication*	*Dose*	*Adverse effects*
Beta-blocker	Propranolol	40–120 mg twice daily	Reduced energy, tiredness, postural symptoms, contra-indicated in asthma
	Metoprolol	25–100 mg twice daily	
Anticonvulsant	Valproate	500–1000 mg twice daily	Drowsiness, weight gain, tremor, hair loss, fetal abnormalities, hematological or liver abnormalities
	Divalproex	500–1000 mg twice daily	Diarrhea, drowsiness, dizziness, tremor, hair loss, tinnitus
	Topiramate	50–200 mg twice daily	Paresthesia, cognitive dysfunction, weight loss, glaucoma, nephrolithiasis
Tricyclic antidepressant	Amitriptyline	10–100 mg daily	Hypersomnolence, xerostomia, urinary retention, poor concentration, EKG changes
	Nortriptyline	10–100 mg daily	Hypersomnolence, xerostomia, urinary retention, poor concentration, EKG changes

Source: Adapted from Goadsby and Sprenger.[7]

(e.g. caffeine) and limiting foods with tyramine, is effective in some patients. Reploeg and Goebel showed complete resolution of migraine-associated vertigo symptoms in 13 of 81 patients with diet modification.[8] For those who do not respond to diet modification alone, the addition of a tricyclic antidepressant improves treatment efficacy.[8] Some patients require addition of a second medication (beta-blocker or calcium channel blocker) or a neurology referral.

For the treatment of acute symptoms, a triptan can be tried with some help[4]; for preventive treatment, migraine headache medications are tried and used in a particular patient depending more on their side effect profile than their efficacy, since migraine preventive medications have not been studied in vestibular migraine extensively, and only case series exist.[4] For the prevention of migraines, three main classes of medications exist, including the antihypertension group (such as propranolol), antidepression group (such as nortriptyline/amitriptyline), and antiepileptic medications group (valproic acid, topiramate, gabapentin, lamotrigine). Therefore, in patients with blood pressure or heart rate that are on the high side, propranolol starting at 60 mg per day can be tried and increased as tolerated; for patients with concomitant insomnia, a tricyclic antidepressant can be tried starting at 10 mg at night and titrating up as tolerated up to 100 mg at night (amitriptyline has more sedative effect, but also more side effects such as dry mouth or urine retention, than nortriptyline); an electrocardiogram should be ordered with each tricyclic antidepressant dose increase. For those with obesity, topiramate at 25 mg per day and titrating up to 50 mg twice daily can be considered (since it may promote weight loss). Valproic acid at 250 or 500 mg/day is typically avoided in childbearing age females due to teratogenicity. Lamotrigine (starting at 25 mg per day and increasing slowly by 25 mg every 2 weeks till 50 mg twice daily) has been shown to help the dizziness in vestibular migraine, but is not helpful for headache. Gabapentin starting at 100 mg per day and titrating up is used in patients with polypharmacy since it does not interact with other medications. For evidence-based medicine review of migraine headache treatment, *see* Silberstein et al.[9] Physical (vestibular) therapy has been anecdotally found to help vestibular migraine.[4]

The prognosis for migraine-associated vertigo is excellent. The only blinded, placebo-controlled trial of migraine-associated vertigo examined the effect of zolmitriptan compared to placebo.[10] The most compelling finding of this study was the large number of patients who had to be excluded due to lack of vertigo attacks after enrollment. This suggests that a large number of patients with migraine-associated vertigo experience spontaneous resolution, and for many of the remainder, diet modification and/or medical therapy suffice.

VASCULAR CAUSES OF VERTIGO

Vascular causes are also a relatively common source of central vertigo, especially in the elderly. For a detailed review of vascular causes of vertigo, see that of Karatas.[11] Around 20% of TIAs and strokes involve the posterior circulation and may present with vertigo.[12] Seventeen percent of patients with TIA/stroke present with isolated dizziness.[13] The vascular supply to the vestibular system is via the vertebrobasilar circulation that includes the paired vertebral arteries, which arise from their respective subclavian arteries and merge to form the basilar artery, the basilar artery, and the three main cerebellar branches: the posterior inferior cerebellar artery (PICA), anterior inferior cerebellar artery (AICA), and the superior cerebellar artery (Fig. 30.1).[14] The PICA supplies the vestibular nuclei as well as the lateral medulla and cerebellum. The AICA supplies

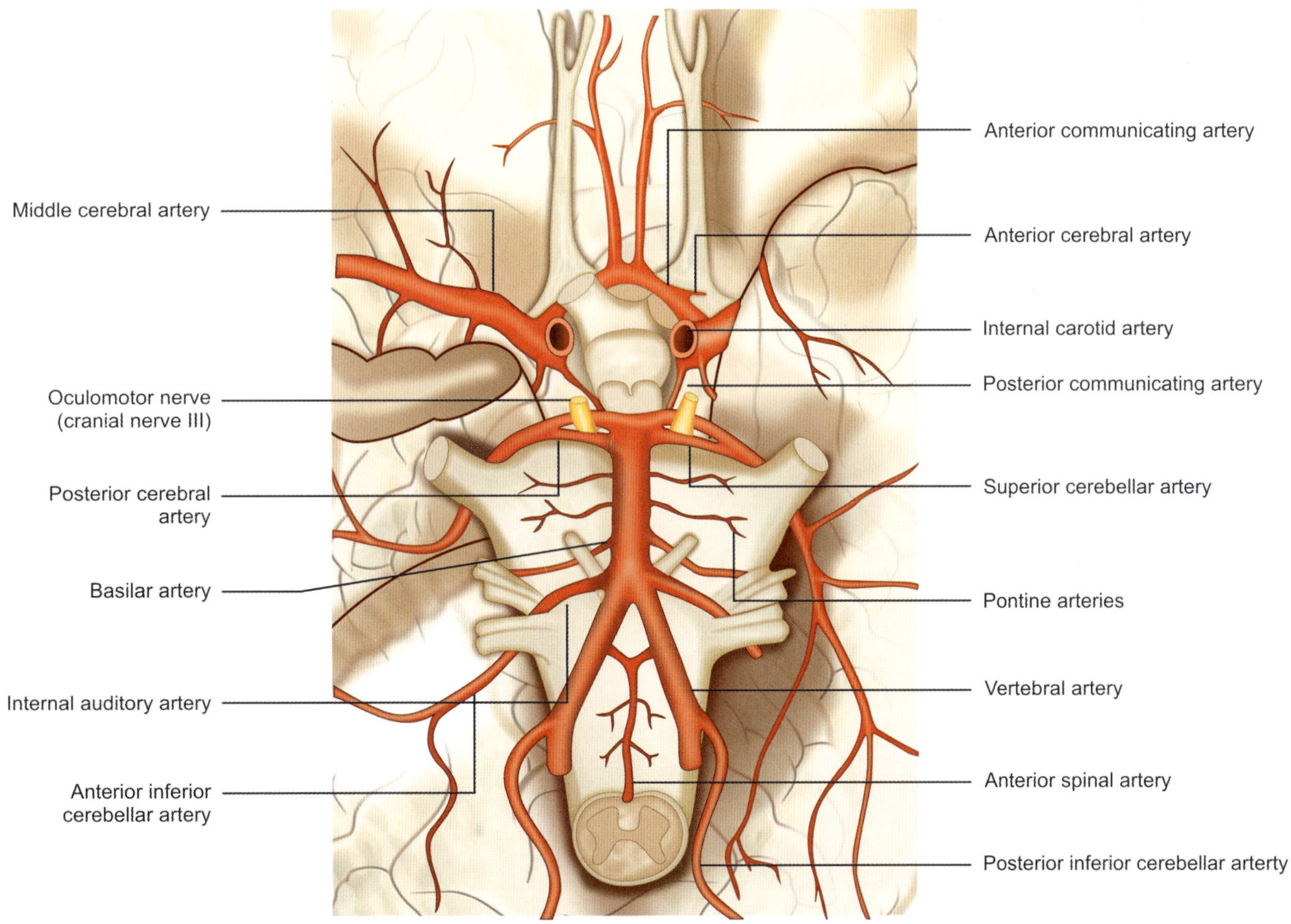

Fig. 30.1: The vascular supply to the vestibular system is via the vertebrobasilar circulation that includes the paired vertebral arteries, which arise from their respective subclavian arteries and merge to form the basilar artery, the basilar artery, and the three main cerebellar branches: the posterior inferior cerebellar artery (PICA), anterior inferior cerebellar artery (AICA), and the superior cerebellar artery.

the labyrinth as well as portions of the pons and cerebellum. The superior cerebellar artery supplies the cerebellum. Vascular compromise anywhere in this system can result in vertigo. This can be from hypotension, vascular spasm, or atherosclerotic, embolic or hemorrhagic stroke. The inner ear is particularly vulnerable to ischemia because its main blood supply, the labyrinthine artery, is an end artery. In the case of vascular disruption, no collateral flow exists for the inner ear, which is not the case for the pons or cerebellum where redundancy exists in vascular supply.[15] Therefore, an embolic event in the labyrinthine artery generally leads to infarction.

Relative posterior circulation ischemia leading to TIA occurs due to the presence of atherosclerotic disease in the vertebrobasilar circulation, which causes narrowing of the vascular lumen predisposing to ischemia with relative interruptions in blood flow leading to vestibular symptoms. This transient posterior circulation compromise is common in the elderly and typically presents with vertigo that lasts minutes. The key to differentiating transient posterior circulation compromise from other types of central and peripheral vertigo is to look for concomitant neurologic signs as isolated vertigo is uncommon. Grad and Baloh characterized the most common nonvestibular neurologic symptoms associated with transient posterior circulation compromise. These include vision changes (69%), drop attacks (33%), incoordination (21%), extremity weakness (21%), confusion (17%), headache (14%), hearing loss (14%), loss of consciousness (10%), extremity numbness (10%), dysarthria (10%), tinnitus (10%), and perioral numbness (5%).[16] The time course of symptoms also helps distinguish transient posterior circulation compromise from other causes of vertigo as transient posterior circulation ischemia typically lasts minutes and fully reverses between episodes. In addition, it may be precipitated by head position. In the setting of luminal narrowing due to atherosclerotic disease, changes in head position, especially turning and extension, can provoke vertiginous symptoms.[17]

Generally, vascular causes of vertigo occur in individuals with underlying atherosclerotic disease. Such patients often have predisposing medical conditions including hypertension, diabetes, and hypercholesterolemia. In addition, smoking is also a risk factor for disease.

Typically, the diagnosis of vascular causes of vertigo can be made after a thorough history and clinical examination. Confirmation in cases of stroke can be made with intracranial imaging such as head computed tomography (CT), in the acute setting, or magnetic resonance imaging (MRI). Specifically, CT is used to rule out hemorrhage, but it is unlikely to find the cause of dizziness; e.g., in a study of 200 dizzy patients, CT had a diagnostic yield of zero.[18] The brain MRI detects strokes acutely in the brainstem and cerebellum, but has a false negative rate of 8–19% within the first 24 hours (Figs. 30.2A and B).[19] In an elderly patient with atherosclerotic risk factors, there should be a low threshold for obtaining intracranial imaging. Generally neurotologic testing is not needed for diagnosis.

When patients present to the emergency room with acute vertigo, especially elderly patients, the clinician must

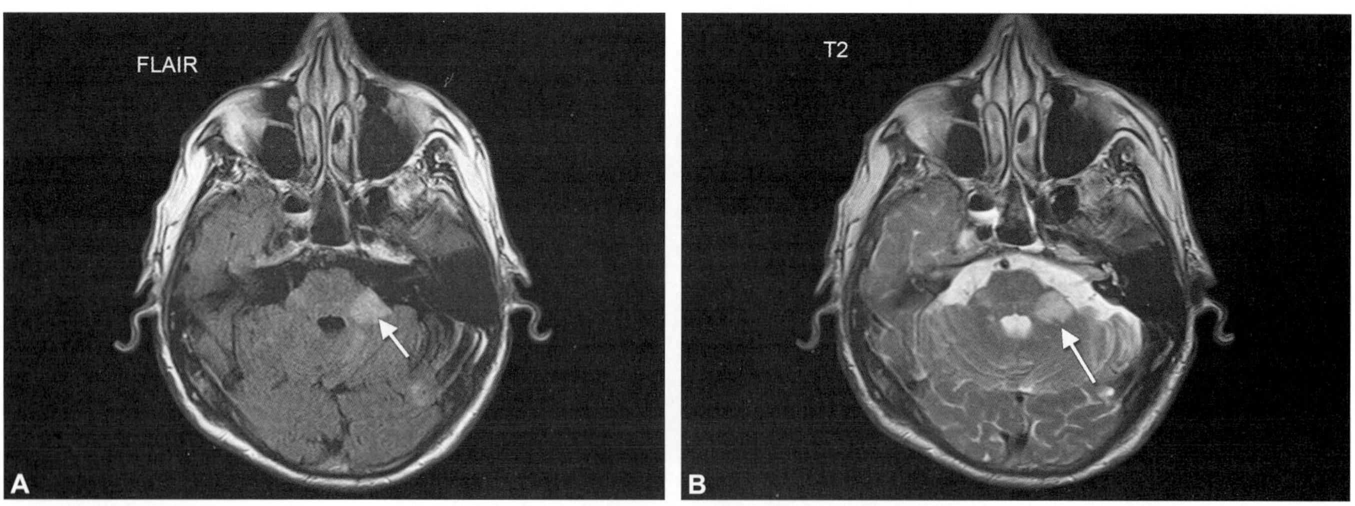

Figs. 30.2A and B: Magnetic resonance imaging of a 75-year-old man presenting with altered mental status, vertigo, and nystagmus diagnosed with acute ischemic stroke of the brachium pontis, occipital lobe, and cerebellum likely from posterior cerebral artery embolic infarcts. Images demonstrate areas of restricted diffusion on fluid attenuation inversion recovery (FLAIR) and T2 sequences.

have a high index of suspicion for stroke. There should be a low threshold for evaluation with a head CT to assess the possibility of stroke. If positive, prompt evaluation by a neurologist for consideration of thrombolytic agents should be considered.

An important set of neurotologic signs that distinguishes central versus peripheral causes of vertigo is the triad of head impulse, skew deviation, and central nystagmus.[20] For example, the presence of normal horizontal head impulse test, direction-changing nystagmus in eccentric gaze, or skew deviation (vertical ocular misalignment) was 100% sensitive and 96% specific for stroke, better than MRI within the first 24 hours.

Treatments of vascular causes of vertigo generally include treating the underlying cause. If the underlying cause is an acute thromboembolic cerebrovascular accident, then treatment with tissue plasminogen activator (TPA) should be considered. The patient should be followed by a neurologist and is often begun on chronic anticoagulative therapy with aspirin, clopidogrel, or warfarin. In addition, the patient should be evaluated for risk factors for atherosclerotic disease and medical therapy should be optimized. This includes identifying and treating HTN, hyperlipidemia, and hypercholesterolemia and encouraging smoking cessation.

The prognosis for patients with vascular causes of vertigo caused by vertebrobasilar stenosis or disruptions in the posterior cerebral circulation is typically worse than for patients with other forms of stenosis such as carotid stenosis and worse than those with TIA/CVA of other intracranial territories.[21] If a patient has a TIA involving the vertebrobasilar circulation, they are at high risk of repeat events and future cerebral infarctions.[21] Therefore, prompt referral after a presenting event is important so that risk factors can be modified to decrease the risk of further events.

Patterns of Vascular Disruption

There are several patterns of vascular disruption that result in recognizable patterns of neurologic deficits. When recognized, prompt imaging and consultation of a neurologist should be pursued. These will be briefly discussed.

Lateral Medullary Syndrome

Infarction of the ipsilateral vertebral artery or the PICA results in a classic constellation of neurologic deficits termed lateral medullary syndrome or Wallenberg syndrome (Fig. 30.3).[14] This results from infarction of the dorsolateral aspect of the medulla. The classic syndrome involves ipsilateral cranial nerve deficits, including ipsilateral facial numbness due to involvement of the spinal trigeminal nucleus and tract and contralateral body sensory loss (spinothalamic tract involvement). In addition,

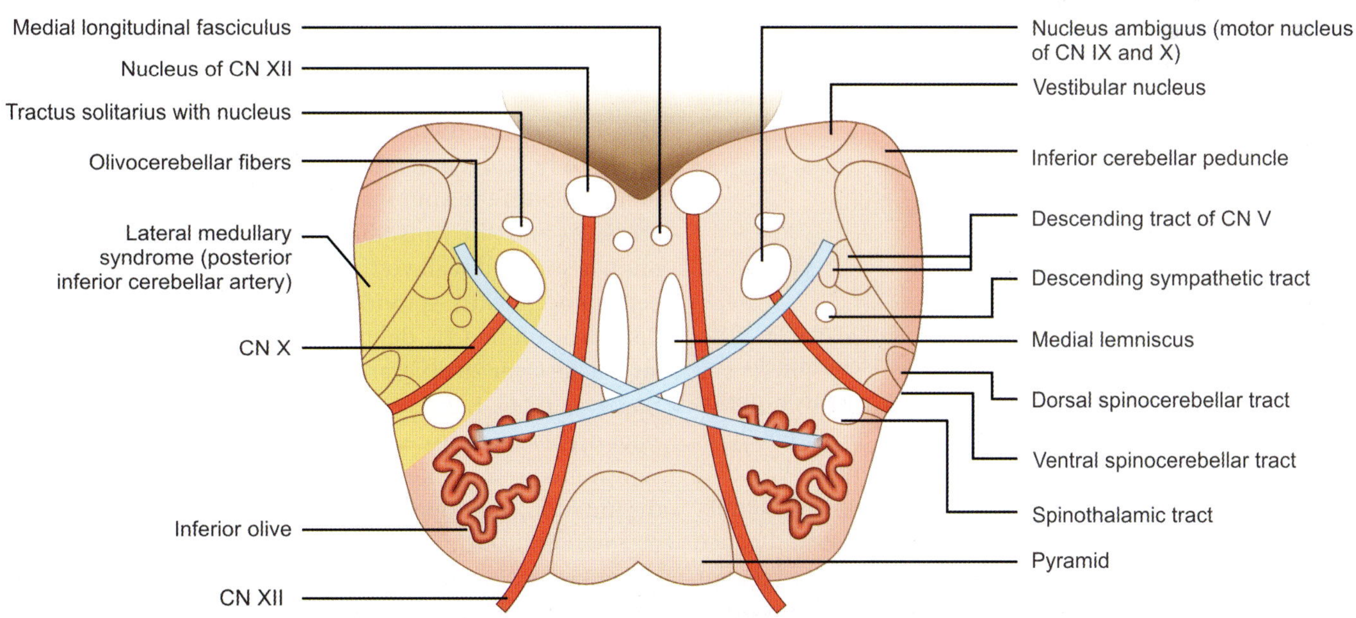

Fig. 30.3: Lateral medullary syndrome. The classic syndrome involves ipsilateral cranial nerve deficits including ipsilateral facial numbness due to involvement of the spinal trigeminal nucleus and tract, and contralateral body sensory loss (spinothalamic tract involvement). In addition, there is associated vertigo, ataxia, nausea, nystagmus, Horner's sign, dysphagia, and hoarseness.

there is associated vertigo, ataxia, nausea, nystagmus, Horner's sign, dysphagia, and hoarseness. The vertigo occurs secondary to infarction of either the vestibular nuclei or cerebellar infarction. The dysphagia and dysphonia result from infarction of the nucleus ambiguous. Ataxia is ipsilateral and is usually present if there is concomitant cerebellar involvement.

Dorsolateral Pontine Syndrome

Vascular disruption of the AICA can result in dorsolateral pontine syndrome due to infarction of the dorsolateral pons region as well as cerebellum. In most cases of AICA infarction, the labyrinthine artery suffers vascular compromise often resulting in inner ear infarction, so that 98% of patients have vertigo and 63% will have hearing loss.[22] Importantly, about 5% of patients present with isolated vertigo.[22] Other associated symptoms including ipsilateral face and contralateral body sensory loss (pain and temperature due to involvement of the spinal trigeminal and spinothalamic tracts respectively) and ipsilateral facial paralysis if the facial nucleus are involved. Vertigo generally persists until contralateral vestibular compensation occurs and hearing loss is permanent if infarction occurs. These patients often benefit from vestibular rehabilitation and a contralateral routing of sound hearing aid or osseointegrated auditory prosthesis to rehabilitate the unilateral deafness.

A similar constellation of symptoms can occur with AICA distribution TIA, however, symptoms resolve within minutes. Again it should be stressed that those presenting with TIA should have a thorough risk factor assessment so that risk factor modification can take place. These patients may also benefit from vestibular rehabilitation.

Cerebellar Stroke

Any of the above patterns of ischemia can have concomitant involvement of the cerebellum, as ischemia in the distribution of the vertebral, PICA, AICA, or the superior cerebellar artery can result in infarction of the cerebellum. Cerebellar stroke can also happen in isolation by vascular disruption in these territories. It is important to identify cerebellar infarction as the event can progress and cause brainstem compression and herniation. Pure cerebellar strokes may be distinguished from peripheral and other central causes by the characteristic gaze-evoked nystagmus, which changes directions and limb ataxia. Gait ataxia also points to cerebellar involvement; in fact 72% of patients are unable to walk independently.[23] Hemorrhagic stokes affecting the cerebellum can result in rapid patient decompensation due to brainstem herniation and must be recognized promptly, as surgical decompression can be lifesaving in some cases.

CEREBELLAR ATAXIA SYNDROMES

There are many genetic and sporadic syndromes that affect the cerebellum and result in central vertigo or nystagmus. For a review of cerebellar ataxias, the reader is referred to Manto and Marmolino [24] or Jayadev and Bird.[26]

Autosomal Recessive Ataxias

There are many ataxias that are inherited in an autosomal recessive manner and encompass a heterogeneous group of disorders with diverse neurologic presentations. The most common inherited ataxia, Friedreich's ataxia, results from an intronic GAA repeat in the *FXN* gene, encoding the frataxin protein, and is inherited in an autosomal recessive fashion. Like many other trinucleotide repeat disorders, ataxia is delayed in onset and typically presents before the third decade of life. It generally presents with gait disturbance and falling. Neurologic examination typically demonstrates areflexia, distal weakness, impaired proprioception, dysarthria, cardiomegaly, and diabetes mellitus. VOR testing typically reveals decreased gain and saccades have increased latency and square wave jerks.[25]

Autosomal Dominant Ataxias

The autosomal dominant ataxias encompass another group of heterogenous disorders. This group of disorders includes both the spinocerebellar ataxias, which are progressive, and the episodic ataxias. These disorders are often associated with vertigo and nystagmus suggestive of central origin. The spinocerebellar ataxias are a group of disorders unified by delayed onset, progressive cerebellar ataxia. Over 28 different subtypes have been identified; however, types 1, 2, 3, 6, and 7 are the most common. The phenotypes include cerebellar ataxia but other neurologic symptoms are variable and may include seizures, cognitive dysfunction, neuropathy, ocular involvement, and other movement disorders depending on the subtype. Some of the subtypes involve trinucleotide repeats. For a detailed review, the reader is referred to Jayadev and Bird.[26]

The episodic ataxias, which are also dominantly inherited, are characterized by the episodic nature of attacks, which involve ataxia and vertigo and can be triggered by stress. Several subtypes of the episodic ataxia disorders have been identified. These episodes are usually short-lived and respond to therapy with acetazolamide.[27]

MULTIPLE SCLEROSIS

Multiple sclerosis (MS) is a disease that causes demyelination of axon tracts in the central nervous system (CNS). MS can result in vertigo if the vestibular nuclei are involved in demyelination (Figs. 30.4A to D). Vertigo is common among patients with MS; however, it is a rare presenting symptom. In fact, the most common cause of vertigo in patients with MS is BPPV. Given that peripheral causes of vertigo such as BPPV are common in patients with MS, it is important to be able to distinguish central from peripheral causes of vertigo. Usually, central and peripheral entities can be distinguished by the type of nystagmus. With BPPV the nystagmus is provoked by position change and is typically geotropic and fatigable; however, central nystagmus caused by MS is often multidirectional. VEMPs can be a useful adjunct for diagnosing central vertigo caused by MS as the latency can be increased.[28] Vertigo caused by a flare of MS can be treated with steroids; however, treatment should be initiated with consultation of a neurologist with experience treating MS.

CERVICAL VERTIGO

Cervical vertigo is an uncommon cause of vertigo that is not well accepted. Cervical vertigo includes conditions where manipulation of the cervical spine results in dizziness or vertigo. One potential mechanism for cervical

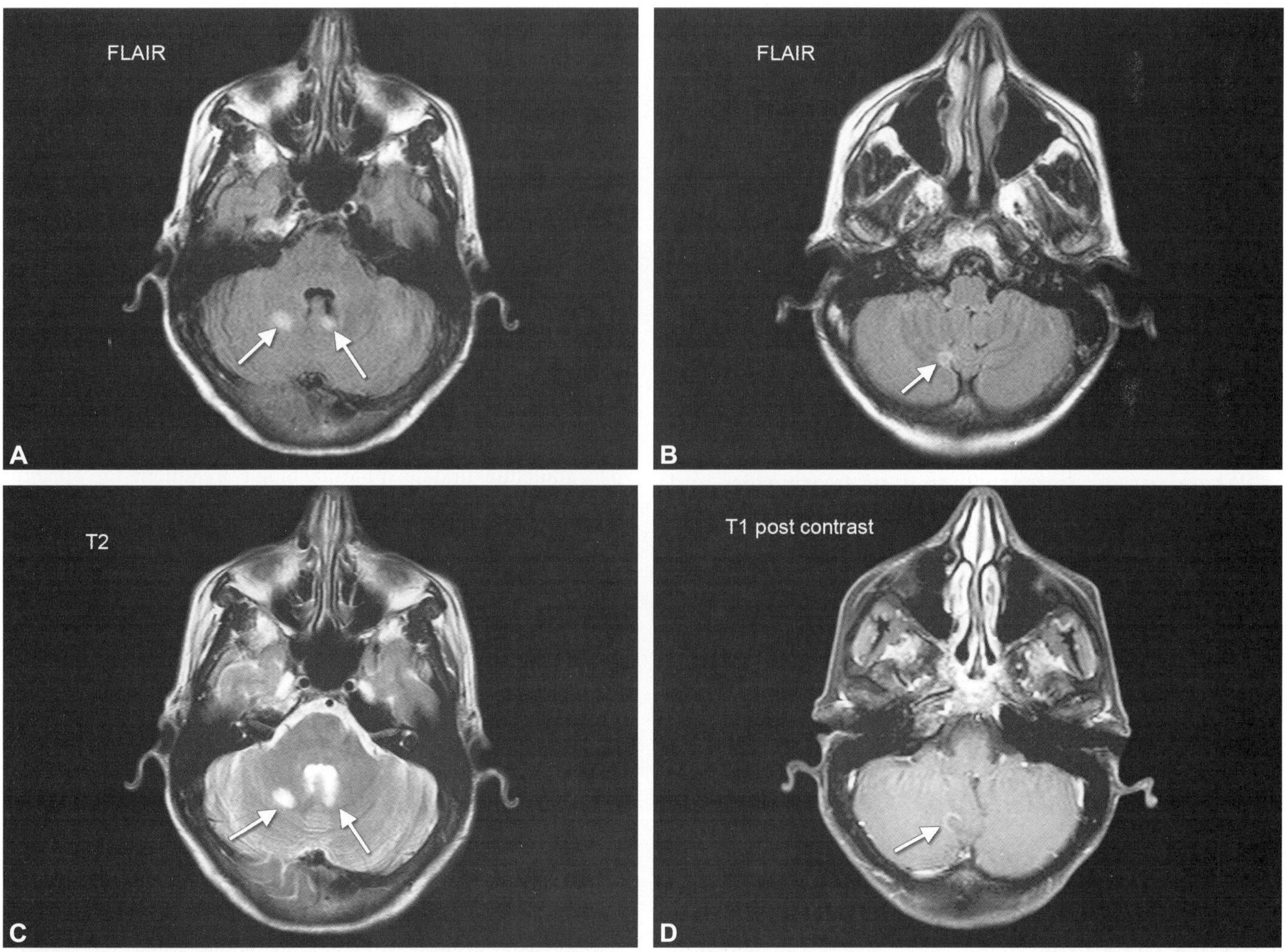

Figs. 30.4A to D: Magnetic resonance imaging of a 50-year-old woman presenting with nausea, vertigo, and vertical nystagmus diagnosed with multiple sclerosis. Images demonstrate areas of abnormal T2/FLAIR signal prolongation in the cerebellum one of which enhances on T1 postcontrast images suggesting an acute plaque. The patient had multiple other lesions in the white matter, mostly periventricular, of the parietal lobes.

vertigo is anatomic compression of the cerebellum or brainstem by variants in cranial base or cervical anatomy. Examples of this include Chiari malformations and upper cervical spine abnormalities. In Chiari malformations, herniation of the cerebellar tonsils through the foramen magnum can result in vertigo. The presence of downbeating (or upbeating) nystagmus or other neurologic abnormalities such as ataxia, headache, motor, and sensory deficits provides clues that the vertigo is central in nature. Another mechanism of cervical vertigo is due to ischemia caused by vertebrobasilar compression during cervical extension. There have been case reports of neck extension, as during a shampoo at a hair salon, resulting in vertigo.[29] Despite these reports, cervical vertigo is extremely rare and a difficult diagnosis to establish.

TUMORS

Tumors and other intracranial masses of various types have the ability to cause vertigo. In addition, tumors may result in vertigo without concomitant other CNS symptoms as can be the case of vestibular schwannomas, or with other lesions there may be many other neurologic sequelae. The variability in sequelae from tumors not only is predicated on the behavior of the tumor cell type but is equally important in determining the clinical course, the size, and the location of the lesion. Vestibular schwannomas are benign tumors of Schwann cell origin, which arise on the vestibular nerves. They are usually slow growing and often asymptomatic for many years. They are most commonly found in the internal auditory canal and cerebellopontine angle (CPA) and usually present with tinnitus, hearing loss, and/or disequilibrium. They rarely cause true vertigo. The nystagmus, if present, can mimic other causes of peripheral vertigo. Larger tumors may present with other neurologic findings including facial numbness or headaches. Other tumors of the CPA can present in similar fashion, and may also result in abducens and/or lower cranial neuropathies. Tumors that originate in the posterior fossa or cerebellum typically can be distinguished with cerebellar signs such as ataxia. Patients often have spontaneous nystagmus, which is another defining feature. Gliomas are particularly aggressive and rapidly progress to involve brainstem compression and associated neurologic findings.

CONCLUSION

Causes of central vertigo are varied but share features that are usually able to be distinguished from peripheral vertigo by proficient history and examination. In some cases, as in vascular causes, prompt diagnosis is paramount. Vestibular testing and imaging are useful adjuncts. Otolaryngologists should be familiar with central causes of vertigo, as they are common reasons for referral.

REFERENCES

1. Newman-Toker DE, Cannon LM, Stofferahn ME, et al. Imprecision in patient reports of dizziness symptom quality: a cross-sectional study conducted in an acute care setting. Mayo Clin Proc. 2007;82(11):1329-40.
2. Kerber KA, Brown DL, Lisabeth LD, et al. Stroke among patients with dizziness, vertigo, and imbalance in the emergency department: a population-based study. Stroke. 2006; 37(10):2484-7.
3. Neuhauser HK, Radtke A, von Brevern M, et al. Migrainous vertigo: prevalence and impact on quality of life. Neurology. 2006;67(6):1028-33.
4. Furman JM, Marcus DA. Migraine and motion sensitivity. Continuum (Minneap Minn). Neuro-otology. 2012;18(5): 1102-17.
5. Thakar A, Anjaneyulu C, Deka RC. Vertigo syndromes and mechanisms in migraine. J Laryngol Otol. 2001;115(10): 782-7.
6. Polensek SH, Tusa RJ. Nystagmus during attacks of vestibular migraine: an aid in diagnosis. Audiol Neurootol 2010; 15(4):241-6.
7. Goadsby PJ, Sprenger T. Current practice and future directions in the prevention and acute management of migraine. Lancet Neurol. 2010;9(3):285-98.
8. Reploeg MD, Goebel JA. Migraine-associated dizziness: patient characteristics and management options. Otol Neurotol. 2002;23(3):364-71.
9. Silberstein SD, Holland S, Freitag F, et al. Evidence-based guideline update: pharmacologic treatment for episodic migraine prevention in adults: report of the Quality Standards Subcommittee of the American Academy of Neurology and the American Headache Society. Neurology. 2012; 78(17):1337-45.
10. Neuhauser H, Radtke A, von Brevern M, et al. Zolmitriptan for treatment of migrainous vertigo: a pilot randomized placebo-controlled trial. Neurology. 2003;60(5):882-3.
11. Karatas M. Vascular vertigo: epidemiology and clinical syndromes. Neurologist. 2011;17(1):1-10.
12. Cloud GC, Markus HS. Diagnosis and management of vertebral artery stenosis. QJM. 2003;96(1):27-54.
13. Kerber KA, Brown DL, Lisabeth LD, et al. Stroke among patients with dizziness, vertigo, and imbalance in the emergency department: a population-based study. Stroke. 2006; 37(10):2484-7.
14. Flint PW, Cummings CW. Cummings Otolaryngology Head & Neck Surgery, Fifth edition. Philadelphia, PA: Mosby/ Elsevier; 2010.
15. Konishi T, Butler R, Fernandez C. Effect of anoxia on cochlear potentials. J Acoust Soc Am. 1961;33:349-55.

16. Grad A, Baloh RW. Vertigo of vascular origin. Clinical and electronystagmographic features in 84 cases. Arch Neurol. 1989;46(3):281-4.
17. Ishiyama G, Ishiyama A. Vertebrobasilar infarcts and ischemia. Otolaryngol Clin North Am. 2011;44(2):415-35, ix-x.
18. Wasay M, Dubey N, Bakshi R. Dizziness and yield of emergency head CT scan: is it cost effective? Emerg Med J. 2005; 22(4):312.
19. Oppenheim C, Stanescu R, Dormont D, et al. False-negative diffusion-weighted MR findings in acute ischemic stroke. AJNR Am J Neuroradiol. 2000;21(8):1434-40.
20. Kattah JC, Talkad AV, Wang DZ, et al. HINTS to diagnose stroke in the acute vestibular syndrome: three-step bedside oculomotor examination more sensitive than early MRI diffusion-weighted imaging. Stroke. 2009;40(11):3504-10.
21. Flossmann E, Rothwell PM. Prognosis of vertebrobasilar transient ischaemic attack and minor stroke. Brain. 2003; 126(Pt 9):1940-54.
22. Lee H. Neuro-otological aspects of cerebellar stroke syndrome. J Clin Neurol. 2009;5(2):65-73.
23. Edlow JA, Newman-Toker DE, Savitz SI. Diagnosis and initial management of cerebellar infarction. Lancet Neurol. 2008;7(10):951-64.
24. Manto M, Marmolino D. Cerebellar ataxias. Curr Opin Neurol. 2009;22(4):419-29.
25. Fahey MC, Cremer PD, Aw ST, et al. Vestibular, saccadic and fixation abnormalities in genetically confirmed Friedreich ataxia. Brain. 2008;131(Pt 4):1035-45.
26. Jayadev S, Bird TD. Hereditary ataxias: overview. Genet Med. 2013;15(9):673-83.
27. Harno H, Hirvonen T, Kaunisto MA, et al. Acetazolamide improves neurotological abnormalities in a family with episodic ataxia type 2 (EA-2). J Neurol. 2004;251(2): 232-4.
28. Alpini D, Caputo D, Pugnetti L, et al. Vertigo and multiple sclerosis: aspects of differential diagnosis. Neurol Sci. 2001; 22 Suppl 2:S84-7.
29. Endo K, Ichimaru K, Shimura H, et al. Cervical vertigo after hair shampoo treatment at a hairdressing salon: a case report. Spine. 2000;25(5):632-4.

CHAPTER

31

Aural Rehabilitation and Hearing Aids

Jaclyn B Spitzer, Dean M Mancuso, Joseph J Montano

INTRODUCTION

The management of hearing loss in adults is neither ordinary nor predictable. We can often be misled when looking at an audiogram by making assumptions that are frequently proven false. While we have the capability of classifying hearing loss as either sensorineural, conductive, or mixed and determining its severity, standard audiometric evaluation does not provide any information about the impact of this loss on a person's quality of life. How one reacts to the presence of hearing loss is a personal process that must be explored in order to provide the necessary tools for effective management. For example, one person with a mild high-frequency sensorineural hearing loss may report that he/she has no difficulties in any listening conditions; while, another, who perhaps works as a waitress in a restaurant, may find it impossible to continue her employment. The circumstances in one's life influence the reaction to hearing loss and largely contribute to the decision to pursue rehabilitation.

FORMULATING AN AUDIOLOGIC REHABILITATION PLAN

Acknowledging that some patients will reject options for surgery (where such options exist) that might improve or restore hearing, other methods must be available to assist with the management of hearing loss. The terms aural/audiologic/auditory rehabilitation (AR) have been used interchangeably in the literature to describe a process that aims to improve the communication skills of people with hearing loss. This process has been defined as the "services and procedures for facilitating adequate receptive and expressive communication in individuals with hearing impairment...."[1] Since the publication of this ASHA statement, literature abounds with articles on the psychosocial and emotional impact that hearing loss has on a person's functioning. Publications such as the World Health Organization's landmark *International Classification of Functioning, Disability and Health* (2001)[2] highlight the importance of understanding the impact of impairment on a person's activities and participations. As a result, authors have redefined the process of AR in order to highlight the influence of hearing loss not only on communication but also on function. Montano refers to AR as "...a person-centered approach to the assessment and management of hearing loss that encourages the creation of a therapeutic environment conducive to a shared decision process necessary to explore and reduce the impact hearing loss has on communication, activities and participations...."[3]

AR services fall under the scope of practice for both audiologists and speech-language pathologists (SLPs). ASHA[4] delineates the skills and knowledge specific to both disciplines. While services can be provided by either professional to patients of any age, given the impact hearing impairment has on speech and language development, the SLP is crucial for the management of this loss in children. The goal of AR services is not merely the management of hearing loss, but rather the facilitation of adjustment to it. This is best accomplished through patient self-management.[5] Therefore, therapeutic intervention should foster self-efficacy. The belief behind self-efficacy is that the person has the ability and skills necessary to manage a task or behavior successfully.[6,7] In this case, a person with hearing loss is capable of improving his/her communication ability and adjusting to life's circumstances. It is a goal to be able to establish an environment of care conducive to shared decision making that takes into account the role of the patient in the therapeutic interaction. Commonly, we refer to this as patient-centered care (PCC).

It is apparent that change in the provision of health care is causing a shift toward more patient-centered approaches. The recently enacted Patient Protection and Affordable Care Act[8] and the emphasis on patient-centered outcomes by third party insurers are evidence of the shift currently underway. That shift may, in some instances, force us to rethink the models we use to practice medicine. These models of service delivery have been described as the medical/biomedical or the rehabilitation/biopsychosocial.[5,9]

The medical/biomedical model implies a top-down system. The model is largely curative in nature, consisting of assessment, diagnosis, and treatment. The treatment, therefore, is meant to resolve the impairment. Here, the clinician can be described as "doing" something to/for the patient. The patient is primarily passive and is instructed by the clinician. It makes the assumption that, in this case, hearing loss is treated more like a disease with the outcome of a result of medication, surgery, or hearing aids. However, this model is primarily directed toward acute medical conditions. Hearing loss that is the object of AR, on the other hand, is generally not acute, but rather chronic.

The rehabilitative/biopsychosocial model is more horizontal in nature, meaning that it is more interactive and encourages patient participation in the treatment decisions. The clinician identifies the problems associated with the hearing loss and looks to the patient for direction when determining the treatment options. The patient takes a more active role in the decisions regarding their individualized care.

When using a PCC approach to intervention, both the medical and biopsychosocial models have their place. In fact, since the treatment in a PCC model revolves around the needs of the patient, he/she should determine the desired method of service delivery. Regardless, pivotal to any method of intervention is the need to establish a relationship with the patient and build the necessary rapport to encourage successful outcomes.

Montano[10] reported that AR treatments tend to emphasize the technological aspects of patient care; that is, the concept that the hearing aid will be the solution to living with hearing loss. As a result, more time is spent talking about hearing aids and assistive technology systems than on the impact the hearing loss may have on psychosocial functions. The process becomes overly dependent on instrumentation.[11] As seen in Figure 31.1, the technocentric model of audiology service delivery[10] highlights the influence of technology on the provision of service. Almost every aspect of patient care is technology driven. The assessment performed results in the audiogram that most people use as the basis for recommending hearing aids. Subsequent treatment emphasizes choices in hearing aids, fitting, dispensing, and orientation. Real-ear verification, as well, is a technological means to determine the performance of hearing aids using a prescriptive target. Essentially, the patient has little input to the process other than wearing the hearing aid and using the ear canal for probe microphone measurements. Verification of hearing aid performance should not be confused with personal adjustment to hearing loss. Finally, the patient is offered accessories to help the hearing aids work more effectively in various listening conditions. All of these steps are technology driven.

The Person-Centered Model[11] places the treatment emphasis on counseling with the patient at the core of the process. It highlights the importance of the patient

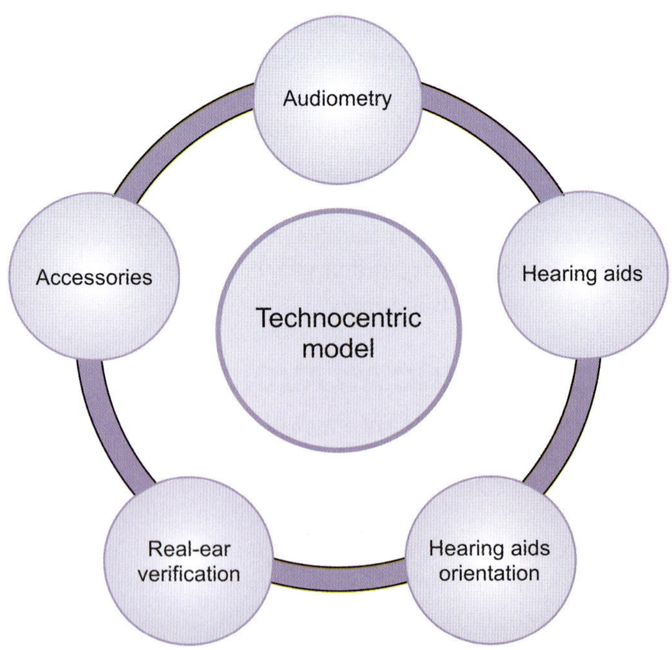

Fig. 31.1: Model representing a technology-focused delivery of audiologic rehabilitation services.

story, an important component of narrative medicine. The patient's story is the basis for shared decision making allowing the clinician to get a glimpse of the patient's needs, his/her self-perceptions, and values.[12] Unlike the history form that elicits primarily yes/no responses, patient narratives provide a better understanding of the unique problems that occur as a result of hearing loss.

Montano[10] emphasized the inclusion of self-assessment in addition to the audiogram when trying to determine the impact of hearing loss. Self-assessment measures have been used to quantify healthcare service and provide important outcome information.[13] In addition, self-assessment questionnaires can be useful in the counseling process. A tool such as the Hearing Handicap Inventory for the Elderly[14] can provide both a level of patient self-perceived handicap and a basis for counseling. Such questionnaires can spark conversation and guide a patient into areas that may be in need of remediation. It provides valuable information to the clinician while reinforcing the establishment of the caring relationship. Self-assessment is an underutilized approach in both audiology[15] and otolaryngology.

Upon further review of Figure 31.2, the technological aspects critical to rehabilitation are not eliminated but rather become part of the counseling realm instead of the core of treatment. Hearing aids, assistive technology systems, and verification measures remain important

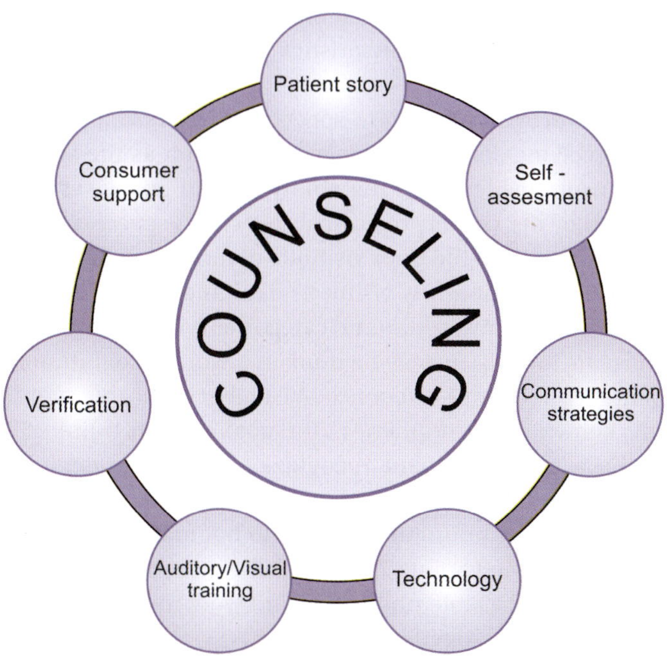

Fig. 31.2: Model representing a person-centered delivery of audiologic rehabilitation services.

components of this rehabilitation process, as do areas such as communication strategy training, auditory–visual interventions, and the availability of consumer support. Counseling, however, is the emphasis of this model.

COUNSELING PATIENTS WITH HEARING LOSS

Many clinicians are uncomfortable with the concepts of counseling, thinking they may not have adequate training to provide such services. In reality, the audiologist is uniquely qualified to provide the support needed to help patients adjust to living with hearing loss. Counseling allows the audiologist to help individuals adjust and make the changes necessary in order to develop a more positive approach to living with hearing loss, accepting the limitations, and embracing the technologies presented to them.[16]

Clark and English[17] describe two components of counseling common in practice. These include patient education and personal support counseling. Patient education stresses the importance of teaching; providing the information necessary so patients can effectively manage such things as hearing aid/sensory aids troubleshooting and communication strategies. Personal support counseling, on the other hand, enters the realm of feelings and affect. It requires important listening skills on the part of the audiologist and the need to address effectively the issues raised by the patient. It requires matching a response that is aligned with the affect presented by the individual with hearing loss.

Counseling skills are also an important component of motivational engagement. Clark et al.[18] describe methods that can be used to help the patient with hearing loss move toward greater self-awareness of the issues related to the impairment and foster efficacy. The idea behind motivational engagement is that a patient will have the greatest success when he convinces himself of the need for the given interventions. The process can be individual or include input from the communication partners. Preminger and Lind[19] likewise emphasize the importance of including communication partners in the rehabilitation process.

Prochaska and DiClemente[20] described the transtheoretical approach to behavior change. Often referred to as the Readiness for Change Model, it is believed that one goes through a series of adjustments in order to achieve change, progressing from a point when the existence of the problem is not recognized to gradually preparing to take action. While this approach was not designed with the management of hearing loss as its inspiration, it can easily be seen how patients may take years before they finally agree to wear hearing aids or amplification. During that period of time, they are progressing through the changes until they reach the point when they finally agree to take action. The audiologist can more effectively counsel their patients by having an understanding of where the person's beliefs lie within the change process.

The importance of counseling cannot be overemphasized. It is at the heart and soul of PCC and shared decision making. But one must remember the ultimate goal is not that a patient agrees to obtain hearing aids or a sensory aid, but rather, that he/she takes control of the hearing loss and does whatever is necessary to manage communication successfully. For some, it is clear that hearing aids are the solution, but for others, an amplified telephone or infrared system for the television may be the only technology that is needed. Still, for others whose audiogram suggests candidacy for amplification, there is likelihood that the hearing aid will remain in the nightstand drawer if the patient has not reached the stage in his/her life that will allow him/her to proceed. The rehabilitation plan established must include a process that enables the audiologist and patient to develop a therapeutic relationship that will enable PCC. That means establishing rapport, obtaining patient trust, eliciting a narrative, demonstrating empathy and, probably most important, listening to what the patient says. Once this critical foundation is created, the rehabilitation plan can progress to include sensory aids, hearing assistive technology systems, communication repair strategies, individual and group interventions, auditory training, speechreading, and, of course, continued counseling.

GOALS OF COMMUNICATION THERAPY

The overall goal of AR is improvement in communication. The audiologist or SLP, in working with the person with hearing loss, will provide a number of tools to assist in the development of skills toward improvement in coping with communication breakdown. In order to combat the combined deleterious effects of a sensory deficit with an often adverse acoustic environment, suboptimal lighting, distance from a speaker, conversational challenges stemming from poor speaker habits, or situational disadvantages, a person with a hearing loss must be prepared to use a variety of techniques to make the best of bad circumstances to attempt to communicate successfully. Learning these skills under the guidance of an audiologist and implementing them on a daily basis will lead to reduction in stress in communication and greater confidence in entering into conversations.

The categories of communication therapy include maximizing visual cues (speechreading/lipreading), improving utilization of the auditory channel (auditory training), training in how to respond in the event of communication failures (communication therapy), and, when applicable, therapy for those who suffer from tinnitus (tinnitus management). These types of therapy may be provided in individual or group settings, but the interpersonal or communication treatments especially lend themselves to a group model and have been widely applied in self-help programs, such as Hearing Loss Association of America (*see* hearingloss.org).

UTILIZATION OF VISION: SPEECHREADING/LIPREADING

Acquiring information from the visual channel entails reading gestures, body language, facial expression, contextual cues, environmental information, and speechreading. The person attempting to speechread must combat a host of factors that degrade the visibility of the visual communication signal. As seen in Table 31.1, these factors relate to the environment in which the conversation takes place as well as to the characteristics of the communication partner.

Boothroyd[21] referred to speechreading as "...a process of perceiving spoken language using vision as the source of sensory evidence...". The ability to read lips is severely limited by the rapidity of normal speech (13 speech sounds per second) and the poor visibility of most speech sounds (only 29% of speech is visible).[22] Training in the recognition of easily confused sound categories (visemes), such as those in Table 31.2, may be done in a word recognition or sentence recognition context. Visually confusable words are known as homophenes. The goal of such training is to have the participant recognize the visual categories and understand that some confusions may be resolved by eliminating homophenes that do not make sense from a linguistic viewpoint. Therapy will proceed from highly visible to less visible phonemes and work toward increasing recognition speed and accuracy.

The act of speechreading draws upon a larger linguistic knowledge for an adult with a background of having had hearing and language learning in the past. So, using

Table 31.1: Factors that adversely affect visual communication

Factors	
Environmental variables	• Poor lighting • Lighting that places the speaker's face in shadow • Sun or light source in speechreader's face • Positioning at an unfavorable angle (>45°) • Distance >20 feet • Visual barriers
Speaker variables	• Facial hair (beards or moustaches) • Chewing gum • Smoking • Extraneous gestures or putting hands near/in front of mouth • Holding hand(s) in front of mouth • Exaggerated articulation • Insufficient mouth movement • Foreign accent • Rapid speech • Thin lips • Facing or turning away from communication partner • Speaking from the side of the mouth • Gender of the speaker (females better perceived) • Complex sentence structure

contextual cues, it is possible to understand the sentence "Fry the egg in the *pan*" without confusing the word "pan" with its homophenes (from Table 31.2) "*man*" and "*ban*". For the child acquiring language through an impaired auditory system, and using vision as a modality to supplement diminished input through sensory device(s), the task is entirely different because he or she is in the process of learning a lexicon and the rules of syntax simultaneously while learning the process of lipreading.

Training methods involve encouraging the speechreader to follow the gist of the conversation, rather than relying on a word-for-word understanding. This is referred to as a synthetic approach. At the same time, this dynamic method is supplemented by drills that increase the patient's speed and accuracy of comprehension, both for single words and for sentences, which is a more analytic approach.

A practice technique that has gained wide use is speechtracking[23] in which the speechreader shadows the clinician and must repeat read materials accurately; records are kept of the number of words per minute that the patient is able to repeat in a trial, which may consist of

Table 31.2: Examples of visemic sounds and homophenous words. These sounds or words will appear equivalent on the lips when spoken without voice or below the level of a person's threshold of hearing

Visemes	*Homophenous words*
/m, b, p/	Baby, maybe
/f,v/	Rope, robe
/n, t, d/	Man, ban, pan
/l,r,w/	Mom, bomb
/k,g/	Mail, pail, bail
	Lab, lamb

lipreading-only stimulation, and other modalities as well (auditory-only, or combined auditory-visual stimulation). Speechtracking is a vehicle for teaching the patient and communication partner repair strategies (*see* below and Table 31.5) to cope with a situation when there is a failure to lipread accurately. After experiencing several sessions of speechtracking, the speechreader becomes more efficient and increases the number of words per minute that can be tracked.

MAXIMIZING THE AUDITORY CHANNEL: AUDITORY TRAINING

The act of applying a sensory aid (be it a hearing aid, osseointegrated device, cochlear implant or something as yet to be conceived) does not imply that the person using it will be able to obtain full benefit from the signal provided for a variety of reasons. Though we often talk about limitations in the neural survival that may impose restrictions on signal encoding, auditory training may allow improvement in performance with a device despite distortions imposed by the auditory system. There is strong evidence that auditory training is effective in changing behavior (*see* Sweetow & Palmer[24] for a comprehensive review of the literature.)

The levels of function that are targeted in an auditory training program are outlined and defined in Table 31.3. As seen in this hierarchy, a person with a hearing loss may initially have poor sound awareness on a reliable basis despite the signals being presented at a loud enough (i.e. suprathreshold) level. With training, however, the reliability of that awareness will increase and it is possible to proceed through the hierarchy to be able to discriminate stimuli, such as two-syllable versus three-syllable words reliably. Once that level of skill is mastered, recognizing words in isolation or in sentences would be the next goal. Finally, comprehending connected discourse would be the long-term objective.

Table 31.3: Levels of auditory function and auditory training progression

Easy	Awareness	Can tell that a sound is present; cannot necessarily describe its characteristics
↓	Discrimination	Can tell that two sounds are different from each other; may not be able to recognize or repeat either sound
↓	Identification	Can tell what the sound is
Difficult	Comprehension	Can understand the sound and its implications

Many persons with hearing loss begin at a level that is apparently initially higher than described in the scenario above. Such individuals may have satisfactory function in quiet, but experience significantly reduced performance in adverse listening situations (as well as perceiving significant activity restrictions and participation limitations or handicap). As indicated in Table 31.4, well-recognized factors that degrade the auditory signal are background noise, reverberation (echo), and competing speech, among others. An auditory training program teaches the patient (1) to manipulate the environment to reduce these adverse conditions whenever possible and (2) through practice, to perform better under such challenges as progressively increasing signal-to-noise ratios.

Individualized, one-on-one therapy may be supplemented by the use of materials that have been generated to permit the person with hearing loss to develop or practice skills independently. Programs for practicing lipreading or auditory skills are widely available for use with home computers. Among these programs, Seeing and Hearing Speech[25] Read My Quips[26] and Conversation Made Easy[27] provide training in both auditory and visual domains.

One of the most widely used and validated programs is the Listening and Communication Enhancement (LACE).[28] As initially described by Sweetow and Henderson Sabes,[29] this program has the goal of "...better comprehension of degraded speech, enhancement of cognitive skills, and improvement of communication strategies" (p. 243). The recommended practice regimen is 30 minutes per day for 5 days per week for 4 weeks (10 hours total). During the LACE program, the patient listens to three types of degraded signals: time compressed speech, as a practice for rapid conversation; speech with a multitalker babble background; and speech with a single competing speaker background. The program also contains routines for increasing auditory memory and processing speed, as well as developing improved communication strategies.

Table 31.4: Factors that adversely affect auditory signal transmission

Factors	
Environmental variables	• Background noise • Competing speech • Reverberation (echo) • Distance (affects intensity of direct signal and, thereby, signal-to-noise ratio) • Physical barriers • Sun or fluorescent light source (may affect performance of assistive listening device)
Speaker variables	• Fundamental frequency of voice • Spectrum of speech (females or children may be poorly perceived in high-frequency hearing loss) • Habitual loudness of voice • Rapid speech • Complex sentence structure • Foreign accent • Inadequate/substandard articulation

Use of music in auditory training has been discussed by several authors.[30-32] Music may be a means of teaching rhythm or intonation to children with hearing loss.[30] Musical timbre is poorly represented in current cochlear implants[33-36] while temporal envelope cues are more accessible.[37] Gfeller et al.[33] showed that timbre recognition was amenable to training, leading to the possibility that patients motivated to improve aspects of their musical perception may be able to do so with intervention. Musical enjoyment is also of great importance to adult cochlear implant users in enhancing quality of life.[38,39] Less systematic research has explored the satisfaction of hearing aid users in regard to music.

COMMUNICATION TRAINING

Given a successful fitting with a hearing aid or other sensory device and active engagement with counseling about methods to improve communication, one of the dimensions that will be addressed is how to deal with occurrences of communication failure. Given the limited visibility of speech sounds, the environmental and speaker variables that may limit the visibility (*see* Table 31.2) or the acoustic transmission (Table 31.4) of the communication signals, it is understandable that instances of inadequate reception or misunderstanding may occur multiple times during any conversation. It is necessary for the person with a hearing loss and his/her communication partner to learn methods to "work through" such misunderstandings.

Table 31.5 summarizes a series of techniques that may be used to repair communication breakdowns.[40] These strategies are used in a communication partnership in which a cooperative speaker is modifying his/her message, not in its content, but in its method of presentation, when the partner with hearing loss indicates misunderstanding or responds inappropriately in conversation. Thus, when there has been a communication failure, the speaker has options other than only repeating verbatim what was just said. She might, e.g. simplify the sentence or rephrase it, or give a key word in order to get meaning to be clarified.

Another component of communication training is teaching Clear Speech[41] to communication partners, as well as training the person with hearing loss how to instruct others in what actions enhance the clarity of speech. As listed in Table 31.6, Clear Speech is a sensible approach to communication with a person with hearing loss. It entails slow presentation rate, normal articulation, and phrasing in reasonable length sentences.

Suggesting to a communication partner, sometimes a stranger, that he/she modifies speaking style as an accommodation for your hearing loss demands assertiveness. Requesting such accommodations is not natural to most people. Asking a speaker to face you or rephrase a difficult sentence requires the person with hearing loss to be willing to engage with both familiar and unknown persons about what modifications in conversational behavior will make it easier to communicate. Therefore, one aspect of communication therapy is reinforcing the use of appropriate assertiveness, a difficult change in behavior that requires practice in many venues, and which the audiologist will guide in development. In most instances, patients with hearing loss who are seen for therapeutic communication training typically use some form of amplification.

Table 31.5: Repair strategies

Repair strategies
Repeat the sentence
Simplify
Rephrase
Give a keyword
Select a more visible alternative word
Provide a definition of the difficult word
Break information up into two sentences

Source: Based on Tye-Murray.[40]

AMPLIFICATION IN REHABILITATION

In many cases, amplification is an integral step in the treatment of hearing loss. More so than at any other time in history, there is a greater variety of amplification options available. This includes not only a tremendous array of hearing aid styles, circuit types, and processing schemes from a wide variety of manufacturers but also a proliferation of assistive listening devices (ALDs) that function either independently of, or in conjunction with hearing aids, often employing either FM or Bluetooth technology. Hearing aid technology is continually changing, and the last 10 years have been no exception. From smaller physical size to better, more sophisticated processing algorithms, the ultimate goal is always to provide greater benefit for the hearing aid user.[42]

Hearing Aids

Generally speaking, hearing aid styles are named on the basis of how they are worn and their physical size. The choice of hearing aid style should be made based on factors such as gain/power requirements, physical features of the ear canal (size, contour, etc.), ease of insertion and manipulation, need for specific features (directional

Table 31.6: Elements of clear speech

Element	*Error made in uncontrolled conversation*	*Clear speech approach*
Rate	Rapid	Slowed (not labored) presentation
Phrasing	May ignore sentence breaks or continue with run-on sentences	Pauses interjected at ends of phrases or sentences
Articulation	Slurred or exaggerated	Natural articulation with an aim at clear pronunciation
Loudness	Too soft, or when attempting to compensate for a person with hearing loss, too loud	Natural presentation at a moderately loud level but not shouted
Emphasis on key points in sentences	Emphasis may be haphazard	Emphasis on key words

microphones, telecoil, etc.), physical comfort and occlusion considerations, and cosmetic concerns.[43] Currently, the most common styles of hearing aids are behind-the-ear (BTE), in-the-ear (ITE), and over-the-ear (OTE) types. Although eyeglass and body aid style devices are still available, they account for a minor percentage (<1%) of hearing aids sold.[44]

The circuitry for the BTE style hearing aid (Fig. 31.3) is contained in an instrument behind the ear, and is usually offered in an assortment of colors, shapes, and sizes. This case is attached via a small length of tubing to a custom-shaped earmold. Currently, hearing aid manufacturers also offer a "mini-BTE", a somewhat smaller and more cosmetically appealing variant. BTE hearing aids are frequently preferred when working with young children because, as the child grows, only the earmold needs to be replaced periodically to accommodate the change in the physical dimensions of the growing ear.[42] This is a significant cost advantage as compared to replacing an entire custom hearing aid every few months. Additionally, the physical size of the BTE permits the use of larger components, making them capable of fitting the widest range of all the styles.[42] Therefore, they are often the best choice for severely- or profoundly impaired patients, although they are suitable for all magnitudes of impairment. The BTE's larger physical size as well (as the larger size of the battery) may also be easier to handle than smaller styles for patients who have limited manual dexterity or who suffer from visual deficits. Some patients, however, may find BTE hearing aids more difficult to manipulate because they are composed of three components (hearing aid, earmold, and tubing) instead of one component, as is the case for other styles.[45] Additionally, there are many FM and direct auditory input options (to be discussed later) available on BTEs.[42] Patients with cosmetic concerns may be dissatisfied with the larger size of BTE hearing aids.

The ITE style hearing aid (Fig. 31.4) is one piece and fits directly into the external ear. The circuitry is contained in the concha in the case of a full shell or half shell size instrument. For smaller sized instruments, the circuitry is contained in the canal portion. Ongoing reduction in the size of circuit components makes it possible to manufacture hearing aids today that are smaller than ever and rest completely in the ear canal (completely-in-the-canal, or CIC). CIC instruments are typically considered by many to be more cosmetically acceptable than BTE or full ITE instruments.[42] Additionally, the deeper receiver placement possible in many of these hearing aids may result in increased sound pressure level at the eardrum compared with other styles.[42,46] For some patients, the ITE style may be easier to handle than the BTE style, because all components are integrated into a one-piece shell.[45] However, individual variations in ear canal anatomy and size may preclude some patients from wearing ITEs comfortably, if at all. Furthermore, it is not possible to use accessories such as FM boots with ITE hearing aids.

The OTE style hearing aid (Fig. 31.5) is a relatively new contender in the marketplace, coming into popularity in the last 10 years. This style is also referred to as an "open-fit" hearing aid, since it is does not occlude the external auditory canal. The OTE hearing aid is a mini-BTE, with its smaller body positioned closer to the top of

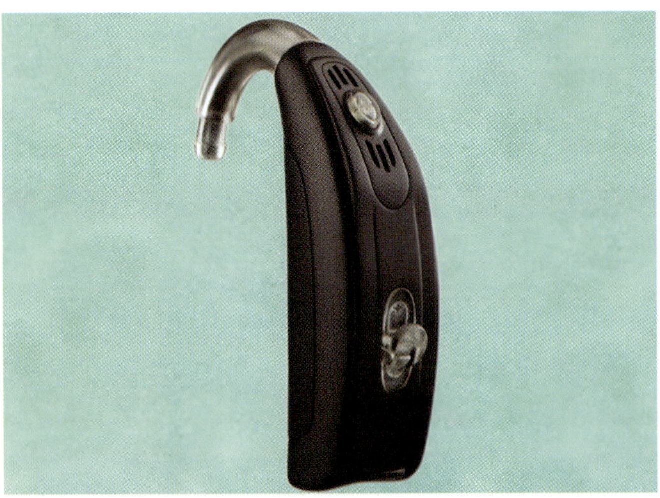

Fig. 31.3: Behind-the-ear (BTE) hearing aid. Photo courtesy of Unitron Hearing.

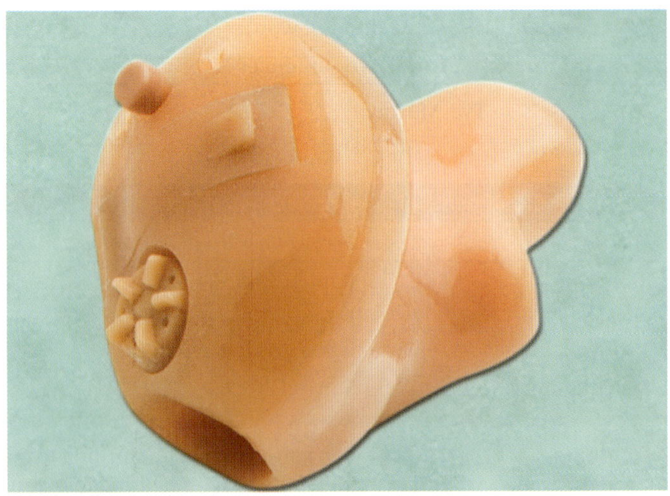

Fig. 31.4: In-the-ear (ITE) hearing aid. Photo courtesy of Unitron Hearing.

the pinna. Instead of using tubing to attach an earmold to the main housing of the device, the OTE uses a very thin wire with an active receiver attached (receiver-in-the-ear, RITE) or a slim-tube at the end that is positioned in the external auditory canal. The receiver's position in the ear canal is maintained with a soft, lightweight and typically non-occluding dome. This style has several advantages. First, since the ear canal usually remains open, more low-frequencies escape the ear canal, including the patient's own voice, and the patient experiences less occlusion effect.[47] Secondly, the receiver wire element is usually modular and can be replaced in-office rather than being sent to the factory for repair. Third, these devices are smaller and lighter than the other styles, and are usually the least conspicuous. However, they are not suitable for severely or profoundly impaired patients due to their relatively limited power.[48] It is worth noting, however, that many manufacturers now offer higher power receivers as an option. These receivers, in combination with more occluding dome styles or earmolds, can in many cases allow more severely impaired patients to use this style hearing aid.

Nearly all hearing aids available today employ digital signal processing. Most manufacturers have discontinued the production of analog circuits because it is cheaper to produce and repair digital circuits.[44] Digital signal processing has several advantages over analog. For example, advancements in chip technology have allowed a reduction in circuit size and faster processing speeds than ever before.[42] Another advantage is that current digital devices have lower power consumption than their predecessors.[49] Most significantly, and in contrast to their analog counterparts, digital hearing aids use algorithms to perform complex manipulations of the signal, allowing virtually unlimited flexibility without a change in hardware. These manipulations, which can often be performed within multiple individual channels, include gain adjustment, compression or expansion, feedback reduction, digital noise reduction (filtering), frequency shifting, and speech enhancement or extraction. This flexibility allows for digital hearing aids to be customized to specific hearing losses and specific environments.[42] Finally, data logging features enable hearing aids to compile and store information about hearing aid usage time, listening environments, percentage of time each program has been used, characteristics of input signals, and user adjustments. These data may be useful for improving fitting outcomes and troubleshooting, although there remains little objective evidence to support this notion.

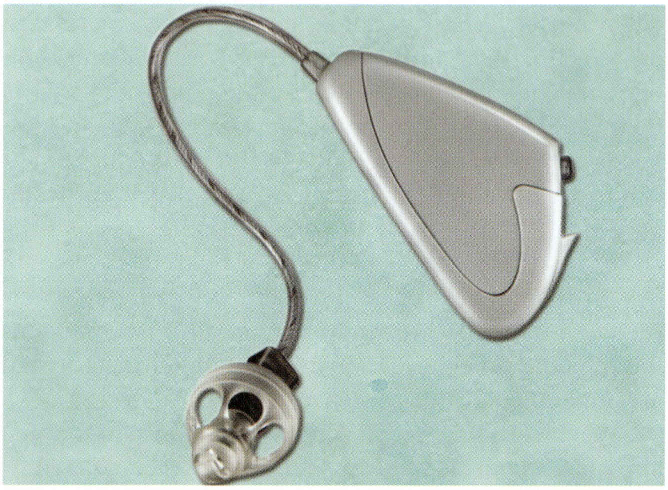

Fig. 31.5: Over-the-ear (OTE) hearing aid. Photo courtesy of Unitron Hearing.

One of the most prevalent issues reported by hearing aid users is difficulty understanding speech in noisy situations.[50,51] Despite initial expectation and promise, digital noise reduction has not been shown to improve speech intelligibility scores in noise.[51] Therefore, in an attempt to address this persistent problem, most modern hearing aids include directional microphone technology, which has been shown to improve signal-to-noise ratio.[52] The primary exception to this is the CIC style instrument, whose faceplate is physically too small to accommodate the requisite two-microphone array. Directional microphone technology is recommended for patients who experience difficulty understanding speech in noise because it maintains sensitivity to sounds coming from in front of the listener while reducing sensitivity to sounds arising from other directions.[53] By contrast, the omnidirectional microphone does not improve signal to noise ratio because it has the same sensitivity for sounds from all directions, and is therefore incapable of favoring sounds from the front. It is important to remember that directional microphone technology also has some disadvantages. For example, they are more sensitive to wind noise, and can reduce available volume in the hearing aid. Therefore, there will be some situations for which each of the two microphone technologies is preferred, and many hearing aids are designed to switch between them either manually or automatically.

Acoustic feedback occurs when the amplified sound output from a hearing aid receiver reenters the microphone port of the hearing aid. As a consequence, the signal received by the microphone is re-amplified and will begin to oscillate. Leakage of the feedback signal can be either acoustic through the vent or poor fit, or electrical through the components of the hearing aid.[54] In the past, reducing feedback in hearing aids usually entailed some combination of high-frequency gain reduction, decreasing vent size, remaking or recoating the earmold or shell. These measures often substantially limited the amount of amplification available to the hearing aid user, and resulted in a reduction of benefit from the aid. Modern digital circuitry attempts to prevent feedback by reducing gain more selectively around the offending frequency through notch filtering, frequency shifting, negative feedback/phase cancellation, and other adaptive measures.[47] While acoustic feedback remains problematic in some cases, it is now much less a limiting factor.

CROS/BiCROS Hearing Aids

A contralateral-routing-of-signals (CROS) hearing aid system consists of a pair of hearing aids where one aid contains only a microphone and transmitter, and the other contains the amplifier, signal processing circuitry, and receiver. A cable connected older style CROS instruments, but in recent years the transmission is accomplished wirelessly. A patient is considered a candidate for a CROS hearing aid system if he or she has one good hearing ear and one ear where the loss is so great or the word recognition so poor that the ear is considered "unaidable", that is, a hearing aid will provide no benefit.[55] The principle of the CROS system is to bring sounds arriving at the poorer ear to the better ear. A BiCROS system also features a microphone and amplifier on the receiver side, and is used in cases where the better ear also has some degree of impairment.

ALDs/Bluetooth Options

ALDs are a broad category of devices designed to either expand the functionality of hearing aids, or provide assistance independently of hearing aids. These devices exist to help hearing-impaired listeners overcome difficulties such as hearing distant speech, understanding speech in noisy environments, listening in environments with poor room acoustics or reverberation, or some combination of these.[4] Examples of ALDs include amplified telephones, TV listeners, and alerting devices such as specialized smoke alarms, doorbells, and alarm clocks. Currently, the most development has been in the area of Bluetooth wireless technology, which uses radio waves to transmit and receive information within the user's personal space, up to 164 feet. This relatively small operating distance is in contrast to other types of radio technology, such as FM, cellular phones, and television, which are designed to broadcast many people over much greater distances.[56] Applications of Bluetooth technology with hearing aids include wireless "streaming" of cell phone signals to hearing aids, the use of remote wireless microphones to overcome problems of distant speech or speech in noise, and wireless transmission of TV sound to hearing aids. In addition to Bluetooth technology, FM, infrared, and induction or hearing loop systems are available. These technologies use radio waves, light waves, or magnetic fields, respectively, to transmit the desired signal to the hearing instruments.

Another application of wireless technology is binaural linkage wherein two hearing aids fitted bilaterally are in communication with one another. The goal of this application is to improve binaural hearing and sound quality through synchronization and comparison of sound arriving at each ear, and also to facilitate ease of use by enabling simultaneous activation of controls such as volume, and program adjustments.

EVALUATION

Evaluation for hearing instrument candidacy typically involves the completion of diagnostic testing (i.e. tonal and speech audiometry, immittance measures), procurement of medical clearance against contraindications for amplification (abnormalities of the external auditory canal, infections, etc.), and a thorough counseling session to assess the patient's individual needs.[57] In the past, the "Carhart method" was used; however, this method of briefly auditioning several different BTE circuits has largely fallen out of favor. Nowadays, more emphasis is placed on selecting hearing instruments and assistive technology that will allow the patient to function to the best of their ability given their particular hearing loss, lifestyle needs and demands, and in consideration of any physical or cognitive limitations that exist with that particular patient. Handicap scales and questionnaires, such as the HHIE and the Abbreviated Profile of Hearing Aid Benefit (APHAB)[58] may be used, or the examining audiologist may prefer an interview format. Items typically discussed during the hearing aid evaluation appointment include, but are not limited to, those listed in Table 31.7.

When selecting amplification, it is important that the audiologist consider each patient's needs as indicated by personal preference, lifestyle demands, and the individual's physical and cognitive limitations. This is often best accomplished by eliciting input and comments from the patient's family members or friends, who should be encouraged to attend all hearing aid-related appointments. These individuals are often helpful to the audiologist in addressing and overcoming any objections, resistance, or uncertainties that the patient may have about hearing aids. The items listed in Table 31.7 should, ideally, serve as a springboard for further discussion and elaboration, and should not be used simply as a checklist of topics to be discussed during the hearing aid evaluation.

FITTING

The hearing aid fitting session is where the actual programming, orientation, and dispensing of the hearing aids takes place. The audiologist will input the patient's audiometric data into the hearing aid manufacturer's fitting software and configure the instruments to the patient's individual needs. This configuration includes the provision of one or more program variations (i.e. a "quiet" listening program, a "restaurant", or noisy environment program), activation of the telecoil, activation of various auditory indicators (signals for low battery, program change, etc.), and activation of the feedback reduction parameters. After this takes place, the audiologist may ask the patient several questions about the sound quality and comfort of the hearing instruments. These questions will address such issues as the sound of their own voice (the occlusion effect), overall loudness of the instruments, relative loudness of one hearing instrument to the other, physical comfort of the devices, etc. Depending on the patient's responses to these questions, various adjustments will typically be made in the programming software, and possibly to the physical device itself (e.g. changing venting, physical alteration of the shell or earmold, and changing dome size or receiver wire length). At this time, a demonstration of the various auditory indicators for low battery status, program changes, and other functions will also take place.

Next, the patient will be trained in the use and daily care of the hearing instruments. Topics typically discussed at this time include: a review of the basic components of the hearing aid, insertion and removal of the battery, differentiation of right versus left instruments, cleaning and maintenance the hearing aids, insertion and removal of

Table 31.7: Items to be discussed at hearing aid evaluation appointment

The patient's hearing loss	• A review of the type, magnitude, and severity of the patient's hearing loss as shown on the audiogram • Review of the patient's word recognition scores • Discussion of how the patient's hearing loss may limit outcomes (i.e. realistic expectations and size or style of instrument that is appropriate)
Preconceived notions about amplification	• Does the patient have past experience with amplification? • Does the patient have any opinions about amplification? • Has the patient talked to friends or family about amplification? • Does the patient have past experience with amplification?
The patient's individual needs/lifestyle issues	• Does the patient have difficulty hearing at work? • Does the patient have difficulty with TV? • Does the patient have difficulty talking on the telephone? • Does the patient have difficulty in noisy environments, such as restaurants? • Is there a particular group of people that the patient has more difficulty hearing than others? • Does the patient believe they have a hearing problem, or are they primarily discussing amplification at the urging of family members or friends? • Does the patient have trouble understanding distant speech? • Are there any other problems the patient is experiencing, such as reduced enjoyment of music? • Does the patient have any physical limitations that may affect the type of hearing aid that will fit into the ear (i.e. physical size of pinna or ear canal)? • Does the patient have any limitations with vision or manual dexterity that might make it difficult to handle the hearing aid or the batteries? • Is the patient's comfort level with technology a limiting factor in the selection of accessories for the hearing aid, or selection of the hearing aid style itself?
Price levels and technology	• An overview of the benefits of technology available at different price levels • A recommendation of which technology level/price level of instrument would be the most suitable for the patient's needs • A recommendation of whether or not additional assistive accessories are warranted at this time

instruments into the ear, battery safety, and storage, and strategies for troubleshooting. Training on the use of other assistive equipment that accompanies the hearing aids should also take place at this time.

Lastly, a discussion of acclimatization to the new hearing instruments and realistic expectations regarding outcomes must occur. Despite the numerous advances in hearing aids and assistive technology as described above, there are still limitations that exist when fitting this equipment. While it is safe to assume that most patients will benefit from such technology, it is nonetheless important to remember that outcomes will still typically be at least somewhat suboptimal when compared to normal hearing. For example, for most patients, hearing and comprehension of speech in the presence of background noise remains a challenge.[50,51] so that other strategies, such as speechreading, must be employed. Additionally, many hearing aid wearers still complain of loudness recruitment, direction dependent performance, and unnatural sound quality from their hearing instruments. For these and many other reasons, it is important to counsel patients that their expectations must be realistic.

FOLLOW-UP/PROBLEMS

A significant portion of the cost of hearing aids is due to the intensive research and development on the part of the manufacturers, who, among other things, attempt to assure a comfortable and effective initial fitting of the hearing instruments. Despite this, most follow-up appointments for hearing aid fittings will include adjustments to the sound quality and behavior of the hearing aids that are based on comments, complaints, and concerns voiced by the patient. Although the initial fitting parameters are generally within an accepted range of efficacy, it is unrealistic to expect that a single formula will be suitable for all patients. Differences in personality, expectations, physiology, and etiology of hearing impairment, lifestyle, and other factors all influence the patient's level of satisfaction and success with the initial fitting. Therefore, due to these factors, as well as other problems that may occur, the follow-up session after the initial fitting will usually involve making further refinements in the manufacturer's fitting software to address the patient's needs. Real-ear measures, as well as soundfield testing, and other verification measures can assist the audiologist with the decision making behind these adjustments. Furthermore, the patient may report issues such as physical discomfort of the hearing instruments in the ear canal, problems or difficulties with cleaning and maintenance, changes in motivation or attitude towards hearing instruments, frustration or disappointment with early outcomes, or the arising of other issues or circumstances that were unforeseen previously. Often times, these issues can be resolved in one or two follow-up sessions, although for a smaller percentage of the patient population, multiple visits may be required to arrive at a satisfactory outcome. The hearing aid fitting process does not end with technical adjustments. Ongoing counseling and support, albeit time consuming, is central to the continued success.

TINNITUS MANAGEMENT

Audiologic rehabilitation for tinnitus may take many forms. (The reader is also referred to Chapter 20, which addresses tinnitus treatment from many perspectives.) The audiologic component of a tinnitus treatment program should be seen in a team approach that entails medical, dental, psychological, neurologic, physical therapy, and other specialists.[59] It is assumed that all of these assessments take place following a comprehensive audiologic evaluation including pure tone and speech audiometry, immittance measurements (i.e. tympanometry, acoustic reflex thresholds, and reflex decay), otoacoustic emissions, and auditory brainstem response measurement and such neurotologic evaluation as demanded by the presentation.

Assessment of the severity of tinnitus annoyance and the components of a tinnitus evaluation are summarized in Table 31.8. It is necessary to determine a description of the patient's functional disruption by his tinnitus. This may be accomplished through in-depth interview that touches on the impact that tinnitus has on the individual's lifestyle, hearing, emotional status, and general health. Previous attempts to address tinnitus therapeutically should be revealed during the interview as well. The impact of these issues can be probed further through measurement of his or her activity restrictions and participation limitations using questionnaires that have known psychometric qualities, such as the Tinnitus Handicap Inventory (THI)[60] or the Tinnitus Functional Index (TFI).[61] Due to its ease of administration and high test-retest reliability, the THI is the most widely used tinnitus questionnaire, translated and validated into a number of languages.[62] An extensive review of tinnitus handicap measurement can be found in Newman et al.[63] Magnitude estimation of tinnitus is often performed using direct estimation or visual analog scales for loudness (e.g. ranging from 0 for "very quiet" to 10 for "very loud") or for pitch. This approach has been suggested as a step to allow the patient a means to quantify his symptom in a manner that is understandable from his perspective.[64]

A formal tinnitus evaluation is composed of audiologic measures under earphones. The components of a tinnitus evaluation include pitch matching, loudness matching, determining a minimum masking level, trials to determine if, in addition to masking, residual inhibition can be achieved, and, finally, measurement of loudness discomfort levels for pure tones or broadband stimuli including speech. Such evaluation is complicated by the likelihood that the patient's tinnitus is not a tonal signal but instead a complex combination that is not precisely comparable to that produced by audiometric equipment. Additionally, there is the possibility the evaluation may reveal that the tinnitus believed to be unilateral was in fact bilateral of asymmetric loudness or nonequivalent in some other dimensions, As a result, judgments are difficult for the patient. Failure to obtain residual inhibition during the formal tinnitus assessment does not preclude effective use of sound therapies.

Sound therapy refers to application of a wide range of devices that provide an enriched sound environment and relief from tinnitus. It has been known for many years that, for people with hearing loss and tinnitus, wearing a hearing aid may provide relief from tinnitus annoyance. There are many other devices and strategies that can substantially improve the tinnitus sufferer's day-to-day experience. Some of these devices are generic sound generators while others, like hearing aids, tinnitus maskers and tinnitus habituation devices, can only be obtained by audiologist prescription. The selection of the most appropriate device for a given individual is the outcome of intensive counseling and the review of options. The options will also include the type of masker to be employed, which may vary from noises to natural sounds to modified musical applications.

Two trends in customized sound therapy exist for motivated persons with severe tinnitus. These two trends, the use of tinnitus masking versus the approach of tinnitus habituation or retraining, employ signals to be present at the same time as the person's tinnitus. Both of these

Table 31.8: Components of tinnitus evaluation

Component	*Purpose*
Interview	Determine tinnitus-related impact on: • *Lifestyle*: sleep, persistence of tinnitus, pattern, relationship to noise exposure (past and current), impact on social relationships, current practices relating to quiet environments; • Hearing effects, such as speech understanding; • Emotional consequences, such as frustration, depression, changes in concentration, confusion, worry; • *Impact on general health*: use or dependence on drugs, headaches
Handicap assessment or assessment of participation limitations	• Use of self-report questionnaires for detailed review of impact of tinnitus on activities of daily life Examples: • Tinnitus Handicap Inventory (THI)[60] • Tinnitus Functional Index (TFI)[61]
Magnitude estimation of loudness	• Use of visual analog scales to quantity patient's degree of perceived loudness
Tinnitus evaluation under earphones	• Pitch matching entails use of pure tones or noise stimuli to derive a match or near match to perceived tinnitus • Loudness matching involves establishing an intensity which the patient states is comparable to the loudness of his/her tinnitus, usually within 10 dB of his threshold at that frequency • Minimal masking level involves a trial attempting to mask the person's tinnitus with an effective masker, usually a narrow band or broad band signal produced by the audiometer • Trial to measure residual inhibition is an attempt to measure whether the masker produces a time period of cessation (inhibition) or reduction in perceived tinnitus after withdrawal of the masker • Measurement of loudness discomfort levels is assessment of maximal levels that should not be exceeded in employing sound therapy devices

approaches employ sound generators in their therapeutic techniques, but there are essential differences in intent. In the application of tinnitus masking, sound generators are worn with the purpose of covering the person's tinnitus either completely or partially. The expectation in this approach is that the tinnitus sufferer will obtain relief from his symptom as soon as he begins to wear the masker device. This is to be contrasted with tinnitus habituation or retraining therapy[65] in which a process of adjustment to a (lower level or partial) masking is required over a period of 18–24 months. Through counseling, the patient learns that tinnitus is a nonthreatening signal and emotional responses are diminished; during this time, the brain is thought to readjust its limbic responses to the negative stimulation of the tinnitus.

Decades of experience with cochlear implants have opened the tantalizing possibility of the use of electrical stimulation specifically for the treatment of tinnitus. Whereas we have seen electrical stimulation provide relief in many instances, there is still uncertainty as to the proper selection criteria for candidates that will permit the maximal desired effect for this treatment modality. As audiologists will be involved in evaluation, postimplantation programming, and research to determine such elements as efficacious stimulation parameters, this may be a future tinnitus management that has promise of providing relief for many people.

SUMMARY

The rehabilitation plan for patients with hearing loss varies from individual to individual. Regardless of the degree or nature of hearing loss, it is important to establish a relationship with the patient. This should be conducive to shared decision making so that a rehabilitative plan can be developed. Whether it is a hearing aid fitting, speechreading, or group therapy, goals must be established early in the process and this can only be accomplished by having an understanding of the patient's needs and expectations. The audiogram is merely a start of a sometimes complex patient journey with the audiologist and physician as guiding partners.

REFERENCES

1. ASHA. Definition of and competencies for aural rehabilitation. ASHA. 1984; May:37-41.
2. World Health Organization. International classification of functioning, disability and health. Geneva: World Health Organization; 2001.
3. Montano JJ. Defining audiologic rehabilitation. In: Montano JJ, Spitzer J (Eds.). Adult Audiologic Rehabilitation. San Diego: Plural Publications; 2014; p.23-34.
4. ASHA. Knowledge and skills required for the practice of audiologic/aural rehabilitation. ASHA desk reference. c2001; cited June 4, 2013. Available at http://www.asha.org/uploadedFiles/aud/InfoSeriesAssistiveTechnology.pdf#search=%22ald%22.
5. Erdman SA. The biopsychosocial approach in patient and relationship centered care: Implications for audiologic counseling. In: Montano JJ, Spitzer J (Eds.). Adult Audiological Rehabilitation. San Diego: Plural Publishing; 2014; p.159-206.
6. Bandura A. Social Foundations of Thought and Action: A Social Cognitive Theory. Englewood Cliffs:Prentice Hall; 1986.
7. Bandura A. Self-Efficacy: The Exercise of Control. New York: Freeman; 1997.
8. Patient Protection and Affordable Care Act, 201. Pub. L. No. 111-148, §2702, 124 Stat.; 119:318-9.
9. Erdman SA, Wark D, Montano JJ. Implications of service delivery models in audiology. J Acad Rehabilitat Audiol. 1994;27:45-60.
10. Montano JJ. Building relationships: An important component to the aural rehabilitation process. ENT and Audiology. 2011;20:91-2.
11. Montano JJ. Overdependence on technology in the management of hearing loss. In: Goldfarb R (Ed.). Translational Speech-Language Pathology and Audiology. San Diego: Plural Publishing Inc.; 2012, p.97-106.
12. Gregory M, Jones L, Erdman S, et al. Managing hearing loss: A shared decision making process. ENT Audiol. 2013; 22(2):84-86.
13. Abrams H, Chisolm T. Measuring health-related quality of life in audiologic rehabilitation. In: Montano J, Spitzer J (Eds). Adult Audiologic Rehabilitation. San Diego: Plural Publishing; 2014; p.103-16.
14. Ventry I, Weinstein B. The Hearing Handicap Inventory for the Elderly: A new tool. Ear Hea. 1982;3:128-34.
15. Pietrzyk, P. Counseling Comfort Levels of Audiologists. University of Cincinnati, Capstone Project; 2009 (unpublished).
16. Clark JG, English KE. Effective Counseling in Audiology. Boston: Allyn & Bacon; 2004.
17. Clark JG, English K. Counseling-Infused Audiologic Care. Boston: Allyn & Bacon; 2014.
18. Clark JG, Maatman C, Gailey L. Moving patients forward: motivational engagement. Semin Hear. 2012;33:35-45.
19. Preminger J, Lind C. Assisting communication partners in the setting of treatment goals: The development of the Goal Sharing for Partners Strategy. Semin Hear. 2012;33: 53-64.
20. Prochaska J, DiClemente CC. Self change processes, self efficacy and decisional balance across five stages of smoking cessation. Prog Clin Biol Res. 1984;156:131-40.

21. Boothroyd A. Linguistic factors in speechreading. Volta Review. 1987;90(5):77-88.
22. Jeffers J, Barley M. Speechreading (lipreading). 5th ed. Springfield, IL: Bannerstone. 1971.
23. DeFilippo CL, Scott BL. A method for training and evaluating the reception of ongoing speech. J Acoust Soc Amer. 1978;63:1186-92.
24. Sweetow RW, Palmer CV. Efficacy of individual auditory training in adults: A systematic review of the evidence. J Am Acad Audiol. 2005;16(7):494-504.
25. Boothroyd A. Seeing and hearing speech: lessons in lipreading and listening. Ear Hear. 2003;24(1):96.
26. Sensesynergy. (Read my quips. http://www.sensesynergy.com/, accessed 5/23/2013).
27. Tye-Murray N. Conversation Made Easy: Speechreading and Conversation Strategies Training for People With Hearing Loss. Available at: http://www.cid.edu/Libraries/Misc_Documents/TestCurriculaOrderForm.sflb.ashx Accessed April 30, 2013.
28. Neurotone, Inc. [Internet]. Redwood City: Neurotone, Inc; 2013 [cited May 23, 2013]. Available form :http://www.neurotone.com/
29. Sweetow RW, Sabes J. The need for and development of an adaptive Listening and Communication Enhancement (LACE) Program. J Amer Acad Audiology. 2006;17:538-58.
30. Barton C, Robbins A, Trautwein P. Bringing music to their bionic ears: Nurturing music development in children with cochlear implants. Loud Clear News Adv Bion. 2006;1-6.
31. Chermak G. Music and auditory training. Hearing J. 2010; 63:57-58.
32. Plant G. Music and cochlear implants in audiologic rehabilitation. In: Montano JJ, Spitzer JB (Eds). Adult Audiologic Rehabilitation. San Diego:Plural Publishing, 2014; p.415-30.
33. Gfeller K, Christ A, Knutson JF, et al. Musical backgrounds, listening habits, and aesthetic enjoyment of adult cochlear implant recipients. J Am Acad Audiol. 2000;11: 390–406.
34. Heng J, Cantarero G, Elhilali M, et al. Impaired perception of temporal fine structure and musical timbre in cochlear implant users. Hear Res. 2011;280(1-2):192-200.
35. McDermott HJ, Looi V. Perception of complex signals, including musical sounds, with cochlear implants. In: Miyamoto RT (Ed). Proceedings of the VIII International Cochlear Implant Conference; Indianapolis, IN: Indiana University 2004;201-04.
36. Nimmons GL, Kang RS, Drennan WR, et al. Clinical assessment of music perception in cochlear implant listeners. Otol Neurotol. 2008;29:149-55.
37. Cheng MY, Spitzer JB, Shafiro V, et al. Reliability measure of a clinical test: Appreciation of music in cochlear implantees (AMICI). J Amer Acad Audiol. 2013;24:969-79.
38. Looi V, Winter P, Anderson I, et al. A musical quality rating test battery for cochlear implant users to compare the FSP and HDCIS strategies for music appreciation. Intern J Audiol. 2011;50:503-18.
39. Tyler RS, Gfeller K, Mehr MA. A preliminary investigation comparing one and eight channels at fast and slow rates on musical appraisal in adults with cochlear implants. Cochlear Implants Intern. 2000;1:82-7.
40. Tye-Murray N. Repair strategy usage by hearing-impaired adults and changes following communication therapy. J Speech Hear Res. 1991;34:921-28.
41. Schum DJ. Intelligibility of clear and conversational speech of young and elderly talkers. J Am Acad Audiol. 1996;7(3): 212-18.
42. Bentler R, Wu YH. Developments in hearing aid technology and verification techniques. In: Montano JJ, Spitzer JB (Eds). Adult Audiologic Rehabilitation. San Diego: Plural, 2014; pp.145-67.
43. Valente M, Abrams H, Benson D, et al. Guidelines for the audiologic management of adult hearing impairment. Amer Acad Audiol Task Force, 2007;13-19.
44. Strom K. Hearing aids are not only for old people. Hear Rev. 2007;14(11):8.
45. Singh G. The aging hand and handling of hearing aid: A review. In: Hickson L (Ed). Hearing Care for Adults 2009—The Challenge of Aging. Proceeding of 2nd International Adult Conference. Staefa, Switzerland: Phonak AG. 265-76.
46. Martin R. Deep canal fittings: Acoustics and comfort. Hear J. 2003;56(10):52.
47. Schum, DA. Broader View of Open Fittings. Audiology Online, Course: #19226, recorded August 25, 2011; accessed June 1, 2013.
48. Edwards B. The future of hearing aid technology. Trends Amplif. 2007;11(1):31-46.
49. Stetzler T, Magotra N, Gelabert P, et al. Low-power real-time programmable DSP development platform for digital hearing aids. Texas Instruments Application Report, SPRA 657 2000; (April): 1-20.
50. Chung K. Noise reduction algorithms. Trends Amplif. 2004;8(3):83-124.
51. DiGiovanni JJ, Davlin EA, Nagaraj NK. Effects of transient noise reduction algorithms on speech intelligibility and ratings of hearing aid users. Am J Audiol. 2011;20:140-50.
52. Bentler RA. Effectiveness of directional microphones and noise reduction schemes in hearing aids: A systematic review of the evidence. J Am Acad Audiol. 2005;16(7):473-84.
53. Agnew J. Acoustic feedback and other audible artifacts in hearing aids. Trends Amplif. 1996;1:45-82.
54. Stach B. Comprehensive Dictionary of Audiology. Clifton Park, NY:Thomson Delmar Learning. 2003; p.82.
55. Bluetooth.com, http://www.bluetooth.com/Pages/Fast-Facts.aspx, accessed June 4, 2013.
56. Spitzer JB, Mancuso DM, Cellum IP. Non-surgical alternatives for treatment of single-sided deafness. In: Lalwani LK, Pfister M (Eds). Recent Advances in Otolaryngology—Head and Neck Surgery (Vol.2). New Delhi: Jaypee Publishers; 2013;52-65.
57. American Academy of Audiology. Pre-purchase assessment guideline for amplification devices. Audiol Today. 2000; 12(3):39.

58. Cox RM, Alexander GC. The abbreviated profile of hearing aid benefit. Ear Hear. 1995;16:176-83.
59. Newman CW, Sandridge SA. Tinnitus management. In: Montano JJ, Spitzer JB (Eds). Adult Audiologic Rehabilitation. San Diego:Plural Publishing; 2014.
60. Newman C, Jacobson J, Spitzer JB. Development of the Tinnitus Handicap Inventory. Arch Otolaryng. 1996;122: 143-47.
61. Meikle MB, Henry JA, Griest SE, et al. The Tinnitus Functional Index: development of a new clinical measure for chronic, intrusive tinnitus. Ear Hear. 2012;32: 153-76.
62. Langguth B, Searchfield GD, Biesinger E, et al. History and questionnaires. In: Moller AR, Langguth B, DeRidder D, Kleinjung T (Eds). Textbook of Tinnitus. New York: Springer. 2011;387-404.
63. Newman CW, Sandridge SA, Jacobson GP. Assessing outcomes of tinnitus intervention. J AM Acad Audiol. 2014;25 (1):76-105.
64. Stouffer JL, Tyler RS. Characterization of tinnitus by tinnitus patients. J Speech Hear Dis.1990;55:439-53.
65. Jastreboff PJ, Hazell JW. Tinnitus Retraining Therapy: Implementing the Neurophysiological Model. New York: Cambridge University Press, 2004.

CHAPTER

Implantable Middle Ear and Bone Conduction Devices

32

Alejandro Vázquez, Robert W Jyung

IMPLANTABLE MIDDLE EAR DEVICES

It is estimated that 34.25 million Americans suffer from hearing loss; however, only one in four of these individuals use hearing aids. Although rates of hearing aid adoption have been steadily increasing, the majority of those who could benefit from hearing aid use do not take advantage of it.[1] Even among hearing aid users, dissatisfaction is high (17.3%), and as many as 12.4% of users keep their hearing aids in devices in a drawer.[2] Despite technological advances, conventional hearing aids remain subject to several limitations. The degree of sound amplification, or gain, is limited by acoustic feedback. Tightly fitted hearing aids can minimize feedback, albeit at the expense of canal occlusion, which may result in pain or discomfort, autophony, and otitis externa. Sound fidelity, moreover, is suboptimal, in part because of the occlusion phenomenon and in part because of the sound processing characteristics of the hearing aid itself. Conventional hearing aids are typically optimized to function in the 500- to 2000-Hz range, which corresponds to speech; the lack of upper and lower register amplification, however, can give sounds an artificial, hollow or "tin can" sound. Other important limitations to conventional hearing aids include cost, maintenance, appearance/visibility, and the social or psychological stigma associated with hearing aid use.

The designs of implantable middle ear devices address many of these limitations specifically. Direct coupling to the ossicular should theoretically improve functional gain, reduce distortion, and eliminate the adverse acoustic and clinical effects of canal occlusion. Moreover, in the case of fully implantable devices, the possibility of total implant concealment may overcome the aforementioned psychosocial stigma. One of the major disadvantages of implantable hearing aids, however, is the need to undergo a surgical procedure. In addition to the risks inherent to ear surgery, in some cases the procedure may entail significant surgical alterations to the native middle ear anatomy.

Vibrant Soundbridge (MED-EL Corporation, Innsbruck, Austria)

The Vibrant Soundbridge (VSB), a semi-implantable middle ear device, was invented by Geoffrey Ball, a biomedical engineer with sensorineural hearing loss (SNHL) since childhood (Fig. 32.1). Motivated by his dissatisfaction with

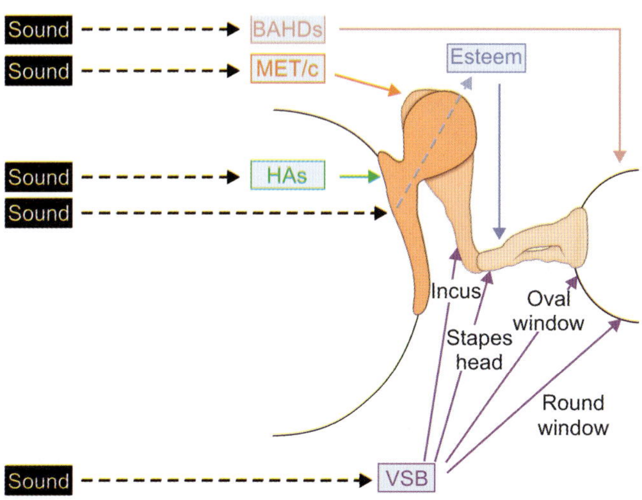

Fig. 32.1: Mechanisms of action of different assistive hearing devices. (BAHDs, bone-anchored hearing devices; HAs, conventional hearing aids; MET/c, middle ear transducer and MET Carina devices. VSB, vibrant Soundbridge).

conventional hearing aids, he developed the concept of a miniature transducer to mimic the vibrations within the middle ear, called "direct drive". This led to his invention of the floating mass transducer (FMT) in 1992, which was patented in 1993. Ultimately, he was one of the first recipients of the VSB and later had a second device implanted in the contralateral ear.[3] The VSB was introduced in Europe in the year 1997 and the United States in 2000. The VSB was initially manufactured by Symphonix Devices, Inc. (San Jose, CA, USA), which declared bankruptcy in 2002 and was subsequently acquired by the MED-EL Corporation (Innsbruck, Austria).

The VSB device consists of an external component, called the audio processor (AP), and an implanted component, termed the vibrating ossicular prosthesis (VORP) (Fig. 32.2A). The AP consists of a microphone, a digital signal processor, and a battery; it is worn on the head behind the ear, where it is held in place by a magnet. The VORP consists of a receiver/stimulator unit, a conductor link, and an electromagnetic FMT. The FMT consists of a coil, a magnet, and an attachment clip designed to clamp onto the long process of the incus. Sound traveling in air is registered by the AP unit, much like a conventional hearing aid. The processed signal is transferred to the VORP via induction, in a manner similar to that of a cochlear implant. The signal then travels along the conductor link to the FMT, which vibrates in a controlled fashion, causing the middle ear structure to which it is coupled to vibrate as well.

The device may be implanted by one of two approaches: a posterior tympanotomy through the facial recess, or a transmeatal approach. The facial recess approach is carried out in a standard fashion, taking care to create an aperture wide enough to accommodate the FMT, a drum-shaped structure 2.3 mm in length and 1.8 mm in diameter. In the transmeatal approach, a tympanomeatal flap is elevated and a longitudinal groove drilled along the inferior aspect of the external auditory canal; the conductor link is laid into the groove, and the redundant length coiled once within a shallow partial mastoidectomy cavity. In both cases, a well (or seat) for the VORP demodulator is drilled using a template, and the unit is secured with sutures (Figs. 32.2B and C).[4,5] Figure 32.3 summarizes the manufacturer's clinical and audiometric selection criteria for implantation.

In 2002, results from the US phase III clinical trial demonstrated statistically significant improvement in functional gain at all frequencies (and >10 dB at 2000, 4000,

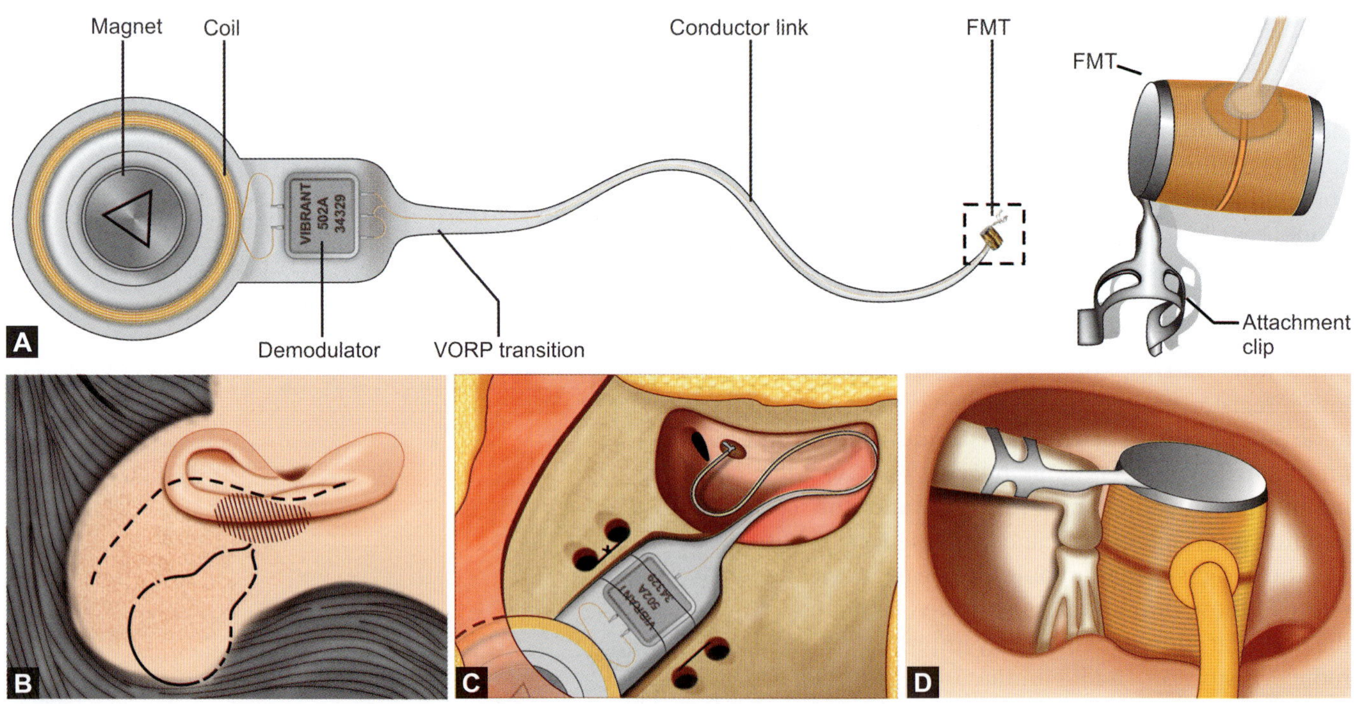

Figs. 32.2A and B: Vibrant Soundbridge. (A) Vibrating ossicular prosthesis (VORP) schematic with close-up view of floating mass transducer (FMT). (B) Approximate location of VORP and standard S-shaped incision. (C) VORP in situ. (D) Placement of FMT in incus vibroplasty.

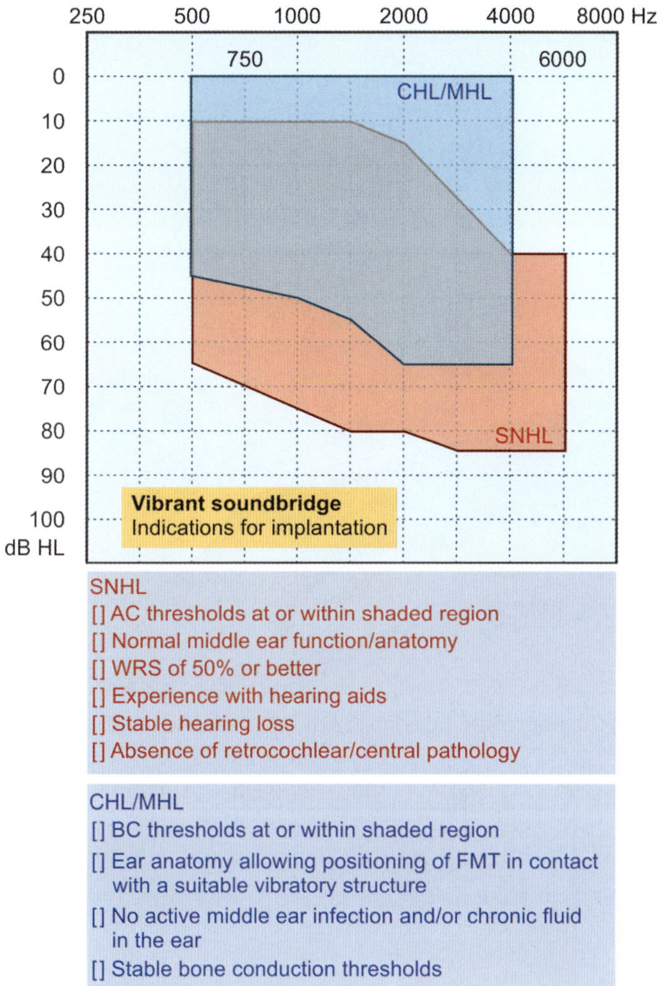

Fig. 32.3: Vibrant Soundbridge: Manufacturer's clinical and audiometric criteria for implantation. (CHL, conductive hearing loss; FMT, floating mass transducer. MHL, mixed hearing loss; SNHL, sensorineural hearing loss).

and 6000 Hz) relative to presurgery-aided hearing for all 53 subjects. Feedback and occlusion were essentially eliminated. Further statistically significant improvements were noted in terms of patient satisfaction and device preference.[6] A 2008 study by Mosnier et al. aimed to provide long-term follow-up data by examining the first 125 patients in France at 5 to 8 years postimplantation (compared with initial follow-up). This study found no change in functional gain for the frequency range of 500 to 4000 Hz and a high satisfaction rate of 77%. Seven patients in this study required reimplantation for device failure; however, failures were only observed in patients implanted before 1999, the year in which the device underwent redesign.[7] In a review of 1000 cases by the manufacturer published in 2005, device failure rates were reported to be 0.3%.[8]

The application of direct vibratory stimulation to middle ear structures (i.e. by way of a middle ear implant) has been termed vibroplasty. Although incus vibroplasty was the intended purpose of the VSB device (Fig. 32.2D), several variations have proved successful. In round window vibroplasty, the FMT is placed against the round window membrane and stimulates it directly. In a retrospective study of 50 patients from 2013, Colletti et al. have demonstrated the safety and efficacy of this technique in patients with moderate to severe mixed hearing loss resulting from a variety of ossicular chain and other middle ear pathologies.[9] A third variation on the vibroplasty involves the use of surgical devices termed couplers. Coupler vibroplasty involves the interposition of a metallic device optimally shaped to fit the round window, oval window, or head of the stapes.[10]

Given the magnetic nature of the FMT, concerns regarding the safety of magnetic resonance imaging (MRI) have been raised. A retrospective questionnaire study by Todt et al. has found noise, middle ear pain, and pressure at the receiver bed to be frequent complaints among VSB implantees undergoing MRI. In two (of thirteen) cases, alterations in FMT position required surgical repositioning via a transtympanic approach. None of the patients experienced SNHL after MRI scanning.[11] Wagner et al. in a review of the literature, found no evidence of injury to middle or inner ear structures as a result of MRI scanning. Furthermore, no cases of FMT demagnetization have been reported. In their review, the authors argue that 1.5 Tesla MRI can be carried out at calculated risk, provided that a clear and compelling indication exists.[12]

Middle Ear Transducer (MET) and MET Carina (Otologics, LLC, Boulder, CO, USA)

The MET, also known as the MET Ossicular Stimulator, was a semi-implantable middle ear device manufactured by Otologics, LLC (Boulder, CO, USA).[13] Eventually, it came to be replaced by a fully implantable version, the MET Carina (Fig. 32.4A).[14] The two devices share a common actuator but differ in that the MET Carina's microphone and rechargeable battery are placed beneath the skin.

The origin of the MET dates back to the 1970s, when Dr. John M. Fredrickson induced vibrations of a magnet implanted onto the stapes of rhesus monkeys using an electromagnetic coil. By the 1990s, Drs. Fredrickson, Coticchia, and Khoslaat (Washington University, St Louis) had demonstrated that safe stimulation could be accomplished using an electromechanical, motorized transducer

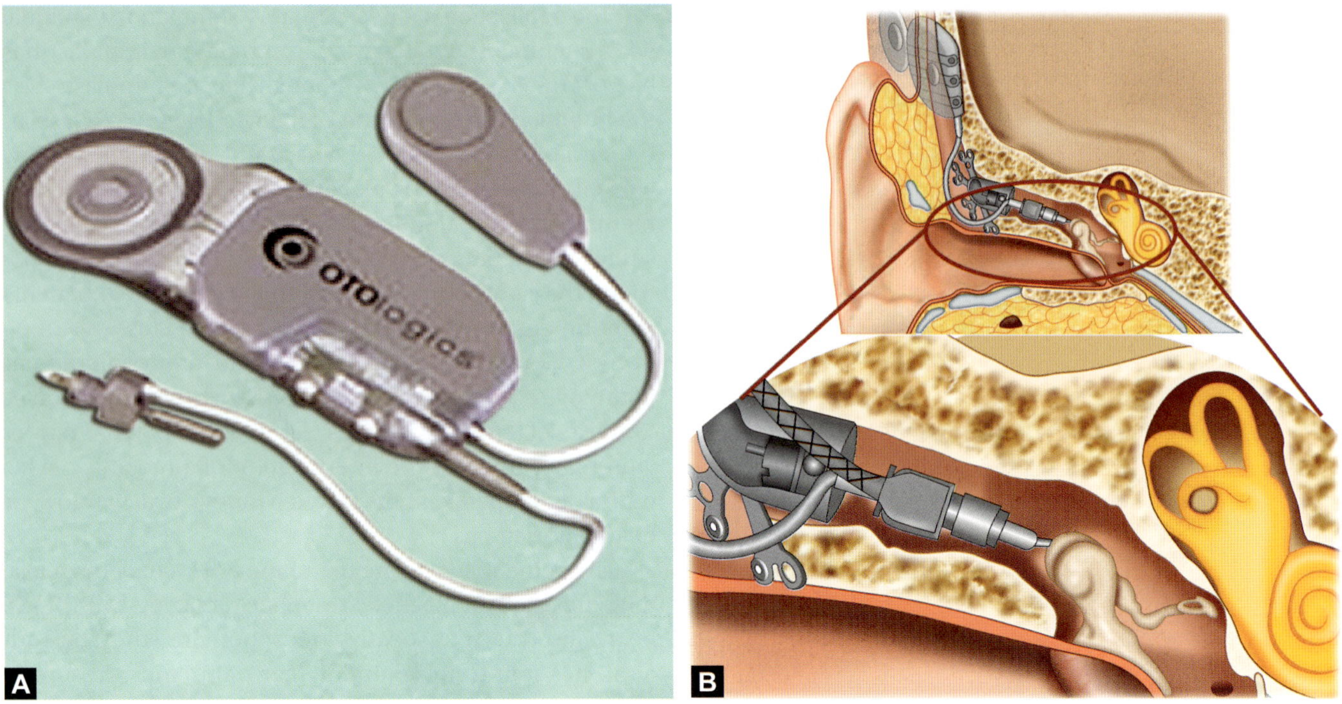

Figs. 32.4A and B: (A) Otologics MET Carina fully-implantable system. (B) Diagram of MET Carina in situ. (MET, middle ear transducer).

placed into a laser-drilled sleeve in the incus of rhesus monkeys. In 1996, the MET technology was sold to Otologics, LLC, which relocated to Boulder, CO, USA. The Food and Drug Administration (FDA) evaluation began in 1998 and by 2000 a semi-implantable version of the device was available in Europe. In 2006 the Otologics fully implantable MET received the European CE-mark.

For both devices, the implantation procedure begins by exposing the mastoid cortex through a postauricular incision. The middle ear is approached through a limited mastoidectomy, essentially a modified posterior atticotomy fashioned by tunneling between the external auditory canal and the tegmen mastoideum until exposure of the incus body and malleus head is achieved (Fig. 32.4B). A metallic stage is affixed to the ledge of cortical bone surrounding the cavity. A KTP laser incudotomy is then performed, targeting the posterosuperior aspect of the incus; then, the transducer probe is embedded into the orifice. In the case of the MET Carina, the receiver and transducer are positioned into a well drilled on the retromastoid cortical bone, and the microphone may be placed at the mastoid tip or in the retroauricular region.[14] At least one case of successful round window implantation via a facial recess approach has been reported.[15] Figure 32.5 summarizes the audiometric selection criteria for implantation.

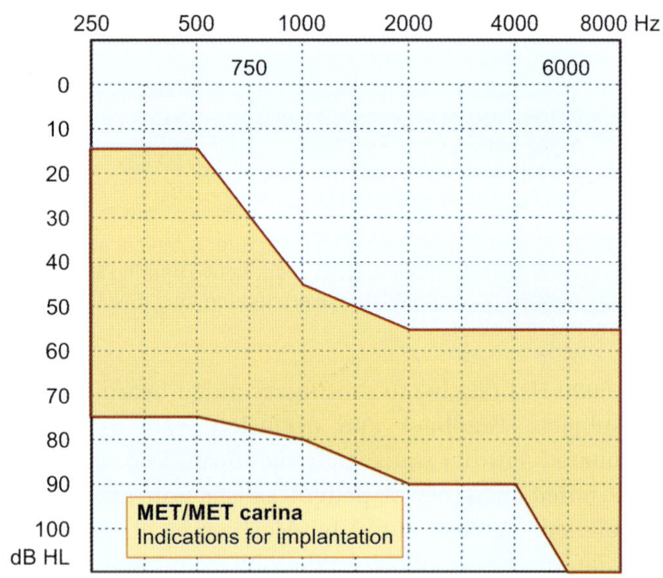

Fig. 32.5: MET/MET carina. Manufacturer's audiometric criteria for implantation.

Bruschini et al. studied outcomes of MET Carina implantation in eight adult patients with moderate to severe sensorineural and one with mixed hearing loss. All patients showed improvements in speech perception abilities and reported subjective benefits. The main adverse effect identified consisted of feedback noise in seven patients. This problem resolved with minor fitting adjustments in all but one patient, who required surgical repositioning of the microphone unit. Two cases required revision surgery: one because of microphone extrusion, the other because of device failure.[16] A prior study of five patients by the same author had shown improvements in hearing thresholds, speech perception, and also reported subjective benefits. Although no complications were noted, four patients had trouble with feedback noise, but most resolved with minor fitting adjustments.[14] Tringali et al., moreover, have reported a benefit over conventional hearing aids (39 dB mean functional gain versus 29 dB) in patients with severe SNHL (range of 71–90 dB HL).[17]

Some reports have suggested that the standard implantation approach may be especially susceptible to peculiarities of the patient's anatomy.[18] For instance, in a retrospective case series of 22 patients receiving either the standard MET or MET Carina implants, a dural–meatal distance of <8 mm was associated with dural exposure in nine cases.[19]

In 2012, Otologics LLC, Boulder, CO, USA, filed for bankruptcy.[20] Previously, Cochlear Corporation, Sydney, Australia, had acquired patent rights to Otologics LLC technologies and entered into joint development activities with the company, with the stated intent of developing a fully implantable cochlear implant.[21] However, at present, the future of the MET and MET Carina implants remains uncertain.

Esteem Hearing Implant (Envoy Medical Corporation, St. Paul, MN, USA)

Envoy Medical Corporation (St. Paul, MN, USA) was originally founded as St. Croix Medical in 1995, with the mission to develop and market the first fully implantable hearing aid that did not require a microphone or speaker. In 2004, clinical trials began in the United States and in Europe, with subsequent European CE Mark approval in 2006. In 2010, the FDA approved the Esteem Hearing Implant for commercial distribution.[22]

The Esteem Hearing Implant is a fully implantable device with a piezoelectric actuator. In contrast to other implantable hearing devices, the Esteem uses the tympanic membrane and malleus as a microphone. A piezoelectric sensor surgically fixed to the incus detects vibrations of the tympanic membrane. It then routes these signals to the processor, which amplifies them before delivering them to the piezoelectric actuator, which vibrates the stapes directly (Figs. 32.6A and B). To avoid feedback, implantation requires the disarticulation of the ossicular chain at the incudostapedial joint, along with resection of a 2-mm segment of the long process of the incus. The approach is performed through wide-field canal wall up mastoidectomy with extended facial recess dissection. The device is powered by a nonrechargeable battery, which may last 4.5 to 9 years, depending on usage. A significant disadvantage is that replacement of the battery requires surgical intervention. Figure 32.7 summarizes the manufacturer's clinical and audiometric selection criteria for Esteem implantation. Disarticulation of the ossicular chain is another significant drawback, since it introduces a maximal conductive hearing loss. Following implantation, a patient is obligated to keep the device turned on to hear, in contrast to other devices, which preserve the ossicular chain and therefore maintain patients' baseline, albeit impaired, hearing.

In a prospective, nonrandomized, multicenter FDA phase 2 trial, 57 subjects with bilateral, mild to severe SNHL were implanted. Improvements were noted in terms of speech reception threshold (29.4 dB compared with 41.2 under best-fit aided conditions, $p < 0.001$) and word recognition scores at 50 dB HL (68.9% with Esteem, compared with 46.3% under best-fit aided conditions). Adverse effects reported included wound infections in two cases (one requiring explantation), delayed facial paralysis in one case (resolved with conservative management) and three cases requiring revision surgery due to insufficient benefit.[23] A similarly designed phase 2 trial evaluated the Esteem in five patients with profound

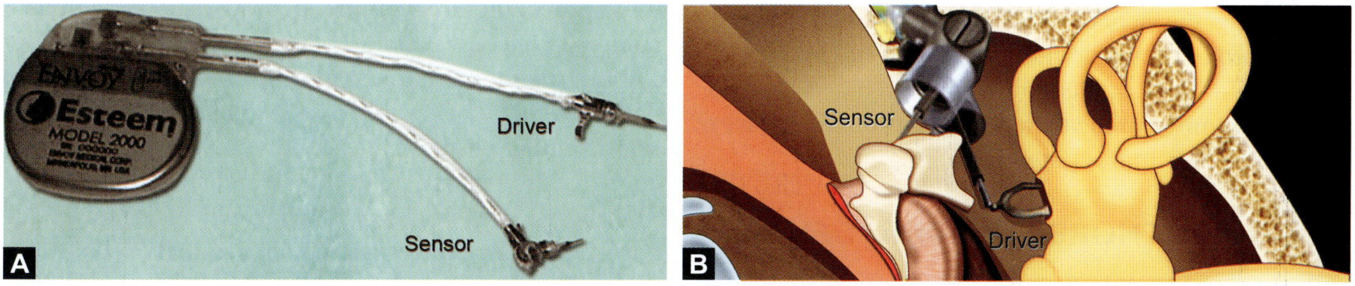

Figs. 32.6A and B: (A) Envoy Esteem system. (B) Schematic representation of Esteem in situ.

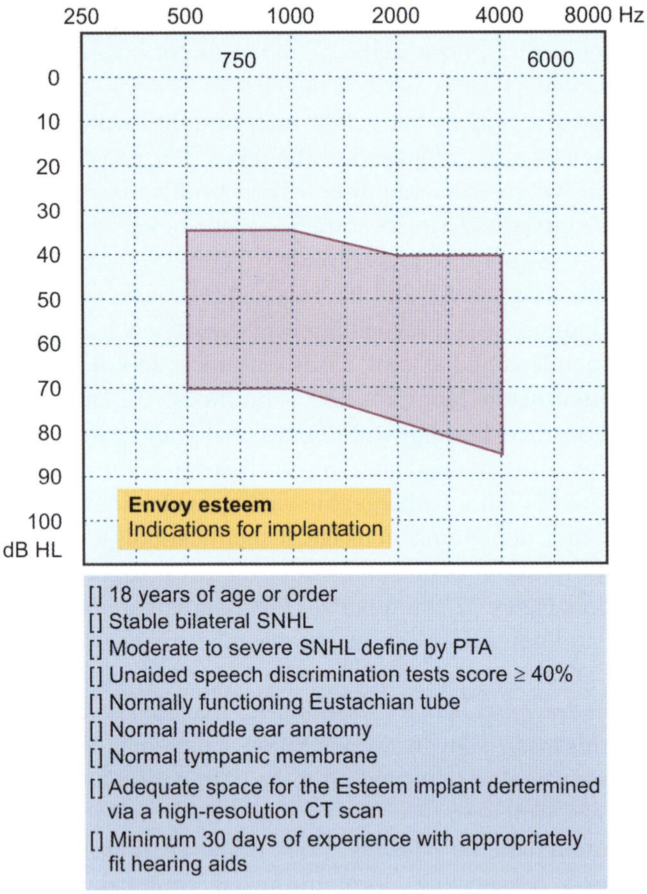

Fig. 32.7: Envoy Esteem: manufacturer's clinical and audiometric guidelines for implantation. (CT, computed tomography; PTA, pure tone audiometry; SNHL, sensorineural hearing loss).

high-frequency SNHL. Results showed an improvement in speech reception threshold (26 dB with the Esteem at 12 months, compared with 48 dB under best-fit aided conditions and 65 dB unaided). Word recognition score at 50 dB improved significantly, from an average of 23% under best-fit aided conditions to 78% postimplantation.[24]

The manufacturer's indications for implantations are as follows: ≥ 18 years of age; stable bilateral SNHL; moderate to severe SNHL defined by Pure Tone Average; unaided speech discrimination tests score ≥40%; normally functioning Eustachian tube; normal middle ear anatomy; normal tympanic membrane; adequate space for the Esteem implant determined via a high-resolution computed tomographic scan; and a minimum 30 days of experience with appropriately fit hearing aids.

BONE-ANCHORED HEARING DEVICES

Unlike conventional hearing aids, bone-conduction hearing devices bypass the apparatus of the middle ear to stimulate the inner ear directly. In general, these devices are indicated for patients with conductive or mixed hearing loss not amenable to surgical reconstruction and patients with single-sided deafness. An externally worn processor unit functions as a receiver and transducer, registering acoustic energy, amplifying it, and transferring it through the bones of the skull to the cochlea. Nonimplanted versions of these devices are typically held against the skull with a soft headband and transmit sound energy transcutaneously. However, the skin and soft tissues interposed between transducer and bone limit the efficiency of sound transduction.

Implantable bone-conduction devices, or bone-anchored hearing devices (BAHDs), on the other hand, take advantage of osseointegration to achieve more efficient transduction of sound energy. Osseointegration, a concept described by Branemark in 1983, refers to the formation of a direct functional and structural connection between a load-bearing implant and living bone tissue.[25] To date, three BAHDs have been approved by the US FDA: the Baha (Cochlear Corporation, Sydney, Australia), Ponto (Oticon Medical, Askim, Sweden), and Alpha 2 (Sophono, Inc., Boulder, CO, USA) systems. The Baha and Ponto systems both utilize a surgically implanted percutaneous abutments (a titanium screw affixed into the skull) to which a sound processor attaches externally. In contrast, the implantable portion of the Alpha 2 device lies entirely beneath the skin, and the external processor is held in place by magnets.

Baha (Cochlear Corporation, Sydney, Australia)

The Baha systems (Cochlear Corporation, Sydney, Australia) consist of three components: a screw-shaped titanium fixture, a percutaneous abutment, and a sound processor unit. Implantation of the Baha may be carried out under sedation or general anesthesia. Typically, the operation is performed in a single stage; however, a two-stage procedure is recommended for patients with soft, compromised or thin bone (< 3 mm in thickness).[26]

The traditional implantation procedure for the Baha device begins by elevating a square flap of thin, hairless skin from the postauricular region. The flap is placed far enough from the auricle to avoid contact with it once the externally worn processor is attached. Elevation of the flap may be carried out with either a scalpel or a specially designed dermatome. In an effort to reduce the potential dampening effects of subcutaneous soft tissues contacting the implant, all soft tissues between the skin and periosteum are excised, and the outer layer of the periosteum is thinned. The periosteum is then incised and a guide hole is drilled into the hole beneath. Osseointegration requires viable osteocytes at the implant site; for that reason, guide hole drilling during Baha surgery is performed in short sequences (of a few seconds at a time) and at low speeds (approximately 2000 rpm), which limits thermal damage. The self-tapping fixture is screwed into the guide hole. After attaching the abutment, the skin flap is laid over the implant and sutured closed. Finally, a hole is made in the skin using a skin biopsy punch and the abutment is passed through the skin.[27]

The so-called "punch method", as described by Goldman et al. in 2013, represents a simpler and less invasive method of BAHD implantation. This approach foregoes the creation of skin flaps; instead, a 12-mm disposable skin punch is used to create a cut through the full thickness of the scalp. The resulting soft tissue cylinder is excised, the periosteum elevated, and the cortical bone beneath exposed. In patients with thick scalps (e.g. males), limited soft tissue thinning is performed in a circumferential fashion. Drilling of the guide hole and fixture placement are carried out as described above. However, longer abutments are used (i.e. 8.5 mm for the Baha device and 9 mm for the Oticon Ponto device, discussed below). Among its advantages over the traditional procedure are faster healing, decreased operative times and improved appearance.[28]

Indications for Baha system implantation fall under two broad categories: (1) conductive and/or mixed hearing losses (e.g. from chronic otitis media, COM, congenital malformations, ossicular fixation, otosclerosis) and (2) single-sided deafness (e.g. from trauma, sudden SNHL, vestibular schwannoma).[29]

The Baha system has been evaluated extensively in the context of conductive and mixed hearing loss. An early study of 34 patients with bilateral conductive/mixed hearing loss and chronic ear disease showed that Baha was superior to conventional air-conduction hearing aids in terms of speech recognition in noise. The improvement was more pronounced with wider air-bone gaps. Moreover, patients expressed a preference for the Baha system; this preference was related to a decrease in the frequency of ear infections.[30]

Two particular clinical scenarios merit mention in this category: external auditory canal (EAC) atresia and COM. In the setting of EAC atresia, Baha implantation has been shown to achieve excellent hearing results. Moreover, compared with surgical atresia repair, Baha implantation is associated with fewer postoperative visits and complications; it is also significantly more cost-effective on a decibel-for-decibel basis.[31]

Baha placement may be indicated in COM when traditional tympanoplasty techniques have failed or when a conventional hearing aid is not feasible because of persistent otorrhea. One retrospective study evaluated the role of EAC closure (with and without Baha implantation) in patients with chronically draining ears; although limited by a small sample size, the study demonstrated this to be a feasible and safe option.[32] Another study followed patients with COM exacerbated by behind-the-ear hearing aids over a 5-year period; this study documented a significant decrease in the number of monthly treatments and visits required, which resulted in a considerable reduction in costs associated with medical care.[33]

Single-sided deafness is a relatively newer indication for device implantation. Patients with single-sided deafness and normal hearing in the contralateral ear have been shown to have improved speech reception thresholds and speech recognition in noise, though not necessarily sound localization.[34,35]

Recent modifications to the Baha implant include a wider diameter (4.5 mm versus 3.75 mm), intended to increase implant stability; smaller size thread at the implant neck, to improve optimum load distribution, and a roughened intraosseous surface, designed to increase the rate and strength of osseointegration. These innovations were found to result in a higher stability quotient and accelerated osseointegration relative to the older model in a prospective trial of 77 patients.[36]

The Baha Attract system, available since late 2013, represents the company's first effort to create a fully subcutaneous implant. Similar to the traditional Baha systems, the Baha Attract uses an osseointegrated screw-like titanium fixture; however, instead of a percutaneous abutment, the fixture is connected to an implanted magnet. Externally, a sound processor is coupled to an outer magnet, which keeps the implant in place and is available in several different strengths. This design is conceptually similar to the Alpha 2 system (Sophono, Inc., Boulder, CO, USA, discussed below) but differs in that it uses a single attachment point rather than a five-point configuration (Fig. 32.8).

Ponto (Oticon Medical, Askim, Sweden)

The Ponto system (Oticon Medical, Askim, Sweden), introduced in 2009, shares a very similar design with the Baha system, and consequently very similar strategies for

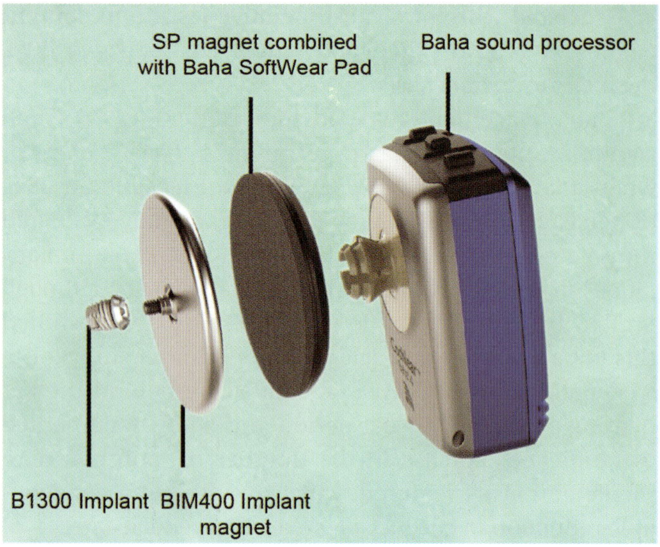

Fig. 32.8: Baha Attract system.

implantation (Figs. 32.9A to D).[37] An affiliate of Oticon (Smørum, Denmark), the world's second largest hearing aid manufacturer, Oticon Medical cites access to Oticon's sound processing technologies and fitting software as a distinct advantage over the competition. According to manufacturer estimates, more than 3000 Ponto implantations have been performed since its introduction. Early clinical data from the manufacturer have been positive, both in terms of performance and safety.[38] An independent, comparative study of 12 first-time users of BAHDs from Denmark showed that 67% of users preferred the Ponto Pro over the Baha BP100, and cited a nicer look, ease of use, and better speech intelligibility as their reasons.[39] The Ponto Pro system, the latest generation of Ponto implants, features automatic adaptive multiband directionality, noise reduction, and learning volume control.[40] The abutment, moreover, is available at a 10° inclination if needed.

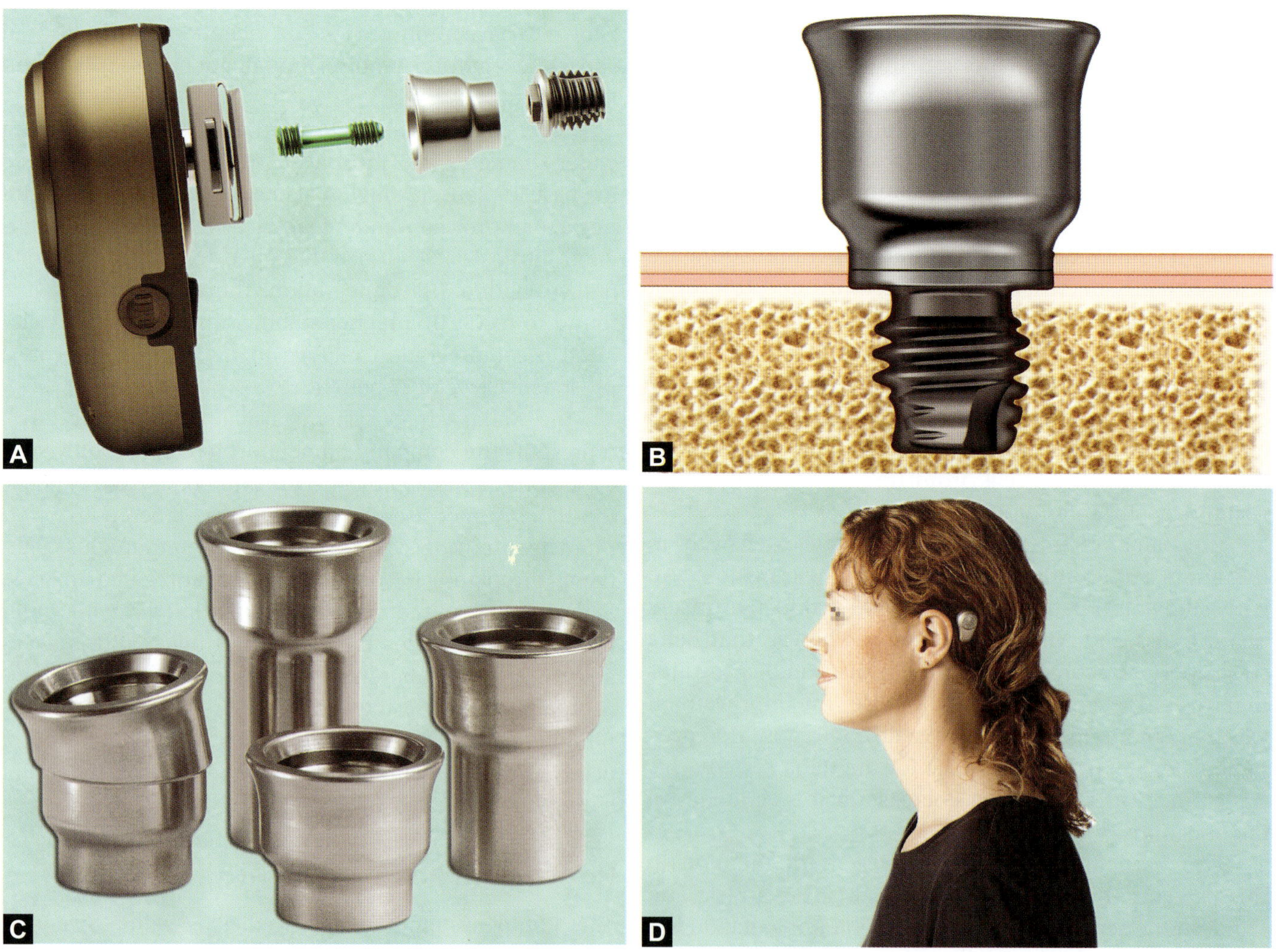

Figs. 32.9A to D: Ponto system. (A) Diagram of Ponto system in situ. (B) Ponto system components. Ponto receiver (C) in place and (D) after removal from abutment.

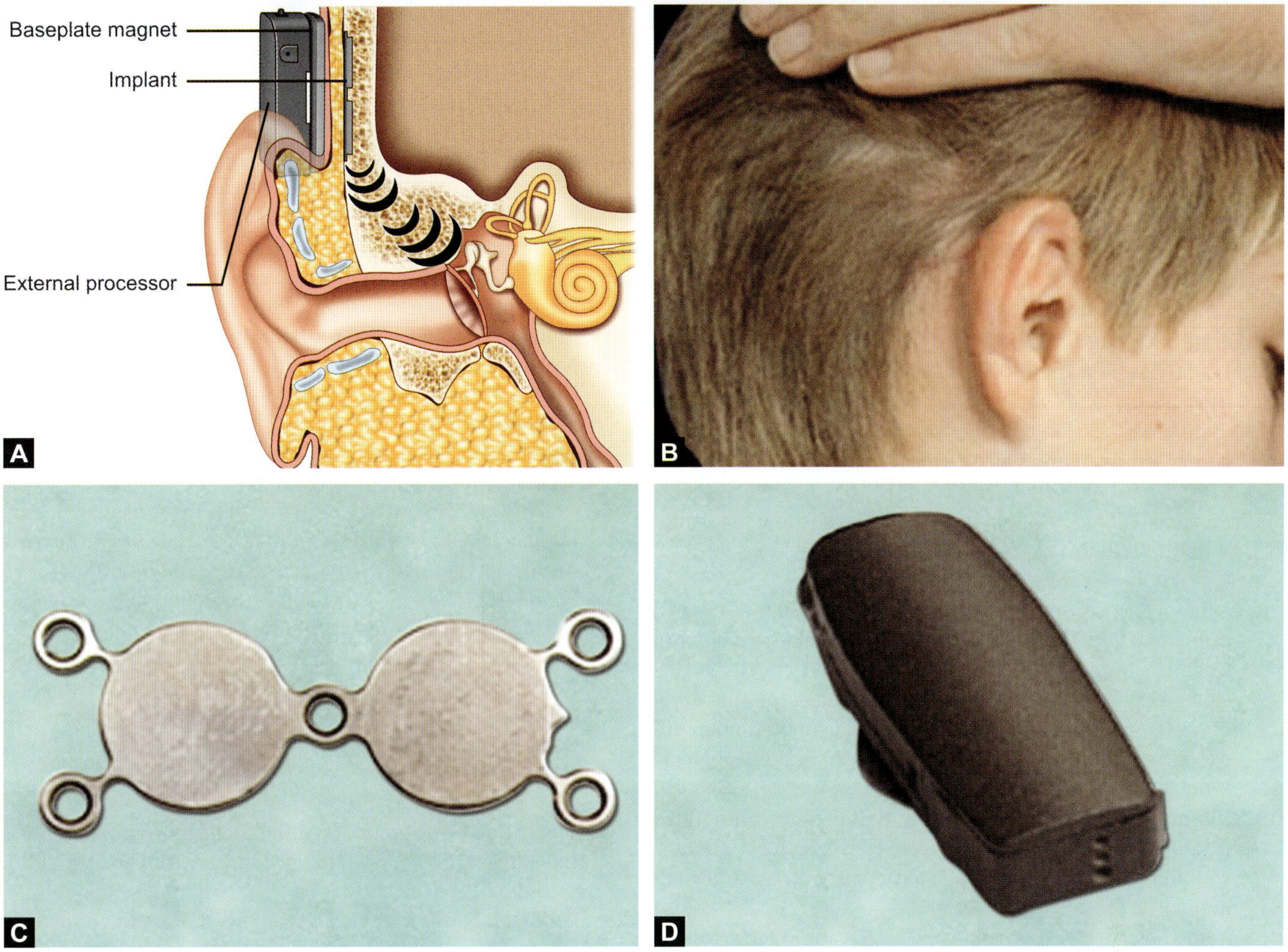

Figs. 32.10A to D: (A) Alpha 2 system in situ. (B) Photograph of implant site showing fully subcutaneous placement. (C) Magnetic implant. (D) Receiver unit.

Alpha 2 (Sophono, Inc., Boulder, CO, USA)

The Alpha 2 (Sophono, Inc., Boulder, CO, USA) system consists of an externally worn sound processor and a surgically implanted magnetic implant. In contrast to the Baha and Ponto systems, the implanted portion does not use an abutment: it lies entirely subcutaneously and is affixed to the skull with five titanium screws, which undergo osseointegration (Figs. 32.10A to D). The sound processor is held in place by magnetic force.[41] In theory, the fully subcutaneous placement would avoid adverse skin reactions related to the percutaneous abutment. However, a comparative study of 12 patients showed no difference in skin reactions between the subcutaneous Sophono implant and the percutaneous Baha system. Moreover, the study showed slightly worse performance with regard to thresholds in sound field, speech reception thresholds, and speech comprehension at 65 dB.[42] As of 2013, the FDA approved the Alpha 2 for use with MRI.[43]

CONCLUSION

Implantable hearing devices represent a synthesis of cutting-edge biotechnological and surgical innovation. Many of these devices offer considerable advantages over conventional means of sound amplification. However, in many cases, their cost and need for specialized surgical training currently limit their widespread availability. Nevertheless, the therapeutic promise of these technologies will likely outweigh these obstacles in the future.

REFERENCES

1. Kochkin S. MarkeTrak VIII: 25-year trends in the hearing health market. Hear Review. 2009;16:12-31.

2. Kochkin S. MarkeTrak VIII: Consumer satisfaction with hearing aids is slowly increasing. Hearing J. 2010;63: 19-32.
3. Geoffrey Ball: Inventor of the VIBRANT SOUNDBRIDGE. http://www.medel.com/us/support-user-stories-geoff-ball/?titel=Geoff,%20Inventor%20VSB&. (Last accessed January 25, 2014.)
4. Fisch U, Cremers CW, Lenarz T, et al. Clinical experience with the Vibrant Soundbridge implant device. Otol Neurotol. 2001;22:962-72.
5. Vibrant Soundbridge: Surgical Guide. http://www.medel.com/data/pdf/20933.pdf. (Last accessed May 2013.)
6. Luetje CM, Brackman D, Balkany TJ, et al. Phase III clinical trial results with the Vibrant Soundbridge implantable middle ear hearing device: a prospective controlled multicenter study. Otolaryngol Head Neck Surg. 2002;126: 97-107.
7. Mosnier I, Sterkers O, Bouccara D, et al. Benefit of the Vibrant Soundbridge device in patients implanted for 5 to 8 years. Ear Hearing. 2008;29:281-4.
8. Labassi S, Beliaeff M. Retrospective of 1000 patients implanted with a vibrant Soundbridge middle-ear implant. Cochlear Implants Int. 2005;6(Suppl 1):74-7.
9. Colletti L, Mandala M, Colletti V. Long-term outcome of round window Vibrant SoundBridge implantation in extensive ossicular chain defects. Otolaryngol Head Neck Surg. 2013;149(1):134-41.
10. Vibrant Soundbridge: Vibroplasty Couplers for more Surgical Flexibility. http://www.medel.com/products-vibrant-soundbrige-vibroplasty-coupler-vibroplasty/. (Last accessed May 2013.)
11. Todt I, Wagner J, Goetze R, et al. MRI scanning in patients implanted with a Vibrant Soundbridge. Laryngoscope. 2011;121:1532-5.
12. Wagner JH, Ernst A, Todt I. Magnet resonance imaging safety of the Vibrant Soundbridge system: a review. Otol Neurotol. 2011;32:1040-6.
13. Kasic JF, Fredrickson JM. The Otologics MET ossicular stimulator. Otolaryngol Clin N Am. 2001;34:501-13.
14. Bruschini L, Forli F, Santoro A, et al. Fully implantable Otologics MET Carina device for the treatment of sensorineural hearing loss. Preliminary surgical and clinical results. Acta Otorhinolaryngologica Italica. 2009;29: 79-85.
15. Tringali S, Pergola N, Berger P, et al. Fully implantable hearing device with transducer on the round window as a treatment of mixed hearing loss. Auris Nasus, Larynx. 2009;36:353-8.
16. Bruschini L, Forli F, Passetti S, et al. Fully implantable Otologics MET Carina(TM) device for the treatment of sensorineural and mixed hearing loss: Audio-otological results. Acta Otolaryngol. 2010;130:1147-53.
17. Tringali S, Perrot X, Berger P, et al. Otologics middle ear transducer with contralateral conventional hearing aid in severe sensorineural hearing loss: evolution during the first 24 months. Otol Neurotol. 2010;31:630-6.
18. Louvrier C, Montalban A, Lietin B, et al. Surgical pitfalls encountered with the semi-implantable middle ear transducer ossicular stimulator (MET-Otologics). Revue de laryngologie—otologie—rhinologie. 2010;131:193-7.
19. Kontorinis G, Lenarz T, Schwab B. Anatomic limitations in implantation of middle ear transducer and carina middle ear implants. Laryngoscope. 2010;120:2289-93.
20. Miller P. Otologics files for bankruptcy. St. Louis Business Journal. St. Louis, Missouri; 2012.
21. Cochlear buys patent rights for Otologics Herald Sun. Melbourne, Australia, 2009.
22. About Envoy. http://envoymedical.com/about-envoy/. (Last accessed January 25, 2014.)
23. Kraus EM, Shohet JA, Catalano PJ. Envoy Esteem totally implantable hearing system: phase 2 trial, 1-year hearing results. Otolaryngol Head Neck Surg. 2011;145:100-9.
24. Shohet JA, Kraus EM, Catalano PJ. Profound high-frequency sensorineural hearing loss treatment with a totally implantable hearing system. Otol Neurotol. 2011;32:1428-31.
25. Branemark PI. Osseointegration and its experimental background. J Prosthet Dent. 1983; 50:399-410.
26. Baha Surgery Guide. http://www.professionals.cochlearamericas.com/taxonomy/term/67/all. (Last accessed June 2013.)
27. Tjellström A. The bone-anchored cochlea stimulator (Baha). In: Brackman D (ed), Otologic surgery. Philadelphia, PA: Saunders Elsevier; 2010.
28. Goldman RA, Georgolios A, Shaia WT. The punch method for bone-anchored hearing aid placement. Otolaryngol Head Neck Surg. 2013;148:878-80.
29. Cochlear Baha System: Indications. http://www.cochlear.com/wps/wcm/connect/us/for-professionals/baha/candidacy/indications/indications. (Last accessed January 25, 2014.)
30. Mylanus EA, van der Pouw KC, Snik AF, et al. Intraindividual comparison of the bone-anchored hearing aid and air-conduction hearing aids. Arch Otolaryngol Head Neck Surg. 1998;124:271-6.
31. Evans AK, Kazahaya K. Canal atresia: "surgery or implantable hearing devices? The expert's question is revisited". Int J Pediatr Otorhinolaryngol. 2007;71:367-74.
32. Yoshida N, Cunningham CD, 3rd, McElveen JT, Jr. External auditory canal closure: an alternative management for the refractory chronically draining ear. Otolaryngol Head Neck Surg. 2007;137:766-71.
33. Watson GJ, Silva S, Lawless T, et al. Bone anchored hearing aids: a preliminary assessment of the impact on outpatients and cost when rehabilitating hearing in chronic suppurative otitis media. Clin Otolaryngol. 2008;33:338-42.

34. Bosman AJ, Hol MK, Snik AF, et al. Bone-anchored hearing aids in unilateral inner ear deafness. Acta Otolaryngol. 2003;123:258-60.
35. Niparko JK, Cox KM, Lustig LR. Comparison of the bone anchored hearing aid implantable hearing device with contralateral routing of offside signal amplification in the rehabilitation of unilateral deafness. Otol Neurotol. 2003;24:73-8.
36. Dun CA, de Wolf MJ, Hol MK, et al. Stability, survival, and tolerability of a novel Baha implant system: six-month data from a multicenter clinical investigation. Otol Neurotol. 2011;32:1001-7.
37. Westerkull P. The Ponto bone-anchored hearing system. Adv Otorhinol. 2011;71:32-40.
38. The Ponto bone anchored implant system: a survey of clinical outcomes. http://www.oticonmedical.com/~asset/cache.ashx?id=11513&type=14&format=web. (Last accessed June 2013).
39. Olsen SO, Glad H, Nielsen LH. Comparison of two bone anchored hearing instruments: BP100 and Ponto Pro. Int J Audiol. 2011;50:920-8.
40. Doshi J, Sheehan P, McDermott AL. Bone anchored hearing aids in children: an update. Int J Pediatr Otorhinol. 2012;76:618-22.
41. Mulla O, Agada F, Reilly PG. Introducing the Sophono Alpha 1 abutment free bone conduction hearing system. Clin Otolaryngol. 2012;37:168-9.
42. Hol MK, Nelissen RC, Agterberg MJ, et al. Comparison between a new implantable transcutaneous bone conductor and percutaneous bone-conduction hearing implant. Otol Neurotol. 2013;34(6):1071-5.
43. Sophono Alpha 2 Hearing System Receives FDA Clearance for Use With MRI. http://sophono.com/2013/04/sophono-alpha-2-hearing-system-receives-fda-clearance-for-use-with-mri/. (Last accessed June 2013).

CHAPTER

33

Cochlear Implants

Maura K Cosetti, Divya Chari, Anil K Lalwani

INTRODUCTION

Since their approval by the US Food and Drug Administration (FDA) in 1985, multichannel cochlear implants (CIs) have become an accepted, well-recognized treatment for severe-to-profound sensorineural hearing loss (SNHL) in adults and children. While SNHL can result from malfunction or injury to any portion of the auditory pathway, damage to the inner hair cells accounts for the majority of severe-to-profound deafness. In these patients, a CI restores varying amounts of auditory function by bypassing the inner hair cells and transmitting electrical impulses directly to the auditory nerve through a surgically implanted, intracochlear electrode.

In the last 25 years, nearly all aspects of cochlear implantation have undergone significant evolution ranging from technological improvements to surgical technique to broadened candidacy criteria. This chapter will address available CI technology, including hardware and software, candidacy and patient selection, operative technique, and outcomes in both adults and children.

COCHLEAR IMPLANT TECHNOLOGY

Worldwide, there are four manufactures of CI systems: Advanced Bionics Corp (CA, USA), Cochlear Ltd (Sydney, Australia), MED-EL and the Neurelec, SA, recently purchased by Oticon Medical (Gothenburg, Sweden.) All CI systems, regardless of manufacturer, have certain basic components: an externally worn processor and a surgically implanted internal device. The external component includes a microphone, power source, speech processor, and a radiofrequency transmitter coil. The internal device contains a receiver coil, stimulator, and a multichannel electrode array. Briefly, acoustic information is received by the external microphone, encoded by a speech processor (based on various strategies described below), and transcutaneously transmitted to the internal device via electromagnetic induction. The surgically implanted receiver-stimulator receives and converts the transmitted acoustic information to electrical impulses, which are then able to directly stimulate remaining auditory neurons within the cochlea through a multichannel intracochlear electrode. In the United States, there are primarily three currently available CI devices: the Advanced Bionics HiRes 90K with a 16-electrode array (Valencia, CA, USA), the Cochlear Ltd. Nucleus Freedom with a 22-electrode array (Sydney, Australia) and the MED-EL Concert (Innsbruck, Austria) with a 24-electrode array (Figs. 33.1A to C) (the Neurelec SP is not currently available in the United States). The following section will include a more in-depth description of currently available, manufacturer-specific hardware and software.

Software Technology: Sound Processing and Stimulation Strategies

The overall goal of all sound processing strategies is to create a coded signal that most accurately represents the original acoustic information. In general, the default strategies for each manufacturer are, respectively, high resolution (HiRes) for the Advanced Bionics device, the advanced combination encoder (ACE) for the Cochlear device, and fine structure processing (FSP) for the MED-EL device.[1] While a full discussion of sound processing strategies is

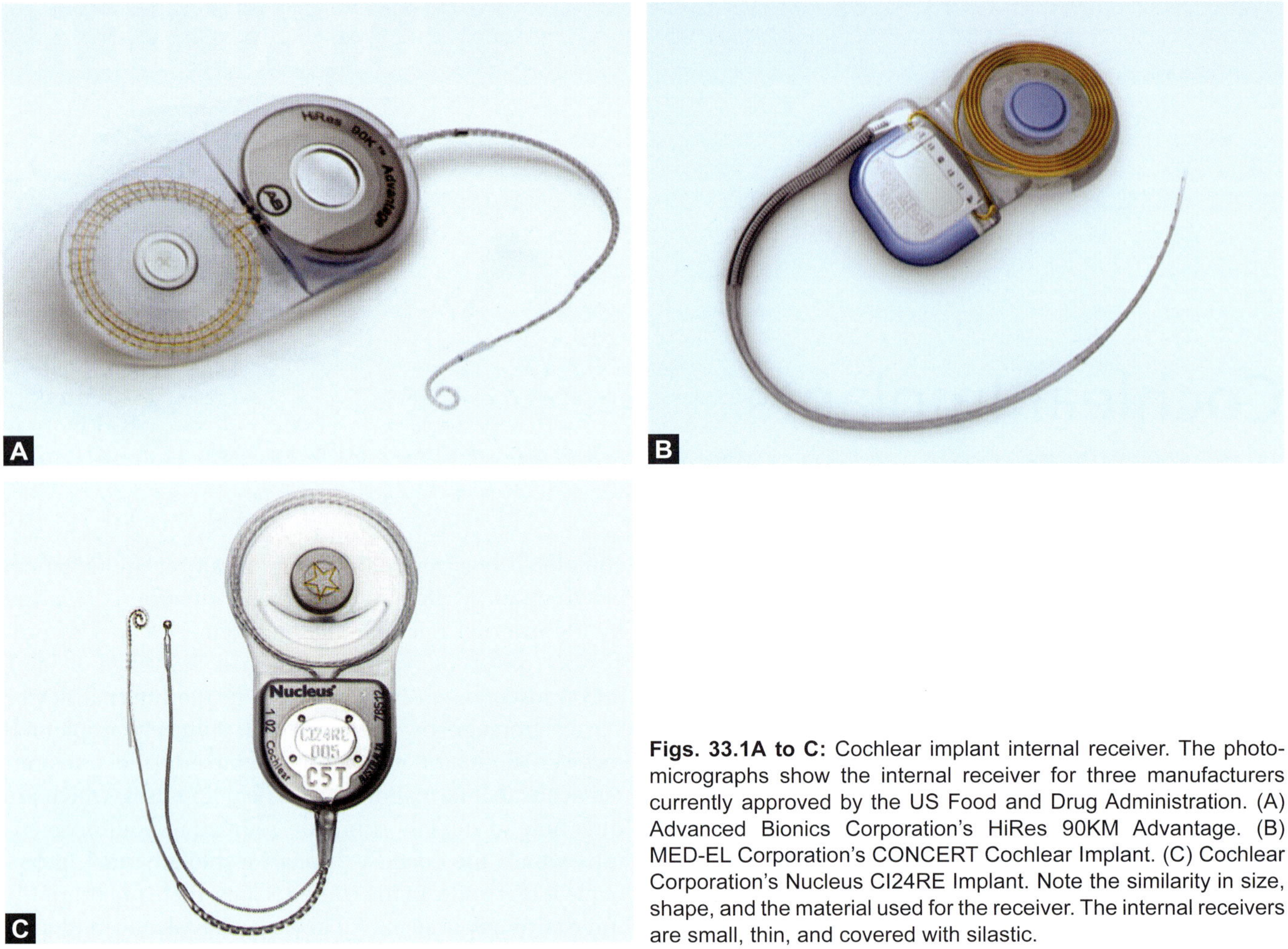

Figs. 33.1A to C: Cochlear implant internal receiver. The photomicrographs show the internal receiver for three manufacturers currently approved by the US Food and Drug Administration. (A) Advanced Bionics Corporation's HiRes 90KM Advantage. (B) MED-EL Corporation's CONCERT Cochlear Implant. (C) Cochlear Corporation's Nucleus CI24RE Implant. Note the similarity in size, shape, and the material used for the receiver. The internal receivers are small, thin, and covered with silastic.

beyond the scope of this chapter, basic approaches to speech coding focus on spectral information, temporal cues or a combination of these. Currently available strategies are manufacturer specific; however, all involve a combination of amplification, compression, filtering or extraction of the encoded acoustic information. In addition, all share a similar attempt to mimic the innate tonotopic organization of the organ of Corti. Specifically, higher-frequency bands are associated with electrodes in the basal cochlea, resulting in the perception of higher pitches, while lower-frequency bands to electrodes are positioned more deeply in the direction of the apex, creating the perception of successively lower pitches. Advancements in CI software have led to increasingly complex sound processing strategies that attempt to not only allow speech understanding in quiet environments but also permit hearing in noise, music appreciation, and improved speech perception of tonal languages.

FSP, developed by MED-EL, provides CI users with improved pitch perception, which in theory enhances speech perception in noise, melody recognition, music appreciation, and sound localization.[2] Improving on prior strategies, FSP allows both temporal and tonotopic coding of sounds in CIs by using filters with a bell-shaped frequency response. In addition, the FSP strategy is thought to provide temporal fine structure by using stimulations at the one to three most apical electrodes that are elicited at a variable rate that corresponds to the fine structure of the signal in the specific filter band. Studies comparing the FSP to previous strategies in the MED-EL system have demonstrated variable clinical effects on speech intelligibility and music sound quality and appreciation. One study, in which 14 CI users received new speech processors with FSP in exchange for their old continuous interleaved sampling (CIS) processors, showed significant improvements on speech and music perception tests as well as higher satisfaction with the FSP strategy.[3] Notably, however, a 1-year follow-up of eight of the 14 subjects from the previous study demonstrated nonsignificant differences between the baseline CIS results and the FSP results.[4] A blinded paired comparison between FSP and CIS performed for subjective speech intelligibility demonstrated that although most individuals showed no significant preference, more individuals rated CIS as significantly better at the first two annual visits, but after 2 years, more individuals rated FSP as significantly better.[5]

To improve processing of the fine structure of acoustic information, the HiRes speech processing software from Advanced Bionics employs virtual channel (VC) technology. Through either simultaneous or sequential stimulation of more than one electrode, an intermediate pitch can be conveyed that corresponds to a "virtual" channel. Given the lack of space for more electrodes in the cochlea, research has investigated using focused stimulation to increase spectral resolution and VCs to increase the number of functional channels. Prior research suggests that while only four frequency bands are necessary for speech understanding in a quiet environment, eight bands are required for speech perception in a noisy environment, and an even greater number of bands are required for effective music perception.[6] Modern CIs typically have 12–22 intracochlear electrodes, but most CI users do not demonstrate significant improvement beyond the use of 4–8 channels, perhaps because of the broad current spread from stimulated electrodes and the resulting channel interaction from overlapping neural populations.[7] Multiple methodologies attempting to minimize current interactions between electrodes have been investigated, including the use of monopolar, tripolar, and even quadrupolar techniques for VC creation. Landsberger and Srinivasan[7] found better VC discrimination with quadrupolar VCs than with monopolar VCs. Srinivasan et al.[8] found that there was a sharper peak in the spread of excitation (measured with psychophysical forward masked excitation curves) with quadrupolar VCs than with monopolar VCs, which may explain better VC discrimination with quadrupolar VC stimulation.[7,8]

While some studies report clinical benefit in speech perception and music appreciation with HiRes, others suggest that benefits may be limited to a small number of users. A study conducted by Firszt et al.[9] of eight postlingually deafened adults demonstrated a small but significant clinical benefit in both speech perception and music appreciation with the HiRes 120 current steering technology.[9] However, Donaldson et al. showed no clear evidence that HiRes 120 supports improved sentence recognition in noise.[10] Current steering via monopolar VCs has not been shown to significantly improve speech perception, despite the increased number of single-channel pitch percepts.[11] Multichannel metrics, such as spectral modulation detection and spectral ripple resolution, tend to be more strongly correlated with speech perception, likely because multichannel metrics more accurately account for channel interactions across electrodes than do single-channel measures.[12] Given these discrepancies, ongoing research is necessary to assess effectively the clinical implications of current steering technology.

ACE is the default speech processing strategy available from Cochlear Corp. This high-rate spectral analysis strategy combines elements of both the temporal and spectral approaches with reliable results. In the feature extraction component of this strategy, speech is analyzed for specific characteristics such as the fundamental frequency, formant information, voicing cues, and acoustic energy peaks, and only the information related to those features is extracted and ultimately conveyed to appropriate electrode. Used alone, this strategy would sequentially stimulate various appropriate electrodes for a given acoustic signal. In ACE, this spectral strategy is combined with a high-rate temporally based strategy, a process that conveys the entire spectrum of auditory detail through simultaneous stimulation of electrodes.

Hardware

External Components

As with software, significant technological advances have improved on the basic external hardware of CIs (Figs. 33.2A to C). Overall trends among all devices include miniaturization and incorporation of preprocessing strategies. Directional microphones have been heavily used in hearing aids to decrease the signal-to-noise ratio, but they have been only recently incorporated into external CI components, in particular with SmartSound Beam (Cochlear Corporation) and UltraZoom in the recently released Naida CIQ70 (Advanced Bionics). Directional microphones allow increased sensitivity to sounds emanating from a specific location, such as in front of the listener, and have been demonstrated to reduce background noise, improve sound quality, and enhance listening comfort in hearing aid users. There is enthusiasm surrounding the application of this hearing aid technology to the CI speech processor, and data on its effect on performance is emerging. In 2009, Chung and Zeng found improved speech

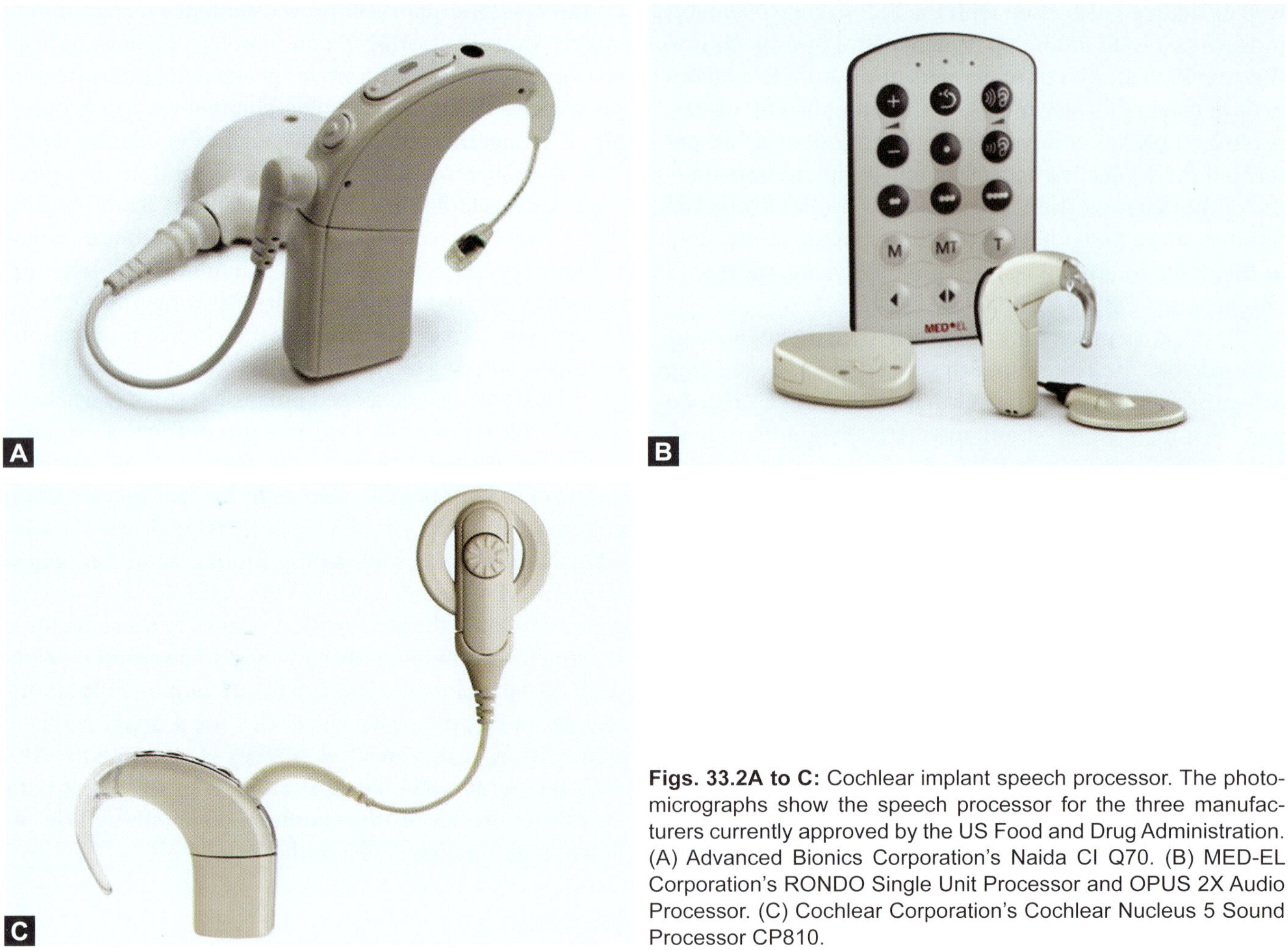

Figs. 33.2A to C: Cochlear implant speech processor. The photomicrographs show the speech processor for the three manufacturers currently approved by the US Food and Drug Administration. (A) Advanced Bionics Corporation's Naida CI Q70. (B) MED-EL Corporation's RONDO Single Unit Processor and OPUS 2X Audio Processor. (C) Cochlear Corporation's Cochlear Nucleus 5 Sound Processor CP810.

recognition in 18 postlingually deafened CI users when an adaptive directional microphone was used over fixed directional and omnidirectional microphones.[13]

ClearVoice, developed by Advanced Bionics Corporation, is a preprocessing strategy that uses a digital signal analysis algorithm to distribute the incoming signal among frequency channels and to estimate each channel's signal-to-noise level. Channels with lower signal-to-noise levels are reduced, emphasizing those more likely to contain speech signals. Results obtained in Europe show improvement in speech perception in noise in a group of 13 experienced HiRes 120 users immediately following ClearVoice activation.[14]

Med-EL recently introduced a single-unit processor (Figs. 33.2A to C), the RONDO. This is the first and only currently available external device that combines the coil, control unit, battery pack, and sound processor into a single component.

Electrode Array

The electrode array interfaces directly between the electrical output of the speech processor and the auditory neural tissue. Over the past few decades, these electrode arrays have undergone improvements; originally single-channel and positioned near the lateral wall of the scala tympani, they are now multiple channels with 12–22 active contacts and typically placed closer to the modiolus (Figs. 33.3A to C).[15] Depth of insertion of a multichannel CI has been suggested as a clinical variable that may correlate with word recognition, perhaps because deeper insertion may allow stimulation of spiral ganglion cells serving lower frequencies.[16] Current literature regarding the optimal depth of insertion is divided, with some studies arguing for longer MED-EL electrodes to obtain complete cochlear coverage, others suggesting that deep insertion yields poorer performance.[17] In a study conducted by Lee et al., examination

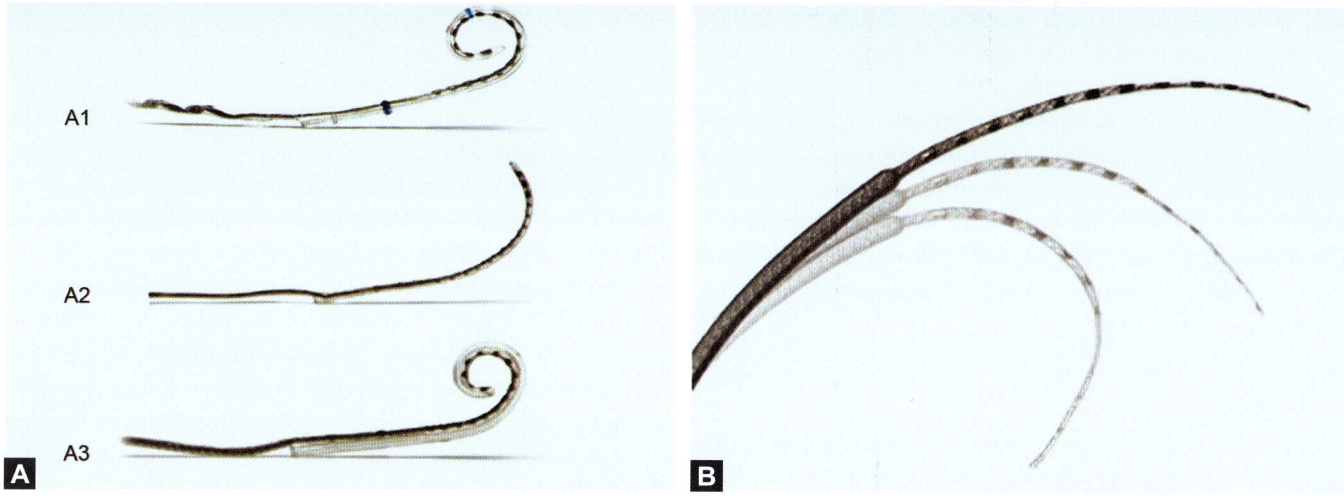

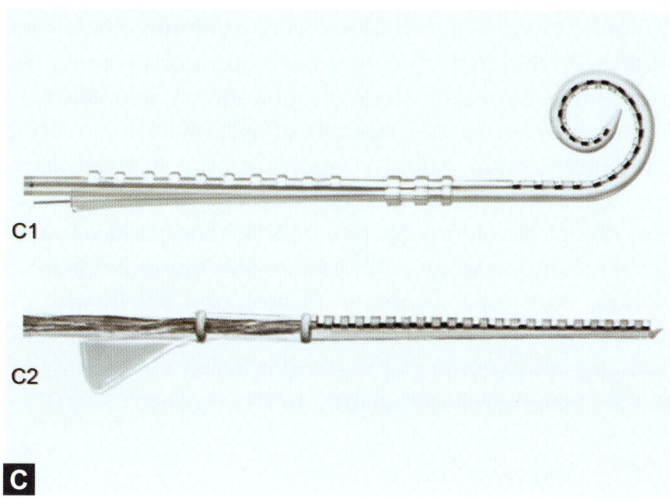

Figs. 33.3A to C: Cochlear implant electrode array. The photomicrographs show the electrodes available for the three manufacturers currently approved by the US Food and Drug Administration. (A) Advanced Bionics Corporation's HiFocus Mid-Scala Electrode (A1), HiFocus 1J Electrode (A2), HiFocus Helix Electrode (A3). (B) MED-EL Corporation's FLEX Electrode. (C) Cochlear Corporation's Contour Advance Electrode (C1), and Slim Straight Array Electrode (C2).

of cadaveric temporal bones with CIs found no correlation between histologically documented depth of insertion and last recorded measures of speech perception.[18] Length, configuration, and number of electrodes within the implanted array vary by manufacturer and to date, there have been no randomized controlled trials comparing available CI device and electrode features.

CANDIDACY ASSESSMENT AND PATIENT SELECTION

Audiologic Assessment

Adults

Comprehensive audiologic assessment is the foundation of CI candidacy evaluation. Overall, the assessment should quantify the patient's audiologic baseline, speech understanding, and use of prosthetic devices (i.e. hearing aids) to determine if expected results with a CI will improve on their present functional hearing. In adults, this consists of behavioral audiometry, including pure tone air and bone conduction thresholds, and speech discrimination testing using consonant–nucleus–consonant words. If not currently in use, a trial period of appropriate amplification may be indicated in some patients. Speech perception information, specifically open-set word or sentence recognition in the best-aided condition, is a crucial element of candidacy evaluation. In general, patients who perform below what would be expected with a CI should be considered for implantation. In the past 25 years, audiometric candidacy criteria have expanded from postlingually, profoundly deafened adults to patients with significant residual hearing. Therefore, specific scores cited here are guideposts at best and may become obsolete with future advances in CI technology. At present, scores of ≤ 60% on tests of hearing in noise (such as the Hearing-in-Noise

Test, HINT, or the Arizona Biodesign sentences, AzBio) in the best-aided condition typically suggest CI candidacy. Current Medicare guidelines require stricter criteria and cover CIs for patients with scores of ≤ 40% correct in the best-aided listening condition on tape-recorded tests of open-set sentence recognition. It is important to note, however, that ultimate candidacy determination remains at the discretion of the treating clinicians and should attempt to identify those individuals in whom a CI will provide better hearing.

Children

Audiometric testing in prelingual children requires a different set of techniques than those used in older children and adults (described above). The gold standard for behavioral evaluation of hearing in infants is visual reinforcement audiometry (VRA). VRA can reliably be applied to children who have reached 6 months' developmental age, but its efficacy decreases in cases of prematurity or neurocognitive delay. Older children may be evaluated by play audiometry or standard behavioral techniques used with adults. Immittance testing, including tympanometry and acoustic reflex testing, is another important component of the objective audiometric evaluation of infants and children with suspected hearing loss. Unique mechanical properties of the infant ear require the use of a high-frequency 1 KHz probe tone versus a 226 Hz tone typically used in older children and adults.

In children, objective audiometric assessments include otoacoustic emissions, auditory brainstem response, and auditory steady-state response. Otoacoustic emissions are generated from the outer hair cells of the cochlea in response to an auditory stimulus, while auditory brainstem response and auditory steady-state response assess the afferent neural connections between the inner hair cells, the vestibulocochlear nerve, and the brainstem. In general, the audiometric component of pediatric CI candidacy evaluation employs a combination of behavioral and electrophysiologic testing.

Speech perception testing of infants remains challenging, as most tests are based on speech production. For the youngest children, the Infant-Toddler Meaningful Auditory Integration Scale (IT-MAIS), a parental survey of early speech development, has been employed reliably to measure speech perception and linguistic development. This 10-question structured interview assesses the frequency of specific auditory behaviors, including vocalization, alerting to sound, and deriving meaning from sound. Also acceptable for children under 24 months of age is the Meaningful Auditory Integration Scale or Early Speech Perception Test. For children older than 2 years of age, open set word and sentence testing can be used, including the Lexical Neighborhood test, Multisyllabic Lexical Neighborhood test, Banford-Kowl-Bench sentences, Glendonald Auditory Screening procedures, Ling Sound test, and Phonetically Balanced Kindergarten word list.

An important aspect of the pediatric candidacy assessment includes the infant or child's response to amplification. An increase in early diagnosis afforded by the advent of universal newborn hearing screening has allowed greater opportunities for early intervention. Regardless of age at diagnosis or degree of hearing loss, attempts should be made to provide all hearing-impaired children access to amplification. Even children with profound SNHL traditionally undergo a hearing aid trial prior to implantation. Long-term data suggest that auditory rehabilitation commenced prior to 6 months of age, including hearing aid amplification, leads to significant gains in vocabulary, speech intelligibility, general language abilities, social–emotional development, parental bonding, and parental grief resolution when compared to late-identified peers.[19] Infants with bilateral severe-to-profound SNHL who do not benefit from a trial of conventional amplification (and who meet anatomic and medical criteria) are considered for cochlear implantation prior to 1 year of age.

Other Audiovestibular Testing

Promontory stimulation may be an adjunctive test used in the candidacy evaluation of CI. This testing can be performed either at the promontory via a needle electrode inserted through the tympanic membrane or at the round window via a round window electrode. A positive response is obtained when the patient can perceive sound with stimulation. Once routinely applied to all CI recipients, it is now uncommonly included in routine CI evaluation as patients with a negative response to stimulation at the promontory will often responds to intracochlear stimulation. Current applications of promontory stimulation include choosing a side for implantation in cases of a long-deafened ear. Vestibular evaluation, including vestibular nystagmography, is not routinely applied in candidacy evaluation for CI.

Medical Evaluation

A complete history and physical evaluation are crucial in CI evaluation and should identify any factors that influence a patient's ability to undergo general anesthesia or postoperative rehabilitation. In patients with significant comorbidities, additional preoperative consultation from medical specialists such as cardiology or nephrology may be indicated. Laboratory studies appropriate to each patient's medical condition should be obtained prior to general anesthesia, but are not unique to the procedure itself. If otologic disease is suspected on physician exam, patients should undergo otomicroscopy to better assess the middle ear for chronic otitis media or cholesteatoma. Mastoid disease can be further evaluated on computed tomography (CT), described in more depth below. When discovered, middle ear or mastoid disease is an important factor to consider and may influence the timing or laterality of cochlear implantation. Ideally, purulent drainage should be treated maximally prior to implantation. Once thought to be an absolute contraindication for cochlear implantation, unique surgical techniques such as staged surgery or the creation of a blind sac may be employed to create a safe ear for implantation in certain cases.

In addition to the above, medical evaluation in the pediatric population involves a detailed perinatal and immunization history, as well as serologic investigation for infectious and genetic causes of SNHL. If syndromic hearing loss is known or discovered, additional testing appropriate for that particular syndrome (such as electrocardiography, ophthalmologic exam) should be pursued.

Genetic mutations account for approximately 50% of cases of nonsyndromic, hereditary congenital hearing loss. Of these, 30% of these are associated with clinical features from a known syndrome, while 70% are considered "nonsyndromic".[20] Among children with nonsyndromic profound SNHL, approximately half have mutations in the gene GJB2, which codes for a gap junction protein involved in cell-to-cell diffusion and recycling of ions such as potassium in the inner ear.[21] In 2005, Preciado et al. suggested early GJB2 testing for infants with indications of severe to profound deafness to assist with early intervention, including cochlear implantation.[22]

Radiologic Evaluation

Assessment of cochlear anatomy is an important component of the CI candidacy evaluation and can be accomplished using high-resolution CT (HRCT) of the temporal bones and/or magnetic resonance imaging (MRI) of the otic capsule and internal auditory canal. Careful examination of the inner ear anatomy is important for identification of cochleovestibular abnormalities that could account for SNHL and influence surgical planning. Preoperative identification of partial or complete ossification of the scala tympani, congenital malformations of the inner ear, and ossification or fibrous occlusion of the round window are not contraindications to implantation, but will influence surgical planning and technique as well postoperative outcome and expectations. Aeration of the mastoid, course of the facial nerve (FN), and presence of otologic disease (such as chronic otitis media or cholesteatoma) should also be noted as they may influence timing of implantation and/or surgical technique. Overall, MRI is superior in identification of early labyrinthine ossification and luminal patency of the cochlea as well as soft tissue abnormalities, including the cochlear nerve aplasia or cochlear agenesis (contraindications for cochlear implantation).[23] HRCT, on the other hand, is superior for diagnosis of bony abnormalities, including estimation of the caliber of the cochlear canal and enlarged vestibular aqueduct. [24] Studies suggest a high specificity and negative predictive value for each modality independently and no benefit with dual-modality screening.[25] At present, choice of radiologic modality is institution or physician dependent.

Patient Counseling and Expectations

Preoperative counseling should include the surgical procedure, choice of ear or bilateral implantation and, postoperative rehabilitative process, specifically programming sessions. A commitment to postoperative rehabilitation by the patient and/or family is a crucial part of preimplantation counseling and the informed consent process. Once routine, a formal psychological evaluation is no longer common in routine CI evaluation; however, if may be indicated in rare cases. While finite predictions for postimplantation outcomes are not possible, realistic expectations should be discussed with patients and their families. To the greatest extent possible, these expectations should be individualized, and for unique populations such as prelingually deafened adolescents/adults or patients with developmental disabilities or multiple handicaps, this discussion should address the range of outcomes and the limitations of cochlear implantation.

SURGICAL CONSIDERATIONS

Surgical Procedure for Patients with Normal Cochlear Anatomy

CI surgery is performed under general anesthesia with continuous intraoperative electromyographic monitoring of the FN. In the standard surgical technique, the implant is inserted via a transmastoid facial recess approach to the scala tympani and may utilize a cochleostomy or round window insertion. Other uncommon techniques, such as the suprameatal approach, have been described but will not be discussed here.

Overall, optimal electrode placement is a prerequisite for maximizing postimplantation success. While numerous modifications to the CI procedure exist, full minimally traumatic scala tympani electrode placement is the goal of each surgery. Incorrect or suboptimal placement, damaged, or kinked electrodes can lead to suboptimal CI function, poor postoperative outcomes, and may subject the patient to additional or revision surgery.

Using a postauricular incision, a standard mastoidectomy is performed using microsurgical techniques. Unlike mastoidectomy performed in chronic ear surgery, saucerization of the mastoid borders is not emphasized in CI surgery. Instead, creation of an overhang of bone around the mastoid borders is encouraged to provide an additional layer of protection for the implant as it courses from the cochlea to the receiver-stimulator.

Placement of the receiver-stimulator is commonly 2 cm posterior to the postauricular incision and with its inferior border approximating the superior border of the external meatus or tragus. To avoid postoperative wound complications, the internal device should be placed far enough from the periauricular region so as not to contact the externally worn speech processor. While multiple techniques exist for internally securing the receiver-stimulator, most agree that some attempt to eliminate device migration and its potential impact on superficial wound complications or electrode extrusion is important. At present, two methods for securing the CI predominate: drilling a device-specific bony well or creation of a subperiosteal pocket. In the former, a custom-fit bony "seat" (or "well") is created to fit the specific CI device, often using manufacturer-specific operative templates. Variations in the depth or configuration of the bony seat are device or surgeon dependent and may also be influenced by patient age or anatomy. Creation of a central bony island with circumferential dural exposure to better recess the CI device and its profile in the skull have been described for use in young children. In contrast, the subperiosteal or "t-pocket" technique secures the device using anatomical fixation points and does not require drilling.[26] These anatomical landmarks include the condensation of the temporalis fascia and pericranium at the temporal–parietal suture (anteriorly) and the pericranial attachment at the lambdoid suture (posteriorly.) A subperiosteal pocket is created using blunt dissection to match the disposable silicon template included with each implant device. The receiver-stimulator can be secured with nonabsorbable suture to the bone (using custom-drilled suture retaining holes) or to the periosteum. Modifications to both techniques can be expected to parallel technological advances that allow further miniaturization of the internal device.

Knowledge of facial recess anatomy is crucial to a safe and adequate cochlear visualization and ideal cochleostomy position. Anteriorly, thinning of the posterior external auditory canal is the first step in creation of an ideal facial recess. A thin posterior canal wall will improve identification of, and thus minimize injury to, the chorda tympani nerve. This anterior border will also maximize the amount of light entering the facial recess, ultimately improving visualization of the cochlea and middle ear structures. To begin the facial recess, the descending or mastoid portion of the FN is identified. As mentioned above, although thorough review of preoperative imaging of can alert and prepare the surgeon for anatomic aberrations such as an abnormal course of the FN or presence of chronic ear disease, a high level of intraoperative vigilance and precise identification of anatomic landmarks remains critical to safe CI surgery.

Superiorly, the fossa incudis is enlarged until the short process of the incus can be seen, keeping a thin bone bridge or incus bar intact. Anatomically, the short process points toward the center of the facial recess and this relationship can be especially helpful in poorly developed or minimally aerated temporal bones where identification of the facial recess may be more challenging. Although the integrity of the incus bar is typically maintained, this bone bridge (and the incus itself) can be removed for increased visualization of the middle ear, if needed. Next, the chorda tympani nerve is identified from its origin at the FN to the chorda iter posterior, where it enters the middle ear. Bone in the facial recess, between the chorda tympani anteriorly, the FN posteriorly and the incus bar superiorly, is then carefully removed using serially smaller diamond burs. An adequate facial recess includes good visualization of the stapedial tendon, round window and cochlear promontory. To achieve full access to the round window niche and inferior cochlea, bone anterior to the FN and inferior to the stapedial tendon must be carefully removed. (Fig. 33.4) Integrity of the chorda tympani can be preserved in nearly all cases and maintenance of this landmark can protect against damage to the annular ligament of the tympanic membrane that lies more anteriorly. Damage to the FN or chorda tympani can result from the

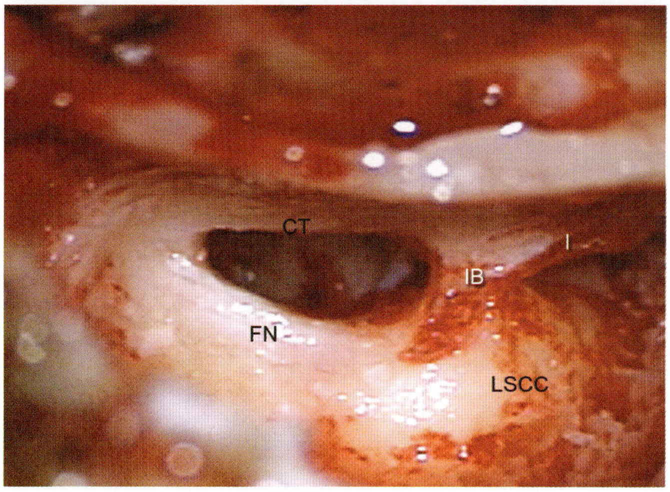

Fig. 33.4: Facial recess. The facial recess is bordered by the chorda tympani (CT) anteriorly, the facial nerve (FN) posteriorly, and the incus bar (IB) superiorly. (I, incus; LSCC, lateral semicircular canal).

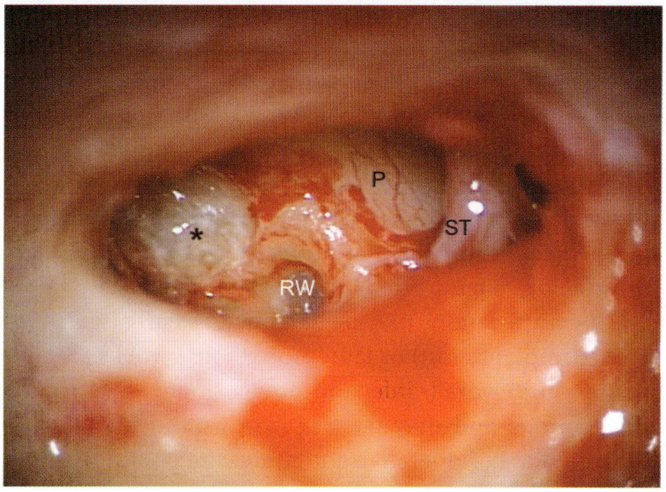

Fig. 33.5: Electrode insertion: cochleostomy and round window approach. Electrode insertion can proceed via an anterior, inferior cochleostomy, or via the round window (RW). Choice of technique may be influenced by surgeon preference, patient anatomy, electrode choice, or some combination of the above. An adequate facial recess includes good visualization of the stapedial tendon (ST), round window (RW), and cochlear promontory (P). Asterisk indicates the location of the cochleostomy.

bur itself, as well as the heat or pressure from the drill shaft. Copious irrigation and vigilant monitoring of both the drill and burr position during creation of the facial recess and cochleostomy are vital to minimize injury.

In general, fixation of the receiver/stimulator is desirable before electrode insertion. The reverse may result in extrusion of a perfectly placed electrode and require reinsertion. Electrode insertion can proceed via an anterior, inferior cochleostomy or via the round window. (Fig. 33.5) Choice of technique may be influenced by surgeon preference, patient anatomy, electrode choice or some combination of the above. Both approaches attempt to maximize scala tympani insertion with minimal trauma to the intracochlear structures, specifically spiral ligament, basilar membrane and modiolus. As discussed above, optimal CI position in the scala tympani requires a thorough understanding of the cochlear orientation through the facial recess. The lumen of the basal turn is oriented in a plane virtually parallel to that of the external auditory canal wall. Therefore, regardless of insertional method, the direction of electrode insertion should be down the midportion of the proximal turn, avoiding both the outer wall and the medial modiolar wall. Unlike creation of the facial recess and cochleostomy, electrode insertion is best accomplished on low power with a wide view of the mastoid cavity and cochleostomy in the distance. This view allows complete visualization of the entire electrode array and insertion instrument. A variety of tools specific to each electrode type and company are available. Regardless of electrode choice, however, gentle, smooth insertion and avoidance of excessive force are universal principles. Tactile feedback during insertion is important: the perception of resistance indicates a problem and stopping to reassess and evaluate anatomic circumstances may prevent electrode tip rollover or malposition. Complete insertion is dictated by electrode type and brand. Packing of the cochleostomy or round window can be done with fascia or periosteum around the electrode array. This enhances scar tissue formation around the electrode and seals the cochleostomy, thereby minimizing perilymph leakage and preventing resultant vertigo, infectious complications and electrode extrusion.

Following electrode insertion, intraoperative monitoring of the implanted device may be performed, including electrode impedances, neural response telemetry and radiologic imaging. While not standard in all centers, these tests provide information on the patient's auditory system response to electrical stimulation. They may also serve as a baseline for postoperative device programming in some difficult to program populations. Radiologic confirmation via X-ray may provide confirmation of intracochlear electrode location and position.[27]

A unique surgical modification to the above technique has been described for cochlear implantation in patients with cochleovestibular abnormalities, a full discussion of which is beyond the scope of this chapter.

Complications

In both adults and children, cochlear implantation is both safe and effective and major complications are rare. Complications common to all ear and mastoid surgery include FN injury, cerebrospinal fluid (CSF) drainage, infection, meningitis, and all risks associated with general anesthesia. Additional risks unique to cochlear implantation include device failure and need for reimplantation.

CI complications may be classified as early (within 14 days of implantation) or late (more than 2 weeks postimplantation.) Overall, infection predominates in the both time periods and may present as a wound infection or otitis media. Perioperative antibiotics are commonly prescribed to all CI patients to prevent these sequelae. FN injury, either paresis or paralysis, is a rare complication of CI surgery. Multiple surgical steps should be taken to avoid damage to the FN during implantation, including routine use of electromyographic monitoring of the FN, copious irrigation during creation of the facial recess, and attempted identification of abnormal FN anatomy or location preoperatively. Chorda tympani injury has been reported in up to 20% of pediatric CI recipients.[28] CSF leaks can occur as a result of iatrogenic injury to the tegmen during mastoidectomy or the squama of the temporal bone during bony fixation of the receiver-stimulator. A high preoperative suspicion for CSF gusher is appropriate for pediatric patients with congenital inner ear malformations as these individuals are at increased risk of intraoperative CSF gusher. Device failures can occur with any device and may occur early or late following implantation. Overall rates of device failure are reported at 2%.[28,29]

Meningitis, historically of great significance following use of an electrode with positioner, is now rare. Voluntarily discontinued by the manufacturer in 2002, the risk of meningitis >96 months after implantation with that device is significantly reduced. [30,31] Currently, stringent following of immunization protocols for *Streptococcus pneumoniae* and *Haemophilus influenzae* is the cornerstone of prevention of bacterial meningitis following cochlear implantation.

OUTCOMES FOLLOWING COCHLEAR IMPLANTATION

Success following cochlear implantation can be assessed across a wide variety of quantitative and qualitative domains, such as speech reception and production, quality of life, and socioeconomic impact. While this chapter will primarily address speech performance outcomes, technological advances in CI hardware and software (described above) have made previously unattainable goals, such as hearing in noise and music appreciation, a reality for some CI recipients.

Table 33.1: Variables affecting outcomes following cochlear implantation

1. Neuronal cell physiology and function
a. Age at implantation
b. Duration of deafness/auditory deprivation
c. Auditory neuroplasticity
2. Binaural hearing
3. Presence of multiple disabilities
a. Autism
b. Auditory neuropathy spectrum disorder
4. Medical/surgical issues
a. Cochleovestibular anatomic malformations
b. Meningitis
c. CHARGE
5. Cochlear implant technology
a Processing strategy
b. Electrode design
6. Preoperative hearing level and speech performance
7. Rehabilitative environment
a. Mode of communication
b. Postimplantation rehabilitative services
8. Auditory training
9. Social factors
a. Socioeconomic status
b. Parent/family expectations and motivations

Research outcomes have identified a wide spectrum of variables known to affect postimplantation performance (Table 33.1). These variables relate to the device itself, including electrode design, speech processing strategies, and device reliability, as well as individual patient characteristics such as cochleovestibular anatomy, presence of associated disabilities, or etiology of deafness. On a cellular level, factors believed to affect spiral ganglion cell survival and function have been shown to influence postoperative performance, including auditory deprivation, duration of deafness, and age at implantation. Social and educational factors, such as mode of communication, parent/family expectations, postimplantation rehabilitation, and socioeconomic status, are additional variables shown to affect postoperative performance. Novel variables capable of affecting performance, such as auditory training and focused attention, continue to emerge with increased understanding of auditory pathway development and neural plasticity.

In all, the most consistent variable affecting performance is duration of deafness. Adults and children with postlingual deafness (i.e. hearing decrement after language development) generally have more consistent success following cochlear implantation than prelingually deafened individuals who receive a CI after a prolonged period of deafness. In general, cochlear implantation allows most average, postlingually deafened pediatric, and adult CI recipients to achieve meaningful auditory sensation and speech understanding. Age at implantation is also an important variable affecting performance, especially in children with congenital hearing loss. In those children, the data on receptive and expressive language development support early implantation (discussed in more detail below).

Open set tests of speech perception used during candidacy evaluation can be readministered postoperatively to specifically assess the impact of on electrical stimulation on a particular individual's speech perception. There is considerable variability in postoperative performance across populations and this remains incompletely understood. As mentioned above, estimation of postimplantation benefit should be individualized and based on comprehensive preoperative assessment, with attention to the complex interplay of the aforementioned patient and device characteristics.

OUTCOMES IN CHILDREN UNDER 1 YEAR OF AGE

Since the advent of pediatric cochlear implantation, formal candidacy criteria have included increasingly younger patients, a trend influenced by the correlation of earlier implantation with improved communication outcomes.[32] In a study by Miyamoto et al., a comparison of receptive and expressive language skills of children who received a CI before 1 year of age to those who received an implant between 1 and 3 years of age showed higher language scores for children implanted at a younger age.[33] In 2010, Houston et al. found that children implanted during the first year of life had larger vocabularies than children implanted between 16 and 23 months after birth; however, there was no significant difference in speech perception.[34] These results suggest that there may be a sensitive period for speech and language development. Ideally, cochlear implantation should occur before this window is closed to prevent impaired development. Currently, cochlear implantation is FDA approved for children 1 year of age and older, but some centers implant younger children. Studies support the safety and efficacy of the procedure, and preliminary data seem to indicate language growth rates comparable to those of normal-hearing children.[35,36]

Perioperative safety, particularly anesthetic risk, is an important consideration in very young children. Epidemiological studies of anesthesia-related complications found the incidence of morbidity, mortality, and life-threatening adverse events in children younger than 12 months to be significantly higher than in older children.[37] Closer evaluation of these population-based studies, however, reveals that the greatest risk factors of anesthetic-related complications include emergency surgery and inadequate fasting period, neither of which applies to a scheduled CI surgery. Growing data support safety in children implanted under 1 year of age, with complication rates comparable to those of older children and adults.[35,38,39]

Over the past decade, there has been a growing body of literature supporting improved auditory and linguistic outcomes in children implanted before 12 months of age. In a study conducted by Lesinski-Schiedat, children implanted prior to 12 months of age demonstrated superior speech understanding compared to children implanted between 1 and 2 years of age.[39] Using IT-MAIS, Waltzman and Roland and Roland et al. found speech perception scores of children implanted prior to 12 months of age were comparable to those of their normal-hearing peers.[35,40] In 2005, Colletti et al. showed that 10 children implanted under 12 months of age had significantly better outcomes than children implanted at an older age, as measured by the Category of Auditory Performance, a global measure of auditory receptive abilities.[41] Dettman et al. used the Rosetti Infant-Toddler Language Scale (RI-TLS) to examine communication abilities of 19 children implanted before 12 months of age; these children achieved receptive and expressive language growth rates comparable to their normal-hearing peers and significantly greater than rates achieved by children implanted between 12 and 24 months of age.[36] Notably, Holt and Svirsky found improved receptive language skills in children implanted under 1 year of age, but negligible differences in expressive ability between those implanted before 12 months and between 12 and 24 months.[42]

Given that multiple studies suggest benefit in areas of receptive and expressive language development and speech perception, and current data support minimal anesthetic and long-term complications to young children, early implantation may maximize a child's ability to achieve full linguistic potential with minimal risk.

Outcomes in Elderly Patients

Hearing loss is one of the most common disabilities in the aging and can negatively impact quality of life and overall health status. Studies suggest that limited or minimal access to acoustic information can lead to social isolation, loss of self-esteem, depression, personality changes, cognitive impairment and reduced functional status.[43,44] Unfortunately, elderly patients remain underserved by cochlear implantation due to concerns about perioperative safety and rehabilitative outcomes.

Cochlear implantation in geriatric patients has long faced concerns about anesthetic risk and surgical complications, in particular flap necrosis, infection, FN injury and CSF leak. However, recent research on anesthetic risk supports safety and efficacy of CI in the elderly and contradicts the pervasive myth that advanced age is an important risk factor for anesthesia-related perioperative complications. In a retrospective review of 70 CI recipients over 70 years of age, Coelho et al. found that general anesthesia was well tolerated by elderly patients, with only 4 patients requiring intraoperative pressor support for hypotension and only 3 patients suffering from postoperative anesthesia-related complications. These complications included urinary retention, delayed extubation and congestive heart failure. No long-term morbidity or perioperative mortality was noted.[45] Eshraghi et al. found no long-term medical or surgical complications or mortality in 21 patients of ages 79–89 following CI.[46]

Other concerns about candidacy include the age-related degeneration of the peripheral and central auditory systems and the overall cognitive deterioration and decreased neural plasticity associated with aging.[47] Successful cochlear implantation requires an intact and functional auditory processing pathway, from spiral ganglion cells to auditory cortex. Dickstein et al. demonstrated an overall decrease in the number of dendrites and dendritic spines in the elderly brain, suggesting a decrease in synaptic activity and neural plasticity.[48]

Despite concerns related to age-related degeneration, multiple studies have documented improved speech perception outcomes in older adults after cochlear implantation. Budenz et al. compared speech perception outcomes in postlingually deafened adults implanted at age 70 and older with those from postlingually deafened adults implanted between ages 18 and 70. Although younger patients outperformed elderly subjects, differences correlated with duration of deafness rather than age.[49] Vermeire et al. and Eshraghi et al. reported improved social life, confidence, and overall quality of life after implantation in the elderly population.[46,50] Furthermore, increased communicative ability of elderly CI recipients allows many individuals to continue or return to full-time employment, a measure of the global societal impact of CI in this expanding population.[51]

EMERGING AND UNIQUE POPULATIONS

Candidacy and Outcomes in Auditory Neuropathy Spectrum Disorder

The diagnosis and management of auditory neuropathy spectrum disorder (ANSD) remains controversial. CI candidacy in individuals with ANSD continues to be hotly debated. ANSD describes a heterogenous group of auditory processing abnormalities typically characterized by presence of otoacoustic emissions and/or cochlear microphonic potentials with a greatly abnormal or absent auditory brainstem response. In ANSD, the outer hair cells function normally, but sound is not properly transmitted from the outer hair cells to the auditory cortex due to desynchronized action potentials in the auditory nerve. For children and adults with ANSD and minimal auditory capacity, multiple studies have confirmed CI outcomes commensurate with those of peers with other forms of SNHL. Rance and Barker reported significant improvement in speech ability (consonant-nucleus-consonant phoneme scores) of children diagnosed with ANSD after cochlear implantation.[52] A recent longitudinal study by Teagle et al. followed the largest cohort of participants receiving CI interventions to date. Of the 52 participants studied, 11 did not have sufficient pre- and postdata for analyses; the remaining 41 demonstrated improved speech perception abilities.[53] Rance and Barker suggested that outcomes for a selected group of children with ANSD treated with hearing aid amplification may equal or exceed outcomes for those managed with CI.[52]

Current literature is inconclusive regarding audiologic treatment of ANSD in children. While some studies indicate that children with ANSD benefit from acoustic amplification, other studies focus on the effect of cochlear implantation on individuals with ANSD. Studies thus far have focused on the ability to perceive and recognize sounds or words, but further work is needed to address other functional aspects, including speech, language, learning, and social/emotional development in patients with ANSD.

Patients with Single-Sided Deafness

Historically, patients with unilateral severe-to-profound deafness were not surgical candidates for cochlear implantation. In patients with single-sided deafness (SSD), rehabilitation of hearing on the deaf side traditionally was accomplished with specialized hearing aids allowing contralateral routing of sound (CROS) and bone-anchored hearing systems (BAHS), allowing contralateral routing of signal through the skull base bone. However, recent literature has investigated the outcomes of cochlear implantation in patients with unilateral profound SNHL. A review of these studies shows a modest, but significant improvement in sound localization and speech perception after cochlear implantation in patients with SSD, as compared to CROS and BAHS strategies.

Arndt et al.[54] assessed speech perception in unilateral hearing loss patients utilizing CROS, BAHS, and cochlear implantation. The patients were tested in three listening conditions: (1) sound and noise presented directly in front of the patient, (2) sound on the normal-hearing side and noise on the deaf side, and (3) sound on the deaf side and noise on the normal-hearing side. The study demonstrated significant improvement in sound localization ability and in speech comprehension in CI patients over those with CROS, BAHS, and unaided strategies.[54] Stelzig et al.[55] evaluated four patients with unilateral deafness months following cochlear implantation. Monaural (unilateral normal hearing) and binaural (normal and CI) hearing were tested. The study demonstrated a modest, but significant improvements in speech intelligibility on the Hochmair-Schulz-Moser sentence test [4.6 and 6.3% at speech reception thresholds of 0 and –5 dB, respectively].[55]

In addition, patients with SSD have reported improvement in quality of life after cochlear implantation. Vermeire and Van de Heyning[56] used the Speech Spatial and Qualities of Hearing Scale, a scale composed of questions addressing speech understanding, spatial hearing, and hearing quality, to evaluate quality of life in patients after implantation. The authors reported a significant improvement in both the contralateral normal hearing and contralateral hearing aid groups in the speech understanding and hearing quality components of the scale following cochlear implantation.[56]

Patients with Low-Frequency Residual Hearing

Expanding CI candidacy criteria now include individuals with low-frequency residual hearing. These individuals undergo cochlear implantation with specifically designed electrodes and surgical techniques designed to preserve and minimize damage to the native acoustic function of the apical region. The FlexEAS electrode from MED-EL and the Nucleus Hybrid-L24 electrode from Cochlear Corporation are promising new devices that are currently being investigated for low-frequency hearing preservation surgery. Postoperatively, these patients undergo electroacoustic stimulation (EAS) in which high frequencies are stimulated electrically using the implanted electrode, while a hearing aid is used for acoustic stimulation of the preserved low-frequency hearing.

Normal-hearing individuals utilize various cues, including pitch, timing, and localization, to separate background speech from the speech of a target individual in a competing talkers condition. Systematic variation in these cues in normal-hearing individuals suggested that pitch resolution may be the most important skill in eliminating the distracting effects of multitalker background speech.[57] Thus, when low-frequency residual hearing is preserved following implantation, fine pitch discrimination, and thus speech perception in noise, would be expected to improve. Data suggests that maintenance of residual low-frequency hearing improves speech understanding in noise and music appreciation, although rates of hearing preservation are inconsistent. Using round window insertion and partial implantation of a standard length electrode, Kiefer et al. accomplished some degree of low-frequency hearing preservation in 11 of 13 patients; the remaining 2 patients experienced total hearing loss.[57] A study conducted by Lorens et al. includes data on 11 of 17 total EAS subjects; two subjects were excluded for total hearing loss occurring between 1 month and 2 years postoperatively, and an additional four could not utilize combined EAS.[58] More recently, Skarzynski and Lorens reported improved rates of speech perception in quiet and noisy environments following EAS in 15 children.[59]

CONCLUSION

Since the introduction of cochlear implantation, changes in CI candidacy, hardware, software, and speech processing technology have allowed greater numbers of adults and children with various degrees of hearing impairment access to sound. Electrode design and atraumatic insertion techniques appear to allow some preservation of low-frequency residual hearing. Advances in the technology related to CI hardware, software, and speech processing strategies demonstrate improved hearing in noise and may afford some music appreciation. Expanding candidacy criteria now allows an increasing number of hearing-impaired individuals, including infants, the elderly, and patients with ANSD, SSD, and those with some residual hearing access to cochlear implantation. Ongoing research in CI technology, candidacy, and outcomes is on the horizon and future research in these areas will ultimately affect clinical practice.

ACKNOWLEDGMENTS

Images courtesy of Advanced Bionics Corporation, MED-EL Corporation, and Cochlear Corporation.

REFERENCES

1. Wilson BS, Dorman MF. Cochlear implants: a remarkable past and a brilliant future. Hear Res. 2008;242:3-21.
2. Hochmair I, Nopp P, Jolly C, et al. MED-EL Cochlear implants: state of the art and a glimpse into the future. Trends Amplif. 2006;10:201-19.
3. Arnoldner C, Riss D, Brunner M, et al. Speech and music perception with the new fine structure speech coding strategy: preliminary results. Acta Otolaryngol. 2007;127: 1298-1303.
4. Riss D, Arnoldner C, Reiss S, et al. 1-year results using the Opus speech processor with the fine structure speech coding strategy. Acta Otolaryngol. 2009;129:988-91.
5. Magnusson L. Comparison of the fine structure processing (FSP) strategy and the CIS strategy used in the MED-EL cochlear implant system: speech intelligibility and music sound quality. Int J Audiol. 2011;50:279-87.
6. Fu QJ, Nogaki G. Noise susceptibility of cochlear implant users: the role of spectral resolution and smearing. J Assoc Res Otolaryngol. 2005;6:19-27.
7. Landsberger DM, Srinivasan AG. Virtual channel discrimination is improved by current focusing in cochlear implant recipients. Hear Res. 2009; 254:34-41.
8. Srinivasan AG, Landsberger DM, Shannon RV. Current focusing sharpens local peaks of excitation in cochlear implant stimulation. Hear Res. 2010; 270:89-100.
9. Firszt JB, Holden LK, Reeder RM, ET AL. Speech recognition in cochlear implant recipients: comparison of standard HiRes and HiRes 120 sound processing. Otol Neurotol. 2009;30:146-52.
10. Donaldson GS, Dawson PK, Borden LZ. Within-subjects comparison of the HiRes and Fidelity120 speech processing strategies: speech perception and its relation to place-pitch sensitivity. Ear Hear. 2011;32:238-50.
11. Berenstein CK, Mens LH, Mulder JJ, et al. Current steering and current focusing in cochlear implants: comparison of monopolar, tripolar, and virtual channel electrode configurations. Ear Hear. 2008;29:250-60.
12. Litvak LM, Spahr AJ, Emadi G. Loudness growth observed under partially tripolar stimulation: model and data from cochlear implant listeners. J Acoust Soc Am. 2007;122: 967-81.
13. Chung K, Zeng FG. Using hearing aid adaptive directional microphones to enhance cochlear implant performance. Hear Res. 2009;250:27-37.
14. Buechner A, Brendel M, Saalfeld H, et al. Results of a pilot study with a signal enhancement algorithm for HiRes 120 cochlear implant users. Otol Neurotol. 2010;31:1386-90.
15. Zeng FG, Rebscher S, Harrison W, et al. Cochlear implants: system design, integration, and evaluation. IEEE Rev Biomed Eng. 2008;1:115-42.
16. Geier LL, Norton SJ. The effects of limiting the number of Nucleus 22 cochlear implant electrodes programmed on speech perception. Ear Hear. 1992;13:340-48.
17. Finley CC, Holden TA, Holden LK, et al. Role of electrode placement as a contributor to variability in cochlear implant outcomes. Otol Neurotol. 2008;29:920-28.
18. Lee J, Nadol JB, Jr., Eddington DK. Depth of electrode insertion and postoperative performance in humans with cochlear implants: a histopathologic study. Audiol Neurootol. 2010;15:323-31.
19. Yoshinaga-Itano C. Early intervention after universal neonatal hearing screening: impact on outcomes. Ment Retard Dev Disabil Res Rev. 2003;9:252-66.
20. Genetics Evaluation Guidelines for the Etiologic Diagnosis of Congenital Hearing Loss. Genetic Evaluation of Congenital Hearing Loss Expert Panel. ACMG statement. Genet Med 2002; 4:162-71.
21. Steel KP, Kros CJ. A genetic approach to understanding auditory function. Nat Genet. 2001;27:143-9.
22. Preciado DA, Lawson L, Madden C, et al. Improved diagnostic effectiveness with a sequential diagnostic paradigm in idiopathic pediatric sensorineural hearing loss. Otol Neurotol. 2005;26:610-15.
23. Parry DA, Booth T, Roland PS. Advantages of magnetic resonance imaging over computed tomography in preoperative evaluation of pediatric cochlear implant candidates. Otol Neurotol. 2005;26:976-82.
24. Trimble K, Blaser S, James AL, et al. Computed tomography and/or magnetic resonance imaging before pediatric cochlear implantation? Developing an investigative strategy. Otol Neurotol. 2007;28:317-24.
25. Gleeson TG, Lacy PD, Bresnihan M, et al. High resolution computed tomography and magnetic resonance imaging in the pre-operative assessment of cochlear implant patients. J Laryngol Otol. 2003;117:692-5.
26. Balkany TJ, Whitley M, Shapira Y, et al. The temporalis pocket technique for cochlear implantation: an anatomic and clinical study. Otol Neurotol. 2009;30:903-7.

27. Cosetti MK, Troob SH, Latzman JM, et al. An evidence-based algorithm for intraoperative monitoring during cochlear implantation. Otol Neurotol. 2012;33:169-76.
28. Bhatia K, Gibbin KP, Nikolopoulos TP, et al. Surgical complications and their management in a series of 300 consecutive pediatric cochlear implantations. Otol Neurotol. 2004;25:730-39.
29. Loundon N, Blanchard M, Roger G, et al. Medical and surgical complications in paediatric cochlear implantation. Cochlear Implants Int. 2010;11 Suppl 1:192-4.
30. Lalwani AK, Cohen NL. Does meningitis after cochlear implantation remain a concern in 2011? Otol Neurotol. 2012;33:93-5.
31. Lalwani AK, Cohen NL. Longitudinal risk of meningitis after cochlear implantation associated with the use of the positioner. Otol Neurotol. 2011;32:1082-5.
32. Niparko JK, Tobey EA, Thal DJ, et al. Spoken language development in children following cochlear implantation. JAMA. 2010; 303:1498-1506.
33. Miyamoto RT, Hay-McCutcheon MJ, Kirk KI, et al. Language skills of profoundly deaf children who received cochlear implants under 12 months of age: a preliminary study. Acta Otolaryngol. 2008;128:373-7.
34. Houston DM, Miyamoto RT. Effects of early auditory experience on word learning and speech perception in deaf children with cochlear implants: implications for sensitive periods of language development. Otol Neurotol. 2010;31:1248-53.
35. Roland JT, Jr., Cosetti M, Wang KH, et al. Cochlear implantation in the very young child: Long-term safety and efficacy. Laryngoscope. 2009;119:2205-10.
36. Dettman SJ, Pinder D, Briggs RJ, et al. Communication development in children who receive the cochlear implant younger than 12 months: risks versus benefits. Ear Hear. 2007;28:11S-18S.
37. Morray JP, Geiduschek JM, Ramamoorthy C, et al. Anesthesia-related cardiac arrest in children: initial findings of the Pediatric Perioperative Cardiac Arrest (POCA) Registry. Anesthesiology. 2000;93:6-14.
38. Valencia DM, Rimell FL, Friedman BJ, et al. Cochlear implantation in infants less than 12 months of age. Int J Pediatr Otorhinolaryngol. 2008;72:767-73.
39. Lesinski-Schiedat A, Illg A, Heermann R, et al. Paediatric cochlear implantation in the first and in the second year of life: a comparative study. Cochlear Implants Int. 2004;5: 146-59.
40. Waltzman SB, Roland JT, Jr. Cochlear implantation in children younger than 12 months. Pediatrics. 2005;116: e487-493.
41. Colletti V, Carner M, Miorelli V, et al. Cochlear implantation at under 12 months: report on 10 patients. Laryngoscope. 2005;115:445-9.
42. Holt RF, Svirsky MA. An exploratory look at pediatric cochlear implantation: is earliest always best? Ear Hear. 2008;29:492-511.
43. Mulrow CD, Aguilar C, Endicott JE, et al. Association between hearing impairment and the quality of life of elderly individuals. J Am Geriatr Soc. 1990;38:45-50.
44. Cacciatore F, Napoli C, Abete P, et al. Quality of life determinants and hearing function in an elderly population: Osservatorio Geriatrico Campano Study Group. Gerontology. 1999;45:323-8.
45. Coelho DH, Yeh J, Kim JT, et al. Cochlear implantation is associated with minimal anesthetic risk in the elderly. Laryngoscope. 2009;119:355-8.
46. Eshraghi AA, Rodriguez M, Balkany TJ, et al. Cochlear implant surgery in patients more than seventy-nine years old. Laryngoscope. 2009;119:1180-83.
47. Mahncke HW, Bronstone A, Merzenich MM. Brain plasticity and functional losses in the aged: scientific bases for a novel intervention. Prog Brain Res. 2006;157:81-109.
48. Dickstein DL, Kabaso D, Rocher AB, et al. Changes in the structural complexity of the aged brain. Aging Cell. 2007; 6:275-84.
49. Budenz CL, Cosetti MK, Coelho DH, et al. The effects of cochlear implantation on speech perception in older adults. J Am Geriatr Soc. 2011;59:446-53.
50. Vermeire K, Brokx JP, Wuyts FL, et al. Quality-of-life benefit from cochlear implantation in the elderly. Otol Neurotol. 2005;26:188-95.
51. Francis HW, Chee N, Yeagle J, et al. Impact of cochlear implants on the functional health status of older adults. Laryngoscope. 2002;112:1482-8.
52. Rance G, Barker EJ. Speech and language outcomes in children with auditory neuropathy/dys-synchrony managed with either cochlear implants or hearing aids. Int J Audiol. 2009;48:313-20.
53. Teagle HF, Roush PA, Woodard JS, et al. Cochlear implantation in children with auditory neuropathy spectrum disorder. Ear Hear. 2010;31:325-35.
54. Arndt S, Laszig R, Beck R, et al. Spectrum of hearing disorders and their management in children with CHARGE syndrome. Otol Neurotol. 2010;31:67-73.
55. Stelzig Y, Jacob R, Mueller J. Preliminary speech recognition results after cochlear implantation in patients with unilateral hearing loss: a case series. J Med Case Rep. 2011; 5:343.
56. Vermeire K, Van de Heyning P. Binaural hearing after cochlear implantation in subjects with unilateral sensorineural deafness and tinnitus. Audiol Neurootol. 2009;14: 163-71.
57. Kiefer J, Pok M, Adunka O, et al. Combined electric and acoustic stimulation of the auditory system: results of a clinical study. Audiol Neurootol. 2005;10:134-44.
58. Lorens A, Polak M, Piotrowska A, et al. Outcomes of treatment of partial deafness with cochlear implantation: a DUET study. Laryngoscope. 2008;118:288-94.
59. Skarzynski H, Lorens A. Electric acoustic stimulation in children. Adv Otorhinolaryngol. 2010;67:135-43.

CHAPTER

34

Auditory Brainstem Implants

Eric P Wilkinson, Steven R Otto, Marc S Schwartz, Derald E Brackmann

INTRODUCTION

The auditory brainstem implant (ABI) for patients was originally developed for patients with neurofibromatosis type 2 (NF2) in order to electrically stimulate the cochlear nucleus complex. Drs. William House and William Hitselberger first used the ABI in such a patient in 1979,[1,2,3] who continues to use it daily. Patients with NF2 usually have bilateral vestibular schwannomas (VS) necessitating tumor removal, which often results in profound deafness, and cochlear implants (CIs), which electrically activate peripheral neural processes within the cochlea, are usually not an option for patients with NF2 because of their loss of integrity of the auditory nerve. The ABI is introduced into the lateral recess of the fourth ventricle and placed over the area of the ventral and dorsal cochlear nuclei after tumor removal. The ABI is similar in design and function to multichannel CIs, except for differences in the design of the stimulating electrode arrays.[4,5,6] Multichannel CIs and ABIs were developed to capitalize on the frequency tuning of neurons in the human cochlea and cochlear nucleus complex, respectively. The programming of ABI devices, however, differs in several important aspects from CI programming.

In multichannel CIs, the electrode is placed into the cochlea. Consistent placement of the electrode carrier and its depth of insertion are assured in normal cochleas. However, in ABI recipients, anatomical landmarks that are used in electrode array placement may be altered or obscured due to the presence of tumors making electrode array placement more challenging. This chapter describes the surgical anatomy of the cochlear nucleus complex, our experience, and results with ABI placement in individuals with and without NF2.

NEUROFIBROMATOSIS TYPE 2

NF2 is an autosomal dominant condition. Bilateral acoustic neuromas (VS) are the hallmark of this disease and are pathognomonic for NF2. The diagnostic criteria for NF2, redefined by the US National Institutes of Health Consensus Development Conference, are met if a person has (1) bilateral eighth-nerve masses seen with computed tomographic scanning or magnetic resonance imaging (MRI) or (2) a first-degree relative (parent or sibling) with NF2 and either unilateral eighth-nerve masses or one of the following: neurofibroma, meningioma, glioma, schwannoma, or juvenile posterior subcapsular lenticular opacity. The incidence of NF2 is one in 33,000–40,000 live births.[7,8] Patients with NF2 present complex and challenging management problems. Previously, delayed diagnosis, growth of tumor, or surgical removal of the acoustic tumors usually resulted in total hearing loss. Early diagnosis using gadolinium-enhanced MRI and refinements in hearing preservation surgery has improved our ability to prevent total hearing loss while achieving complete tumor removal. Appropriate family screening and DNA analysis have helped early diagnosis. For patients with larger tumors or no useful hearing, the ABI allows restoration of some auditory function when the tumor is removed.

PATIENT SELECTION

The nucleus ABI (Cochlear Corporation, Centennial, CO) (Fig. 34.1) is approved by the US Food and Drug Administration (FDA) for implantation at the time of VS removal. Suitable candidates are patients undergoing translabyrinthine VS removal who have (1) nonaidable hearing or an only-hearing ear with a symptomatic tumor or (2) serviceable hearing in the contralateral ear but a contralateral tumor of sufficient size to indicate that hearing will likely be lost in a short period. Criteria for patient selection for receiving an ABI are as follows: evidence of bilateral eighth-nerve tumors, competency in the English language, age 12 years or older, psychological suitability, willingness to comply with the follow-up protocol, and realistic expectations.

While there are some exceptions, the large majority of patients to have received the ABI at the House Clinic have NF2 and bilateral acoustic neuromas. In these patients, the goal is to restore some auditory function in order for these individuals to continue to be a part of the hearing world and to improve their quality of life. The ABI may be implanted during removal of either the first- or second-side tumor, even if some hearing remains on the other side, which is often the case. This approach allows patients to become familiar with the use of the device and prepares them for when all hearing is lost.[9-11]

More recently, other potential indications for ABI placement have developed. Postlingually deafened adults with cochlear ossification following meningitis or with cranial trauma resulting in bilateral cochlear nerve transection or avulsion have been implanted. In Europe, congenitally deaf young children who are deemed not to be candidates for CI due to severe cochlear malformation or cochlear nerve aplasia have been implanted with very good results. FDA-approved trials of patients with these diagnoses are now beginning in the United States.[12-14]

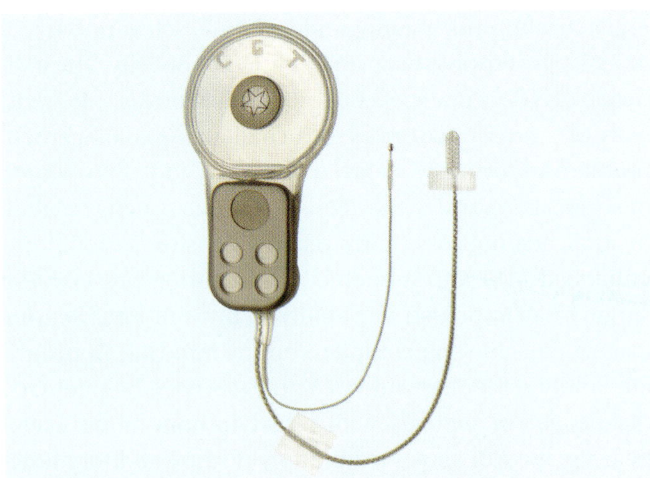

Fig. 34.1: Nucleus auditory brainstem implant.

SURGICAL TECHNIQUE AND ANATOMY OF THE COCHLEAR NUCLEUS

The cochlear nucleus complex (dorsal and ventral cochlear nuclei) lies in the lateral recess of the fourth ventricle. It is partially obscured by the cerebellar peduncles. A surface electrode array introduced in the lateral recess crossing the taenia choroidea will stimulate viable cochlear nucleus structures.

At the House Clinic, we have almost exclusively used the translabyrinthine approach for placement of the ABI. Typically, we use a C-shaped incision that starts behind the pinna and is approximately 2 cm away from the postauricular fold at the level of the mastoid tip, as shown in Figure 34.2. It allows the placement of the internal receiver and magnet under the scalp. It is important that the incision not directly cross the area of the receiver/stimulator.

The translabyrinthine approach provides direct access to the cochlear nuclei. The jugular bulb is skeletonized to provide the widest access to this area (Fig. 34.3). Anatomical landmarks used for placement include the stump of the eighth nerve, the glossopharyngeal nerve, the facial nerve, and the taenia choroidea as well as the mouth of the lateral

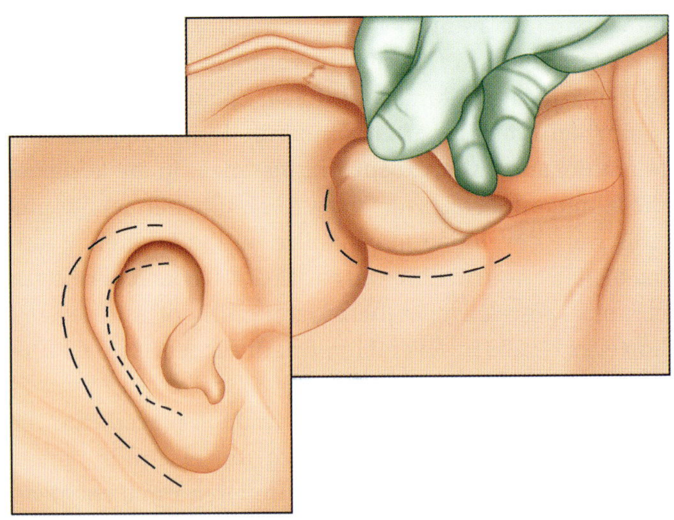

Fig. 34.2: C-shaped incision currently used for the placement of an auditory brainstem implant (ABI). The incision starts behind the pinna and is approximately 2 cm away from the postauricular fold at the level of the mastoid tip.

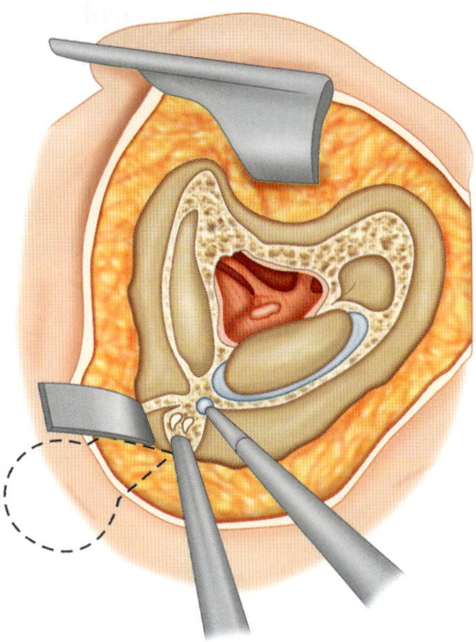

Fig. 34.3: The bed for the internal receiver/stimulator and placement of the magnet under the periosteum. The seat for the receiver is connected to the translabyrinthine craniotomy. The trough created allows running the electrodes into the CPA.

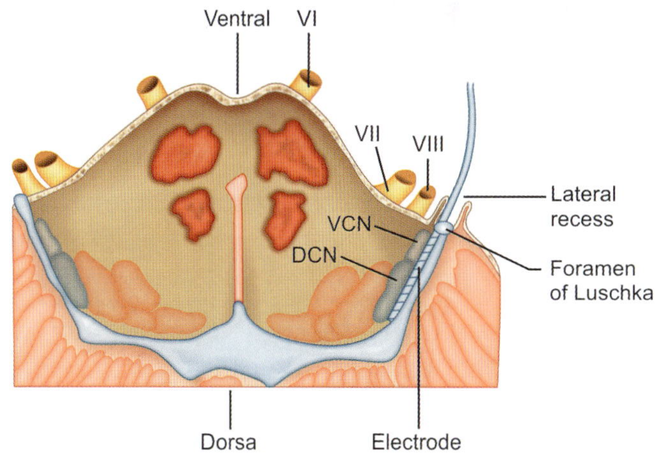

Fig. 34.4: A histological section showing the area of the lateral recess of the fourth ventricle, cranial nerves VI, VII, VIII, and the relationship between ventral cochlear nucleus (VCN), dorsal cochlear nucleus (DCN), inferior cerebellar peduncle, and the vestibular nuclei. The cerebellum (CE) is also shown.

recess where all of these structures converge (Fig. 34.4). Two features frequently used to identify the lateral recess are its relationship to the ninth nerve and the position of the jugular bulb. In the surgical setting where there is almost always distortion of the brain stem from the tumor, the lateral recess is superior to the ninth nerve. The ninth nerve is generally in a fixed anatomic position, and going from there, the lateral recess may be identified in almost every case. The jugular bulb is important because its position may vary. Indeed, with a contracted mastoid and a high jugular bulb, the exposure may be more difficult although it should not be an impediment to placement of the ABI electrode.

Location of the ventral cochlear nucleus, the main target for placement of the ABI, can be problematic. After clearly identifying the basic anatomic landmarks of the lateral recess, including the choroid plexus and the more reflective ependymal surface, dissection is temporarily stopped and the posterior fossa is occluded with Gelfoam. At this point, a subgaleal pocket is created superior and posterior to the mastoidectomy site. A seat is then drilled in the outer table of the skull to secure the position of the ABI receiver. Next, dissection continues in the posterior fossa with the ABI on the operative field. After placing the ground electrode under the temporalis muscle, the ABI electrode array is carefully inserted into the lateral recess. Correct anatomic placement is confirmed using electrophysiological monitoring. Electrically evoked auditory brainstem responses are elicited by stimulation of the nucleus, and the position of the ABI electrode array is optimized using information derived from electrophysiological monitoring, as determined by an experienced auditory physiologist.[15] In addition to facial nerve monitoring, the lower cranial nerves are also monitored to avoid side effects and nonauditory sensations.

Once the optimal position is determined, Teflon felt or muscle is used to secure the electrode in the lateral recess of the fourth ventricle. In patients with NF2 who will require frequent MRIs, the magnetic disc in the receiver/stimulator is replaced with a nonmagnetic plug. The receiver is then placed in the subgaleal pocket prior to filling the mastoid cavity with abdominal fat, carefully inserting a titanium mesh cranioplasty, and closing the scalp (Fig. 34.5).

In other centers, the retrosigmoid approach has been used to implant ABIs with similar success. Both supine/lateral and semi-sitting positions have been used. The latter may offer some benefit in terms of brain relaxation and ease of access to the lateral recess. In young children, the retrosigmoid approach is used universally.[14]

In the case of the previously investigational penetrating ABI (PABI), after establishing landmarks and identifying the cochlear nuclei, the penetrating electrode was placed first into the ventral portion of the nucleus, which is then followed by placement of the surface electrode as in a regular ABI surgery (Fig. 34.6).

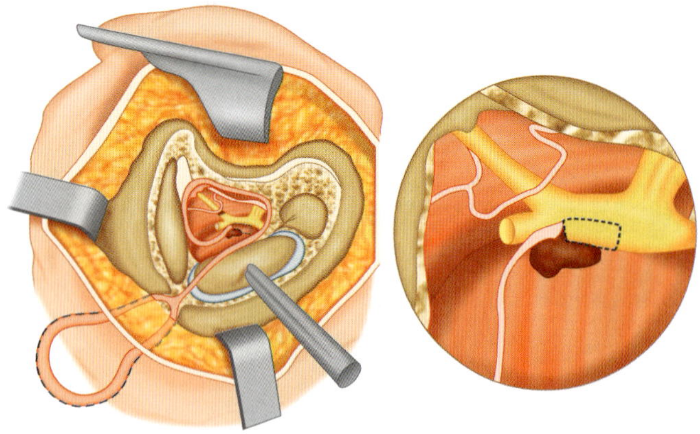

Fig. 34.5: Placement of the electrode in the lateral recess and the mastoid. The facial nerve, cochleovestibular nerve stump, lower cranial nerves, and the choroid plexus emerging from the lateral recess of the fourth ventricle are shown.

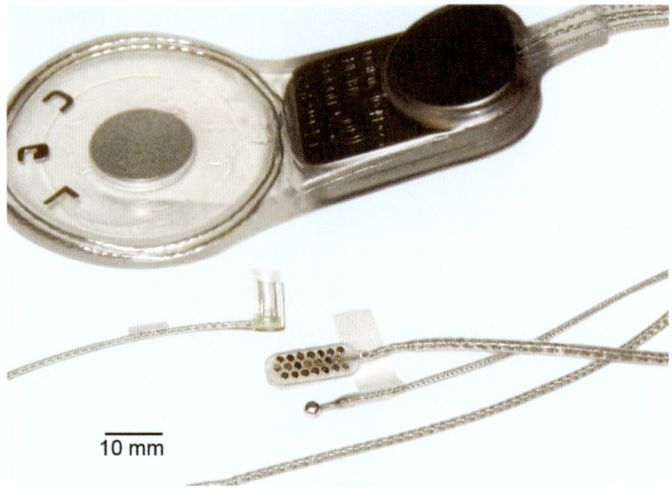

Fig. 34.6: Penetrating auditory brainstem implant (ABI) device with both surface and penetrating electrode arrays.

Implantation is facilitated by preservation of landmarks during tumor resection. Great care is also taken during exposure of the lateral recess, which may be obstructed by arteries, veins or a thin membrane, and during device placement. Very gentle manipulation of brainstem, tumor, and surrounding neurovascular structures may lead to improved audiologic results. With the largest tumors, this may be very difficult or impossible. [12]

DEVICE

We use the current-generation nucleus ABI, manufactured by Cochlear Corporation (Centennial, CO, USA). This device, which is the only one approved for commercial use by the FDA, consists of 21 electrodes embedded in a silicone carrier that is fixed to a fabric mesh, connected to an implantable internal receiver/stimulator. A competing device manufactured by MedEl Corporation is of similar construction and has an array of 12 electrodes. This device has not been approved by the FDA but is in use in Europe and elsewhere. The external equipment for both devices consists of an external transmitter coil held in place by a tape and metal disk placed on the scalp over the receiver/stimulator coil and connected to a microphone and sound processor, which contains the battery power source. All of this is similar to a CI. As long as the magnet is removed from the implanted receiver/stimulator, follow-up serial MR imaging scans (1.5 Tesla maximum) can be obtained with minimal artifact. The MedEl implant does not have a removable magnet, and therefore further MR imaging requires externally securing the implant in place. Presence of the magnet may further affect ability to assess ipsilateral disease, and coronal MR imaging may be more able to assess the cerebellopontine angle in such situations.[16]

The sound processing unit (speech processor) requires appropriate programming and must be fitted to individual users. Programming speech processors involves psychophysical assessment of electrically induced auditory (and nonauditory) percepts including threshold, comfort level, and pitch. The outcomes of these measures are used to program the sound processor appropriately and control the amplitude and the sequential patterns of stimulation.

In multichannel auditory implants, different sites of stimulation can often generate different pitch percepts for the listener. Changes in the frequency spectrum of sound can therefore be coded by appropriate changes in the patterns of electrode activation. CIs can usually employ a relatively standard pattern of neural stimulation because of the homogeneous tuning of neurons in the cochlea. ABI recipients, however, have variations in brainstem anatomy, electrode array placement, and tumor effects that require the use of more individualized stimulus patterns to code frequency cues and manage any nonauditory sensations. Therefore, special techniques and additional time are usually required to program ABI sound processors.

Initial testing and activation of the ABI is typically carried out 1–2 months after the surgery. Any nonauditory sensations are reduced or, if possible, eliminated by altering the electrical parameters of stimulation (particularly pulse duration and reference ground electrode). Nonuditory sensations have included dizziness, sensation of vibration in the eye, throat sensations, and ipsilateral tingling sensations in the head or body. Generally, non-auditory sensations have decreased in magnitude when longer pulse duration stimuli are used.

RESULTS

Auditory outcomes and speech perception performance have generally improved significantly since initial development of the ABI. The first 25 patients implanted prior to 1992 at the House Research Institute (HRI) received a single-channel system.[4] Since 1992, we have used the nucleus multichannel ABI device that has resulted in improved performance.[9] The nucleus multichannel ABI completed clinical trials and received approval from the FDA for commercial release on October 20, 2000.

A number of articles have been published detailing results obtained with the ABI. To date, more than 280 patients have been implanted at HRI, with more than 1250 total recipients worldwide. The safety of this device has been comparable to the safety of CIs. At our institution, only two patients (early users of the "single-channel" ABI) were explanted due to infection, and this was likely related to the percutaneous connector in use at the time rather than the ABI electrode array.

Presently, 80% of the patients are device users, and 92% have received auditory sensations from their ABIs. Approximately 25% of ABI users have achieved open-set speech discrimination (at least 20% correct without lipreading cues on the CUNY Sentence Test).[4,5,9,10] Ten of our patients have scored 65% or better, and three patients have scored 82% or better on this test. The majority of patients recognize a high percentage of environmental sounds, and speech understanding ability has enhanced an average of 35% when ABI sound is combined with lipreading. This enhancement has reached as high as 75% in some individuals.

Initially, most of our patients with NF2 were implanted at the time of surgery to remove second side VS, but in the mid-1990s application was made to the FDA to begin implanting when first side acoustic tumors were being removed. This can assist in easing the transition of patients to hearing exclusively with the ABI after becoming completely deaf. Now, about a third of our patients have received ABIs on their first tumor sides, and their ABIs have been activated soon after surgery. Even though usable hearing may remain on the second-tumor side, this experience has resulted in as much as a 25% "headstart" in speech perception when patients ultimately become completely reliant on ABI sound. Most first-side recipients have commented on practical advantages of this approach, including avoiding any substantial period of complete deafness, being able to remain on the job, and maintaining some ability to hear and monitor their children's activities.

Since about 9% of our NF2 cases do not ultimately obtain hearing sensations from their ABIs, another advantage of first-side implantation is that it can provide a valuable second opportunity to achieve a hearing result when needed. Usually, the second opportunity has resulted in beneficial hearing outcomes; however, in about 20% of these patients, the second ABI did not provide substantially better outcomes than the first. This suggests that whatever affected outcomes on the first side can also influence outcomes on the second side.

In our NF2 cases, we have found that very large acoustic tumors can sometimes distort or damage brainstem anatomy, complicate device implantation, and impact ABI outcomes. Some treatments of acoustic tumors, including surgery, also may affect the stimulability of brainstem auditory structures. For example, we have noted that patients with a history of "gamma knife" radiation therapy for acoustic tumors have had a higher rate of not getting hearing from their ABIs than patients without this history (about 30% vs. 9%). However, there are many examples of patients with large acoustic tumors, or a history of gamma knife, who have experienced great benefit from their ABIs.

EXPANDED APPLICATIONS FOR THE ABI

The PABI,[17] developed at HRI and Huntington Medical Research Institute (Pasadena, CA) in collaboration with Cochlear Corporation, was an effort to improve the efficiency of the ABI through microstimulation with needle electrodes, and to increase access to the subsurface tonotopic organization of the ventral cochlear nucleus. We hoped that this would contribute to higher levels of speech understanding. The PABI was studied in clinical trials the under the auspices of the FDA. Patients had both needle electrode arrays and conventional surface arrays.

Ten patients were implanted, and we found that microstimulation resulted in hearing sensations at much lower electrical levels than conventional surface electrodes, that a wide range of pitch percepts could be elicited depending on the location and depth of the penetrating electrodes, and that sound quality and speech perception performance were better with sound processor maps that used a combination of penetrating and surface electrodes. In two PABI recipients, we also found that stimulation on longer electrodes (2 mm in length) could result in uncomfortable facial sensations, possibly related to activation of trigeminal tracts. Unfortunately, microstimulation with the PABI alone did not substantially improve speech recognition over the conventional surface electrodes. This may have been due to difficulty in identifying the precise location of the subsurface cochlear nucleus structures in NF2 patients with distorted brainstem anatomy, and thus obtaining a high percentage of useable penetrating electrodes. Once placed, the position of the penetrating array could not be adjusted if needed. Clear EABR waveforms also could not be observed when recording from scalp electrodes to assist with accurate placement of the penetrating array. Therefore, the PABI is not in current clinical use. Given their demonstrated advantages, however, newer penetrating electrode array designs are continuing to be studied.

While the original purpose of the ABI was to treat deafness in adults with NF2, we anticipated that it could be useful in treating deafness in non-NF2 cases without viable auditory nerves or implantable cochleas. Recently, many of these cases have been implanted, primarily in Europe. Positive outcomes have led to renewed interest in the ABI as an effective treatment of deafness resulting from traumatic transection or avulsion of the auditory nerve, cochlear ossification after meningitis, and congenital cochlear aplasia/agenesis.

Such non-NF2 cases, both adult and pediatric, were first implanted by Vittorio Colletti in Verona, Italy.[18] While outcomes have been variable, in general results have exceeded those in the historic NF2 population. Many of these cases also were reported to have substantial "sound-only" word recognition ability. Such patients are implanted without concurrent tumor resection and generally have more normal brainstem anatomy, which helps preserve neural function and facilitates the identification of important anatomical landmarks used in device implantation. This may be particularly important in maximizing ABI outcomes in pediatric cases.

ABIs are now being used in the treatment of deafness in pediatric cases with cochlear malformations or cochlear nerve aplasia. In 2004, we reported on ABI outcomes in 21 children with NF2 implanted as young as age 12.[19] We found that these individuals could experience substantial communication benefit. A key factor was appropriate family and other support. Several years ago, we also conducted device programming and comprehensive evaluation of a 3-year-old non-NF2 case implanted with an ABI in Verona,[20] and then subsequently four other very young children implanted at the age of 2–3 years (also in Verona). Our findings have demonstrated that considerable, and in some cases remarkable, benefit is possible. Some of these children have developed a substantial level of auditory function, including discrimination of environmental sounds, some open set recognition of speech, and development of useful speech and language, and in some cases have been able to attend a normal hearing classroom with appropriate support services.

Generally, pediatric cases without concurrent developmental delay or syndromic problems have been reported to perform best.[21] Of course, benefits of ABI implantation must be weighed against the risk of surgery in this group of patients in whom craniotomy is performed solely for ABI placement. In the pediatric population, a retrosigmoid surgical approach is typically used, as the mastoid is less developed. As with pediatric CIs, early implantation seems to provide the best outcomes with generally diminishing returns as duration of deafness increases.

In a recent retrospective cohort study,[22] a group of children were studied who initially underwent CI and failed to progress with auditory perception. Before CI, all of the children had severe-to-profound sensorineural hearing loss and a diagnosis of cochlear nerve deficiency. Explantation of the CI and simultaneous ABI on the same side was performed, and all patients demonstrated an absent cochlear nerve at surgery.

Performance as measured by the categories of auditory performance scale was significantly improved after ABI. Patients with cognitive deficits did gain performance benefits from the ABI, but the difference in performance compared to children without cognitive impairment was significant. Additionally, children implanted before age 3 also performed better than children implanted at an older age.

Cases of a small cochlear nerve on imaging may in reality represent an absent cochlear nerve. The decision on whether to place a CI in a patient with cochlear nerve deficiency is never an easy one, and currently both imaging and electrophysiology are not fully predictive of outcome with CI. Although this cohort was selected from patients with failed CI, ABI is a potential alternative to CI in select cases. In patients who fail to progress with intensive rehabilitation with CI, ABI may be considered as an alternative. While in this study the CI was explanted, we may see more situations where an ABI is considered on the contralateral side, if any CI benefit has been obtained, to allow for continued use of both a CI and an ABI. After more than 33 years of experience with ABIs in adults, we have initiated our own pediatric ABI clinical trials under the auspices of the FDA. Ten children aged 2–5 years will be implanted and their auditory performance tracked on an extensive battery of tests.

Since the beginning of our ABI program in 1979, we have utilized a team approach to maximize patient benefit, satisfaction, and safety. We feel that this is particularly necessary in pediatric ABI implantation given the possibility for eliciting nonauditory sensations, and the much more limited ability of young children to provide detailed feedback about the effects of electrical stimulation. They also are not typically capable of making precise judgments regarding the psychophysical parameters (e.g. electrical threshold, comfortable loudness, and electrode-specific pitch) that are normally considered necessary to properly program ABI sound processors. Initially, best estimates of these perceptual effects and parameters must be determined by skilled clinicians using age-appropriate behavioral testing. The efficacy of the ABI depends on the accuracy of the processor settings that must be objectively verified by further sound-field testing and close observation of the child at home and at school. Regular follow-ups for further behavioral testing and device reprogramming are critical in achieving maximum benefit. Since hearing with the ABI can change over time, some electrodes may become useable that could not be used initially.

Electrophysiological measures in sedated young children have been used, mostly in Europe, to program ABI sound processors[23]; however we have found that these tests can significantly underestimate required stimulation levels. Therefore, we do not consider electrophysiological measures as a substitute for reliable behavioral responses in programming sound processors in pediatric ABI recipients. One area where both electrophysiological and behavioral measures fall short in pediatric cases is in the assessment of electrode-specific pitch sensations. In very young deaf children, the concept of perceptual pitch may not exist, or at least may not be reliably testable. In adults, such testing is used to sensibly assign electrodes to processor frequency analysis bands so that lower and higher frequency spectral cues are sent to electrodes that generate appropriate-sounding pitch percepts. Of course, each adult ABI user is somewhat different in this respect. In pediatric cases, the lack of this data has not been a serious obstacle, and both a generally increasing and a generally decreasing assignment of frequency information across electrodes have resulted in good performance. With little if any prior auditory experience, pre- or perilingually deafened young children appear to have adapted to either electrode-assignment strategy. We feel, however, that a reasonable practice for very young children is to apply the predominant pitch pattern seen in adults, which is a tendency for pitch percepts to rise in a lateral to medial direction across the electrode array.[9] Despite these psychophysical complexities, it is clear that experienced pediatric ABI teams can safely implant and program the devices with very beneficial outcomes.

Recently, there have been encouraging data regarding the long-term safety of ABI use.[24] Histological sections through the cochlear nuclei on both sides were obtained from an adult patient who used his ABI daily for 15 years. This individual demonstrated very high levels of speech recognition performance up until the time of his death from complications of NF2. The analysis showed good and comparable populations of auditory neurons on both implanted and unimplanted sides with no deleterious effects from long-term electrical stimulation. Also in this regard, the very first recipient of an ABI initially implanted in 1979 continues in 2013 to use her ABI daily with benefit. This is a very encouraging finding for pediatric cases potentially facing a lifetime of ABI use.

Recent ABI results in patients with NF2 also have been encouraging. Performance improvements were first seen in patients operated via the retrosigmoid approach in the semisitting position with the 12-electrode MedEl ABI device. In this group, reports indicated that about 30% of patients were experiencing some degree of "sound-only" word recognition ability. Due to concerns of other possible intraoperative complications, such as air embolism, the sitting position is not typically used for VS resection in the United States. When taking care to achieve meticulous tumor resection and brainstem handling via the translabyrinthine approach, our group is also achieving about a 25% incidence of "sound-only" speech understanding ability.

CONCLUSION

The ABI has been utilized to provide auditory benefit to deaf patients who are not candidates for cochlear implantation due to loss or absence of the cochlear nerves or abnormalities of the cochlea itself. By far the most common indication for ABI is NF2. The safety of the stimulation of the cochlear nuclei using this device has been established. Most patients perceive beneficial auditory sensations and improve their communication abilities over lipreading only. A smaller number achieve substantial speech discrimination using only ABI sound, and nontumor patients may achieve greater average benefit. A key factor is regular device use, and with that improvements can occur for 10 years or more. More recent ABI results demonstrate the possibility of achieving improved auditory results even in patients with NF2. Additionally, ABI implantation in prelingually deafened children who are not CI candidates holds much promise for providing auditory stimulation and allowing for language and speech development.

REFERENCES

1. Edgerton BJ, House WF, Hitselberger W. Hearing by cochlear nucleus stimulation in humans. Ann Otol Rhinol Laryngol Suppl. 1982;91(2 Pt 3):117-24.
2. Eisenberg LS, Maltan AA, Portillo F, et al. Electrical stimulation of the auditory brain stem structure in deafened adults. J Rehabil Res Dev. 1987;24(3):9-22
3. Portillo F, Nelson RA, Brackmann DE, et al. Auditory brain stem implant: electrical stimulation of the human cochlear nucleus. Adv Otorhinolaryngol. 1993;48:248-52.
4. Brackmann DE, Hitselberger WE, Nelson RA, et al. Auditory brainstem implant: I. Issues in surgical implantation. Otolaryngol Head Neck Surg. 1993;108(6):624-33.
5. Shannon RV, Fayad J, Moore J, et al. Auditory brainstem implant: II. Postsurgical issues and performance. Otolaryngol Head Neck Surg. 1993;108(6):634-42.
6. Schwartz MS, Otto SR, Brackmann DE, et al. Use of a multichannel auditory brainstem implant for neurofibromatosis type 2. Stereotact Funct Neurosurg. 2003;81(1-4):110-4.
7. Evans DG, Huson SM, Donnai D, et al. A genetic study of type 2 neurofibromatosis in the United Kingdom. II. Guidelines for genetic counselling. J Med Genet. 1992;29 (12):847-52.
8. Evans DG, Huson SM, Donnai D, et al. A genetic study of type 2 neurofibromatosis in the United Kingdom. I. Prevalence, mutation rate, fitness, and confirmation of maternal transmission effect on severity. J Med Genet. 1992;29 (12):841-6.
9. Otto SR, Brackmann DE, Hitselberger WE, et al. Multichannel auditory brainstem implant: update on performance in 61 patients. J Neurosurg. 2002;96(6):1063-71.
10. Otto SR, Brackmann DE, Hitselberger W. Auditory brainstem implantation in 12- to 18-year-olds. Arch Otolaryngol Head Neck Surg. 2004;130(5):656-9.
11. Nevison B, Laszig R, Sollmann WP, et al. Results from a European clinical investigation of the Nucleus multichannel auditory brainstem implant. Ear Hear. 2002;23(3): 170-83.
12. Colletti V, Carner M, Miorelli V, et al. Auditory brainstem implant (ABI): new frontiers in adults and children. Otolaryngol Head Neck Surg. 2005;133(1):126-38.
13. Colletti V, Shannon RV. Open set speech perception with auditory brainstem implant? Laryngoscope. 2005;115(11): 1974-8.
14. Colletti V, Sacchetto L, Giarbini N, et al. Retrosigmoid approach for auditory brainstem implant. J Laryngol Otol Suppl. 2000(27):37-40.
15. Waring MD. Intraoperative electrophysiologic monitoring to assist placement of auditory brain stem implant. Ann Otol Rhinol Laryngol Suppl. 1995;166:33-6.
16. Heller JW, Brackmann DE, Tucci DL, et al. Evaluation of MRI compatibility of the modified nucleus multichannel auditory brainstem and cochlear implants. Am J Otol. 1996;17(5):724-9.
17. Otto SR, Shannon RV, Wilkinson EP, et al. Audiologic outcomes with the penetrating electrode auditory brainstem implant. Otol Neurotol. 2008;29(8):1147-54.
18. Colletti V, Shannon R, Carner M, et al. Outcomes in nontumor adults fitted with the auditory brainstem implant: 10 years experience. Otol Neurotol. 2009;30(5):614-18.
19. Otto SR, Brackmann DE, Hitselberger, WH. Auditory brainstem implantation in 12-to-18-Year-Olds. Arch Otolaryngol Head Neck Surg. 2004;130:656-9.
20. Eisenberg LS, Johnson KC, Martinez AS, et al. Comprehensive evaluation of a child with an auditory brainstem implant. Otol Neurotol. 2008;29(2):251-7.
21. Sennaroglu L, Colletti V, Manrique M, et al. Auditory brainstem implantation in children and non-neurofibromatosis type 2 patients—a consensus statement. Otol Neurotol. 2011;32(2):198-1.
22. Colletti L, Wilkinson EP, Colletti V. Auditory brainstem implantation after unsuccessful cochlear implantation of children with clinical diagnosis of cochlear nerve deficiency. Ann Otol Rhinol Laryngol. 2013;122(10):605-12.
23. Colletti L and Zoccante L. Nonverbal cognitive abilities and auditory performance in children fitted with auditory brainstem implants: preliminary report. Laryngoscope. 2008;118:1443-8.
24. Otto SR, Moore J, Linthicum F, et al. Histopathological analysis of a 15-year user of an auditory brainstem implant. Laryngoscope. 2012;122:645-8.

CHAPTER

35

Inner Ear Molecular Therapies

Manohar Bance, Anil K Lalwani

INTRODUCTION

This is a particularly interesting time for inner ear therapies. In recent years, there has been a move toward locally directed rather than systemic therapies, which has opened up new possibilities for achieving high drug concentrations in the ear without systemic toxicity. The mechanisms of injury for many otologic insults are being elucidated, and found to share many commonalities, which can be exploited in otoprotection. Cell regulation mechanisms are becoming understood, opening up exciting potential in cell repair and replacement. New drugs are being tested, and pharmacokinetic manipulation to target various compartments in the inner ear is becoming possible.

The inner ear is relatively isolated from the rest of the body, which presents both challenges and opportunities for drug delivery. It contains many delicate structures that respond to mechanical stimuli, and which can be easily damaged by numerous toxic factors. These factors include noise, ototoxic drugs, various chemicals, bacterial toxins, ischemia, infectious agents, aging, physical trauma, surgical trauma, barotrauma, and various genetic problems. Unlike avian ears, mammalian inner ear hair cells do not show any capacity for regeneration or cell division and are terminally differentiated.[2] Similarly, spiral ganglion cells, in keeping with other neurons, also do not regenerate, although the peripheral nerve processes contacting hair cells may regrow.[3]

Several inner ear therapies are already in use. To date, these have mostly consisted of generalized therapies that affect the whole inner ear, such as otoprotective therapy centered around the time of an insult to prevent continued inner ear damage (e.g. steroids after sudden sensorineural hearing loss), anti-inflammatory therapies (e.g. steroids for autoimmune inner ear disease), or therapies centered around treatment of Meniere's disease (e.g. gentamicin or steroids). Some therapies attempt to target one part of the inner ear more than another, e.g. ablative gentamicin therapy for vestibular ablation in Meniere's disease. More recently, other targeted therapies are emerging, specifically certain cell types, e.g. neuropeptides to preserve spiral ganglion neurons (SGNs) after hair cell trauma, or specific gene replacements, at least in experimental models. Therapeutic advances have occurred not only in new classes of drugs but also more rapidly in new delivery systems, and in controlling the pharmacokinetics of existing drugs in the inner ear.

The presence of a blood–labyrinth barrier[4] (BLB) presents a challenge for inner ear drug delivery. This barrier means that systemic therapy is only moderately effective in reaching the inner ear. The BLB is maintained by the tight endothelial junctions in the capillaries of the inner ear.[4] In fact, there are really two BLBs, one being from the capillaries of the stria vascularis to the endolymph and the other from the nonstrial capillaries, such as those in the spiral limbus, basilar membrane, and spiral ligament, to the perilymph. There is evidence that some drugs when given systemically, such as aminoglycosides, preferentially enter hair cells directly via the endolymph, rather than through the perilymph.[5] Another hurdle for systemic therapy is the limited inner ear blood supply, means that systemic or regional intra-arterial therapy provides only limited access. One option is to increase inner ear concentrations is to try and make the BLB more "leaky". For instance, Li et al.[5] used acoustic stimulation to change permeability of the BLB. This approach, however, is fraught with problems. Altering the BLB may also change the blood–brain barrier, and still has all the downsides of exposing the whole body to various active chemicals, whose action is desired only in the inner ear.

The relative isolation of the cochlea also offers some advantages. Chief among them is therapy directed locally at the inner ear can be relatively sequestered from the rest of the body, without systemic side effects. The inner ear is accessible for local therapy through semipermeable membranes that connect it to the middle ear space, which itself is relatively accessible. These membranes are primarily the round window membrane (RWM), but to some extent also the stapedio vestibular ligament in the oval window (OW).

To a large extent, the rational design of inner ear drug delivery depends on the tissues being targeted. Drugs can be intended for a specific tissue (e.g. vestibular versus cochlear), or as very general therapy to all of the inner ear (e.g. in protection against nonspecific ototoxic agents). Targeting a specific tissue depends on manipulating the relative activity of the molecular agent against the target tissue versus other tissues, and also in manipulating the pharmacokinetics of the delivered therapy to increase exposure to the target versus nontarget tissues. Actually getting the drug into the inner ear can be a challenge, and the best route may again depend on the tissue being targeted. For instance, if a vasculitis is suspected in the inner ear, then systemic therapy would make more sense, as an intact BLB (which in actual fact might be compromised by the disease) would prevent high perilymph concentrations achieved through RWM therapy reaching the intravascular compartment. If the target is in the inner ear tissues, the RWM is likely to be more permeable than the BLB for many drugs.

The ability to directly access the inner ear through the tympanic membrane, primarily via the semipermeable RWM, has led to a great interest in directing therapy directly to the inner ear for a host of inner ear disorders, including sudden and autoimmune hearing loss, Meniere's disease, tinnitus, autoimmune disorders and also to mitigate injury from insults such as acoustic trauma, chemotherapy, or cochlear implantation. The exact mechanisms of action of many, if not most drugs in the inner ear, are largely unknown. Drugs may have effects on inflammation, electrochemical gradients, blood flow, or inner ear fluid composition or pressure. How most diseases affect these different aspects of inner ear function is also unknown. The ear only has a limited range of responses, either vertigo, pain or pressure, imbalance, hearing loss or tinnitus, so the etiologic cause of symptoms is often difficult to identify. These uncertainties result in much of our current drug therapy being, in essence, "a shot in the dark". We do not have the interrogation tools available currently to understand how various drugs interact with the myriad of complex processes in the inner ear. Targets could be as diverse as electrochemical gradients, blood flow, electrolyte composition, fluid dynamics, or actual transduction processes in the hair cells.

In this chapter, we will focus on molecular therapies for the inner ear, particularly locally directed therapy. In practice, the current tools for administration are fairly crude. In general, the drug and carrier is simply injected into the middle ear until it is full, and left in contact with the RWM (and perhaps the OW) for some small amount of time. The main parameters controlled are drug concentration, frequency of injections, and how long the patient is left lying down after injection. Potentially, a multitude of other parameters could be manipulated. Examples are sustained release devices or carriers, agents to increase permeability of the RWM, agents to increase the permeability of the BLB, and agents to carry the drug, protein, or gene toward a specifically targeted tissue. We will review some of these current and future therapeutic options for the inner ear, many only tested so far in animal models.

ANATOMY AND PHYSIOLOGY OF THE ROUND WINDOW MEMBRANE

The RWM is the primary route for drugs to enter the inner ear in topically directed therapy; hence, it is important to appreciate its anatomy and physiology. This structure is recessed in a bony niche and the round window niche. There are species differences in the RWM, which mitigates the ability to extrapolate from animal studies on drug absorption from the middle ear to human applications. In humans, the area of the RWM is approximately 2.5 mm^2. Its thickness varies by species, being approximately 10–14 μm in chinchillas, 20–40 μm in cats, 40–60 μm in rhesus monkeys, and 40–70 μm in humans (for review, including description of cross species ultrastructure, *see* ref. 6). (Fig. 35.1).

The ultrastructure of the RWM follows that of most biological membranes, with an inner and other epithelial layer with intervening connective tissue. The outer layer is probably the most important in determining permeability.

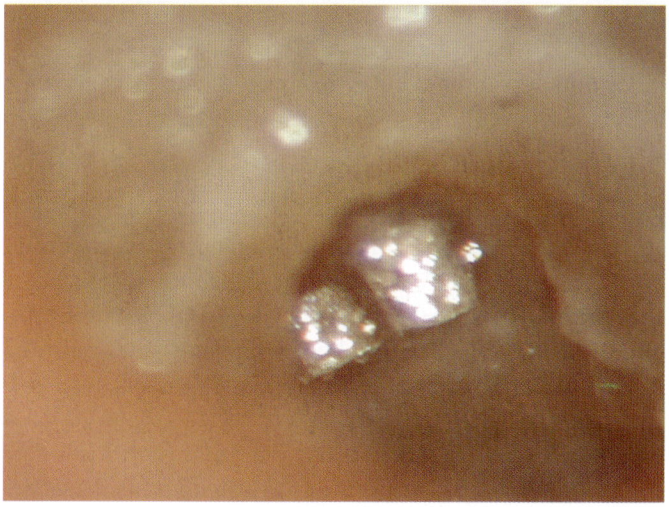

Fig. 35.1: Round window bony recess, with the actual round window membrane highlighted with silver stickers. Notice the membrane is recessed from the bony niche, and may often have mucosal folds covering it. The degree of recessing and orientation of the membrane is very variable.

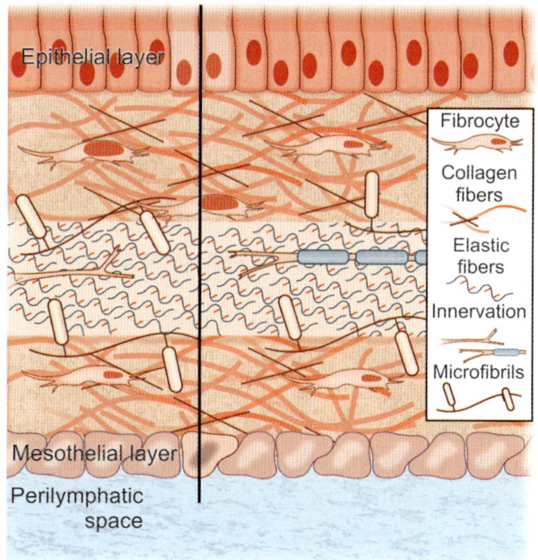

Fig. 35.2: Schematic representation of the microanatomy of the round window membrane, showing the complexity and multiple layers in the membrane. Redrawn from Pritz et al.[227]

It consists of extensively interdigitating low cuboidal cells, with a continuous basement membrane. These cells also have well-developed endoplasmic reticulum, and Golgi complexes and occasional microvilli. These point to potential active transport mechanisms.

The middle connective tissue layer contains collagen and elastic fibers, with fibroblasts, blood vessels, lymphatic vessels, and nerve endings whose function is undefined. The connective tissue layer is divided approximately into thirds, with a gradient of increasing fibroblasts, collagen, and elastic fibers toward the inner surface. The outer third contains primarily loosely arranged collagen fibers without elastic fibers, which first appear in the middle layer along with fibroblasts and blood vessels. The blood vessels are concentrated at the edges of the RWM, and some traverse the whole thickness of the RWM.[6] These are more densely packed closest to the inner surface.

The inner layer consists of squamous cells with long lateral extensions and large spaces between the cells. Hence, some of the middle layer can be in contact with the perilymph directly. Figure 35.2 depicts the histologic complexity of the RWM.

The accessibility of the RWM is variable from ear to ear, which leads to considerable variability in the ability of drugs to cross this membrane. For instance, the degree of bony recessing of the RWM is variable, with shallow niches with exposed RWMs and deep recesses in which it is not visible. Other factors limiting access to the RWM are adhesions, scarring, and mucosal folds that obscure the true RWM. Alzamil and Linthicum found some form of obstruction in about one-third of cadaveric temporal bones,[7] being either a false RWM (21%), a fibrous plug (10%), or a fatty plug (1.5%) in this particular study. Of bilaterally available bones, 22% had bilateral obstruction and 21% had only unilateral obstruction.[7] In living patients, Silverstein et al.[8] found partial RWM obstruction in 17%, and total obstruction in 12%. Obviously this will affect the ability of drugs to access the RWM, and may be the cause of failure of therapy in some cases. For instance, Crane et al.[9] explored eight ears in patients who had failed intratympanic (IT) gentamicin for Meniere's disease, and found that all eight had obstructions that they removed prior to reapplying gentamicin directly on the RWM, with successful results in 6/8 of the subjects. Not all authors agree, however, on the extent of the problem in RWM access. For instance, Banerjee and Parnes[10] report that at endoscopy in 68 consecutive ears, they found complete RW obstruction in only one ear (1.4%). The very high rates of resolution of vertigo in IT gentamicin administration (about 80–90%, see below) would also argue that in most ears, the RWM is relatively accessible to small molecules. The development of microendoscopes may allow better visualization of the RW area, and lysis of adhesions in the outpatient clinic.[11]

Variability in the RWM thickness, orientation, and access is thought to play a role in interpatient variability in drug absorption across this membrane. There is a large variability in the human RWM in vivo, as shown by gadolinium uptake studies from the middle ear in living humans.[12]

PERMEABILITY OF THE RWM

The RWM, like other membranes, is physiologically active and participates in body responses such as those to pathogens and inflammatory mediators, and to bacterial toxins. For instance, in otitis media, the epithelial cells and fibroblasts become hyperplastic with dilation of the capillaries allowing extravasation of fluid, neutrophils, and macrophages, with resulting edema in the membrane.[13,14] The largest inflammatory reactions are seen in the subepithelial layer near the basement membrane.[14] Bacterial toxins can have a pronounced effect on the RWM, e.g. pseudomonas exotoxin results in a doubling in RWM thickness,[15] and in contrast, streptolysin O breaks down the RWM, increasing markedly its permeability.[16]

For small molecules, the RWM essentially acts as a semipermeable membrane, with passive diffusion of most molecules. For larger molecules, active processes may be involved. Many substances have been demonstrated to cross the RWM. These include gentamicin, steroids, anesthetics, albumin, horseradish peroxidase, latex spheres, water, bacterial toxins and other macromolecules, and, of note recently, various nanoparticles (NPs) (*see* section below on nanoparticles, p. 600). Many factors determine the ability of molecules to cross the RWM. These include size, molecular weight, electrical charge, lipid solubility, and the condition of the membrane. The effect of particle size was explored in some of the earliest studies in this area by Goycoolea et al.,[6] who showed that 1 μm microspheres could cross the RWM, but 3 μm microspheres could not. Examples of the effect of molecular weight are that horseradish peroxidase (MW 45,000) can cross the RWM,[17] but albumin (MW 75,000) cannot, unless there is inflammation in the RWM.[18] Molecular charge is also important; cations cross the RWM preferentially to anions as evidenced by cationic ferritin entering the inner ear better than anionic ferritin.[6]

Various mechanisms have been shown to increase RWM permeability, including drugs such as histamine,[19] bacterial endotoxins and exotoxins,[20] drying of the RWM, osmotically active compounds and benzyl alcohol—a preservative in many drugs,[21] and various collagenase enzymes.[22] Newer exciting ways to transport larger molecules include viral vectors such as adenovirus, various NPs, and microbubble-based ultrasound techniques.[23]

OVAL WINDOW PERMEABILITY

It is usually widely assumed that drug entry into the inner ear is through the RWM alone, and that any drugs found in the scala vestibuli (SV) arise because of local communication channels at the basal cochlear region between the scala tympani (ST) and the SV, a process that has been well demonstrated.[24,25]

The OW, however, can also act as an entry point to the inner ear. This is important to appreciate, as drugs are usually widely instilled in the middle ear, and will usually contact both windows. Where exactly the entry point in the OW is, is not clear. Possibilities include the annular ligament and the thin bone of the stapes footplate. As early as 1981, Tanaka and Motomura[26] reported that horseradish peroxidase could pass through both the RWM and the OW in guinea pigs. More recently, with human imaging of the inner ear using with IT injections of gadolinium (a magnetic resonance imaging contrast agent), Zou et al.[27] have shown that the vestibule and semicircular canals show enhancement less than 2 hours after injection, which can only be explained with direct uptake from the stapes region. Indeed, a guinea pig study suggests that 90% of the inner ear uptake of gadolinium is from the OW, rather than the RWM.[28] In an elegant guinea pig study, Salt et al.[29] showed that the ionic marker trimethylphenylammonium (TMPA) was likely absorbed about 65% from the RW, and 35% from the OW. Drug loading of the vestibule through the OW is also important in that it prevents the large volume of the vestibule and labyrinth from acting as a "sink" for drugs in the cochlear basal turn.

For vestibular therapy, OW drug entry would be ideal. Indeed, in drug-loaded NP therapy, many NPs have been shown to enter the inner ear via the OW,[28-31] which could be therapeutically utilized to direct therapy to the vestibular structures.

BASIC CONCEPTS IN INNER EAR DAMAGE

The most common injury to the cochlea is loss of the hair cells and the supporting cells. A variety of insults can cause this. Once hair cells are lost, the remaining hair cells have to seal the interface between endolymph and perilymph to avoid toxicity from the high potassium endolymph. With severe scarring, the range of cells can be lost, and are replaced by a simple epithelial monolayer.[32,33]

There are two classic mechanisms of cell death: apoptosis and necrosis, although the situation in the last few years has turned out to be substantially more complex than this simple dichotomous scenario. Which pathway is primarily activated may depend on the magnitude of the insult; e.g. noise at high levels will activate apoptotic pathways, but at very high toxic levels may result in necrotic cell death.

Readers are referred to reviews such as Vanlangenakker et al.[34] for details of this complex process of cell death. Necrotic cell death can be thought of as due to unexpected and unplanned physical or chemical trauma, radiation, heat, hypoxia, and similar insults. It is usually thought of as an uncontrolled cell death, as apposed to the active, controlled, and programmed cell death mechanisms in apoptosis. However, there is evidence that some aspects of necrosis may also be controlled.[34] In necrosis, the cell structure is disrupted, the membranes become porous, and intracellular structures and materials are released outside the cell. Calcium is able to flood the cells from its high extracellular concentration, and this in turn changes the actions of numerous intracellular enzymes.

Apoptosis is thought of as a programmed active cell death, and indeed is normal during the developmental stages of an organism as structures are resorbed and reformed. Various insults can start this apoptotic process. Two such pathways are the formation of reactive oxygen species (ROS) or free nitrogen species.[35-38] Apoptosis is executed by a cascade of proteins called caspases, which can be "upstream" initiator caspases, or "downstream" executioner caspases. The process is actually hugely complex, and research is rapidly evolving our understanding of the mechanisms of cell death and survival. Readers are referred to recent reviews of this very complex process, such as that by Portt[39] or Elmore[40] for more details.

Below is a basic description of this complicated pathway; in fact many more families of proteins are involved. The apoptotic pathway can be activated by a variety of insults, both by an intrinsic pathway and an extrinsic pathway. More recently, a third granzyme a and b pathways used by killer T cells have been mapped out.[41,42] The intrinsic pathway starts inside the cell, and is governed by a family of proteins termed Bcl-2. This family of proteins is crucial to maintaining a balance of proapoptotic and antiapoptotic signals, and when unbalanced, can result in cell death, or abnormal cell survival despite cell damage. When a cell undergoes severe DNA damage or oxidative stress, proapoptotic proteins (e.g. Bax) are increased and cause mitochondria to become "leakier" allowing cytochrome c to leak into the cell cytosol. This binds to other proteins (Apaf-1 and dATP) to form an "apoptosome", and so activates an upstream caspase, caspase 9. This in turn activates downstream effector caspases (caspase 3 and 7) to initiate the process of cell death.

In addition to the mitochondrial pathway, another parallel signaling pathway is mediated by mitogen-activated protein kinases. Oxidative stress and cell damage can activate phosphorylation of c-jun N-terminal kinase (JNK) that then phosphorylates c-jun, a transcription factor modulating apoptosis induction.

An extrinsic pathway begins outside the cell, by activated proapoptotic ligands on the cell surface. These then ultimately create a death inducing signaling complex, which then feeds into a common final pathway with the intrinsic system. Extrinsic pathways (either pro or antiapoptotic) maybe activated by toxins, hormones, growth factors, cytokines, or nitric oxide.

IONIC INNER EAR MECHANISMS

A large part of the physiologic function of the inner ear depends on maintaining ion and voltage gradients between different compartments. The inner ear has many ion transport mechanisms. The scala media endolymph has a unique high potassium content, similar to intracellular fluid, which surrounds the stereocilia. The hair cell bodies are surrounded by perilymph, which is high in sodium, and low in potassium, and is similar to extracellular fluid. These ion gradients also generate the +80 to 90 mV potential inside the cochlear duct.

To maintain these ion gradients, there is constant recycling of potassium (and of sodium in the opposite direction) from endolymph, through the hair cell bodies (which it enters as part of the transduction process), and back to the lateral wall to be resecreted back to the endolymph by the stria vascularis (for reviews, *see* ref. 43–45). The stria vascularis is specialized to achieve this, with basal and marginal cells and capillary endothelial cells having tight junctions to control the movement of ions and solutions. Numerous genes control these ion transport mechanisms, and many disorders of hearing have been attributed to malfunction of these channels.

Indeed, one of the ways that many insults will damage hearing mechanisms is by triggering inflammatory processes in the endothelial cells, which open up the tight gap junctions, and so disrupt the ion and voltage gradients that allow transduction (for review see ref.46). One method by which drugs such as glucocorticoids affect the inner ear is through stabilizing these processes, both by their anti-inflammatory mechanisms and by their mineralocorticoid actions.

Also involved in ion and water hemostasis are the family of aquaporin channels, in addition to hormones aldosterone and vasopressin (antidiuretic hormone), which regulate numerous genes in the inner ear.[47] This is also a rapidly evolving area of research, and may become a therapeutic window in the future for many inner ear disorders. Certainly, currently used drugs such as diuretics affect these ion channels, and drugs such as furosemide affect the vascular permeability of the inner ear, potentiating other ototoxic drugs.[48]

PHARMACOKINETICS

Despite the complex three-layered structure of the RWM, it acts primarily as a semipermeable membrane, with most small molecules entering by passive diffusion.[25] Before proceeding, it is worth pointing out that almost all studies on inner ear pharmacokinetics have been performed in animals, and extrapolation of these results to humans has to proceed with caution. Most substances applied to the inner ear will lead to much lower concentrations in human cochleae than is reported in animal cochleae. There are many reasons for this. For instance, there are major differences in the thickness of the RWM, with human RWM begin much thicker than murine models (*see* RW anatomy section), which will limit diffusion. The human cochlear duct is much longer than most experimental animals, which will limit apical concentrations arising though diffusion into the basal turn from the RWM, even more so than is already seen in animals with smaller cochleae. The volume of perilymph in the guinea pig ST is in the order of 4–6 µL, with about 10 µL in total volume,[23],[49] compared to human perilymph volumes of about 160 µL, and endolymph volumes of 35 µL.[24,50] There is also passage of drug directly through the very thin otic capsule in small animals, which does not happen in humans.[51]

In general, bioavailability of drugs applied to the RWM to the inner ear is generally low, and very variable, depending on many factors. These factors include how much drug escapes via the Eustachian tube, accessibility and permeability of the RWM, concentration and time of delivery, and efficacy of removal by middle ear mucosa. It has been estimated in guinea pigs that the basal turn of the cochlea experiences only about 2.5% of the gentamicin and 1.4% of the applied dexamethasone concentration with round window irrigation.[52,53] The ST concentration has been calculated to be in a range of 0.005–2.9% of the applied concentration of various tested drugs.[54]

Once drugs are inside the cochlea, there is little active flow of endolymph or perilymph to distribute the drug, and substances are primarily distributed by passive diffusion, a process that is affected by their molecular weight.[25] Therapeutic agents applied to the RW area tend to show a strong concentration gradient in the cochlea, with the highest concentrations in the basal turn area next to the RWM, and progressively less concentration as the apical low frequency cochlear areas are approached.[55-58] This makes it difficult to treat these apical regions. While there maybe some uptake through the otic capsule in small animals,[18,52] this is unlikely in humans because of the much thicker otic capsule, despite the presence of microfissures in the otic capsule in histological specimens in human temporal bones.[6] Primarily, drug absorption is through the RWM, although the OW is certainly a site of absorption of some substances.[29]

Salt and Plontke[51] have calculated some actual fluid flow rates in the guinea pig cochlea, to explain the slight variance in apical concentrations predicted from passive diffusion alone, and estimate these flow rates to be in the order of 0.01–0.002 µL/min. The lack of stirring and flow in the intact cochlea results in a very slow diffusion (approximately 4.4nl/min) of the drug from basal turn to the apex.

Figure 35.3 shows concentration gradients along the ST of the guinea pig.[51] Figure 35.3 also shows the rapid fall in concentration of drug from basal to apical turns, and the large interanimal variation in drug concentrations, which can be 10-fold, and is attributed to variations in RWM permeability. In these experiments, the drug was applied for 2–3 hours to the RWM. Salt and Ma,[56] in simulations based on fluid kinetic models based on data recorded using RWM application of a small ion called TMPA, calculate that altering RWM permeability would be predicted to increase basal concentrations, but not flatten the base to apical gradient very much as the diffusion out of the

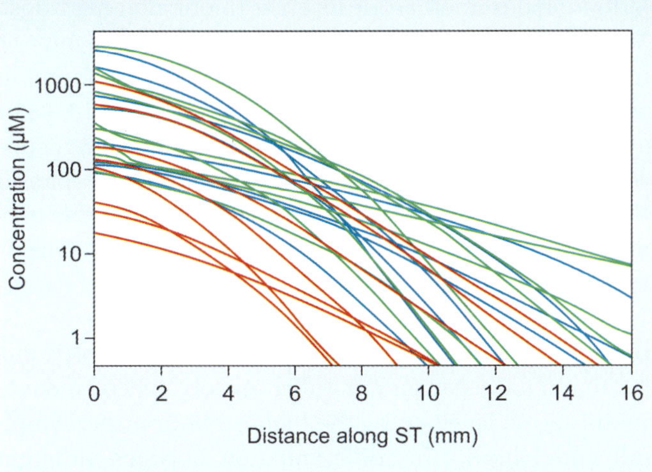

Fig. 35.3: Concentration gradients along the scala tympani by distance from RWM, following application of various drugs to the RWM for 2-3 hours, measured in guinea pigs. Results are shown for the ion TMPA (blue lines), gentamicin (green lines), and dexamethasone (red lines). This shows the steep concentration gradients from base to apex and the marked variability between animals, particularly in the basal turn.
Source: Redrawn from Salt and Plontke.[51]

cochlea is much more rapid than the diffusion to the apex. For ions such as TMPA, the apical region would be difficult to load even with prolonged RWM exposure.

A confounding factor in animal studies is that most experimental animals have a much more patent cochlear aqueduct than humans. In experiments where there is a leak at the infusion site or in which a perforation is made somewhere in the inner ear to sample fluid, this will drastically change the diffusion of drugs as cerebrospinal fluid (CSF) through the patent cochlear aqueduct rapidly replaces the lost perilymph. This will result in much faster apparent "diffusion" flow inside the cochlea than really exists. Another confounding factor in many studies is that the sampling volumes are so great (typically 10 µL) that they overwhelm the 4.6 µL of perilymph volume in the ST of the guinea pig, and if sampled from the basal cochlea (as in many studies), have been estimated to consist about 85% of CSF flowing through the cochlear aqueduct rather than perilymph.[51]

Inside the cochlea, drugs can easily diffuse through from the ST next to the RWM through the spiral lamina and basilar membrane to the SV, or through the canaliculi perforantes into the modialus.[51] Indeed, for many drugs, the primary route of access to the vestibule and SV is not via diffusion all the way around the apical turns through the helicotrema, but rather direct diffusion across the spiral ligament into the SV that results in levels in the SV and vestibule rising almost as fast as the ST, and certainly higher than the apical levels in the ST.

Diffusion into the endolymph compartment, the scala media, is greatly affected by the charge of the molecule because of the large endolymphatic positive charge, so that cationic markers are excluded,[44,59] and anionic ones being able to enter and accumulate.[51,60]

Many factors determine the distribution of a drug inside the cochlea. Primarily these affect the loading rate and the clearance rate. Loading mechanisms determine the dose delivered to the cochlea. If loading is through the RWM, this will depend on the species or individual permeability of the RWM (human RWMs are some of the thickest), the specific permeability of the RWM to the particular drug being tested, the permeability of the OW to the same drug (this also effects the clearance, as if the vestibule is loaded, it doesn't act as much of a "sink" from the cochlea), time of contact with drug (i.e. sustained release versus bolus), and the concentration of the drug solution. Elimination mechanisms that affect the concentration gradient at any part of the cochlea include the interscala permeability (i.e. ST to SV diffusion), uptake by cells, metabolism by cochlear tissues, and clearance to blood. In the inner ear, it is not clear where clearance to blood would take place; there are few blood vessels directly in contact with the perilymph. The most likely sites for indirect clearance are through the capillary beds of the spiral ligament and the modialus.[51,56] A recent study suggests the spiral ganglion vascular bed is the most important site for drug elimination, as the ST eliminates drugs far faster than the SV,[61] and the ST is connected to the open spaces of the spiral ganglion.[62]

Factors affecting inner ear concentrations are summarized in Figure 35.4. Measurements of drug kinetics for some common drugs used for inner ear therapy have been made. Although difficult to measure for technical reasons, the elimination half times have been estimated to be 500 minutes for gentamicin in chinchilla perilymph, and 130 minutes for prednisolone in guinea pig perilymph.[61]

Duration of contact with the RWM seems to be an important factor in determining the basal to apical concentration gradient. This is because most of the drop along the ST occurs because of distribution to other parts of the inner ear, and continuous or long-term delivery will load the other parts of the ear, so that apical regions can also be

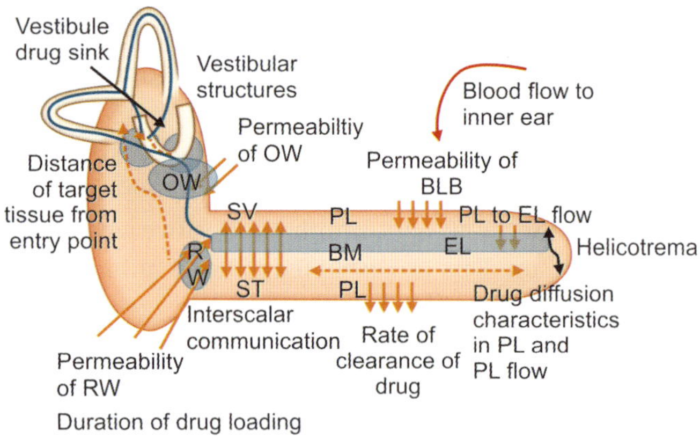

Fig. 35.4: Factors affecting drug concentration in different parts of the inner ear.

loaded. Simulations and calculations suggest that repeated applications or continuous application result in both higher basal concentrations and somewhat higher apical concentrations for some drugs.[63] This can be exploited, e.g. if steroids are required to reach the cochlear apex, a gel-based 24 hour delivery system for steroids results in a more even concentration from base to apex in the cochlea than a 30-minute bolus injection.[64] Conversely, if cochlear dosing is to be minimized, e.g. for gentamicin ablation, then a single shot IT dose will maximize the ratio of vestibular to cochlear dose, as not much drug will reach the cochlear apex, although the maximal vestibular dose will be lower than for repeated or continuous delivery. Also, sustained release results in a more even (less peaks and troughs) then a 30-minute bolus injection.[64]

Despite these potential mechanisms to exploit inner ear drug delivery, it is still difficult to get larger molecules to some segments of the inner ear. For instance, only very small quantities of neurotrophins (NTs) infused directly into the ST reach the SGN bodies in Rosenthal's canal.[65] Below we will review pharmacokinetics of the two most commonly used drugs in IT therapy of the inner ear, steroids, and gentamicin.

STEROIDS IN INNER EAR THERAPY

Pharmacokinetics of Steroids

IT delivery of steroids is attractive because of the higher concentrations achieved in the perilymph when compared to systemic administration, as shown in several studies.[19,66-68] One of the earliest such studies, performed in guinea pigs, was by Parnes et al.[66] In this study, the perilymph dexamethasone levels at 1 hour after high-dose IV injection were much higher (1.5 mg/mL) then after IT injection (0.22 mg/mL). Even higher levels were found in simultaneous sampling of the endolymph (9 mg/L). Later authors, primarily Salt and Plonke, found much lower concentrations of dexamethasone in the endolymph than in the perilymph, and these authors speculate that this may be because Parnes et al. used a cationic salt that is concentrated in the positively charged endolymph.[64] The Parnes study also compared three different types of steroids, methylprednisolone, dexamethasone and hydrocortisone, and found (adjusted for anti-inflammatory effects) methylprednisolone levels to be the highest, both in perilymph and endolymph. This differentiation between different steroid groups has not been re-examined in other studies, to our knowledge. Salt and Plontke have pointed out some caveats to this study, in that the basal repeated sampling volume was equal to or greater than the total perilymph volume in the inner ear, and that most of the sample was in fact CSF; it has been estimated that the true methylprednisolone concentration in the inner ear must have been at least 10x greater than that reported in the samples in the Parnes study.[25]

While many early studies were contaminated by sampling from the ST basal region, with the resulting influx of CSF from the cochlear aqueduct, later studies using more sophisticated protocols have, in general, shown similar qualitative results. These confirm the basal to apical drug gradient, and peaking of the perilymph concentration of steroids at approximately one hour after delivery (this was true for both for IT and for systemic administration), with elimination by around 6 hours. There is almost complete elimination by of the steroid by 24 hours.[66-69]

The elimination half-life of steroids in the inner ear is not clear. There are many divergent studies. In most studies (primarily by Salt and Plontke), a parameter-fitting algorithm has been used to fit experimental data, and elimination half-lives calculated. Based on this technique, fitting the data reported in various studies has yielded cochlear perilymph half-lives of 130 minutes[70] when fitting to a guinea pig prednisolone dosing study,[71] and 27 minutes[72] when fitting to a previously published human methylprednisolone study.[68] In a dexamethasone guinea pig study,[64] the cochlear perilymph half-life was estimated to be 85 minutes. In all the above studies, the elimination includes all routes of elimination, including redistribution to other parts of the inner ear as well as elimination by blood.

To measure the half-life of blood elimination alone, Salt et al.[61] loaded the inner ear with dexamethasone, fluorescein and TMPA via the lateral canal until all inner compartments were loaded. They were then able to measure elimination by the blood route alone, without contamination by redistribution to other parts of the cochlea. They found an elimination half-life in the ST of 22.5 minutes and in the SV of 111 minutes for dexamethasone. For fluorescein and TMPA, the half-lives in ST were 54.1 and 24.5 minutes, respectively. All of these are far faster than previously appreciated, and more consistent with the human data of Bird et al.,[68] who Plontke et al.[72] calculated to have a 27-minute half-life for methylprednisolone. Because of this rapid elimination, the basal to apical concentration gradient is for dexamethasone is likely to be even more pronounced than previously thought.

One way to decrease the variability of dexamethasone levels in the inner ear is to have a prolonged release formulation. Salt et al.[64] tested and confirmed this using a gel based poloxamer hydrogel sustained release formulation. They showed a flatter base to apex gradient for the drug compared to non sustained release formulations. Based on this, they developed a model to predict base to apex gradients with differing durations of exposure to drug at the RWM (*see* Figs. 35.5A and B below). Again they found lower levels in the endolymph than the perilymph for dexamethasone.

Hahn et al.[73] compared injection of dexamethasone directly into the ST via the RWM (using hyaluronic acid to prevent leakage,) versus RWM application for 2–3 hours. They found concentrations in the ST were up to 10 times higher using the injection, and, perhaps because of the flow created by the injection, a much less pronounced base to apex gradient for the drug if injected directly, resulting in much higher apex concentrations. The drug was also detectable for much longer, up to 220 minutes. One method for reaching the apex, then, might be to consider direct injections through the RWM.

Whilst basal to apical gradients are understandable for applications to the RWM, an interesting recent study[74] has suggested that these gradients apply even for systemic administration of steroids. These authors did not measure perilymph concentrations directly, but rather used an antibody to dexamethasone in sectioned tissue after steroid IT and IV administration. Interestingly, they report the same basal to apical gradient for systemic delivery as for IT delivery, unless extremely high systemic doses were used. Also, this study found a much higher affinity for dexamethasone by inner hair cells than outer hair cells. This is unfortunate, as most insults seem to damage outer hair cells more than inner hair cells. In this study, there was labeling of cochlear tissues at 24 hours from the IT group, but not the systemic intraperitoneal group. This might be explained if hair cells retain dexamethasone after perilymph levels are undetectable.

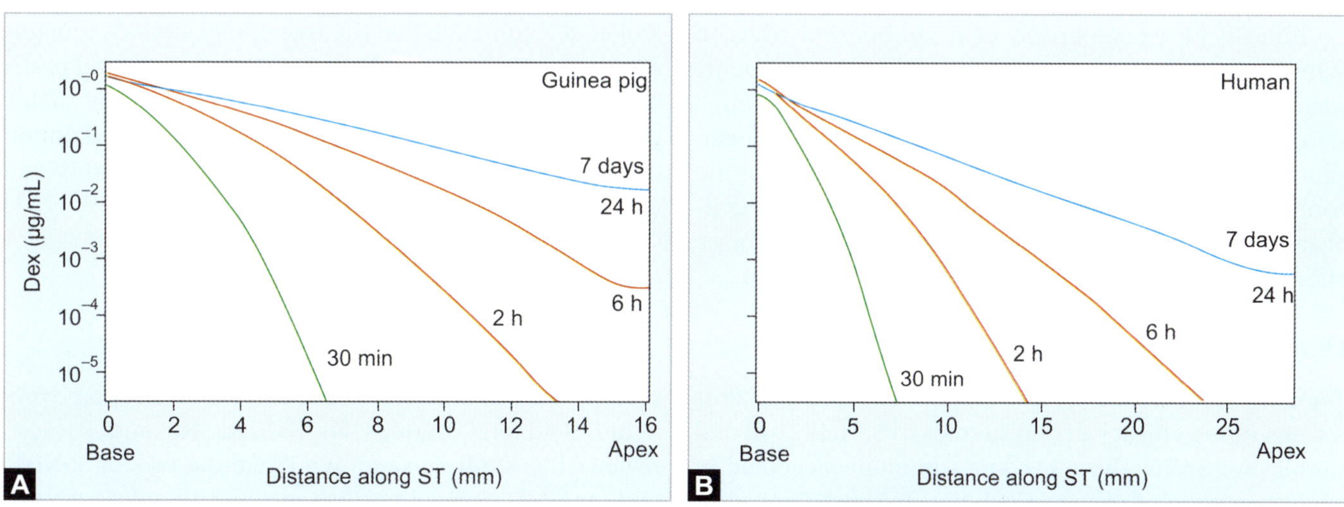

Figs. 35.5A and B: Using a diffusion model for dexamethasone, these are the concentration gradients from the RWM, after application to the RWM for various time durations, calculated by Salt et al.[64] Gradients are calculated both for the guinea pig (A) and for the human (B) ear. Redrawn from Salt et al.[64]

Overall, while there is much variability in the various studies, but all seem to point to a marked basal to apical gradient for steroids, and higher perilymph concentrations with IT versus systemic steroids. The apical low-frequency regions of the cochlea are difficult to provide with high levels of drug.

Clinical Usage of Steroids

Steroids have been recognized treatment option for sudden SNH,[75,76] autoimmune hearing loss[77] and Meniere's disease.[78] There are varying degrees of evidence for these indications. We will briefly overview use in sudden hearing loss and Meniere's disease

Steroids in Sudden Sensorineural Hearing Loss (SSNHL)

There are various treatment regimens that have been reported, either oral steroids alone, IT steroids alone, combined therapy, or salvage therapy with IT steroids after failed oral therapy.

There are numerous confounding variables in all such studies, because of various factors that have been shown in one study or another to affect recovery prognosis for hearing loss. These include different times from onset of loss to treatment, configuration of hearing loss, number of "dead" ears in the study, presence of absence of vertigo or tinnitus, dosage and duration of steroids. Because of these confounders, it still remains unclear if firstly oral steroids are effective, and secondly, if they are, for which subgroups of patents are they most effective.

Indeed, in a comparison of 6 randomized trials of active versus placebo controls, using diverse treatments such as Realogic agents (prostacyclin or hydroxyethyl starch) and steroids, Labus et al.[79] found that the mean gain in hearing for the active arm was 15.8 dB and for the control arm was 14.3 dB, which was not statistically significant. It is possible therefore, that no treatment is more effective than spontaneous recovery for this condition.

Oral Steroids

There are many relatively low quality retrospective studies suggesting efficacy of oral steroids in SSNHL, and oral steroids for SSNHL have become commonly accepted in clinical practice. A recent Cochrane Review[80] looked at this treatment option, with an intention to perform meta-analysis. They found that steroid doses and populations treated were too heterogeneous to perform a meta-analysis, and only three trials,[76,81,82] met their inclusion criteria for high quality evidence, representing 267 subjects. Of these studies, Cinamon et al.[81] found a response rate of 60% in the steroid group, and 63% in the control group, using a criterion of improvement of 15 dB or more in the pure-tone average. They concluded that steroids showed no benefit over placebo, in any measure including speech discrimination outcomes or acute or delayed hearing outcomes in their 41 patients. This trial treated only for 5 days at 1 mg/kg prednisolone.

Nosrati-Zarenoe et al.[82] studied 103 subjects treated using prednisolone 60 mg/day for 3 days, and then a tapering dose for total of 8 days. They found a mean improvement in hearing of 25.5 dB in the prednisolone group, and 26.4 dB in the control group at day 8, and at 3 months improvements of 39.1dB in the steroid group, and 35.1dB in the control group. They conclude there was no significant difference in the groups. Both of the above studies used relatively short duration therapy.

The only randomized trial of the three finding a positive effect of steroids was the Wilson et al.[76] study with 123 subjects, and had many methodological flaws; it was conducted over two sites, who reported very different outcomes, but are pooled overall. Complete recovery was defined as recovery to within 10 dB of the normal hear, with various partial recovery criteria. The treatment consisted either of dexamethasone tapering over 10 days or methylprednisolone tapering over 12 days. In this study, the overall improvement rate was 61% in the steroid treated group, and 32% in the control group, suggesting a large effect size. Wei et al.[80] conclude that the role of oral steroids remains unclear, partly because of conflicting protocols, and partly because of small numbers in each sample. The only study that has shown definitive benefits[76] used a longer duration of treatment of oral steroids, and it is possible that this is an important factor, but not proven.

IT Steroids for SSNHL

Because the inner ear concentration that can be reached with IT steroids is higher than that for oral steroids (*see* section above), it is feasible that IT steroids may work better than oral steroids for SSNHL. Hu and Parnes[83] reviewed 25 studies examining IT steroid use for SSNHL, and found 22 showed positive results and only 3 showed negative results. They comment on the lack of well-controlled studies in this area.

A more recent systematic review by Spear and Schwartz.[84] also examined studies in this area, finding very few high-quality ones. Of these, only two were "Tier 1" studies. The majority looked at IT steroids as salvage therapy (21/32), with only eight looking at IT steroids as initial therapy. The steroids used varied, e.g. dexamethasone in 18 studies, methylprednisolone in 10 studies, and both in 4 studies. Interestingly, despite the guinea pig data from Parnes et al.,[66] there was no difference found overall in results between methylprednisolone and dexamethasone groups. When examining the use of IT steroids as initial therapy for SSNHL, there was only one Tier 1 study, and it did show any benefit of IT steroids over conventional oral steroids,[85] similar to the findings in the two Tier 2 studies,[86,87] although mean PTA improvement couldn't be calculated from these.

As salvage therapy, there were five Tier 2 studies, all of which demonstrated some benefit of IT therapy. There was only one Tier 1 study,[88] which showed no benefit, was deemed to be underpowered and methodologically flawed. A random effects meta-analysis combining these Tier 1 and 2 studies suggested a significant effect of salvage therapy, with an improvement of salvage therapy over controls of 13.3 dB, which was highly significant. Another subsequent randomized double blind study looking at injection of 4 shots of IT steroids over 2 weeks as salvage therapy compared to saline injections,[89] also found a higher rate of improvement, in the active arm, with PTA increase of 9.8 dB with greater than 10 dB improvement in 44% of subjects, compared a recovery of 4.5 dB and greater than 10 dB improvement in only 10.7% of subjects in the control arm.

As first line treatment for SSNHL, a recent study[90] was a large randomized multicenter trial with 250 subjects comparing a high dose of oral prednisone (60 mg/day) for a long time interval (14 days, tapering over 5 days) to four injections methylprednisolone 40 mg/mL over 14 days. It could be said that the dosage was "maximized" for practical purposes for each arm. The average PTA improvement in the oral group was 30.7dB, and 28.7dB in the IT group, which was concluded to be essentially equivalent.

With regard to combined IT and oral versus mono-route therapy for first line treatment of SSHL, the literature is again unclear. Battaglia et al, in a well-designed study[85] with a placebo control group, report combined therapy outcomes to be better than monotherapy, but two other studies showed no benefit from combined therapy over monotherapy.[86,91] A more recent randomized study[92] used fairly maximal oral therapy for 14 days alone, and compared this to combined therapy using both oral therapy with the addition of four injections of IT methylprednisolone over 2 weeks. At 4 weeks, they found a PTA improvement of 44 dB in the combined group, compared to 27.7dB for the oral steroids alone group, which was highly significant in favor of combined therapy. It is interesting that the recovery for steroids alone was similar to that in the Rauch et al.[90] study, which also used long duration oral therapy.

At this time, it is difficult to conclude definitively for the superiority of one treatment regimen over another in SSNHL. IT steroids seem to be at least as efficacious as oral steroids, but with little evidence of superiority for first line treatment. The use of IT steroids as salvage therapy for failed oral therapy has some supporting evidence and maybe worth considering. Combined IT and oral therapy also has some supporting evidence for being more efficacious than either modality alone, recognizing there are some contrary studies.

In practice, oral steroids are much easier to administer logistically than repeated IT injections, which has been the IT paradigm in most high quality studies. There are no high quality studies that we are aware of that used logistically simpler single shot IT steroids alone or in combination with oral steroids. There is also the risk of tympanic membrane perforation and otitis media with IT injections, as well as the patient discomfort. On the other hand, systemic steroids can have a plethora of side effects, which will not be reviewed here, although these are much reduced for short-term therapy compared to long-term therapy.

IT Steroids for Meniere's Disease

The mechanism of action, if any, of steroids in Meniere's disease is unclear. Despite this, they have become accepted, in the IT form especially, as a form of therapy for this disorder. Again, this field also has little high quality evidence to form a definitive recommendation.

Hu and Parnes[83] reviewed published studies on IT steroids for Meniere's disease, and found that of the 13 studies they reviewed, 8 showed a positive effect, and 5 showed a negative effect, although few had any controls.

A Cochrane review[94] of IT steroids for Meniere's disease with Shea grade 3[93] Meniere's disease identified only one study that met criteria for being placebo controlled and of sufficient quality to review. In this study, by Garduno-Anaya et al.,[95] patients with definite Meniere's disease were treated with either IT dexamethasone (4 mg/mL) or placebo injections for 5 days. There was a significant difference in outcomes at 24 months between the control and active arms, with complete control of vertigo in 82% or the IT steroid group versus 57% of controls, and also a significant effect on aural fullness and tinnitus (but exact reporting is a bit ambiguous for these symptoms). However, there was no significant difference in the pure tone average hearing outcomes.

The only other randomized double-blind study was performed by Silverstein et al.[96] This group, however, used a crossover design at 3 weeks, in which the drug and control groups switched over. This leads to difficulties in assessing residual effects of the drug. In this study the active group received of 8 mg/mL dexamethasone and the control group saline. Another problem with this study is that the patient group were Shea grade 4, i.e. mostly not experiencing attacks of vertigo anymore, but having aural fullness, hearing loss and tinnitus. There were no differences in the outcomes for these measured variables between the two groups.

Steroid effects could be dose dependent, but it could be argued that limits of steroid effectiveness were tested with a study by Shea et al.,[97] who used high-dose IT dexamethasone (16 mg/mL) with the patient lying with ear up for 3 hours, in addition to IV dexamethasone given concurrently for 3 consecutive days, followed by 0.25 mg of oral dexamethasone for 30–90 days. This intense treatment resulted in vertigo control in 77%, hearing improvement in 35.4%, and hearing loss in 6.3% of subjects. Overall, using the 6 point function level score from the AAOHNS,[98] 61% of patients were improved, 32% unchanged, and 6 % worse. With no control arm, it is difficult to assess how much was steroid effect, but these kinds of doses put an upper limit on the possible effectiveness of steroid therapy.

While not related to the effectiveness of steroids alone, an interesting study by Casani et al.[99] used a randomized protocol to compare outcomes at 2 years of patients with definite Meniere's disease injected via the IT route, either with gentamicin (maximum of two injections) or with dexamethasone (4 mg/mL, three injections every 3 days). The study was unblinded. Complete control of vertigo rates were 82% in the gentamicin arm, versus 43% in the steroid arm. In terms of the hearing results, there was a clear tendency for slightly worse hearing results over the 2 years with gentamicin, compared to IT steroids, but this did not achieve statistical significance. The authors do not comment on dizziness or balance outcomes that might have resulted from gentamicin vestibular deafferentation.

GENTAMICIN IN INNER EAR THERAPY

Pharmacokinetics of Gentamicin

As with steroids, various clearance rates of gentamicin from the perilymph have been reported, but half-lives in the inner ear are all reported to be longer than for steroids. These range from 505 minutes[24] to between 360 and 5000 minutes in rats following systemic infusion.[100] Salt et al.[63] pooled a number of studies to derive a half-life of 1500 minutes to use in their simulations.

While Salt et al. have shown that gentamicin will diffuse through the spiral ligament and rapidly access the SV and the vestibular structures if applied to the RWM,[51] recent reports also indicate that drugs can potentially access vestibular structures directly through the stapedial ligament.[28,29] The differential toxicity often attributed to gentamicin for vestibular rather than cochlear structures may be as much a manifestation of its IT pharmacokinetics as any intrinsic predilection, as it does not reach the apical cochlea well, and may reach the vestibule through the OW as well as through the spiral ligament.

The method of delivery will have a profound impact on how much of the drug reaches various cochlear regions. In general, higher and more sustained dosing will result in more of the drug reaching the apical regions of the cochlea. A very interesting simulation study using cochlear microfluidics modeling is shown below in Figure 35.6, from Salt et al.[63] It can be seen, if these simulations are correct, that with more frequent dosing, there is increasing dose delivery to the more apical regions of the cochlea.

Also of great interest is the analysis in the same paper, in which the cumulative area under the curve (AUC) for differing gentamicin infusion protocols is compared with the risk of hearing loss (Fig. 35.7). Several features are important to note in this figure, which summarizes results for 568 patients in 19 studies. The authors calculated the peak dose and AUC based on their models. Firstly, there is a huge spread in the hearing loss rates. Secondly, while the single IT dose protocols (open circles) had the lowest rates of hearing loss, it should be noted that, in fact, most protocols showed low hearing loss rates. Important to note, however, is that the protocols with higher total dose or peak dose, had the highest incidence of dead ears (black filled circles).

Not shown here is the microdose study by Hoffer et al.[101] This study used a lower gentamicin dosing (10 mg/mL), so called microdosing by continuous catheter infusion. With

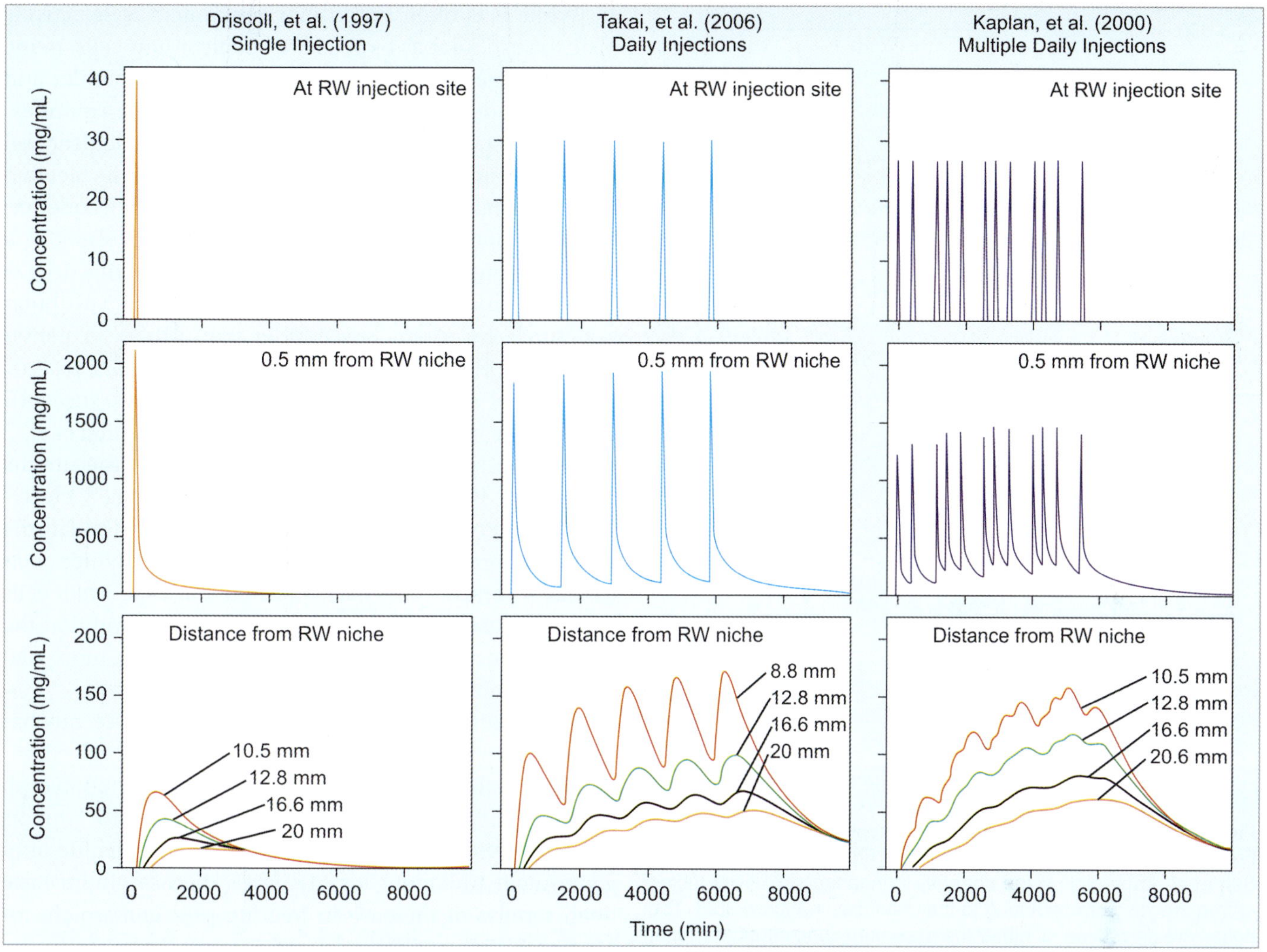

Fig. 35.6: Calculated effects of dosing regimens at the RWM on gentamicin concentrations at different sites along the scala tympani. Calculated graphs are shown for studies using single injection (Driscoll et al.), daily injections (Takei et al.), and three-times-daily injections (Kaplan et al.).[116] The top row shows the dose at the RW niche, the middle at 0.5 mm from the base, and the bottom row the concentration with time at various cochlear locations by distance.
Source: Redrawn from Salt et al.[63]

this protocol, they authors report hearing loss in only 1 of 27 subjects. Interestingly, they report almost no caloric loss signifying no vestibular ablation in this subject group, and hence the mechanism of action of the drug is not clear. It is possible that different levels of the gentamicin activate different pathways. These authors investigating microdosing further in a chinchilla study,[102] in which they compared the pharmacokinetics and morphologic changes in the inner ear for the microdose continuous microcatheter infusion versus a single dose IT injection. The main findings were that when compared to continuous infusion, single IT injection lead to a higher peak dose, much more variability in perilymph levels and more hearing damage than the microcatheter dosing. However, the microcatheter dosing was not free of audiovestibular damage, and with increasing duration of exposure, the incidence of hearing loss increased accordingly even with this protocol. In this study, there was no immunity from hearing low using this low-dose gentamicin, unlike their in their clinical study, and this microdosing protocol, to our knowledge, has not been reported by other authors for comparison.

Gentamicin may take a few days to become maximally active in inner ear cells, and then seems to have quite a prolonged washout time in the order of weeks. Lopez et al.[103] described severe vestibular cell damage in chinchillas from IT gentamicin administration, with signs of

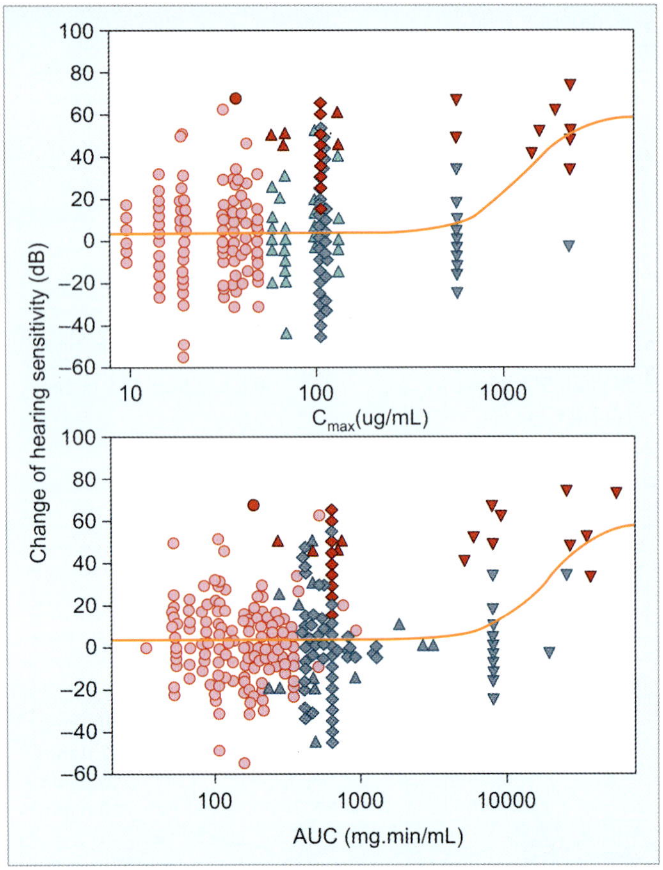

Fig. 35.7: Effect of gentamicin dosing regimen on hearing loss. From the same data from Salt et al.[63] in Figure 35.6, in this case Salt et al. have plotted the changes in hearing sensitivity tested at frequencies corresponding to the distances in Figure 35.6. The doses are calculated as either the maximum concentration (upper plot, C_{max}) or as the cumulative dose (lower plot, area under the curve or AUC). The symbols represent the four delivery protocols depicted in Figure 35.6 (pink circles: one shot; blue triangles: one or two × daily; red diamonds: 3 × daily; inverted red triangles: continuous). Solid red circles indicate patients who were deaf after the gentamicin treatment.
Source: Redrawn from Salt et al.[63]

recovery of some cells at 28 days. Hirvonen et al.[104] also using IT administration in chinchillas, described maximal head tilt at 5–25 days. In the cochlea, the greatest uptake was in outer hair cells and peaked at 3 days, with retention for at least 3 weeks.[105] A recent study by Zhang et al.[106] used immunofluorescence in guinea pigs after IT injection of gentamicin, and found peak uptake in cells, most intense in the saccule, between 3 and 14 days. This had decreased significantly by day 28, but was still present at this time. Other authors have reported that gentamicin is retained in inner ear tissues for up to 6 months.[107,108]

While it is often stated that gentamicin is selectively toxic to vestibular as opposed to cochlear hair cells, many studies suggest that damage to both organs is similar and dose dependent.[109,110] Differential effects may be a manifestation of pharmacokinetics, and access to the cochlear and vestibular compartments. This is keeping with the fact that most hearing loss with IT gentamicin, is high frequency, and the pharmacokinetics of IT gentamicin results in a large gradient in base to apex concentration of this drug.[53]

Some authors have suggested that some vestibular structures are mores susceptible than others to gentamicin. For instance, based on patient vestibular testing, De Waele et al.[111] suggested the saccule is more susceptible than the lateral semicircular canal, and Helling et al.[112] suggest the saccule is more susceptible than the utricle. Supporting this, a recent study in guinea pigs[106] clearly shows higher affinity for gentamicin binding in the saccule than in other vestibular structures. Within the semicircular canals, several authors have reported that Type 1 hair cells are more susceptible than Type II hair cells, and that the central zones of the crista and otolith organs are more susceptible (for a review see Zhang et al.[106]

Some authors[113-115] have suggested that one mechanism of action of aminoglycosides is to preferentially damage dark cells, which are thought to regulate endolymph production. This theory has been advance to support some reports of actual recovery of inner ear function after gentamicin treatment for Meniere's disease. There have been reports of increase in hearing post gentamicin for Meniere's disease,[116-118] and in a microcatheter perfusion treatment study, 78% of patents actually recovered some vestibular function.[119] This has led to a theory that by reducing secretion by dark cells, the inner ear is restored toward normal in Meniere's disease patients.[120,121] However, the findings of dark cell damage have not been borne out in actual animal studies. For instance, Chen et al.[109] did not find any evidence in a chinchilla model for dark cell damage, nor do human temporal bones examined shortly after a short course of systemic gentamicin treatment show any evidence of dark cell damage.[122] In addition, a recent study in humans with IT gadolinium to demonstrate hydrops did not show any evidence of reversal of hydrops after IT gentamicin.[123]

Clinical Use of Gentamicin

Aminoglycosides have long been known to ablate vestibular function as a side effect of their therapeutic use. As early as 1948, Fowler[124] described the use of systemic streptomycin to treat Meniere's disease. Shuknecht[125] first described IT injection of streptomycin in 1957 to treat Meniere's disease, with a high rate of hearing loss. Later, lower dose IT gentamicin strategies were adopted that allowed preservation of hearing with resolution of symptoms.[126]

Different treatment philosophies for Meniere's disease have been espoused, from a goal of total ablation of the vestibular labyrinth using a fixed maximal dose protocol, to minimal therapy to control symptoms without necessarily ablating the labyrinth, i.e. titrating to effect.

There have been several systematic reviews on the use of gentamicin for Meniere's disease.[127-131] For instance, Chia et al.[129] reviewed 27 studies, most retrospective, and found an overall vertigo control score of 73.6%. They found lower dose studies tended to have lower vertigo control scores. In the same study, they found overall hearing loss rates of about 25.1%, and in this review they also included multiple daily dosing regimens, which had a hearing loss rate of 34.7% versus about 24% for other types of delivery. In general, the proportion of profound hearing loss subjects was also higher in the multiple daily dosing studies. They report that patients that achieved complete vestibular ablation, tended to have a higher rate of complete vertigo control (92%) than those with partial ablation (75%).

Cohen-Karem et al.[128] in the same year (2004), reviewed 15 studies, of which about half were retrospective studies and half prospective studies. The AAOHNS Committee has published a scoring system for control of Meniere's disease vertigo, ranging from A to F, which is based on dividing the number of attacks of vertigo from 18 to 24 months post treatment by the number in the 6 months prior to treatment. Class A (total control) or B (substantial control) is usually considered successful treatment. Cohen-Karem et al. found an overall vertigo control rate of 74.7% for class A control, and 92.7% for class A or B control in gentamicin studies. The overall reduction in hearing was 1.5 dB, which was not statistically significant from zero in their analysis.

The most recent systematic review, by Huon et al. in 2012,[131] included over 559 patients in 14 studies that were all prospective, of which two were placebo controlled and double blinded. These studies covered a variety of protocols, but none of the ones reviewed were the very high-dose multiple daily injections protocols. The mean dose was 2.1 injections. These authors found that control of vertigo in the total population was class A in 71.4%, Class B in 16.1%, Class C in 4.3%, Class D in 2.4%, Class E in 2.9% and Class F in 2.9%. Overall successful treatment (Class A and B) was found in 87.5% of patients. The mean weighted PTA and SDS score did not change significantly from before to after treatment, although 1.8% of subjects experienced total deafness. This is similar to the findings in the review by Cohen-Kerem et al.[128]

In the Huon et al.[131] review, tinnitus improved in 12.4% of patients, which was significant, but the improvement in aural fullness in 7.7% did not achieve significance. There was no difference in vertigo control or hearing loss outcomes between the fixed dose and titration protocols, although titration protocols had a significantly higher tinnitus improvement rate (43.5% versus 15.5%) than fixed dose protocols. Huong et al. interestingly put forward a subanalysis, based on a much smaller group, that suggests that the minimal dose required for effective control is 13.4 mg of gentamicin sulphate.

It is worth examining in more detail the only two randomized double-blind placebo controlled studies of gentamicin in Meniere's disease. These are by Postema et al. in 2008,[132] and Stokroos et al. in 2004.[133] These are reviewed in a Cochrane review by Pullens et al.[130] Both were small studies, of 22[133] and 28[132] patients, with relatively low power to show effect, and many ambiguities in the reporting, as outlined by Pullens et al.[130] Stokroos et al.[133] used a 30 mg/mL buffered gentamicin solution, repeated every 6 weeks with the end points being either control of vertigo, a cumulative does of >360mg, or hearing loss. On average, they used 1.5+/- 0.51 injections. The Postema[132] study used a dose of 30 mg/mL of gentamicin once a week for 4 weeks. In both groups, vertigo control was superior in the gentamicin group than the control group. In the Stokroos study, vertigo spells fell from a very high 74 events/6 months to 0 events/6months in the gentamicin group, and from 25 to 11 events/6 months in the placebo group. Clearly the starting point of severity was very different in the active and placebo arms, but despite the higher severity, apparently the gentamicin group did much better. In the Postema study, a visual analogue vertigo score was used, and scores fell 2.1 to 0.5 in the gentamicin group, with no change (2.0 to 1.8) in the placebo group. Confusingly, despite the 100% control for the gentamicin arm in the Stokroos study, the same group seems to have published a retrospective review of their vertigo control, presumably including some of the same data set, of only 61.4% in 2007.[134]

In the Stokroos study, neither active or control groups showed significant hearing loss. The Postema study reported a fairly high incidence of hearing loss, the average hearing loss was 8.1dB in the gentamicin group, with 4 patients (25%) showing a hearing loss greater than 25 dB.

None of the studies really comment on overall health of the patients. For instance, Boleas-Aguirre et al.[135] note that 15.5% of patients experienced dizziness after gentamicin injections, which may not be captured with vertigo reporting alone. Also, if there is vestibular damage, there maybe long-term consequences as this patient population ages, with aging related vestibular, vision and proprioceptive losses. It is not clear, however, that gentamicin in low-dose protocols causes significant vestibular damage, caloric results from these studies are difficult to assess, but do not always show evidence of vestibular loss, and it may be possible that gentamicin in low doses may control vertigo without a necessarily a vestibular ablative effect. For instance in the Stokroos study,[133] there was no change in the cumulative caloric response in either the active or the control group.

Otoprotection

Acquired hearing loss occurs in various insults that can interact with each other. The most commonly identified ototoxic insults are noise, aging, and drugs, most often cisplatin and aminoglycosides. There are many compounds that have been shown to be otoprotective, if given around the time of a major insult, but primarily these have only been proven in animal studies. Almost all agents work much better if given in a pre-exposure phase, as opposed to a postexposure phase; it remains a challenge to find agents that are effective when administered significantly delayed after exposure. If the damage is primarily to hair cells, then the fact that SGN death is much delayed after hair cell loss[3] allows a window of opportunity for salvaging SGNs after hair cell damage has already occurred.

A common mechanism for damage in many tissues is through the side effects of aerobic respiration, which generates ROS. Many ototoxic insults cause damage by increasing the generation of ROS through oxidative stress in all compartments and cell types in the cochlea, which are a strong activator for apoptosis pathways. The apoptotic cascade itself can also generate ROS, rather than being the initiator of these pathways. For instance, Shulz et al.[15] found that blocking caspases, in addition to mitigating apoptosis, also blocked ROS formation, and similar findings have been reported for BDNF (a NT) inhibition of apoptosis.[136] Most drug strategies are either antioxidant in nature and act to block ROS, or are anti-inflammatory, which encompasses many effects, some of which are also antiapoptotic. Experimental drugs are available to specifically block elements of the apoptotic pathway.

The literature in the field of otoprotective agents is rather muddied, with many conflicting studies, with a large number of agents found to be effective in animal studies. Few or these translate to human studies, and often these are not of sufficient quality or power to show efficacy. For noise-induced damage studies, a precaution is that the mechanisms for temporary threshold shift (such as mechanical buckling of the stereocilia) are different from those of permanent threshold shift, and drugs effective against one may not be effective against the other. Despite this, many human studies focus on the effects of drugs on temporary threshold shifts. Some compounds found effective in vitro cannot cross the RWM, but may be induced to do so in the future with novel drug delivery agents, and this field is rapidly evolving. Otoprotective drugs tested in human clinical trials (for review see ref.137) can be categorized into:

Antioxidants

This is probably the largest category of otoprotective drugs. Here we can only briefly touch on a few examples. The most important cellular antioxidant is reduced glutathione (GSH). Some drugs such as *N*-acetylcysteine (NAC) and D-methionine are prodrugs for replenishing glutathione, others are exogenous antioxidants.

A clinically used antioxidant is sodium thiosulfate for cisplatin toxicity. This thiol containing compound unfortunately also binds cisplatin, and inactivates it.[138] This is its major limitation, as it decreases the antitumor efficacy of the cisplatin. This is a large molecule compound, and does not seem to be effective administered IT.[139] D-methionine, which raises antioxidant levels, has also been studied extensively in cisplatin induced toxicity[140,141] and found to reduce toxicity, and also has been studied in noise induced hearing loss.[142] However, it also binds cisplatin and may reduce its efficacy.

NAC has been shown to protect against many types of inner ear damage in animal studies, and particularly studied is its effect against noise.[143,144] It has been shown to be effective in industrial noise settings in humans[145] in some trials, but not in others,[146] and trials are ongoing testing its otoprotective effects against cisplatin.[137] For a review of NAC mechanisms of action and animal data, *see* Kopke et al.[147] A recent trial of IT 2% NAC for cisplatin ototoxicity did not find significant hearing preservation benefit overall in the whole group (using the contralateral ear as a control,[148] but did show a significant effect in two of the tested patients. A similar study using IT 10% NAC found a mild benefit at 8 kHz, but this mild effect at this frequency is clinically not meaningful.[149] NAC has been used in military settings.

Other antioxidants studied include Gingko Biloba, found to be effective against cisplatin ototoxicity in rat studies,[150] and Alpha Lipoic Acid, which also shows efficacy against a variety of insults in rat.[151-153] A human trial testing protection against cisplatinum is ongoing.[137] Ringers lactate has shown protective activity in some studies,[154] but not in others.[155]

Some vitamins and dietary supplements are also powerful antioxidants. Animal studies suggest that antioxidant vitamins such as A, C, and E can act to reduce noise induced hearing loss,[156] sometimes in combination with magnesium. Resveratrol (found in red grapes) has also been shown to protect against hearing loss in rats.[151] Other supplements variably found to be protective in animal studies include melatonin,[157] acetyl-L-carnitine, and lazaroid.[142,157]

Other potent antioxidants studied have been ebselen, in combination with allopurinol, and found in animal studies to reduce cisplatinumdamage[158] and noise induced damage.[159] Lecithin has also been reported to be active in otoprotection.[160] Also very intriguing are the various classes of flavonoids that seem to have numerous neuroprotective effects, a large portion of which are through preventing ROS formation.[48] Despite these advances, what is missing is a potent oral antioxidant that has been well studied in humans, and shown to be effective against a wide variety of insults.

ANTI-INFLAMMATORY DRUGS

In animal studies, salicylates have been found to be otoprotective in cisplatin toxicity,[161] in noise-induced hearing loss,[162] and in humans in a Chinese study on gentamicin-induced hearing loss.[163]

Steroids are used extensively in otology, and will be reviewed in more detail here. The inner ear contains receptors for both glucocorticoids, and mineralocorticoids, the affinity of the mineralocorticoid receptor is much higher than the glucocorticoid receptor, and the mineralocorticoid receptor is probably fully saturated at basal body levels, whereas the glucocorticoid receptor is not.[164] Several studies in animals and cochlear implants have shown mitigation of hearing loss,[165-167] both in terms of cell preservation and in terms of hearing recovery post cochlear implantation (for review *see* ref.168). In various models, including tumor necrosis factor alpha (TNF-α) challenged explant hair cells, steroids have been found to be very effective in reducing apoptotic cell death.[169]

Glucocorticoid receptors are found in hair cells, spiral ligament, and SGNs, and seems to work via both the classic described action of genomic nuclear binding via the GR receptor and controlling transcription of genes, as well as via a much more rapid nongenomic pathway that regulates immune responses (for review, *see* ref.170).

Indeed, the mechanisms of action of steroids are complex and multifold. At a systemic level, they reduce circulating white cells and inflammatory mediators and prevent release of many proinflammatory agents such as cytokines, TNF-α, interferon, interleukins and many others.[171] These will reduce systemic inflammatory responses, including those that might affect the inner ear. Some authors have proposed[172] that the majority of effects of autoimmune inner ear disease are not due to inflammation in the inner ear, but rather on the vasculitis that results from systemic inflammation, which results in loss of the endolymphatic potential by damaging the ion-flow limiting action of normal epithelial tight junctions, leading to inner ear cell damage. There is some data supporting this, as inner ears of subject temporal bones with immune mediated inner ear disease rarely show evidence of direct inflammation.[173-175]

Glucocorticoids can help restore the BLB[172] by limiting this vasculitis. To support this hypothesis, a inflammatory response created with lipopolysaccharide (which results in a vasculitis and tissue damage) can be mitigated with dexamethasone.[176]

In addition, steroids may change ion gradients in the inner ear by affecting Na-K-ATPase and potassium secretion by marginal cells, as well as up regulating genes associated with other ion channels and aquaporins.[177,178] Indeed, combination therapy with mineralocorticoids and glucocorticoids may be efficacious when either alone is not, as shown in an animal model of autoimmune inner ear disease.[179]

In the inner ear, while glucocorticoids may bind to the high affinity mineralocorticoid receptor, blocking binding to the GR receptor causes increased susceptibility to noise damage in mice, dexamethasone administration reduces it, and blocking binding to the mineralocorticoid receptor has little effect,[180] suggesting that the mineralocorticoid effect is not important in protection from acoustic trauma. Modulation of steroids in the hypothalamic pituitary axis is also thought to be the mechanism for sound conditioning, in which prior exposure to low levels of sound protect animals against later acoustic trauma.[170]

As seen above, how exactly glucocorticoids protect the cochlea is not well understood, their effects on the inner ear are extremely complex. In an Affymetrix gene array study, steroids were found to alter the expression of over 8000 of the 17,500 genes identified in the mouse ear within 6 hours.[181] Many of these are genes controlling inner ear hemostasis and the BLB, which may be a more important function than any direct anti-inflammatory effect.

TNF-α inhibitors have also been used in inner ear otoprotection. Many forms of damage lead to proinflammatory cytokine release, and TNF-α antibodies such as infliximab or etanercept can provide protection from cisplatinum ototoxicity in[66,182] animals, and in autoimmune hearing loss.[67,183]

Apoptosis inhibitors would be very useful in many cell death pathways. Inhibitors of the JNK cascade by drugs such as AM-111 and SPB00125 by IT injection have been found to show effective otoprotection in animals.[70-72,184-186] AM-111 has been used IT in a small group of human subjects and found protective against noise-induced hearing loss, but this study was without a control group.[187] In other experimental approaches, inhibitors of caspase 3 and 9 protected against cisplatin ototoxicity[188] in guinea pigs. Rolipram is another promising agent that prevents apoptosis by downstream upregulation of cAMP and BDNF and TRKB targets.[189]

NEUROTROPHINS (NTS)

Because there is continuous NT support of the SGNs by hair cell secretion of NT-3 and BDNF, hair cell loss can lead to subsequent SGN loss. This has been noted in numerous studies (*see* ref.190 for review). Sometimes loss of SGNs can occur alone, without hair cell loss, e.g. through excitotoxicity by prolonged stimulation. In a later section, we will review the role of NTs in hair cell differentiation and as growth factors, but here we will review their otoprotective role.

Neurotrophic support seems crucial to prevent apoptotic cell death. This has been demonstrated for various cell types in various studies.[191] NTs seem to provide tonic suppression of proteins in the apoptotic cascade.[192] Withdrawal of NT support seems to increase intracellular ROS in cultured auditory neurons,[193] and interestingly, blocking caspases not only blocked apoptosis, but also ROS formation.[15] NTs have a host of effects in neuronal and hair cells, including calcium homeostasis,[194] and regulation of endogenous free radical scavengers.[15,136,193]

NTs have been shown to protect inner ear cells from a variety of insults, e.g. noise, ototoxicity,[195] and aminoglycoside toxicity.[196] Why hair cells, NT secretors, are also protected is not clear. It maybe that hair cells also require trophic support from SGNS, and there may be complex local NT recycling networks.

In humans there is a window of opportunity between hair cell loss and SGN loss in which NTs may have utility as therapeutics. This has been studied extensively for NT-3 and BDNF, and to a lesser extent with GGNF, and much less so with nerve growth factor (NGF).[190] Unfortunately, this protective effect requires an ongoing supply of NTs, so requires some ongoing source of NT delivery or production.[197] Other studies have not shown such a dramatic loss of protection after NTs were stopped,[198-200] and it has been speculated that this is because electrically stimulated eABRs were used to measure hearing function, which could have acted as SGN protectant. A few authors[190,201] have shown that continued electrical stimulation could preserve SGNs after exogenous NTs were stopped. Another possibility is that SGNs take on an autocrine mechanism and can start to secrete their own NTs. It is at present unclear if electrical stimulation is adequate in humans to preserve SGNs if they were prevented from dying by temporary NT support initiated soon after hair cell loss. This would be a useful strategy in cochlear implantation if proven to be effective.

Almost all types of NTs, whether expressed in the adult cochlea or not, seem to have a protective effect on SGNs. It seems, however, that the morphology and functional aspects of response may vary by NT.[202,203] NTs have been delivered through a variety of approaches. The most effective route is intracochlear injection (including through cochlear implants), other somewhat less effective methods are IT injections, and IT infusion with hydrogels, Gelfoam (Upjohn, Kalamzoo, MI), and alginate beads.[204-206]

In addition to SGN survival, NTs can also increase axonal sprouting of peripheral processes of SGNs toward the hair cells.[207] This could be used to bring peripheral processes closer to cochlear implant electrodes for instance.

INNER EAR DRUG DELIVERY METHODS

Inner ear drug delivery mechanisms have been devised to provide drugs over a longer period of time, to control drug release, or to increase drug concentration inside the inner ear.

Essentially, drug delivery mechanisms can be divided into those that bypass barriers to entry (such as direct inner ear injection and some NP carriers) and those that provide sustained drug concentrations, such as pumps or drug eluting compounds. Of course these mechanisms interact in that a higher concentration (whether by increase in applied drug concentration or increase in RWM permeability) will provide active drug for longer before elimination (i.e. prolonged exposure in the inner ear), and sustained release will result in higher concentrations if the RWM is not normally very permeable to the drug, i.e. increased concentration. Some technologies, such as cochlear implants can combine direct access with longer term drug delivery.

Injections or Bolus Administrations

Intratympanic Injections

The commonest method to deliver drugs directly to the inner ear, apart from systemic administration, is via direct IT injections. These are simple and cost effective, even with multiple injections, and well proven.

IT injections provide a "bolus" of drug, but have little or no sustained delivery of the drug. IT injections are plagued by various limitations. Firstly, the solutions are usually low viscosity, and easily run down the Eustachian tube. The dose delivered is unpredictable, and may vary from patient to patient, or from injection to injection. More viscous or gel formulations may stay in the middle ear for longer, and provide a more controlled and repeatable dosing scheme. Secondly, bolus administration results in high peak concentrations over a short time, but low plateau concentrations. These high peaks may be harmful so some inner ear tissue that it would be advantageous to preserve. Sustained release formulations may result in better-targeted or more potent effects on the target tissue. Thirdly, the primary entry point to the inner ear is the RWM, which has varying degrees of permeability to various compounds. Carriers maybe able transport the drug across the RW, or the RW can be made more permeable to the drug.

Despite these limitations, as of yet, there is little convincing evidence in humans that any other drug delivery mechanism outperforms direct IT injection for common drugs such as steroids or gentamicin. However, there are many drugs that will likely not achieve adequate concentrations inside the inner ear by IT injection alone, and this limits the scope of IT therapy to only a few drugs currently.

Direct Inner Ear Injection

Otologic surgeons have long experience in opening the inner ear and preserving hearing through operations such as stapedotomy or lateral canal fenestration. More recently, the cochlea itself has been opened for cochlear implantation in hearing preservation short electrode implants, and it is now accepted that hearing preservation is possible despite insertion of an implant into the ST. Direct injection is likely to result in the greatest concentration of drug in the inner ear. However, cochlear opening (e.g. for cochlear implantation) is rarely, if ever, performed in the presence of good residual hearing in the high frequencies that reside at the basal region near the RWM. If intracochlear therapies are used to address ears that are still hearing well, there is understandably concern as to the hearing risks. This has led to development of new technologies and drug injection techniques that are less traumatic to the inner ear.

Methods to access the inner ear directly include stapedotomy, round window injection, endolymphatic sac (ELS) injection, lateral canal fenestration and cochleostomy. Gadolinium injected into the human ELS was shown to reach all areas of the cochlea without residual hearing damage,[208] and in animal studies, ELS dexamethasone injections were able to modulate aquaporin 3 expression.[209]

Access to some compartments maybe preferentially achieved by injecting in specific areas, e.g. injection via stapedotomy will allow better access of vestibular compartments than round window injection. To minimize the hearing loss risk inherent in opening the cochlea, some researchers have tested accessing cochlear fluids by opening the vestibule instead, e.g. Praetorius et al. were able to show expression of viral particles introduced into the vestibular system in both the vestibular and cochlear organs.[210] The semicircular canals have also been reported for injections for inner ear gene transfection, but there was loss of vestibular function in the tested mice.[211]

Depot Injections

Various polymers or depot compounds can be use to hold and elute drugs more slowly. The release of the drug is due to slow degradation of the material, drug diffusion or a combination of these. Polymers can be biostable or biodegradable, depending on the function required.

Hydrogels and Polymers

Hydrogels are promising for short term (in the order of days) delivery of drugs, but not for chronic long-term delivery. The best clinically known hydrogel is probably Gelfoam. Gelfoam, and similar products, are biodegradable polymers, which have been used clinically, e.g. to deliver gentamicin[212] on the RWM. It has been used also in many animal studies to deliver various substances, including BDNF.[205] In the BDNF study, the BDNF effect was mainly noted in the basal cochlear region. Certainly other carriers have been shown to perform better for specific applications. For instance, comparing radioactive NT3 concentrations in he inner ear with delivery on Gelfoam pledgets versus alginate polymer microspheres, Noushi et al.[206] found higher concentrations with the alginate. Alginate is a polysaccharide polymer, which can incorporate bioactive peptides, and is broken down into harmless metabolites.

Another commonly used hydrogel is hyaluronic acid, an anionic nonsulfated glycosaminoglycan polysaccharide. A commercial preparation of this is Seprapack (Genzyme, Boston MA), which has been used to deliver dexamethasone[205] and NAC[213] to the inner ear via IT injection, and has been reported to reduce the hearing loss seen following cochlear implantation when used in this manner.[214] Seprapack has been shown to provide a higher and more sustained concentration of dexamethasone in the cochlea after IT injection than injecting the dexamethasone alone drug alone.[215] This has also been reported with other hydrogels.[216] Various other hydrogels have been studied[204,217] and found to be effective in delivering drug to the inner ear, including bioadhesive chitosans.[218] Chitosan is a glucosamine polysaccharide, and have been used in animal experiments to deliver steroids[219] and neomycin[218] to the cochlea.

Of particular interest are hydrogels that are temperature sensitive polymers. These can be injected as liquids, but transition into gels at body temperature, allowing sustained delivery. These types of hydrogels can be formulated from chitosan, or other polymers, e.g. Poloxamer. In animal models, Poloxamer provided a better concentration gradient along the cochlea from base to apex through its sustained release action than IT injections of drug alone.[64]

Microwicks

Wicks act to channel externally applied drug or molecules to the RWW, i.e. they act as a refillable reservoir. One such example is the Silverstein Microwick, (Micromedics, Minnesota), made from polyvinyl acetate. This is introduced through a ventilation tube and placed in the round window niche. Whilst there do not appear to be any controlled studies comparing the Microwick to IT injection alone, it has been shown to be effective in various treatment regimens. Gentamicin applied to the wick (10 mg/mL) was shown to control vertigo in 76.8% of Meniere's disease patients,[220] and with self-applied steroids also for Meniere's disease an improvement was reported in 67% of subjects.[221] As noted, it is unclear at this point if this method of delivery outperforms weekly IT injections.

Pumps

Various types of pumps, primarily osmotic mini-pumps, have been used to deliver drugs over a longer time period to the cochlea. Previously the IntraEar Microcatheter (Durect, Cupertino, CA) was available as device for longer term delivery of drugs to the inner ear, and several publications showed efficacy of this system in delivering gentamicin and steroids to the inner ear.[222] This has been used in the past in interesting "micro-dose" paradigms for gentamicin, in which it is claimed that vestibular function was not compromised, and perhaps even enhanced.[101] This particular pump is no longer available commercially, and at present there are no micro-pumps that are available for widespread clinical use.

Other types of pumps are reciprocating perfusion systems, which have zero net fluid volume change, through a process of pulsed drug injection, and perilymph fluid withdrawal, incorporating a recirculation element.[223,224] By mixing perilymph with a reservoir of drug, these systems could potentially provide drug delivery for months or years. These can be programmed for complex dosing schedules. Because there is zero net fluid flow, there is less likelihood of spread of material to the CNS and contralateral ear.

Other investigators have also proposed bone anchored subcutaneous micropumps, and shown proof of concept in rat models.[225]

Nanoparticles

Various kinds of NPs have been studied for inner ear drug delivery, and numerous publications have shown in animal models that they can increase drug delivery and the sustained release of compounds to the inner ear, when compared to free drug alone. As of yet, however, none have been applied for clinical use in the inner ear, and their safety in the inner ear in humans has yet to be established, although most NPs seem safe in animal studies to date. NPs can increase transport across the RW, and increase solubility, as many compounds have low aqueous solubility. NPs can also provide sustained release of their cargo drugs or compounds. They can also be coated with surface compounds such as peptides or antibodies, which allow them to target-specific structures. For instance, Zhang et al.[226] used NP coated with TET1 peptide, and compared with non-TET1 coated particles, only TET1 coated ones were taken up by the cochlear nerve. However, this surface modification also changed the RWM permeability for the particles, and this may be a difficult additional challenge. All the NPs described below have been shown to cross the RWM, by both a paracellular and an intracellular route involving endocytosis (for a recent review, *see* ref.227). RWM transition efficiency decreases with increasing NP diameter.[228] Interestingly, the OW maybe a site of entry for some NPs, allowing preferential treatment of vestibular structures. Some of the major categories of NPs are reviewed below:

Poly(lactic-co-glycolic acid) (PGLA): This is a biodegradable lactic acid/glycolic acid copolymer, which breaks down into naturally occurring metabolites. It is a versatile carrier, able to accept both hydrophilic and hydrophobic loads, and has been used for a wide variety of loads, including protein, steroids, antibiotics and nucleic acids.[227,229] PGLA NPs are endocytosed and their packaging can modulate their release characteristics. They have been shown to distribute inside the cochlea when applied to the RWM, and could provide a way to provide sustained release inside the cochlea.[230] They offer a safe and versatile way to deliver a variety of compound to the inner ear.

Lipid nanocapsules: These contain a hydrophobic lipid (usually triglyceride) core, and a nonionic surfactant shell. They are cheap and very stable, for up to 1.5 years, and are very good for hydrophobic cargo. They have been used for a variety of purposes in the body, and in the inner ear to successfully deliver rolipram to the SGNs.[231,232] They have been shown to penetrate the RWM and reach spiral ganglion cells in the rat, within 30 minutes of application.[233]

Polymersomes: Also known as polymeric vesicles, they are biomimetic structures that overcome the body's natural defenses, are stable and their membrane properties can be configured for specific targets. They can accept both hydrophilic and hydrophobic loads, and drug delivery is through diffusion though the membrane, depending on a concentration gradient. They have been successfully used to deliver peptides to the cochlear nerve in rats.[226]

SPIONs: Magnetically active ferrous Fe3O4 particles can be coated with polymers such as PGLA, and made to enter the inner ear by external magnetic fields, by so called "magnetic injection" in guinea pigs, rats, and human temporal bones.[234] Du et al. delivered dexamethasone to guinea pig cochleae using this technique.[235] PGLA NPs encapsulated within iron oxide NPs can be made to cross the RWM when a magnetic field is applied. There are some safety concerns, however, with these ferrous particles, with reports of neural activity disruption even at low concentrations.[236]

Cochlear Implants as Drug Delivery Devices

Cochlear implants enter the inner ear perilymph space anyway, and could be designed as a portal to deliver drugs.[237,238] Primarily the interest in there use has been to preserve SGNs from any implantation trauma, and to prevent their ongoing degeneration. SGNS will degenerate without trophic support from hair cells, over time.[190] If neurotrophic supporting factors such as NT3 or BDNF can be applied, however, SGNs survive, and these neuropeptides can be made to elute from CI coatings.[239] These have to be continuously supplied, however, as their SGN supportive actions cease a few weeks after their supply ceases. There is some evidence, however, that electrical stimulation alone may provide some preservation of SGNs (see section above on neuropeptides). Steroids may also be supplied via the CI, and may reduce hearing loss from the trauma of implant insertion.[240-243]

REGENERATIVE AND GENE THERAPIES

Cell Cycle Regulation

It has long been appreciated that hair cell recovery can occur after cochlear damage in avian cochleae,[244,245] but that this does not seem to happen spontaneously in the adult mammalian inner ear. In birds, hair cell regeneration can occur using two mechanisms, mitosis and transdifferentiation. Mitosis does not occur in adult mammals, but does in adult birds. In this process, actual hair cells divide, providing new hair cells. Another mechanism, which adult birds also exhibit, is transdifferentiation of supporting cells directly into hair cells.

In general, cells in mammalian cochleae cells are prevented from reentering the mitotic cell cycle by various factors, such as the tumor suppressor gene p27kip1.[246] Other cell cycle regulation genes such as p19/ink4d and Rb1 can also be manipulated to cause mammalian cochlear cells to divide, but the cells seem to enter programmed cell death soon after being produced.

In transdifferentiation, certain transcription factors bind to cell DNA and code for specific types of inner ear cells. One powerful such factor is Atoh 1 (also called Math1) that signals undifferentiated cells to become hair cells. Another important transcription factor is Sox 2. The Atoh1 factor is only one present in the developing cochlea, and but is turned off in the adult mammalian cochlea.

Cells in the cochlea also exhibit lateral inhibition, in which local signals from neighboring cells prevent an overabundance of one cell type. With death of certain cell types, cell differentiation pathways are turned on in neighboring cells. This local control pathway is partly regulated by a receptor protein called Notch, and signals transcription factors Hes 1 and Hes 5.[247,248]

Cells in the adult organ of Corti are postmitotic, and there has been much research to try to induce these cells to proliferate. For an overview, the reader is directed to Raphael et al, and Okano et al.[249,250] Cell phase transitions are controlled by cyclins and cyclin dependant kinases, which are controlled by many factors including the lnk4 cyclin-dependant inhibitor family, and Cip/Kip factors.[251] It appears that p27kip1(also know as Cdkn1b) is highly expressed in supporting cells, but not in hair cells, and maybe a major reason for lack of regeneration in hair cells. For instance, mice lacking p27kip1 exhibit supernumerary cochlear hair cells and supporting cells, although function of the cochlea is disrupted by this overabundance.[246,252] Raphaels' group showed that inhibiting p27kip1 leads to division of the auditory epithelium, but not to the production of hair cells.[33] Hence, inhibition of p27kip1 is not sufficient, by itself, for hair cell generation. Numerous other factors are known to be involved, including Rb, Rb12, Cdkn2d, Cdkn1a, and Cyclin D.[250]

The final step in cochlear development is the commitment of the prosensory cells to their hair or supporting cell fate. This is where Atoh 1 has been shown to be a crucial factor in driving cells toward a hair cell fate. Indeed Atoh 1 seems both necessary and sufficient to drive these cells in the early development phase toward hair cell differentiation. Atoh 1 is itself regulated through a complex mechanism that involves the transcription factor Sox2. Atoh 1 is not the only regulator of hair cell differentiation, however, as Notch signaling, through lateral inhibition, also determines the quantity of Atoh-1 positive cells that become hair cells; disrupting Notch signaling increases the number of hair cells.[250] Despite these possibilities, generating actual new cells rather than transdifferentiating existing ones is important, as the population of supporting cells is not depleted, and it also allows the opportunity to insert large genes during into the genome, e.g. using retroviruses that is only possible during mitosis.

ROLE OF CELL DEATH AND CELL REPLACEMENT

Many of the common ototoxic agents, such as aminoglycosides, cisplatinum and noise exposure, have their effect on hair cells by an apoptotic pathway, often by generating ROS (for review *see* section on cell death above, and ref.253).

SGN cell death is often apoptotic as well, but occurs later than hair cell death in most insults. However, it can also occur by direct neuronal insult (as can happen from aminoglycosides), but more often from loss of neurotrophic support from hair cells.[254]

Neurotrophins

In addition to their role in otoprotection, reviewed above, NTs have also been studied as growth factor proteins, and are involved in neurogenesis and synaptic and neuronal differentiation. They are generally produced by the innervation target cells, and then affect more central neurons. Four types of NTs have been identified in mammals. These include NGF, brain-derived neurotrophic factor (BDNF), neurotrophin-3 (NT-3), and neurotrophin 4 (NT-4). In the greater family of neurotrophic factors, other important proteins in the nervous system are glial-line derived neurotrophic factor [CDNF0, ciliary neurotrophic factor (CNTF) and fibroblast growth factor (FGF)]. These proteins activate extensive intracellular signaling pathways,[190] and are known to be essential for the differentiation and survival of cochlear neurons. Hair cells secrete BDNF and NT-3, and these factors can act to stimulate formation of synapses with nerves attracted to the cells.[255,256] Expression of these NTs by various cells (vestibular and cochlear), however, varies during developmental and mature phases. NT-3, e.g. is expressed by inner hair cells throughout development and adulthood, but not in outer hair cells in adulthood.[190] This regulation of secretion of all the NTs, and expression of their target receptors is modified throughout the embryonal, early developmental and mature phases of the animal's life in a highly complex and regulated manner. Null-mutation studies show that mice lacking BDNF only show a mild loss of type II SGNs, which innervate outer hair cells, primarily at the apical turn,[257] whereas NT-3 null mutation mice show lack of inner and outer hair cell innervation, but primarily in the basal turn.[258]

When any of the four NT receptors are activated, they initiate a complex intracellular cascade that affects cell differentiation, proliferation, plasticity, axonal growth, and sometimes apoptosis (for review *see* references190,259,260).

NT3 and BDNF have a vital role in maintaining SGNs in the mature cochlea, and their loss results in secondary degeneration of SGNs in various animal models, and the time course of the loss varies from species to species, occurring within a month in guinea pigs, and taking possibly years in humans. Conversely, SGN loss can actually occur without hair cell loss,[261,262] presumably by excitatoxicity by overstimulation of the SGNs, e.g. by prolonged or intense acoustic stimulation.

Many of the NTs have been found to be protective against ototoxic and acoustic trauma. However, they are relatively large molecules and difficult to get into the cochlea.

Small Molecule Regulation

Tissue differentiation in many tissues is controlled partly by the Notch signaling pathway,[263] including in the inner ear, which controls progenitor cell differentiation into hair cells and supporting cells by a process of lateral inhibition.[264-266] Supporting cells are prevented from becoming hair cells, by Notch signaling from adjacent hair cells. Blocking Notch receptors diminishes activation of Hes1 and Hes5, which are a bHLH (basic helix-loop-helix) family of transcription factors and negative regulators of hair cell differentiation, and suppress Atoh 1.[267] Notch inhibition could result in transdifferentiation of nonsensory cells to hair cells by increasing Atoh1 expression. Direct transfection of Atoh1 leading to cochlear hair cell generation directly has only been proven to be successful in embryonic or newborn ears tissues.[268-270] Izumikawa et al.[271] used adenoviral transfection of Atoh 1 in adult damaged cochlea, and shown some hair cell differentiation, but it is unclear if these were cells that had recovered from trauma, or truly newly transdifferentiated hair cells.[272]

In a breakthrough recent study, Mizutari et al.[272] were clearly able to restore hair cells damaged by noise, by transdifferentiation of supporting cells in adult mice, instead of newborn mice, by using a Notch inhibitor selected for potency from a range of gamma secretase inhibitors. These mice showed both hair cell numbers increase and a functional increase in hearing ability. This may not be possible in long term deafened individuals when the Notch signaling pathway has returned to baseline levels, as opposed to the recently deafened animal model. Notch inhibitors such as gamma secretase inhibitors are small molecules that could be delivered to the inner ear through the round window, as proven by Mizutari et al.[272] Other methods would be by the use of siRNA to block Hes gene product formation. These are exciting, as drug delivery to the inner ear is potentially easier to deliver than gene therapies, but at the expense of shorter term effects.

Another small molecule that has exciting potential is DAPT, a molecule that inhibits gamma secretase and increases Atoh1 expression. Using this approach, various authors have shown generation of new hair cells in vitro[273] and in vivo.[274]

GENE THERAPY

The relative isolation of the cochlea makes it a difficult target for pharmacotherapy, but the same isolation makes it a very good candidate for gene therapy. Gene therapy can provide ongoing, perhaps lifetime, sources of molecules that are necessary for inner ear health, make the ear less susceptible to various insults by overexpressing protective factors, replace missing factors, down regulate or inhibit harmful factors, and potentially regenerate the inner ear. Gene therapy requires some kind of vector to deliver the gene cargo. The reader is referred to papers from Raphael's group recent reviews on gene therapy.[275]

Gene Therapy Vectors

Gene therapy holds great potential for inner ear regeneration, and has been studied for decades. Some of the earliest work was from the Lalwani group.[276] Various vectors have been proposed, and they differ in their ability to cross the round window, transfect various types of cells, the size of the gene they can carry, their potential pathogenicity, and the duration of transgene expression that occurs. In general, they can be divided into viral and nonviral vectors. Nonviral vectors include nonpackaged plasmids, or cationic liposomes or dendrimer carrier structures.[275] While these induce less inflammation than viral vectors, they are generally less effective at gene transfection as well.

Many different viruses are available for transfection in the inner ear, including adenovirus, adeno-associated virus (AAV), herpes simplex virus (HSV), vaccinia virus, lentivirus, and Sendai virus. For various reasons, among them concern about possible toxicity and unwanted transfection and pathogenicity in human use, and considering those most investigated to date, the most likely vectors for human use in the near term are adenovirus and AAV.

Adenovirus crosses the RWM well, and is expressed within 2 days across a wide variety of tissue types. However, its limitations are its possible toxicity and host immune responses to the adenovirus, and the transient gene expression.[275] AAV shows long-term expression of genes, but can only carry relatively small genes, and is more difficult to transfect the inner ear with across the RWM.[277]

Among candidate vectors, AAV are unique in that the wild type virus does not cause any known human disease, and is probably the most promising viral vector for human use for small gene payloads.

Genes can be delivered via the RWM using gel foam, partial digestion of the RWM,[22] cochleostomy, injection through the RWM, or via infusion pumps. Other reported routes are via the semicircular canals and the ELS. For ears that are already deafened, cochleostomy openings may ensure efficient delivery with little additional risk to the inner ear, but for hearing ears, the risks of cochleostomy include hearing loss and damage, and other portals are more attractive.

Most gene therapy to date has focused on hair cell regeneration, or on chronic delivery of NTs. For instance, Staecker et al.[278] used a Herpes Simplex virus to deliver BDNF. After neomycin injection, the gene therapy group showed a 94.7% cell salvage rate, versus a 64.3% rate in control animals. Lalwani et al.[279] showed a significant protective effect using an AAV to deliver BDNF, although the expression was very low, and far from the optimal dose. Since then, there have been several other studies showing effective gene transfer of NT-3[280,281] showing protection against cisplatinum, as well as adenovirus mediated transfection of BDNF,[282-284] which was protective against a variety of otologic insults. More recent work has shown that in addition to hair cell protection, NTs can induce auditory fiber growth toward the basilar membrane.[285,286]

Of particular interest are genes such as the X-linked inhibitor of apoptosis (XIAP), because they should be effective against many apoptotic processes. These genes have been studied by Wang's group in mice, and found to show impressive protection against aging and noise,[22,287,288] and shown by Cooper et al.[289] when transfected with AAV, to prevent cisplatinum toxicity to hair cells.

Once damage has occurred, the "holy grail" is hair cell and neuronal regeneration. So far, it seems that cochlear hair cell transdifferentiation from supporting cells is primarily effective in the neonatal period.[290,291] A particularly well-studied gene is that Atoh/Math 1 gene, which seems particularly heavily involved in transdifferentiation of supporting cells into hair cells. Using a plasmid vector expressing Math 1 to transfect neonatal organ of Corti cultures resulted in supernumerary hair cells.[292] A similar study using a human homologue of Math 1, with adenovirus transfection resulted in regeneration of vestibular neuroepithelium in vitro.[293] Similarly, Kawamoto et al. delivered Math 1 to mature guinea pigs and showed production of ectopic hair cells that attracted some innervation,[294] and in ears deafened with kanamycin and ethacrynic acid; this treatment was also shown to produce some recovery of hearing suggesting functional regrowth.[271] However, in general the effects of transfection of Atoh 1 into wild type animals (as opposed to transgenic mice models overexpressing Atoh 1) have shown limited success in the mature cochlea, although they seem to be more successful in vestibular regeneration.[275]

Another exciting application of gene therapy is in hereditary disease. In these cases, hair cell regeneration is likely to lead to renewed death of the hair cells, as the underlying defect is still present. However, replacement of the faulty gene or supplementation may be possible. An example of this is that hearing was successfully restored in VGLUT3 mice mutants with AAV1-VGLUT3 gene delivery in knockout mice, improving hearing thresholds.[295]

Certainly, there are numerous obstacles to overcome before gene therapy becomes a reality. Not least of these are safety concerns, both with the pathogenicity and toxicity of the vector, and of uncontrolled expression of the gene. Genes may migrate to nontarget tissues, e.g. Lalwani et al.[276] for AAV, and Stover et al.[296] showed expression of the Adenoviruses in the contralateral cochlea.

RNA Therapies

At the interface of peptide and gene incorporation strategies are strategies that involve the RNA interface. RNA strategies involve inactivating faulty messenger RNA (mRNA) by particles called small interfering RNAs, (siRNA), made from cleaving double strand RNA and incorporating them in a protein complex.[297,298] These siRNAs are 20–30 nucleotides in length, and can "silence" specific genes by binding to mRNA to inactivate it. In the serum, siRNAs have a short life span, but in the cochlea, their life span maybe more prolonged. They are particularly suited to silencing aberrant mRNA in dominant-negative types of disorders. The GJB2 protein, e.g. has been silenced by this mechanism in the mouse inner ear.[299] In other uses siRNA therapy has been used in the rat to prevent cisplatin ototoxicity.[300,301] Other uses have been in the inhibition of NOX3, which is one of the primary sources of ROS in the cochlea. siRNA directed against NOX3 prevented SGN and HC damage from cisplatinum, for instance.[301]

Stem Cell Therapies

Although stem cell therapies are not strictly molecular therapies, they will be briefly reviewed here. Stem cells are defined by their ability to proliferate into multiple distinct cell lines. Stem cell research overcame a huge hurdle in 2006, when it was demonstrated that expressing only 4 genes (Sox2, Pou5fl, Klf4, and Myc) was sufficient to induce many adult cell types to become pluripotent,[302,303] avoiding the need for embryonal stem cells.

Ito et al.[304] showed, as early as 2001, that hippocampal cells injected into the neonate rat cochlea took on morphologies similar to cochlear cells. Work since then has shown that some stem/progenitor cells are present in the mammalian inner ear, but after birth, their numbers drop rapidly.[250] Various authors[250] have shown that isolated stem cells can be made to develop into hair cell like structures with the right growth and transcription factors, but the yields have been low, and much still is unknown about this process. While stimulating endogenous stem cells to differentiate into hair cells, neural cells and supporting cells would be the ideal solution, the population of such cells is likely very low in the adult inner ear.

This has led to investigations into the use of transplanted stem cells into the inner ear. Numerous authors have investigated various types of stem cell transplants into the inner ear, and have shown that they can develop into neural cells, supporting cells and hair cells, but the yield is low and the cells population seems to fall within several weeks. The functional status of the cells is also not clear in most reports. It is also difficult to get cells into various inner ear compartments, because of the tight junctions between cells to maintain the electrochemical gradient in the scala media. The high potassium in the scala media is also likely toxic to cells. Cells must also attract innervation once differentiated into hair cells. Also, in many ears, both the hair cells and neural cells have been lost, and both would have to be replaced in a coordinated manner to achieve auditory function.

Another target, perhaps more advanced in terms of research, has been replacement of spiral ganglion cells using stem cells. Many investigators have successfully derived neural cells from implanted stem cells, and shown that they will extend processes toward the organ of Corti. To date, no study has clearly shown that these cells will sense auditory function (for review *see* ref. 250) The relative accessibility of the spiral ganglion makes this a promising area of research however.

Other targets have been to implant cells that secrete various neurotrophic or growth factor that maintain health of the inner ear, or promote repair. This is another promising approach, and one that may be functionally easier to achieve, and may help improve function of devices such as cochlear implants.

CONCLUSION

This is an exciting time in inner ear molecular therapy. The ability to target the inner ear directly through the RWM and OW will increase even further with new carriers that allow drugs to cross these windows more efficiently, and with little risk to residual inner ear function. These carriers and vectors will also allow us to manipulate the pharmacokinetics of drugs to target various tissues, and avoid injury to other sensitive tissues. They will also allow us to get classes of drugs into the inner ear that currently are unable to access it efficiently.

We are only beginning to understand the complexities of inner ear homeostasis, and the actions of various drugs in the inner ear, and indeed the actions of various diseases in the ear. This may allow us to develop new types of drugs to specifically address deficits caused by specific otologic diseases. Some drugs may prove to be nonspecific protectants against a wide variety of insults. One such insidious damaging factor is simple aging. It may be possible to make the inner ear generally more "robust" to any inner ear insult, so protecting against noise, ototoxicity, and other traumas for a lifetime.

Of course, the most exciting development would be the ability to completely regenerate healthy, functioning and stable inner ear tissue in damaged ears. Significant strides have been made in this area, but there are numerous hurdles, both scientific, safety related and regulatory before such treatments become feasible. These regenerative treatments could be combined with artificial implants to improve function of the implants, or perhaps even to improve function beyond human "normal" auditory and vestibular abilities.

REFERENCES

1. Goycoolea MV. Clinical aspects of round window membrane permeability under normal and pathological conditions. Acta Otolaryngol. 2001;121(4):437-47.
2. Cotanche DA, Kaiser CL. Hair cell fate decisions in cochlear development and regeneration. Hear Res. 2010;266(1-2): 18-25.
3. Miller JM, Miller AL, Yamagata T, et al. Protection and regrowth of the auditory nerve after deafness: neurotrophins, antioxidants and depolarization are effective in vivo. Audiol Neurootol. 2002;7(3):175-9.
4. Jahnke K. The blood-perilymph barrier. Arch Otorhinolaryngol. 1980;228(1):29-34.
5. Li H, Wang Q, Steyger PS. Acoustic trauma increases cochlear and hair cell uptake of gentamicin. PloS One. 2011;6(4):e19130.
6. Goycoolea MV, Muchow D, Schachern P. Experimental studies on round window structure: function and permeability. Laryngoscope. 1988;98(6 Pt 2 Suppl 44):1-20.
7. Alzamil KS, Linthicum FH, Jr. Extraneous round window membranes and plugs: possible effect on intratympanic therapy. Ann Otol Rhinol Laryngol. 2000;109(1):30-2.
8. Silverstein H, Rowan PT, Olds MJ, et al. Inner ear perfusion and the role of round window patency. Am J Otol. 1997;18 (5):586-9.
9. Crane BT, Minor LB, Della Santina CC, et al. Middle ear exploration in patients with Meniere's disease who have failed outpatient intratympanic gentamicin therapy. Otol Neurotol. 2009;30(5):619-24.
10. Banerjee A, Parnes LS. The biology of intratympanic drug administration and pharmacodynamics of round window drug absorption. Otolaryngol Clin North Am. 2004;37(5): 1035-51.
11. Plontke SK, Plinkert PK, Plinkert B, et al. Transtympanic endoscopy for drug delivery to the inner ear using a new microendoscope. Adv Otorhinolaryngol. 2002;59:149-55.
12. Yoshioka M, Naganawa S, Sone M, et al. Individual differences in the permeability of the round window: evaluating the movement of intratympanic gadolinium into the inner ear. Otol Neurotol. 2009;30(5):645-8.
13. Goycoolea MV, Lundman L. Round window membrane. Structure function and permeability: a review. Microsc Res Tech. 1997;36(3):201-11.
14. Yoon YJ, Hellstrom S. Ultrastructural characteristics of the round window membrane during pneumococcal otitis media in rat. J Korean Medical Sci. 2002;17(2):230-5.
15. Schulz JB, Bremen D, Reed JC, et al. Cooperative interception of neuronal apoptosis by BCL-2 and BAG-1 expression: prevention of caspase activation and reduced production of reactive oxygen species. J Neurochem. 1997;69(5): 2075-86.
16. Engel F, Blatz R, Kellner J, et al. Breakdown of the round window membrane permeability barrier evoked by streptolysin O: possible etiologic role in development of sensorineural hearing loss in acute otitis media. Infect Immun. 1995;63(4):1305-10.
17. Kim CS, Cho TK, Jinn TH. Permeability of the round window membrane to horseradish peroxidase in experimental otitis media. Otolaryngol Head Neck. 1990;103(6): 918-25.
18. Hamaguchi Y, Morizono T, Juhn SK. Round window membrane permeability to human serum albumin in antigen-induced otitis media. Am J Otolaryngol. 1988;9(1):34-40.
19. Chandrasekhar SS, Rubinstein RY, Kwartler JA, et al. Dexamethasone pharmacokinetics in the inner ear: comparison of route of administration and use of facilitating agents. Otolaryngol Head Neck Surg. 2000;122(4):521-8.
20. Hoft J. [The permeability of the round window membrane and its changes by pantocaine (tetracaine)]. Archiv fur klinische und experimentelle Ohren- Nasen- und Kehlkopfheilkunde. 1969;193(2):128-37.
21. Mikulec AA, Hartsock JJ, Salt AN. Permeability of the round window membrane is influenced by the composition of applied drug solutions and by common surgical procedures. Otol Neurotol. 2008;29(7):1020-6.
22. Wang H, Murphy R, Taaffe D, et al. Efficient cochlear gene transfection in guinea-pigs with adeno-associated viral vectors by partial digestion of round window membrane. Gene Ther. 2012;19(3):255-63.
23. Shih CP, Chen HC, Chen HK, et al. Ultrasound-aided microbubbles facilitate the delivery of drugs to the inner ear via the round window membrane. J Control 2013;167(2): 167-74.
24. Plontke SK, Wood AW, Salt AN. Analysis of gentamicin kinetics in fluids of the inner ear with round window administration. Otol Neurotol. 2002;23(6):967-74.
25. Salt AN, Plontke SK. Local inner-ear drug delivery and pharmacokinetics. Drug Discov Today. 2005;10(19):1299-306.
26. Tanaka K, Motomura S. Permeability of the labyrinthine windows in guinea pigs. Arch Otorhinolaryngol. 1981;233 (1):67-73.
27. Zou J, Pyykko I, Bjelke B, et al. Communication between the perilymphatic scalae and spiral ligament visualized by in vivo MRI. Audiol Neurootol. 2005;10(3):145-52.
28. King EB, Salt AN, Eastwood HT, et al. Direct entry of gadolinium into the vestibule following intratympanic applications in Guinea pigs and the influence of cochlear implantation. J Assoc Res Otolaryngol.: JARO. 2011;12(6): 741-51.
29. Salt AN, King EB, Hartsock JJ, et al. Marker entry into vestibular perilymph via the stapes following applications to the round window niche of guinea pigs. Hear Res. 2012; 283(1-2):14-23.
30. Zhang Y, Zhang W, Johnston AH, et al. Comparison of the distribution pattern of PEG-b-PCL polymersomes delivered into the rat inner ear via different methods. Acta Otolaryngol. 2011;131(12):1249-56.
31. Zou J, Yoshida T, Ramadan UA, et al. Dynamic enhancement of the rat inner ear after ultra-small-volume administration of Gd-DOTA to the medial wall of the middle ear cavity. ORL. 2011;73(5):275-81.
32. Kim YH, Raphael Y. Cell division and maintenance of epithelial integrity in the deafened auditory epithelium. Cell Cycle. 2007;6(5):612-9.

33. Minoda R, Izumikawa M, Kawamoto K, et al. Manipulating cell cycle regulation in the mature cochlea. Hear Res. 2007;232(1-2):44-51.
34. Vanlangenakker N, Vanden Berghe T, Krysko DV, et al. Molecular mechanisms and pathophysiology of necrotic cell death. Curr Mol Med. 2008;8(3):207-20.
35. Forge A, Li L. Apoptotic death of hair cells in mammalian vestibular sensory epithelia. Hear Res. 2000;139(1-2):97-115.
36. Ohlemiller KK, Dugan LL. Elevation of reactive oxygen species following ischemia-reperfusion in mouse cochlea observed in vivo. Audiol Neurootol. 1999;4(5):219-28.
37. Rybak LP, Whitworth C, Somani S. Application of antioxidants and other agents to prevent cisplatin ototoxicity. Laryngoscope. 1999;109(11):1740-4.
38. Schacht J. Antioxidant therapy attenuates aminoglycoside-induced hearing loss. Ann N Y Acad Sci. 1999;884:125-30.
39. Portt L, Norman G, Clapp C, et al. Anti-apoptosis and cell survival: a review. Biochimica et biophysica acta. 2011;1813(1):238-59.
40. Elmore S. Apoptosis: a review of programmed cell death. Toxicol Pathol. 2007;35(4):495-516.
41. Ewen CL, Kane KP, Bleackley RC. A quarter century of granzymes. Cell death and differentiation. 2012;19(1):28-35.
42. Martinvalet D, Zhu P, Lieberman J. Granzyme A induces caspase-independent mitochondrial damage, a required first step for apoptosis. Immunity. 2005;22(3):355-70.
43. Fettiplace R. Defining features of the hair cell mechanoelectrical transducer channel. Pflugers Archiv: Eur J Physiol. 2009;458(6):1115-23.
44. Gillespie PG, Muller U. Mechanotransduction by hair cells: models, molecules, and mechanisms. Cell. 2009;139(1):33-44.
45. Couloigner V, Sterkers O, Ferrary E. What's new in ion transports in the cochlea? Pflugers Archiv: Eur J Physiol. 2006;453(1):11-22.
46. Trune DR. Ion homeostasis in the ear: mechanisms, maladies, and management. Curr Opin Otolaryngol Head Neck Surg. 2010;18(5):413-9.
47. Marshall AF, Jewells VL, Kranz P, et al. Magnetic resonance imaging of guinea pig cochlea after vasopressin-induced or surgically induced endolymphatic hydrops. Otolaryngol Head Neck Surg. 2010;142(2):260-5.
48. Jones QR, Warford J, Rupasinghe HP, et al. Target-based selection of flavonoids for neurodegenerative disorders. Trends Pharmacol Sci. 2012;33(11):602-10.
49. Shinomori Y, Spack DS, Jones DD, et al. Volumetric and dimensional analysis of the guinea pig inner ear. Ann Otol Rhinol Laryngol. 2001;110(1):91-8.
50. Buckingham RA, Valvassori GE. Inner ear fluid volumes and the resolving power of magnetic resonance imaging: can it differentiate endolymphatic structures? Ann Otol Rhinol Laryngol. 2001;110(2):113-7.
51. Salt AN, Plontke SK. Principles of local drug delivery to the inner ear. Audiol Neurootol. 2009;14(6):350-60.
52. Mikulec AA, Plontke SK, Hartsock JJ, et al. Entry of substances into perilymph through the bone of the otic capsule after intratympanic applications in guinea pigs: implications for local drug delivery in humans. Otol Neurotol. 2009;30(2):131-8.
53. Plontke SK, Mynatt R, Gill RM, et al. Concentration gradient along the scala tympani after local application of gentamicin to the round window membrane. Laryngoscope. 2007;117(7):1191-8.
54. Bowes AK, Wiet RJ, Monsell EM, et al. Brain herniation and space-occupying lesions eroding the tegmen tympani. Laryngoscope. 1987;97(10):1172-5.
55. Saijo S, Kimura RS. Distribution of HRP in the inner ear after injection into the middle ear cavity. Acta Otolaryngologica. 1984;97(5-6):593-610.
56. Salt AN, Ma Y. Quantification of solute entry into cochlear perilymph through the round window membrane. Hear Res. 2001;154(1-2):88-97.
57. Plontke SK, Siedow N, Wegener R, et al. Cochlear pharmacokinetics with local inner ear drug delivery using a three-dimensional finite-element computer model. Audiol Neurootol. 2007;12(1):37-48.
58. Mynatt R, Hale SA, Gill RM, et al. Demonstration of a longitudinal concentration gradient along scala tympani by sequential sampling of perilymph from the cochlear apex. J Assoc Res Otolaryngol. 2006;7(2):182-93.
59. Salt AN, Ohyama K, Thalmann R. Radial communication between the perilymphatic scalae of the cochlea. I: Estimation by tracer perfusion. Hear Res. 1991;56(1-2):29-36.
60. Salt AN, DeMott JE. Endolymph volume changes during osmotic dehydration measured by two marker techniques. Hear Res. 1995;90(1-2):12-23.
61. Salt AN, Hartsock JJ, Gill RM, et al. Perilymph pharmacokinetics of markers and dexamethasone applied and sampled at the lateral semi-circular canal. J Assoc Res Otolaryngol. 2012;13(6):771-83.
62. Rask-Andersen H, Schrott-Fischer A, Pfaller K, et al. Perilymph/modiolar communication routes in the human cochlea. Ear Hear. 2006;27(5):457-65.
63. Salt AN, Gill RM, Plontke SK. Dependence of hearing changes on the dose of intratympanically applied gentamicin: a meta-analysis using mathematical simulations of clinical drug delivery protocols. Laryngoscope. 2008;118(10):1793-800.
64. Salt AN, Hartsock J, Plontke S, et al. Distribution of dexamethasone and preservation of inner ear function following intratympanic delivery of a gel-based formulation. Audiol Neurootol. 2011;16(5):323-35.
65. Richardson RT, Wise A, O'Leary S, et al. Tracing neurotrophin-3 diffusion and uptake in the guinea pig cochlea. Hear Res. 2004;198(1-2):25-35.
66. Parnes LS, Sun AH, Freeman DJ. Corticosteroid pharmacokinetics in the inner ear fluids: an animal study followed by clinical application. Laryngoscope. 1999;109(7 Pt 2):1-17.

67. Yang J, Wu H, Zhang P, et al. The pharmacokinetic profiles of dexamethasone and methylprednisolone concentration in perilymph and plasma following systemic and local administration. Acta Otolaryngol. 2008;128(5): 496-504.
68. Bird PA, Begg EJ, Zhang M, et al. Intratympanic versus intravenous delivery of methylprednisolone to cochlear perilymph. Otol Neurotol. 2007;28(8):1124-30.
69. Tobita T, Senarita M, Hara A, et al. Determination of prednisolone in the cochlear tissue. Hear Res. 2002;165(1-2): 30-4.
70. Plontke SK, Salt AN. Quantitative interpretation of corticosteroid pharmacokinetics in inner fluids using computer simulations. Hear Res. 2003;182(1-2):34-42.
71. Bachmann G, Su J, Zumegen C, et al. [Permeability of the round window membrane for prednisolone-21-hydrogen succinate. Prednisolone content of the perilymph after local administration vs. systemic injection]. Hno. 2001;49(7): 538-42.
72. Plontke SK, Mikulec AA, Salt AN. Rapid clearance of methylprednisolone after intratympanic application in humans. Comment on: Bird PA, Begg EJ, Zhang M, et al. Intratympanic versus intravenous delivery of methylprednisolone to cochlear perilymph. Otol Neurotol. 2007;28:1124-30. Otol Neurotol. 2008;29(5):732-3; author reply 3.
73. Hahn H, Salt AN, Biegner T, et al. Dexamethasone levels and base-to-apex concentration gradients in the scala tympani perilymph after intracochlear delivery in the guinea pig. Otol Neurotol. 2012;33(4):660-5.
74. Grewal AS, Nedzelski JM, Chen JM, et al. Dexamethasone uptake in the murine organ of Corti with transtympanic versus systemic administration. J Otolaryngol Head Neck Surg. = Le Journal d'oto-rhino-laryngologie et de chirurgie cervico-faciale. 2013;42(1):19.
75. Gianoli GJ, Li JC. Transtympanic steroids for treatment of sudden hearing loss. Otolaryngol Head Neck Surg.: Official Journal of American Academy of Otolaryngology-Head and Neck Surgery. 2001;125(3):142-6.
76. Wilson WR, Byl FM, Laird N. The efficacy of steroids in the treatment of idiopathic sudden hearing loss. A double-blind clinical study. Arch Otolaryngol. 1980;106(12):772-6.
77. Hughes GB, Freedman MA, Haberkamp TJ, Guay ME. Sudden sensorineural hearing loss. Otolaryngol Clin North Am. 1996;29(3):393-405.
78. Silverstein H, Isaacson JE, Olds MJ, et al. Dexamethasone inner ear perfusion for the treatment of Meniere's disease: a prospective, randomized, double-blind, crossover trial. Am J Otol. 1998;19(2):196-201.
79. Labus J, Breil J, Stutzer H, et al. Meta-analysis for the effect of medical therapy vs. placebo on recovery of idiopathic sudden hearing loss. Laryngoscope. 2010;120(9):1863-71.
80. Wei BP, Stathopoulos D, O'Leary S. Steroids for idiopathic sudden sensorineural hearing loss. Cochrane Database Syst Rev. 2013;7:CD003998.
81. Cinamon U, Bendet E, Kronenberg J. Steroids, carbogen or placebo for sudden hearing loss: a prospective double-blind study. Eur Arch Otorhinolaryngol. 2001;258(9):477-80.
82. Nosrati-Zarenoe R, Arlinger S, Hultcrantz E. Idiopathic sudden sensorineural hearing loss: results drawn from the Swedish national database. Acta Otolaryngol. 2007;127(11): 1168-75.
83. Hu A, Parnes LS. Intratympanic steroids for inner ear disorders: a review. Audiol Neurootol. 2009;14(6):373-82.
84. Spear SA, Schwartz SR. Intratympanic steroids for sudden sensorineural hearing loss: a systematic review. Otolaryngol Head Neck Surg. 2011;145(4):534-43.
85. Battaglia A, Burchette R, Cueva R. Combination therapy (intratympanic dexamethasone + high-dose prednisone taper) for the treatment of idiopathic sudden sensorineural hearing loss. Otol Neurotol. 2008;29(4):453-60.
86. Ahn JH, Yoo MH, Yoon TH, et al. Can intratympanic dexamethasone added to systemic steroids improve hearing outcome in patients with sudden deafness? Laryngoscope. 2008;118(2):279-82.
87. Hong SM, Park CH, Lee JH. Hearing outcomes of daily intratympanic dexamethasone alone as a primary treatment modality for ISSHL. Otolaryngol Head Neck Surg. 2009;141(5):579-83.
88. Plontke SK, Lowenheim H, Mertens J, et al. Randomized, double blind, placebo controlled trial on the safety and efficacy of continuous intratympanic dexamethasone delivered via a round window catheter for severe to profound sudden idiopathic sensorineural hearing loss after failure of systemic therapy. Laryngoscope. 2009;119(2):359-69.
89. Wu HP, Chou YF, Yu SH, et al. Intratympanic steroid injections as a salvage treatment for sudden sensorineural hearing loss: a randomized, double-blind, placebo-controlled study. Otol Neurotol. 2011;32(5):774-9.
90. Rauch SD, Halpin CF, Antonelli PJ, et al. Oral vs intratympanic corticosteroid therapy for idiopathic sudden sensorineural hearing loss: a randomized trial. JAMA. 2011;305 (20):2071-9.
91. Lautermann J, Sudhoff H, Junker R. Transtympanic corticoid therapy for acute profound hearing loss. Eur Arch Otorhinolaryngol.: Official Journal of the European Federation of Oto-Rhino-Laryngological Societies. 2005;262(7): 587-91.
92. Gundogan O, Pinar E, Imre A, et al. Therapeutic efficacy of the combination of intratympanic methylprednisolone and oral steroid for idiopathic sudden deafness. Otolaryngol Head Neck Surg. 2013;149(5):753-8.
93. Shea JJ, Jr. Classification of Meniere's disease. Am J Otol. 1993;14(3):224-9.
94. Phillips JS, Westerberg B. Intratympanic steroids for Meniere's disease or syndrome. Cochrane Database Syst Rev. 2011(7):CD008514.
95. Garduno-Anaya MA, Couthino De Toledo H, Hinojosa-Gonzalez R, et al. Dexamethasone inner ear perfusion by intratympanic injection in unilateral Meniere's disease: a two-year prospective, placebo-controlled, double-blind, randomized trial. Otolaryngol Head Neck Surg. 2005;133(2): 285-94.
96. Silverstein H, Smouha E, Jones R. Natural history vs. surgery for Meniere's disease. Otolaryngol Head Neck Surg. 1989;100(1):6-16.

97. Shea JJ, Jr. The role of dexamethasone or streptomycin perfusion in the treatment of Meniere's disease. Otolaryngol Clin North Am. 1997;30(6):1051-9.
98. Committee on Hearing and Equilibrium guidelines for the diagnosis and evaluation of therapy in Meniere's disease. American Academy of Otolaryngology-Head and Neck Foundation, Inc. Otolaryngol Head Neck Surg. 1995;113(3):181-5.
99. Casani AP, Piaggi P, Cerchiai N, et al. Intratympanic treatment of intractable unilateral Meniere disease: gentamicin or dexamethasone? A randomized controlled trial. Otolaryngol Head Neck Surg. 2012;146(3):430-7.
100. Tran Ba Huy P, Bernard P, et al. Kinetics of gentamicin uptake and release in the rat. Comparison of inner ear tissues and fluids with other organs. J Clin Invest. 1986;77(5):1492-500.
101. Hoffer ME, Kopke RD, Weisskopf P, et al. Use of the round window microcatheter in the treatment of Meniere's disease. Laryngoscope. 2001;111(11 Pt 1):2046-9.
102. Hoffer ME, Allen K, Kopke RD, et al. Transtympanic versus sustained-release administration of gentamicin: kinetics, morphology, and function. Laryngoscope. 2001;111(8):1343-57.
103. Lopez I, Honrubia V, Lee SC, et al. Quantification of the process of hair cell loss and recovery in the chinchilla crista ampullaris after gentamicin treatment. Int J Develop Neurosci. 1997;15(4-5):447-61.
104. Hirvonen TP, Minor LB, Hullar TE, Carey JP. Effects of intratympanic gentamicin on vestibular afferents and hair cells in the chinchilla. J Neurophysiol. 2005;93(2):643-55.
105. Zhai F, Liu JP, Dai CF, et al. Evidence-based modification of intratympanic gentamicin injections in patients with intractable vertigo. Otol Neurotol. 2010;31(4):642-8.
106. Zhang R, Zhang YB, Dai CF, et al. Temporal and spatial distribution of gentamicin in the peripheral vestibular system after transtympanic administration in guinea pigs. Hear Res. 2013;298:49-59.
107. Roehm P, Hoffer M, Balaban CD. Gentamicin uptake in the chinchilla inner ear. Hear Res. 2007;230(1-2):43-52.
108. Lyford-Pike S, Vogelheim C, Chu E, et al. Gentamicin is primarily localized in vestibular type I hair cells after intratympanic administration. J Assoc Res Otolaryngol.: JARO. 2007;8(4):497-508.
109. Hilton M, Chen J, Kakigi A, et al. Middle ear instillation of gentamicin and streptomycin in chinchillas: electrophysiological appraisal of selective ototoxicity. Clin Otolaryngol Allied Sci. 2002;27(6):529-35.
110. Wanamaker HH, Slepecky NB, Cefaratti LK, et al. Comparison of vestibular and cochlear ototoxicity from transtympanic streptomycin administration. Am J Otol. 1999;20(4):457-64.
111. De Waele C, Meguenni R, Freyss G, et al. Intratympanic gentamicin injections for Meniere disease: vestibular hair cell impairment and regeneration. Neurology. 2002;59(9):1442-4.
112. Helling K, Schonfeld U, Clarke AH. Treatment of Meniere's disease by low-dosage intratympanic gentamicin application: effect on otolith function. Laryngoscope. 2007;117(12):2244-50.
113. Park JC, Cohen GM. Vestibular ototoxicity in the chick: effects of streptomycin on equilibrium and on ampullary dark cells. Am J Otolaryngol. 1982;3(2):117-27.
114. Ge X, Shea JJ, Jr. Scanning electron microscopic observation of dark cells after streptomycin perfusion of the vestibule in guinea pigs. Scanning Microsc. 1995;9(1):283-8.
115. Pender DJ. Gentamicin tympanolysis: effects on the vestibular secretory cells. Am J Otolaryngol. 1985;6(5):358-67.
116. Kaplan DM, Nedzelski JM, Chen JM, et al. Intratympanic gentamicin for the treatment of unilateral Meniere's disease. Laryngoscope. 2000;110(8):1298-305.
117. Atlas JT, Parnes LS. Intratympanic gentamicin titration therapy for intractable Meniere's disease. Am J Otol. 1999;20(3):357-63.
118. Youssef TF, Poe DS. Intratympanic gentamicin injection for the treatment of Meniere's disease. Am J Otol. 1998;19(4):435-42.
119. Hoffer ME, Kopke RD, Weisskopf P, et al. Microdose gentamicin administration via the round window microcatheter: results in patients with Meniere's disease. Ann NY Acad Sci. 2001;942:46-51.
120. Abou-Halawa AS, Poe DS. Efficacy of increased gentamicin concentration for intratympanic injection therapy in Meniere's disease. Otol Neurotol. 2002;23(4):494-502; discussion -3.
121. Wang J, Dib M, Lenoir M, et al. Riluzole rescues cochlear sensory cells from acoustic trauma in the guinea-pig. Neuroscience. 2002;111(3):635-48.
122. Cureoglu S, Schachern PA, Paparella MM. Effect of parenteral aminoglycoside administration on dark cells in the crista ampullaris. Arch Otolaryngol Head Neck Surg. 2003;129(6):626-8.
123. Fiorino F, Pizzini FB, Barbieri F, et al. Magnetic resonance imaging fails to show evidence of reduced endolymphatic hydrops in gentamicin treatment of Meniere's disease. Otol Neurotol. 2012;33(4):629-33.
124. Fowler EP, Jr. Streptomycin treatment of vertigo. Transactions—American Academy of Ophthalmology and Otolaryngology American Academy of Ophthalmology and Otolaryngology. 1948;52:293-301.
125. Schuknecht HF. Ablation therapy in the management of Meniere's disease. Acta Oto-laryngologica Supplementum. 1957;132:1-42.
126. Beck C, Schmidt CL. 10 years of experience with intratympanally applied streptomycin (gentamicin) in the therapy of Morbus Meniere. Arch Otorhinolaryngol. 1978;221(2):149-52.
127. Diamond C, O'Connell DA, Hornig JD, et al. Systematic review of intratympanic gentamicin in Meniere's disease. J Otolaryngol. 2003;32(6):351-61.
128. Cohen-Kerem R, Kisilevsky V, Einarson TR, et al. Intratympanic gentamicin for Meniere's disease: a meta-analysis. Laryngoscope. 2004;114(12):2085-91.
129. Chia SH, Gamst AC, Anderson JP, et al. Intratympanic gentamicin therapy for Meniere's disease: a meta-analysis. Otol Neurotol. 2004;25(4):544-52.
130. Pullens B, van Benthem PP. Intratympanic gentamicin for Meniere's disease or syndrome. Cochrane Database Syst Rev. 2011(3):CD008234.

131. Huon LK, Fang TY, Wang PC. Outcomes of intratympanic gentamicin injection to treat Meniere's disease. Otol Neurotol. 2012;33(5):706-14.
132. Postema RJ, Kingma CM, Wit HP, et al. Intratympanic gentamicin therapy for control of vertigo in unilateral Meniere's disease: a prospective, double-blind, randomized, placebo-controlled trial. Acta Otolaryngol. 2008;128(8):876-80.
133. Stokroos R, Kingma H. Selective vestibular ablation by intratympanic gentamicin in patients with unilateral active Meniere's disease: a prospective, double-blind, placebo-controlled, randomized clinical trial. Acta Otolaryngol. 2004;124(2):172-5.
134. De Beer L, Stokroos R, Kingma H. Intratympanic gentamicin therapy for intractable Meniere's disease. Acta Otolaryngol. 2007;127(6):605-12.
135. Boleas-Aguirre MS, Sanchez-Ferrandiz N, Guillen-Grima F, et al. Long-term disability of class A patients with Meniere's disease after treatment with intratympanic gentamicin. Laryngoscope. 2007;117(8):1474-81.
136. Gabaizadeh R, Staecker H, Liu W, et al. BDNF protection of auditory neurons from cisplatin involves changes in intracellular levels of both reactive oxygen species and glutathione. Brain Res Mol Brain Res. 1997;50(1-2):71-8.
137. Mukherjea D, Rybak LP, Sheehan KE, et al. The design and screening of drugs to prevent acquired sensorineural hearing loss. Expert Opin Drug Discov. 2011;6(5):491-505.
138. Otto WC, Brown RD, Gage-White L, et al. Effects of cisplatin and thiosulfate upon auditory brainstem responses of guinea pigs. Hear Res. 1988;35(1):79-85.
139. Wimmer C, Mees K, Stumpf P, et al. Round window application of D-methionine, sodium thiosulfate, brain-derived neurotrophic factor, and fibroblast growth factor-2 in cisplatin-induced ototoxicity. Otol Neurotol. 2004;25(1):33-40.
140. Korver KD, Rybak LP, Whitworth C, et al. Round window application of D-methionine provides complete cisplatin otoprotection. Otolaryngol Head Neck Surg. 2002;126(6):683-9.
141. Campbell KC, Meech RP, Rybak LP, et al. The effect of D-methionine on cochlear oxidative state with and without cisplatin administration: mechanisms of otoprotection. J Am Acad Audiol. 2003;14(3):144-56.
142. Kopke RD, Coleman JK, Liu J, et al. Candidate's thesis: enhancing intrinsic cochlear stress defenses to reduce noise-induced hearing loss. Laryngoscope. 2002;112(9):1515-32.
143. Kopke RD, Weisskopf PA, Boone JL, et al. Reduction of noise-induced hearing loss using L-NAC and salicylate in the chinchilla. Hear Res. 2000;149(1-2):138-46.
144. Fetoni AR, Ralli M, Sergi B, et al. Protective effects of N-acetylcysteine on noise-induced hearing loss in guinea pigs. Acta Otorhinolaryngologica Italica. 2009;29(2):70-5.
145. Lin CY, Wu JL, Shih TS, et al. N-Acetyl-cysteine against noise-induced temporary threshold shift in male workers. Hear Res. 2010;269(1-2):42-7.
146. Dolgin E. Sound medicine. Nat Med. 2012;18(5):642-5.
147. Kopke RD, Jackson RL, Coleman JK, et al. NAC for noise: from the bench top to the clinic. Hear Res. 2007;226(1-2):114-25.
148. Yoo J, Hamilton SJ, Angel D, et al. Cisplatin otoprotection using transtympanic L-N-acetylcysteine: A pilot randomized study in head and neck cancer patients. Laryngoscope. 2013.
149. Riga MG, Chelis L, Kakolyris S, et al. Transtympanic injections of N-acetylcysteine for the prevention of cisplatin-induced ototoxicity: a feasible method with promising efficacy. Am J Clin Oncol. 2013;36(1):1-6.
150. Huang X, Whitworth CA, Rybak LP. Ginkgo biloba extract (EGb 761) protects against cisplatin-induced ototoxicity in rats. Otol Neurotol.: Official Publication of the American Otological Society, American Neurotology Society [and] European Academy of Otology and Neurotology. 2007;28(6):828-33.
151. Seidman MD, Khan MJ, Bai U, et al. Biologic activity of mitochondrial metabolites on aging and age-related hearing loss. Am J Otol. 2000;21(2):161-7.
152. Pouyatos B, Gearhart C, Nelson-Miller A, et al. Lipoic acid and 6-formylpterin reduce potentiation of noise-induced hearing loss by carbon monoxide: preliminary investigation. J Rehabil Res Dev. 2008;45(7):1053-64.
153. Rybak LP, Husain K, Whitworth C, et al. Dose dependent protection by lipoic acid against cisplatin-induced ototoxicity in rats: antioxidant defense system. Toxicol Sci. 1999;47(2):195-202.
154. Choe WT, Chinosornvatana N, Chang KW. Prevention of cisplatin ototoxicity using transtympanic N-acetylcysteine and lactate. Otol Neurotol. 2004;25(6):910-5.
155. Munguia R, Sahmkow SI, Funnell WR, et al. Transtympanic Ringer's lactate application in the prevention of cisplatinum-induced ototoxicity in a chinchilla animal model. Otolaryngol Head Neck Surg. 2010;143(1):134-40.
156. Le Prell CG, Hughes LF, Miller JM. Free radical scavengers vitamins A, C, and E plus magnesium reduce noise trauma. Free Radic Biol Med. 2007;42(9):1454-63.
157. Seidman MD. Effects of dietary restriction and antioxidants on presbycusis. Laryngoscope. 2000;110(5 Pt 1):727-38.
158. Lynch ED, Gu R, Pierce C, et al. Combined oral delivery of ebselen and allopurinol reduces multiple cisplatin toxicities in rat breast and ovarian cancer models while enhancing anti-tumor activity. Anticancer Drugs. 2005;16(5):569-79.
159. Pourbakht A, Yamasoba T. Ebselen attenuates cochlear damage caused by acoustic trauma. Hear Res. 2003;181(1-2):100-8.
160. Seidman MD, Khan MJ, Tang WX, et al. Influence of lecithin on mitochondrial DNA and age-related hearing loss. Otolaryngol Head Neck Surg. 2002;127(3):138-44.
161. Hyppolito MA, de Oliveira JA, Rossato M. Cisplatin ototoxicity and otoprotection with sodium salicylate. Eur Arch Otorhinolaryngol. 2006;263(9):798-803.
162. Adelman C, Freeman S, Paz Z, et al. Salicylic acid injection before noise exposure reduces permanent threshold shift. Audiol Neurootol. 2008;13(4):266-72.
163. Sha SH, Qiu JH, Schacht J. Aspirin to prevent gentamicin-induced hearing loss. N Engl J Med. 2006;354(17):1856-7.
164. De Kloet ER, Reul JM. Feedback action and tonic influence of corticosteroids on brain function: a concept arising from the heterogeneity of brain receptor systems. Psychoneuroendocrinology. 1987;12(2):83-105.

165. Himeno C, Komeda M, Izumikawa M, et al. Intra-cochlear administration of dexamethasone attenuates aminoglycoside ototoxicity in the guinea pig. Hear Res. 2002;167 (1-2):61-70.
166. Park SK, Choi D, Russell P, et al. Protective effect of corticosteroid against the cytotoxicity of aminoglycoside otic drops on isolated cochlear outer hair cells. Laryngoscope. 2004;114(4):768-71.
167. Paksoy M, Ayduran E, Sanli A, et al. The protective effects of intratympanic dexamethasone and vitamin E on cisplatin-induced ototoxicity are demonstrated in rats. Med Oncol. 2011;28(2):615-21.
168. van de Water TR, Dinh CT, Vivero R, et al. Mechanisms of hearing loss from trauma and inflammation: otoprotective therapies from the laboratory to the clinic. Acta Otolaryngol. 2010;130(3):308-11.
169. Dinh CT, Haake S, Chen S, et al. Dexamethasone protects organ of corti explants against tumor necrosis factor-alpha-induced loss of auditory hair cells and alters the expression levels of apoptosis-related genes. Neuroscience. 2008;157(2):405-13.
170. Meltser I, Canlon B. Protecting the auditory system with glucocorticoids. Hear Res. 2011;281(1-2):47-55.
171. Ryan AF, Pak K, Low W, et al. Immunological damage to the inner ear: current and future therapeutic strategies. Adv Otorhinolaryngol. 2002;59:66-74.
172. Trune DR, Canlon B. Corticosteroid therapy for hearing and balance disorders. Anat Rec. 2012;295(11):1928-43.
173. Arnold WJ. Oto-immunology. Facts or fantasy? In: Veldman JE (ed.), Immunobiology, Histophysiology, Tumor Immunology in Otorhinolaryngology. Amsterdam: Kugler Publications; 1987. p. 39-45.
174. Nadol JB, McKenna MJ. Histopathology of Meniere's disease and otosclerosis. In: Veldman JE (ed.), Immunobiology, Histophysiology, Tumor Immunology in Otorhinolaryngology. Amsterdam: Kugler Publications; 1987. p. 165-84.
175. Keithley EM, Chen MC, Linthicum F. Clinical diagnoses associated with histologic findings of fibrotic tissue and new bone in the inner ear. Laryngoscope. 1998;108(1 Pt 1):87-91.
176. Gloddek B, Lamm K, Arnold W. Pharmacological influence on inner ear endothelial cells in relation to the pathogenesis of sensorineural hearing loss. Adv Otorhinolaryngol. 2002;59:75-83.
177. Curtis LM, ten Cate WJ, Rarey KE. Dynamics of Na,K-ATPase sites in lateral cochlear wall tissues of the rat. Eur Arch Otorhinolaryngol. 1993;250(5):265-70.
178. Lee JH, Marcus DC. Nongenomic effects of corticosteroids on ion transport by stria vascularis. Audiol Neurootol. 2002;7(2):100-6.
179. Trune DR, Kempton JB. Low dose combination steroids control autoimmune mouse hearing loss. J Neuroimmunol. 2010;229(1-2):140-5.
180. Tahera Y, Meltser I, Johansson P, et al. NF-kappaB mediated glucocorticoid response in the inner ear after acoustic trauma. J Neurosci Res. 2006;83(6):1066-76.
181. Trune D, Delaney K, Hausman F, editors. Transtympanically delivered steroids impact thousands of inner ear genes over conventional systemic delivery. Meeting of the Association Research Otolaryngology; 2012; San Diego, CA.
182. Van Wijk F, Staecker H, Keithley E, et al. Local perfusion of the tumor necrosis factor alpha blocker infliximab to the inner ear improves autoimmune neurosensory hearing loss. Audiol Neurootol. 2006;11(6):357-65.
183. So H, Kim H, Lee JH, et al. Cisplatin cytotoxicity of auditory cells requires secretions of proinflammatory cytokines via activation of ERK and NF-kappaB. J Assoc Res Otolaryngol.: JARO. 2007;8(3):338-55.
184. Pirvola U, Xing-Qun L, Virkkala J, et al. Rescue of hearing, auditory hair cells, and neurons by CEP-1347/KT7515, an inhibitor of c-Jun N-terminal kinase activation. J Neurosci.: The Official Journal of the Society for Neuroscience. 2000;20(1):43-50.
185. Wang J, Van De Water TR, Bonny C, et al. A peptide inhibitor of c-Jun N-terminal kinase protects against both aminoglycoside and acoustic trauma-induced auditory hair cell death and hearing loss. J Neurosci. 2003;23(24):8596-607.
186. Dinh CT, Van De Water TR. Blocking pro-cell-death signal pathways to conserve hearing. Audiol Neurootol. 2009; 14(6):383-92.
187. Suckfuell M, Canis M, Strieth S, et al. Intratympanic treatment of acute acoustic trauma with a cell-permeable JNK ligand: a prospective randomized phase I/II study. Acta Otolaryngol. 2007;127(9):938-42.
188. Wang J, Ladrech S, Pujol R, et al. Caspase inhibitors, but not c-Jun NH2-terminal kinase inhibitor treatment, prevent cisplatin-induced hearing loss. Cancer Res. 2004;64 (24):9217-24.
189. Asanuma M, Nishibayashi S, Iwata E, et al. Alterations of cAMP response element-binding activity in the aged rat brain in response to administration of rolipram, a cAMP-specific phosphodiesterase inhibitor. Brain Res Mol Brain Res. 1996;41(1-2):210-5.
190. Ramekers D, Versnel H, Grolman W, et al. Neurotrophins and their role in the cochlea. Hear Res. 2012;288(1-2): 19-33.
191. Malgrange B, Rigo JM, Coucke P, et al. Identification of factors that maintain mammalian outer hair cells in adult organ of Corti explants. Hear Res. 2002;170(1-2):48-58.
192. Rong P, Bennie AM, Epa WR, et al. Nerve growth factor determines survival and death of PC12 cells by regulation of the bcl-x, bax, and caspase-3 genes. J Neurochemistry. 1999;72(6):2294-300.
193. Dugan LL, Creedon DJ, Johnson EM, Jr., et al. Rapid suppression of free radical formation by nerve growth factor involves the mitogen-activated protein kinase pathway. Proceedings of the National Academy of Sciences of the United States of America. 1997;94(8):4086-91.
194. Blakley BW. Update on intratympanic gentamicin for Meniere's disease. Laryngoscope. 2000;110(2 Pt 1):236-40.
195. Duan M, Agerman K, Ernfors P, et al. Complementary roles of neurotrophin 3 and a N-methyl-D-aspartate antagonist in the protection of noise and aminoglycoside-induced ototoxicity. Proceedings of the National Academy of Sciences of the United States of America. 2000;97(13):7597-602.
196. Ruan RS, Leong SK, Mark I, et al. Effects of BDNF and NT-3 on hair cell survival in guinea pig cochlea damaged by kanamycin treatment. Neuroreport. 1999;10(10):2067-71.

197. Gillespie LN, Clark GM, Bartlett PF, et al. BDNF-induced survival of auditory neurons in vivo: Cessation of treatment leads to accelerated loss of survival effects. J Neurosci Res. 2003;71(6):785-90.
198. Maruyama J, Miller JM, Ulfendahl M. Glial cell line-derived neurotrophic factor and antioxidants preserve the electrical responsiveness of the spiral ganglion neurons after experimentally induced deafness. Neurobiol Dis. 2008;29(1):14-21.
199. Agterberg MJ, Versnel H, van Dijk LM, et al. Enhanced survival of spiral ganglion cells after cessation of treatment with brain-derived neurotrophic factor in deafened guinea pigs. J Assoc Res Otolaryngol.: JARO. 2009;10(3):355-67.
200. Fransson A, Maruyama J, Miller JM, et al. Post-treatment effects of local GDNF administration to the inner ears of deafened guinea pigs. J Neurotrauma. 2010;27(9):1745-51.
201. Shepherd RK, Coco A, Epp SB. Neurotrophins and electrical stimulation for protection and repair of spiral ganglion neurons following sensorineural hearing loss. Hear Res. 2008;242(1-2):100-9.
202. Davis RL. Gradients of neurotrophins, ion channels, and tuning in the cochlea. Neuroscientist. 2003;9(5):311-6.
203. Adamson CL, Reid MA, Davis RL. Opposite actions of brain-derived neurotrophic factor and neurotrophin-3 on firing features and ion channel composition of murine spiral ganglion neurons. J Neurosci. 2002;22(4):1385-96.
204. Endo T, Nakagawa T, Kita T, et al. Novel strategy for treatment of inner ears using a biodegradable gel. Laryngoscope. 2005;115(11):2016-20.
205. Havenith S, Versnel H, Agterberg MJ, et al. Spiral ganglion cell survival after round window membrane application of brain-derived neurotrophic factor using Gelfoam as carrier. Hear Res. 2011;272(1-2):168-77.
206. Noushi F, Richardson RT, Hardman J, et al. Delivery of neurotrophin-3 to the cochlea using alginate beads. Otol Neurotol. 2005;26(3):528-33.
207. Shibata SB, Budenz CL, Bowling SA, et al. Nerve maintenance and regeneration in the damaged cochlea. Hear Res. 2011;281(1-2):56-64.
208. Mandala M, Colletti L, Carner M, et al. Induced endolymphatic flow from the endolymphatic sac to the cochlea in Meniere's disease. Otolaryngol Head Neck Surg.: Official Journal of American Academy of Otolaryngology-Head and Neck Surgery. 2010;143(5):673-9.
209. Kitahara T, Fukushima M, Uno Y, et al. Up-regulation of cochlear aquaporin-3 mRNA expression after intra-endolymphatic sac application of dexamethasone. Neurolog Res. 2003;25(8):865-70.
210. Praetorius M, Knipper M, Schick B, et al. A novel vestibular approach for gene transfer into the inner ear. Audiol Neurootol. 2002;7(6):324-34.
211. Kawamoto K, Oh SH, Kanzaki S, et al. The functional and structural outcome of inner ear gene transfer via the vestibular and cochlear fluids in mice. Mol Ther. 2001;4(6):575-85.
212. Silverstein H, Arruda J, Rosenberg SI, et al. Direct round window membrane application of gentamicin in the treatment of Meniere's disease. Otolaryngol Head Neck Surg. 1999;120(5):649-55.
213. Eastwood H, Pinder D, James D, et al. Permanent and transient effects of locally delivered n-acetyl cysteine in a guinea pig model of cochlear implantation. Hear Res. 2010;259(1-2):24-30.
214. Eastwood H, Chang A, Kel G, et al. Round window delivery of dexamethasone ameliorates local and remote hearing loss produced by cochlear implantation into the second turn of the guinea pig cochlea. Hear Res. 2010;265(1-2):25-9.
215. James DP, Eastwood H, Richardson RT, et al. Effects of round window dexamethasone on residual hearing in a Guinea pig model of cochlear implantation. Audiol Neurootol. 2008;13(2):86-96.
216. Borden RC, Saunders JE, Berryhill WE, et al. Hyaluronic acid hydrogel sustains the delivery of dexamethasone across the round window membrane. Audiol Neurootol. 2011;16(1):1-11.
217. Inaoka T, Nakagawa T, Kikkawa YS, et al. Local application of hepatocyte growth factor using gelatin hydrogels attenuates noise-induced hearing loss in guinea pigs. Acta Oto-laryngol. 2009;129(4):453-7.
218. Saber A, Strand SP, Ulfendahl M. Use of the biodegradable polymer chitosan as a vehicle for applying drugs to the inner ear. Eur J Pharm Sci. 2010;39(1-3):110-5.
219. Paulson DP, Abuzeid W, Jiang H, et al. A novel controlled local drug delivery system for inner ear disease. Laryngoscope. 2008;118(4):706-11.
220. Hill SL, 3rd, Digges EN, et al. Long-term follow-up after gentamicin application via the Silverstein MicroWick in the treatment of Meniere's disease. Ear Nose Throat J. 2006;85(8):494, 6, 8.
221. Van Wijck F, Staecker H, Lefebvre PP. Topical steroid therapy using the Silverstein Microwick in sudden sensorineural hearing loss after failure of conventional treatment. Acta Otolaryngol. 2007;127(10):1012-7.
222. Hoffer ME, Balough B, Henderson J, et al. Use of sustained release vehicles in the treatment of Meniere's disease. Otolaryngol Clin North Am. 1997;30(6):1159-66.
223. Chen Z, Kujawa SG, McKenna MJ, et al. Inner ear drug delivery via a reciprocating perfusion system in the guinea pig. J Control Release. 2005;110(1):1-19.
224. Sewell WF, Borenstein JT, Chen Z, et al. Development of a microfluidics-based intracochlear drug delivery device. Audiol Neurootol. 2009;14(6):411-22.
225. Praetorius M, Limberger A, Muller M, et al. A novel microperfusion system for the long-term local supply of drugs to the inner ear: implantation and function in the rat model. Audiol Neurootol. 2001;6(5):250-8.
226. Zhang Y, Zhang W, Johnston AH, et al. Targeted delivery of Tet1 peptide functionalized polymersomes to the rat cochlear nerve. Int J Nanomed. 2012;7:1015-22.
227. Pritz CO, Dudas J, Rask-Andersen H, et al. Nanomedicine strategies for drug delivery to the ear. Nanomedicine. 2013;8(7):1155-72.

228. Zou J, Sood R, Ranjan S, et al. Size-dependent passage of liposome nanocarriers with preserved post-transport integrity across the middle-inner ear barriers in rats. Otol Neurotol. 2012;33(4):666-73.
229. Danhier F, Ansorena E, Silva JM, et al. PLGA-based nanoparticles: an overview of biomedical applications. J Control Release. 2012;161(2):505-22.
230. Eshraghi AA, Adil E, He J, et al. Local dexamethasone therapy conserves hearing in an animal model of electrode insertion trauma-induced hearing loss. Otol Neurotol. 2007;28(6):842-9.
231. Meyer H, Stover T, Fouchet F, et al. Lipidic nanocapsule drug delivery: neuronal protection for cochlear implant optimization. Int J Nanomed. 2012;7:2449-64.
232. Lamprecht A, Ubrich N, Yamamoto H, et al. Design of rolipram-loaded nanoparticles: comparison of two preparation methods. J Control Release. 2001;71(3):297-306.
233. Ye Q, Tillein J, Hartmann R, et al. Application of a corticosteroid (Triamcinolon) protects inner ear function after surgical intervention. Ear Hear. 2007;28(3):361-9.
234. Kopke RD, Wassel RA, Mondalek F, et al. Magnetic nanoparticles: inner ear targeted molecule delivery and middle ear implant. Audiol Neurootol. 2006;11(2):123-33.
235. Du X, Chen K, Kuriyavar S, et al. Magnetic targeted delivery of dexamethasone acetate across the round window membrane in guinea pigs. Otol Neurotol. 2013;34(1):41-7.
236. Gramowski A, Flossdorf J, Bhattacharya K, et al. Nanoparticles induce changes of the electrical activity of neuronal networks on microelectrode array neurochips. Environ Health Perspect. 2010;118(10):1363-9.
237. Hochmair I, Nopp P, Jolly C, et al. MED-EL Cochlear implants: state of the art and a glimpse into the future. Trends Amplif. 2006;10(4):201-19.
238. Ibrahim HN, Bossard D, Jolly C, et al. Radiologic study of a disposable drug delivery intracochlear catheter. Otol Neurotol. 2011;32(2):217-22.
239. Richardson RT, Wise AK, Thompson BC, et al. Polypyrrole-coated electrodes for the delivery of charge and neurotrophins to cochlear neurons. Biomaterials. 2009;30(13):2614-24.
240. Niedermeier K, Braun S, Fauser C, et al. A safety evaluation of dexamethasone-releasing cochlear implants: comparative study on the risk of otogenic meningitis after implantation. Acta Otolaryngol. 2012;132(12):1252-60.
241. Krenzlin S, Vincent C, Munzke L, et al. Predictability of drug release from cochlear implants. J Control Release. 2012;159(1):60-8.
242. Eshraghi AA, Dinh CT, Bohorquez J, et al. Local drug delivery to conserve hearing: mechanisms of action of eluted dexamethasone within the cochlea. Cochlear Implants Int. 2011;12 Suppl 1:S51-3.
243. Farahmand Ghavi F, Mirzadeh H, Imani M, et al. Corticosteroid-releasing cochlear implant: a novel hybrid of biomaterial and drug delivery system. J Biomed Mat Res Part B, Appl Biomater. 2010;94(2):388-98.
244. Corwin JT, Cotanche DA. Regeneration of sensory hair cells after acoustic trauma. Science. 1988;240(4860):1772-4.
245. Ryals BM, Rubel EW. Hair cell regeneration after acoustic trauma in adult Coturnix quail. Science. 1988;240(4860):1774-6.
246. Lowenheim H, Kil J, Gultig K, et al. Determination of hair cell degeneration and hair cell death in neomycin treated cultures of the neonatal rat cochlea. Hear Res. 1999;128(1-2):16-26.
247. Kelley MW. Determination and commitment of mechanosensory hair cells. ScientificWorldJournal. 2002;2:1079-94.
248. Zine A, de Ribaupierre F. Notch/Notch ligands and Math1 expression patterns in the organ of Corti of wild-type and Hes1 and Hes5 mutant mice. Hear Res. 2002;170(1-2):22-31.
249. Shibata SB, Raphael Y. Future approaches for inner ear protection and repair. J Commun Disord. 2010;43(4):295-310.
250. Okano T, Kelley MW. Stem cell therapy for the inner ear: recent advances and future directions. Trends Amplif. 2012;16(1):4-18.
251. Sherr CJ, Roberts JM. CDK inhibitors: positive and negative regulators of G1-phase progression. Genes Dev. 1999;13(12):1501-12.
252. Kanzaki S, Beyer LA, Swiderski DL, et al. p27(Kip1) deficiency causes organ of Corti pathology and hearing loss. Hear Res. 2006;214(1-2):28-36.
253. Cheng AG, Cunningham LL, Rubel EW. Mechanisms of hair cell death and protection. Curr Opin Otolaryngol Head Neck Surg. 2005;13(6):343-8.
254. Hansen MR, Zha XM, Bok J, et al. Multiple distinct signal pathways, including an autocrine neurotrophic mechanism, contribute to the survival-promoting effect of depolarization on spiral ganglion neurons in vitro. J Neurosci. 2001;21(7):2256-67.
255. Despres G, Romand R. Neurotrophins and the development of cochlear innervation. Life Sci. 1994;54(18):1291-7.
256. Medd AM, Bianchi LM. Analysis of BDNF production in the aging gerbil cochlea. Exp Neurol. 2000;162(2):390-3.
257. Bianchi LM, Conover JC, Fritzsch B, et al. Degeneration of vestibular neurons in late embryogenesis of both heterozygous and homozygous BDNF null mutant mice. Development. 1996;122(6):1965-73.
258. Farinas I, Jones KR, Tessarollo L, et al. Spatial shaping of cochlear innervation by temporally regulated neurotrophin expression. J Neurosci. 2001;21(16):6170-80.
259. Teng KK, Felice S, Kim T, et al. Understanding proneurotrophin actions: recent advances and challenges. Develop Neurobiol. 2010;70(5):350-9.
260. Greenberg ME, Xu B, Lu B, et al. New insights in the biology of BDNF synthesis and release: implications in CNS function. J Neurosci. 2009;29(41):12764-7.
261. Kujawa SG, Liberman MC. Acceleration of age-related hearing loss by early noise exposure: evidence of a misspent youth. J Neurosci. 2006;26(7):2115-23.
262. Kujawa SG, Liberman MC. Adding insult to injury: cochlear nerve degeneration after "temporary" noise-induced hearing loss. J Neurosci. 2009;29(45):14077-85.
263. Baron M. An overview of the Notch signalling pathway. Semin Cell Dev Biol. 2003;14(2):113-9.

264. Brooker R, Hozumi K, Lewis J. Notch ligands with contrasting functions: Jagged1 and Delta1 in the mouse inner ear. Development. 2006;133(7):1277-86.
265. Lanford PJ, Lan Y, Jiang R, et al. Notch signalling pathway mediates hair cell development in mammalian cochlea. Nat Genet. 1999;21(3):289-92.
266. Kelley MW. Regulation of cell fate in the sensory epithelia of the inner ear. Nat Rev Neurosci. 2006;7(11):837-49.
267. Zine A, Aubert A, Qiu J, et al. Hes 1 and Hes 5 activities are required for the normal development of the hair cells in the mammalian inner ear. J Neurosci. 2001;21(13):4712-20.
268. Doetzlhofer A, Basch ML, Ohyama T, et al. Hey 2 regulation by FGF provides a Notch-independent mechanism for maintaining pillar cell fate in the organ of Corti. Dev Cell. 2009;16(1):58-69.
269. Gubbels SP, Woessner DW, Mitchell JC, et al. Functional auditory hair cells produced in the mammalian cochlea by in utero gene transfer. Nature. 2008;455(7212):537-41.
270. White PM, Doetzlhofer A, Lee YS, et al. Mammalian cochlear supporting cells can divide and trans-differentiate into hair cells. Nature. 2006;441(7096):984-7.
271. Izumikawa M, Minoda R, Kawamoto K, et al. Auditory hair cell replacement and hearing improvement by Atoh1 gene therapy in deaf mammals. Nat Med. 2005;11(3):271-6.
272. Mizutari K, Fujioka M, Hosoya M, et al. Notch inhibition induces cochlear hair cell regeneration and recovery of hearing after acoustic trauma. Neuron. 2013;77(1):58-69.
273. Lin V, Golub JS, Nguyen TB, et al. Inhibition of Notch activity promotes nonmitotic regeneration of hair cells in the adult mouse utricles. J Neurosci. 2011;31(43):15329-39.
274. Hori R, Nakagawa T, Sakamoto T, et al. Pharmacological inhibition of Notch signaling in the mature guinea pig cochlea. Neuroreport. 2007;18(18):1911-4.
275. Fukui H, Raphael Y. Gene therapy for the inner ear. Hear Res. 2013;297:99-105.
276. Lalwani AK, Walsh BJ, Reilly PG, et al. Development of in vivo gene therapy for hearing disorders: introduction of adeno-associated virus into the cochlea of the guinea pig. Gene Ther. 1996;3(7):588-92.
277. Jero J, Mhatre AN, Tseng CJ, et al. Cochlear gene delivery through an intact round window membrane in mouse. Human Gene Ther. 2001;12(5):539-48.
278. Staecker H, Kopke R, Malgrange B, et al. NT-3 and/or BDNF therapy prevents loss of auditory neurons following loss of hair cells. Neuroreport. 1996;7(4):889-94.
279. Lalwani AK, Jero J, Mhatre AN. Current issues in cochlear gene transfer. Audiol Neuro-otol. 2002;7(3):146-51.
280. Bowers WJ, Chen X, Guo H, et al. Neurotrophin-3 transduction attenuates cisplatin spiral ganglion neuron ototoxicity in the cochlea. Mol Ther. 2002;6(1):12-8.
281. Chen X, Frisina RD, Bowers WJ, e al. HSV amplicon-mediated neurotrophin-3 expression protects murine spiral ganglion neurons from cisplatin-induced damage. Mol Ther. 2001;3(6):958-63.
282. Yagi M, Magal E, Sheng Z, et al. Hair cell protection from aminoglycoside ototoxicity by adenovirus-mediated overexpression of glial cell line-derived neurotrophic factor. Hum Gene Ther. 1999;10(5):813-23.
283. Suzuki M, Yagi M, Brown JN, et al. Effect of transgenic GDNF expression on gentamicin-induced cochlear and vestibular toxicity. Gene Ther. 2000;7(12):1046-54.
284. Yagi M, Kanzaki S, Kawamoto K, et al. Spiral ganglion neurons are protected from degeneration by GDNF gene therapy. J Assoc Res Otolaryngol. 2000;1(4):315-25.
285. Wise AK, Fallon JB, Neil AJ, et al. Combining cell-based therapies and neural prostheses to promote neural survival. Neurotherapeutics. 2011;8(4):774-87.
286. Wise AK, Hume CR, Flynn BO, et al. Effects of localized neurotrophin gene expression on spiral ganglion neuron resprouting in the deafened cochlea. Mol Ther. 2010;18(6):1111-22.
287. Wang J, Menchenton T, Yin S, et al. Over-expression of X-linked inhibitor of apoptosis protein slows presbycusis in C57BL/6J mice. Neurobiol Aging. 2010;31(7):1238-49.
288. Wang J, Tymczyszyn N, Yu Z, et al. Overexpression of X-linked inhibitor of apoptosis protein protects against noise-induced hearing loss in mice. Gene Ther. 2011;18(6):560-8.
289. Cooper LB, Chan DK, Roediger FC, et al. AAV-mediated delivery of the caspase inhibitor XIAP protects against cisplatin ototoxicity. Otol Neurotol. 2006;27(4):484-90.
290. Kelly MC, Chang Q, Pan A, et al. Atoh1 directs the formation of sensory mosaics and induces cell proliferation in the postnatal mammalian cochlea in vivo. J Neurosci. 2012;32(19):6699-710.
291. Liu Z, Dearman JA, Cox BC, et al. Age-dependent in vivo conversion of mouse cochlear pillar and Deiters' cells to immature hair cells by Atoh1 ectopic expression. J Neurosci.: The Official Journal of the Society for Neuroscience. 2012;32(19):6600-10.
292. Zheng JL, Gao WQ. Overexpression of Math1 induces robust production of extra hair cells in postnatal rat inner ears. Nat Neurosci. 2000;3(6):580-6.
293. Shou J, Zheng JL, Gao WQ. Robust generation of new hair cells in the mature mammalian inner ear by adenoviral expression of Hath1. Mol Cell Neurosci. 2003;23(2):169-79.
294. Kawamoto K, Ishimoto S, Minoda R, et al. Math1 gene transfer generates new cochlear hair cells in mature guinea pigs in vivo. J Neurosci. 2003;23(11):4395-400.
295. Akil O, Seal RP, Burke K, et al. Restoration of hearing in the VGLUT3 knockout mouse using virally mediated gene therapy. Neuron. 2012;75(2):283-93.
296. Stover T, Yagi M, Raphael Y. Transduction of the contralateral ear after adenovirus-mediated cochlear gene transfer. Gene Ther. 2000;7(5):377-83.
297. Behlke MA. Progress towards in vivo use of siRNAs. Mol Ther. 2006;13(4):644-70.
298. Hildebrand MS, Newton SS, Gubbels SP, et al. Advances in molecular and cellular therapies for hearing loss. Mol Ther. 2008;16(2):224-36.
299. Maeda Y, Fukushima K, Nishizaki K, et al. In vitro and in vivo suppression of GJB2 expression by RNA interference. Hum Mol Genet. 2005;14(12):1641-50.

300. Mukherjea D, Jajoo S, Whitworth C, et al. Short interfering RNA against transient receptor potential vanilloid 1 attenuates cisplatin-induced hearing loss in the rat. J Neurosci. 2008; 28(49):13056-65.
301. Mukherjea D, Jajoo S, Kaur T, et al. Transtympanic administration of short interfering (si)RNA for the NOX3 isoform of NADPH oxidase protects against cisplatin-induced hearing loss in the rat. Antioxid Redox Signal. 2010;13(5):589-98.
302. Takahashi K, Tanabe K, Ohnuki M, et al. Induction of pluripotent stem cells from adult human fibroblasts by defined factors. Cell. 2007;131(5):861-72.
303. Takahashi K, Yamanaka S. Induction of pluripotent stem cells from mouse embryonic and adult fibroblast cultures by defined factors. Cell. 2006;126(4):663-76.
304. Ito J, Kojima K, Kawaguchi S. Survival of neural stem cells in the cochlea. Acta Otolaryngol. 2001;121(2):140-2.

CHAPTER

36

Anatomy and Physiology of the Facial Nerve

Ruwan Kiringoda, John K Niparko, Lawrence R Lustig

INTRODUCTION

The facial nerve is uniquely complex in terms of its form, function, and physiology. The facial nerve, the seventh cranial nerve, is involved in congenital anomalies and degenerative disorders and affected by a range of acquired pathology, from infectious to neoplastic conditions. A thorough understanding of its embryology, anatomy, and physiology enables the physician to accurately diagnose and treat disorders of the facial nerve.

EMBRYOLOGY

Intratemporal Development

The facial nerve (Figs. 36.1A to C and Table 36.1) begins to form near the end of the first month of gestation. A collection of neural crest cells gives rise to the acousticofacial primordium that develops adjacent to the primordial inner ear, the otic placode, and eventually gives rise to the facial and acoustic nerves.[1] As the facial and acoustic portions differentiate, the otic placode invaginates, forming the otocyst, a precursor to the eventual membranous labyrinth of the inner ear. Anlagen of the geniculate ganglion appears early in the second month of gestation. Adjacent to the geniculate ganglion, the distal segment of the acousticofacial primordium differentiates into caudal and rostral trunks, which represent the eventual main trunk of the facial nerve and chorda tympani nerve, respectively. The complex, tortuous course of the facial nerve and chorda tympani is explained by their separate origin and subsequent intersection.[2] During the sixth week of gestation, the motor division of the facial nerve establishes its position in the middle ear between the membranous labyrinth (an otic placode structure) and the developing stapes (a second arch structure). During this time, the chorda tympani nerve becomes associated with the trigeminal nerve, which carries the chorda tympani on its way to the tongue via the lingual nerve. The greater superficial petrosal nerve, which carries preganglionic parasympathetic fibers toward the pterygopalatine ganglion, also develops during this time period.[3]

Anatomic relationships of the facial nerve are established by the end of the second month; when the cartilaginous otic capsule forms around the membranous labyrinth, while the facial nerve travels in a sulcus within the cartilaginous capsule. The otic capsule begins to ossify at the end of the fourth month, while the fallopian canal, the bony canal that transmits the facial nerve through the temporal bone, begins ossification in the fifth gestational month, in a process that is not complete until several years after birth.[3-5] Formation of the fallopian canal occurs when two periosteal shelves of bone surround the facial nerve. Fusion of the shelves occurs in an anterior to posterior direction, concluding postpartum in the region of the oval window.[6] Incomplete development of the fallopian canal in this model represents normal anatomic variation, rather than a congenital anomaly. These natural dehiscences may contribute to facial palsies associated with otitis media or barotrauma, while also placing the facial nerve at risk during middle ear surgery.[7-9]

Extratemporal Development

During the sixth gestational week through the end of the second gestational month, all five divisions of the

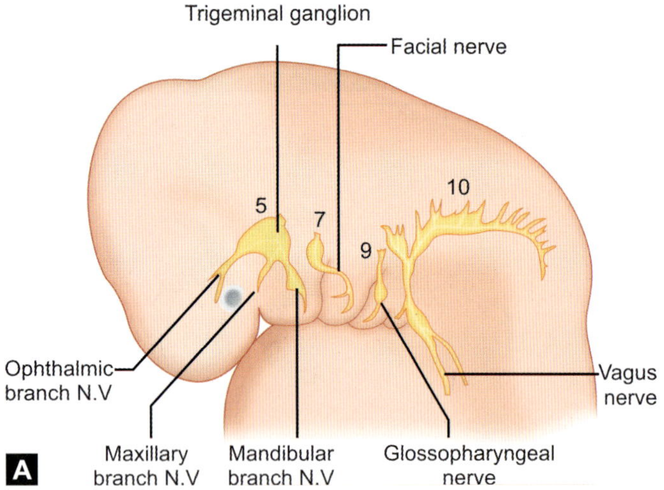

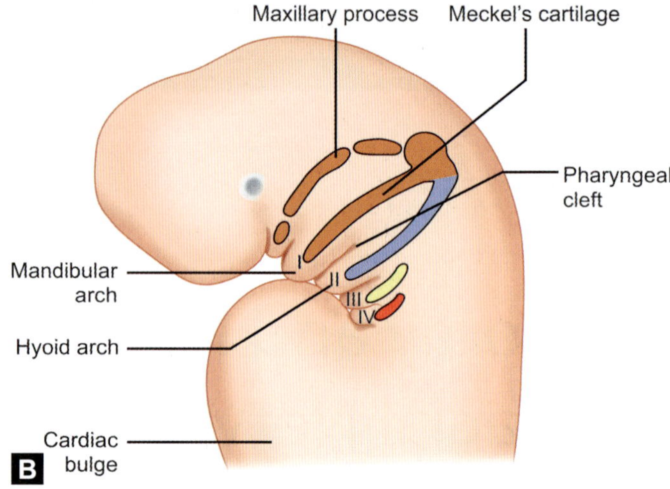

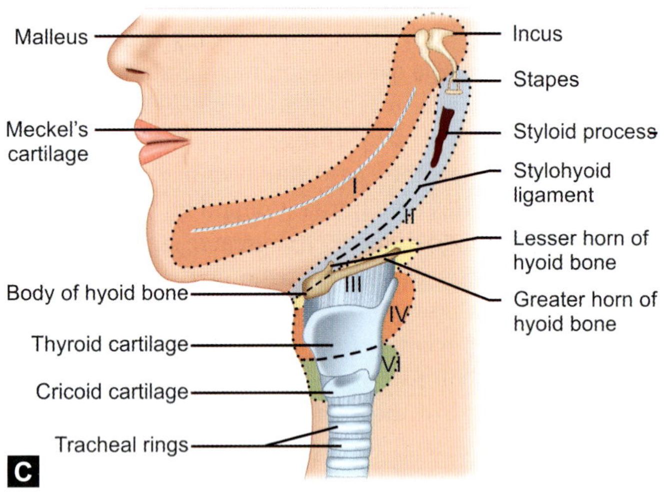

Figs. 36.1A to C: A schematic illustration demonstrating the embryology of the facial nerve. (A) The location of the facial nerve in the developing embryo is shown in relation to the other important nerves in the head and neck. The trigeminal nerve (5) supplies the first pharyngeal arch and has three branches: the ophthalmic, maxillary, and mandibular. The nerve of the second arch is the facial nerve (7); that of the third is the glossopharyngeal nerve (9). The musculature of the fourth arch is supplied by the superior laryngeal branch of the vagus nerve (10), and that of the sixth arch by the recurrent branch of the vagus nerve. (B) The location of the second branchial arch, giving rise to the main trunk of the facial nerve, is shown in relation to the other branchial arches. (C) Other derivatives of the second branchial arch are shown, which help explain the complex innervation pattern of the facial nerve. Labels I-V represent the first through fifth branchial arch derivatives, respectively.
Source: Adapted with permission from Sadler TW. Langman's Medical Embryology, fifth edition. Baltimore: Lippincott, Williams and Wilkins; 2006.

extratemporal nerve—the temporal, zygomatic, buccal, mandibular, and cervical branches—are present. With time, interconnections develop between peripheral branches of the facial nerve, while communications also develop between extratemporal facial nerve branches and branches of the cervical plexus and trigeminal nerve.[10,11]

During the third month, the parotid bud enlarges and engulfs the facial nerve.[10] Gland ductules grow between the developing nerve branches, resulting in myriad connections between the superficial and deep portions of the gland, without any discrete capsule separating these two aspects. The facial muscles (Fig. 36.2), developing independently, are formed at 7–8 weeks' gestation and must be innervated by the distal facial nerve branches or else the muscle will degenerate, although this critical time period before degeneration is not currently known. By the end of the third gestational month, a majority of the facial musculature is identifiable and functional.[5]

Postnatal Development

At birth, the facial nerve is located just beneath the skin near the mastoid tip as it emerges from the temporal bone, and is vulnerable to the postauricular incision in a young child. As the mastoid tip forms and elongates during childhood however, the facial nerve assumes its more medial and protected position. Individual axons of the facial nerve also undergo myelination until the age of 4 years, an important consideration during electrical testing of the nerve during this time period.[12]

CENTRAL NEURONAL PATHWAYS

Supranuclear Pathways

The primary somatomotor cortex of the facial nerve, controlling the complex motor function of the face, is located in the precentral gyrus, corresponding to Brodmann areas

Table 36.1: Facial nerve development

Gestational month	*Development*
1	Acousticofacial (AF) primordium gives rise to both the facial and acoustic nerves
2	Geniculate ganglion develops Caudal trunk of AF primordium develops into main trunk of facial nerve (FN) Rostral trunk of AF primordium develops into chorda tympani nerve Motor division of FN establishes position between labyrinth and stapes Chorda tympani nerve becomes associated with trigeminal nerve Greater superficial petrosal nerve develops Five extratemporal branches develop Facial muscles develop independently
3	FN elongates Fallopian canal develops, continuing through birth Parotid bud engulfs extratemporal FN Facial musculature is identifiable and functional
4-Birth	FN elongates Fallopian canal continues to develop
Postnatal	FN axon myelination, continuing through age 4 years Lateral location of extratemporal FN gradually medializes under developing mastoid tip

4, 6, and 8 (Fig. 36.3). Neural projections from this area making up the corticobulbar tract descend through the internal capsule and then through the pyramidal tracts within the basal pons. In the caudal pons, most of the facial nerve fibers cross the midbrain to reach the contralateral facial nucleus. A small number of facial nerve fibers innervate the ipsilateral facial nucleus, a majority of which are destined for the temporal branch of the nerve.[13] This innervation pattern explains why central nervous system lesions spare the forehead muscle, since they receive input from both cerebral cortices, whereas peripheral lesions involve all branches of the facial nerve.[14-17] More recent somatotopic primate studies suggest an alternate explanation: upper facial motor neurons receive little direct cortical input, while lower facial muscles depend heavily on cortical innervation. Thus, the forehead-sparing aspect of cortical lesions may in fact be explained by this regions relatively lower dependence on cortical innervation.[18]

In addition to these voluntary neural projections to the facial nerve, there is also an extrapyramidal cortical input to the facial nucleus from the hypothalamus, the globus pallidus, and the frontal lobe, all of which control involuntary facial expression associated with emotion. Additional projections to the facial nuclei from the visual system are involved in the blink reflex. Projections from the trigeminal nerve and nuclei contribute to the corneal reflex, whereas those from the auditory nuclei help the eye close involuntarily in response to loud noises.

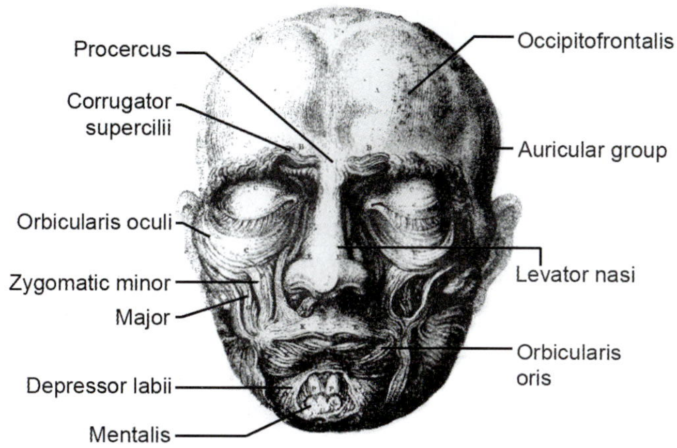

Fig. 36.2: An adaptation of Sir Charles Bell's classic illustration of the muscles of facial expression, with the muscles labeled. *Source*: Reproduced from Bell C. Essays on the Anatomy of Facial Expression, 2nd edition. London: Murray; 1824.

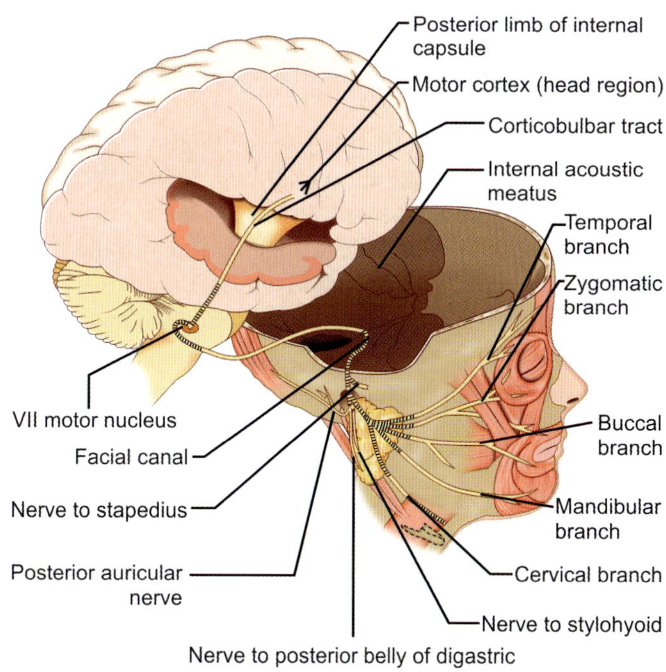

Fig. 36.3: A schematic illustration of the complete pathway of the motor division of the facial nerve.
Source: Redrawn with permission from Sadler TW. Langman's Medical Embryology, 12th ed. Baltimore: Lippincott Williams & Wilkins; 2012.

Facial Nucleus and Brainstem

The efferent projections from the facial motor nucleus emerge dorsomedially to form a compact bundle that loops over the caudal end of the abducens nucleus beneath the facial colliculus or internal genu (or turn). The neurons then pass between the facial nerve nucleus and the trigeminal spinal nucleus, emerging from the brainstem at the pontomedullary junction (Fig. 36.4).

Nervus Intermedius

The nervus intermedius, or Wrisberg's nerve, mediates taste, cutaneous sensation of the external ear, proprioception, lacrimation, and salivation. The nervus intermedius exits the brainstem adjacent to the motor branch of the facial nerve (Table 36.2 and Fig. 36.5). The nerve commonly clings to the adjacent cochleovestibular nerve complex rather than the facial nerve and crosses back to the seventh nerve as it approaches the internal auditory meatus.[19]

General visceral efferent fibers of the nervus intermedius are preganglionic parasympathetic neurons that innervate the lacrimal, submandibular, sublingual, and minor salivary glands. The cell bodies of these nerves arise in the superior salivatory nucleus and join the facial nerve after it has passed the abducens nucleus. They travel together until reaching the geniculate ganglion in the temporal bone. At this point, the greater superficial petrosal nerve branches off, composed of neurons destined for the pterygopalatine ganglion. The greater superficial petrosal nerve ultimately innervates the lacrimal, minor salivary, and mucosal glands of the palate and nose. Remaining fibers form part of the chorda tympani nerve, proceed to the submandibular ganglion, and eventually proceed to the submandibular and sublingual salivary glands.

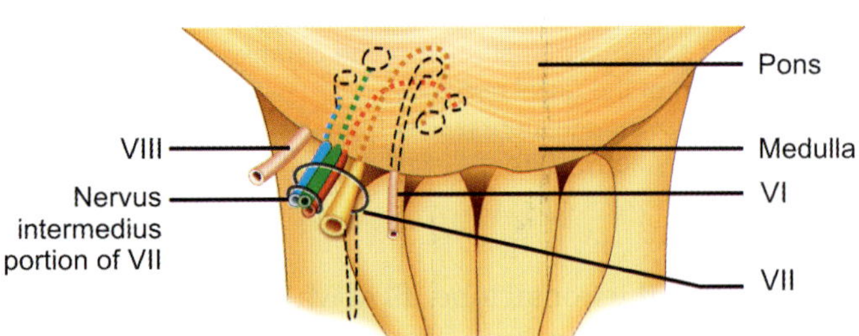

Fig. 36.4: The anatomy of the facial nerve (CN VII) and cochleovestibular nerve (CN VII) as they exit the brainstem at the level of the pontomedullary junction.
Source: Redrawn with permission from Sadler TW. Langman's Medical Embryology, 12th ed. Baltimore: Lippincott Williams & Wilkins; 2012.

The special visceral afferent fibers, which also form a portion of the chorda tympani nerve, receive input from the taste buds of the anterior two-thirds of the tongue, as

Table 36.2: Subdivisions and functions of the facial nerve

Facial nerve subdivision	*Function*
Branchial motor	Muscles of facial expression Posterior belly of the digastric muscle Stylohyoid muscle Stapedius muscle
Visceral motor	Salivation—lacrimal, submandibular, and sublingual glands Nasal mucosa or mucous membrane
General sensory	Sensory to auricular concha External auditory canal Tympanic membrane
Special sensory	Chorda tympani nerve—taste to anterior two-thirds of tongue

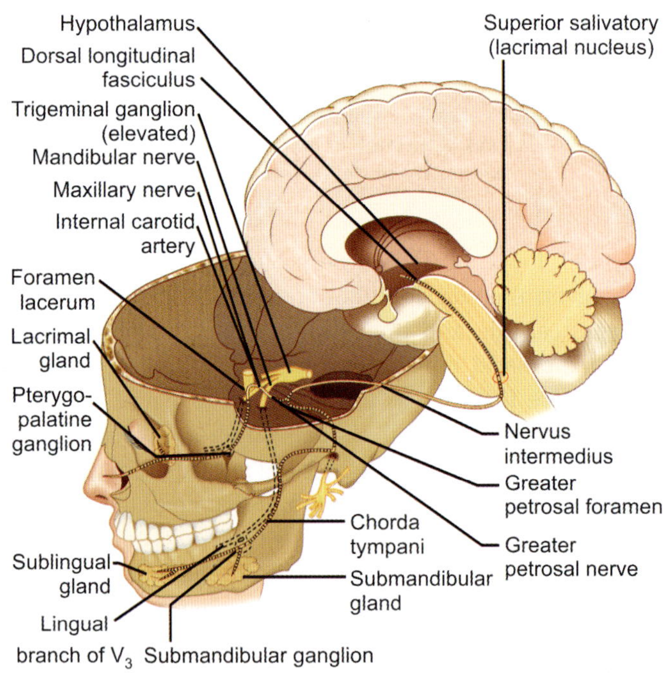

Fig. 36.5: The anatomy of the visceral motor portion of the facial nerve, making up the *nervus intermedius*, or nerve of Wrisberg. The preganglionic, parasympathetic portions of this nerve have cell bodies located in the abducens nucleus. From there they travel toward the geniculate ganglion in the temporal bone, located at the first genu of the facial nerve on the floor of the middle cranial fossa. Fibers from this nerve are destined to innervate the lacrimal gland, minor salivary glands, and mucosal glands of the palate and nose.
Source: Redrawn with permission from Sadler TW. Langman's Medical Embryology, 12th ed. Baltimore: Lippincott Williams & Wilkins; 2012.

well as the hard and soft palates (Fig. 36.6). The sensory afferents for taste have their cell bodies in the geniculate ganglion and will eventually synapse in the medulla, in the nucleus solitarius.

The general sensory afferent neurons of the nervus intermedius are responsible for cutaneous sensory information from the external ear canal and postauricular region. These cutaneous sensory fibers enter the spinal trigeminal tracts without synapsing in the geniculate ganglion.

Cerebellopontine Angle

The facial nerve leaves the brainstem at the pontomedullary junction, where it lies in close approximation to the vestibulocochlear nerve (*see* Fig. 36.4). This intimate relationship takes on critical importance when lesions arise in the region of the cerebellopontine angle (CPA), a common location for central nervous system tumors. In this location, the facial nerve is placed in jeopardy both during the growth of the tumor and during attempted surgical resection in this area. During its lateral course through the CPA and internal auditory canal (IAC), the relative positions of the facial and cochleovestibular nerves change by rotating 90°.[20] In the CPA, the facial nerve is covered with pia, is bathed in cerebrospinal fluid, and is devoid of epineurium, leaving it susceptible to manipulation trauma during intracranial surgery.

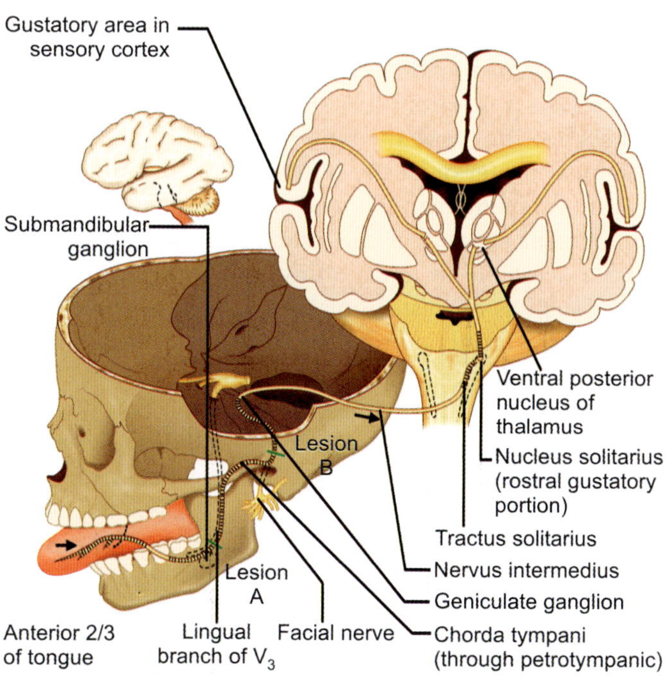

Fig. 36.6: The anatomy of the special sensory component of the facial nerve, comprising the chorda tympani nerve.
Source: Redrawn with permission from Sadler TW. Langman's Medical Embryology, 12th ed. Baltimore: Lippincott Williams & Wilkins; 2012.

Lesions involving the CPA commonly include vestibular schwannomas, meningiomas, and primary cholesteatomas. Larger lesions can cause compression of the CPA that leads to deficits affecting more than just the vestibulocochlear nerve, involving the fifth, then ninth, tenth, and eleventh cranial nerves. Also of note, the presence of coursing arteries in proximity to the facial nerve at the CPA has been implicated as one cause of hemifacial spasm; treatment with microvascular decompression at the facial nerve root is a well described.[21]

INTRATEMPORAL NERVE PATHWAYS

After traversing the CPA, the facial nerve enters the temporal bone along the posterior face of the petrous bone. Within the temporal bone, the facial nerve successively passes through four regions before its exit out of the stylomastoid foramen: (1) the IAC, (2) the labyrinthine segment, (3) the intratympanic segment, and (4) the descending segment (Figs. 36.7 to 36.9). From the lateral end of the IAC to its exit out the stylomastoid foramen, the nerve travels approximately 3 cm within the fallopian canal.

Internal Auditory Canal

The facial nerve enters the temporal bone along the posterior face of the petrous bone, piercing the internal auditory meatus. At the lateral end of the IAC, the traverse crest divides the IAC into superior and inferior portions. The superior portion is in turn further divided by the smaller and more laterally located vertical crest or "Bill's bar". At this lateral portion of the IAC, the anatomy is most consistent: The superior portion is occupied by the facial nerve anteriorly and the superior vestibular nerve posteriorly (Fig. 36.8). Within the IAC, the dural covering of the facial nerve transitions to epineurium.

Labyrinthine Segment

At the lateral portion of the IAC, the facial nerve pierces the meatal foramen to enter the labyrinthine segment. This portion of the nerve runs beneath the middle cranial fossa, passing posterior to the cochlea and anterior and medial to the ampulated ends of the horizontal and superior semicircular canals. The distance between the facial nerve and basal turn of the cochlea that is less than the standard size of the smallest diamond drills (0.6 mm) in

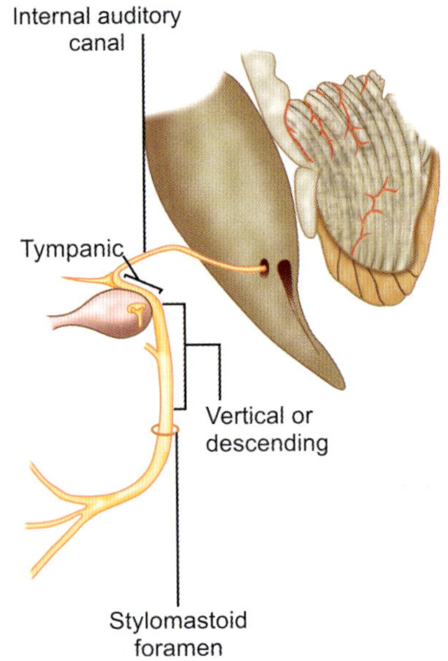

Fig. 36.7: The intratemporal divisions of the facial nerve. After passing through the internal auditory meatus on the posterior face of the petrous temporal bone, the nerve enters its canalicular segment, as it traverses between the cochlea and the vestibular labyrinth. After making its first genu (bend) at the genicular ganglion, it becomes the tympanic segment, coursing through the middle ear space, just superior to the oval window. It then makes its second major genu at the level of the horizontal semicircular canal, and becomes the vertical or descending segment. After passing through the stylomastoid foramen, it becomes extracranial.

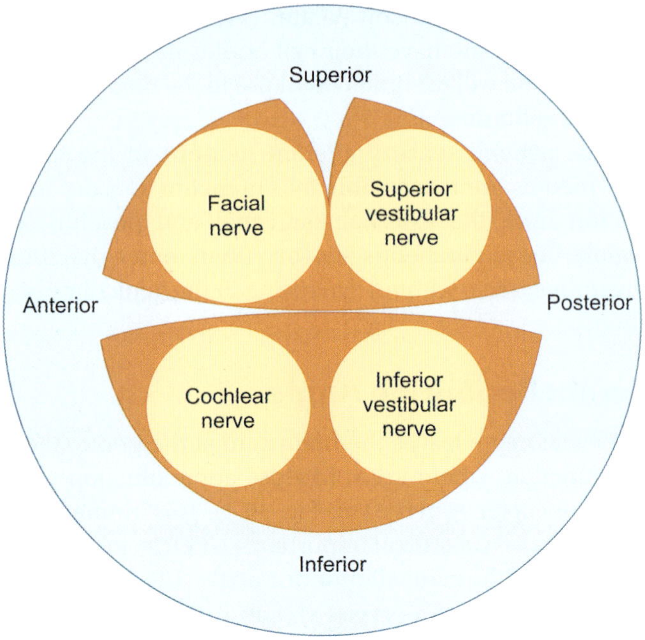

Fig. 36.8: A stylized representation of the lateral aspect of the internal auditory canal. The facial nerve lies at the most anterior and superior location at this level.

the vast majority of patients, underscoring the importance of meticulous dissection of the facial nerve during middle cranial fossa approaches.[22]The geniculate ganglion is considered the end of the labyrinthine segment of the nerve and lies just superior to the nerve. Arising from the geniculate ganglion is the greater superficial petrosal nerve, containing preganglionic parasympathetic fibers destined for the lacrimal gland, as well as for the nasal and palatine mucosal glands. The nerve also contains some minor taste neurons that supply the posterior palate.

The labyrinthine segment is further notable in that it is the narrowest portion of the fallopian canal, where it averages < 0.7 mm in diameter, occupies the canal to the greatest proportional extent, and is lined by a fibrous annular ligament.[23] As a result, it is believed that infections or inflammations causing edema of the facial nerve within this region can lead to temporary or permanent paralysis of the nerve, such as in Bell palsy.

Tympanic Segment

At the geniculate ganglion, the facial nerve makes its first genu and becomes the tympanic segment of the facial nerve, so called because it travels within the middle ear space. This portion of the nerve is approximately10 mm long. Landmarks for the nerve at this location include the cochleariform process, which gives rise to the tensor tympani muscle, and the "cog", a small bony prominence projecting from the roof of the epitympanum. The facial nerve then travels posteriorly, just superior to the oval window and stapes. The nerve then curves inferiorly at its second genu, just posterior to the oval window, pyramidal process, and stapedial tendon, and anterior to the horizontal semicircular canal. It is this portion of the nerve that is most susceptible to injury during surgery because processes such as cholesteatoma frequently erode the bone covering the facial nerve in this region, leaving it precariously exposed.

In addition to bony dehiscence from pathology, natural fallopian canal dehiscences have also been described in cadaver specimens, a majority of which occurred in the tympanic segment. In more than 80% of cases, the dehiscences involved the portions of the canal adjacent to the oval window.[24]

Vertical, Descending, or Mastoid Segment

After the second genu, the nerve traverses the synonymously named vertical, descending, or mastoid segment

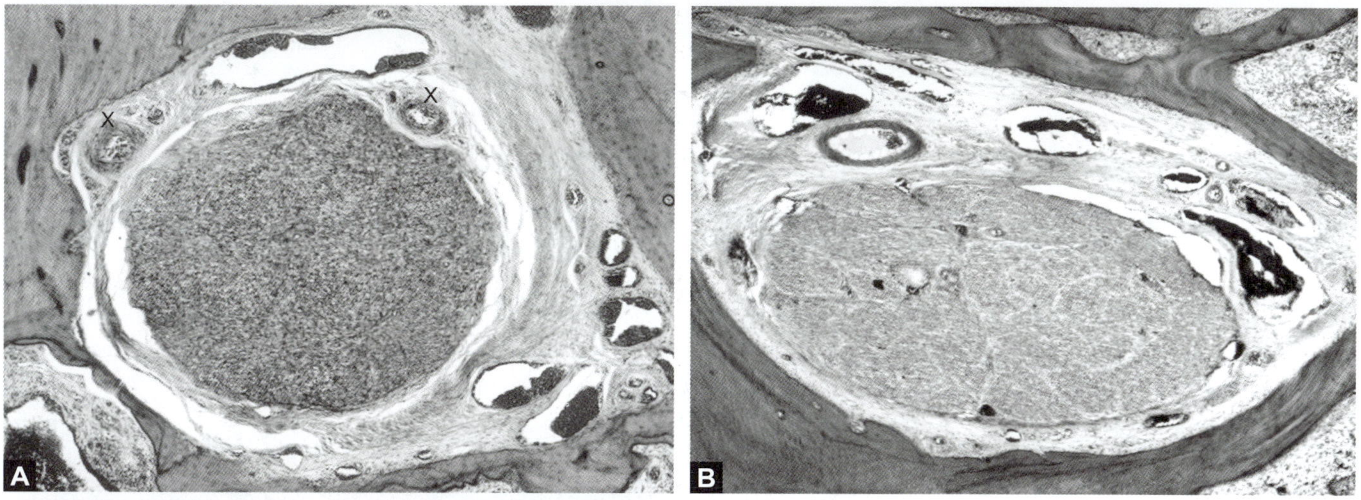

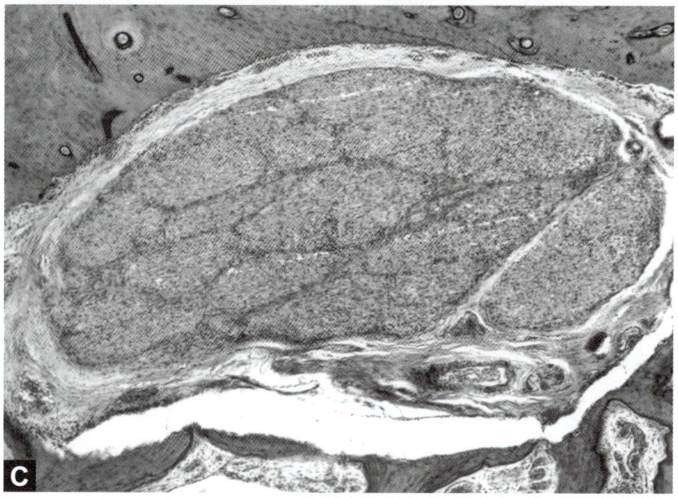

Figs. 36.9A to C: Histologic cross sections of the facial nerve at three points along its course within the temporal bone. Proximally within the temporal bone at the level of the internal auditory canal (A), the individual nerve fascicles are not defined, and nerve elements appear homogeneous. (B) As the nerve proceeds through the tympanic segment and (C) at the level of the stylomastoid foramen, individual nerve fascicles become increasingly defined.

en route to the stylomastoid foramen. As the facial nerve descends inferiorly in this portion, it gradually assumes a more lateral position. Important branches of the nerve in this segment include the nerve to the stapedius muscle and the chorda tympani nerve. As it arises from the facial nerve, the chorda tympani nerve makes an approximately 30° angle and delineates a triangular space known as the "facial recess", an important surgical route of entry into the middle ear space.

In its most inferior portion, the facial nerve takes on a close proximity to the digastric ridge and muscle, where the nerve is consistently medial and anterior to these structures. On exiting the stylomastoid foramen, the nerve becomes encased in the thick fibrous tissue of the cranial base periosteum and digastric muscle.

Although the facial nerve most commonly descends in its vertical segment as a single nerve, bifurcations, trifurcations, and hypoplasia of the facial nerve have been found within the mastoid segment.[7] In addition, the chorda tympani nerve has been noted to arise from the facial nerve anywhere from the stylomastoid foramen to the geniculate ganglion.[25]

Peripheral Facial Nerve Anatomy

The facial nerve exits the skull base through the stylomastoid foramen, between the mastoid tip laterally and the styloid process medially (Fig. 36.10). At the stylomastoid foramen, the facial nerve passes into the parotid gland, typically as a single large trunk. The nerve then divides within the parotid gland into its temporofacial and cervicofacial branches. Rarely, this division can occur within the temporal bone and exit the stylomastoid foramen as separate branches.

Within the parotid gland, the nerve can assume numerous configurations, with frequent anastomoses between branches. However, generally five main branches of the nerve can be identified: (1) the temporal, (2) the zygomatic,

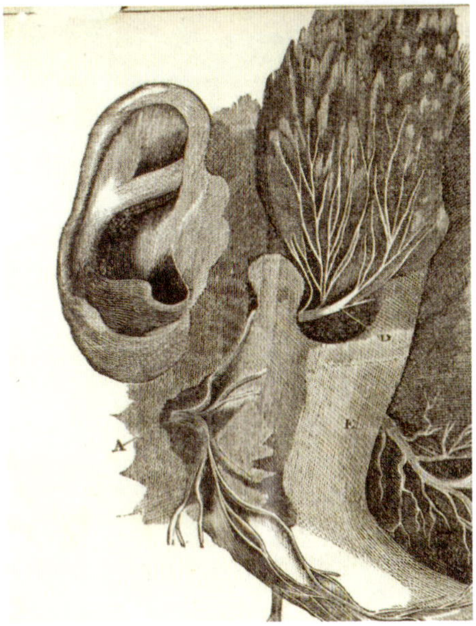

Fig. 36.10: A portion of an illustration from Sir Charles Bell, demonstrating the exit of the facial nerve from the stylomastoid foramen. *Source*: Reproduced from Bell C. The Nervous System of the Human Body. Longman; 1830.

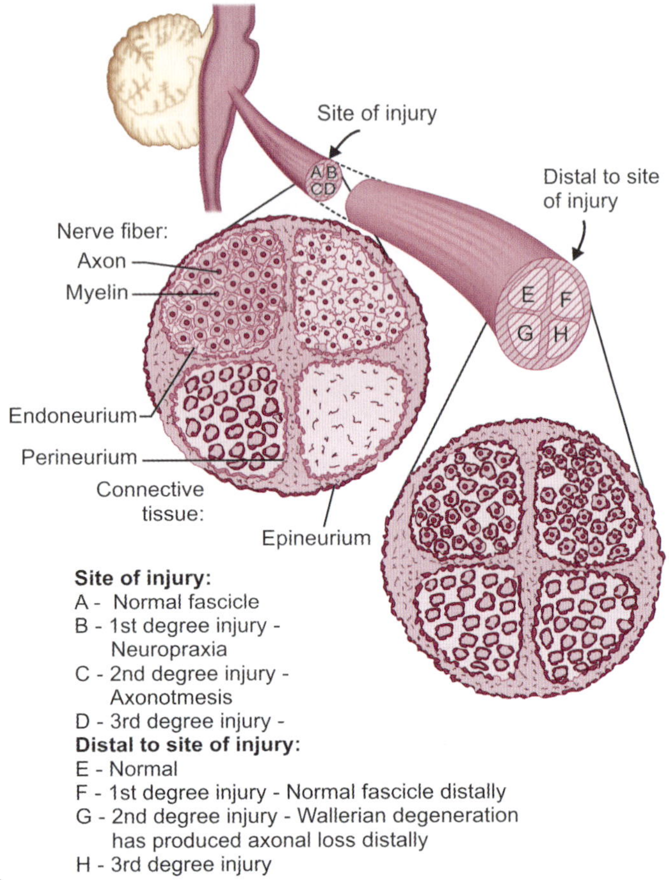

Fig. 36.11: A model of graded neural injury that details clinical–pathologic classifications. Microanatomic changes in cranial nerve injury are demonstrated in cross section. The potential for approximate axonal regeneration across the site of injury is dictated principally by the status of connective tissue elements.

(3) the buccal, (4) the mandibular, and (5) the cervical. The temporal branch innervates the frontalis muscle, which allows for the voluntary raising of eyebrows. The zygomatic branch innervates the orbicularis oculi muscle and is critical for proper eye closure. The buccal nerve innervates the buccinator and orbicularis oris, allowing for proper mouth closure and cheek muscle activity. The mandibular branch innerves the platysma. The posterior auricular nerve, arising just after the exit of the facial nerve from the stylomastoid foramen, sends branches to the occipitalis muscle posteriorly on the skull.

FACIAL NERVE PHYSIOLOGY

Anatomic Considerations

The facial nerve trunk consists of approximately 10,000 nerve fibers, approximately 7000 of which are myelinated motor fibers. The facial nerve sheath consists of several layers. The endoneurium, closely adherent to the layer of Schwann cells of the axons, surrounds each nerve fiber. The perineurium, which is the intermediate layer surrounding groups of fascicles, provides tensile strength to the nerve and is believed to represent the primary barrier to the spread of infection. The outermost layer of the nerve is the epineurium. This outer layer contains the vasa nervorum, which provides the blood supply to the nerve.

Classification of Facial Nerve Degeneration

If the facial nerve is injured, various degrees of injury may result.[26] The most widely used model of clinicopathologic classification of nerve injury is the classification originally proposed by Sunderland (Fig. 36.11):

1. First-degree injuries are characterized by *compression* causing the blockage of axoplasmic flow (neuropraxia). There are no morphologic changes. Although an action potential cannot be propagated across the lesion site, a stimulus applied distal to the lesion will conduct normally to produce an evoked response. Complete recovery is expected.
2. Second-degree injuries entail axonal and myelin disruption distal to the injury site as a result of the progression of a first-degree injury (axonotmesis). *Wallerian*

degeneration occurs distal to the site of injury, which eliminates the propagation of an externally applied stimulus. Axon regeneration occurs at 1 mm per day; near complete recovery is expected, except in fibers that suffer progression to third degree injury.

3. Third-degree injuries involve complete disruption of the endoneurial tube, including the axon plus its surrounding myelin and endoneurium (neurotmesis). Axonal regrowth may occur, but is susceptible to synkinesis, the contraction of multiple muscle fibers simultaneously with voluntary movement, e.g. mouth movement with eye closure.
4. Fourth-degree injuries entail the disruption of the perineurium (partial transection). Profound long-term weakness is expected.
5. Fifth-degree injuries entail the disruption of the epineurium (complete transection). No recovery is expected without intervention.
6. Sixth-degree injuries, a proposed addition to the Sunderland classification by later authors, take into account the observed patterns of blunt and penetrating injuries of the nerve. These injuries are characterized by normal function through some fascicles and varying degrees of injury (first-degree through fifth-degree injuries), differentially involving fascicles across the nerve trunk.

Central to the Sunderland classification is the notion that axonal recovery depends on the integrity of the connective tissue elements of the nerve trunk. This model predicts a high likelihood for the complete recovery of peripheral innervation when endoneurial tubules remain intact to support reinnervation, as is the case with first- and second-degree injuries. In contrast, disruption of the endoneurium—a third-degree injury or worse in this model—increases the likelihood of irreversible axonal injury and aberrant patterns of regeneration.

An example of abnormal neural regrowth is "crocodile tears", or increased lacrimation associated with eating. It occurs when efferent fibers normally targeted to travel with the chorda tympani nerve to the submandibular and sublingual glands are misdirected through the greater superficial petrosal nerve to the lacrimal gland. This results in parasympathetic innervation of the lacrimal gland as well as the normal target, the salivary glands.

REFERENCES

1. Vidic B. The anatomy and development of the facial nerve. Ear Nose Throat J. 1978;57(6):236-42.
2. Gasser RF, May M. Embryonic development of the facial nerve. M M, editor. New York: Thieme Straton; 1987.
3. Vidic B, Wozniak W. The communicating branch of the facial nerve to the lesser petrosal nerve in human fetuses and newborns. Arch Anat Histol Embryol. 1969;52:369-70.
4. Gasser R. The development of the facial nerve in man. Ann Otol Rhinol Laryngol. 1967;76:37-56.
5. Gassser, RF. The development of the facial nerve muscles in man. The American journal of anatomy. 1967;120:357-76.
6. Spector JG, Ge X. Ossification patterns of the tympanic facial canal in the human fetus and neonate. Laryngoscope. 1993;103(9):1052-65.
7. Nager GT, Proctor B. Anatomic variations and anomalies involving the facial canal. Otolaryngol Clin North Am. 1991;24(3):531-53.
8. Nager GT, Proctor B. The facial canal: normal anatomy, variations and anomalies. II. Anatomical variations and anomalies involving the facial canal. Ann Otol Rhinol Laryngol Suppl. 1982;97:45-61.
9. Antonelli PJ, Parell GJ, Becker GD, et al. Temporal bone pathology in scuba diving deaths. Otolaryngol Head Neck Surg. 1993;109(3 Pt 1):514-21.
10. Gasser RF. The early development of the parotid gland around the facial nerve and its branches in man. Anat Rec. 1970;167(1):63-77.
11. Gasser RF, Shigihara S, Shimada K. Three-dimensional development of the facial nerve path through the ear region in human embryos. Ann Otol Rhinol Laryngol. 1994; 103(5 Pt 1):395-403.
12. Waylonis GW, Johnson EW. Facial nerve conduction delay. Arch Phys Med Rehabil. 1964;45:539-47.
13. Crosby EC, Dejonge BR. Experimental and clinical studies of the central connections and central relations of the facial nerve. Ann Otol Rhinol Laryngol. 1963;72:735-55.
14. Radpour S. Organization of the facial nerve nucleus in the cat. In: Fisch U (ed.) Facial Nerve Surgery. Birminghan: Aesculapius Publishing; 1977. pp. 71-81.
15. Radpour S, Gacek RR. Facial nerve nucleus in the cat. Further study. Laryngoscope. 1980;90(4):685-92.
16. Radpour S, Gacek RR. Anatomic organization of the cat facial nerve. Otolaryngol Head Neck Surg. 1985;93(5): 591-6.
17. Nelson JR. Facial paralysis of central nervous system origin. Otolaryngol Clin North Am. 1974;7(2):411-24.
18. Jenny AB, Saper CB. Organization of the facial nucleus and corticofacial projection in the monkey: a reconsideration of the upper motor neuron facial palsy. Neurology. 1987;37(6):930-9.
19. Rhoton AL, Jr., Kobayashi S, Hollinshead WH. Nervus intermedius. J Neurosurg. 1968;29(6):609-18.
20. Silverstein H, Norrell H, Smouha EE. Retrosigmoid-internal auditory canal approach vs. retrolabyrinthine approach for vestibular neurectomy. Otolaryngol Head Neck Surg. 1987; 97(3):300-7.
21. McLaughlin MR, Jannetta PJ, Clyde BL, et al. Microvascular decompression of cranial nerves: lessons learned after 4400 operations. J Neurosurg. 1999;90(1):1-8.

22. Redleaf MI, Blough RR. Distance from the labyrinthine portion of the facial nerve to the basal turn of the cochlea. Temporal bone histopathologic study. Ann Otol Rhinol Laryngol. 1996;105(4):323-6.
23. Fisch U, Esslen E. Total intratemporal exposure of the facial nerve. Pathologic findings in Bell's palsy. Arch Otolaryngol. 1972;95(4):335-41.
24. Baxter A. Dehiscence of the Fallopian canal. An anatomical study. J Laryngol Otol. 1971;85(6):587-94.
25. Fowler EP, Jr. Variations in the temporal bone course of the facial nerve. Laryngoscope. 1961;71:937-46.
26. Sunderland S. Anatomical features of nerve trunks in relation to nerve injury and nerve repair. Clin Neurosurg. 1970; 17:38-62.

CHAPTER

37

Facial Nerve Testing

Sachin Gupta, Brandon Isaacson

FACIAL NERVE DEVELOPMENT AND ANATOMY

The facial nerve is a complex nerve composed of motor, sensory, and parasympathetic fibers that develop at 3 weeks of gestation. Complete separation of the facial and acoustic nerves occurs at 5–6 weeks, at which time the nervus intermedius also develops. At 8 weeks, the fallopian canal begins to develop and by the 16th week, the neural connections are completely developed. The fallopian canal continues to develop after the 16th week until birth, enclosing the facial nerve in bone throughout its course except at the facial hiatus in the floor of the middle cranial fossa.[1] Dehiscence of the fallopian canal is most commonly seen adjacent to the oval window, at a reported rate of 25–55%.[2] At birth, the facial nerve's anatomy is similar to that of an adult, except in the region of the stylomastoid foramen. This area continues to develop after birth as the mastoid tip develops.

Motor fibers originate from cell bodies located in the precentral and postcentral gyri of the frontal motor cortex. These fibers travel in the posterior limb of the internal capsule inferiorly to the caudal pons. There, the motor fibers supplying the facial musculature beneath the brows cross the midline to reach the contralateral motor nucleus in the reticular formation of the lower pons anterior to the fourth ventricle. The majority of motor fibers that supply the musculature of the forehead also cross the midline; however, a few fibers do not, instead traversing in the ipsilateral motor nucleus. Thus, muscles of the forehead receive innervation from both sides of the motor cortex, and so forehead-sparing facial paralysis raises suspicion of a central etiology. The motor fibers then pass dorsally, loop in a medial-to-lateral manner around the abducens nucleus, and create a bulge in the floor of the fourth ventricle (the facial colliculus). This loop of the facial nerve forms the internal genu of the facial nerve.[3-4]

The nervus intermedius contains sensory, special sensory, and parasympathetic fibers. The nervus intermedius provides sensation to the posterior concha and external auditory canal. The nervus intermedius special sensory fibers supply taste sensation to the anterior two-thirds of the tongue. Afferent sensory fibers synapse with cell bodies in the geniculate ganglion at the first genu of the facial nerve. These sensory afferents then join the parasympathetic fibers, passing via the nervus intermedius to the nucleus tractus solitarius in the medulla. The parasympathetic portion of the nervus intermedius originates in the superior salivatory nucleus in the dorsal pons and innervates the lacrimal, submandibular, sublingual, and minor salivary glands.

Both the motor root of the facial nerve and the nervus intermedius leave the brainstem near the dorsal pons at the pontomedullary junction (the cisternal segment of the facial nerve). Within the cerebellopontine angle (CPA), the nerve travels anterolaterally into the porus acusticus of the internal auditory canal (IAC), anterior to the vestibulocochlear nerve. The cisternal segment is typically 24 mm in length.[5] The nervus intermedius either integrates with the facial nerve as they emerge from the brainstem or joins near the meatus of the IAC.[6] The facial nerve runs in the anterosuperior quadrant of the IAC. This intracanalicular segment of the facial nerve is approximately 8 mm in length. At the lateral end of the meatus, a horizontal segment of bone (the transverse or falciform crest) separates the facial nerve from the cochlear nerve that lies inferiorly. Vertically, a segment of bone (Bill's bar) separates the facial nerve from the superior vestibular nerve (which lies posteriorly).

The fallopian canal begins as the facial nerve exits the IAC at the fundus. The major blood supply for the facial nerve proximally within the canal is the superficial petrosal artery, a branch of the middle meningeal artery, while the stylomastoid artery supplies the fallopian canal distally.[7-8] The fallopian canal has three segments: labyrinthine, tympanic, and mastoid. The labyrinthine segment runs from the fundus of the IAC to the geniculate ganglion. It is both the narrowest (<0.7 mm diameter) and shortest segment (3–5 mm in length). The labyrinthine segment travels anterolaterally from the IAC, superior to the cochlea up to the geniculate ganglion.

While the geniculate ganglion is typically covered by bone, in up to 18% of cases the ganglion is instead in direct contact with the dura of the middle cranial fossa.[6,9] The first branch of the facial nerve, the greater superficial petrosal nerve (GSPN), exits the anterior aspect of the geniculate ganglion. The GSPN carries preganglionic parasympathetic fibers from the superior salivatory nucleus, and runs along the superior surface of the temporal bone into the pterygoid canal (Vidian canal). It then synapses at the pterygopalatine ganglion in the pterygopalatine fossa. Postganglionic parasympathetic fibers then join the maxillary nerve to innervate the lacrimal gland and minor salivary glands in the nose and palate. At the geniculate ganglion (first or anterior genu), the facial nerve makes a 75° turn posteriorly to become the tympanic segment.

The tympanic segment is 10 mm in length and runs from the geniculate ganglion to the second (or posterior) genu.[10] Within the tympanic cavity, the facial nerve passes medial to the incus. It runs posterosuperior to the cochleariform process, superolateral to the oval window, and then inferior to the lateral semicircular canal. Bony dehiscence of the facial nerve canal is common in this segment 41–74%).[7,8,10] At the pyramidal process, the tympanic segment turns inferiorly at a 95-125° angle to become the mastoid, or vertical, segment.[10]

The mastoid segment of the facial nerve runs from the second genu posteromedial to the external auditory canal to its exit from the temporal bone at the stylomastoid foramen (a course measuring approximately 13 mm).[10] Two branches arise from the mastoid segment: the nerve to the stapedius muscle and the chorda tympani. The stylomastoid foramen arises between the styloid process anteriorly and the mastoid process posteriorly. The nerve exits the temporal bone at the stylomastoid foramen, entering the substance of the parotid gland.

Extratemporally, the facial nerve separates into two main branches at the pes anserinus: the temporofacial branch and the cervicofacial branch. Within the parotid gland, these branches further divide into five main branches that supply the facial musculature: temporal (or frontal), zygomatic, buccal, marginal mandibular, and cervical (Fig. 37.1).

FACIAL NERVE PHYSIOLOGY

As stated previously, the facial nerve is composed of motor, sensory, and parasympathetic fibers. Peripherally, the facial nerve sheath is composed of three layers: endoneurium, perineurium, and epineurium. Endoneurium surrounds each nerve fiber, and is adherent to Schwann cells of the axons. Perineurium is an intermediate layer surrounding fascicles of nerve fibers, providing tensile strength and a barrier to infection. Epineurium is the outermost layer, and contains vasa nervorum. Centrally, the intracranial and intracanalicular segments of the facial nerve lack perineurium and epineurium, making these segments more susceptible to injury.

Sunderland devised a classification that is widely used to describe degrees of nerve injury. First-degree injuries, also known as neuropraxia, are characterized by blockage of axonal flow. Second-degree injuries, also known as axonotmesis, are characterized by disruption of the axon and distal Wallerian degeneration. In both first- and second-degree injuries, the endoneurium is intact and thus there is a high likelihood of complete recovery. Third-degree injuries are characterized by disruption of the endoneurium. Fourth-degree injuries are characterized by disruption of the perineurium. Lastly, fifth-degree injuries are characterized by disruption of the epineurium. In third-, fourth-, and fifth-degree injuries, there is injury to the neural connective tissue and thus a high likelihood of aberrant regeneration.

FACIAL NERVE TESTING

Facial nerve testing provides information about the extent of injury and prognosis for recovery. Early detection of nerve degeneration may permit interventions that can optimize facial nerve recovery. The facial nerve can be affected by a number of disorders resulting in weakness or paralysis of the facial musculature. One of the critical steps

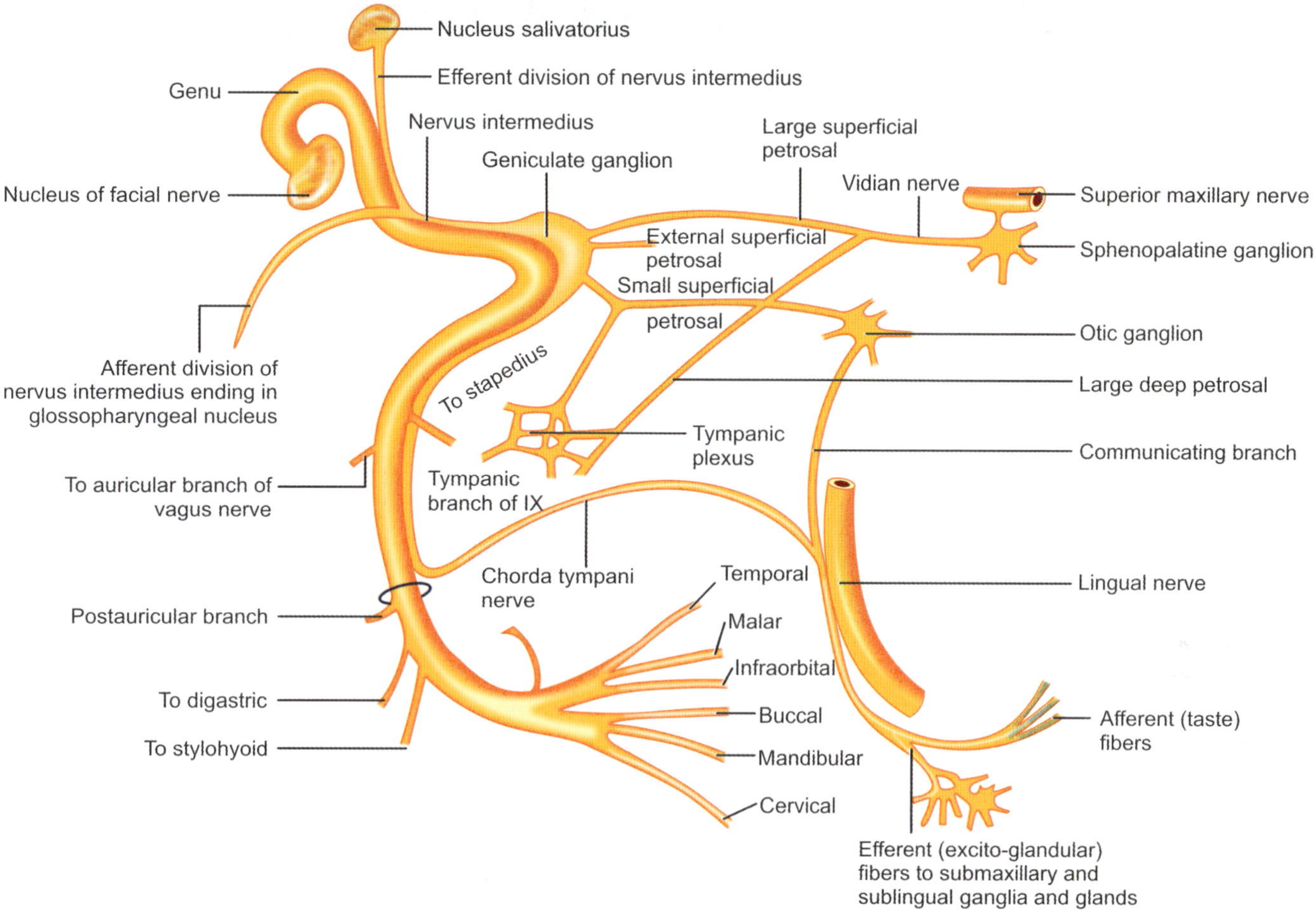

Fig. 37.1: Facial nerve anatomy.
Source: Redrawn from Gray H. Anatomy of the Human Body. Philadelphia: Lea & Febinger; 1918.

in the clinical evaluation of facial paralysis is discerning whether a central nervous system process (e.g. cerebrovascular accident and multiple sclerosis) or peripheral disease (e.g. Bell's palsy and middle ear cholesteatoma) is the cause of the weakness.

TOPOGRAPHIC TESTING

Topographic testing aims to identify the location of facial nerve injury by testing specific branches of the facial nerve (Table 37.1). The Schirmer test assesses lacrimal flow, which depends on the presence of an intact geniculate ganglion, where the GSPN arises. The GSPN supplies autonomic, parasympathetic fibers to the lacrimal gland. The test is performed by administering a topical anesthetic, and placing a piece of filter paper in the lower lid conjunctival fornix. After 5 minutes, normal lacrimal flow should yield at least 5 mm of wet filter paper. Also, the tested side should have at least one-half the amount of lacrimation seen on the healthy side, as shown by Fisch.[11] Decreased lacrimation suggests injury to the GSPN, the geniculate ganglion, or the facial nerve proximal to the geniculate ganglion.

Other topographic testing modalities include stapedial reflex testing, electrogustometry, and salivary secretion testing. Stapedial reflex testing is typically performed during audiological evaluation, and tests the stapedius branch of the facial nerve. This branch arises from the mastoid segment, just distal to the second genu. A loud tone is presented to the ipsilateral or contralateral ear, which results in simulation of the stapedius branch of the facial nerve and contraction of the stapedius muscle. The tension of the tympanic membrane increases, causing a change in the impedance of the ossicular chain. Absence of the stapedial reflex with an intact vestibulocochlear nerve suggests injury to the facial nerve proximal to the stapedius branch.

Electrogustometry is utilized to assess taste, which in the anterior two-thirds of the tongue is dependent on the chorda tympani nerve. A controlled, anode current is

Table 37.1: Topographic tests of the facial nerve

Topographic test	*Facial nerve function tested*	*Facial nerve site tested*
Schirmer test	Lacrimation	Greater superficial petrosal nerve
Stapedial reflex	Stapedius muscle contraction	Stapedius branch of facial nerve
Electrogustometry	Taste	Chorda tympani
Salivary secretion testing	Salivary flow	Chorda tympani

Table 37.2: Electrophysiologic tests of the facial nerve

Electrophysiologic test	*Measure*	*Prognostic significance*
Nerve excitability test	Lowest stimulus that elicits a facial twitch	Threshold difference of 3.5 mA or greater predicts incomplete recovery with 80% accuracy
Maximal stimulation test	Stimulus that elicits maximal facial twitching	Markedly diminished facial contraction (<25% of healthy side) within first 2 weeks of facial paralysis predicts 75% chance of incomplete recovery
Electroneuronography	Compound muscle action potential (CMAP) elicited by a supramaximal stimulus	CMAP<10% of healthy side within first 2–3 weeks of facial paralysis may predict poor recovery, decompression can be considered
Electromyography	Spontaneous and voluntary muscle action potentials	Fibrillation potentials within first 2 weeks of facial paralysis predict incomplete recovery in 81% of patients

passed through the tongue, resulting in the perception of a metallic or sour taste. The lowest thresholds necessary to elicit the change in taste are recorded. Patients with injury to the chorda tympani have increased thresholds on electrogustometry, as has been shown following injury during middle ear surgery.[12,13] Salivary secretion testing is performed by cannulating the submandibular ducts and measuring salivary flow over 5 minutes. A flow rate of 25% or less than that of the normal side is considered significant, indicating an injury to the facial nerve proximal to the chorda tympani.[14]

ELECTROPHYSIOLOGIC TESTING

Electrophysiologic testing is based on the principle that electric stimulation produces an electromyographic response in intact nerve fibers. Testing can help delineate the severity of nerve injury in complete facial paralysis, and is useful for determining prognosis and optimal treatment (Table 37.2). Electrophysiologic testing indirectly evaluates injury to the intratemporal facial nerve, as nerve stimulation is performed in branches of the extratemporal, peripheral facial nerve. Thus, for testing to be valid, degeneration has to progress from the intratemporal to the extratemporal nerve. This process of Wallerian degeneration requires 48–72 hours. Testing performed before Wallerian degeneration has ensued can underestimate the degree of facial nerve injury.

Nerve excitability testing (NET), maximal stimulation testing (MST), electroneuronography (ENoG), and electromyography (EMG) are most commonly utilized. NET was first introduced by Laumans and Jonkees,[15] and is performed by placing a stimulating electrode on the skin over the stylomastoid foramen or a peripheral nerve branch, and a return electrode on the forearm (Figs. 37.2A and B). Electrical pulses are delivered at increasing current levels until a facial twitch is elicited. The healthy side is simulated first, and the lowest current level that elicits a facial twitch is set as the normal threshold. The injured side is then tested, and a 2.0–3.5 mA difference between the sides' thresholds is considered abnormal. A difference of 3.5 mA has been used to predict complete versus incomplete recovery from facial paralysis with 80% accuracy.[15] In terms of absolute threshold values, abnormal thresholds are considered to be ≥1.25 mA in the upper divisions and 2.0 mA in the lower divisions of the extratemporal facial nerve.[16] Advantages of NET are that the equipment is portable and the test itself causes less patient discomfort as compared to other tests. A disadvantage is that the test is subjective, relying on visual detection of facial twitches.

MST measures the stimulus that elicits the greatest amplitude of facial movement. Beginning with the healthy side, facial nerve branches are simulated with increasing current levels until the maximal facial twitch is elicited (Fig. 37.3). This maximal current level is then used to stimulate the injured side, and the degree of facial contraction

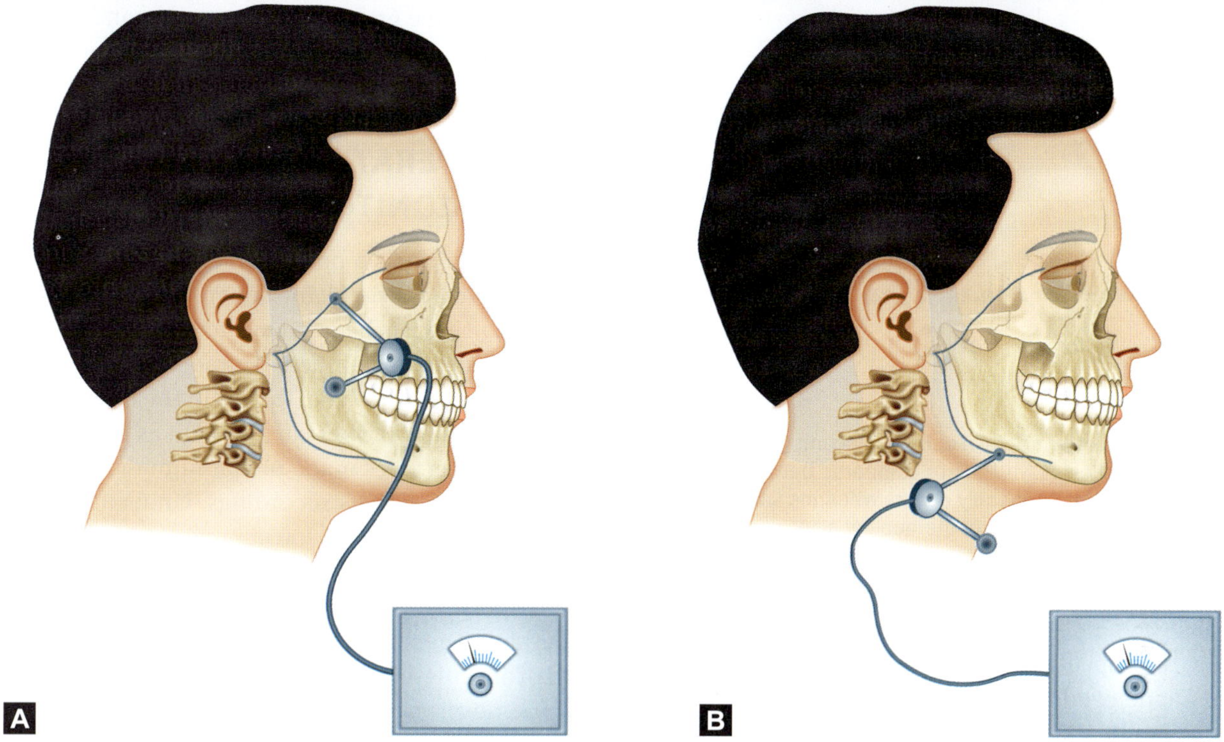

Figs. 37.2A and B: Nerve excitability testing. (A) Electrode placement for testing of upper divisions. (B) Electrode placement for testing of lower divisions. A threshold difference between the two sides of >2.0–3.5 mA is considered abnormal.
Source: Redrawn from Gates GA. Nerve excitability testing: technical pitfalls and threshold norms using absolute values. Laryngoscope. 1993;103:379-85.

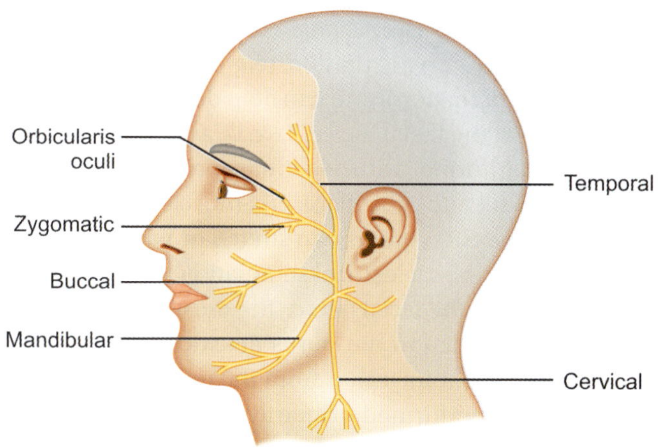

Fig. 37.3: Maximal stimulation testing electrode placement. Facial contraction is expressed as a fraction of the healthy side: equal, minimally diminished (50%), markedly diminished (<25%), or absent.
Source: Redrawn from Jackler R. Neurotology. Philadelphia: Mosby; 2005.

is expressed in relation to the healthy side's contraction as equal, minimally diminished (50%), markedly diminished (<25%), or absent. When MST results are normal in facial paralysis, 88% of patients recover completely.[17] Conversely, when the injured side has markedly diminished function within the first 2 weeks of facial paralysis, it has been shown that there is a 75% chance of incomplete recovery.[18] Like NET, this test is also subjective, relying on visual detection of maximal facial twitches.

ENoG is useful within the first 2–3 weeks of facial paralysis by providing information on prognosis as well as candidacy for facial nerve decompression. In ENoG, a bipolar simulating electrode is placed on the skin at the stylomastoid foramen, and a bipolar recording electrode is placed in the nasolabial groove (Fig. 37.4). A supramaximal stimulus is used, and the evoked compound muscle action potential (CMAP) is measured. The CMAP amplitudes are then compared between the healthy and injured sides. More than 50% of patients with idiopathic facial paralysis who exhibit CMAP amplitude reductions to <10% of the healthy side (>90% degeneration) have incomplete recovery.[18,19] In these cases, authors have shown that decompression of the facial nerve medial to the geniculate ganglion within the first 2 weeks of paralysis significantly improves the chances of complete or near-complete recovery.[20] When the CMAP amplitude is >10% of the healthy side (<90% degeneration), excellent recovery generally occurs. In those patients with complete facial paralysis and <90% degeneration, it has been recommended

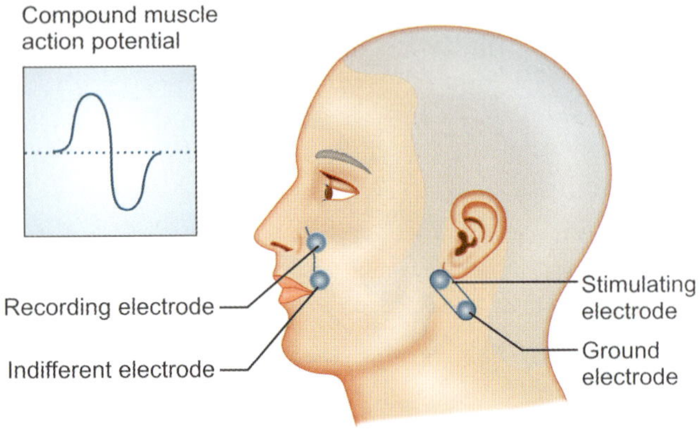

Fig. 37.4: Electroneuronography electrode placement. Compound muscle action potentials (CMAPs) are compared between the two sides. Excellent recovery generally occurs when the CMAP amplitude of the injured side is >10% of the healthy side.
Source: Redrawn from Jackler R. Neurotology. Philadelphia: Mosby; 2005.

that ENoG be repeated every other day during the first 2–3 weeks to detect degeneration that progresses to >90%. Once degeneration is >90%, decompression can be considered.

EMG records spontaneous and voluntary muscle potentials using needles introduced into facial muscles. EMG is particularly useful for assessing facial motor units after Wallerian degeneration has occurred. Testing should be performed in at least two muscle groups to accurately assess the degree of denervation.[21] Prior to 10 days after the onset of facial paralysis, electrical evidence of nerve degeneration is absent. After 10–14 days, denervated muscle membrane undergoes changes that cause spontaneous depolarizations. On EMG, these fibrillation potentials indicate the degeneration of facial motor units. In 81% of these patients, incomplete recovery will occur.[22] Absence of volitional potentials serves as confirmation of a severe injury and supports the decision to offer facial nerve decompression. Surgeons often use EMG as a confirmatory test of denervation in addition to a finding of >90% degeneration on ENoG after 2–3 weeks.[20] However, if reinnervation begins at 4–6 weeks, polyphasic potentials replace fibrillations. This portends a higher likelihood of recovery.

After long-term facial paralysis, EMG is also useful for determining the best procedure for facial reanimation. If fibrillation potentials are still present, nerve grafting is a viable option as the motor units are available. However, if the paralysis has been present for over 12 months, muscle atrophy can occur, and EMG recordings become silent. In these cases, nerve grafting is inadequate, and neuromuscular transfers (e.g. gracilis muscle microneurovascular transfer) are necessary for reanimation.

INTRAOPERATIVE FACIAL NERVE MONITORING

Facial nerve injury is a potential complication of otologic and neurotologic surgery. Intraoperative facial nerve integrity monitoring has been advocated to reduce the risk of facial nerve injury. A number of intraoperative nerve monitoring systems are available for use in the operating room. Current stimulator probes can be set to as low as 0.01 mA. Subdermal electrodes made of platinum or stainless steel are often used for EMG recordings. Uninsulated needles are preferred, as they have lower impedance and the larger surface area can record activity from a larger amount of muscle fibers.[23] It is important that the patient is not given any paralytic agents during nerve monitoring. An adequate depth of anesthesia must be achieved such that the patient does not move, yet still has spontaneous and evoked EMG activity. In addition, care must be taken to ensure that local anesthetic is not infiltrated near the stylomastoid foramen, as the facial nerve can then be anesthetized and not provide spontaneous or stimulated EMG activity.

In neurotologic surgery, intraoperative facial nerve monitoring can detect any changes in the spontaneous EMG that occur with nerve irritation (e.g. vestibular schwannoma tumor dissection), and can help determine the functional status of the facial nerve. Two channels are typically used for monitoring, with electrode pairs placed in the orbicularis oculi and orbicularis oris muscles. In the posterior fossa, large CPA tumors can stretch or widen the facial nerve. In these cases, electrical stimulation assists in identifying and tracing the facial nerve. The most common site of injury is just medial to the porus acusticus, where it can be difficult to separate tumor from the nerve.[24] Tumor dissection is thus performed primarily in a medial-to-lateral direction, so as to avoid a distal conduction block that would prohibit stimulation of the nerve at the brainstem. Following tumor resection, it has been suggested that the ability to elicit an EMG response with low-threshold stimulation at the brainstem can predict long-term facial nerve function.[25] At 1 year postoperatively, Lalwani et al. found that 98% of patients with electrical thresholds of 0.2 volts (V) or less had House-Brackmann grade 1 or 2 facial nerve function, as compared to only 50% of patients with thresholds between 0.21 and 0.6 V.[26] Selesnick et al. found that at 1 year postoperatively, 90% of patients with thresholds of

0.1 mA had grade 1 or 2 function, as compared to 58% of patients with thresholds of 0.2 mA.[27] Fenton et al. demonstrated in their series that all patients with an elicited EMG response after tumor resection recovered to at least grade 3 function at 2 years' follow-up. They contended that the best predictor of long-term facial nerve function was the level of early postoperative function, which had a sensitivity of 95% and positive predictive value of 96%.[28]

The routine use of facial nerve monitoring in otologic surgery is controversial. However, the current evidence suggests that facial nerve monitoring can be useful when the nerve is dehiscent and at higher surgical risk. In a prospective study of 260 consecutive otologic surgeries performed for chronic ear disease, monitoring identified 93% of dehiscent facial nerves prior to visual identification. This early detection could help identify facial nerves at risk of injury, particularly in the residency training setting.[29]

DIFFUSION TENSOR TRACTOGRAPHY IMAGING

In cases of large vestibular schwannomas, it can be difficult to distinguish between the facial nerve and the tumor on magnetic resonance imaging (MRI). Both the facial nerve and the schwannoma have similar signal intensities, and larger tumors cause thinning of the facial nerve. Additionally, there is typically no intervening cerebrospinal fluid.[30] In these cases, diffusion tensor (DT) tractography has proven useful for assessing facial nerve course and displacement. Taoka et al.[30] evaluated the accuracy of facial nerve DT tractography in eight patients. MRI was performed using a 1.5 Tesla scanner, and DT images were obtained using a single-shot echo-planar sequence. Tracts of the facial nerve were constructed from the pons to the internal auditory meatus, and compared with the facial nerve course visualized on high-resolution, heavily T2-weighted sequence of the brainstem. Tractography images were also compared with the facial nerve course observed intraoperatively. In seven of eight patients, all of whom had tumors >20 mm in size and for whom MRI was unable to distinguish facial nerve from tumor, DT tractography accurately localized the facial nerve from the pons to the internal auditory meatus.[30]

Chen et al. used a 3 Tesla scanner to obtain three-dimensional (3D) visualization of the facial nerve in cases of vestibular schwannoma. DT images were acquired with an echo-planar/spin-echo sequence.[31] T1 anatomic axial images were used to construct a 3D tumor model. Detailed anatomy of the fibers was better visualized in larger tumors, with small fibers seen coursing inferior to the tumor from the porus acusticus to the brainstem. For the smallest tumor, the VII/VIII complex was visualized at the porus, but the cisternal segment of the facial nerve could not be visualized with as much detail. The authors' ability to distinguish between cranial nerves VII and VIII was limited due to their proximity and similar size. Thus, even further technical improvement is needed to better distinguish between individual nerve fibers using MRI tractography.[31]

CONCLUSION

Facial nerve testing can provide critical information about the extent of nerve injury and the prognosis for recovery. Topographic testing can help localize the site of facial nerve injury. Electrophysiologic testing in the form of ENoG and EMG can help predict which patients with facial paralysis will benefit from surgical decompression. EMG is also helpful when planning facial reanimation procedures. DT tractography is a new imaging modality that shows promise for 3D visualization of facial nerve fibers, potentially lowering the risk of facial nerve injury during treatment of vestibular schwannomas.

REFERENCES

1. Raghavan P, Mukherjee S, Phillips CD. Imaging of the facial nerve. Neuroimaging Clin N Am. 2009;19:407-25.
2. Cisneros A, Orozco JR, Nogues JA, et al. Development of the stapedius muscle canal and its possible clinical consequences. Int J Pediatr Otorhinolaryngol. 2011;75:277-81.
3. Curtin H, Sanelli P, Som P. Head and Neck Imaging. Missouri, USA: Mosby; 2003.
4. May M. The Facial Nerve. New York: Thieme; 2000.
5. Al-Noury K, Lotfy A. Normal and pathologic findings for the facial nerve on magnetic resonance imaging. Clin Radiol. 2011;66:701-7.
6. Jager L, Reiser M. CT and MR imaging of the normal and pathologic conditions of the facial nerve. Eur J Radiol. 2001;40:133-46.
7. Swartz JD, Harnsberger HR. Imaging of the Temporal Bone. New York: Thieme; 1998.
8. Harnsberger H, Osborn A, Macdonald A, et al. Diagnostic and Surgical Imaging Anatomy: Brain, Head and Neck, Spine. Utah: Amirsys; 2006.
9. Isaacson B, Vrabec JT. The radiographic prevalence of geniculate ganglion dehiscence in normal and congenitally thin temporal bones. Otol Neurotol. 2007;28:107-10.
10. Nager GT, Proctor B. Anatomic variations and anomalies involving the facial canal. Otolaryngol Clin North Am. 1991; 24(3):531-53.

11. Fisch U. Facial Nerve Surgery. Alabama: Aesculapius Publishing; 1977.
12. Stillman JA, Morton RP, Hay KD, et al. Electrogustometry: strengths, weaknesses, and clinical evidence of stimulus boundaries. Clin Otolaryngol. 2003;28:406-10.
13. Saito T, Manabe Y Shibamori Y, et al. Long-term follow-up results of electrogustometry and subjective taste disorder after middle ear surgery. Laryngoscope. 2001;111:2064-70.
14. May M, Hawkins CB. Bell's palsy: salivation test vs. nerve excitability as a basis of treatment. Laryngoscope. 1972;82: 1337.
15. Laumans EP, Jonkees LB. On the prognosis of peripheral facial paralysis of endotemporal origin. Ann Oto Rhino Laryngol. 1963;72:621.
16. Gates GA. Nerve excitability testing: technical pitfalls and threshold norms using absolute values. Laryngoscope. 1993;103:379-95.
17. May M, Hardin WB, Sullivan J, et al. Natural history of Bell's palsy: the salivary flow test and other prognostic indicators. Laryngoscope. 1976;86:704.
18. May M, Blumenthal F, Klein SR. Acute Bell's palsy: prognostic value of evoked electromyography, maximal stimulation, and other electrical tests. Am J Otol. 1983;5:1-7.
19. Sillman J, Niparko JK, Lee SS, et al. Prognostic value of evoked and standard EMG in acute facial paralysis. Otolaryngol Head Neck Surg. 1992;107:377.
20. Gantz BJ, Rubinstein JT, Gidley P, et al. Surgical management of Bell's palsy. Laryngoscope. 1999;109:1177.
21. Lalwani A. Current Diagnosis and Treatment in Otolaryngology-Head and Neck Surgery. New York: McGraw-Hill; 2008.
22. Sittel C, Stennert E. Prognostic value of electromyography in acute peripheral facial nerve palsy. Otol Neurotol. 2001;22:100.
23. Jackler R. Neurotology. Philadelphia: Mosby; 2005.
24. Bacciu A, Falcioni M, Pasanisi E, et al. Intracranial facial nerve grafting after removal of vestibular schwannoma. Am J Otolaryngol. 2009;30:83-8.
25. Isaacson B, Kilen PR, El-Kashlan H, Gadre AK. Intraoperative monitoring and facial nerve outcomes after vestibular schwannoma resection. Otol Neurotol. 2003;24:812-7.
26. Lalwani AK, Butt FY, Jackler RK, et al. Facial nerve outcome after acoustic neuroma surgery: a study from the area of cranial nerve monitoring. Otolaryngol Head Neck Surg. 1994;111:561-70.
27. Selesnick SH, Carew JF, Victor JD, et al. Predictive value of facial nerve electrophysiologic stimulation thresholds in cerebellopontine-angle surgery. Laryngoscope. 1996;106: 633-8.
28. Fenton JE, Chin RY, Fagan PA, et al. Predictive factors of long-term facial nerve function after vestibular schwannoma surgery. Otol Neurotol. 2002;23:388-92.
29. Pensak ML, Willging JP, Keith RW. Intraoperative facial nerve monitoring in chronic ear surgery: a resident training experience. Am J Otolaryngol. 1994;15:108-10.
30. Taoka T, Hirabayashi H, Nakagawa H, et al. Displacement of the facial nerve course by vestibular schwannoma: preoperative visualization using diffusion tensor tractography. J Magn Reson Imag. 2006;24:1005-10.
31. Chen DQ, Quan J, Guha A, et al. Three-dimensional in vivo modeling of vestibular schwannomas and surrounding cranial nerves with diffusion imaging tractography. Neurosurgery. 2011;68:1077-83.

CHAPTER

38

Facial Nerve Paralysis

Elizabeth H Toh

INTRODUCTION

Facial paralysis may result from a variety of central and peripheral disorders (Table 38.1). Although Bell's palsy is the commonest cause of peripheral facial paralysis, it remains a diagnosis of exclusion. Since treatment and

Table 38.1: Causes of facial paralysis

Congenital
Möbius syndrome
Hemifacial microsomia
Congenital lower lip palsy
Traumatic
Penetrating injuries to the face and temporal bone
Skull base fracture
Barotrauma
Iatrogenic trauma
Neoplastic
Parotid tumors
Facial nerve tumors
Acoustic neuroma
Meningioma
Intratemporal glomus tumors
Sarcoma
Squamous cell carcinoma
Metastatic carcinoma
Leukemia
Infectious
Otitis media
Malignant otitis externa
Mastoiditis
Herpes zoster oticus
Infectious mononucleosis
Lyme disease
Leprosy
Syphilis
Human immunodeficiency virus
Coxsackie virus
Meningoencephalitis
Poliomyelitis (type I)
Mucormycosis
Botulism
Metabolic
Pregnancy
Diabetes mellitus
Hyperthyroidism
Renal osteodystrophy
Toxic
Alcoholic neuropathy
Thalidomide toxicity
Tetanus
Diptheria
Lead poisoning
Carbon monoxide
Vascular
Sigmoid anomaly
Petrous carotid aneurysm
Benign intracranial hypertension
Hypertension
Cerebrovascular thromboembolism
Neurologic
Opercular syndrome (cortical lesion in facial motor area)
Millard-Gubler syndrome (ventral pontine syndrome)
Guillain-Barré syndrome
Multiple sclerosis
Others
Bell's palsy
Melkersson-Rosenthal syndrome
Sarcoidosis
Hyperostoses
Myasthenia gravis
Amyloidosis
Hereditary hypertrophic neuropathy
Autoimmune syndromes
Eosinophilic granuloma

Contd...

prognosis for facial paralysis is dictated primarily by the etiology of the paralysis, an effort must be made to seek other causes of facial palsy. Traumatic injuries are typically obvious to diagnose whether they be due to penetrating injuries, barotrauma, temporal bone fractures, or iatrogenic events. Determining if the paralysis is a single episode, recurring, bilateral, or alternating gives clues to the etiology as well. Lesions affecting the intratemporal facial nerve pose a unique challenge from a diagnostic and management perspective due to our inability to accurately assess the structural and functional integrity of the nerve at the site of injury, and therefore prognosticate recovery. The functional and aesthetic sequelae resulting from facial paralysis can have a devastating impact on one's psychological and emotional well-being. Proper diagnosis and treatment offers the best opportunity to minimize unwanted long-term sequelae. This chapter will review common causes of facial paralysis, clinical evaluation of these patients, and management options for specific causes of the condition. Facial nerve tumors are covered in detail in a separate chapter, as facial nerve rehabilitation.

PATHOGENESIS

A basic knowledge of the anatomy and physiology of the facial nerve is imperative for understanding the pathophysiologic mechanism for facial paralysis and recovery. These topics are covered extensively in earlier chapters.

Fundamentally, most diseases causing facial paralysis do so by interfering with electrical conduction of nerve impulses through some or all of the myelinated motor axons innervating the facial muscles. The Sunderland classification system for peripheral nerve injuries elegantly summarizes the pathologic changes occurring within the injured nerve and correlates these to anticipated functional outcomes (Fig. 38.1).[1]

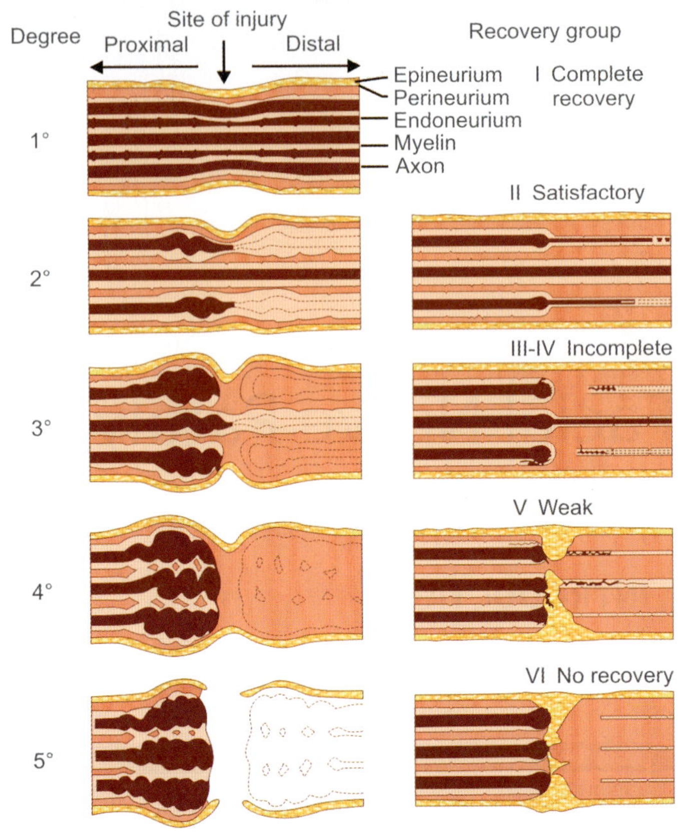

Fig. 38.1: Sunderland classification system for peripheral nerve injuries correlates degree of injury, histopathologic changes in the nerve, and expected functional recovery. First-degree injury—compression without structural violation; expect normal recovery. Second-degree injury—axonal degeneration with consistent regeneration and satisfactory recovery. Third-degree injury—disruption of endoneurium; incomplete recovery with synkinesis. Fourth-degree injury—disruption of endoneurium and perineurium; recovery is poor. Fifth-degree injury—nerve transection; no recovery.
Source: Redrawn from May M, Schaitkin BM. (eds). The facial nerve, 2nd edn. New York: Thieme; 2000.

First-degree injuries (neuropraxia) result in a temporary conduction block, which reverses rapidly and completely with relief of the compressive insult. In these cases, the nerve distal to the site of compression retains normal electrical excitability. Evoked electromyography (EMG) tests therefore remain normal through the course of the disease. Functional recovery is usually complete within days to weeks.

Second-degree injuries (axonotmesis) result from moderate to severe nerve compression. Incremental nerve compression results in proximal and distal nerve edema. This in turn causes vascular strangulation and axonal degeneration distal to the site of injury, a process referred to as Wallerian degeneration. Electrical testing distal to the site of injury will demonstrate some muscular denervation correlating to the degree of neural degeneration and gradual onset of muscle reinnervation potentials. Since the neural support structures remain intact in second-degree injuries, subsequent axonal regeneration is complete and functional outcomes, although delayed in comparison to neuropraxic injuries, are generally good.

In third to fifth-degree injuries (neurotmesis), progressively more neural support structures are violated. As such, axonal regeneration is expected to be incomplete and inconsistent. The long-term functional implications of this are residual facial paresis and synkinesis, respectively. Recovery occurs in a delayed manner and may take many months in third- and fourth-degree injuries. A fifth-degree injury is essentially a complete nerve transection, necessitating surgical intervention as the only hope for any functional recovery. Electrical testing with third- and fourth-degree injuries will reveal similar findings to second-degree injuries with progressive degrees of muscle denervation, reflecting increased severity of neural degeneration. Electrical silence is noted with fifth-degree injuries on evoked EMG [ENoG (electroneurography)] testing, followed 3 weeks later by fibrillation potentials.

Facial nerve injury associated with Bell's palsy, Herpes zoster oticus (HZO), otitis media, tumors, and most blunt traumatic injuries (temporal bone fractures and birth injuries) are first- to third-degree injuries. Extent of nerve injury with surgical and penetrating trauma can vary.

CLINICAL FINDINGS

A detailed history and physical examination of the patient presenting with facial paralysis are vital in making the appropriate diagnosis. Clinical features helpful to some extent in determining the underlying etiology of facial paralysis include onset, rate of progression, unilateral versus bilateral involvement, segmental facial involvement, recurrence, and associated symptoms and signs.[2] It is important to remember that none of these characteristics singularly offer any diagnostic clue on the etiology of facial paralysis. However, severity of paresis, time course for progression of paresis, and onset of recovery are very helpful in prognosticating functional recovery. A comprehensive physical examination must include examination of the ears, parotid gland, neck, eyes, skin, and cranial nerves. The degree of facial weakness involving all the nerve branches must be carefully assessed and documented.

Grading Facial Function

Several standardized global and regional grading systems have been used to report facial function. In 1985, the House-Brackmann scale was endorsed as the universal standard for reporting facial function recovery by the American Academy of Otolaryngology–Head and Neck Surgery (Table 38.2). Other commonly used grading systems such as the Sunnybrook and Yanagihara grading systems rely on a more comprehensive regional assessment of facial function for increased accuracy and reduced interobserver and intraobserver variability. These descriptive grading systems continue to be used in clinical practice, but efforts are being made to develop more accurate computer-based video approaches to quantify facial function.

Bell's Palsy

Bell's palsy accounts for the vast majority of cases of acute onset unilateral facial palsy in all ages, affecting 15–40 per 100,000 individuals per year. The condition affects males and females equally and has been found to occur more commonly between age 15 and 45 years. The risk of Bell's palsy appears to be increased with pregnancy, severe preeclampsia diabetes, and hypertension.[3] Bell's palsy is usually self-limited with spontaneous recovery of normal facial function in 71% of patients.[4]

Table 38.2: House-Brackmann facial nerve grading system

Grade	*Description*	*Characteristics*
I	Normal	Normal facial function in all nerve branches
II	Slight weakness	*Gross*: Slight weakness on close inspection, slight synkinesis *At rest*: Normal tone and symmetry *Motion*: Forehead—good to moderate movement; eye—complete closure with minimum effort; mouth—slight asymmetry
III	Moderate weakness	*Gross*: Obvious but not disfiguring facial asymmetry. Synkinesis is noticeable but not severe. May have hemifacial spasm or contracture *At rest*: Normal tone and symmetry *Motion*: Forehead—slight to moderate movement; eye—complete closure with effort; mouth—slight weakness with maximum effort
IV	Moderate to severe weakness	*Gross*: Asymmetry is disfiguring and/or obvious facial weakness *At rest*: Normal tone and symmetry Motion: Forehead—no movement; eye—incomplete closure; mouth—slight movement
V	Severe weakness	*Gross*: Only slight, barely noticeable movement *At rest*: Asymmetrical facial appearance *Motion*: Forehead—no movement; eye—incomplete closure; mouth—slight movement
VI	Total paralysis	No facial function

Table 38.3: Clinical features atypical for Bell's palsy
Progression of palsy beyond 3 weeks
Absence of recovery after 6 months
Hyperkinetic function (twitching, spasm)
Segmental paresis
Recurrent ipsilateral palsy
Bilateral simultaneous palsy
Involvement of multiple cranial nerves
Presence of other neurologic symptoms
Presence of mass in parotid or ear
Presence of vesicular lesions

The isolation of herpes simplex virus (HSV) genomic material in the perineural fluid of patients affected with Bell's palsy has led to the prevailing notion that the condition is a result of an HSV viral infection.[5] The resulting inflammatory response results in neural edema and vascular compromise of the facial nerve within the fallopian canal. This entrapment neuropathy is most evident in the labyrinthine segment of the facial nerve where the fallopian canal is narrowest in diameter.

In 50% of patients with Bell's palsy, the onset is rapidly progressive over the course of 72 hours. Weakness peaks within the first 10 days and does not progress beyond then. Progression beyond 3 weeks should alert one's suspicion for an underlying tumor and prompt further investigation. Paralysis may be complete or incomplete with Bell's palsy. In the remaining 50% of patients, unilateral facial paralysis is sudden and complete. These patients tend to have a less favorable prognosis for recovery. Ipsilateral otalgia is a common complaint preceding or associated with Bell's palsy as well, reported in 60% of patients. Other associated symptoms may include hyperacusis, dry mouth, dysgeusia, and decreased tearing or dry eye. With Bell's palsy, spontaneous recovery begins within 3 weeks after onset of paralysis in 85% of patients and is complete in over two thirds of patients within a few months.[4] The absence of any sign of recovery 4–6 months after onset of paralysis should elicit further diagnostic evaluation for other etiologies of facial paralysis. Clinical features atypical for Bell's palsy are listed in Table 38.3.

Bell's palsy may recur in 10–12% of patients. Contralateral recurrence is more common. A positive family history is present in 14% of cases, leading one to consider the diagnosis of Bell's palsy if the affected individual has other family members with a history of facial paralysis.

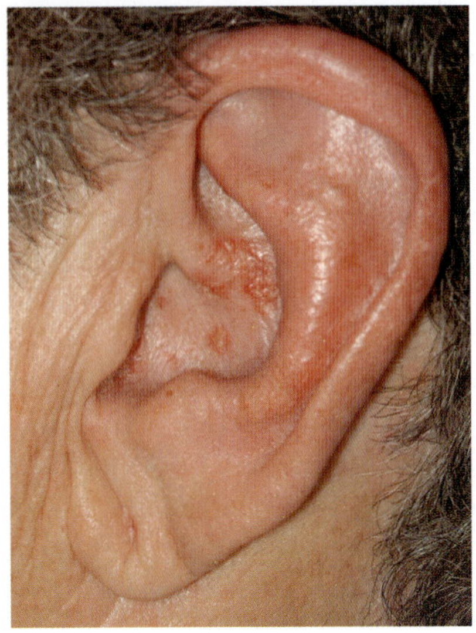

Fig. 38.2: Cutaneous manifestations in the external meatus in herpes zoster oticus.

Herpes Zoster Oticus (Ramsey Hunt Syndrome)

Herpes zoster oticus is the second most common cause of acute facial paralysis after Bell's palsy. It occurs most commonly in adults with an increasing incidence with age, presumably due to decreased cell-mediated immunity in older adults. Serologic and epidemiologic data suggest that the reactivation of a latent varicella zoster virus, as opposed to a reinfection, is the mechanism of infection.

The condition is characterized by acute unilateral facial paralysis accompanied by severe pain and vesicular eruptions over the dermatome(s) innervated by the involved sensory afferent nerve fibers, including the pinna, ear canal, face, neck, and oral cavity (Fig. 38.2). Unlike Bell's palsy, facial weakness may continue to evolve over a 3-week period. A viral prodrome is not uncommon. The vesicular eruptions may sometimes precede the onset of facial paralysis, in which case, the diagnosis of herpes zoster infection may be confirmed on serologic or cerebrospinal fluid analysis for antibodies to varicella zoster virus.[6]

Unlike Bell's palsy, the clinical course of HZO tends to be more aggressive and may sometimes involve of other cranial nerves. Peitersen's series reported complete facial paralysis in 88% of patients with HZO.[6] Sensorineural hearing loss and vestibular symptoms occur more often in HZO.[6] Hearing loss is generally irreversible and recovery from vestibular symptoms is often protracted. Postherpetic neuralgia and persistent facial dysfunction are also more likely. Satisfactory recovery of facial function is

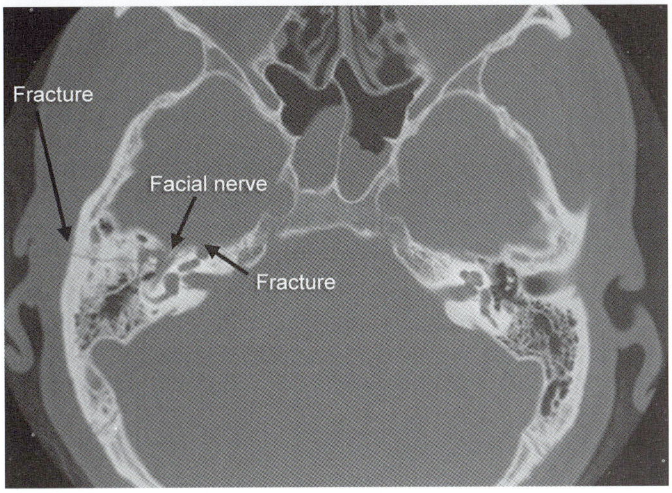

Fig. 38.3: Longitudinal temporal bone fracture through the perigeniculate region of the fallopian canal.

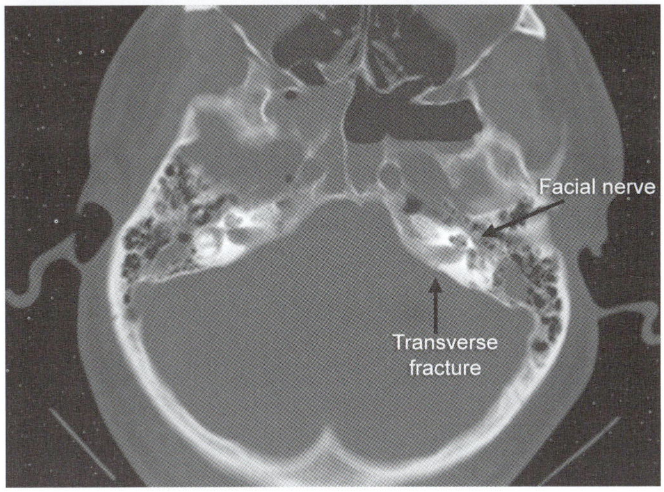

Fig. 38.4: Transverse temporal bone fracture through the internal auditory canal, cochlea, and labyrinthine facial nerve.

often reported in over 80% of Bell's palsy patients but only in <50% of patients diagnosed with HZO.[6] Fortunately, recurrence of HZO is rare.

TRAUMA

Birth Injuries

Approximately, 90% of all congenital peripheral facial nerve paralysis improves spontaneously and most can be attributed to difficult deliveries, cephalopelvic disproportion, high forceps delivery, or intrauterine trauma. These types of congenital facial paralyses are often unilateral and partial, especially involving the lower division of the facial nerve.

Blunt Head Trauma

Blunt trauma resulting in temporal bone fracture is another cause of facial paralysis or paresis in all ages. The pathogenesis of facial paralysis in such cases is either direct injury with nerve transection or traction injury with resulting nerve edema and entrapment neuropathy. Rarely, the facial nerve may be compressed by a bony spicule within the fallopian canal. Temporal and parietal blows to the head result in longitudinal fractures of the temporal bone. This is the most common type of temporal bone fracture (approximately 90%) and is also the most common type of fracture associated with facial nerve injury. The geniculate ganglion region of facial nerve is most frequently injured (Fig. 38.3).

Frontal and particularly occipital blows to the head tend to result in transverse fractures of the temporal bone. More severe head injury is usually required to cause these fractures. Since these fractures often extend through the internal auditory canal or across the otic capsule, sensorineural hearing loss and vertigo are common (Fig. 38.4). Although only 10–20% of temporal bone fractures are transverse in orientation, they cause facial nerve injury in approximately 50% of patients. The anatomic region of the facial nerve most commonly injured is the labyrinthine segment.

Immediate complete facial paralysis in the setting of temporal bone fractures is concerning for nerve transection or severe traction injury. This should prompt urgent exploration for confirmation of neural violation and early repair or nerve decompression, especially if a bony spicule is found to impinge the facial nerve on temporal bone computed tomography (CT) imaging. In many such cases, significant intracranial trauma coexists and takes priority over surgical management of the facial nerve. Incomplete paralysis and delayed onset facial paralysis, even if progressive to complete paralysis, carry a good prognosis for recovery of function and can therefore be managed conservatively. Other clinical findings associated with temporal bone fractures include hearing loss, dizziness, bleeding from the ear or hemotympanum, ear canal laceration, tympanic membrane perforation, postauricular ecchymosis, and cerebrospinal fluid otorrhea or rhinorrhea. These are further reviewed in a separate chapter.

Penetrating Injuries

Penetrating injuries to the extratemporal facial nerve are easily diagnosed by history and clinical presentation. Nerve transection is common in such cases. Gunshot wounds to the head can violate the facial nerve in its intratemporal course and usually cause immediate onset facial paralysis.

Iatrogenic Injuries

The facial nerve may be injured in surgery of the parotid gland, neck, ear, or skull base. The most straightforward mechanism of injury in otologic surgery, and the one most easily recognized intraoperatively, is when the nerve is injured directly by the dissecting instrument, otologic drill, laser, or electrocautery instrument. The incidence of iatrogenic injury is highest with parotid surgery since nerve dissection is commonly part of the procedure. However, clinical evaluation and management is incrementally more challenging with facial nerve trauma in temporal bone surgery since the injury may not be evident at the time of surgery. Such direct injury may occur in the mastoid cavity, the facial recess, the second genu, or the tympanic segment. The facial nerve is naturally dehiscent in the tympanic segment in up to 30% of patients and therefore prone to injury when dissecting cholesteatoma or granulation tissue in this region.[7] The risk of otologic surgical injury of the facial nerve is also particularly high in children with congenital ear malformations and cases where the disease has significantly distorted or obscured normal temporal bone anatomy. More subtle mechanisms of nerve damage include heat injury and possible viral reactivation. These mechanisms may lead to delayed nerve paresis through progressive neural edema following intraoperative nerve trauma.

INFECTION

Bacterial

Infections involving the ear that may cause facial paralysis include acute suppurative otitis media, chronic otitis media, mastoiditis, and malignant otitis externa. In suppurative otitis media, a natural dehiscence in the fallopian canal serves as a portal of entry for bacterial invasion and inflammatory products to cause neural edema. Facial paralysis often progresses rapidly over the course of 2–3 days and is preceded by severe ear pain with or without otorrhea, hearing loss, and sometimes dizziness.

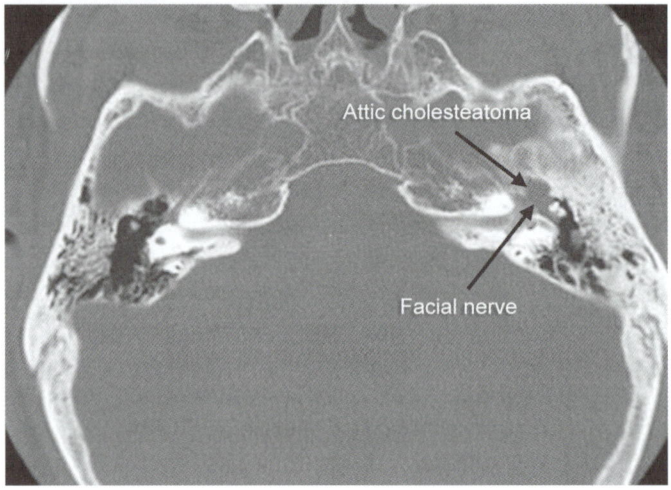

Fig. 38.5: Attic cholesteatoma with erosion of the fallopian canal in the tympanic segment.

Chronic Otitis Media

Facial paralysis complicating mastoiditis or cholesteatoma is usually secondary to inflammation, edema, and subsequent entrapment neuropathy. Alternatively, extraneural and intraneural compression may also result from an enlarging cholesteatoma or abscess. The tympanic segment and second genu are most often the site of involvement. A history of ear infections, prior ear surgery, hearing loss, and dizziness must be sought. Facial paresis is usually gradual in onset and slowly progressive. Clinical examination of the ear is revealing and extent of disease should be confirmed with a high-resolution temporal bone CT scan (Fig. 38.5). Resolution is rapid and complete with eradication of the inflammatory tissue or cholesteatoma. Patients with chronic suppurative otitis media without cholesteatoma appear to have a better functional outcome compared with those with cholesteatoma.[8] The prognosis for recovery of facial function in these patients is related to the time of intervention.[9]

Malignant Otitis Externa

Facial paralysis may occur with advanced malignant otitis externa. The patient is usually an older adult, diabetic, or immunocompromised. A history of severe ear pain and purulent discharge is obtained. The finding of painful inflammatory swelling of the external auditory canal with fleshy granulation tissue along the inferior aspect of the canal at the bony–cartilaginous junction is characteristic. *Pseudomonas aeruginosa* is the most common pathogen, accounting for up to 98% of documented cultures. In rare cases, methicillin-resistant *Staphylococcus aureus* or fungal pathogens may be found. The nidus of disease originates in the external auditory canal but spreads into adjacent tissues. The temporal bone, parotid gland, and lower cranial nerves may become involved. Involvement of the facial nerve is indicative of advanced disease and associated with a mortality rate of over 50%.[10] Complete recovery of facial nerve function is unlikely in these cases.

Lyme Disease

Infection with the spirochete *Borrelia burgdorferi* can result in facial paralysis. This tickborne infection is endemic to the Northeast and is named for the town of Lyme, CT, USA. Widespread infections have been reported in the West Coast, Midwest, and East Coast as well as throughout Europe and Australia. As is the case with other spirochete infections, the clinical manifestations of Lyme disease are protean. In the early stage of the disease, flu-like symptoms are reported, along with a characteristic maculopapular rash which extends outward with central clearing (erythema chronicum migrans) lasting up to 3 weeks. Neurologic manifestations occur in 10–20% of patients. Facial paralysis is the most common of these. Bilateral involvement has been reported but is uncommon.

BENIGN AND MALIGNANT NEOPLASMS

Facial nerve tumors are reviewed in detail in a separate chapter. A history of malignant neoplasms involving the parotid gland, skin, breast, lung, thyroid, upper aerodigestive tract, kidney, ovary, or prostate with unilateral facial paralysis is suspicious for metastatic disease as a cause of the palsy. Imaging studies are needed to confirm this suspicion and determine extent of disease, even if clinical evaluation reveals an obvious site of facial nerve involvement.

BILATERAL FACIAL PARALYSIS

The onset of simultaneous bilateral facial paralysis suggests Guillain-Barré syndrome, sarcoidosis, Lyme disease, HIV infection, or some other systemic disorder (Table 38.4).

Table 38.4: Causes of bilateral simultaneous facial palsy
Guillain-Barré syndrome
Möbius syndrome
Sarcoidosis
Lyme disease
Skull base trauma
Infectious mononucleosis
Cytomegalovirus infection
Human immunodeficiency virus
Botulism

Guillain-Barré syndrome is an acute inflammatory polyradiculoneuropathy that progresses to varying degrees of paralysis. The etiology remains unknown; however, autoimmune or viral mechanisms have been considered. Classical histopathologic features of the syndrome include a lymphocytic cellular infiltration of peripheral nerves and destruction of myelin. The facial paralysis seen in these cases is typically bilateral and often resolves spontaneously after a prolonged course of paralysis.

Sarcoidosis is a granulomatous disease of unknown etiology affecting multiple organ systems. Facial paralysis may be unilateral or bilateral and is the most common neurologic finding in sarcoidosis. Perineural inflammation is the postulated underlying pathology causing neuropathy. Since the integrity of the facial nerve is maintained, treatment of sarcoidosis with systemic steroids usually results in complete functional recovery. Other associated clinical findings may include bilateral tender parotid enlargement, cervical lymph node enlargement, and uveitis.

RECURRENT FACIAL PARALYSIS

Differential diagnoses for recurring facial palsy include Bell's palsy and Melkersson-Rosenthal syndrome. Recurrence more commonly affects the contralateral side in both of these conditions. Multiple recurrences with progressive residual palsy can occur.

Melkersson-Rosenthal syndrome is a neuromucocutaneous disease with a classic triad of recurrent facial (labial) edema and recurrent facial paralysis associated with a fissured tongue. Patients with Melkersson-Rosenthal syndrome may not present with the complete triad, and although facial paralysis is the most common neurologic symptom, it is not mandatory for the diagnosis. Headache, granular cheilitis, trigeminal neuralgiform attacks, dysphagia, laryngospasm, and a variety of cranial nerve and cervical autonomic dysfunctions may also occur. The patient with Melkersson-Rosenthal syndrome may present at any age and with any variety of classic and associated features, which may wax and wane. Approximately one third of the patients have recurrent facial paralysis as part of their syndrome. Bilateral facial paralysis has been reported as well.[11] The underlying etiologic factor has been thought to be a neurotropic edema causing compression and paralysis of the facial nerve as it passes through the fallopian canal. Recurrent paralysis over a prolonged period of time usually results in increasing residual dysfunction. If evidence of residual paresis exists, total facial nerve decompression is recommended at the time of the next episode of paralysis.[12]

CONGENITAL DISORDERS

Möbius Syndrome (Congenital Facial Diplegia)

This is a rare congenital disorder presenting with congenital bilateral facial paralysis and unilateral or bilateral abducens nerve paralysis. It is inherited in an autosomal dominant manner with variable penetrance. The inheritance pattern is thought to be no higher than 1 in 50 families in whom myopathies or other extremity anomalies such as club foot, arthrogyposis, or digital anomalies are not present.

The etiology of Möbius syndrome is unclear. Neuropathologic studies have noted that the nuclei of cranial nerves 6, 7, and 12 are abnormal, with lesser abnormalities being found in the nuclei of cranial nerves III and XI. Other authors have reported that the facial nerves are smaller or absent at autopsy.[13] Alternatively, primary failure of facial muscle development has been proposed as a possible etiology since normal facial nuclei were found in postmortem studies.[14]

Magnetic resonance imaging (MRI) reveals no structural abnormalities or masses. Ophthalmologic consultation and management is mandatory. Reinnervation procedures such as cross-face grafts or hypoglossal-facial nerve anastomosis yield poor results, either due to the paucity of motor endplates or the atrophic seventh nerves. Significant improvements in resting tone and voluntary facial movement can be achieved with temporalis muscle transposition, which brings in a new neuromuscular system.

Hemifacial Microsomia

Hemifacial microsomia refers to patients with unilateral microtia, macrostomia, and mandibular hypoplasia, resulting in underdevelopment of the lower half of the face on one side. This can occur bilaterally in 31% of cases with one side being more affected than the other. Goldenhar's syndrome (oculoauriculovertebral dysplasia) is considered to be a variant of this complex and is characterized by vertebral anomalies and epibulbar dermoids. The occurrence of hemifacial microsoma is 1 in 3000–4000 live births. It is the second most common birth defect after cleft lip and cleft palate. The cause of the condition is thought to be multifactorial, including a small genetic predisposition. Twenty-five percent of patients with hemifacial microsomia have facial paralysis as well. Management of this condition requires a multidisciplinary approach for craniofacial repair of jaw and ear abnormalities, and lower facial reanimation using free muscle transfer.

Osteopetrosis

Osteopetrosis is a generalized bone dysplasia, which may have an autosomal dominant or recessive inheritance pattern. The recessive form is more rapidly progressive and causes hepatosplenomegaly and severe neural atrophy secondary to bony overgrowth at neural foramina. Optic atrophy, facial paralysis, sensorineural hearing loss, and mental retardation are common in the recessive form, and death usually occurs by the second decade.

The dominant form causes progressive enlargements of the cranium and mandible and clubbing of the long bones. Increased bone density is seen radiographically. Progressive optic atrophy, trigeminal hypesthesia, recurrent facial paralysis, and sensorineural hearing loss are common, and result from cranial nerve compression. Complete decompression of the intratemporal facial nerve may be performed in patients with recurrent facial paralysis and radiographic evidence of osteopetrosis.

EVALUATION

Electrodiagnostic Testing

Electrical testing of the facial nerve is helpful in prognosticating recovery and planning treatment when facial paralysis becomes complete. Patients with incomplete paralysis have a favorable prognosis for recovery and therefore do not require electrical testing. A full description of the tests is found in an earlier chapter.

Evoked EMG (ENoG) and EMG testing are most valuable for prognosticating spontaneous recovery and guiding management. In assessing diseases affecting the intratemporal facial nerve, electrical testing measures downfield potentials, and results are interpreted with the assumption that the extent of facial muscle denervation is closely related to the extent of neural degeneration. This basic assumption introduces a small degree of predictive variability with functional outcomes and should therefore be interpreted with caution. Within the first 72 hours after onset of complete paralysis, before Wallerian degeneration is complete, downfield electrical testing may be normal. The subsequent rate of decline in evoked responses is predictive of severity of nerve injury. In addition, evoked compound muscle action potentials measured on evoked EMG/ENoG testing rely on synchronous firing of the facial nerve, which may be absent in the early phases of neural regeneration. ENoG results may therefore underestimate extent of recovery and must be correlated with spontaneous EMG activity.

EMG testing is valuable at any point after the onset of complete facial paralysis. After 2–3 weeks, the presence of polyphasic potentials is indicative of neural regeneration and hint of favorable recovery, whereas fibrillations suggest muscle denervation and poor recovery.

Imaging Studies

Imaging studies may be helpful in some patients with facial paralysis. The clinical history and physical examination will often times dictate, which scan should be obtained. Gadolinium-enhanced MRI scan of the facial nerve is valuable when the clinical presentation is atypical for Bell's palsy. This includes progressive paresis beyond 2–3 weeks, selective paralysis of isolated branches of the facial nerve, no sign of recovery by 4 months, recurrent palsy, hyperkinesis, multiple cranial nerve involvement and presence of a mass lesion or underlying malignancy. Routine imaging for Bell's palsy is much more controversial since it does not prognosticate recovery or impact clinical management decision making. Most clinicians agree that imaging should be obtained for Bell's palsy only if the patient shows no signs of recovery 4–6 months after onset of palsy.

In Bell's palsy, enhancement of the perigeniculate and labyrinthine facial nerve is visualized (Fig. 38.6).[15] The severity of enhancement has no prognostic implications and enhancement typically lags behind clinical recovery.[16,17] MRI scan of the facial nerve and brain is also indicated if concurrent intracranial injury or infection is suspected or being evaluated.

In patients with a history of trauma, ear infection, cholesteatoma, or prior ear surgery, a dedicated temporal bone CT scan without contrast is helpful. Intravenous

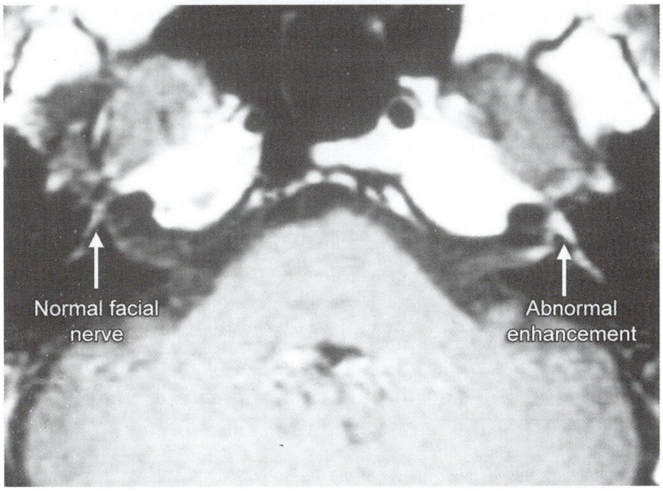

Fig. 38.6: Gadolinium-enhanced magnetic resonance imaging scan of the facial nerve demonstrating enhancement of the left perigeniculate facial nerve extending into the internal auditory canal in Bell's palsy.

contrast is indicated only if an abscess suspected. In some instances, both CT and MR imaging may be indicated.

Other imaging studies that may be relevant for evaluating facial paralysis based on clinical history or examination include chest X-ray for sarcoidosis, and technetium radioisotope and gallium scans for malignant otitis externa.

Audiometric Testing

Since hearing loss can occur with a variety of diseases causing facial paralysis, routine audiometric testing is prudent for both diagnosis and management of these patients. When surgical treatment is being entertained, the status of hearing in the affected ear influences the selection of surgical approach used.

Laboratory and Miscellaneous Testing

Laboratory testing is indicated only when specific diagnoses are suspected based on presenting clinical features. A complete blood count and metabolic profile are helpful for evaluating systemic diseases and extensive infections. Specialized testing for erythrocyte sedimentation rate (malignant otitis externa), Lyme titers, angiotensin converting enzyme (sarcoidosis), cerebrospinal fluid analysis (sarcoidosis, Guillain-Barré syndrome) may be obtained as indicated.

Tissue biopsy is often indicated if clinical examination reveals an obvious head and neck masses. Diagnosis of sarcoidosis can be readily confirmed by the presence of typical noncaseating granulomas with multinucleate giant cells. Inflammatory ear disease can be differentiated from malignant diseases as treatment varies considerably.

TREATMENT

Medical Treatment

Eye Care

Eye care remains a priority in the management of patients with facial paralysis who experience incomplete eye closure. The lagophthalmos along with reduced blink, decreased tearing, and sometimes lower lid ectropion, often result in dry eye symptoms, which may include eye pain, itching, redness, discomfort, and visual impairment. Exposure keratopathy, corneal abrasion, and corneal ulceration may lead to corneal scarring and permanent loss of vision.[18] Aggressive eye lubrication and use of a moisture chamber are recommended to maintain hydration of the corneal surface. Caution should be exercised with patching of the eye as corneal abrasion is possible, especially if concurrent trigeminal nerve dysfunction exists. If early recovery is not anticipated, consideration should be given to placing an eyelid spring, upper eyelid weight, or temporary tarsorrhaphy. Any hint of exposure keratitis should prompt an immediate ophthalmology consultation for definitive management.

Steroids

The use of systemic steroids in treatment of Bell's palsy has been supported by several randomized controlled trials demonstrating reduced recovery time, improved functional outcomes, and reduced long-term sequelae compared with placebo treatment when administered early in the course of the disease.[19-24] The presumed mechanism of action is its anti-inflammatory effect on neural edema. With steroid treatment alone, up to 94.4% of patients with Bell's palsy had full recovery of function at 9 months, compared with 81.6% of patients who did not receive steroids.[19] Treatment should be initiated within 72 hours of onset of paralysis/paresis.

With HZO, systemic steroids are thought to relieve acute pain, reduce vertigo, and minimize postherpetic neuralgia despite their questionable role in reversing the disease process. Unless otherwise contraindicated, systemic steroids may also be used for treatment of acute facial palsy associated with otitis media, trauma, and systemic diseases, although literature supporting such treatment is less robust. Regardless of etiology, similar dosing schedules are used for treatment of acute facial palsy. A 10–14 day taper starting with a dose of 60 mg/day is typically prescribed.

Known risks of systemic steroid treatment include blood glucose and blood pressure elevation, mood swings, acute psychosis and rarely, avascular necrosis of the femoral head. Systemic steroids should be used with caution in diabetics and immunocompromised patients. Such patients should be management in consultation with their internists to assure close monitoring for adverse effects of treatment.

Antiviral Therapy

Antiviral therapy in combination with oral steroids early in the course of the Bell's palsy result in shorter recovery times, although the improvement in functional outcomes compared with steroid therapy alone are controversial.[19,20,22,23] Some reports suggest a small but statistically insignificant long-term functional outcome with combination therapy in Bell's palsy. Antiviral monotherapy has not been found to improve recovery compared with placebo and is inferior to steroids alone for Bell's palsy.[20,25] Combination therapy with steroids and antivirals has been found to improve clinical outcomes in HZO.[26] Valcyclovir 500 mg, given three times a day for 7 days, is preferred over acyclovir since it is a prodrug, which achieves a bioavailability level 3–5 times that of acyclovir. Side effects related to antiviral therapy are predominantly gastrointestinal including nausea, vomiting, diarrhea, but can occasionally include renal failure and hepatic failure.[27]

Antibiotics

Antibiotic therapy directed at the appropriate organism is indicated in infectious bacterial etiologies for facial palsy. Broad-spectrum coverage with augmented penicillins or cephalosporins is appropriate for acute suppurative otitis media where the common pathogens include *Haemophilus influenzae*, *Streptococcus pneumoniae*, and *Moraxella catarrhalis*. In chronic otitis media, quinolone therapy is appropriate for suspected *Pseudomonas aeruginosa* infections. Quinolone-associated tendinopathy and arthropathy may occur in older patients and those who are undergoing concurrent therapy with systemic steroids. Confirmed Lyme disease requires treatment with a 4-week course of doxycycline to prevent late complications of the disease.

Analgesics

Postherpetic neuralgia is known to occur with HZO and can be prolonged and incapacitating. It is treated with opioid analgesics, gabapentin, tramadol, and pregabalin.[28] Pain management may also be necessary with other causes of facial paralysis such as Bell's palsy, suppurative otitis media, malignant otitis media, trauma, and metastatic malignancies.

Adjunctive Therapies

There is no high-quality evidence to support the clinical benefit of massage therapy, facial exercises, acupuncture, or electrical stimulation for facial paralysis.[29] However, given the concomitant lack of evidence demonstrating harm with these treatment modalities, any of these adjunctive measures may be offered to the patient if skilled therapists are available for these therapies.

Surgical Treatment

Bell's Palsy

Surgical decompression of the facial nerve for Bell's palsy remains controversial. Response to treatment with systemic steroids assumes that neural edema and subsequent entrapment neuropathy result in facial nerve dysfunction in Bell's palsy. This has led to the theory that surgical decompression would be of some benefit. Esslen and Fisch demonstrated that when 95% of the facial nerve had degenerated, the patient had a 50% chance of poor outcome with residual facial weakness and synkinesis.[30] Proponents for surgical decompression endeavor to improve the odds of favorable recovery in this subset of patients.

The site of pathology in Bell's palsy has evolved over the decades from the mastoid segment to the meatal segment of the facial nerve. Earlier efforts focused on transmastoid decompression of the facial nerve for Bell's palsy.[31] This approach has fallen out of favor since several randomized controlled studies have reported lack of improved outcomes.[32] Fisch reported intraoperative findings of nerve edema proximal to the geniculate ganglion in 94% of patients who underwent combined transmastoid and middle fossa facial nerve decompression.[33] In 1999, Gantz reported on a prospective multi-institutional trial supporting middle fossa decompression of the facial nerve reported improved functional outcomes in surgically treated patients with poor prognostic indicators for recovery.[34] Patients who had >90% degeneration on ENoG and had no spontaneous EMG activity within 14 days of onset of paralysis were offered surgical decompression. Ninety-one percent of 34 surgically treated patients achieved House-Brackmann grade I-II function. Of the 36 control subjects with similar electrical test results who elected not to undergo surgery, 58% had persistent weakness at 7 months (House-Brackmann grades III-IV).

Middle fossa decompression of the meatal foramen and labyrinthine facial nerve is now advocated by many for Bell's palsy patients who have ≥90% degeneration on ENoG testing within the first 14 days of onset of complete paralysis and absence of motor unit action potentials on voluntary EMG testing. In those with poor or no hearing in the affected ear, a translabyrinthine approach is used. The risk of iatrogenic facial nerve injury, sensorineural hearing loss, dizziness, cerebrospinal fluid leak, meningitis, and cerebrovascular events related to craniotomy surgery and facial nerve decompression must be weighed heavily against the potential benefit of improved long-term functional outcomes. The lack consensus on the role of surgical decompression for Bell's palsy is mostly attributed to the paucity of high-quality evidence supporting this treatment.[35]

Otitis Media

In acute suppurative otitis media associated with acute facial palsy, a wide field myringotomy with or without tube placement, is indicated for drainage of middle ear purulence, in addition to medical treatment with steroids, systemic antibiotics, and topical antibiotics. Cultures of fluid aspirated from the middle ear help direct antibiotic therapy in the course of treatment.

In chronic otitis media with or without cholesteatoma, definitive surgery for removal of cholesteatoma and granulation tissue is the treatment of choice. In addition, decompression of the affected facial nerve segment may be necessary. Rarely, when cholesteatoma extensively involves the facial nerve, exteriorization of the cholesteatoma is indicated.

Tumors

The most common neoplasms causing facial paralysis are malignant tumors of the parotid gland. Facial nerve neuroma, acoustic neuroma, and primary brain tumors are less common causes of facial paralysis. Surgical management is dictated by tumor pathology and is described in detail in other chapters of this textbook.

Temporal Bone Trauma

In temporal bone fractures, the facial nerve is most commonly violated in the perigeniculate region with temporal bone fractures. When facial paralysis is immediate and complete, nerve transection is suspected and surgical exploration for repair is indicated when the patient is clinically stable. The location of the fracture largely determines the surgical approach in these cases.

Iatrogenic Trauma

Iatrogenic facial nerve trauma is best prevented by acquiring a thorough knowledge of its anatomical course. Injuries to the facial nerve detected at the time of surgery should be addressed immediately. Surgical decompression of the fallopian canal 1 cm proximal and distal to the site of an injury is usually adequate if the nerve is intact but contused. The epineurium may be incised if the significant neural edema is noted. If > 50% of the nerve has been transected, repair is warranted using primary neurorrhaphy or interposition grafting. If facial nerve paralysis is unexpected and noted immediately in the recovery room, any packing in the ear should be removed and the patient should be observed for several hours to allow for any effect of lidocaine used during the procedure to dissipate. Operative trauma to the facial nerve must be suspected if the facial paralysis persists beyond this observation period. Neural integrity can also be confirmed by the presence of voluntary motor unit action potentials on needle EMG testing in the immediate postoperative period. Surgical exploration for suspected iatrogenic trauma should be performed within 24–48 hours.

Delayed facial paralysis occurring after any surgery is usually a result of neural edema and secondary entrapment neuropathy. Packing should be removed from the ear canal and mastoid cavity to relieve any compressive effects on the facial nerve. Since the prognosis for recovery with delayed facial paralysis following surgery, additional exploratory surgery is not required.

Every effort should be made to restore the continuity of a severed nerve. A tension-free primary anastomosis is the preferred neurorrhaphy technique. If any tension occurs at the anastomotic site, an interposition nerve graft has a better chance of providing facial movement. All nerve repair techniques produce synkinesis, but sphincteric function of the mouth and eye are usually restored. When an interposition graft is required, the greater auricular nerve or sural nerve is the preferred graft donor sites.

PROGNOSIS

Although acute facial paralysis can be frightening for patients, with proper diagnosis and treatment, the long-term functional outcomes are generally good with minimal or no sequelae. Bell's palsy remains a diagnosis of exclusion and due diligence must be exercised when evaluating patients with facial paralysis.

Regardless of etiology, incomplete facial paralysis portends a favorable prognosis. Close clinical surveillance is essential if facial paresis progresses. Serial electrical testing over the first 2 weeks after onset of complete paralysis will help guide patient management and counseling. If no functional recovery is evident 3–6 months after onset of complete paralysis, imaging should be done to rule out an underlying tumor. Long-term follow-up is recommended for patients with facial paralysis so that any remaining sequelae of facial nerve dysfunction may be appropriately managed.

REFERENCES

1. Sunderland S. A classification of peripheral nerve injuries producing loss of function. Brain. 1951;74(4):491-516.
2. Baugh RF, Basur GJ, Iahii LE, et al. Clinical practice guideline: Bell's palsy. Otolaryngol Head Neck Surg. 2013;149 (3 Suppl):S1-27.
3. Adour KK, Byl FM, Hilsinger RL, et al. The true nature of Bell's palsy: analysis of 1,000 consecutive patients. Laryngoscope. 1978;88:787-801.
4. Peitersen E. The natural history of Bell's palsy. Am J Otol. 1982;4:107-11.
5. Murakami S, Mizobuchi M, Nakashiro Y, et al. Bell palsy and herpes simplex virus; identification of viral DNA in endoneural fluid and muscle. Ann Intern Med. 1996;124 (1 pt 1):27-30.
6. Peitersen E. Bell's palsy: the spontaneous course of 2,500 peripheral facial nerve palsies of different etiologies. Acta Otolaryngol. 2002;(Suppl 549):4-30.
7. Di Martino E, Sellhaus B, Haensel J, et al. Fallopian canal dehiscences: a survey of clinical and anatomical findings. Eur Arch Otorhinolaryngol. 2005;262(2):120-6.
8. Makeham TP, Croxson GR, Coulson S. Infective causes of facial nerve paralysis. Otol Neurotol. 2007;28(1):100-3.
9. Quaranta N, Cassano M, Quaranta A. Facial paralysis associated with cholesteatoma: a review of 13 cases. Otol Neurotol. 2007;28(3):405-7.
10. Soudry E, Hamazany Y, Preis M. Malignant external otitis: analysis of severe cases. Otolaryngol Head Neck Surg. 2011; 144(5):758-62.
11. Rivera-Serrano CM, Man LX, Klein S, et al. Melkersson-Rosenthal syndrome: a facial nerve center perspective. J Plast Reconstr Aesthet Surg. 2014;67(8):1050-4.

12. Graham MD, Kemink JL. Total facial nerve decompression in recurrent facial paralysis and the Melkersson-Rosenthal Syndrome: a preliminary report. Am J Otol. 1986;7(1):34-7.
13. Hanissian AS, Fuste F, Hayes WT, et al. Moebius syndrome in twins. Am J Dis Child. 1970;120:472-5.
14. Pitner SE, Edwards JE, McCormick WF. Observations on the pathology of the Möbius syndrome. J Neurol Neurosurg Psychiat. 1965;28:362-74.
15. Schwaber MK, Larson TC, Zealear DL, et al. Gadolinium-enhanced magnetic resonance imaging in Bell's palsy. Laryngoscope. 1990;100:1264-9.
16. Engstrom M, Abdsaleh S, Ahlstrom H, et al. Serial gadolinium-enhanced magnetic resonance imaging and assessment of facial nerve function in Bell's palsy. Otolaryngol Head Neck Surg. 1997;117(5):559-66.
17. Jonsson L, Tien R, Engstrom M, et al. Gd-DPTA enhanced MRI in Bell's palsy and herpes zoster oticus: an overview and implications for future studies. Acta Otolaryngol. 1995;115(5):577-84.
18. Bhatti MT, Schiffman JS, Pass AF, et al. Neuro-ophthalmologic complications and manifestations of upper and lower motor neuron facial paresis. Curr Neurol Neurosci Rep. 2010;10:448-58.
19. Sullivan FM, Swan IRC, Donnan PT, et al. Early treatment with prednisolone or acyclovir in Bell's palsy. N Engl J Med. 2007;357:1598-607.
20. Engstrom M, Berg T, Stjernquist-Desatnik A, et al. Prenisolone and valaciclovir in Bell's palsy: a randomized, double-blind, placebo-controlled, multicenter trial. Lancet Neurol. 2008;7:993-1000.
21. Berg T, Bylund N, Marsk E, et al. The effect of prednisolone on sequelae in Bell's palsy. Arch Otolaryngol Head Neck Surg. 2012;138(5):445-9.
22. Axelsson S, Berg T, Jonsson L, et al. Bell's palsy-the effect of prednisolone and/or valacyclovir versus placebo in relation to baseline severity in a randomized controlled trial. Clin Otolaryngol. 2012;37:283-90.
23. Grogan PM, Gronseth GS. Practice parameter: steroids, acyclovir, and surgery for Bell's palsy (an evidenced-based review): report of the Quality Standards Subcommittee of the American Academy of Neurology). Neurology. 2001;56(7):830-6.
24. Gronseth GS, Paduga R. Evidence-based guideline update: steroids and antivirals for Bell's palsy: report of the Guideline Development Subcommittee of the American Academy of Neurology. Neurology. 2012;79:2209-13.
25. Lockhart P, Daly F, Pitkethly M, et al. Antiviral treatment for Bell's palsy (idiopathic facial paralysis). Cochrane Database Syst Rev. 2009;(4):CD001869.
26. De Ru, JA, van Bentham PP. Combination therapy is preferable for patients with Ramsey Hunt Syndrome. Otol Neurotol. 2011;32(5):852-5.
27. Allen D, Dunn. Aciclovir or valaciclovir for Bell's palsy (idiopathic facial paralysis. Cochrane Database Syst Rev. 2004;(3):CD001869.
28. Hempenstall K, Nurmikko TJ, Johnson RW, et al. Analgesic therapy in postherpetic neuralgia: a quantitative systematic review. PLoS Med. 2005;2(7):e164.
29. Teixeira LJ, Valbuza JS, Prado GF. Physical therapy for Bell's palsy (idiopathic facial paralysis). Cochrane Database Syst Rev. 2011;7(12):CD006283.
30. Fisch U. Surgery for Bell's palsy. Arch Otolaryngol. 1981;107:1-11.
31. May M, Blumenthal F, Taylor FH. Bell's palsy: surgery based on prognostic indicators and results. Larygoscope. 1981;91:2092-103.
32. McAllister K, Walker D, Donnan PT, et al. Surgical interventions for the early management of Bell's palsy. Cochrane Database Syst Rev. 2013;(10):CD007468.
33. Fisch U, Esslen E. Total intratemporal exposure of the facial nerve. Pathologic findings in Bell's palsy. Arch Otolaryngol. 1972;95:335-41.
34. Gantz BJ, Rubenstein JT, Gidley P, et al. Surgical management of Bell's palsy. Laryngoscope. 1999;109(8):1177-88.
35. Smouha E, Toh E, Schaitkin BM. Surgical treatment of Bell's palsy: current attitudes. Laryngoscope. 2011;121:1965-70.

CHAPTER 39

Facial Nerve Tumors

Gregory J Basura, H Alexander Arts

INTRODUCTION

Facial nerve tumors are quite rare and often not considered as a potential etiology of facial paralysis. As a result, delays in diagnosis and treatment of patients afflicted with these lesions are frequent. It is critical that neoplasms, either arising from or affecting the facial nerve, be included in the differential diagnosis of facial paralysis.

Neoplasms affecting the facial nerve present in multiple ways. Progressive facial weakness is the most common physical finding, followed by hearing loss, often secondary to lesion extension into the middle ear. In patients with facial nerve tumors, approximately 97% present with some degree of insidious facial nerve deficit.[19] The spectrum of motor deficit ranges from barely perceptible to complete facial paralysis, and can also include hemifacial spasm. The facial weakness is always ipsilateral to the lesion, and is typically slow and insidious in onset. On occasion, the facial weakness can spontaneously recover, and may even present as a recurrent, ipsilateral paralysis. Slow, insidious onset of weakness, or recurrent weakness, clinically distinguishes a paralysis from a facial nerve tumor from Bell's palsy (idiopathic peripheral facial paralysis), by far the most common cause of facial paralysis. While the majority of patients with Bell's palsy show spontaneous and near complete facial recovery within 8–12 weeks, those with facial nerve tumors rarely experience spontaneous recovery.

The facial nerve can be affected by neoplasms at any location along the course of the nerve. It is convenient to subdivide facial nerve tumors by their relationship to the nerve (*intrinsic or extrinsic*) and by its general location (*intracranial, intratemporal, or extratemporal*).

Intrinsic tumors arise from the facial nerve itself and are virtually always schwannomas or neurofibromas. Tumors primarily arising from the facial nerve are referred to as *peripheral nerve sheath tumors.* These usually arise from Schwann cells, but can arise from fibroblast supporting cells of the endoneurium or the epithelial-like cells of the perineurium. Terms like *neuroma* or *neurinoma* are nonspecific and have no histopathologic correlate.

Extrinsic facial nerve tumors arise from nonfacial nerve tissues and secondarily infiltrate the nerve. These lesions can include primary tumors adjacent to the facial nerve, metastases, or systemic or diffuse malignancies such as leukemia or carcinomatous meningitis.

PATHOPHYSIOLOGY

Neoplasms Intrinsic to the Facial Nerve

Facial nerve *schwannomas* or neuromas are tumors that arise from the Schwann cell or supporting structures.[52] It has been traditionally considered that these tumors arise from sensory fibers within the facial nerve, yet no histopathologic evidence directly supports this hypothesis. These tumors often appear as interlacing bundles of spindle-shaped cells arranged in palisades with two patterns commonly recognized: Antoni A (comprising densely cellular areas with cohesive cells arranged in regular patterns) and Antoni B (demonstrating areas of vacuolation between cells secondary to accumulation of extracellular matrix). Regardless of type, Schwann cells can undergo many cytologic configurations called "ancient change" whereby many nuclear pleomorphisms and changes in hyperchromicity without mitotic changes can be seen. Whorled arrangements of cells called Verocay bodies are sometimes seen. None of these histologic features appear to have any clinical prognostic value. S-100 is a calcium-binding protein that is found in both normal and neoplastic Schwann cells, and immunostaining for this protein is a helpful and is often used for pathological confirmation.

Facial nerve schwannomas can involve any segment of the facial nerve from the pontomedullary junction to the parotid gland,[44] with the highest incidence in the internal auditory canal (IAC) and cerebellopontine angle (CPA). Certainly "atypical" facial nerve tumors may arise involving a variety of facial nerve segments and consist of diverse histology.[50] Schwannomas typically grow very slowly. When measured by tumor diameter, growth rates range from 0 to 3 mm/year on average.[22] Spontaneous involution has been rarely seen.[22] They typically arise eccentrically on the facial nerve compressing the adjacent nerve trunk that can often be surgically removed. While almost entirely benign in presentation, malignant varieties have been reported. Janeck and Conley[25] reported that of 30 facial nerve schwannomas they encountered, 26 (87%) were benign, while 4 (13%) were malignant.

In addition to direct facial nerve involvement along the entire course, schwannomas of the temporal bone may also invade adjacent bony structures. Of 48 patients with schwannomas a mass behind the tympanic membrane was seen in 14 (29%). Diagnostic imaging of these patients revealed that the tumors typically involved more than one segment of the facial nerve and eroded otic capsule bone also in 14 (29%) patients. Schwannomas have not classically been shown to erode adjacent otic capsule bone to produce asymptomatic fistulas of either the cochlea or the labyrinth. Saito[51] reported a small tympanic segment schwannoma that had autodecompressed the surrounding fallopian canal with erosion and extension into the middle ear. The specific locations for tumors occurrence along the course of the facial nerve included the labyrinthine segment (16%), the geniculate ganglion (22%), the tympanic segment (21%), mastoid segment (21%), and were extratemporal (7%).[44] A separate review revealed that intratemporal tumors are the most common while intracranial tumors are the least common.[53] Importantly, facial nerve schwannomas should not be clinically confused with Jacobson's nerve schwannomas that lie in close proximity but maintain distinction from the tympanic portion of the facial nerve.[29] It is also rare that a discrete facial nerve schwannoma will involve the nervusintermedius,[32] the greater superficial branch,[41] or the chorda tympani.[9] Within the temporal bone, facial nerve tumors often display a predilection for the geniculate ganglion.[12,44] One possible explanation is related to the structural reorganization of the nerve that takes place at that location[18] as this area marks the junction between the intracranial portion of the nerve [enclosed in a variable degree of cerebrospinal fluid (CSF)] and the true intratemporal nerve with a fascicular arrangement caused by an ingrowth of connective tissue at the ganglion.

A review of 1400 temporal bones investigating the incidence of facial nerve schwannomas found only one within the labyrinthine segment in a patient who also had a facial paralysis and a concurrent vestibular schwannoma.[26] Facial nerve schwannomas being the most common have been shown in an autopsy series within the temporal bone to be approximately 0.8%.[57]

Neurofibromas are thought to arise from endoneurial connective tissue and infrequently arise from the nerve roots of other cranial nerves, yet are more commonly found on peripheral nerves within the subcutaneous tissues. These lesions are often associated with von Recklinghausen's disease. Because they arise intrinsically within nerves, complete removal usually requires a total nerve resection .[22]

Granular cell tumors originate from Schwann cells and are typically confined within the confines of the nerve sheath, which may serve as a pseudocapsule for the lesion. They have a predilection for the upper respiratory tract with a higher incidence in women and African Americans.[39] The tumor itself consists of multiple sheaths of cells within an eosinophilic granular cytoplasm. The formal diagnosis is made histologically as the tumor granules stain robustly with periodic acid-Schiff.

Traumatic facial nerve neuromas are non-neoplastic proliferations of the facial nerve and typically arise from an aggressive reparative response to neural injury. Histologically, these lesions are composed of disrupted axons, Schwann cells, and endoneurial and epineurial cells within a collagenous matrix. Specific to the facial nerve, neuromas may arise following injury to the face or head. Conversely, traumatic neuromas may result from chronic inflammatory responses adjacent to a dehiscent segment of the nerve resulting in a large proliferation of the connective tissue and neural elements.[59] Other forms may be secondary to granulation tissue from schwannomas or an inflammatory neuroma from complicated chronic suppurative otitis media when there is no documented associated temporal bone trauma.[60]

EXTRINSIC LESIONS

Intratemporal

Facial nerve *hemangiomas* are rare tumors that typically arise from the intracanalicular or geniculate segment of the facial nerve. First described in 1901,[35] these benign vascular tumors are thought to arise from fibrous capillary networks and have been well documented within the geniculate ganglion of the facial nerve.[5] Being characterized as benign venous malformations due to the absence of internal elastic lamina on histological evaluation,[1,7] these tumors are thought to arise directly from cellular hyperplasia versus vascular malformations that originate from errors in vascular morphogenesis.[7] Unlike schwannomas, they are not considered to be true neoplasms; rather, they are vascular hamartomas composed of blood vessels. In human temporal bones, increased vessel counts have been found along the geniculate ganglion with fewer counts located at other facial nerve segments including the labyrinthine.[5] It has therefore been hypothesized that the rich vascular plexus around Scarpa's and geniculate ganglia is the nidus for increased frequency of hemangiomas in these regions.[18] These lesions typically present in midlife with equal distribution between males and females.

Like schwannomas, facial nerve hemangiomas also typically arise eccentrically from the nerve, often allowing for the physical separation of these tumors without compromising the continuity or integrity of the main trunk.[5,56] Unlike schwannomas, hemangiomas can lead to facial paralysis with even very small tumors only millimeters in size. Interestingly, the size of the lesion is not directly correlated to the extent of the facial nerve deficit, with small (<10mm) tumors leading to substantial deficits. This concept supports the "vascular steal" phenomenon and the resultant ischemic changes of the facial nerve trunk in the absence of any compressive forces from small tumors. This is thought to occur from blood flow to the highly vascular facial nerve being detoured toward the tumor leading to ischemia.[7,54] It is this concept that supports the notion that facial nerve schwannomas of comparable size lead to less facial nerve dysfunction.[36] While once considered a rare tumor, these lesions have increasingly been diagnosed and in some reports are more commonly found than facial nerve schwannomas.

Paragangliomas or chemodectomas may directly invade the facial nerve. These lesions arise from derivatives of neural crest cells. They can originate from paraganglionic tissue at the carotid bifurcation (*carotid body tumor*), jugular foramen (*glomus jugulare*), vagus nerve (*glomus vagale*), or tympanic plexus (*glomus tympanicum*;[33]). They often arise sporadically or can be associated with hereditary syndromes including MEN type II, von Hippel-Lindau, and NF1[33] with 80% of hereditary and 20% of sporadic lesions presenting with multiple lesions. These tumors often present with facial paralysis or pulsatile tinnitus. Management is largely based on the size and level of nerve infiltration, with conservative management being a high consideration.[49]

Rare tumors of the facial nerve, including paragangliomas, were presented in a landmark paper by Guild in 1941.[45] The initial theory proposed that tumors arose from Arnold's nerve (auricular branch of the vagus nerve) that merges with the facial nerve near the stylomastoid foramen; a common conduit for glomus jugulare and tympanicum tumors.[13] Other rare causes of facial nerve paresis from tumor infiltration at the intratemporal level include epidermoid (cholesteatoma), metastatic disease, and direct malignant invasion (carcinoma, mucoepidermoid carcinoma, squamous cell carcinoma).[20]

Primary *temporal bone malignancy* typically consists of squamous cell carcinomas of the external ear canal that may infiltrate to the adjacent tympanic and mastoid portions of the facial nerve. Facial paresis or paralysis is typically secondary to frank infiltration of the fallopian canal and nerve with significant destruction of the surrounding periosteal bone, while endochondral bone remains somewhat resistant (Fig. 39.1A). Other potential malignant tumors that may infiltrate the facial nerve include papillary adenocarcinoma,[11] malignant melanoma,[63] lymphoma,[4] and adenoid cystic carcinoma that typically present with perineural invasion.

Chondrosarcoma is a rare and aggressive malignancy that often arises near the petrous bone. It arises from chondrocytes located typically in foramen lacerum or the petroclival synchondrosis, yet can also be located adjacent to the sphenopetrosal, petrooccipital, and spheno-occipital syncondroses. As such, these tumors often arise off of the midline near the parasellar region, petrous apex, or CPA. Because chondrosarcomas arise from these locations, it has been hypothesized that the cartilages at these junctions serve as progenitors for these tumors. Alternatively, it has been postulated that these tumors arise from fibroblasts, or pluripotent cells of the dura or temporal bone. Chondrosarcomas may infiltrate most cranial nerves and affect those typically near their point of origin. Common symptoms that predate the diagnosis include headache, hearing loss, hoarseness, or diplopia. More common

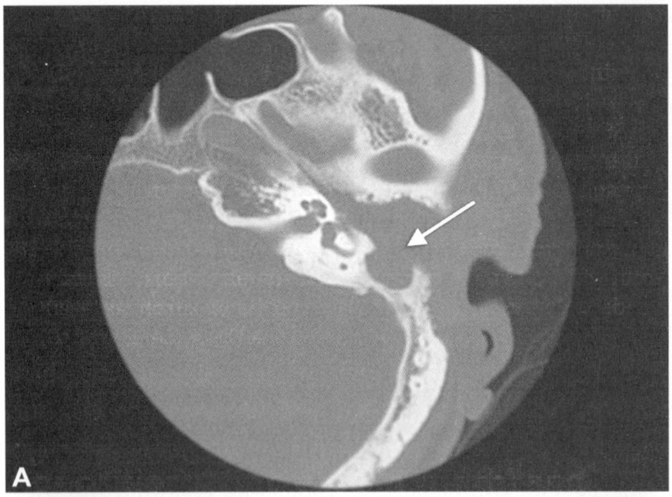

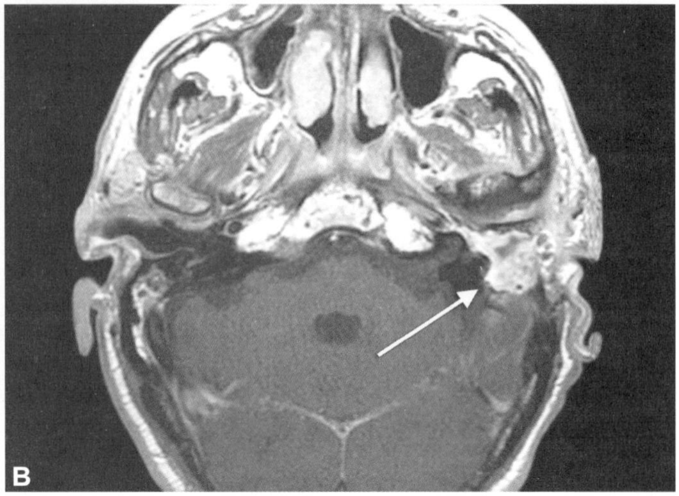

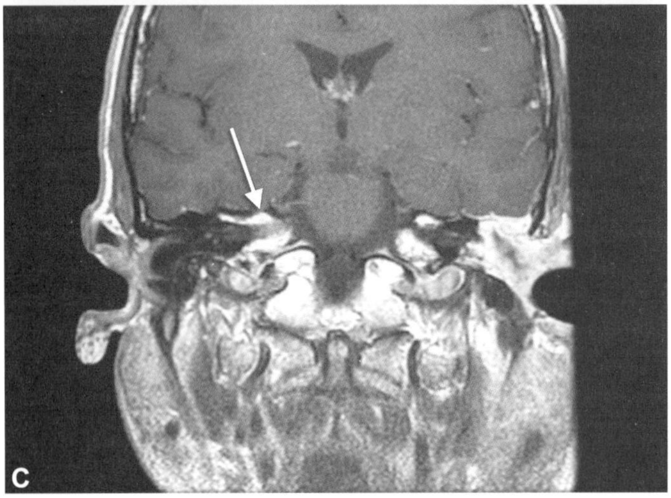

Figs. 39.1A to C: Squamous cell carcinoma of the temporal bone. Part (A) shows an axial sequence through the temporal bone. Note the soft tissue infiltration and frank bone erosion (arrow). While not entirely diagnostic, frank erosion on computed tomography (CT) is often indicative of malignancy. Parts (B) (axial) and (C) (coronal) show T1-weighted magnetic resonance imagings (MRIs) of squamous cell carcinoma of the temporal bone. Note the enhancement of the lesion (B) as well as the infiltration into surrounding structures including the middle fossa dura (C; arrows).

symptoms at the time of diagnosis include decreased visual acuity, facial weakness, tinnitus, and dysphagia. The most commonly affected cranial nerves are the abducens, occulomotor, vagus, and the glossopharyngeal.[22]

With approximately 100 cases of temporal bone chondrosarcoma reported, the natural growth rates are not well documented. Both computed tomography (CT) and magnetic resonance imaging (MRI) are necessary to evaluate a lesion at the skull base. CT scans are superior at illustrating the bony destruction of the skull base and areas of calcification often exemplified by these tumors that give them a classic "popcorn" appearance. MRI is superior for soft tissue structures and chondrosarcomas are typically isodense on T1 and have increased signal intensity on T2. Gadolinium contrast leads to marked enhancement of the lesion that is most commonly heterogeneous in pattern. Surgical extirpation is the main treatment modality and adjunctive radiotherapy has been utilized for residual tumor or microscopic disease. Chemotherapy is unproven and not recommended for these tumors.[21]

Metastatic disease has a particular proclivity for the rich vascularity of the marrow spaces of the petrous apex of the temporal bone. Hematogenous spread of lesions from the breast, kidney, lung, gastrointestinal tract, and rarely from other sites like the prostate and skin may be found in the petrous apex. Interestingly, in approximately half of patients with metastatic lesions involving the fallopian canal, no significant facial paralysis has been observed.[52] However, 6 of 14 patients with metastatic lesions to the temporal bone demonstrated paralysis that directly correlated with a disruption of the nerve sheath or was concurrent with extensive intracranial extension. The most common sites for temporal bone metastatic involvement are the IAC, mastoid, and the tympanic and labyrinthine segments, with the greatest risk of facial paralysis occurring with involvement of the labyrinthine segment.

Leukemia/Lymphoma may also involve the temporal bone and facial nerve. The process by which leukemia affects the temporal bone is through direct infiltration and hemorrhage.[47] Interestingly, inner ear infiltration by leukemia is quite rare.[8] Paparella et al.[47] found that in 19 patients with invasion of the temporal bone by acute leukemia, 9 patients had evidence of facial nerve involvement with only 1 patient showing violation of the labyrinth. This finding is supported by Berlinger et al.[8] who reported that infiltration of the facial and vestibulocochlear nerves is "not rare" in leukemia. Interestingly, facial paralysis has been reported as either the initial presenting sign of leukemia[66] or as a sign of leukemia relapse after treatment.[2]

Similar to patients with leukemia, those suffering from lymphoma often show infiltration within the temporal bone. These patients will also show malignant cellular infiltration, hemorrhage, and edema of the middle ear that can also predispose patients to middle ear effusions and infections. This was confirmed on 16 temporal bones from patients with lymphoma that revealed malignant cell infiltration of the marrow spaces with perivascular invasion and involvement of the facial and vestibulocochlear nerves.[48]

In cases of leukemia or lymphoma, evaluation by hematology/oncology is required for an accurate and specific diagnosis and staging of the disease. The subsequent treatment is then largely based on cell type, symptoms, and disease extent. In the case of facial nerve paralysis, eye protection is paramount while systemic therapy is being rendered. Superimposed diagnosed middle ear infections are commonly treated with antibiotics as they would be without concurrent hematologic malignancy.

Childhood: Neoplastic involvement of the facial nerve is rare in children and when present is largely isolated to lesions including cerebellar astrocytomas, leukemia, and rhabdomyosarcoma.[11a] Facial paralysis in a child may be the presenting symptom in childhood leukemia,[66] while eosinophilic granuloma (Langerhans' cell histiocytosis) rarely leads to facial paralysis, despite extensive temporal bone extension.

Embryonal rhabdomyosarcomas make up approximately 4–8% of all malignant tumors of childhood and is the most common soft tissue sarcoma in children.[22] Within the temporal bone it accounts for approximately 30% of temporal bone sarcomas. In the head and neck rhabdomyosarcoma is almost exclusively a disease of children. It often presents as recalcitrant otitis media/mastoiditis, and physically may be found as an external ear canal aural polyp, frank bloody otorrhea, chronic otalgia and hearing loss. Facial paralysis has only been documented to present in 14% of cases as the tumor is quite aggressive and locally destructive.[22] While regional metastasis is rare, the tumor usually spreads through the temporal bone via the middle era cleft to the fallopian canal with facial nerve infiltration to therefore potentially extend to the IAC and onto intracranial locations. The current treatment for temporal bone rhabdomyosarcoma is surgical intervention for tissue biopsy followed by chemoradiation.[62]

Other less common sarcomas of childhood that may involve the temporal bone and facial nerve include Ewing's sarcoma, fibrosarcoma, osteogenic sarcoma and granulocytic sarcomas (choloromas). Unlike the treatment paradigms for rhabdomyosarcoma, the optimal treatment for nonrhabdomyosarcomas of the head and neck typically includes aggressive surgery with adjunctive radiotherapy reserved for cases of incomplete resection.[22]

EXTRATEMPORAL

Parotid Tumors

Extratemporal tumors involving the facial nerve are often isolated to the parotid gland. Salivary gland tumors as a whole occur fairly infrequently and typically account for only 3–4% of all head and neck neoplasms.[9a] The tendency for a malignancy arising within the parotid gland to involve the facial nerve is partially explained by the close anatomic location and to those tumors with a proclivity for perineural invasion. Tumors that arise within or metastasize to the parotid gland and are most likely to produce facial nerve dysfunction include undifferentiated carcinoma, squamous cell carcinoma, adenoid cystic carcinoma, adenocarcinoma, and high-grade mucoepidermoid carcinoma.[22] Within this group of tumors, the highest percentage leading to facial nerve involvement/dysfunction occurs in undifferentiated tumors (24%) followed by squamous cell tumors (19%), adenoid cystic (17%), adenocarcinoma (11%), and mucoepidermoid carcinomas (9%).[10,15] A more specific discussion about the nature of these tumors and each specific treatment modality is beyond the scope of this chapter.

Intracranial Tumors

Facial nerve *meningiomas* are exceedingly rare[37] and associations between progesterone, breast cancer, and radiation therapy have been made.[23] These lesions typically arise from arachnoid villi along the walls of the dural venous sinuses and near neural foramina of cranial nerves.

Extracranial extension of neural foramina meningiomas is even more rare. Facial nerve meningiomas are likely to arise from the arachnoid villi along the porus acusticus (opening between the CPA cistern and IAC) and embryological is justified in that fibers of the facial nerve exit the neural tube along the sheath of arachnoid and dura at 5 weeks of gestation. The arachnoid has the capacity to grow toward the geniculate ganglion and beyond as it fuses with the endoneurium.[30,43]

Astrocytomas (gliomas) arise from neuroepithelium and are typically found in the cerebral hemispheres, cerebellum or brainstem. They are graded I through IV with the latter being described as an aggressive and essentially uniformly fatal glioblastoma multiforme. Within the CPA, astrocytomas often extend from the fourth ventricle or grossly from the brainstem parenchyma. Exophytic forms can extend into the IAC and subsequent widening of the bony canal may falsely indicate a vestibular schwannoma and is therefore not diagnostic. Typical treatment consists of primary surgical resection with postoperative radiation. Survival rates after treatment are largely based on tumor grade.[22]

CLINICAL FINDINGS

Tumors of the facial nerve are rare and often misdiagnosed as idiopathic or consistent with Bell's palsy. Bell's palsy is the most common acute mononeuropathy affecting a single nerve, and is the most common diagnosis associated with facial nerve paresis (weakness) /paralysis (complete loss of movement).[6] In contrast to the insidious weakness associated with facial nerve tumors, Bell's palsy is a rapid unilateral facial nerve paresis or paralysis of unknown cause. Although typically self-limited, the facial paresis/paralysis that occurs in Bell's palsy may cause significant temporary oral incompetence and an inability to close the eyelid, leading to potential eye injury.

Facial nerve neoplasms generally present with milder symptoms including progressive facial weakness, recurrent palsies, facial twitching, and symptoms consistent with cochleovestibular dysfunction and potentially increased intracranial pressure. Occasionally, facial nerve tumors may present as an asymptomatic middle ear mass. On initial physical examination, patients with neoplasms of the facial nerve may present with a parotid mass or signs based on the specific response and site of the nerve to tumor compression or gross infiltration to adjacent structures (i.e. cochlea). Typically, the facial nerve is seemingly resistant to compressive forces, yet the most common presentation of facial nerve tumors is the insidious facial paralysis, often concurrent with facial musculature twitching. The initial paralysis/paresis may be intermittent and mislabeled as "recurrent Bell's palsy" that typically presents with a sudden facial paralysis, but a similar process is thought to occur in approximately one-third of patients with neoplastic involvement of the facial nerve.[38] In Bell's, a majority of patients show meaningful recovery within 8–12 weeks, therefore a search for a neoplastic process should be carried out if no signs of recovery are evident by that point. Conversely, insidious facial paralysis beyond 3 weeks is indicative of a neoplastic process and warrants a thorough workup. Interestingly, while the positive response to steroids supports a diagnosis of Bell's palsy, facial paralysis caused by a neoplasm may also positively respond to steroids and should not be overlooked and dismissed as an idiopathic cause. The important difference is the rapid (Bell's) versus insidious (facial nerve tumor) affects on the facial nerve when differentiating the two diagnoses.

Other presenting physical findings include sensorineural hearing loss, tinnitus (pulsatile and nonpulsatile) or vertigo if the tumor involves the labyrinthine portion of the facial nerve, leading to cochlear or vestibular symptoms secondary to adjacent structure extension. Aside from facial nerve paresis/paralysis, reports have revealed the most common symptoms being hearing loss (69%), tinnitus (60%), and vertigo (34%). Since Bell's palsy seldom presents with hearing loss, the combination of facial paralysis and hearing loss should heighten the clinical suspicion of a facial nerve lesion. Certainly, more ominous symptoms including facial and ear pain and the accompanying disturbance of facial nerve function warrant a more thorough clinical evaluation and workup. While pain may be a feature of Bell's palsy or Ramsay Hunt syndrome, pain may also be a major feature of malignancy secondary to trigeminal infiltration or extensive bone, dura or other cranial nerve involvement.

EVALUATION: NEUROTOLOGIC TESTING

Diagnosis of facial nerve tumors requires a thorough history and physical examination with specific emphasis on the facial nerve, otologic findings, the head and neck (particularly the parotid gland), and neurologic/cranial nerve status. A comprehensive examination of all facial nerve branches is important, and the House-Brackmann scale is recommended for initial documentation of any facial weakness following an insult. Evaluation of the eye,

eye closure, and protection of the cornea is of paramount importance. In conditions of incomplete eye closure, moisture chambers, artificial tears, and lid tightening procedures should be implemented to protect the underlying cornea from desiccation. Examination of the ear is mandatory during the workup of facial paralysis, and may reveal a mass in the middle ear cleft. Previous studies have demonstrated that a middle ear mass was present in 29% of all cases with facial paralysis, while less frequently a facial nerve tumor may present as an aural polyp, particularly if it arises from the descending portion of the facial nerve that ultimately may erode bone and present as a mass in the ear canal.[67] Gross features such as vascularity may help aid in diagnosis or warrant a transcanal biopsy in some cases. These patients may present with otitis externa or otitis media, resulting in a delayed diagnosis and further complications. Tuning fork examinations are often useful in categorizing the hearing loss into a conductive or sensorineural variety.[44] Thorough examination of the neck with particular attention to the parotid gland should be observed during the routine workup and considered closely in patients with facial paralysis. General examination of the neck, to especially exclude nodal disease, is essential and the use of fine needle aspiration may be beneficial in situations when warranted. Moreover, a comprehensive neurological examination is mandatory in patients with insidious facial paralysis, with particular attention to be paid to the lower cranial nerves and any evidence of cerebellar findings to suggest posterior-fossa involvement.

Formal audiometric testing should be obtained on all patients with facial paralysis, as subtle changes in hearing may not be appreciated by the patient. Typically, Bell's palsy does not present with concurrent hearing loss; therefore, audiology threshold changes in setting of facial nerve paralysis should alert the clinician of an alternative disease process. Certainly, if surgical intervention is planned, evaluation of hearing status is paramount in planning. Stapedial (acoustic) reflex testing should be considered due to the usefulness of the diagnostic information. The presence of a reflex in a patient with significant facial paralysis is suggestive of a lesion distal to the branch to the stapedius muscle and may orient the clinician to the location of the lesion. This measure is not always accurate and should be selectively interpreted in situations with a concurrent conductive hearing loss or with knowing that some fibers may be present and stimulated adequately to maintain the reflex despite a concurrent facial nerve lesion/tumor. Moreover, in those patients with temporal bone/facial nerve tumors with erosion into the otic capsule, formal vestibular testing is indicated.

In terms of facial nerve physiologic testing, electroneuronographic and electromyographic testing has been advocated when patients present with complete facial paralysis. Due to a lack of standardization from center to center and the level for error adversely affecting the interpreted result, some opinions on the utility of this testing differ. Errors with skin impedance, electrode placement, and physiologic artifact may make interpretation of the data difficult. In general, these tests are typically helpful in evaluating the extent of nerve injury and in certain cases may help differentiate between tumors of the other cranial nerves (i.e. vestibular schwannomas) versus facial nerve tumors.

EVALUATION: RADIOLOGIC

A high degree of clinical suspicion is required to make a diagnosis of a facial nerve tumor. This should be considered in any adult who presents with a progressive facial nerve weakness or facial twitching. While imaging modalities have become more sophisticated over the years, they have certainly not replaced the detailed clinical history and evaluation. Two main modalities including thin-section CT with bone algorithms and cranial nerve protocol MRI are highly utilized when investigating the etiologies of facial nerve paralysis.[53] CT scans of the temporal bone may reveal a pathognomonic expansion of the fallopian canal that typically reveals a smooth remodeling of the bone with no frank erosion. MRI studies will reveal a low-intensity lesion on T1 weighting with gadolinium enhancement.

For facial nerve tumors, advances in MRI technology have helped to define the anatomic extent of these lesions and the involvement of adjacent structures.[24,28,53,64] Facial nerve tumors will typically create a smooth but enlarged course along the fallopian canal and therefore may be differentiated from hemangiomas, which often lack clear margins and usually contain bony spicules on fine-cut CT (Fig. 39.2A). They will also enhance on postcontrast T1-weighted MRI (Fig. 39.2B). Limitations of imaging within the petrous apex, where the anatomy may become distorted, may make it more challenging to discern whether the tumor represents a common vestibular schwannoma or a more rare facial nerve tumor. In a review of 30 facial nerve schwannomas, 17 were found to be extracranial (12 involving the main trunk and 5 the peripheral branches) and 13 were intratemporal (10 affecting the horizontal and vertical segments and 3 at the geniculate).[25]

Imaging characteristics of facial nerve hemangiomas are similar to schwannomas and meningiomas. The presence of intralesional calcifications and greater erosion

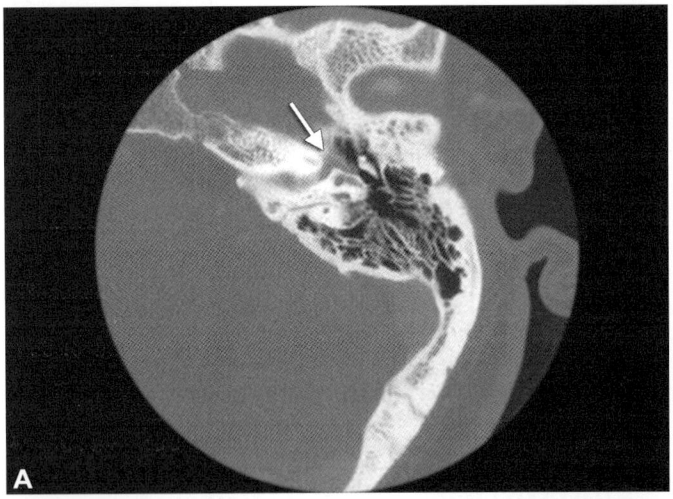
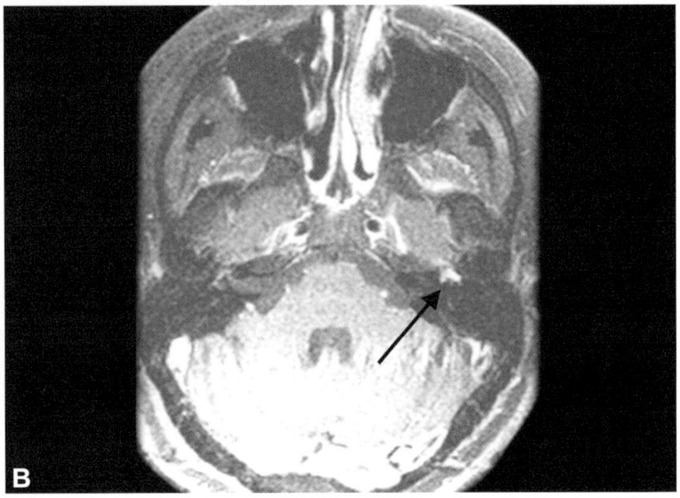
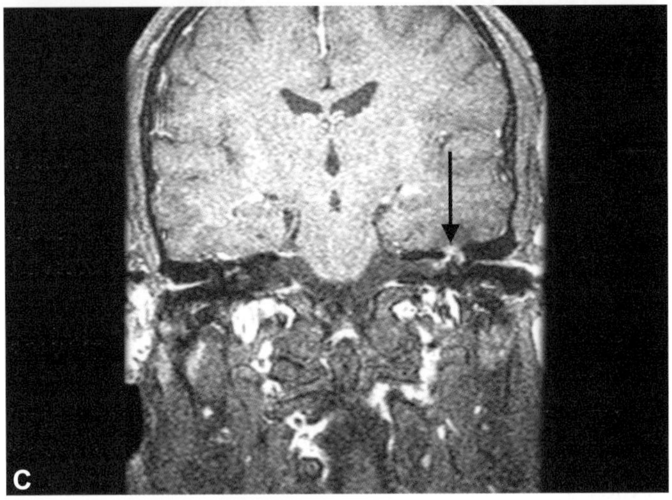

Figs. 39.2A to C: Facial nerve hemangioma. Part (A) shows an axial computed tomography (CT) scan of the temporal bone demonstrating a widened geniculate ganglion and spiculated bone anteriorly consistent with facial nerve hemangioma (white arrow). The presence of intralesional calcifications and greater erosion of the fallopian canal can often help differentiate hemangiomas from other facial nerve tumors. Despite only being present approximately 50% of the time, the honeycomb pattern is important as it is pathognomic for hemangioma and often aids in the differentiation between schwannomas and meningiomas. Parts (B) (axial) and (C) (coronal) T1-weighted magnetic resonance imagings (MRIs) demonstrate the enhanced area (black arrow in B and C) of the geniculate consistent with facial nerve hemangioma. While many lesions will enhance with contrast, the location adjacent to the geniculate ganglion in this case is diagnostically helpful.

of the fallopian canal can often help differentiate hemangiomas from other facial nerve tumors (Fig. 39.2A). In many hemangiomas, the blood vessels are surrounded by newly formed lamellar bone displaying an "ossifying hemangioma" with classic radiologic findings. Ossifying hemangiomas on CT scan will show the typical honeycomb or sunburst appearance as a result of osteoclastic remodeling leading to intralesional lamellar bone trabeculae.[7,42] Despite only being present approximately 50% of the time,[16] the honeycomb pattern is important as it is pathognomic for hemangioma and often aids in the differentiation between schwannomas and meningiomas. Typical facial nerve hemangiomas show enlargement of the fallopian canal with a lesion exhibiting an irregular margin, amorphous shape, and often intratumor bony spicules (Fig. 39.2A). Grossly, hemangiomas have a red sponge-like appearance,[56] and the ossification is thought to represent dystrophic changes to slow tumor growth and from ongoing bone remodeling in response to tumor growth. These imaging characteristics can be helpful in diagnostic properties when these lesions are located away from the geniculate region with presentation within the CPA. A definitive evaluation requires a high-resolution CT scan of the temporal bones to evaluate the tegmen tympani and mastoideum, the extent of potential osseous destruction, and the identification of soft tissue/fluid in the tympanic and mastoid cavities. Smaller defects may not be readily apparent in axial views, underscoring the importance of thin-cut coronal images with the workup.

The often-needed soft-tissue detail of the presumed facial nerve tumor requires concurrent MRI technology in order to delineate. High-resolution MRI with 3 mm sections provides optimal characterization of the fallopian canal, which, when demonstrating circumferential expansion with well-preserved margins and smooth architecture, is consistent with schwannomas (Figs. 39.3A and B).

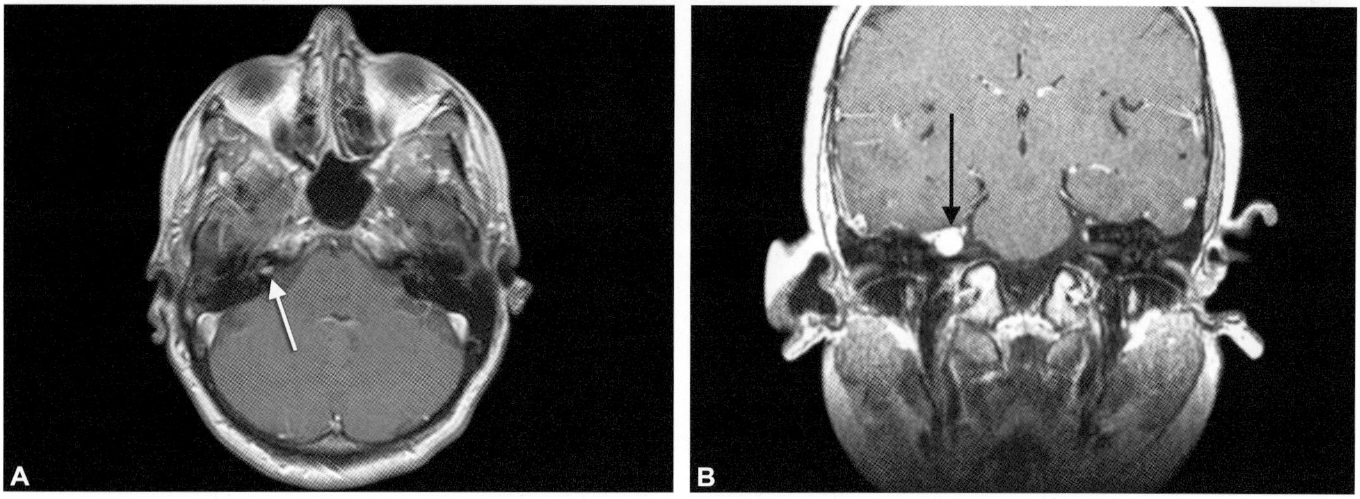

Figs. 39.3A and B: Facial nerve schwannoma. Part (A) is an axial T1-weighted magnetic resonance imaging (MRI) sequences showing a gadolinium-enhancing lesion within the right internal auditory canal (white arrow). Schwannomas involving any cranial nerve typically demonstrate circumferential expansion with well-preserved margins and smooth architecture. Part (B) represents a coronal T1-weighted image following gadolinium again demonstrating the smooth configuration with limited surrounding bone erosion (black arrow).

T2-weighted images will characteristically reveal space-occupying lesions with CSF flow voids (Fig. 39.4). Pathognomonic salt and pepper[46] are described in paragangliomas larger than 2 cm; otherwise these lesions may reveal hypointensity to muscle on T1-weighted imaging and show heterogeneous enhancement with gadolinium contrast. T2-weighted images reveal isointensity to muscle[27] with angiography showing hypervascularity, enlarged feeding arteries, and a potential venous conduit.

Although the second most common tumor of the CPA, facial nerve meningiomas are quite rare. These lesions typically arise from arachnoid villi along the walls of the dural venous sinuses and near neural foramina of cranial nerves. When involving the facial nerve imaging, characteristics on CT scan may show a widening of the fallopian canal (Figs. 39.5A and B) with no significant bone destruction. On MRI, meningiomas of significant size will not only enhance with contrast but may show the characteristic "dural tail" that is often helpful in the diagnostic workup (Figs. 39.6A and B).

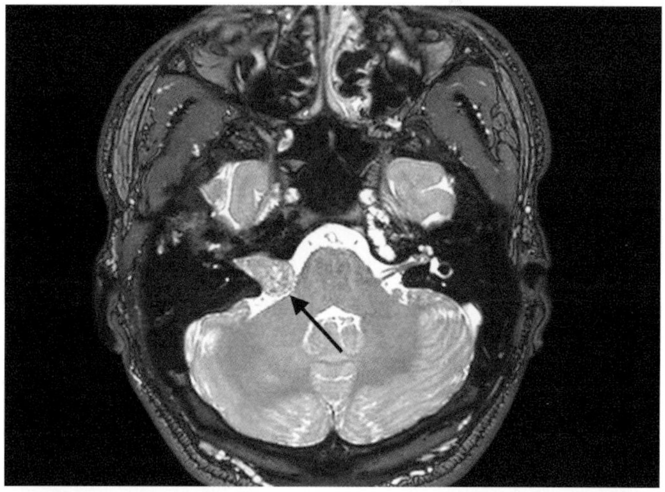

Fig. 39.4: Facial nerve schwannoma. T2-weighted axial magnetic resonance imaging (MRI) through the inner ear. Note the space-occupying lesion of the right internal auditory canal that displaces cerebrospinal fluid (CSF) signal (black arrow). When compared to the noninvolved left side, both the neural planes and CSF flow are completely distorted by tumor burden/mass effect.

TREATMENT

Because they are rare, there is little guidance in the literature that speaks to the appropriate management of facial nerve tumors. Facial nerve tumor management involves weighing the balance between the risks of facial weakness that may often result with primary surgical resection versus the typical slow growing nature of these lesions. The treatment decision should take into consideration the size of the tumor, the current facial nerve function, hearing status in the ipsilateral ear, and any other associated cranial nerve or head or neck signs or symptoms related to the tumor. Treatment strategies include radiological surveillance, gross total resection, bony decompression of the skull casing around the tumor, and radiosurgery. Regardless of approach, a thoughtful and open dialogue between provider and patient must exist to discuss treatment and rehabilitation options.

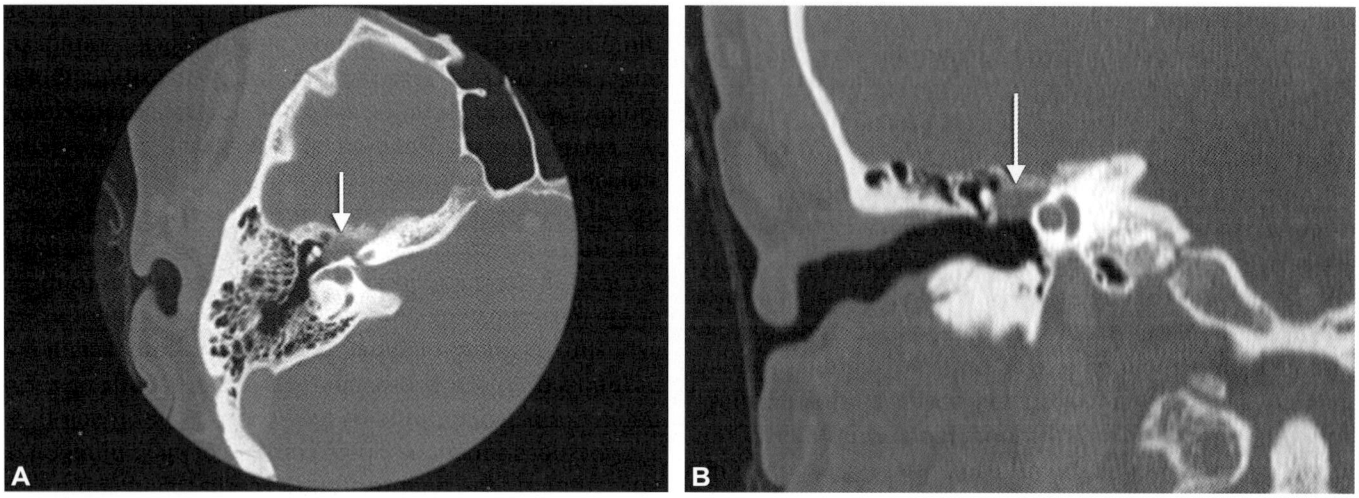

Figs. 39.5A and B: Facial nerve meningioma. Axial (A) and coronal (B) computed tomography (CT) images of the temporal bone demonstrating soft tissue density adjacent to the tympanic, labyrinthine, and geniculate ganglion portions of the facial nerve (white arrows). Note the widening of the fallopian canal with relatively minimal bone involvement. Given the location of the lesion, the differential diagnosis would also include facial nerve hemangioma; however, the pathognomonic spicules of adjacent bone are not present that are often seen with hemangiomas.

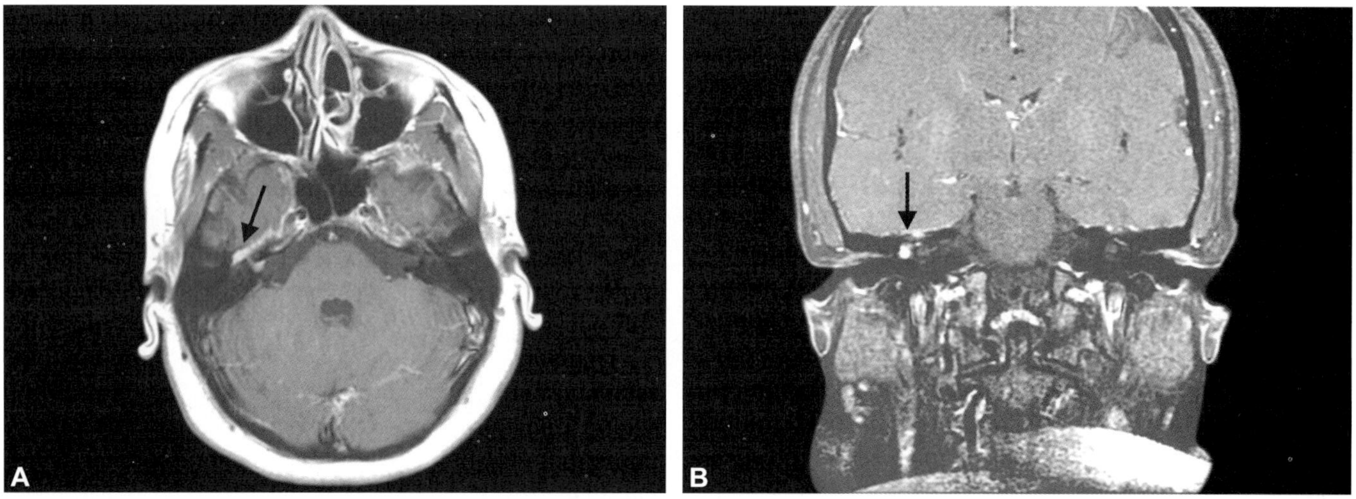

Figs. 39.6A and B: Facial nerve meningioma. Axial (A) and coronal (B) T1-weighted magnetic resonance imagings (MRIs) through the inner ear demonstrating the enhancing lesion within the inner ear (black arrows). Note the extension to the adjacent dural and the characteristic "dural tail" that is often described with meningioma (black arrow in part B).

In patients with small tumors and good facial nerve function, watchful waiting is often advocated.[3,34] Shirazi et al.[58] has recommended conservative management of facial neuromas when patients who present without facial motor or hearing deficits.[31,40] Serial surveillance MRI scans to monitor tumor growth should be implemented. Since surgery undoubtedly carries a risk of significant morbidity to the facial nerve, other adverse events can lead to permanent sensorineural hearing loss, CSF leaks, and tinnitus. Since most benign tumors are slow growing, those patients with normal or near normal facial function are often reticent to undertake major temporal bone surgery. It has been shown that when compared to those patients who underwent surgery, those patients whose tumors were managed conservatively overall fared better.[34] The rationale here is that by delaying surgical resection, patients have an opportunity to enjoy intact facial nerve function.

In symptomatic patients with intact facial nerve function, surgical decompression may help alleviate or prevent worsening of symptoms. Gross surgical resection is warranted when facial weakness progresses to advanced stages, with the surgical approach being dependent on the location and size of the tumor and the current hearing status. Regardless of surgical approach, a comprehensive discussion about the risks of surgery versus the risks of watching the untreated disease needs to be clarified.

The responsiveness of some neoplastic paralyses to high-dose systemic steroids may be the result of the affects of edema exerted on the facial nerve by these tumors. Intratemporal facial nerve schwannomas commonly involve varying degrees of facial paralysis as they exert a compressive effect on the nerve within the bony confines of the fallopian canal. While the facial nerve may be resilient and some reports have documented regenerative capacity during prolonged compression,[51] this is typically only seen with acoustic neuromas. Once the epineurium has been breached (not typically seen in benign tumors), facial function is more likely to be impaired. It has been claimed that >50% of facial nerve fibers require degeneration before the clinical signs of degeneration are seen.

From a clinical perspective, when surgery is indicated, it is important to distinguish an invasive acoustic neuroma from a true facial nerve schwannoma (FNS). Dort and Fisch reported a series of five patients with intracranial FNS with concurrent eighth nerve involvement requiring resection. They determined that the histopathology of intracranial FNS is different from peripheral schwannomas and is akin to an invasive vestibular schwannoma. Given that these tumors are often multicentric, grossly, these tumors often appear as diffuse bulging/multiple-discrete tumors of the facial nerve that may often span many segments. The areas of enlargement have been described as a series of "dumb-bells" that makes resection quite complicated in determining the limits of tumor resection, placing a premium on intraoperative frozen pathological sections. These tumors can reach considerable size and typically follow the anatomic pathway of least resistance and therefore may present as external or middle ear masses or may extend into the CPA or anteriorly and present as a mass within the middle fossa.[28]

A transmastoid or middle fossa approach can be utilized for smaller, localized tumors, while a combined approach may be required for larger tumors in an interest to preserve hearing. If the lesion is confined to the transverse or descending portions of the nerve, a transmastoid approach is advocated. From this approach, ossiculoplasty if warranted or primary facial nerve grafting (from great auricular or lateral sural) is possible and can be easily achieved. It is believed that the chances of meaningful recovery decrease significantly postoperatively if the resection is not completed within the first year of initial clinical facial nerve dysfunction.[17] Frozen tissue pathology margins should always be taken intraoperatively to ensure tumor clearance, as incomplete tumor resection may result in recurrence.[61] This is important to remember in circumstances where the lesion is a facial nerve schwannoma that may present like "beads" along the nerve and extend from the "pons to the parotid" involving several segments of the facial nerve.

Hemangiomas at the geniculate ganglion are best approached through a middle fossa approach. The combined transmastoid-middle cranial fossa approach has been widely used and adopted for primary resection of facial nerve tumors. This combined approach has been used for lesions that involve the genu or the labyrinthine segment of the facial nerve in a setting of the desire to preserve hearing. Also, tumors that may cause a fistula into the labyrinth that require meticulous extirpation and approach to prevent hearing or balance loss may require this approach. Management strategy of the facial nerve hemangioma follows the same principles as outlined for facial nerve schwannomas. Hemangiomas are typically extraneural and as such are more readily dissected off the facial nerve. There is, however, a higher incidence of hearing loss after resection, as these tumors are thought to arise from the vasculature around Scarpa's ganglion.

For those situations where current cochlear function is poor, a translabyrinthine or transcochlear approach may be utilized. These approaches have the benefit of wide exposure to the intracranial and intratemporal segments of the nerve obviating the need for brain retraction, while preserving excellent access for nerve suturing, rerouting, and nerve interposition if needed. It is, however, critical that the defect be closed properly with a fat graft to prevent a postoperative CSF leak.

Lastly, the retrosigmoid approach can be used for tumors of the intracranial segment, and a parotidectomy and facial nerve dissection are useful in extratemporal tumors. In rare cases, the tumor can be surgically removed from the facial nerve; however, the majority of cases require a resection of the involved segment of nerve with a nerve grafting. If a resection is indicated and appropriate, cable grafting with the great auricular or lateral sural nerve may be considered and has been shown to preserve facial nerve function in a range from 50 to 75%.[14]

In situations where the tumor may not be removed in the interest of maintaining normal facial function, wide bony decompression of the nerve may be required, postponing the definitive resection until paralysis progresses.[3] Despite leaving the nerve unmolested, this approach still, depending on approach, carries risks to cochlear and labyrinthine function.

Stereotactic radiosurgery has also been successfully used in the management of these tumors and there have been published rates of increased reliance on this treatment of facial nerve tumors.[65] The attraction of this approach lies in the avoidance of surgery, yet the tumor is not removed and the goal of this treatment paradigm is to "control" the tumor growth. The main risks include the collateral injury to adjacent structures and the potential for malignant transformation of the benign tumor that may not occur for many years.[55] The long-term benefits of radiosurgery to facial nerve tumors remain uncertain.

PROGNOSIS

Given the wide variety of tumor types that are involved with facial nerve dysfunction, the prognosis of survival or disease-free survival after treatment is quite variable and specific to the tumor of interest. A comprehensive description of prognosis stratified for each potential tumor that may infiltrate the facial nerve lies beyond the scope of this chapter. The most important factor determining the efficacy and prognosis lies in the duration of the pretreatment facial paralysis. That being said, patients with long-standing, complete paralysis typically do worse than those with shorter duration of insult. Many have advocated that for the best possible result, that surgery be offered within the first year of diagnosis prior to perineural fibrosis or frank neural infiltration making the resection more challenging.[1] Of those nerves that have required resection and primary grafting, no distinct advantage has been determined in grafting type,[44] while longer grafts appeared to heal better than short grafts, and there was no significant difference in recovery between patients with and without preoperative facial dysfunction.[29] Static and dynamic facial nerve reanimation procedures have also been shown to have utility in rehabilitation. In all cases, early intervention is best, particularly when treating the paralyzed eye in an interest to prevent damage to the exposed cornea.

CONCLUSION

Approximately 5% of facial paralysis is caused by facial nerve tumors and up to 50% of patients with facial nerve tumors present to their clinician with intact facial function. Progressive or recurrent paralysis or twitching of the face is often indicative of a neoplastic process. The most common tumors of the facial nerve are schwannomas and often involve many contiguous segments of the nerve with potential erosion of otic capsule bone. Hemangiomas are the second most common and while they are typically small, they are capable of causing of facial paralysis. A comprehensive history and physical examination and the appropriate use of neuroimaging are paramount in the detection of facial nerve tumors. Once diagnosed, a detailed discussion about treatment options is required to cover the wide range of options from watchful waiting to radiosurgery to definitive surgical excision. Lastly, facial nerve reanimation or restoration should be considered at the time of the primary procedure.

REFERENCES

1. Ahmadi N, Newkirk K, Kim HJ. Facial nerve hemangioma: a rare case involving the vertical segment. Laryngoscope. 2013;123(2):499-502.
2. Almadori G, Del Ninno M, Cadoni G, et al. Facial nerve paralysis in acute otomastoiditis as a presenting symptom of FAB M2, T8:21 leukemia relapse. Int J Ped Otorhinolaryngol. 1996;36:42-52.
3. Angeli SI, Brackmann DE. Is surgical excision of facial nerve schwannomas always indicated? Otolaryngol Head Neck Surg. 1997;117:S144-S147.
4. Angeli SI, Brackmann DE, Xenellis JE. Primary lymphoma of the internal auditory canal. Case report and review of the literature. Ann Otol Rhinol Laryngol. 1998;107:17-21.
5. Balkany T, Fradis M, Jafek BW, et al. Hemangioma of the facial nerve: role of the geniculate capillary plexus. Skull Base Surg. 1991;1:59-63.
6. Baugh R, Basura GL, Ishii L, et al. Clinical practice guideline: Bell's palsy. Otolaryngol Head Neck Surg. 2013;149:656-63.
7. Benoit MM, North PE, McKenna MJ, et al. Facial nerve hemangiomas: vascular tumors or malformations? Otolaryngol Head Neck Surg. 2010;142:108-14.
8. Berlinger NT, Koutroupas S, Adams G, et al. Patterns of involvement of the temporal bone in metastatic and systemic malignancy. Laryngoscope. 1980;90:619-27.
9. Biggs ND, Fagan PA. Schwannoma of the chorda tympani. J Laryngol Otol. 2001;115:50-52.

9a. Chandana SR, Conley BA. Salivary gland cancers: current treatments, molecular characteristics and new therapies. Expert Rev Anticancer Ther. 2008;8(4):645-52.

10. Conley J, Hammaker RC. Prognosis of malignant tumors of the parotid gland with facial paralysis. Arch Otolaryngol. 1975;101:39-41.
11. Dadas B, Alkan S, Turgut S, et al. Primary papillary adenocarcinoma confined to the middle ear and mastoid. Eur Arch Otorhinolaryngol. 2001;258:93-5.

11a. DeLozier H, Spinella MS, Johnson GD. Facial nerve paralysis with benign parotid masses. Ann Otol Rhinol. 1989;98: 644-47.
12. Dort JC, Fisch U. Facial nerve schwannomas. Skull Base Surg. 1991;1:51-6.
13. Dutcher PO Jr, Brackmann DE. Glomus tumor of the facial canal. A case report. Arch Otolaryngol Head Neck Surg. 1986;112:986-7.
14. Eby TL, Fisch U, Makek MS. Facial nerve management in temporal bone hemangiomas. Am J Otol. 1992;13:223-32.
15. Eneroth CM. Facial nerve paralysis-a criterion of malignancy in parotid tumors. Arch Otolaryngol. 1972;95:300-4.
16. Escada P, Capucho C, Silva JM, et al. Cavernous haemangioma of the facial nerve. J Laryngol Otol. 1997;111:858-61.
17. Falcioni M, Russo A, Taibah A, Sanna M. Facial nerve tumors. Otol Neurotol. 2003;24:942-7.
18. Fisch U, Ruttner J. Pathology of intratemporal tumors involving the facial nerve. In: Fisch U (ed.), Facial Nerve Surgery. Birmingham: AlaKugler/Aesculapius. 1977. pp. 448-56.
19. Friedman O, Neff BA, Willcox TO, et al. Temporal bone hemangiomas involving the facial nerve. Otol Neurotol. 2002;23:76066.
20. Gross BC, Carlson ML, Moore EJ, et al: The intraparotid facial nerve schwannoma: a diagnostic and management conundrum. Am J Otolaryngol. 2012;33: 497-504.
21. Jackler RK, Brackmann DE. Neurotology. Second edition. Philadelphia, PA: Elsevier Mosby; 2005.
22. Jackler RK, Driscoll CLW. Tumors of the Ear and Temporal Bone. Philadelphia, PA: Lippincott Williams & Wilkins; 2000.
23. Jabor MA, Amedee RG, Gianoli GJ. Primary meningioma of the fallopian canal. South Med J. 2000;93:717-20.
24. Jager L, Reiser M. CT, MR imaging of the normal and pathologic conditions of the facial nerve. Eur J Radiol. 2001;40: 133-46.
25. Janecka IP, Conley J. Primary neoplasms of the facial nerve. Plastic Reconstr Surg. 1987;79:177-83.
26. Jung TTK, Jun B, Shea D, Paparella MM. Primary and secondary tumors of the facial nerve. a temporal bone study. Arch Otolaryngol Head Neck Surg. 1986;112:1269-73.
27. Kania RE, Bouccara D, Colombani JM, et al. Primary facial canal paraganglioma. Am J Otolaryngol. 1999;20:318-22.
28. Kertesz TR, sheltom C, Wiggins RH. Intratemporal facial nerve neuroma: anatomical location and radiological features. Laryngoscope. 2001;111:1250-56.
29. Kesser BW, Brackmann DE, Ma Y, Weiss M. Jacobsen's nerve schwannoma: a rare middle ear mass. Ann Otol Rhinol Laryngol. 2001;110:1030-34.
30. Kettel K. Peripheral facial palsies due to tumors; pathology and clinical picture: a review of the literature and a report of three cases of intratemporal tumors of the facial nerve. AMA Arch Otolaryngol. 1959;69:276-92.
31. Kim CS, Chang SO, Oh SH, et al. Management of intratemporal facial nerve schwannoma. Otol Neurotol. 2003;24: 312-6.
32. Kudo A, Suzuki M, Kubo N. Schwannoma arising from the intermediate nerve manifesting as hemifacial spasm. Case report. J Neurosurg. 1996;84:277-9.
33. Kunzel J, Zenk J, Koch M, et al. Paraganglioma of the facial nerve, a rare differential diagnosis for facial nerve paralysis: case report and review of the literature. Eur Arch Otorhinolaryngol. 2012;269:693-8.
34. Liu R, Fagan P. Facial nerve schwannoma: surgical excision versus conservative management. Ann Otol Rhinol Laryngol. 2001;110:1025-9.
35. Magliulo G, Alla FR, Colicchio G, et al. Geniculate ganglion meningioma. Skull Base. 2010;20:185-8.
36. Mangham CA, Carberry JN, Brackmann DE. Management of intratemporal vascular tumors. Laryngoscope. 1981;91: 867-76.
37. Maniglia AJ. Intra and extracranial meningiomas involving the temporal bone. Laryngoscope. 1978;88:9 Pt 2 Suppl 121-58.
38. May M. The Facial Nerve. New York: Thieme-Stratton; 1986. pp. 365-99.
39. May M, Beckford NS, Bedetti CD. Granular cell tumor of facial nerve diagnosed at surgery for idiopathic facial nerve paralysis. Otolaryngol Head Neck Surg. 1985;93:122-6.
40. McMonagle B, Al-Sanosi A, Croxson G, et al. Facial schwannoma: results of a large case series and review. J Laryngol Otol. 2008;122:1139-50.
41. Michel O, Wagner M, Guntinas-Lichius O. Schwannoma of the greater superficial petrosal nerve. Otolaryngol Head Neck Surg. 2000;122:302-3.
42. Mijangos SV, Meltzer DE: Case 171: facial nerve hemangioma. Radiology. 2011;260:296-301.
43. Nager GT. Meningioma involving the temporal bone: clinical and pathological aspects. Ir J Med Sci. 1966;41:69-96.
44. O'Donoghue GM, Brackmann DE, House JW, et al. Neuromas of the facial nerve. Am J Otol. 1989;10:49-54.
45. O'Leary M, Shelton C, Giddings N, et al. Glomus tympanicum tumors: a clinical perspective. Laryngoscope. 1991; 101:1038-43.
46. Olsen WL, Dillon WP, Kelly WM, et al. MR imaging of paragangliomas. AJR Am J Roentgenol. 1987;148:201-4.
47. Paparella MM, Berlinger NT, Oda M, et al. Otologic manifestations of leukemia. Laryngoscope. 1973;83:1510-26.
48. Paparella MM, El Fiky FM. Ear involvement in malignant lymphoma. Ann Otol. 1972;81:352-63.
49. Petrus LV, Lo WM. Primary paraganglioma of the facial nerve canal. AJNR Am J Neuroradiol. 1996;17:171-4.
50. Ross L, Drazin D, Eboli P, et al. Atypical tumors of the facial nerve: case series and review of the literature. Neurosurg Focus. 2013;34:1-9.
51. Saito H. Tumor invasion of the facial nerve: a study of 8 temporal bones. In: Graham MD, House WF (eds). Disorders of the Facial Nerve: Anatomy, Diagnosis and Management. New York: Raven Press; 1982.
52. Saito H, Baxter H. Undiagnosed intratemporal facial nerve neurilemmomas. Arch Otolaryngol. 1972;95:415-9.

53. Sartoretti-Schefer S, Kollias S, Valavanis A. Spatial relationship between vestibular schwannomas and facial nerve on three dimensional T2-weighted fast spin echo MR images. Am J Neurorad. 2000;21:810-16.
54. Semaan MT, Slattery WH, Brackmann DE. Geniculate ganglion hemangiomas: clinical results and long-term follow-up. Otol Neurotol. 2010;31:665-70.
55. Shamisa A, Bance M, Nag S. Glioblastoma multiforme developing in a patient treated with gamma knife radiosurgery: case report and review of the literature. J Neurosurg. 2001;94:816-21.
56. Shelton C, Brackmann DE, Lo WMM, et al. Intratemporal facial nerve hemangiomas. Otolaryngol Head Neck Surg. 1991;104:116-21.
57. Sherman JD, Dagnew E, Pensak ML, et al. Facial nerve neuromas: report of 10 cases and review of the literature. Neurosurgery. 2002;50:450-56.
58. Shirazi MA, Leonetti JP, Marzo SJ, et al. Surgical management of facial neuromas: lessons learned. Otol Neurotol. 2007;28:958-63.
59. Snyderman C, May M, Berman MA, et al. Facial paralysis: traumatic neuromas versus facial nerve neoplasms. Otolaryngol Head Neck Surg. 1988;98:53-9.
60. Telischi FF, Arnold DJ, Sittler S. Inflammatory neuroma of the facial nerve associated with chronic otomastoiditis. Otolaryngol Head Neck Surg. 1995;113:319-22.
61. Vrabec JT, Guinto F Jr, Nauta HJ. Recurrent facial neuromas. Am J Otol. 1998;19:99-103.
62. Wells SC. Embryonal rhabdomyosarcoma of the ear: a review of the literature and case history. J Laryngol Otol. 1984;98:1261-6.
63. Whinney D, Kitchen N, Revesz, Brookes G. Primary malignant melanoma of the cerebellopontine angle. Otol Neurotol. 2001;22:218-22.
64. Wiggins RH III, Harnsberger HR, Salzman KL, et al. The many faces of facial nerve schwannoma. AJNR Am J Neuroradiol. 2006;27:694-9.
65. Wilkinson EP, Hoa M, Slattery WH III, et al. Evolution in the management of facial nerve schwannoma. Laryngoscope. 2011;121:2065-74.
66. Zappia JJ, Bunge FA, Koopman CF, et al. Facial nerve paresis as a presenting symptom of leukemia. Int J Pediatr Otorhinolaryngol. 1990;19:259-64.
67. Zhang Q, Jessurun J, Schachern PA, et al. Outgrowing schwannomas arising from tympanic segments of the facial nerve. Am J Otolaryngol. 1996;17:311-5.

CHAPTER 40

Facial Nerve Reanimation

Monica Tadros

INTRODUCTION

The surgical treatment of facial paralysis continues to be extremely challenging. A number of procedures have been described and refined over the past several decades attempting to overcome the limitations of flaccid paralysis, incomplete reinnervation, facial hypertonicity, facial synkinesis, and uncoordinated recovery. Still, the imperfect quality of facial reanimation leaves surgeons and patients seeking new alternatives for a more natural appearance.

The ideal procedure is one that would restore mimetic facial function without aberrant synkinesis or mass movement. The basic goals of reanimation focus on enhancing symmetry at rest and aiding ocular, nasal, and oral sphincter control. Advanced goals seek dynamic reanimation. Preferred treatment plans often differ among surgeons to achieve voluntary reanimation and are continuing to evolve to include restoration of the involuntary emotional smile. It is important to understand the realistic goals, patient timeline, and multifactorial reasons guiding variations in therapeutic management.

The most critical factor in patient management is defining where the patient is on the timeline of his condition in the context of causative factors. If there is any opportunity to restore nerve continuity, the earliest possible intervention is advocated. In cases where the integrity of the nerve is uncertain, conservative management may be employed for 6–12 months. Patients with chronic facial nerve paralysis < 2 years' duration may be candidates for neural substitutions. Beyond this time frame, chronic neuromuscular injury results in atrophy of the motor endplates and the native facial muscles are no longer able to receive neural input. In this case, dynamic reanimation requires the transfer of muscle in some form. This can be accomplished by selecting a pedicle neuromuscular transposition flap or a nerve substitution in combination with a microvascular free muscle flap. Patients who are not candidates for dynamic neuromuscular reanimation may still greatly benefit from static reanimation and ancillary palliative procedures, including autogenous fascia lata and alloplastic Gore-Tex slings to the lower lip and Mitek anchor suspension to the nasal ala and upper lip.

Nerve regeneration relies on the timely activated connectivity of viable axons. Optimal surgical outcomes are seen when donor and recipient nerves are closely matched in terms of axonal load and coapted in tension-free fashion.[1] Superior outcomes are reported from ideal circumstances, including shorter duration of paralysis and younger age.[2-4] This can be attributed to less nerve fibrosis, less muscle atrophy, age-related regenerative potential and cortical adaptation.[5-8]

Faulty regeneration leads to a number of conditions that may confound the traditional picture of facial paralysis, including facial synkinesis, Bogorad's crocodile tears, stapes tendon spasm, hemifacial spasm, and blepharospasm. Synkinesis is the abnormal synchronization of muscle contractions that do not normally contract together. Hyperkinesis is an undesirable hyperexcitable muscle response. It is fundamental to evaluate and characterize the patient-specific sequelae of neural injury as flaccid paralysis, hyperkinetic paralysis, synkinetic paralysis, or most commonly a combined facial paralysis with zonal variation.

In flaccid facial paralysis, there is a clear lack of muscle movement. Hyperkinetic and synkinetic facial paralysis are less obvious. Hyperkinetic paralysis may be equated with chronic spasm, where there is a failure to produce a desired movement due to chronic muscle activation. In this case, some voluntary movement is present but it may be uncoordinated, exaggerated, or uncontrolled. In facial paralysis with synkinesis, there may be undesirable "mass movement" of separate zones during voluntary contraction or involuntary upper and lower division twitching, both due to faulty synchronous nerve reorganization. Facial synkinesis is the most common sequelae of neurotmesis and its debilitating nature should not be underestimated. It is one of the most important issues affecting recovery of function due to the misdirection of regenerating axons to incorrect end targets.[4] Modern day rehabilitation of permanent facial paralysis is best performed through multimodality treatment including surgical intervention, biofeedback physical therapy and chemodenervation.

Evaluation

In all cases of facial reanimation, patient evaluation and selection is critical for optimal outcomes. Evaluation begins with a detailed history and physical examination (Table 40.1). The three most important criteria from the patient's history that help stratify patient management are (1) the time elapsed since the onset of the paralysis, (2) the etiology of the paralysis, and (3) the initial degree of paralysis. Associated symptoms can often help determine the etiology and topographic location of nerve injury. Age of the patient, health status and life expectancy are important considerations in recommending treatment.

Careful patient assessment is required to understand the nature of the nerve injury and its resulting sequelae. Historically, the House–Brackmann scale of facial paralysis has been used to grade facial paralysis and follow recovery. This scale was originally designed to follow the recovery of skull base etiologies of facial paralysis that typically affect the entire nerve profoundly. For this reason, critics caution the grading scale has only "fair" inter-rater reliability and may fail to distinguish many zonal variations in the upper and lower divisions and terminal branches of the facial nerve.[3,9] A thorough zonal assessment should go beyond the House-Brackmann scale and take into account facial asymmetry, compromise of orbital, nasal and oral function, and facial synkinesis or mass movement. Evaluation of seven important parameters are used to qualify facial tone, symmetry at rest and deficits during facial motion:[10] (1) eyebrow raise to evaluate the frontalis muscle and temporal branch, (2) eye closure to evaluate the orbicularis oculi muscle and zygomatic branch, (3) open-mouth smile to evaluate the risorius and zygomaticus muscles and buccal branch, (4) facial snarl to evaluate the levator superioris alaeque nasi and levator labii superioris muscles and buccal branch, (5) lip pucker to evaluate the orbicularis oris muscle and buccal branch, (6) lower lip depression to survey the depressor labii inferioris (DLI) muscle and marginal mandibular branch innervation, and (7) clenching of the jaw to survey platysma muscle involvement, especially as it relates to synkinesis and the cervical branch.

Comprehensive physical examination also includes orbital assessment of visual acuity, corneal examination, eyelid closure, tearing, corneal blink reflex, Bell's phenomenon, lagophthalmos, lower lid position, laxity or ectropion, position of the lacrimal punctum, and eyebrow position and heaviness. Nasal examination highlights airway compromise with emphasis on the nasal septum, nasal valve, and malposition of the nasal ala. Complete cranial nerve examination should also be documented.

Separating intracranial, transtemporal, and extracranial etiologies is important to formulate a differential diagnosis. Supranuclear facial nerve lesions may involve: the cerebral cortex such as those caused by stroke; the midbrain such as those caused by neoplasm, vascular lesions, and Parkinsonism, or the pontine facial nucleus such as those caused by tumor, multiple sclerosis, or infection. These etiologies must be separated from infranuclear facial nerve lesions that may involve: the intracranial cerebellopontine angle such as meningioma or acoustic neuroma; the bony internal auditory canal such as a temporal bone fracture, or transtemporal extension of a meningioma or acoustic neuroma; the temporal bone extending to the labyrinthine and tympanomastoid regions such as Bell's palsy, Ramsay-Hunt (herpes zoster oticus), complications of acute suppurative otitis media, complications of cholesteatoma, or glomus tumors; or extracranial etiologies that originate distal to the stylomastoid foramen such as malignant tumors of the parotid gland and traumatic penetrating wounds of the face.[11]

Additional testing to help determine etiology and prognosis may include computed tomography or magnetic

Table 40.1: Facial paralysis–patient assessment

Patient age:	
Time from onset: Acute injury: 0–21 days/subacute injury: 3 weeks–6 months Chronic neural injury: 6 months–2 years/chronic neuromuscular injury: >2 years	
Degree/etiology:	*PMH:*
Incomplete paralysis	Diabetes: yes or no
Complete paralysis at onset	Neurologic:
Incomplete to complete paralysis: acute	Other:
Incomplete to complete paralysis: progressive	
Trauma	*Prior testing:*
Iatrogenic	CT scan: head, temporal bone
Neoplasm	MRI: head, internal auditory canal
Infectious	Electrical testing: ENoG, EMG
Bell's palsy	Audiogram:
Congenital	Other:
Other/unknown	*Prior treatment:*
Zonal assessment:	
EYE:	*MIDFACE:*
Eye closure: normal, weak, none	Vertical ptosis: yes, no
Brow elevation: normal, no elevation, ptosis at rest	Philtrum shift: yes, no
Palpebral aperture: normal, wider rounding with scleral show, ectropion, smaller	*MOUTH:*
Dry eyes: Schirmer's test normal, hypolacrimation	Resting symmetry: normal, upper lip droop, commissure droop, loss of lip depressors
Poor eye closure, lower lid ectropion	Oral sphincter tone: normal, weak, drooling
Epiphora: normal, hyperlacrimation, lower lid ectropion	Open-mouth smile: normal, asymmetric
Bell's phenomenon/corneal protection: sufficient, insufficient	Pucker: normal, asymmetric
Blink reflex: present, absent, hyperactive	Snarl: normal, weak, retracted incisor show
NOSE:	Speech: normal, articulation defect
Nasal valve collapse/nasalis weak: yes, no	
Cottle maneuver: positive, negative	
Alar malposition: yes, no	
Hyperkinesis/Synkinesis:	
Blink with chewing/voluntary smile: yes, no	
Oral twitch with voluntary eye closure: yes, no	
Other abnormal facial twitching: yes, no	
Hypertonic facial contracture: yes, no	
Teeth clenching/platysma: normal, weak, Hypertonic, causing lower lip synkinesis	
Contralateral facial compensation: yes, no	

resonance imaging and electrical testing. Topographic analysis (Fig. 40.1) may help localize a lesion within the temporal bone. Testing may include audiometry to survey the stapedial reflex (nerve to the stapedius), a Schirmer's test to survey lacrimal gland function (greater superficial petrosal nerve [GSPN]), and a taste test to evaluate the chorda tympani.[12] Decisions regarding facial nerve rehabilitation can only be made after understanding the anatomy of the injury and patient-specific pathogenesis of their condition.

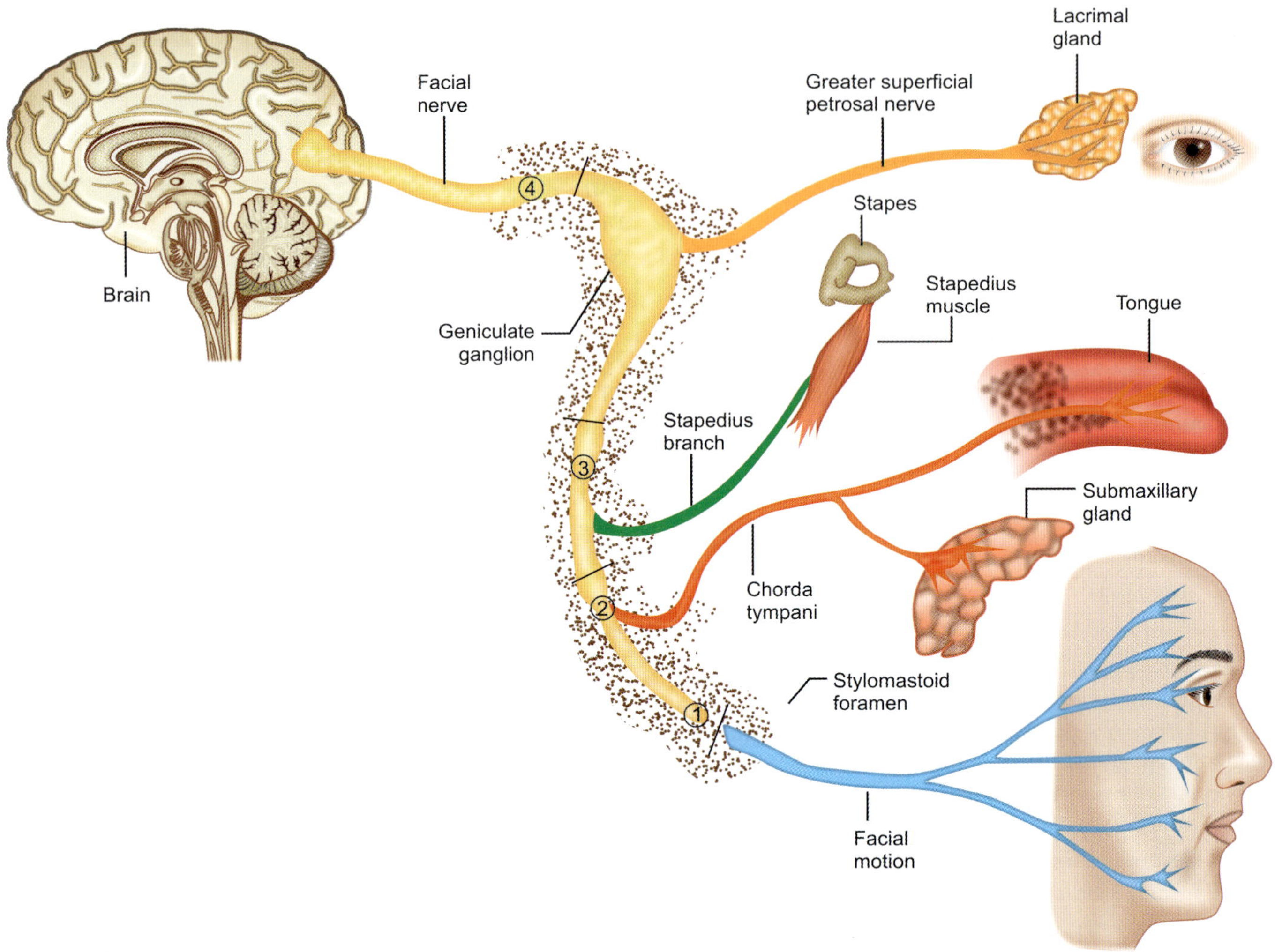

Fig. 40.1: Pathway for topographic analysis of intratemporal facial nerve lesions. (1) Lesion at the stylomastoid foramen will affect facial motion, (2) lesion proximal to the chorda tympani will also affect taste, (3) lesion proximal to the stapedius branch will also affect the acoustic reflex, (4) lesion proximal to the geniculate ganglion will also affect lacrimation.

Surgical Anatomy of the Extratemporal Facial Nerve

The facial nerve is a mixed motor and sensory nerve intracranially. Once it leaves the stylomastoid foramen extratemporally, it is purely a motor nerve that supplies the muscles of the face, scalp, and platysma of the neck. As the facial nerve leaves the skull through the stylomastoid foramen, it gives rise to two branches, the posterior auricular nerve, which supplies the occipitalis muscle, and the nerve to the posterior belly of the digastric. The facial nerve then enters the deep surface of the parotid gland where the pes anserinus then divides into upper and lower divisions within the substance of the gland. Classically, the upper division gives rise to the frontal and zygomatic branches of the facial nerve, and the lower division gives rise to the buccal, marginal mandibular, and cervical branches of the facial nerve. The frontal branch supplies the frontalis and some upper portions of orbicularis oculi muscle. The zygomatic branch has an upper division that passes across the zygomatic bone to innervate the orbicularis oculi muscle and a lower division that passes along the lower border of the zygomatic bone to supply the muscles in the infraorbital and nasal region. Classically, the buccal branch has extensive arborization that may communicate between the upper and lower divisions of the facial nerve, but it predominantly runs toward the angle of the mouth to supply the buccinator, lip elevators, and orbicularis oris muscles. The marginal mandibular branch supplies the muscles to the lower lip and the cervical branch provides motor innervation to the platysma muscle.[13,14]

The preferred point of convergence used to localize the facial nerve is where the tip of the mastoid process, the cartilaginous auditory canal, and the superior border of the posterior belly of the digastric muscle meet.[13] As the facial nerve branches exit the parotid gland, they course just beneath the superficial musculoaponeurotic system (SMAS). The facial nerve branches innervate the facial muscles from their deep surface with three exceptions: the buccinator, levator anguli oris, and mentalis muscles.[14] These three facial muscles are oriented more deeply and innervation emerges from their superficial aspect.

Reliable operative landmarks are essential for peripheral branch explorations (Fig. 40.2). A line drawn from a point 1 cm anterior to the tragus to the tail of the eyebrow demarcates the territory of the superior division of the facial nerve. This division crosses the zygomatic arch within the temperoparietal fascia and gives rise to the frontal branch. The frontal nerve can be found anterior to the superficial temporal artery and vein along Pitanguy's line. Pitanguy's line runs from 0.5 cm below the tragus to 1.5 cm above the lateral eyebrow and more reliably defines the distal course of the frontal nerve.[15] The buccal branch lies superior to the parotid duct, which can be found in the middle third of a line drawn from the antitragal notch to the oral commissure. The complex arborization of the extratemporal facial nerve, especially in the region of the zygomatic and buccal branch distribution, provides additional collateral nerve fibers for donor nerve substitution.[13] The marginal mandibular branch consistently divides into two to three branches innervating the lower lip depressors and mentalis muscles. In 80% of patients, the dominant branch runs above the mandibular ramus; however, in all patients a critical branch that commonly innervates the depressor labii inferioris (DLI) runs 1–3 cm below the ramus of the mandible deep to the platysma, which is continuous with the SMAS. The branch then arcs up over the mandible where it can be found crossing the facial artery and vein at the facial notch along the body of the mandible.[16]

Neurologic Injury of the Facial Nerve

Each neuron is composed of a cell body in the pontine facial nucleus of the brainstem and a myelinated axon that conducts impulses to the neuromuscular junction in the face. Nerves are organized as axonal bundles surrounded by a connective tissue neural sheath composed of

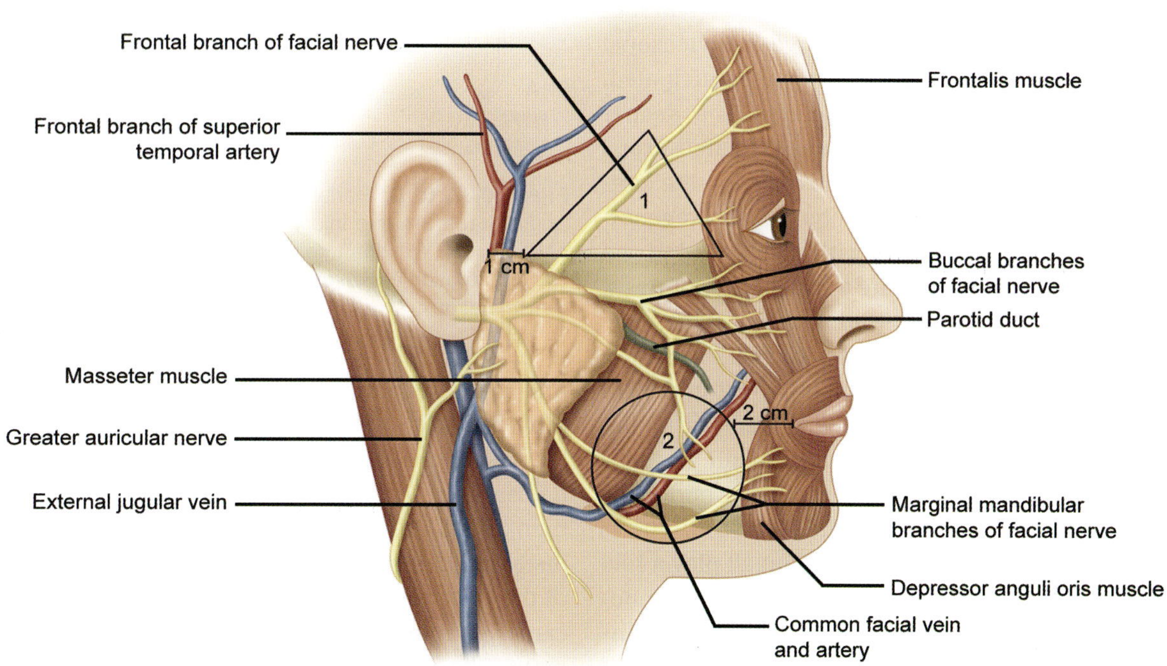

Fig. 40.2: Anatomy of the facial nerve and operative landmarks. (1) zone of the superior division of the facial nerve, (2) zone of the marginal mandibular branches. The marginal mandibular nerve branches become more superficial as they approach a 2-cm radius from the oral commissure.

Table 40.2: Sunderland classification of peripheral nerve injury

Grade	Pathology	Translation	EMG % Normal[23]	Recovery[23]	Recovery begins[23]
1	Neuropraxia	Conduction block	100%	Complete	1–3 weeks
2	Axonotmesis	Sheath intact	25%	Fair	3–4 weeks
3	Neurotmesis	Endoneurium loss	0–10%	Moderate-poor (HB 3-4) with synkinesis	12–16 weeks
4	Neurotmesis	Endoneurium and perineurium loss	0	Profound weakness (HB5) with synkinesis	16 weeks–18 months
5	Neurotmesis/Complete transection	Endoneurium perineurium and epineurium loss	0	None	None

three layers: endoneurium, perineurium, and epineurium. Endoneurial tubules form a loose connective tissue layer around bundles of axons. Multiple endoneurial tubules are organized into a fascicle surrounded by perineurium. Multiple fascicles run within the nerve trunk protected by an outer nerve sheath layer called the epineurium.

Understanding the Sunderland Classification system of peripheral nerve injury[3,17] (Table 40.2) is critical to evaluating the potential and timing for recovery and the likely risk for aberrant nerve regeneration. There are five sequential grades of injury affecting the deepest axons of the nerve first, progressing radially to disrupt the outer epineurial layer last.

Grade 1 injury is a neuropraxia, defined as a conduction block within the core axons of the nerve without axonal disruption, and early complete recovery is anticipated. Grade 2 injury is an axonotmesis, defined as a deeper injury that results in disruption of the myelinated axons and Wallerian degeneration but has no effect on the connective tissue sheath. In this case, axons typically regenerate normally, remaining on course within their sheath as a boundary. Grades 3 to 5 injuries are termed a neurotmesis, describing varying degrees of injury to the connective tissue neural sheath; in addition to the axonal disruption and Wallerian degeneration seen with Grade 2 injury. In Grade 3 injury, the axons and endoneurium are disrupted. In Grade 4 injury the axons, endoneurium, and perineurium are disrupted. In Grade 5 injury, the axons, endoneurium, perineurium, and epineurium are disrupted.

Grade of injury, etiology, and treatment all play a role in the likelihood of misrouting and aberrant nerve regeneration. It is important to realize that once there is full transection of the nerve, recovery will never be complete.[18] The success of nerve regeneration relies on precise axonal routing, using the neural sheath as a guide and boundary. Even with a grade 3 injury, regenerating axonal sprouts may fail to reconnect with the original distal endoneurial tube, leading to incomplete or failed recovery, neuroma formation or may connect with another incorrect endoneurial tube leading to facial synkinesis or mass movement (Figs. 40.3 and 40. 4).[18,19] This is especially true in the distal mastoid and extratemporal facial nerve. The trunk of the facial nerve at its origin from the internal auditory canal is monofascicular until the proximal mastoid segment. The nerve then branches into two to four distinct fascicles in the distal mastoid portion, and ultimately six to ten fascicles in the extratemporal segment.[20,21] Nuclear hyperexcitability with loss of synaptic inhibition at the level

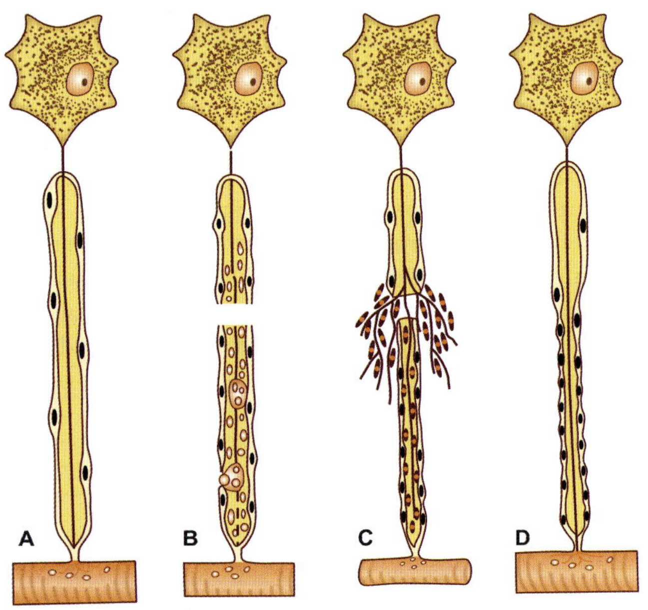

Figs. 40.3A to D: Peripheral nerve injury and regeneration. (A) Acute grade 3 nerve injury disrupting the nerve axon and endoneurium, (B) Wallerian degeneration (at 72 hours), (C) Schwann cell proliferation and axonal sprouting, (D) nerve regeneration and remyelination.

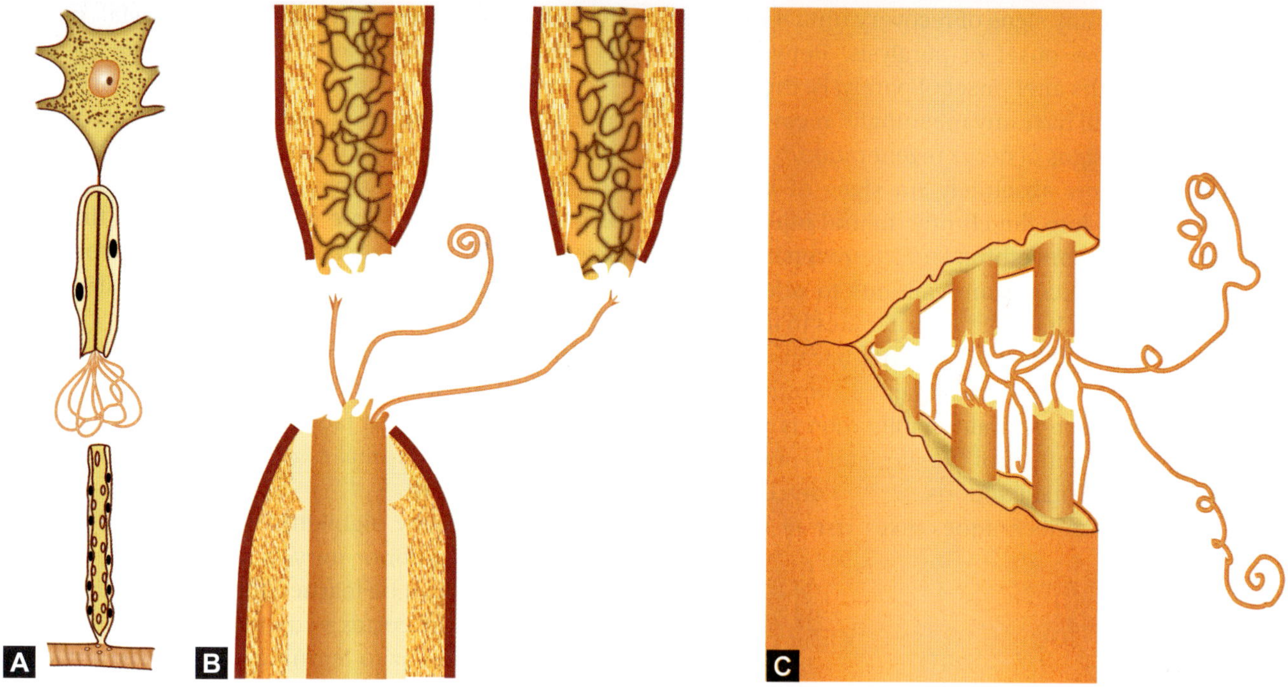

Figs. 40.4A to C: Faulty peripheral nerve regeneration after nerve injury. (A) Failure of axonal sprouts to reconnect leads to nerve fibrosis and neuroma formation. (B) Breach of endoneurium allows axonal regeneration to proceed unguided. Misrouting may lead to synkinesis. (C) Breach of the epineurium allows axonal regeneration to proceed outside the sheath. Axonal misrouting increases the likelihood of neuroma formation, facial synkinesis, or mass movement.

of the pontine facial nerve nucleus, faulty regeneration of myelin and axonal misrouting all contribute to the etiology of mass movement and synkinesis commonly arising from facial nerve injuries, even in the absence of epineurial injury.[13]

Timing

Facial nerve injury should be assessed in four phases based on the duration of the condition: acute neural injury, subacute neural injury, chronic neural injury, and chronic neuromuscular injury.

During acute neural injury, Wallerian degeneration will take place over the first 72 hours after a facial nerve injury. Degeneration starts at the point of injury and extends distally to the motor endplate of the facial muscle and proximally to the first adjacent node of Ranvier.[20] Therefore, more proximal nerve lesions result in longer distal nerve degeneration, greater retrograde insult to the cell body, and are associated with a worse prognosis for recovery.[18,19] During this early 72-hour window, there are no electrophysiologic tests available to separate a grade 1 neuropraxia from higher axonal grades of injury.[12] In this setting, failure to appreciate that Wallerian degeneration may not be complete, can lead to underdiagnosis of a more serious of injury. Once Wallerian degeneration is complete, electroneuronography (ENoG) testing becomes helpful between Day 3 and 21 to quantify the degree of nerve degeneration. This is based on the percentage of viable axons when compared with the contralateral normal facial nerve. It is generally accepted that <50% degeneration on ENoG testing is associated with rapid complete recovery in 97% of patients. While, 90–95% degeneration of the facial nerve on ENoG indicates a neurotmesis with a worse prognosis of incomplete recovery or permanent paralysis in nearly all patients.[22] By 21 days, the cell body and proximal segment reorganize and retain the ability to regenerate for an indefinite period of time. It is only after Day 21 when reorganization is complete, that electromyography (EMG) testing becomes valuable.

The subacute neural injury period marks the early regeneration phase from the period of 3 weeks to 6 months. In this period, the possibility for recovery is greatest and the clinician must take note of the time of onset of any recovery to guide the treatment plan. Onset of recovery is bimodal and corresponds to the degree of injury and hence anticipated outcome. If patients show no signs of any recovery within 3 to 4 weeks, they most likely have experienced a neurotmesis. The nerve will require time to organize and regenerate and accordingly the patient will most likely not show any signs of recovery until 4 months have passed from the onset of paralysis. Between the period of 4 to 6 months after onset of paralysis, the majority of patients who will have any meaningful recovery, will begin to show some signs of nerve regeneration.[23]

Patients who show absolutely no signs of recovery within 6 months fall into the chronic neural injury category and are a deeply concerning and controversial population of patients. Clinicians are cautious to offer nerve reconstructions with indeterminate outcomes to this early chronic neural injury cohort of patients because of the chance of recovery over the subsequent 6 months. Typically, the window where neural rehabilitation is possible is approximately 18 months, but the sooner it is performed the better the outcome in all reports.[13,24,25,26] Early consideration of reinnervation techniques gives rise to the best clinical outcomes.

Explaining the Course of Recovery

The natural course of facial nerve recovery is complicated for a number of reasons.

There are many patient-specific variables, permutations, and inconsistent outcomes from intervention that make the treatment of patients under protocols nearly impossible. The clinician must review several factors and tailor a treatment plan with the mechanism of injury, stage of paralysis, status, goals, and needs of the patient in mind. There are some basic tenets that help guide the discussion.

Reasons for variability: Variation in recovery may stem from axonal misrouting into a dead end, or the wrong muscle leading to weakness, synkinesis, or hypertonicity. Also lesions often display characteristics of mixed injury grades, making electrical nerve testing less reliable. This is especially true of delayed EMG testing. Fibrillation on EMG testing defines the presence of viable muscle with active motor endplates, but it does not quantify the degree of muscle viability nor atrophy.[18] Testing also cannot provide information about the status of the distal nerve branches, which might be fibrosed even in the presence of viable muscle.[18] These reasons may in part explain why more favorable outcomes are seen with earlier reinnervation procedures.

Risk factors: Older age and poor nutritional and metabolic patient status are associated with worse outcomes.[23] The proximity of the injury to the cell body in the brainstem is associated with greater injury to the entire neuronal length through Wallerian degeneration and portends a worse outcome when compared with more distal extratemporal lesions.[19,20] In fact, large series have shown that only 1.5% of patients with immediate facial paralysis after vestibular schwannoma surgery where the facial nerve was anatomically preserved will experience House-Brackmann grade one complete return of function after one year.[19] This is in stark contrast to 71% of patients with Bells Palsy who can anticipate complete recovery.[23] Crush injuries also produce more cell body damage than clean transections and are associated with worse outcomes.[20]

Cerebral plasticity: Proponents of cerebral plasticity assert the ability of the brain to modify its organization to permit postinjury adaptation.[5,6,7,8,13] The hypothesis has been applied to explain the spontaneous recovery of facial nerve function following facial nerve transection and surgical recovery after cranial nerve substitution or dynamic muscle reanimation.

Cortical plasticity highlights the importance of facial rehabilitation and donor nerve selection. New behaviors and associations can be learned through repetitive stimulation of the motor cortex without having to concentrate on the action, similar to learning how to ride a bike.[27] In this way, small desired movements can be practiced until the pattern is learned and becomes automatic.

Cortical adaptation requires the presence of a functional neuromuscular contraction. The more similar the neural input is to normal facial kinetics, the more successful the process. From a practical sense, the donor nerve input that most closely resembles natural facial kinetics will result in more favorable rehabilitation. Aside from the contralateral facial donor nerve, which does not require cortical adaptation, the trigeminal motor nerve arguably has the closest similarity to facial kinetics. This can be explained by the proximity of the motor cortex to that of the facial nerve, and success with unconscious smiling has been reported after masseter nerve substitution.[5,6,28,29] This is in contrast to the hypoglossal nerve, which produces an acceptable volitional smile, but does not share the same cortical properties.

Surgical Planning

Patient assessment must take into account the status of the facial nerve pathway. Evaluation of patients with complete facial paralysis includes a determination of (1) nerve continuity, (2) the viability of cell bodies in the facial nucleus of the brainstem, (3) the presence of an intact proximal facial nerve segment in continuity with the facial nucleus, (4) the presence of a distal segment with intact endoneurial tubules that can accept and transmit regenerating axons to the facial muscles, and (5) the presence of viable facial muscles with intact motor endplates.

Patients fulfilling all of the above criteria should spontaneously regenerate but may need surgical ocular management and physical therapy to minimize aberrant regeneration in the interim. Those with a known nerve transection should undergo early primary nerve repair whenever possible. Early exploration within the first 48 hours of a nerve transection takes advantage of the window of opportunity before Wallerian degeneration is complete. During this time electrical stimulation can still be used to stimulate distal muscles and help locate the terminal transected branch. Iatrogenic injury from exploration of acute injuries medial to an arbitrary line drawn from the lateral canthus to the oral commissure may outweigh the risk of observation. It is generally accepted that traumatic wounds resulting in a distal branch facial nerve transection in this zone may be observed given the high rate of spontaneous recovery from collateral innervation.[30] Circumstances associated with a limited segment of nerve loss, such as oncologic parotid tumor resection, dictate immediate, or early interposition grafting. Patients without an intact proximal nerve segment or viable facial nucleus may qualify for nerve substitutions. Those that do not meet any of the above criteria are candidates for nerve and muscle transfers for dynamic outcomes, or static reanimation to improve gross asymmetries (Table 40.3).

Beyond the few clear-cut scenarios of known transection or early limited segment nerve loss, there are no clear guidelines on how to treat every surgical candidate. This stems from the extensive patient variables, inconsistent outcomes from the same interventions and lack of a sophisticated universal grading system for the purposes of reporting. For this reason, patients with chronic neural injury must be involved in the difficult decision-making process guiding surgical management.

Candidates for classic neural rehabilitation demonstrate fibrillation potentials on EMG testing. This confirms the presence of denervated viable muscle with intact motor endplates that are still able to receive neural input from regenerating nerves but does not quantify the degree of this muscle viability.[18] This is why timing is so important in deciding the best course of action for each patient. For example, the reliance on EMG alone in a patient with facial paralysis of >2 years may fail to quantify the relative muscle atrophy or miss a distal branch nerve fibrosis that cannot be detected on EMG.[18] These occurrences are related to prolonged denervation time and may explain why low axonal load procedures fail in the later stages of chronic neural injury. In this setting, the goal to obtain a symmetric spontaneous smile with a cross-facial only procedure should not cloud the reality that failure is probable.

From scenarios such as this, modern techniques have evolved to improve donor–recipient axonal load matching, minimize the morbidity from cranial nerve substitutions, and treat the upper and lower divisions independently.[1,31] With this goal in mind, the masseter nerve substitution to the lower division of the facial nerve or the combined cross-facial nerve graft (CFNG) (buccal–buccal) and masseter nerve substitution to the lower division of the facial nerve have emerged as front runners. Alternative combined methods use the power of a hypoglossal nerve jump graft to complement the spontaneous reanimation potential of the single-zone CFNG. With these approaches successful static treatment of the upper division is commonly employed.

Electrical silence on EMG indicates muscle atrophy with fibrosis often seen with facial paralysis of >2–3 years duration. In that case, only neuromuscular transfers or static reanimation options remain. Favored neuromuscular procedures include the two-stage gracilis muscle transfer powered by the CFNG,[32,33] the single-stage gracilis muscle transfer powered by the masseter nerve[5,6,28,34] or the single-stage latissimus dorsi muscle transfer powered by the contralateral facial nerve.[35]

TECHNIQUES

Orbital Management

The need for periocular management of patients with complete facial paralysis is universal. Complications of facial paralysis in the eye area with inability to close the eye may lead to exposure keratitis, corneal ulceration, and potential loss of vision. Eyelid weight implants, lower eyelid suspension, and brow lifting procedures should be considered for rehabilitation of this critical zone. Evaluation for a Bell's phenomenon will determine adequate corneal protection in the setting of incomplete eye closure. At the very minimum, corneal protection includes the use of lubricating drops during the day and lubricating ointments at night. Patients should always be surveyed for corneal anesthesia, especially after skull base surgery. If the cornea is insensate, the patient has an even greater risk for significant corneal injury and may need more advanced ancillary procedures, including temporary or permanent tarsorrhaphy.

Eyelid weight implantation is the mainstay in rehabilitation of the paralyzed eye. The use of traditional bulky gold weights has been replaced by thinner low profile gold and platinum implants. Studies have shown that traditional gold weights have nearly a 40% long-term complication rate, most commonly bulging and astigmatism.[36]

Table 40.3: Considerations for neural treatment of permanent complete facial paralysis

Injury	*Timing*	*Special considerations*	*Prox FN*	*Distal FN*	*Motor endplates*	*Neural Rx*	*Alternate Rx*
Facial nerve transection	Acute	Within 48 hours (before Wallerian degeneration)	Normal	Lesion	Normal	Earliest primary repair	Close observation for spontaneous recovery of distal branch injuries medial to line from lateral canthus to oral commissure
FN paralysis w/ temporal bone fracture	Acute	Day 3–14: ENoG > 95% axon loss versus normal side	Normal	Lesion	Normal	Consider early FN decompression	Observation
Resection of parotid neoplasm w/segmental loss of FN	Acute	Oncologic reasons may limit use of greater auricular nerve	Normal	Lesion	Normal	Immediate interposition graft	
Acoustic neuroma resection with FN lesion	6–12 months	Early repair associated with best outcome. Poor long-term prognosis. Intraop factors may elude to likelihood of facial nerve recovery and early two-stage CFNG considered	Lesion	Normal	Normal	Combined CFNG and/or masseter nerve substitution	Modified hypoglossal nerve substitution
Congenital-Mobius syndrome	Any age	Bilateral facial nerve deficit requires alternate cranial nerve substitution	Lesion	Lesion	Abnormal	Bilateral masseter to gracilis Favored	Alternate neuromuscular transfer
Marginal mandibular branch	12 months	Consider lidocaine test to simulate contralateral DLI paresis	Normal	Lesion	Abnormal	Cross-facial graft or direct neurotization	Contralateral DLI chemodenervation or contralateral DLI resection
	>2 years	Anterior digastric pedicle flap requires neuromuscular training	Normal	Lesion	Abnormal	Anterior digastric transfer ± CFNG	
Chronic facial paralysis	12–18 months	Masseter nerve substitutions favored Combined buccal CFNG for spontaneous smile & masseter—lower division FN for power and prevention of mass movement	Uncertain	Lesion	Abnormal	Combined CFNG and/or masseter nerve substitution	Modified hypoglossal nerve substitution
Prolonged facial paralysis	>2 years	Pediatric: CFNG with gracilis favored Advanced age: masseter with gracilis favored	Uncertain	Lesion	Abnormal	Neuromuscular transfer	Static reanimation in poor surgical candidates

(CFNG, cross-facial nerve graft; DLI, depressor labii inferioris; ENoG, electroneuronography; FN, facial nerve).

The extrusion rate of low profile gold weights at 5 years is approximately 10%.[37] The shift in paradigm to thinner profile implants highlights the importance of protecting the cornea without occluding the visual axis. Platinum is less allergenic and more dense than gold, allowing for an even thinner implant of equal weight. Platinum in the shape of links allows better eyelid contouring with substantially lower complication rates and is emerging as the implant of choice.[38,39,40]

Lagophthalmos and tearing abnormalities are debilitating and intervention should not be delayed beyond 3 weeks for the possibility of spontaneous recovery. This is especially true given the ease of reversibility and quality-of-life improvement during the waiting period for return of function.[3,41] In cases of early paresis of uncertain duration, the immediate use of hyaluronic acid gel eyelid injection in lieu of surgical weight implantation is valuable. The technique is beneficial in its efficacy for the treatment of temporary lagophthalmos, low complication rate with careful injection technique, and ease of reversibility with hyaluronidase.[42,43] After placement of topical anesthetic, suborbicularis oculi injections are placed in the pretarsal space in a serial threading pattern following the same principles of eyelid weight implantation. The volume required depends on the degree of lagophthalmos and ranges from 0.3 to 1.0 cc, with the average patient requiring 0.5 cc.[42] Initial pretarsal injections may be started with 0.3 cc in the awake patient in the semifowler (reclining lounge chair) position. Serial injection may be titrated at increments of 0.05 to 0.1 cc as needed until the desired eye closure is reached without obstructing the visual axis. In cases of severe lagophthalmos, additional injections may be placed more superiorly in the prelevator aponeurosis space to achieve the desired endpoint.[43] As with all facial injections, careful injection techniques are required to minimize the risk of complications. Aspirating and checking for hematogenous flashback prior to injection is important to prevent inadvertent intravascular injection. Although the use of other fillers has been described,[43] Restylane (Galderma Laboratories, Fort Worth, TX, USA) may be preferred for initial injection in the eye area because of its less hydrophilic nature and cross-linking pattern that empirically allows for more rapid enzyme reversal in the event of complication or early return of function.

Eyelid Weight Implant Insertion

The weight of the implant may be assessed with sizers preoperatively. Incrementally heavier weights may be taped to the upper eyelid and eyelid closure is then evaluated while the patient is in the upright position. The appropriate weight is selected based on the lightest weight that permits eyelid closure comfortably. Typically, 1-gram weights are used in females and 1.2-gram weights are used in males.

Eyelid weight implantation (Figs. 40.5A to E) can be performed under local anesthesia with the patient in the semi-Fowler position. The incision is approximately 1 cm favoring the medial two thirds of the supratarsal crease. The incision is made through the skin and orbicularis muscle parallel to the orientation of its fibers. Suborbicularis dissection is extended directly over the tarsal plate creating a pocket just above the eyelash margin. The pocket should be dissected so that approximately two thirds of the weight is medial to the mid-pupillary line. The weight should rest on the tarsal plate with the inferior border no more than 2 to 3 mm above the upper lash line. Superiorly, the weight is fixated with partial thickness sutures through the tarsus using a 4-0 clear nylon suture. If contouring links are being used, three sutures are sufficient.[38] If the pocket is precise, suture fixation of the weight to the tarsal plate inferiorly is not necessary. The orbicularis muscle and the skin are closed in layers using interrupted 6-0 plain or fast absorbing suture.

Conforming spring implants have been reported and described in the literature. Their use has fallen out of favor due to a high propensity for extrusion.[44] Despite the appropriate utilization of a weighted implant, there is still a frequent need for ointment during sleep.

Tarsorrhaphy

The tarsorrhaphy procedure (Figs. 40.6A to C) is recommended for facial paralysis patients who fail more conservative methods of corneal protection and for all patients without an intact corneal blink reflex due to trigeminal nerve deficits. The loss of corneal sensation leaves them extremely susceptible to keratitis, corneal abrasions, and serious orbital injury. Tarsorrhaphies may be temporary or permanent and/or reversible. The duration of efficacy for a temporary tarsorrhaphy is approximately 4 to 6 weeks. Soft #4 French red rubber catheters or vessel loops may be cut into 3–4 mm pieces and fashioned as bolsters to buttress the skin in temporary tarsorrhaphy procedures. After local injection, a series of three horizontal mattress sutures are performed using 5-0 Prolene. The sutures are equally positioned staying approximately 5-10 mm in from the medial and lateral canthus.[45] Approximately 5-6 mm above the upper lid margin, a partial thickness suture is placed that exits through the gray line. This then enters the opposite gray line of the lower lid, again exiting approximately 5-6 mm below the lower lid margin. The suture is then passed through the center of the trimmed #4 French red rubber catheter or pierced through a trimmed vessel loop

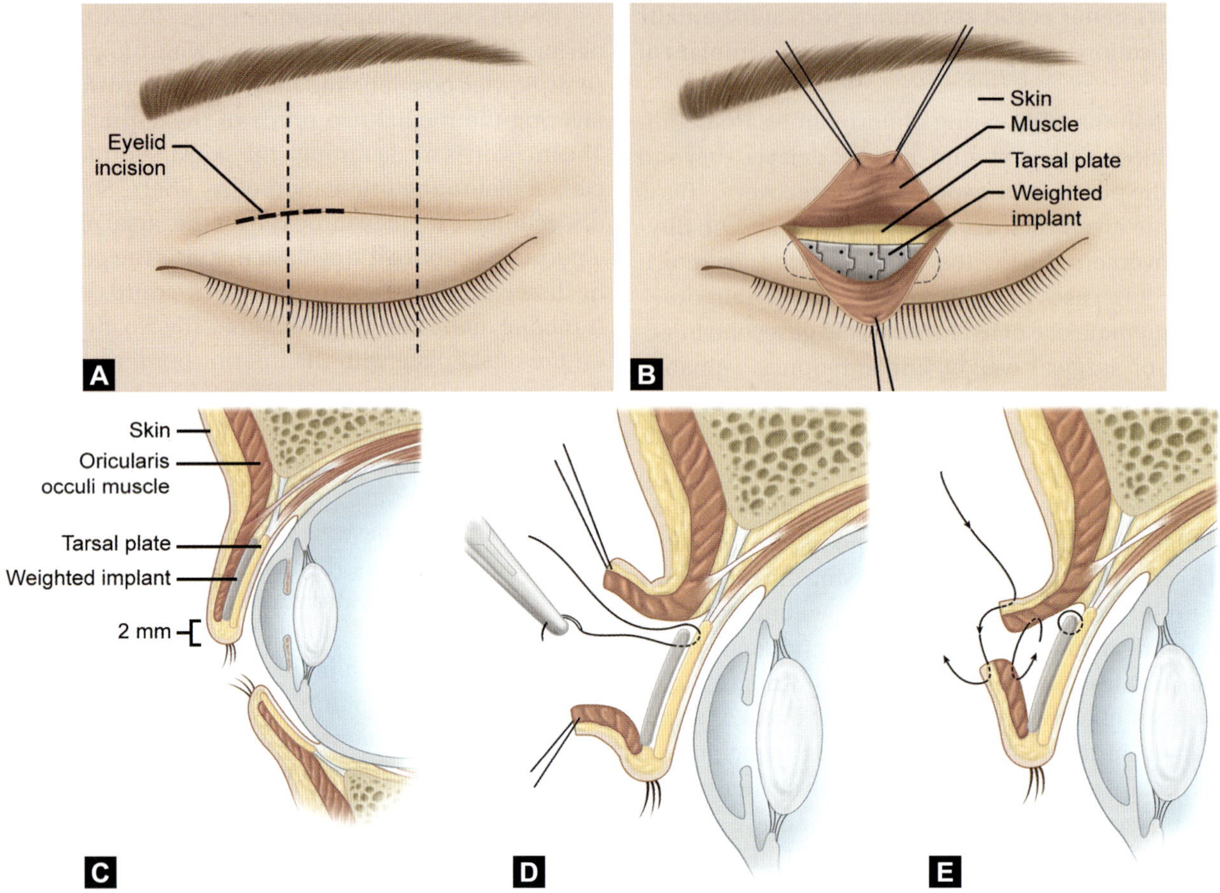

Figs. 40.5A to E: Eyelid weight implantation with platinum links. (A) Incision should be made in the supratarsal crease, centered on the medial two thirds of the upper eyelid. (B and C) A precise suborbicularis pocket is dissected over the tarsus and conforming platinum links are positioned as close as possible to the lid margin. (D) Partial thickness permanent sutures are placed through the tarsus to stabilize the implant. (E) Layered closure of orbicularis muscle and skin with fast-absorbing sutures.

bolster and then passed back in reverse through the lower and upper eyelid and superior bolster completing the horizontal mattress stitch before it is tied down.

A lateral tarsorrhaphy permits long-term corneal protection with less visual obstruction and is easily reversible. Performing a lateral tarsorrhaphy requires the formation of an intermarginal adhesion. A 7–10-mm incision is made along the gray line with a scalpel extending medially from the lateral canthal angle. Westcott scissors may then be used to sharply dissect the anterior skin muscle lamella from the anterior tarsus taking care not to disrupt the eyelash insertion. Next, a strip of epithelium from the tarsal side is cut along the margin. The procedure is repeated along the upper eyelid margin leaving the anterior surface of the upper and lower eyelid tarsus exposed. 6-0 Vicryl sutures are then placed in interrupted fashion and tied. Finally, the lash bearing skin margins are allowed to close over the approximated tarsal plates without additional skin sutures.[46]

Neurorrhaphy

Tension-free primary reattachment of a transected nerve gives the best chance of recovery. Most frequently this is seen in trauma where there is no loss of nerve tissue. The goal of any neurorrhaphy is to unite perineurial fascicles to permit axonal regeneration. All would agree that the best results are seen with the earliest repairs.[13,25] Controversy remains surrounding the best way to accomplish this. Options for primary repair include suture neurorrhaphy or utilization of fibrin glue for coaptation.

Surgeons who prefer to suture only the epineurium argue that excessive suturing of the perineurium may compromise the axonal load.[20] Surgeons who advocate suturing the perineurium argue that epineurial scar tissue and retraction of the fascicles within the outer sheath is one reason for failures of the epineurium only technique. If perineurial suture techniques are employed, the nerve is prepared by trimming back the epineurium until the

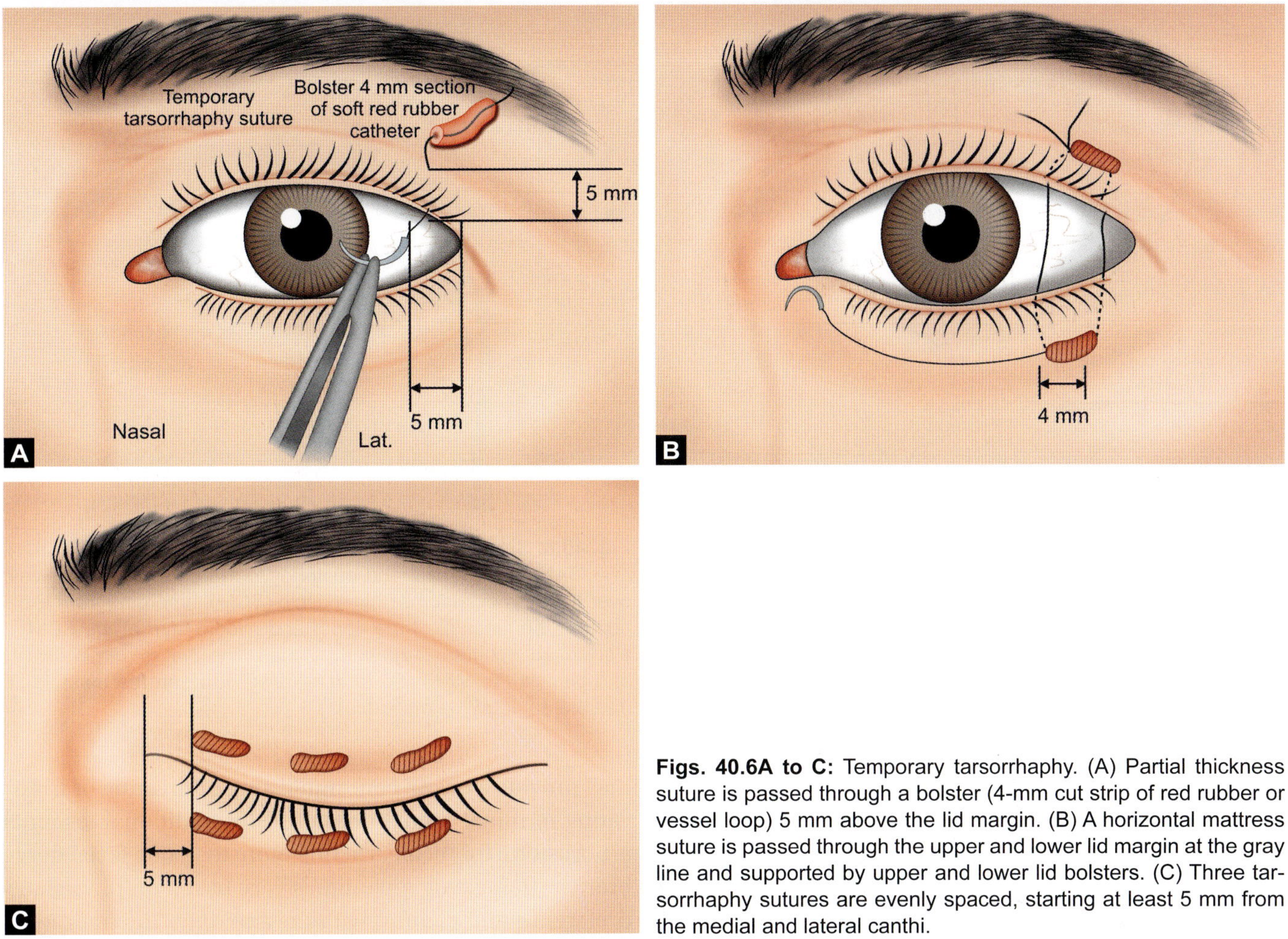

Figs. 40.6A to C: Temporary tarsorrhaphy. (A) Partial thickness suture is passed through a bolster (4-mm cut strip of red rubber or vessel loop) 5 mm above the lid margin. (B) A horizontal mattress suture is passed through the upper and lower lid margin at the gray line and supported by upper and lower lid bolsters. (C) Three tarsorrhaphy sutures are evenly spaced, starting at least 5 mm from the medial and lateral canthi.

fascicles protrude from the cut surface.[47] Most would agree that the fewest number of sutures required to precisely coapt fascicles is preferred if suture techniques are employed.[20]

Nonsuture fibrin glue coaptation has gained recent popularity and studies demonstrate equally effective outcomes.[48] Although there seems to be no additional long-term benefit, proponents argue it is quicker and easier than microsurgical suture techniques, especially in the hands of inexperienced surgeons.[49,50] Future developments involve synthetic nerve sheaths impregnated with neurotropic factors to assist in nerve regeneration and reduce fibrosis at the point of coaptation.[51]

From a practical perspective, and for the purposes of techniques reviewed in this chapter, the caliber of nerves is taken into consideration when selecting a suturing technique. For example, the facial nerve trunk proximal to the pes anserinus has more fascicles and is more amenable to perineurial suturing. Conversely, peeling back the epineurium in a distal monofascicular buccal branch may not be advisable. Another favored approach is the oblique preparation of the nerve providing a greater surface area for any mode of coaptation (Fig. 40.7).[47]

Interposition Grafting

When tension-free primary repair is not possible, the next best option is interposition (cable) grafting. Cable grafting uses an autogenous donor graft as a conduit to permit axonal regeneration to span the lost distance. Unlike primary coaptation, regenerating axons must span two lines of coaptation with cable grafting. Sensory nerves such as the greater auricular nerve and the sural nerve are the most frequently selected grafts because of the low morbidity associated with the loss of sensation at their respective donor sites.[52] Alternative donor nerves less commonly used include the lateral femoral cutaneous nerve, the medial antebrachial cutaneous nerve, and the

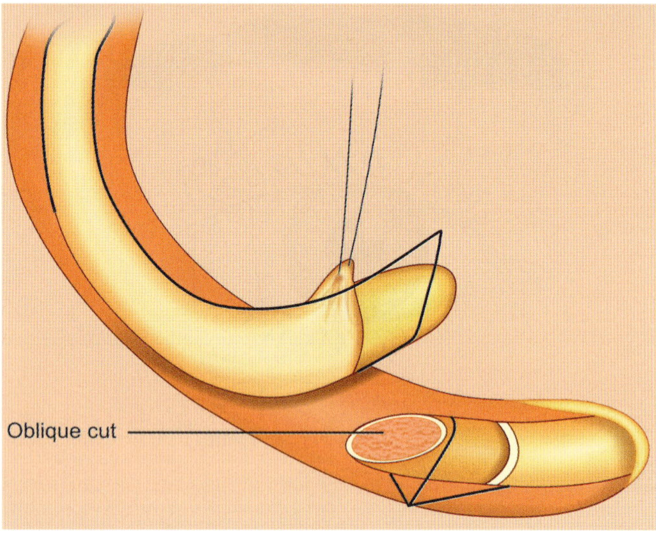

Fig. 40.7: Neurorrhaphy. Oblique preparation of the nerve provides greater surface area for coaptation.

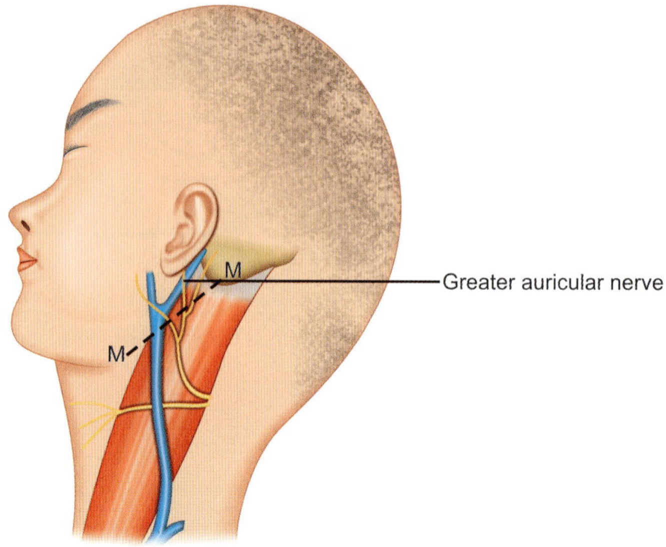

Fig. 40.8: Surgical anatomy of the greater auricular nerve (GAN). The GAN runs parallel and posterior to the external jugular vein over the sternocleidomastoid muscle (SCM), emerging from Erb's point at the junction of the upper and middle third of the SCM. It also reliably courses superiorly along a line that is perpendicular and bisects the M&M line (a line drawn between the mastoid tip and the angle of the mandible).

ansa hypoglossi. In settings of nerve sacrifice for tumor resection, studies have shown that positive margins, perineural invasion, and radiation are not a predictor of the success of regeneration.[53,54]

The greater auricular nerve is limited to 7–8 cm, whereas the sural nerve may provide up to 35–40 cm of donor graft.[40] The length of the graft does not affect graft survival because revascularization occurs segmentally, rather than longitudinally from the adjacent wound bed.[20,55] For this reason, grafts should be longer than the defect because graft contraction can occur. Occasionally, use of the greater auricular nerve may be contraindicated for oncologic reasons.

The greater auricular nerve (C2/C3) is a sensory branch from the cervical plexus. It emerges from Erb's point at the junction of the upper and middle third of the posterior border of the sternocleidomastoid muscle. It traverses the muscle parallel and posterior to the external jugular vein. The three branches of the greater auricular nerve (mastoid, auricular, and facial) can be harvested to bridge mutiple distal facial nerve branches to the main trunk. Sensory loss to the mastoid, ear lobe, and angle of the mandible will result. The greater auricular nerve can be found under a perpendicular line bisecting a line drawn between the mastoid tip and the angle of the mandible (Fig. 40.8).[20]

The sural nerve arises between the two heads of the gastrocnemius muscle and descends with the lesser saphenous vein wrapping posterior to the lateral malleolus and deep to the lesser saphenous vein to branch onto the side of the foot (Fig. 40.9).[20] On occasion, tracing the nerve may provide a useful communicating bifurcating or trifurcating terminal branch that provides additional terminal arborization for reconstructing more than one facial nerve branch. Harvesting techniques vary based on physician's preference and comfort with the anatomy. The traditional longitudinal open approach will provide the greatest exposure. Alternately, harvesting can be performed through a series of small stair step incisions.[33] Others suggest using a nerve stripper through fewer small incisions or harvesting the nerve endoscopically using approaches similar to vein harvesting for coronary artery bypass grafting.[56] In all cases, a pneumatic tourniquet is important to minimize bleeding and the nerve graft should rest in balanced saline solution upon harvest. Sensory loss to the side of the foot will result and in most cases this extends to the outer surface of the fifth toe.[57]

Mobilization of the Mastoid Segment

On rare occasion, additional length to close a very small gap between facial nerve ends for tension-free coaptation may be required. Additional dissection to drill out and mobilize the mastoid segment of the facial nerve provides a limited length advantage of approximately 1 cm and disrupts the blood supply in the process. The risks associated with this approach may be warranted in select cases

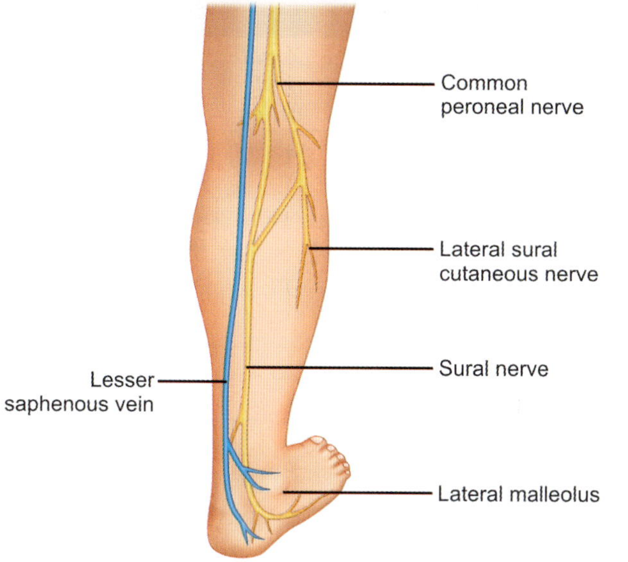

Fig. 40.9: Surgical anatomy of the sural nerve. The sural nerve arises between the two heads of the gastrocnemius, descends with the lesser saphenous vein (LSV) and wraps around posterior to the lateral malleolus and deep to the LSV.

where primary end-to-end coaptation (one suture line) circumvents the need for a cable graft (two suture lines), and thereby may improve outcomes.[20,54]

Cranial Nerve Substitution

A nerve substitution must be considered in facial nerve injuries where the proximal facial nerve is unavailable. This implies redirection of motor axons from the donor nerve into a viable distal facial nerve. It is generally believed that neural techniques may be employed for up to 2 years with reliable outcomes.[33] The high likelihood of distal facial nerve fibrosis and partial facial muscle atrophy limits success beyond this time regardless of technique.[18] If neural procedures are considered without muscle transfer within the 2 to 3 year window, the slow rate of nerve regeneration at 1 mm/day [40,44] must be factored. In these patients cranial nerve substitutions that do not preclude the possibility of future neuromuscular transfers are preferred.

The next issue is the selection of donor nerves (Table 40.4). This has largely been limited by proximity, axonal density, and iatrogenic donor site morbidity. The ipsilateral hypoglossal, spinal accessory, and phrenic nerves have historically been used to supply functional axons to the extratemporal facial nerve trunk. The spinal accessory—facial nerve substitution and phrenic–facial nerve substitution have largely been abandoned because of their relative donor site morbidity and their unnatural relationship to facial kinetics.

The hypoglossal–facial nerve substitution has long been used in dynamic facial reanimation because of its acceptable relationship to facial kinetics. Based on the hypoglossal nerve, learned elevation of the tongue in the mouth helps simulate a smile and some voluntary movements of facial expression. These voluntary actions are countered with undesirable involuntary facial movements that become apparent during eating and talking. Moreover, the morbidity associated with hypoglossal nerve sacrifice should not be underestimated. Many patients with facial nerve paralysis already have difficulty with speech and mastication. Sacrifice of the hypoglossal nerve in this setting may worsen oral motor dysfunction and in many cases is debilitating. The majority of patients with hypoglossal nerve loss will complain of speech and swallowing disturbances that worsen over time.[58] Although still useful in the surgeon's armamentarium, most would agree that complete hypoglossal nerve sacrifice is not a first choice procedure in any patient[4,59] and a relative contraindication in patients with other lower cranial nerve deficits or at high risk for future cranial nerve neuropathy associated with skull base and intracranial etiologies.[3,58] Because of the complexity of facial reanimation and the need for alternatives, several modifications to the classical approach have been successfully employed over the years (1) to minimize complete hypoglossal nerve sacrifice and tongue atrophy with split nerve and jump graft techniques and (2) to decrease mass movement of the face by coaptation to the lower division of the facial nerve only.

The experience with masseter nerve substitution in the reanimation of bilateral congenital facial palsy (Möbius syndrome) has expanded our appreciation of the utility of this donor nerve. From these studies, the trigeminal masseter nerve substitution has gained popularity as the first choice donor nerve in a variety of applications. Proponents highlight its well-matched axonal load, insignificant donor site morbidity, geographic proximity requiring a single line of coaptation and predictable results.[3,6,29] The anatomic relationship between the masseter and facial nerves is more closely related than any other nonfacial cranial nerve substitute. Advocates suggest this adds to the relative ease of cortical adaptation. The initial experiences report rapid reinnervation with return of motion averaging <6 months, and a natural voluntary smile by 8 months. After appropriate rehabilitation, 40% of patients were found to produce an "effortless" smile by 19 months and 75% of patients could produce a smile without bite posturing within two years.[6]

The use of contralateral facial nerve branches to reinnervate the paralyzed face was first described by Scaramella in 1971.[60] The stimulus for emotive expression is

Table 40.4: Comparison of neural substitution procedures

Neural technique	*Suture lines*	*Donor site morbidity*	*Proximity to facial kinetics*	*Success rate*	*Voluntary smile*	*Spont aneous smile*	*Zonal appli-cation*	*Pitfalls*
CFNG (branch-FN trunk)	2	Negligible	Excellent	Poor	Yes	Yes	No	Axonal load mis-match
CFNG (branch-branch)	2	Negligible	Excellent	Variable (ideal 80%)	Yes	Yes	Yes	Donor and recipient nerve selection
Classic 12-7: hypoglossal to FN trunk	1	Tongue atrophy	Acceptable	Good	Yes	No	No	Mass movement
Split hypoglossal to FN trunk	1	Mild-moderate tongue atrophy	Acceptable	Good	Yes	No	No	Interdigitation of nerve fascicles, mass movement
Split hypoglossal to lower Div FN	1	Mild-moderate tongue atrophy	Acceptable	Good	Yes	No	Yes	Interdigitation of nerve fascicles, mass movement
Hypoglossal-jump graft to lower Div FN	2	Low risk of tongue atrophy	Acceptable	Variable (40–45% used alone)	Yes	No	Yes	Primary utility as an adjunct or babysitter procedure
Masseter to FN trunk	1	Negligible	Very good	Excellent (95%)	Yes	No/ maybe	No	Mass movement
Combined CFNG & mas-seter to lower division facial nerve	1 & 2	Negligible	Excellent	Good–excellent	Yes	Yes	Yes	Upper division donor and recipient nerve selection, donor nerve tissue limita-tions

(CFNG, cross-facial nerve graft; FN, facial nerve).

guided naturally by the same muscle group on the contralateral nonparalyzed side. The best surgical outcomes are associated with early cross-facial nerve grafting within the first 6 months of paralysis.[1,26] Good outcomes are still reported with a duration of paralysis up to 2 years, but results are typically less consistent.[3] Critics have faced frustration with poor outcomes, insufficient axonal load of donor nerves to reanimate the paralyzed side, failed neurotization, and decreased risk of synkinesis with prolonged denervation time.[9,59] However, despite mixed surgical outcomes from cross-facial nerve grafting, it is difficult to entirely abandon the concept. Proponents advocate that it enables the most symmetric spontaneous smile because the source of sensory stimulus does not require adaptation.

Modern-day modifications utilize the CFNG to reinnervate a single zone rather than the entire nerve trunk.[33] In this way, the donor–recipient axonal density is better matched and may result in better outcomes. Adjunct procedures, traditionally referred to as "babysitter" procedures involving the hypoglossal nerve[61] or masseter nerve,[62,63] are also commonly employed in cases of paralysis exceeding six months.[2,51] This overcomes the prolonged denervation time required for neurotization of long cross-facial grafts, ensures the delivery of early neurogenic input to the motor endplates, minimizes permanent muscle atrophy, and when used in permanent fashion may allow for permanent zonal treatment to minimize mass movement.[31,59]

Hypoglossal Nerve Substitution

In the classic technique, the hypoglossal nerve is sacrificed, mobilized, and coapted directly to the facial nerve trunk. The classic hypoglossal nerve substitution is straightforward requiring only one point of coaptation ("suture line"). The tongue is related to facial kinetics in a way that learned behavior can permit a voluntary smile and functional disability from nerve loss to the tongue is generally tolerable. The ipsilateral proximity translates to rapid return of function and facial movement may begin within 3 to 6 months.[5,64] The return of meaningful function is approximately 90% when biofeedback physical therapy techniques are employed for rehabilitation.[58] Critics of hypoglossal nerve substitution argue that involuntary tongue movements and those associated with eating and chewing, cause aberrant facial movements in these patients regardless of technique.[31,33]

In the classic technique (Fig. 40.10), a modified Blair incision is made in the preauricular crease. This may be pre or post-tragal. It is carried under the lobule of the ear and extended into the neck 4 cm below the body of the mandible. A skin flap is then elevated over the parotid gland. The anterior border of the sternocleidomastoid and the posterior belly of the digastric are dissected. The main trunk of the facial nerve is identified in the classic triangle formed by the tragal pointer, posterior belly of the digastric muscle, and the sternocleidomastoid. Once the nerve is identified inferomedial to the tragal pointer, it is dissected into the parotid to the level of the pes anserinus. Next, the hypoglossal nerve is identified in the neck at the angle between the posterior belly of the digastric and the sternocleidomastoid muscle. The hypoglossal nerve lies just superior to the carotid bulb and medial to the internal jugular vein. The nerve is then followed deep to the digastric muscle into the submandibular triangle where it is transected as far distally as possible. The hypoglossal nerve is then mobilized superiorly over the posterior belly of the digastric and the distal facial nerve is transected at the stylomastoid foramen and mobilized inferiorly. A perineural repair with three to five 10-0 nylon sutures is then used to coapt the nerves.[47] The surgical wound is irrigated. The site of coaptation is protected by oversewing a superficial layer of tissue. A Hemovac drain is then carefully placed away from the site of coaptation. The wound is closed with 4-0 chromic subcutaneous sutures and 5-0 nylon is used to close the skin. If a post-tragal incision is employed, the preauricular sulcus is redefined with a subdermal longitudinal tacking suture and the post-tragal skin is closed with a running 5-0 plain gut suture.

The hypoglossal split nerve is a modification of the classic technique that preserves a single line of coaptation by mobilizing a longitudinally split segment of the nerve comprising 30–40% of the diameter from the hypoglossal nerve trunk.[33,65] This segment is sectioned, mobilized, and most commonly coapted to the lower division of the facial nerve.[65] In this instance the upper division is rehabilitated separately by additional grafting or static techniques. The theoretic advantage of preserving a portion of the nerve to continue to innervate the tongue however is not observed. This is attributed to the interwoven fascicular anatomy of the hypoglossal nerve whereby the axons do not travel in a linear path through the epineurium. In this way, many more axons are damaged than the percentage sacrificed.[33,65] Patients treated with this technique all have some degree of tongue atrophy, but proponents argue the functional deficit is rarely as extensive as those seen with complete hypoglossal sacrifice.[59,65,66] The success rate of 77% of patients achieving a volitional smile is associated with severe atrophy in only 8%. Split techniques are currently favored over classic hypoglossal nerve transection,[59,65] especially when other alternatives are not available.

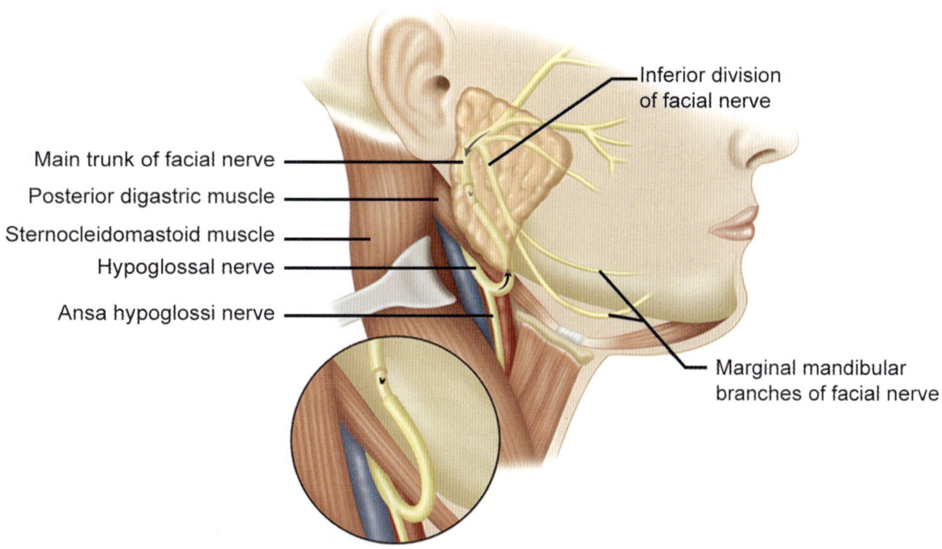

Fig. 40.10: Classic hypoglossal to facial nerve substitution. The hypoglossal nerve can be identified between the posterior digastric and sternocleidomastoid muscle. It courses superior to the carotid bulb and medial to the internal jugular vein. In the classic technique the hypoglossal nerve is sacrificed as far distal as possible in the submandibular triangle. The transected nerve is then mobilized and coapted to the main trunk of the facial nerve. Modifications of this procedure involve splitting the hypoglossal nerve to lessen tongue atrophy and/or coaption to the inferior division of the facial nerve to prevent mass movement.

The hypoglossal jump graft is another modification of this technique that employs an interposition graft to preserve hypoglossal nerve function. This graft can either be directed to the main trunk of the facial nerve or more commonly its lower division. In this technique, a donor graft is required, most often the greater auricular nerve. An end-to-end coaptation between the facial nerve and the interposition graft is performed using 10-0 nylon suture neurorrhaphy. The other end of the graft is sutured to the hypoglossal nerve distal to the ansa hypoglossi in an end-to-side manner by creating a small hypoglossal window transecting the superior 30% of the hypoglossal nerve. The end of the donor graft is fish mouthed to accommodate the hypoglossal window and secured with 10-0 nylon sutures to the epineurium. The fishmouth technique allows the mismatched smaller caliber of the graft to accommodate the larger size of the window.[47] With this technique, creation of a small window does not result in the lengthy interfascicular disruption caused by mobilization of a long split segment, and the risk of any tongue atrophy is minimal.[61] The technique is helpful to provide facial tone, but good facial movement is only seen in 40–45% of patients when used to reinnervate the main trunk of the facial nerve.[58,66] For this reason, the utility of the technique has evolved as a "babysitter" or adjunct to combined nerve substitution procedures.[2]

Another modification includes the minihypoglossal nerve transfer whereby the cervicofacial lower division of the facial nerve may be mobilized and inset in an end-to-side manner directly into the hypoglossal window. This eliminates the need for an interposition graft and requires only one site of coaptation.[61]

Masseter Nerve Substitution

The procedure is initiated with a modified Blair incision and preauricular elevation of a cervicofacial flap is performed. The main trunk of the facial nerve is identified. In cases of complete paralysis this may be ligated and reflected superiorly. In cases of incomplete paralysis, careful dissection is performed preserving the zygomaticotemporal division. The masseter nerve (Fig. 40.11) can be found along the undersurface of the masseter muscle coursing along its posterior border. Surface landmarks 3 cm anterior to the tragus and approximately 1 cm inferior to the zygomatic arch guide the dissection.[5,67] In this location the fascia is spread parallel to the zygomatic arch until the SMAS is released. Blunt dissection is then continued parallel to the muscle fibers in conjunction with a nerve stimulator. Countertraction on the muscle is helpful. Once the nerve is isolated, it can usually be dissected for 1 cm before multiple small branches are encountered. Most commonly the nerve is transected in this location. The nerve generally courses obliquely toward the oral commissure at an angle 50° relative to the zygomatic arch[67] and harvesting the full length of the descending branch has been described if a longer pedicle is required.[6] Conversely, leaving a few proximal branches intact may also prevent total masseter denervation.[3,67] Proponents suggest using the masseter nerve to power the lower division of the facial nerve to prevent mass movement (Fig. 40.12).[6,31] In this case, the frontal and/or zygomatic branches may be concurrently treated with cross-facial interposition nerve grafts[31] or ultimately with static procedures.

Cross-Facial Interposition Grafting

Whereas most cranial nerve substitutions are in close proximity, allowing for a single line of coaptation, the CFNG graft marries the idea of a cranial nerve substitution with a cable graft to bridge the long distance across the face (Fig. 40.13). A single-stage nerve graft procedure is advocated if the paralysis is greater than 1 year and is generally believed to be permanent. In patients with a high probability of permanent paralysis but concern for the possibility of return

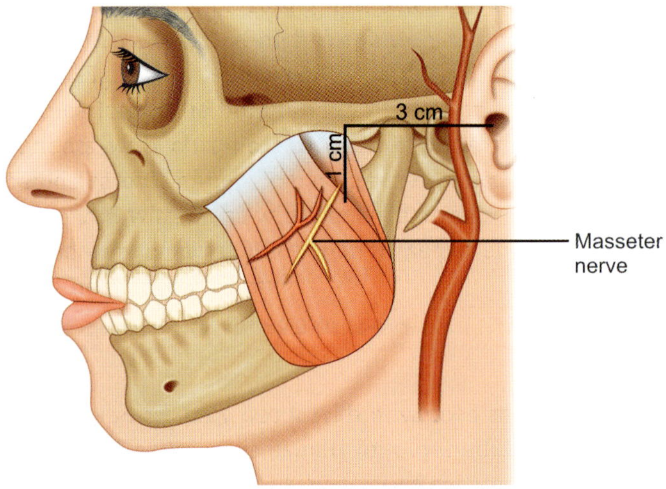

Fig. 40.11: Anatomy of the masseter nerve. Dissection of the masseter nerve can be started at a point 3 cm anterior to the tragus and 1 cm inferior to the zygomatic arch. The nerve usually courses obliquely toward the oral commissure at an angle 50° relative to the zygomatic arch.

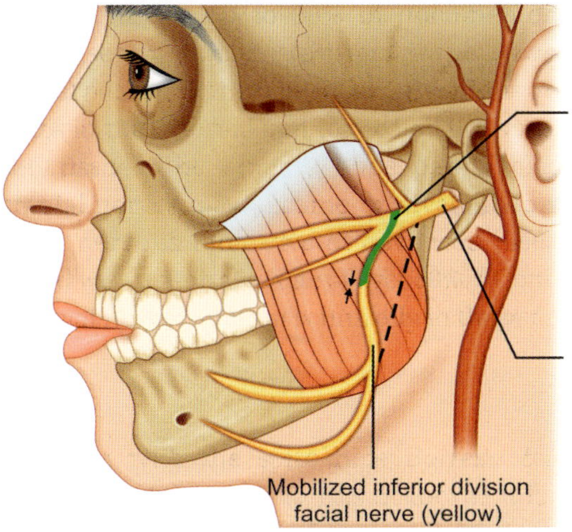

Fig. 40.12: Masseter to facial nerve substitution. The masseter nerve is in close proximity to the main trunk of the facial nerve, allowing for a more limited dissection and a single line of coaptation. (1) Classic masseter to facial nerve substitution involves coaptation to the main trunk of the facial nerve. (2) Modified masseter to inferior division of facial nerve substitution (above) may limit mass movement and facial synkinesis.

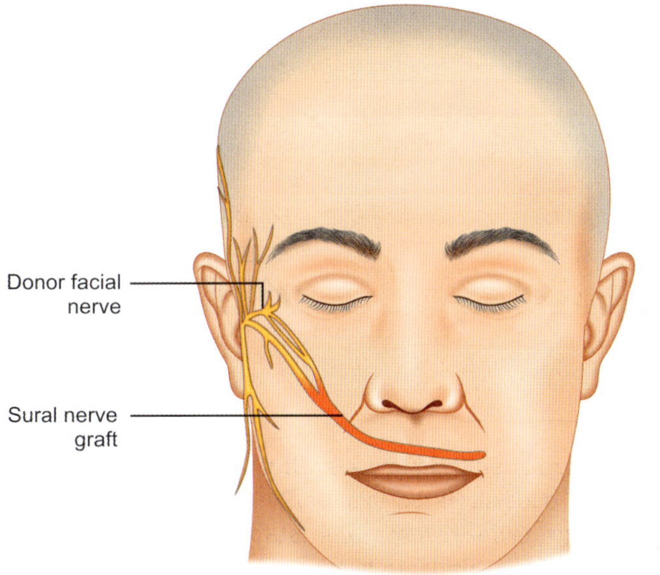

Fig. 40.13: Cross-facial nerve graft (CFNG). The CFNG is an interposition nerve graft between a donor facial nerve branch on the unparalyzed side and a recipient branch (not shown) on the paralyzed side. CFNGs provide a small axonal load because they are powered by small distal facial nerve donor branches and must travel a long distance to regenerate. The CFNG is the only neural substitution that can activate an involuntary emotional smile without adaptation.

of function, a two-stage procedure may be employed.[68] This allows first-stage nerve grafting to be employed with little morbidity as early as 6 months, to begin the slow process of neurotization across a long sural nerve graft. Once the Tinel sign (tingling over the regenerated nerve graft elicited by percussion) is noted or after approximately 4 to 6 months, the absence of polyphasic potentials is again confirmed by EMG. A second-stage procedure may then be performed to coapt the CFNG to the nerve on the paralyzed side.[69] It should also be appreciated that cross-facial interposition grafting does not preclude a neuromuscular transfer, such as a revised cross-facial or masseter nerve with staged gracilis muscle transfer, should the denervated facial muscles fail to recover.[29]

The CFNG procedure utilizes a modified Blair incision to elevate a cervicofacial flap on the nonparalyzed side extending into the deep plane just lateral to the nasolabial fold. Here a nerve stimulator is used to identify functional distal nerve branches mapping the arborization of the zygomatic and buccal nerve branches in this area. Because of significant arborization, it is important to be thoughtful in selection of both the branches for donor sacrifice and the branches that will remain unsacrificed. The largest donor nerve that does not produce a functional deficit on the unparalyzed side and provides optimal lateral oral commissure excursion without simultaneous eye closure should be selected for smile reanimation (Fig. 40.14).[13,24] Careful selection of one or two collateral buccal and zygomatic branches for sacrifice may also help balance facial symmetry,[59] similar in principle to the use of chemodenervation to treat overcompensation on the unparalyzed side. Depending on the situation and the availability of donor branches, the lower division buccal nerve branches are the most critical to provide symmetric reinnervation to the levator muscles of the upper lip. The sural nerve graft is then reversed to maximize the number of axons crossing the CFNG, coapted to the donor nerve(s) and tunneled sublabially to the contralateral side. In the single-stage procedure, the contralateral exposure is similarly obtained and the desired recipient nerve or nerve branches are selected, transected, and coapted.

The limitations imposed by a finite amount of donor nerve and graft material require priority driven decisions to maximize outcomes. In classic CFNG the zygomatic and temporal branches may also be addressed. Historically, upper division CFNGs have been unreliable, whereas upper face static animation procedures are generally

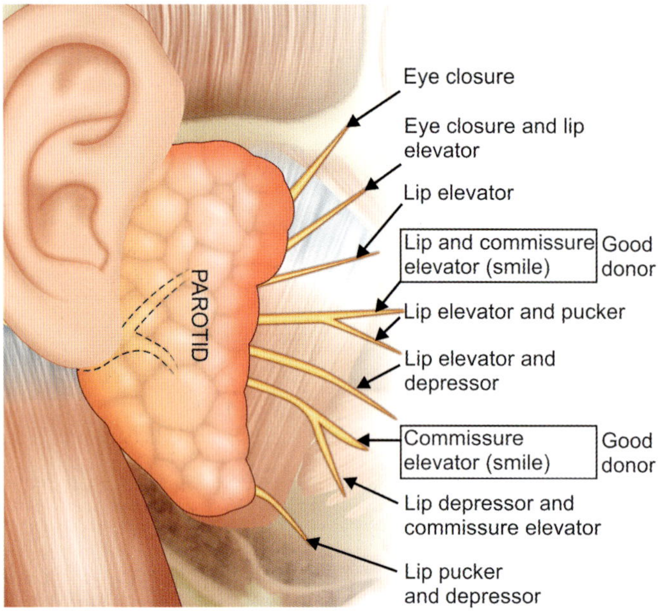

Fig. 40.14: Selection of donor branches for smile reanimation. Careful selection of donor nerve branches involves nerve mapping to select a branch that provides good lateral oral commissure elevation without simultaneous eye closure.

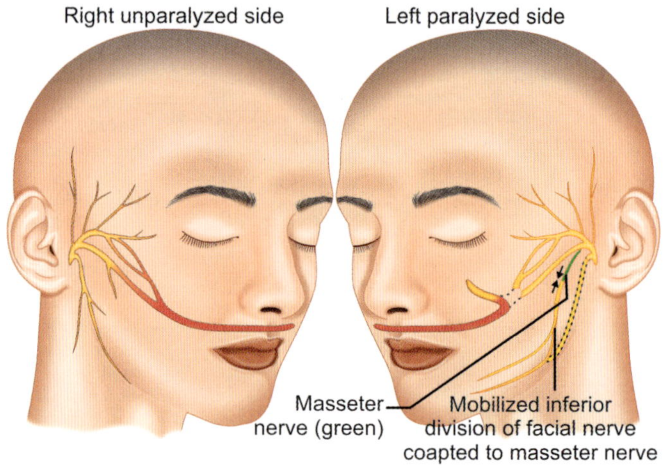

Fig. 40.15: Combined cross-facial nerve graft (CFNG) and masseter to facial nerve substitution. Modification of the CFNG procedure may utilize the benefit of cross-facial neural stimulation (red) in combination with the power of a combined masseter nerve (green) substitution to the lower division of the facial nerve.

satisfactory.[40] For these reasons, many surgeons only perform additional cross-facial upper division grafting in the ideal early cases of facial paralysis. In cases of isolated marginal mandibular branch nerve paralysis, the CFNG has been successful when used alone.[16,70]

On occasion, the sural nerve graft may be harvested with a small accessory terminal branch such that a single sural nerve graft may provide an opportunity for more than one recipient branch coaptation within the same zone. Some authors also suggest the sural nerve graft may be carefully split into two grafts longitudinally to graft geographically separate zones.[31,44] If multiple coaptation is contemplated, then appropriate matching of the diminished axonal load must be considered. The relative outcomes of this method when compared with using two grafts have not been proven and the microscopic dissection required to split the sural nerve into two branches of sufficient length can damage the axons.[9] A modification of this technique involves splitting only the distal end of the sural nerve graft for a short distance to provide multiple branches for mixed innervation, such as a combined CFNG and ipsilateral hypoglossal graft.[71] Although technically easier, the relative efficacy of any nerve splitting interposition graft technique has yet to be established for the purposes of facial reanimation.

Combined CFNG and Masseter Nerve or Hypoglossal Nerve Substitution

The CFNG should be recognized for its unique delivery of neurogenic input to the paralyzed side to prompt a spontaneous smile. Failures are seen when expectations of this graft exceed reality. When used alone, a single-donor facial nerve branch lacks the axonal load to power the entire paralyzed facial nerve trunk through a CFNG and poor outcomes are certain.

Modifications of the cross-facial technique combined with ancillary donor nerve substitutions continue to evolve with the hope that the ideal natural emotive expression may be more consistently achieved. Combination repair techniques involving the CFNG and modifications of the hypoglossal nerve substitution have demonstrated improved results avoiding synkinesis and mass movement between the upper and lower face.[2,4,71] The CFNG has also been described to address zygomatic and buccal deficiencies, coupled with lower division masseter nerve substitution (Fig. 40.15). This technique provides better axonal load matching, provides early facial tone to the lower division, and helps discourage mass movement by addressing zonal reinnervation.[31]

Direct Facial Muscle Neurotization

Heineke first described the procedure of directly implanting motor nerves into muscle in 1914.[72] In cases where no nerve branches are found, a donor nerve graft can be sutured directly to the desired target muscles. This relies on axonal sprouting into the viable motor endplates and seems to work best in cases of early or partial facial nerve paralysis.[73] Donor nerves are ideally selected from well-matched branches from the contralateral unparalyzed facial nerve.[70] More recently, direct muscle neurotization has been employed to augment partially denervated muscle in patients with incomplete paralysis. There are many situations where nerve branch injury may result in loss of partial function with no guarantee of improvement after nerve substitution. These patients may be candidates for direct muscle neurotization without disrupting their intact partially functioning neural connections. Noteworthy, coordinated animation has been shown with good results in the orbicularis oculi and depressor anguli oris (DAO) muscles and fair improvement in the levator anguli oris and orbicularis oris muscles.[16,73]

Neuromuscular Transfers

Within 2 to 3 years of complete facial paralysis, a lack of neuronal information to the motor endplates of facial muscles will result in muscle atrophy. This is characterized by a loss of fibrillation potentials and a finding of electrical silence on EMG evaluation.[18] In this setting, there is no option for nerve substitution or nerve repair. The only surgical options that remain are regional muscle and/or tendon transfers, microvascular free muscle flap transfer with nerve substitution, or static reanimation.

Dynamic muscle transfer requires repositioning of a muscle and a nerve to power that muscle in a meaningful way. Since the first description of free-muscle transfer to the paralyzed face by Harii et al. in 1976,[32] proponents suggest it has become the mainstay of facial paralysis management. In patients who are not free-flap candidates or have poor nerve regeneration potential, muscle transfer techniques can also be considered. Traditional regional temporalis and masseter transposition flaps have the advantage of maintaining their own innervation but continue to be limited by donor site deformity and the vector of pull. These muscles are powered by the trigeminal nerve and require early rehabilitation to condition voluntary reanimation through clenching of the jaw. Even with muscle transpositions, the concept of cerebral plasticity applies, whereby learned associations may lead to animation without conscious posturing of the teeth.[29]

Pedicle Muscle Transfer

Dynamic muscle transfers have long been effective in improving facial symmetry and restoring some lower facial reanimation. Early techniques employed the temporalis muscle and masseter muscle transposition flaps powered by the trigeminal nerve in smile reanimation. Modifications of the original techniques focus on the use of the temporalis muscle because of its desirable vector of pull directed from the zygomatic arch on an oblique to the modiolus. The partial temporalis muscle transfer is one favored approach to minimize tissue bulk and disfigurement. The orthodromic temporalis tendon transfer is another effective adaptation that minimizes donor-site deficit. Alternative muscle transfers have also been effectively employed to treat other regions of the face. Most notably, the anterior digastric muscle has been used in restoration of the lower lip depressors.

Partial temporalis muscle transposition flap: The temporalis muscle remains the best option for pedicle neuromuscular transfer because its vector of pull most closely simulates that of the zygomatic major lip elevator.[30] This technique has the added benefit of improved facial tone and movement without interfering with facial nerve regeneration in patients where the integrity of the facial nerve remains unknown.[33,74] The temporalis muscle is a fan-shaped muscle that arises from the temporal line and inserts into the coronoid process of the mandible. The muscle is innervated by the trigeminal nerve along the undersurface and the vascular supply is from the deep temporal artery, a branch of the internal maxillary artery. Terzis reported on the use of this flap as a secondary procedure to improve outcomes after cross-facial nerve or minihypoglossal nerve grafts in select patients who are not candidates for revision free-muscle transfers for smile restoration.[75]

Modification to the minitemporalis muscle technique described by May[76] minimizes excessive bulk and donor-site morbidity and is a favored approach for pedicled muscle transfer. Concurrent elevation of a temporoparietal. fascia flap as described by Cheney et al.[77] to help fill the donor defect is also popular.[33,74] In this technique, a Doppler probe is used to mark the superficial temporal artery. A modified hemicoronal scalp incision with preauricular extension down to the lobule may be used. The hair may be partitioned in rubber bands and shaving the hair is not required. Local anesthetic is injected. The skin is incised to the level of the temporoparietal fascia. The scalp flap is dissected in the deep subcutaneous plane to prevent damage to the hair follicles. Any bleeding is controlled with a limited use of bipolar cautery. A temporoparietal fascia flap is then elevated on the basis of the superficial temporal artery. The skin incision is then extended either pre or post-tragal, similar to a facelift incision. Subcutaneous dissection is performed above the SMAS layer, and the dissection is continued to the level of the nasolabial fold. The lateral aspect of the orbicularis oris muscle is then identified. The middle third of the temporalis muscle is then incised and elevated with the pericranium attached (Fig. 40.16). A tunnel is created with the help of finger dissection below the zygomatic arch. The tunnel should be at least two finger-breadths wide to prevent flap strangulation. The 2-cm strip of muscle is then rotated through the tunnel as a transposition flap and positioned so that it lays flat. Perioral incisions are made and the muscle is secured to the medial border of the orbicularis oris muscle using 4-0 Vicryl sutures. The patient's smile pattern is surveyed preoperatively and the vector and degree of correction is adjusted accordingly. Stretch relaxation can be anticipated over 4 to 6 weeks and overcorrection is important. The perioral skin incisions are closed primarily, and the donor-site defect is closed by anterior advancement of the posterior temporalis remnant. The temporoparietal fascia flap is then replaced over the remaining temporal defect and secured with 3-0 Vicryl sutures and a Hemovac drain is placed. The scalp flap is closed taking care to avoid hair follicle compromise, relying on galeal re-approximation for the strength of the closure. Antibiotic ointment and a compressive turban dressing are applied.

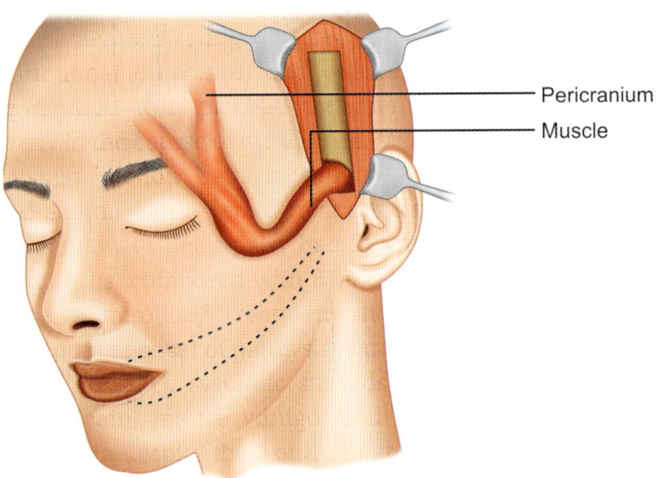

Fig. 40.16: Partial temporalis muscle transposition flap. A 2-cm strip of temporalis muscle is elevated and tunneled below the zygomatic arch to the oral commissure. The distal sling can then be bisected into slips to support the upper and lower orbicularis.

Temporalis tendon transfer: Additional modifications for dynamic regional reanimation have expanded on the temporalis tendon transfer first described by McLaughlin in 1953.[78] These include the lengthening temporalis myoplasty technique developed by Labbe and Hault[79] and the temporalis tendon transfer described by Boahene[80] as alternatives to primarily treat or augment incomplete function in candidates who do not qualify for free muscle transfer. Modern techniques follow the orthodromic modifications described by Boahene, with a single vector of pull that most closely matches the elevation of the zygomaticus major muscle.[59,80,81] This technique allows advancement of the tendon toward the modiolus without reflection over the zygomatic arch and without the donor site defect seen with other temporalis procedures. Preoperatively the smile characteristics and position of the nasolabial fold are surveyed on the unparalyzed side. A 2–3-cm incision is made through the nasolabial fold and blunt dissection is carried into the buccal space. Alternately, a strictly intraoral approach may be used.[59] The coronoid process is identified and a right-angle clamp is positioned deep to this at the sigmoid notch to protect the deep temporal artery blood supply and structures of the infratemporal fossa. A reciprocating saw is used to release the coronoid and attached temporalis tendon. If this anchor complex can reach the modiolus it can be fixated with permanent suture. The bone anchor is helpful to secure a strong hold on the tendon because of its tendency to retract into the infratemporal fossa.[59] Tension-free fixation helps improve contractility by minimizing lengthening of the sarcomeres and decreasing myofilament overlap.[80,81] A modification to this procedure described by Sidle and Simon[81] permits extension with a fascia lata graft. In this case, a fulcrum is created using a 4-mm cutting burr to drill a hole in the center of the coronoid process. The fascia lata extension graft may be passed through the hole creating an extension with two limbs. One limb is sutured to the modiolus and the other limb is secured to the midline of the upper lip. The graft is adjusted to the desired length allowing for exposure of the first premolar.[81] Physical therapy employing mirror biofeedback can help improve the volitional smile through controlled clenching of the jaw. In this way contraction of the temporalis muscle permits lateral commissure excursion.

Digastric muscle transfer: Digastric muscle transfer is one option to treat chronic paralysis of the marginal mandibular nerve.[16,82] In this technique an incision is made in the submandibular triangle to expose the anterior digastric muscle and tendon. The neurovascular bundle emerging from the deep surface of the muscle is carefully freed and the muscle tendon unit is mobilized up to the border of the mandible. The entire tendon is harvested to ensure adequate length to prevent undue tension on the muscle tendon unit. A modification of this procedure described by Terzis and Kalantarian[70] leaves only the vascular pedicle intact and transection of the nerve to the digastric for coaptation to a CFNG is employed. More favorable results have been reported in adults using the CFNG because of difficulty seen with muscular retraining after digastric neurovascular pedicle transfer.[16] The mandibular origin of the muscle is severed and the tendinous insertion is released at the level of the hyoid. Care is taken to preserve the vascular pedicle and the muscle is advanced laterally. The tendon is cut into three or four slits that are subsequently tunneled and secured to the orbicularis oris at various points along the vermillion border. The desired endpoint is a tension-free length that simulates lower lip depression on the normal contralateral side.[16] Caution must be taken to prevent thickening at the margin of the vermillion border.[82]

Neuromuscular Free-Flap Transfer

If a spontaneous smile is the goal in the setting of muscle atrophy of the motor endplates (EMG electrical silence), then options include a two-stage procedure utilizing a CFNG with a microvascular muscle free-flap transfer or a one-stage CFNG combined with a longer pedicle microvascular muscle free-flap transfer. Historically, the CFNG has been inserted into a number of transplanted muscles including the gracilis, pectoralis minor, serratus anterior, and latissimus dorsi muscles.[5] The gracilis muscle is the most commonly selected muscle for free-flap muscle transfer with an emphasis on reanimating the patient's smile and oral competence. The gracilis has a more favorable shape for facial reanimation with a powerful contraction to restore wide oral commissure excursion. However, its pedicle is small limiting its utility for single-stage gracilis procedures.[33] Alternately, many report good results with single-stage reconstructions using the longer pedicle afforded by the latissimus dorsi muscle transfer in conjunction with the contralateral facial nerve donor.[35] Most recently, the single stage gracilis muscle transfer powered by the masseter nerve has gained popularity fueled by predictable results, early return to function and the possibility of cortical adaptation.[5,6,29,34]

The selection of donor nerve substitution again depends on a variety of factors. Classically, the CFNG has been employed as a two-stage procedure. The advantage of the CFNG to power free muscle transfer remains the possibility of reproducing the spontaneous smile. Cross-facial nerve grafting utilizing a two-stage reconstruction with gracilis muscle transfer is preferred in the pediatric and young adult population when there is a lack of viable facial muscle.[24,83] In this population, nerve regeneration across long nerve grafts continues to yield favorable outcomes with a low 11% failure rate and optimizes the chance to regain the spontaneous smile.[83] In the event of failure, salvage surgery with the masseter nerve can still be performed.[29] Disadvantages of the CFNG to power the gracilis muscle transfer are the variability of outcome with a 20% failure rate in the adult population, the need for bilateral dissection and the length of time for nerve regeneration requiring two stages separated by one year.[83] Utilization of the single-stage masseter nerve has gained popularity in the adult population because of the lack of donor site morbidity, rapid reinnervation, close proximity, and its high success rate in >95% of patients.[3,29] Proponents generally site a stronger contraction of the gracilis muscle permitting greater excursion of the commissure when the masseter nerve is selected.[33,34] The disadvantage is the smile created is powered by the fifth cranial nerve and requires rehabilitation for the patient to learn to make it appear more natural. Proponents of this procedure continue to show improved outcomes, including "effortless" or volitional smile with minimal effort in up to 75% of patients though cortical adaptation after 12–18 months of biofeedback physical therapy and training.[5,6,34]

In the classic two-stage CFNG and gracilis muscle transfer (Fig. 40.17), the first stage follows a procedure similar to the CFNG previously described. In this stage the donor nerves are isolated and coapted to the sural nerve on the unparalyzed side. After this, the nerve graft is tunneled through an upper lip sublabial incision to the paralyzed side. Surgeons will ordinarily wait for Tinel's sign to indicate nerve regeneration or wait approximately 9 to 12 months to ensure that the maximum number of axons are available before proceeding with the second-stage muscle transfer.[54,74]

During the second stage, a cervicofacial flap approach to the paralyzed side is elevated and the denervated nerve

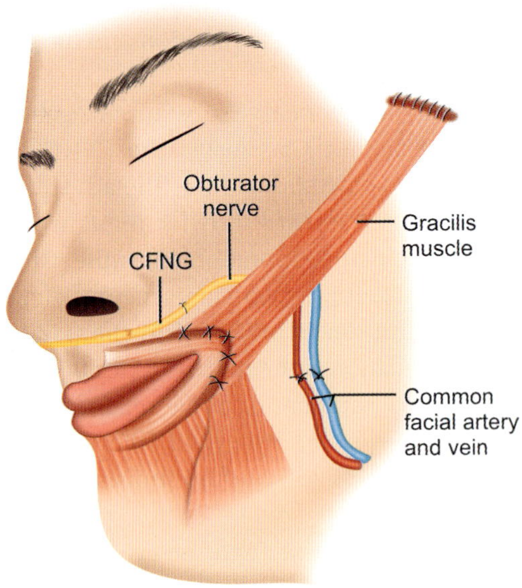

Fig. 40.17: Cross-facial nerve graft (CFNG) and gracilis muscle transfer. A two-stage approach is commonly used. In the first stage, a CFNG is coapted to a donor nerve from the unparalyzed side and tunneled to the contralateral side to permit axonal regeneration through the graft. In the second stage, the gracilis muscle is transferred and the obturator nerve is coapted to the CFNG on the paralyzed side. The transplanted muscle is suspended on the zygomatic arch and inserted on the oral commissure.

branches and the donor sural nerve graft stump are identified. The biggest complication associated with second-stage CFNG is neuroma formation.[13,20] This should be recognized and removed prior to nerve graft coaptation. The gracilis muscle lies between the adductor longus and magnus in the medial aspect of the thigh and can be harvested via a medial thigh incision. The neurovascular bundle is located approximately 8 to 10 cm distal to the origin of the gracilis muscle from the pubic tubercle. The emergence of the neurovascular bundle determines the midpoint of the flap and 50% to 60% of the muscle diameter is then harvested.[84] Typically, the transplanted muscle is aligned at a 30° angle to the horizontal and may be adjusted to counterbalance the patient's normal side. The muscle is inserted into the oral commissure in two limbs with a portion overlying the upper lip and the second portion overlying the lower lip. A third limb may be extended to the alar base and recreation of the nasolabial fold through subdermal suture techniques is performed. The flap is positioned in much the same way as a static sling where the transplanted muscle is inserted into the zygomatic arch and pretragal region. It is important to support the muscle along the inferior border of the zygomatic arch to avoid producing an unsightly bulge from the muscular bulk. Additional bulk may be reduced by removing the adjacent buccal fat pad. After arterial and venous anastomosis to the common facial artery and vein, the obturator nerve is microsurgically sutured with 10-0 nylon to the recipient nerve graft of choice. Careful skin closure and judicious use of drains is important to avoid vascular pedicle compression.

The use of the masseter nerve to power the gracilis free-flap transfer has the advantage of a single-stage surgery. The dissection involves only the affected paralyzed side of the face, and there is minimal donor-site morbidity. The donor nerve is in close proximity to the ideal location for a muscle transplant and a single obturator to masseter nerve coaptation will permit return of function as early as 10 to 12 weeks after the procedure.[29]

Static Reanimation and Ancillary Procedures

Over the past several decades, there has been a shift toward the restoration of dynamic function. However, simple static techniques are still important given the numerous shortcomings of dynamic reanimation. Many patients with facial paralysis are not candidates for neural rehabilitation and may benefit from static reanimation or ancillary procedures. Many more patients have multiple chronic sequelae that cannot be fully ameliorated from a single approach. Patients with incomplete paralysis, poor outcomes after reinnervation surgery and or aberrant regeneration represent the largest segment of facial paralysis patients and their treatment should not be overlooked.

It is important to classify the nature of chronic facial paralysis: flaccid, hyperkinetic, or synkinetic. A full zonal assessment of the face may reveal several areas where static and ancillary procedures are paramount to improve facial symmetry and improve orbital, nasal, and oral function. Brow ptosis, eyelid malposition, hemifacial atrophy and ptosis, hemifacial spasm, blepharospasm, cervical dystonia, and facial synkinesis are frequent sequelae of chronic facial paralysis and many palliative options exist for their management. It is also important to appreciate the compensatory effects of facial paralysis are equally significant on the unparalyzed side. The effort to maintain oral competence and speech or elevate the brow in a futile attempt to maintain vision result in hypercontraction of the normal side, with exaggerated asymmetry and fatigue. Studies have also shown that contralateral reorganization after facial nerve paralysis may increase the hyperexcitability of the contralateral facial nucleus, especially notable in overcompensation of the blink reflex.[85]

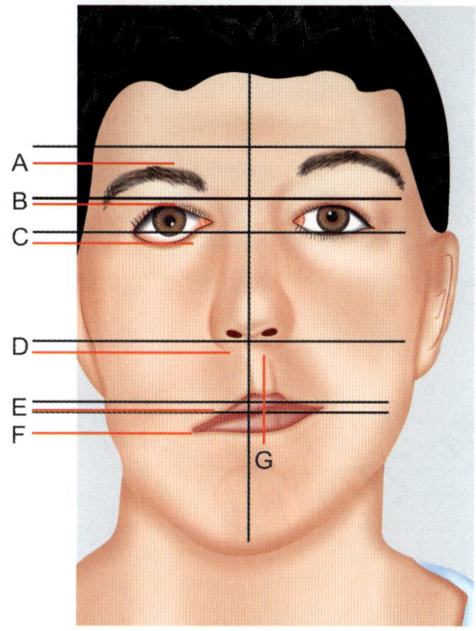

Fig. 40.18: Critical landmarks to assess facial asymmetry. A. Resting brow ptosis. B. Superior eyelid malposition. C. Inferior eyelid malposition. D. Nasal base ptosis. E. Upper lip ptosis. F. Oral commissure droop. G. Philtrum deviation.

Primary areas of asymmetry are evaluated focusing on the eyebrow, ocular region, midface, nasolabial folds, buccal region, philtrum, oral commissure and lower lip, and cervical platysma. Seven critical distances at rest adapted from the FACE software program[86] can be compared with the normal side and used to set goals for static facial reanimation (Fig. 40.18): (1) Resting brow ptosis, (2) superior eyelid malposition, (3) inferior eyelid malposition, (4) nasal base ptosis in the vertical Y-axis, (5) Mid-upper lip ptosis, (6) oral commissure malposition, (7) philtral deviation from the midline along the X-axis.

Brow ptosis may be treated by a direct or minimally invasive brow lift. Orbital restoration may require upper lid or ectropion repair. Mitek anchor suture techniques may be used to adjust the nasal valve, philtrum, and upper lip. Facial asymmetry may be balanced with fascia lata or Gore-Tex facial slings and facial rhytidecotmy. Faulty nerve regeneration may require treatment of synkinesis or hyperkinetic facial spasms with chemodenervation, selective myectomy, selective neurolysis, and biofeedback exercises.

Chronic Orbital Sequelae

There should also be an appreciation of how facial tone (flaccidity versus hypertonic spastic contracture) and synkinesis affect the eye area. The most frequent manifestations of facial synkinesis are an abnormal blink reflex and eye closure with mastication, speech or smiling or conversely twitching of the corner of the mouth with each blink. Hypertonic contraction will manifest as excessive wrinkling and narrowing of the orbital palpebral fissure in addition to prominent bulging of the cheek with a deepened nasolabial fold, loss of lip depressor function, and chin dimpling. This is in contrast to flaccid paralysis where there is effacement of wrinkles, eyebrow droop, and palpebral fissure enlargement, in addition to nasal deviation to the unparalyzed side or flattening of the nasal ala, lip muscle atrophy, flattening of the nasolabial fold, droop of the oral commissure, and dynamic deviation of the lips and philtrum. Long-term flaccid paralysis may lead to significant brow ptosis and paralytic eyelid ectropion requiring static ancillary procedures. Facial synkinesis and hypertonic spastic muscle contracture are commonly seen after faulty facial nerve regeneration. Although appropriate use of physical therapy has proven helpful, there is still a concern that inappropriate use of electrical stimulation may aggravate synkinesis and hypertonicity.[10] Physical therapy in the form of reproducible mirror exercises and biofeedback for muscle relaxation and stimulation remains advocated.[27,82] This is often used in conjunction with surgery and botulinum toxin chemodenervation[87,88] and will be reviewed later in this chapter.

Asymmetric Brow Ptosis Repair

Brow ptosis is commonly seen after frontal branch facial nerve paralysis. This may result in pseudoblepharoptosis due to heaviness of the brow skin. Several procedures are available for the correction of brow ptosis. The patient must be evaluated in the upright position manually elevating the brow to the desired position. Any difficulty with eye closure in the corrected position should be noted, especially if the patient has no return of function. The direct brow lift allows some shaping of the brow contour and gives significant brow elevation, which is often necessary for patients suffering from facial paralysis.[89] One disadvantage of the direct brow lift is the scar along the upper border of the brow. Careful incision, meticulous layered closure, and inversion of the wound edges using vertical mattress sutures will result in an acceptable scar outcome in most patients. Alternate methods have successfully employed minimally invasive suspension techniques[90] for the selective contouring of brows in both the paralyzed and unparalyzed brow.

Direct Brow Lift

With a direct brow elevation procedure (Figs. 40.19A to F), a fusiform crescent-shaped incision is drawn along the brow margin based upon the width of skin to be removed as

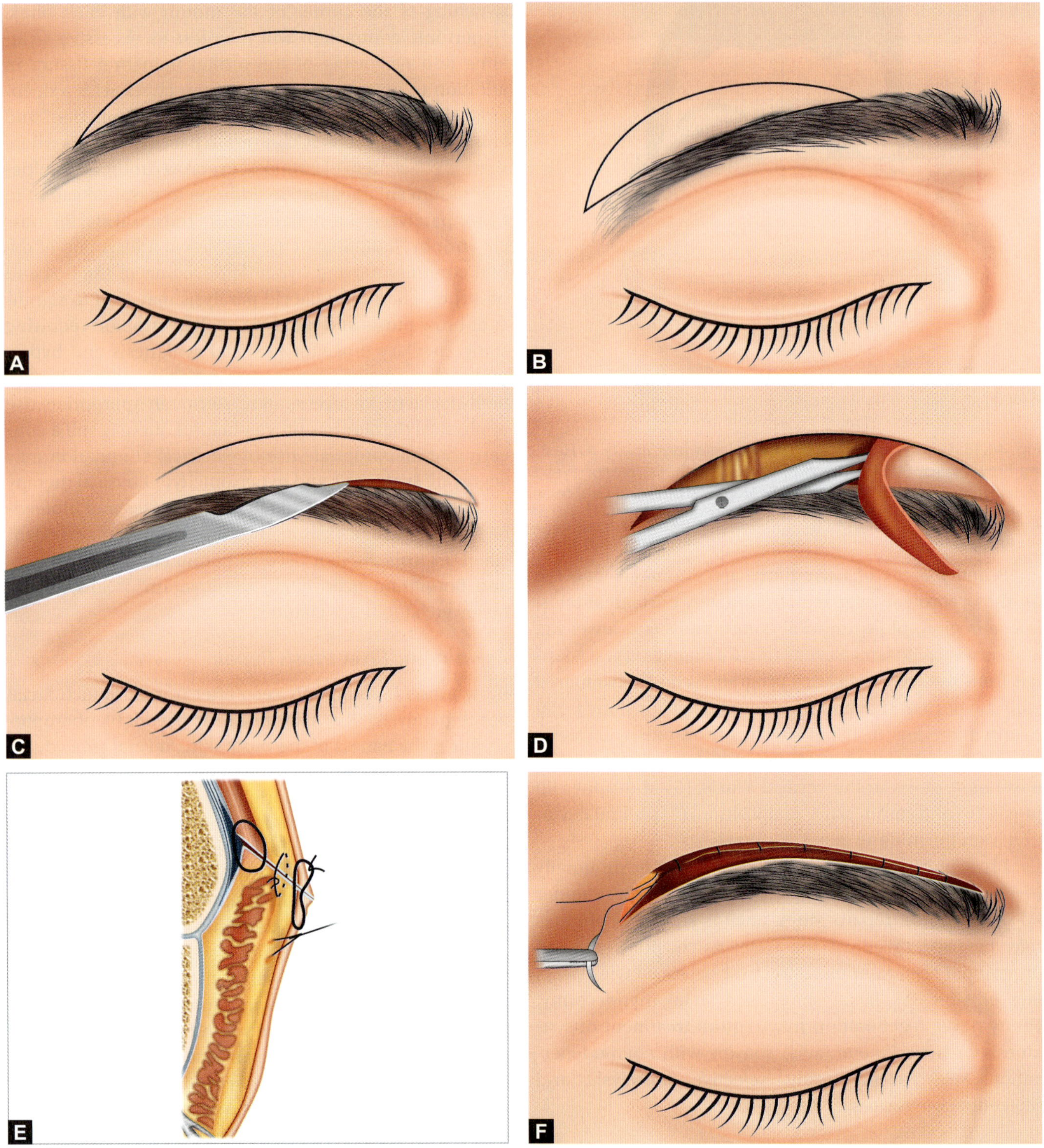

Figs. 40.19A to F: Direct brow lift. (A) Incision planning for medial/middle brow ptosis. (B) Incision planning for lateral brow ptosis. (C) The blade is beveled parallel to the growth of the brow hair follicles. (D) The skin flap is elevated in the subcutaneous plane. (E) The frontalis is suture fixated to the periosteum in the desired position. (F) Meticulous muscle and skin-layered closure.

determined preoperatively. The extent and shape of excision is determined by the pattern of brow ptosis. The supraorbital neurovascular bundle is injected with local anesthetic as it exits the supraorbital notch. Local anesthetic is injected along the skin incision lines. The inferior incision is made orienting the blade parallel to the direction of the hair follicles. Next, the superior incision is made parallel to the bevel used along the inferior incision to permit appropriate wound closure. The skin flap is dissected in the supra-SMAS subcutaneous plane above the frontalis muscle, taking care to remain very superficial in the region of the supraorbital nerve. In the setting of facial paralysis the brow can be suture fixated through the frontalis muscle to the frontal bone periosteum with two to three 4-0 clear nylon sutures to support the repair and shape the arch as desired. The subdermal layer is closed with 5-0 Vicryl sutures. Interrupted vertical mattress sutures are then placed with 5-0 Prolene, carefully everting the wound margin. Antibiotic ointment and a compression dressing are then placed.[91]

Minimally Invasive Brow Suspension

One of the most obvious sequelae of facial paralysis is the involuntary disgusted or angry appearance associated with facial asymmetry and contralateral overcompensation. Selective brow suspension as described by Costantino et al.[90] is a very powerful technique that gives the surgeon complete control over brow contouring on both the paralyzed and unparalyzed sides (Figs. 40.20A to C). Selective suture placement and cinching can be applied like marionette strings to elevate and reshape the brows into a more gentle aesthetic arch. Further the tremendous control in elevation allows for conservative upper lid skin excision as needed to optimize aesthetics without compromising eye closure (Figs. 40.21A to F).

In this procedure, three oblique 0.7-mm brow incisions are demarcated parallel to the orientation of the hair follicles in the eyebrow. The degree of medial, central, and lateral brow suspension desired and thus the ideal placement of the incisions are assessed preoperatively. Care is taken to survey where brow elevation elevates the critical areas of ptosis, without further compromising eye closure. An additional three 1.5-cm incisions are marked approximately 1 cm above the hairline in the desired vector of pull just above the areas where brow elevation is desired. Most commonly, the first vertical scalp incision is made approximately 1.5-cm paramedian, the next is made between the midpoint of the brow and the desired arch point and a third incision is made at or below the lateral temporal fusion line and oriented obliquely (perpendicular to the lateral brow). Dissection is then performed in the subperiosteal plane undermining the soft tissue from the central calvarium and frontal bone around each of the medial incisions. Elevation is continued anteriorly to the supraorbital rim avoiding the region of the supraorbital neurovascular bundle. The use of an endoscope is not required in cases of permanent frontal nerve paralysis as long as the dissection remains mindful of the position of the supraorbital notch and its anatomic relevance. The retaining ligament along the superior orbital rim is released with the dissector until

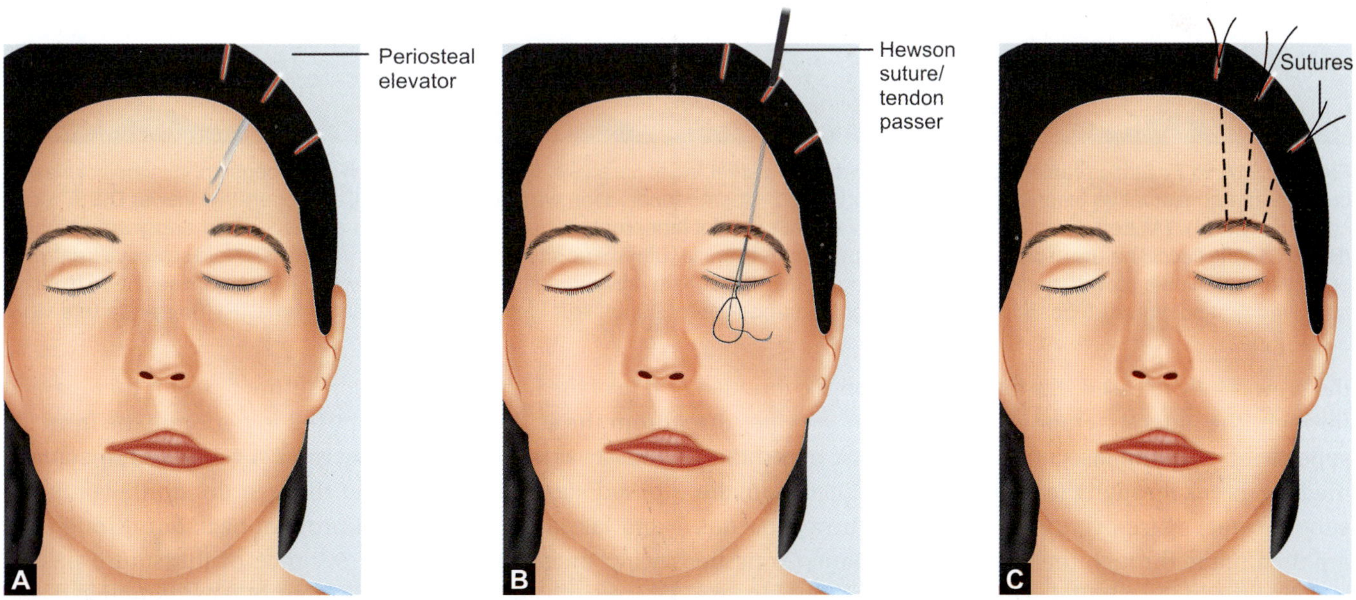

Figs. 40.20A to C: Minimally invasive brow suspension. (A) Subperiosteal elevation is performed until the arcus marginalis is released superiorly. (B) 4-0 clear nylon brow suspension sutures are tunneled out the scalp incisions using a Hewson suture passer. (C) Three suspension sutures are tightened to permit selective brow contouring.

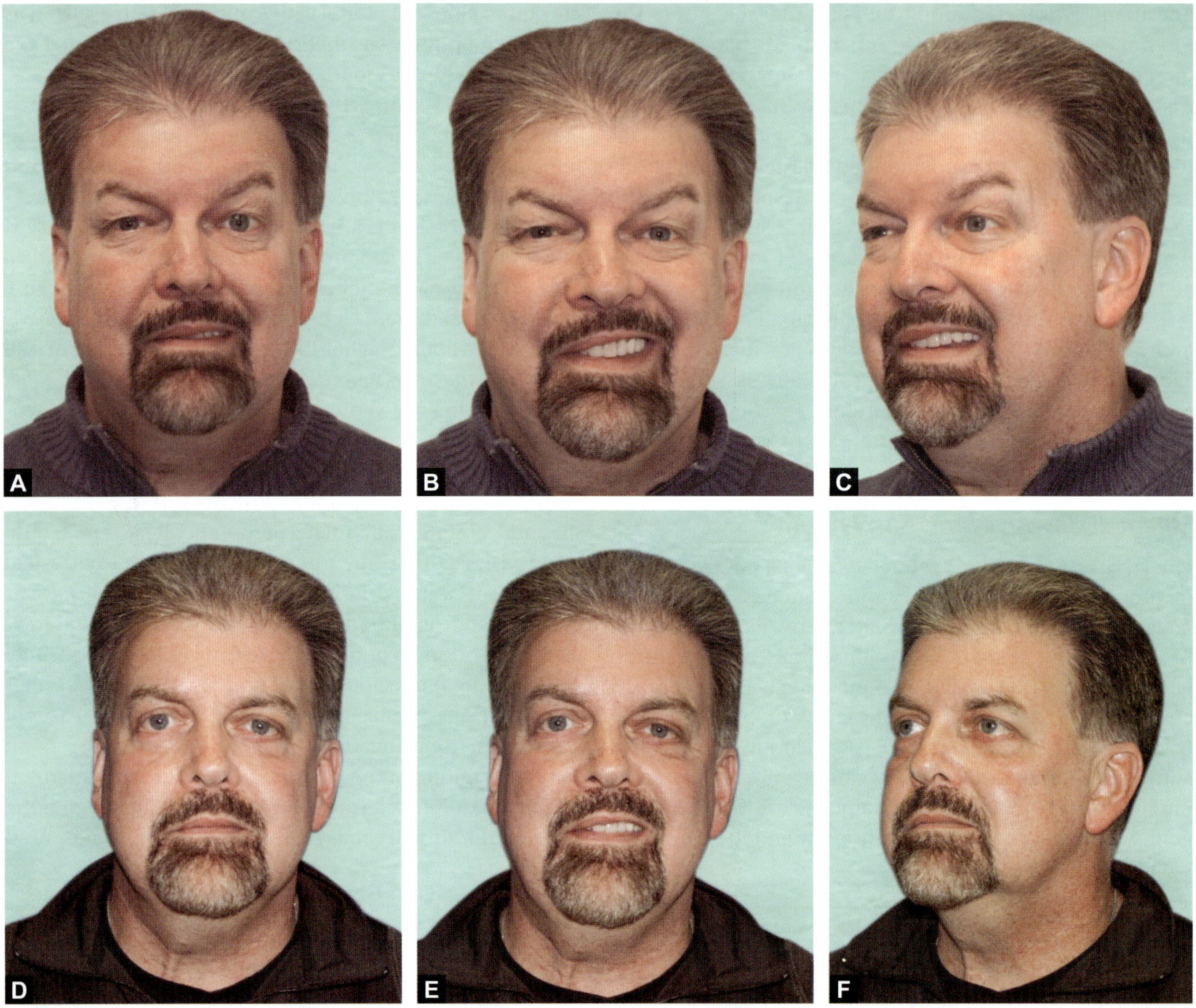

Figs. 40.21A to F: Static reanimation in patient with right partial facial paralysis. Midface Mitek anchor suspension, minimally invasive browlift, and conservative blepharoplasty were performed. Chemodenervation was not used. (A,B,C: preoperative views; D,E,F: postoperative views). (A) Left compensation to improve right pseudoblepharoptosis leaves patient with an involuntary angry appearance. (B and C) Note flaccid nature of partial paralysis on open-mouth smile with limited show of right maxillary teeth. (D) Note selective treatment of medial and middle brow to permit brow reshaping bilaterally. Conservative upper lid skin excision without compromise of eye closure. Improved oral commissure position at rest. (E) Improved position of the philtrum and right upper teeth show. (F) Three-quarters view.

the brow is fully released. The lateral dissection is continued through the lateral temporal incisions to elevate the superficial temporal fascia from the deep fascia and then medially break through the temporal fusion line to join the subperiosteal space over the frontal bone. Brow incisions are then made through the skin and subcutaneous tissue beveling the blade parallel to the hair follicle. The skin and subcutaneous fat are undermined from the underlying frontalis muscle and fascia for a few millimeters on each side of the incision. A Hewson suture passer is then passed from the scalp incision and used to perforate the frontalis muscle as it exits the brow incision. A generous horizontally based suture is then passed through the frontalis muscle and fascia in this area and brought back out through the scalp incisions with the assistance of the suture passer. Care is taken to avoid catchment of subcutaneous tissue in this stitch to prevent brow puckering. A small amount of puckering may be treated with additional subcutaneous

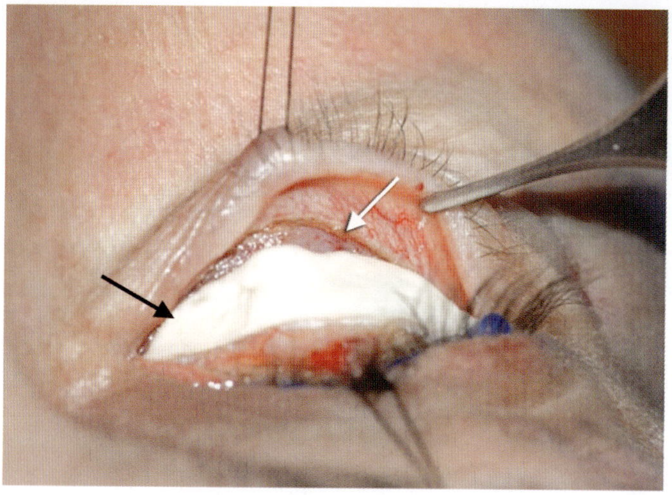

Fig. 40.23: Cadeveric banked sclera used as a lower lid spacer graft in paralytic ectropion repair. Black arrow: scleral graft; white arrow: orbicularis oculi muscle.

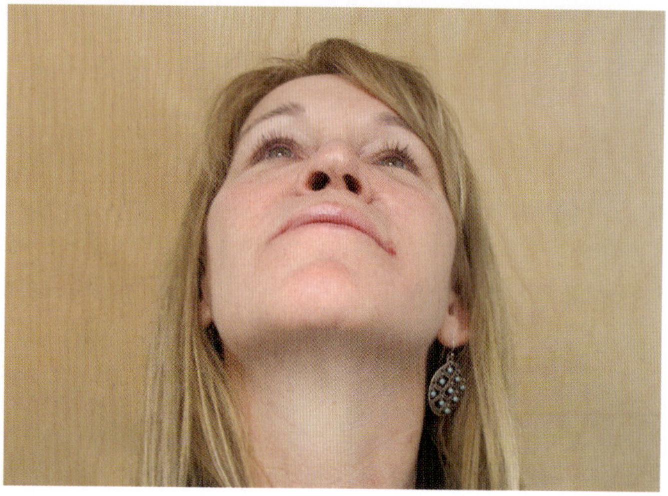

Fig. 40.24: Paralytic nasal valve collapse. Note the downward shift in the left nasal side wall and ala.

suborbicularis plane (Fig. 40.23). The graft is then secured to the periosteum at the level of the arcus marginalis to support the lower lid complex. This procedure can be performed in conjunction with lateral canthal tightening procedures and/or midface suspension to support the repair and prevent recurrence.[93]

Mitek Anchor Suspension for Nasal Valve and Philtrum Adjustment

The effect of paralysis on the nasal airway is frequently neglected. The dominant nonparalyzed side imposes severe deviation of the philtrum and subnasal region (Fig. 40.24). Combined with the progression of midface ptosis and weakening of the nasalis muscles, profound external and internal nasal valve compromise results. Treatment of the alar base with fascia lata slings[33] or Mitek anchor suture techniques[94] have demonstrated good outcomes. Alternative approaches include the use of classic alar batten grafts to stiffen the nasal sidewall.

In addition to nasal valve repositioning, upper lip asymmetry can effectively be treated by a modified subnasal lift that employs the 2.0 mini-Mitek bone anchor system (Dupuy Mitek, Raynham, MA, USA) for soft tissue stabilization (Figs. 40.25A to C).[94] A circum-alar incision is made that may include excision of a crescent-shaped strip of skin as in a subnasal labial lift (Figs. 40.26A to D). The upper skin incision is then taken down and the soft tissue is elevated in the subperiosteal plane. A mini-Mitek anchor custom drill bit is used to drill a hole in the maxilla adjacent to the piriform aperture. The bone anchor is then firmly

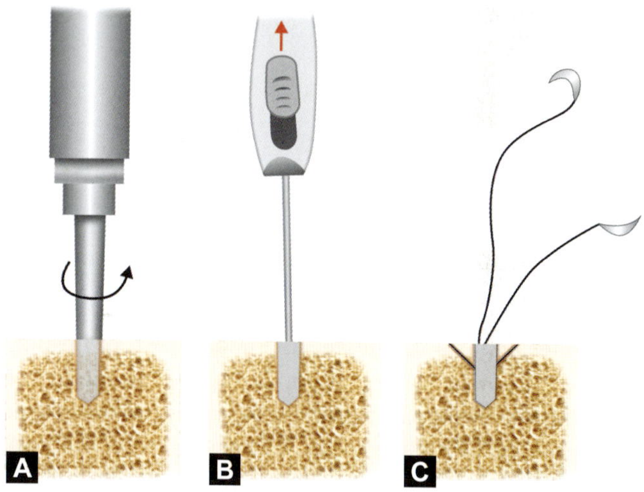

Figs. 40.25A to C: Mitek bone anchor for midface suspension. (A) Drill hole with Mitek custom drill bit. (B) Insert Mitek firmly into predrilled hole. Pull back on the applicator to release sutures and deploy anchor. Remove inserter. (C) Deployed Mitek minianchor fixated to bone with two free suture limbs available for soft tissue repositioning.

inserted into the predrilled hole. The applicator is retracted to release the sutures and deploy the anchor. The two free suture limbs may then be used to reposition the soft tissues. Success with maneuvering soft tissue must not rely solely on the strength of the suture but also in the technique used to plicate or advance the underlying musculature into the desired position. The vector advantage of pull corresponds to the position of anchor placement. Placement at the level of the piriform aperture is reliable to treat the external nasal valve and alar tissue, permit eversion of

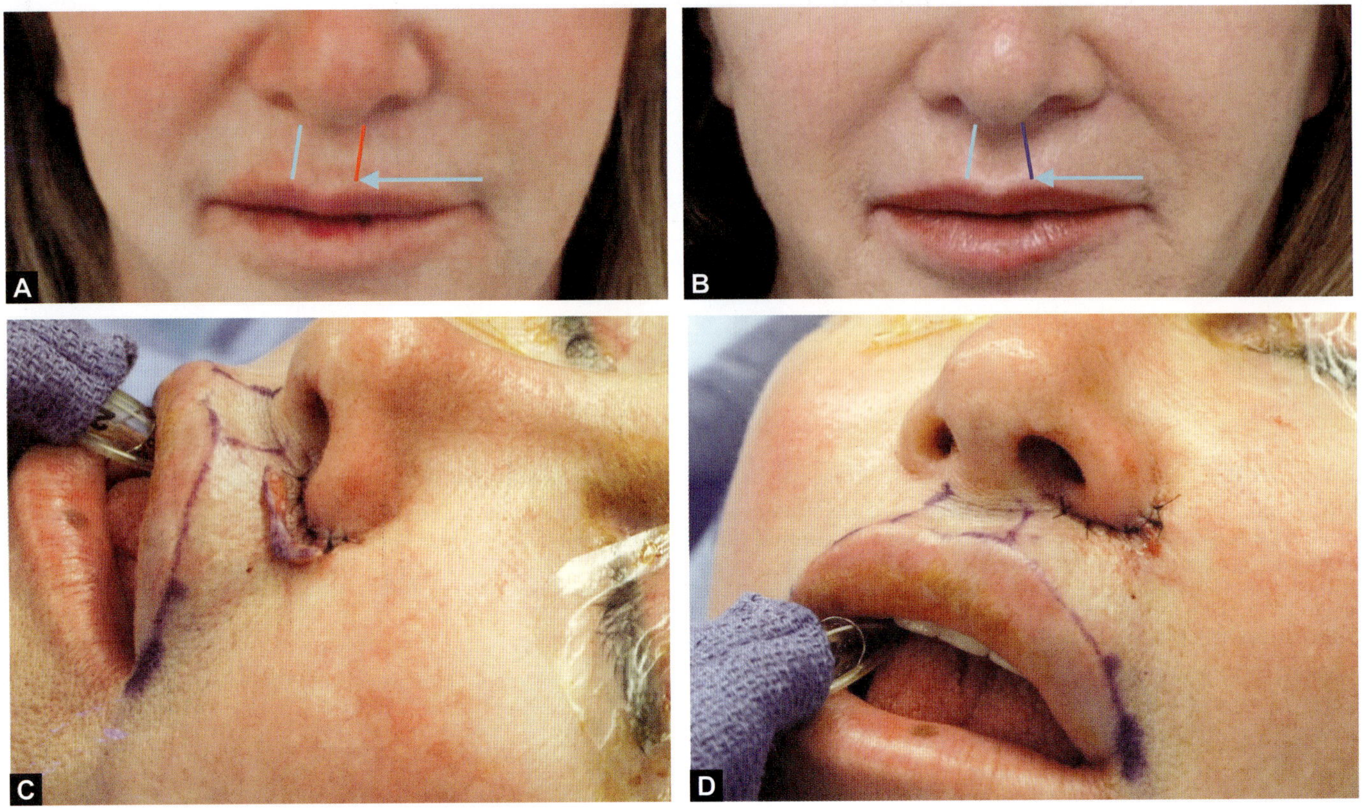

Figs. 40.26A to D: Subnasal lift with Mitek anchor suspension. (A) Preoperative: deviation of philtrum, left upper lip malposition, and elongation. (B) Postoperative: note correction of philtrum position and angle, lip shortening in the X-axis and lip elevation and eversion in the Y-axis. (C) Upper lip circum-alar approach and skin excision. (D) Closure allows for adjustment of nasal ala and philtrum.

the upper lip, and to a lesser degree improve philtral and lateral oral commissure position.[94] After bone stabilization of the Mitek minianchor, one suture arm is passed through the midpoint of the upper lip segment to evert the upper lip and elevate the oral commissure. The second suture limb may then be used to elevate and lateralize the alar base and reposition the philtrum. Moderate overcorrection is recommended because relaxation always occurs.

Lower Facial Suspension and Static Slings

In end-stage cases where the goal is not production of a spontaneous smile, many static reanimation techniques have been successfully employed. Tensor fascia lata or Gore-Tex (W.L. Gore & Associates, Inc., Flagstaff, AZ, USA) reliably provides material to support static facial suspension and improve symmetry at rest. The goal of static techniques is to restore the effacement of the nasolabial fold and the loss of facial domain seen with severe midface and lower face ptosis. An open rhytidectomy approach may be utilized to place slings fashioned into independent slips. The slips are connected to the orbicularis muscle in the area of the oral commissure at the upper and lower lip and suspended to the zygomatic arch to elevate the corner of the mouth at a position slightly higher and more lateral than the resting contralateral unparalyzed side. Overcorrection is required because relaxation always occurs. Gore-Tex alloplastic material has been shown to decrease the risk of attenuation, more commonly seen with fascia lata. But as an alloplastic implant it does carry a greater risk of infection and inflammation.[59]

Alternately, Alam[95] describes the use of a minimally invasive percutaneous sling that addresses recreation of the nasolabial fold and oral commissure suspension with a much smaller Gore-Tex implant (Figs. 40.27A to D). In this technique, a stab incision is made in the superior nasolabial fold at the level of the piriform aperture. A second stab incision is made at the inferior nasolabial fold at the level of the oral commissure. A harvesting liposuction cannula is used to dissect a tunnel releasing the nasolabial attachments. A thin strip of Gore-Tex (4 cm x 5 mm) is then sutured to the cannula and tunneled out the opposite end. Next, a temporal incision is made and taken down to the level

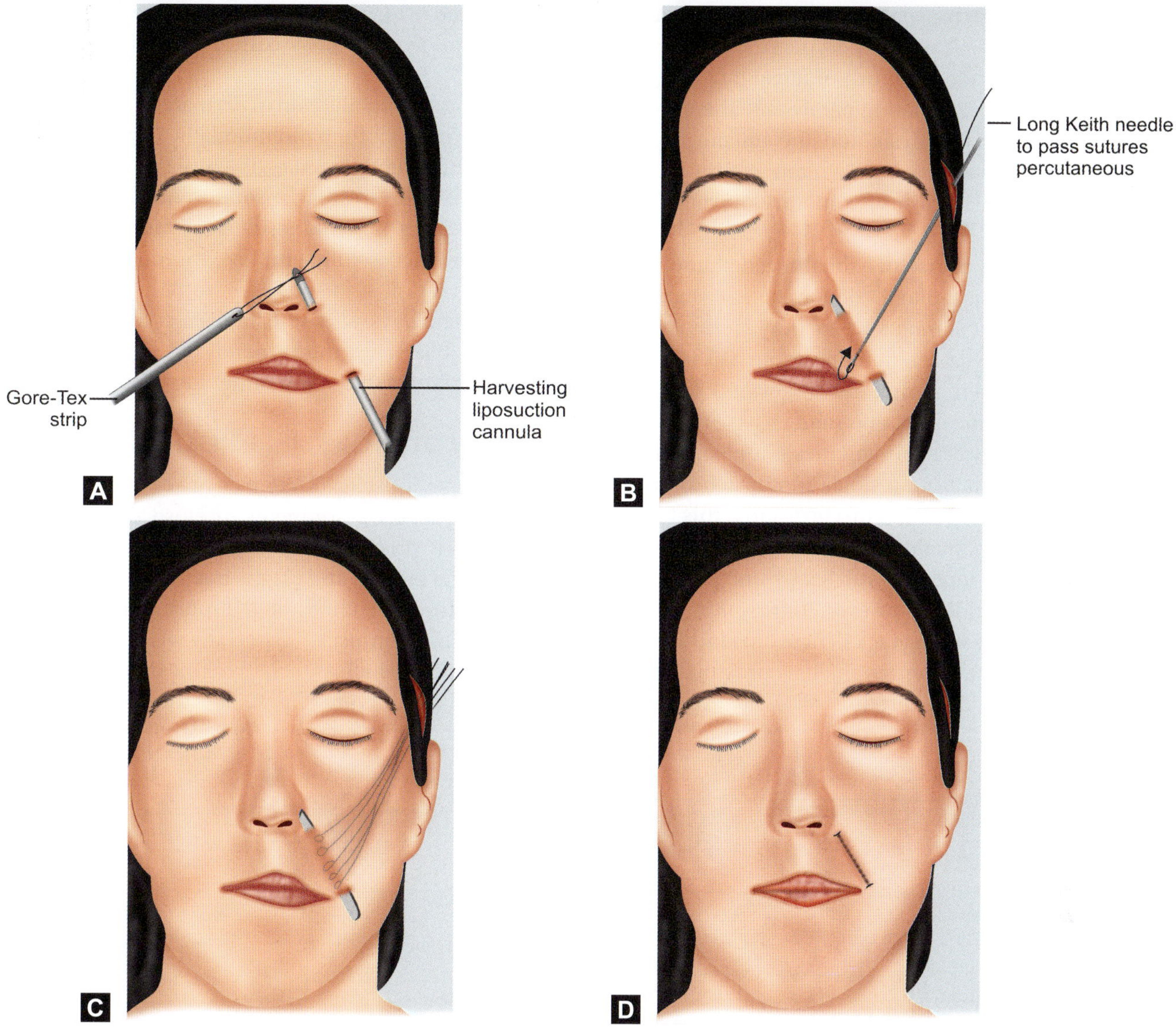

Figs. 40.27A to D: Minimally invasive percutaneous facial sling. (A) A liposuction cannula is tunneled below the nasolabial fold and used to guide a thin strip of Gore-Tex. (B) Each suspension suture is guided on a long Keith needle through the scalp incision. This is then passed through the Gore-Tex and skin and percutaneously reversed back out the scalp incision. (C) Four to five suspension sutures are tied down to the deep temporalis fascia at the desired level of correction. (D) The Gore-Tex implant is trimmed and the incisions are closed.

of the deep temporalis fascia. 4-0 clear nylon or Prolene suture is threaded on a 4 inch abdominal Keith needle and passed from the temporal incision through the implant and passed percutaneously through the nasolabial fold. The pass is reversed taking another bite through the implant and exiting back through the temporal incision. Four to five suspension sutures approximately 7 mm apart are placed along the length of the strip. The sutures are passed through the deep temporal fascia and secured at the desired position. Once stabilized, the ends of the Gore-Tex anchor are trimmed, the facial incisions are closed with 4-0 nylon and the scalp incisions are closed with staples. Antibiotic ointment and a sterile turban pressure dressing are applied.

ABERRANT FACIAL NERVE REGENERATION

Facial synkinesis is the most common sequelae of neurotmesis and its debilitating nature should not be underestimated.[88]

It is important to characterize the recovery of meaningful function in facial paralysis patients. Hyperkinesis and synkinesis often masquerade as return of facial function, but they are still a form of debilitating paralysis.[96] The chronic spasm of hyperkinetic paralysis and the uncoordinated movement of synkinetic paralysis, often confound the uncontrolled and weak return of voluntary movement in recovering patients.

During the normal course of axonal regeneration each parent axon gives rise to up to 25 donor axons.[58] Denervated muscles produce a stimulus to encourage this axonal spreading. Many of these regenerating axons fail to make a connection with their peripheral target and are lost, whereas others reach incorrect end targets (*see* Figs. 40.4A a to C). The pathogenesis of synkinesis and abnormal mass movement results from a single motor neuron activating antagonistic or separate muscle groups. This "polyinnervation" is a maladaptation that results in synchronous activation of different motor endplates by uncoordinated motor neurons.[58] In addition to axonal misrouting at the site of the lesion, the resulting lack of neuronal input leads to hypersensitivity of the pontine nucleus proximal to the lesion and Wallerian degeneration distal to the lesion. With this as the prevailing theory, more proximal lesions are associated with greater nerve damage and a higher incidence and severity of synkinesis and abnormal facial movement.[88]

Modern-day rehabilitation of permanent facial paralysis is best performed through multimodality treatment including surgical intervention, biofeedback physical therapy, and chemodenervation to treat chronic sequelae. In severely debilitating cases of synkinesis, cross-facial nerve grafting has been successfully employed in conjunction with chemodenervation and muscular retraining to override the faulty pathways and re-establish coordinated facial movements based on the unparalyzed side.[88] The commonplace utility of this is still under investigation.

Anatomy of the Facial Muscles

The workhorse muscles of the face are (1) the orbicularis oculi, which forms a sphincter to close the eyelids, (2) the orbicularis oris, which forms a sphincter around the opening of the mouth, and (3) the buccinator, which forms the fleshy part of the cheek. It is important to understand the relationship of muscles especially when attempting to treat disturbances such as facial synkinesis and myofascial spastic facial contracture (Fig. 40.28). The fibers of the buccinator run horizontally from the deeper muscular layer

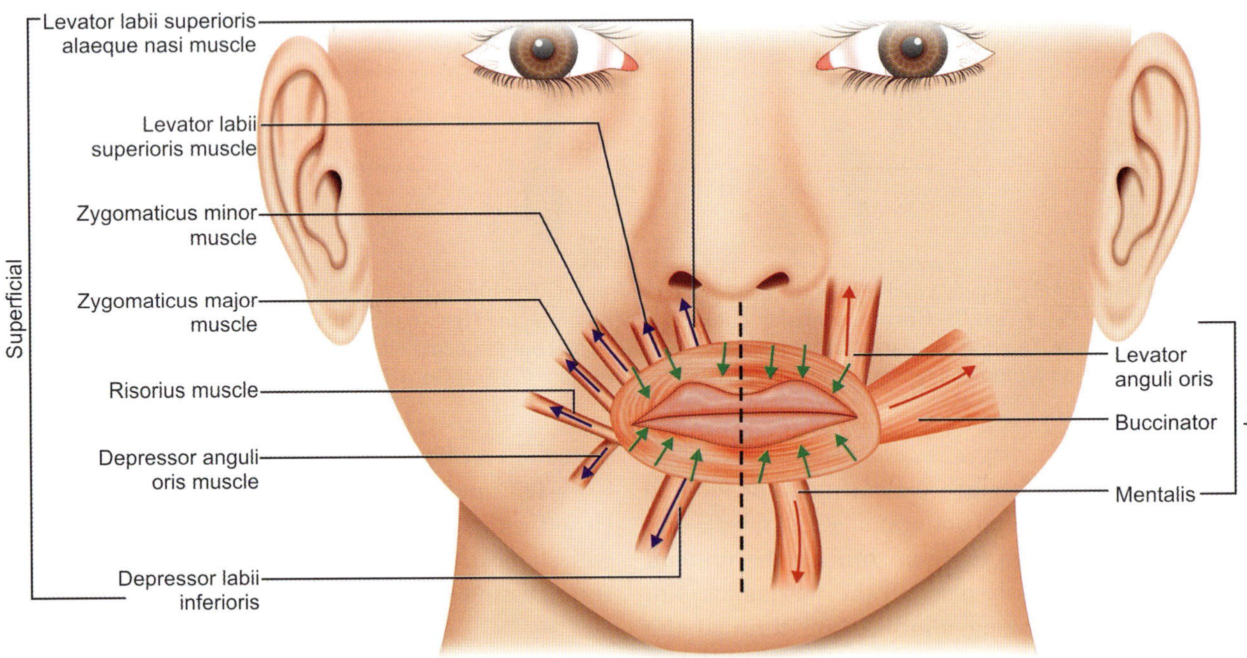

Fig. 40.28: Mimetic muscles that animate the lips. In addition to the sphincter action of the orbicularis oris muscle (green arrows), several muscles act in concert to animate the lips. The right side of the diagram (blue arrows) demonstrates the vector of pull of each of the superficial muscles. These muscles are innervated by the facial nerve branches entering from their deep surface. The left side of the diagram (red arrows) demonstrates the vector of pull of each of the deep muscles. These three muscles are innervated by the facial nerve branches entering from their superficial surface.

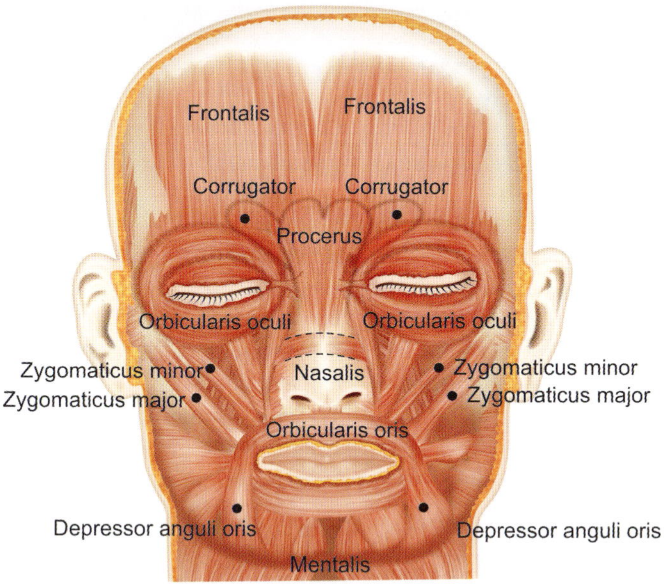

Fig. 40.29: Anatomy of the facial muscles.

toward the angle of the mouth. It additionally gives fibers to the orbicularis oris making these muscles intimately related. The buccinator muscle is required to whistle and more importantly press the cheek against the gums to prevent the escape of food into the vestibule of the mouth during mastication. In cases of buccinator paralysis, partially masticated food or saliva accumulates between the cheeks and the gums and may cause drooling from the corner of the mouth.

The mimetic muscles of the face (Fig. 40.29) work in concert to produce endless variations in facial expression. By definition, these muscles have a bony origin, reside within a superficial fascia, and unlike other muscles they insert only into the skin of the face and lack tendons.[14] The frontalis, procerus, and corrugator supercilii muscles comprise the brow elevators and depressors. The compressor and dilator naris comprise the nasalis musculature. The levator labii superioris, levator labii superioris alaeque nasi, the zygomaticus major and minor muscles, the levator anguli oris, the depressor anguli oris (DAO), the depressor labii inferioris (DLI), mentalis, and risorius muscles are among the many small muscles innervated by the lower division of the facial nerve. The cervical branch of the facial nerve innervates the platysma muscle.

Facial Synkinesis

Facial synkinesis is one of the most important issues affecting recovery of facial nerve function. Facial synkinesis may occur after any form of injury to the facial nerve and full transection of the nerve is not required. Facial synkinesis is commonly seen as a sequelae of Bell's palsy where edema leading to ischemic neurotemesis is the cause. Abnormal movements are usually noted 3 to 4 months after the time of injury due to axonal sprouting but may be seen as early as 6 weeks after facial nerve injury with early failure of pontine synaptic inhibition[13] Facial synkinesis may continue to progress or worsen in parallel with regeneration for two years or more.[4,58]

An uncontrolled disgusted facial grimace is often seen with hypertonic contraction of the nasolabial fold and the patient commonly complains of severe muscle pain and tension in the zygomaticobuccal distribution. Abnormal tonic spasms may also involve narrowing of the palpebral aperture from the orbicularis oculi, popply dimpling of the chin from the mentalis and cervical spasm from the platysma. Over and above this hemifacial spasms commonly exhibit involuntary muscle twitching. EMG findings are pathognomonic for this condition. EMG will commonly reveal synchronized activity of the motor unit of the involved facial muscles. In contrast to a normal maximal firing rate of 50/s, classical hemifacial spasm muscles will reflect a firing rate of up to 350/s.[18]

Botulinum Toxin for Selective Chemodenervation and Ancillary Procedures

Botulinum A toxin has proven an effective temporary treatment for the control of aberrant facial kinetics such as blepharospasm, hemifacial spasm, and facial synkinesis, atonic spasm following faulty regeneration and other dystonic disorders. Chemodenervation with botulinum toxin inhibits the presynaptic release of acetylcholine at the neuromuscular junction. The process of chemodenervation with botulinum toxin produces a paralytic effect that is dose related. Dosages and injection sites must be carefully mapped for each individual patient. Botox (Allergan, Inc., Irvine, CA, USA) and Dysport (Galderma Laboratories, Fort Worth, TX, USA) are popular alternatives. It is important to appreciate that the dosage units are not interchangeable. On average, clinicians accept the conversion ratio of 3 units Dyport (abobotulinum toxin A) to 1 unit Botox (onabotulinum toxin A), and modify the dosages accordingly.[97] To make this easier, a 300-unit vial of Dysport is roughly equivalent to a 100-unit vial of Botox. For the purposes of this chapter, recommended units will be expressed as Botox units. Table 40.5 explains the

Table 40.5: Facial muscles, action, and therapeutic implications for chemodenervation*

Facial nerve	*Muscle*	*Paretic muscle Botox*†	*Normal muscle Botox*†	*Action*	*Common finding*
Frontal	Procerus	—	3–6 unit	Pulls medial brow down	Contralateral hypertonic
Frontal	Corrugator supercilii	—	3–6 unit	Pulls medial brow down and in	Contralateral hypertonic
Frontal	Frontalis	—	8–12 unit	Elevates brow	Contralateral for symmetry
Frontal & zygomatic	Orbicularis oculi	6–8 unit‡	6–8 unit	Closes eyelid, depresses lateral brow	Synkinesis blink, narrow palpebral fissure
Zygomatic & Buccal	Zygomaticus major	1–2 unit‡	1–2 unit‡	Elevates corner of upper lip	Treat hypertonic/ balance smile
Buccal	Zygomaticus minor	1 unit‡	1 unit‡	Elevates upper lip	Treat hypertonic
Buccal	Levator labii superioris	1–2 unit‡	1–2 unit‡	Elevates upper lip & middle nasolabial fold	Upper lip retraction/ incisor show
Buccal	Levator labii superioris alaeque nasi	1 unit	1 unit‡	Elevates medial nasolabial fold and nasal ala	Alar flaring, philtrum deviation
Buccal	Risorius	—	3 unit	Lateral pull on corner of mouth	Balance smile
Buccal	Buccinator	1–2 unit	—	Compresses cheek & lateral pull on corner of mouth	Severe NLF spasm may be associated with buccinator hypertonicity
Buccal	Levator anguli oris	—	—	Pulls corner of mouth up and medial	Injection rarely indicated
Buccal	Orbicularis oris	—	—	Protrudes and puckers lips	Injection rarely indicated
Buccal	Dilator naris	—	—	Flares nostrils	Injection rarely indicated
Buccal	Compressor naris	—	—	Compresses nostrils	Injection rarely indicated
Marginal mandibular	Depressor anguli oris	2–3 unit	2–3 unit	Depresses corner of mouth	Downturned commissure
Marginal mandibular	Depressor labii inferioris	—	2–4 unit	Depresses lower lip	Contralateral only for symmetry
Marginal mandibular	Mentalis	3 unit	3 unit	Pulls chin upward and protrudes lower lip	Chin dimpling
Cervical	Platysma	8–10 unit per band	8–10 unit per band	Depresses corner of the mouth	Downturned commissure, lip synkinesis

*Sample strategy for initial dosing of botulinum toxin during serial titration.
†Only hypertonic or synkinetic target muscles are selected for treatment.
‡High-risk areas for iatrogenic overdosing.

independent actions of each of the facial muscles and sample starting doses for therapeutic intervention. Facial diagrams should be used to document dosing, which can be titrated in serial visits 2–3 weeks apart until the appropriate therapeutic dosage is determined. Denervation persists on average 3 to 4 months, but the duration of action is patient specific depending on collateral sprouting to restore neurotransmitter release at the neuromuscular junction. Prolonged repetitive treatment can produce muscle atrophy and in some cases lengthen the duration of action.[98]

Patients with hyperkinesis frequently exhibit narrowing of the palpebral fissure that worsens with fatigue (Figs. 40.30A to F). This originates from orbicularis oculi spasm and may or may not be seen in tandem with oro-ocular blink synkinesis. In both scenarios, treatment of the

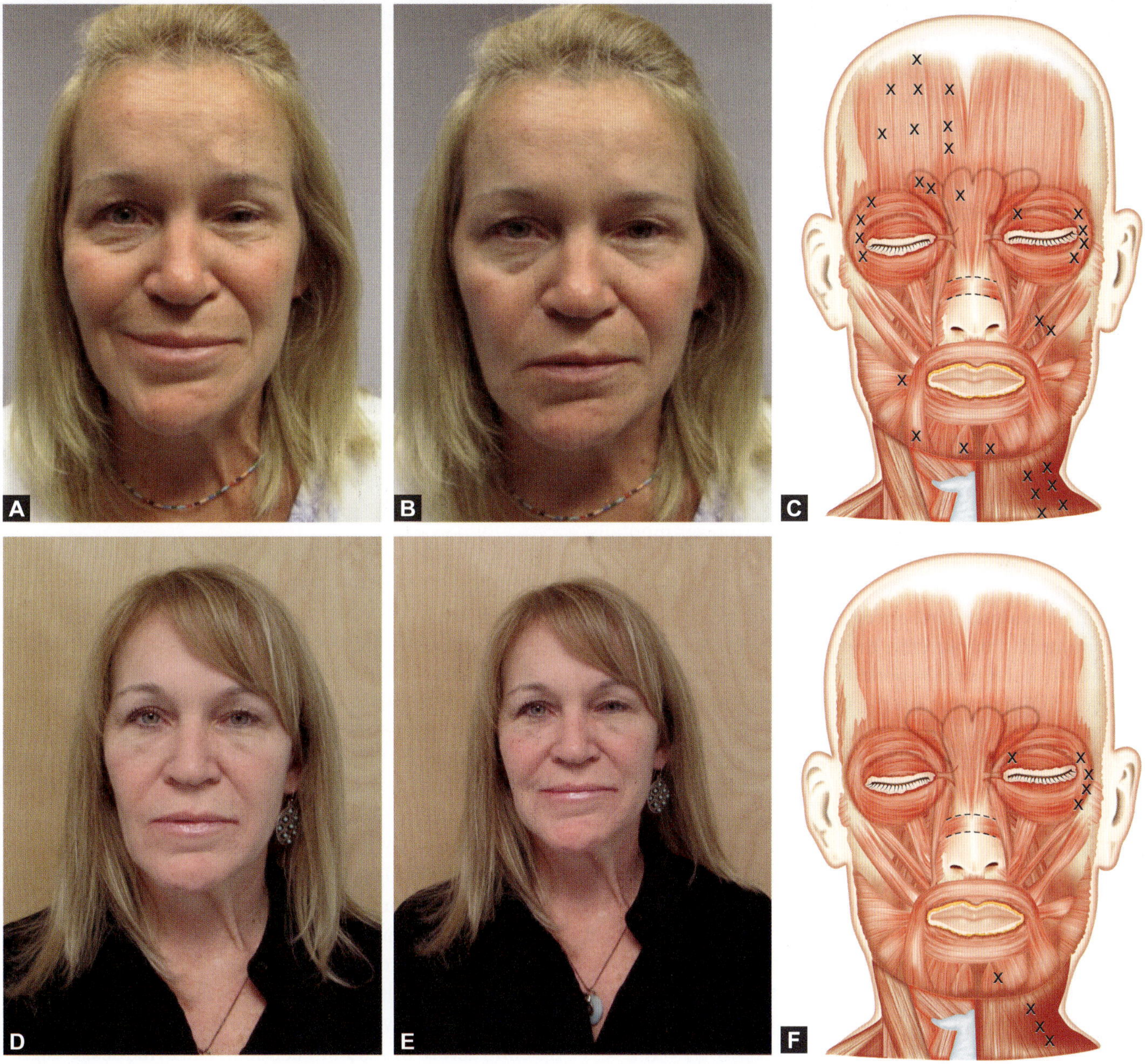

Figs. 40.30A to F: (A to C) Evaluation of patient with left hyperkinetic and synkinetic facial paralysis for serial Botox chemodenervation. (D to F) Follow-up evaluation of left hyperkinetic facial paralysis for serial dosing after first Botox chemodenervation. (A) At rest: note the hyperkinetic left zygomaticus muscles causing severe facial contracture at the nasolabial fold with left upward deviation of the upper lip complex. Normal depressor anguli oris (DAO) activation on the right is perceived as an oral commissure droop. Also note right over-compensation causing shift of the philtrum to the weaker left side. (B) Smile: note the hyperkinetic left orbicularis oculi causing narrowing of the palperbral fissure. The patient also suffers from left smile mediated oro-ocular blink synkinesis. Note the mentalis dimpling on the left and hyperkinetic left platysma muscles. The patient has generalized right over-compensation causing asymmetry in other views (not provided). (C) DOSE TITRATION 1: right frontalis/corrugator/procerus (15 u), bilateral orbicularis oculi (6 u each), left zygomaticus major (3 u), left zygomaticus minor (1 u), bilateral mentalis (3 u each), right DAO (3 u), right risorius (3 u), left platysma (6 u per band × 2). (D) At rest: note improved relaxation of hyperkinetic left zygomaticus muscles with improved upper lip and philtrum position. Right DAO relaxation provides oral commissure symmetry at rest. Orbicularis relaxation with lateral brow elevation at rest. (E) Smile: improved hyperkinetic left orbicularis oculi with incomplete widening of the palpebral fissure. Persistent mentalis dimpling on the left and persistent dominant hyperkinetic left platysma band. Persistent oro-ocular blink synkinesis with modest improvement. (F) DOSE TITRATION 2: left orbicularis oculi (6 u), left mentalis (3 u), left platysma (6 u).

orbital orbicularis oculi (lateral crow's feet) alone may be insufficient to correct the problem. The problem resides in the hyperkinetic pretarsal and preseptal orbicularis, a zone not routinely treated in aesthetic applications. Candidates for this treatment should have a good snap test without laxity. Patients with oro-ocular synkinesis and hyperkinesis are treated cautiously in the preseptal orbicularis oculi to minimize hyperactivity. Care is taken to start with low doses to prevent upper lid ptosis, ectropion, and untoward effects.

It is also important to appreciate the antagonistic paired action of muscles when treating facial zones by chemodenervation. Paralyzing one muscle group invariably has some effect on its antagonistic pair. In facial paralysis, this may be a favorable outcome, but only when used intentionally. Pitfalls are seen with selective treatment of the procerus and corrugator brow depressors leading to rebound hyperactive furrows of the frontalis. Isolated treatment of the DAO may result in unopposed mentalis action with an unnatural upturned smirk.

Treatment of the DAO and the mentalis muscles should be evaluated in concert, especially in patients with hyperkinesis. Popply chin dimpling (peau d' orange) is frequently seen with hyperkinesis on the paralyzed side or over compensation on the unparalyzed side. Injection is usually initiated with 3 units of Botox. It is important to stay below the mental crease in the fleshy part of the mentalis closer to the midline to avoid inadvertent weakening of the adjacent DLI. The permanent mouth frown extending to the marionette lines is caused by the depressor action of the DAO. The DAO partially overlies the DLI and caution must be used to avoid inadvertent injection of both muscles. Safe DAO injection can be performed with a starting dose of 3 units at the posterior aspect of the muscle belly, just above its insertion on the mandible at a point 1 cm lateral to the oral commissure. The contribution of the platysma muscle to facial synkinesis has long been underappreciated.[99] In many individuals, fibers of the platysma muscle interdigitate with the depressor muscles of the lower lip (Figs. 40.31A and B). Hyperkinesis of the platysma may lead to oral commissure droop and exacerbate cervicofacial synkinesis. Vertical bands can be manually palpated and three to four injections are placed along the length of the dominant band at a starting dose of 8–10 units. Additional bands may be treated at the same or lower dose depending on the degree of hyperactivity.

Alternate treatments for hyperkinesis following aberrant regeneration include selective neurectomy or more commonly, myectomy to resect the affected muscle groups and provide permanent release of muscular spasms. The efficacy of myectomy may be surveyed through preoperative planning with selective botulinum toxin treatment. Successful treatment with a paralytic agent is helpful in identifying the ideal treatment algorithm for myectomy in select patients. Considerations may include partial resection of the zygomatic major muscle to correct nasolabial spasm caused by sustained hypertonic contracture of this muscle group.[100] In cases where the upper lip is retracted superiorly, the levator labii superioris muscle may be addressed.[3] This effectively treats the exaggerated canine smile or excessive lateral incisor show (Figs. 40.32A to G). Prominent chin dimpling can be treated by injection or resection of the mentalis muscle. Resection of the DLI may be used to improve symmetry by inhibition of lower lip depression on the normal side, especially in patients seeking a permanent result after success with chemodenervation.[82] Platysma spasm with tonic contracture may worsen lower lip contracture or result in cervicofacial synkinesis.[3] Significant success with platysmectomy is seen in patients who have a good result after platysmal chemodenervation.[99]

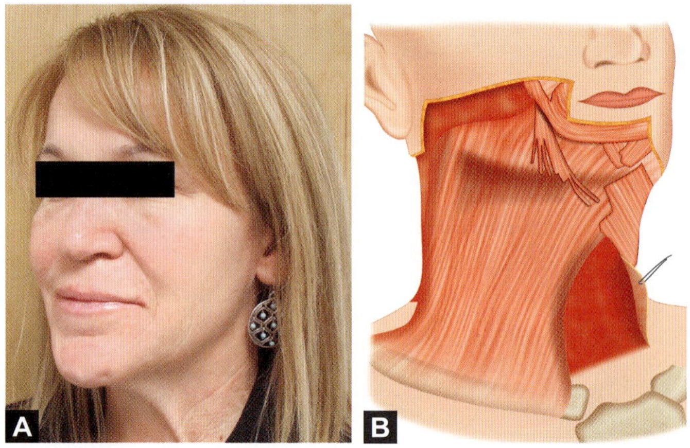

Figs. 40.31A and B: Note the direct contribution of platysma muscle fibers to the depressor anguli oris causing oral commissure droop. Platysma hyperactivity is commonly seen in oro-ocular blink synkinesis. Treatment of the platysma muscle is important to safely and effectively treat this condition.

Treatment of the Contralateral Face

The impact of functional treatment of the contralateral face should not be underestimated. Treatment of the procerus, corrugator, and frontalis muscle on the unparalyzed side is highly effective in treating muscle overcompensation and balancing the upper third of the face. Chemodenervation of the DLI has effectively been used to balance the smile without oral incompetence or speech abnormalities in the majority of patients.[82] However, a small percentage

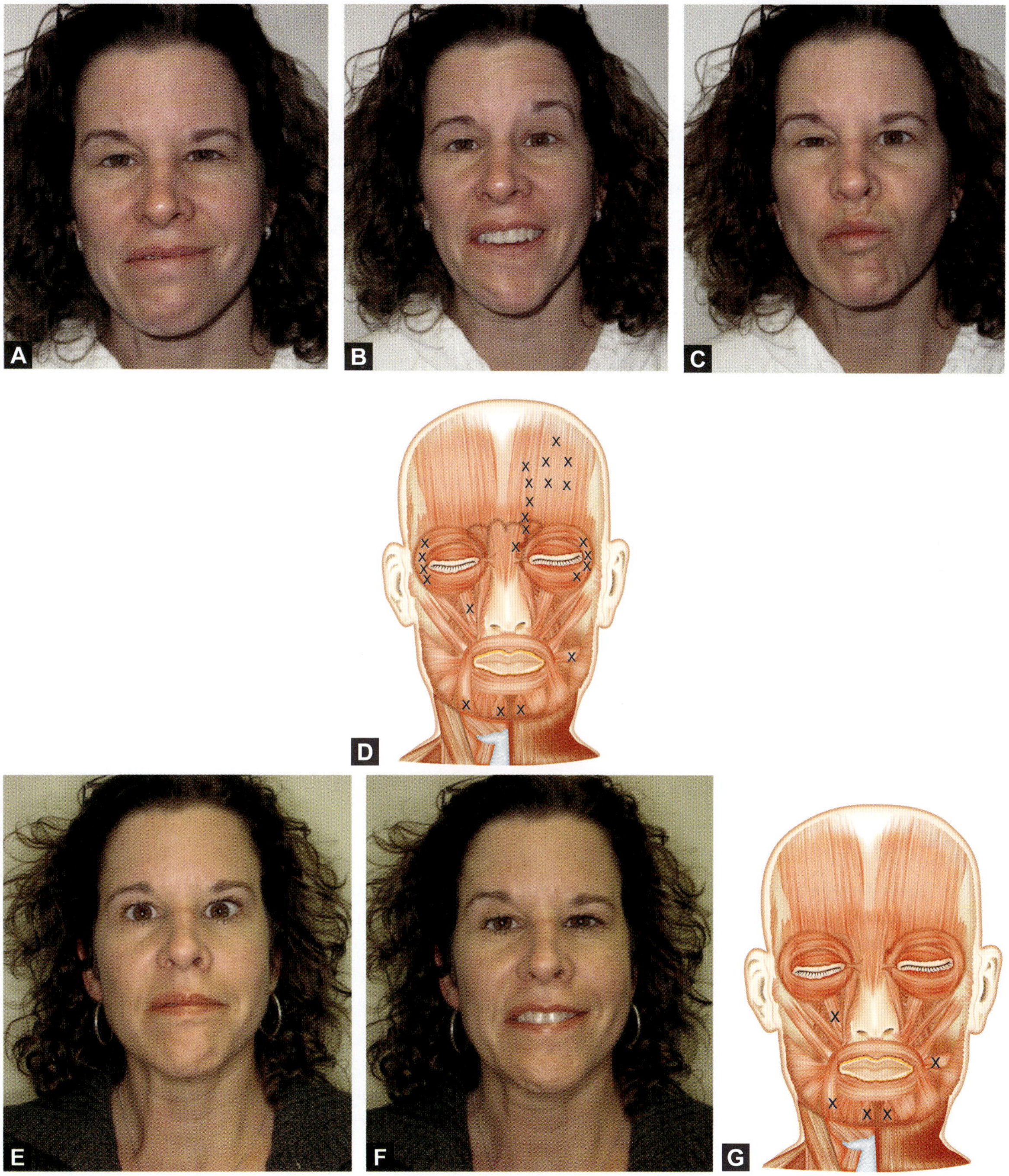

Figs. 40.32A to G: (A to D) Evaluation of patient with right hyperkinetic facial paralysis for serial Botox chemodenervation. (E to G) Follow-up evaluation of right hyperkinetic facial paralysis for serial dosing after first Botox chemodenervation. (A) Smile: Note the hyperkinetic levator labii superioris (LLS) causing upper lateral incisor show, hyperkinetic depressor anguli oris (DAO) causing oral commissure droop, hyperkinetic mentalis muscle causing chin dimpling. (B) Eyebrow raise: Note right paralyzed brow with left facial overcompensation. (C) Lip pucker: Note involuntary narrowing of the right palpebral aperature, failure of the right hyperkinetic mentalis to assist in elevation of the lower lip, left mentalis overcompensation. (D) DOSE TITRATION 1: Left frontalis/corrugator/procerus (15 u), Bilateral orbicularis oculi (6 u each), Right LLS (2 u), Bilateral mentalis (3 u each), Right DAO (3 u), Left risorius (3 u). (E) Smile: Note the hyperkinetic LLS continues to cause upper lateral incisor show, hyperkinetic DAO causing oral commissure droop has partially improved, hyperkinetic mentalis muscle causing chin dimpling has partially improved. (F) Eyebrow raise: Brow symmetry established without causing pseudoblepharoptosis. Relaxation of the right orbicularis oculi with slight lateral brow elevation and widening of the palpebral fissure. Partially improved symmetry with softening of the left risorius and left mentalis muscles. (G) DOSE TITRATION 2: Right LLS (3 u), Bilateral mentalis (3 u), Right DAO (3 u), Left risorius (3 u).

of patients may not find further lip weakening acceptable. A trial injection of approximately 2 mL of 2% lidocaine is commonly used to simulate the effects of contralateral weakening prior to chemodenervation.[82,100] Additional treatment is commonly performed to soften the appearance of the face and optimize symmetry. Caution must be taken when treating the lip elevators on the unparalyzed side for the high risk of speech disturbance that may ensue. Many patients rely on the overcompensation of the uninvolved side to purse their lips, articulate, and maintain oral competence. This is especially true in the central lip, where treatment of the normal labii superioris alaeque nasi and zygomaticus minor may greatly disturb lip compensation. Balancing treatment on the unparalyzed side should be initiated further laterally at 1 unit increments in the area of the zygomaticus major and 2–3 unit increments in the risorius where muscle weakness remains more forgiving.

Physical Therapy and Rehabilitation

The effectiveness of facial exercises and physical rehabilitation for the treatment of facial paralysis has been debated for decades. Objections to facial rehabilitation stem from historic electrical stimulation protocols and maximal effort facial exercises thought to be ineffective and perhaps even harmful, leading to increased facial synkinesis.[10,27]

Reports of modern day success highlight the importance of slower, small movement strategies, and mirror biofeedback to reinforce desired pathways and inhibit the undesirable movements of synkinesis and mass movement. Physical therapy for the optimization of facial movement and facial balance is important in patients with hypertonic paralysis, facial synkinesis, and other forms of incomplete facial paralysis. Most agree that the early stimulation of flaccid muscles in complete facial paralysis is ineffective and not advised.[27,101] Neuromuscular retraining should be deferred until the first sign of recovery is present to reduce the progression of aberrant movements and improve overall function.[3,27,101]

Patients with flaccid facial paralysis and asymmetry at rest should be advised to avoid overuse compensation of the uninvolved side. At the first sign of voluntary movement, EMG and/or mirror biofeedback is used to reinforce small desirable symmetric movements. Re-education strategies are practiced in front of a mirror to help avoid unwanted movement patterns. Patients who have hypertonic contractions are also concurrently treated with deep soft tissue mobilization and meditation-relaxation strategies.[27] Once a regimen is determined, home programs are monitored at regular intervals by a trained physical therapist to re-evaluate progression, impairments, and ongoing goals. Synkinesis and faulty nerve regeneration is a chronic sequelae of facial paralysis that remains responsive to cerebral adaptation through neuromuscular retraining, even decades after the injury.[101]

CONCLUSION

It is difficult to review the outcomes of facial reanimation procedures given the high variability of patient grading systems, low numbers, and inherent biases relating to patient and procedure selection. Controversies remain regarding the best options; however, most would agree no one technique has evolved into the gold standard. Patient and surgeon preferences remain important factors in determining the appropriate course of treatment. Many patients are not candidates for neural or neuromuscular reconstruction for a variety of reasons but may still benefit from static reanimation and other ancillary procedures that should not be overlooked. Treatment of the eye remains universal and corneal protection is paramount.

Trends in neural substitution continue to rely on cross-facial nerve grafting and masseter nerve substitution to provide donor input in a variety of clinical scenarios. Currently, the biggest limitation remains determining when it is safe to intervene early enough to prevent the problems associated with delays in return of function including nerve fibrosis, muscle atrophy, and increased risk of synkinesis.

When prolonged denervation time and axonal load is in question, adjunct or babysitter procedures involving the hypoglossal or masseter nerve are recommended for the prevention of muscle atrophy and improvement of function. The contralateral facial nerve will always be the theoretic first choice for donor nerve because of its ability to provide symmetric, spontaneous neural input. The contralateral facial nerve remains the nerve of choice to power free-muscle transfer in the pediatric population because of better regeneration outcomes seen in this population. In less than ideal scenarios, the axonal load may be insufficient with CFNG and the masseter nerve remains the next best choice. The masseter nerve is able to provide rapid reinnervation and stronger lateral commissure excursion when used to power native or freely transferred muscle. Masseter innervation exhibits close facial kinetics with facial innervation, and cortical adaptation has been shown to result in emotional smile activation after masseter nerve substitution and neuromuscular retraining. Modern day techniques have evolved to reanimate facial zones separately to prevent mass movement and minimize synkinesis. In this scenario, cross-facial nerve grafting and masseter nerve or modified hypoglossal nerve substitution may be used concurrently. The limitations of dynamic reanimation can be addressed by static and ancillary procedures to balance asymmetry and support orbital, nasal, and oral function. In all cases of reanimation, appropriate use of neuromuscular retraining in concert with selective chemodenervation has been shown to suppress undesirable movements, reinforce desired pathways, and significantly improve outcomes.

ACKNOWLEDGMENT

Special thanks to Angelique Petropouleas for her invaluable assistance in preparation of this manuscript.

REFERENCES

1. Terzis JK, Wang W, Zhao Y. Effect of axonal load on the functional and aesthetic outcomes of the cross-facial nerve graft procedure for facial reanimation. Plast Reconstr Surg. 2009;124:1499-512.
2. Terzis J, Konofaos P. Experience with 60 adult patients with facial paralysis secondary to tumor extirpation. Plast Reconstr Surg. 2012;130:51e-66e.
3. Hadlock T. Evaluation and management of the patient with post-operative facial paralysis. Arch Otolaryngol Head Neck Surg. 2012;138(5):505-8.
4. Guntinas-Lichius O, Streppel M, Stennert E. Postoperative functional evaluation of different reanimation techniques for facial nerve repair. Am J Surg. 2006;191:61-7.
5. Manktelow RT, Tomat LR, Zuker RM, et al. Smile reconstruction in adults with free muscle transfer innervated by the masseter motor nerve: effectiveness in cerebral adaptation. Plast Reconstr Surg. 2006;118:885-99.
6. Klebuc MJ. Facial reanimation using the masseter-to-facial nerve transfer. Plast Reconstr Surg. 2011;127:1909-15.
7. Bitter T, Sorger B, Hesselmann V, et al. Cortical representation sites of mimic movements after facial nerve reconstruction: a functional magnetic resonance imaging study. Laryngoscope. 2011;121:699-706.
8. Lifchez SD, Matloub HS, Gosain AK. Cortical adaptation to restoration of smiling after free muscle transfer innervated by the nerve to the masseter. Plast Reconstr Surg. 2005;115:1472-9; discussion 1480-2.
9. Sardesai MG, Moe KS. Recent progress in facial paralysis: advances and obstacles. Curr Opin Otolaryngol Head Neck Surg. 2010;18:266-71.
10. Henkelmann TC, May M. Physical therapy and neuromuscular rehabilitation. In: May M, Schaitkin BM (eds), The facial nerve, 2nd edn. Thieme New York: 2000; 301-318.
11. Veillon F, Taboada LR, Eid MA, et al. Pathology of the facial nerve. Neuroimag Clin N Am. 2008;18(2):309-20.
12. Dobie RA. Tests of facial nerve function. In: Cummings CW, et al. (eds), Cummings otolaryngology - head & neck surgery. Philadelphia, PA: Mosby; 2005:3321-32.
13. May M. Anatomy for the clinician. In: May M, Schaitkin BM (eds), The facial nerve, 2nd edn. New York: Thieme; 2000;19-56.
14. Freilinger G, Gruber H, Happak W, et al. Surgical anatomy of the mimic muscle system and the facial nerve: importance for reconstructive and aesthetic surgery. Plast Reconstr Surg. 1987;80(5):686-90.
15. Babakurban ST, Cakmak O, Kendir S, et al. Temporal branch of the facial nerve and its relationship to fascial layers. Arch Facial Plast Surg. 2010;12(1):16-23.
16. Terzis JK, Tzaffetta K. Outcomes of mini-hypoglossal nerve transfer and direct muscle neurotization for restoration of lower lip function in facial palsy. Plast Reconstr Surg. 2009; 124:1891-904.
17. Sunderland S. Nerve injuries and their repair. New York, NY: Churchill Livingstone; 1991:82-3.
18. Kumar A, Ryzenman J, Barr A. Revision facial nerve surgery. Otolaryngol Clin N Am. 2006;39:815-32.
19. Jain Y, Falcioni M, Agarwal M, et al. Total facial paralysis after vestibular schwannoma surgery: probability of regaining normal function. Ann Otol Rhinol Laryngol. 2004;113: 706-10.
20. Johns ME, Crumley RL. Facial nerve injury, repair and rehabilitation, 2nd edn, Alexandria, VA, AAOHNSF; 1984: 11-58.
21. Gacek R, Radpour S. Fiber orientation of the facial nerve: an experimental study in the cat. Laryngoscope. 1982;92: 547-56.
22. Danielides V, Skevas A, Van Cauwenberge. A comparison of electroneuronoraaphy with facial nerve testing for prognostic accuracy in patients with Bell's palsy. Eur Arch Otorhinolaryngol. 1996;253:35-8.
23. Pietersen E. Bell's palsy: the spontaneous course of 2,500 peripheral facial nerve palsies of different etiologies. Acta Otolaryngol. 2002; (Suppl 549):4-30.
24. Bianchi B, Ferri A, Sesenna E. Facial reanimation after nerve sacrifice in the treatment of head and neck cancer. Curr Opin Otolaryngol Head Neck Surg. 2012;20(2): 114-9.
25. Ozmen OA, Falcioni M, Lauda L, et al. Outcomes of facial nerve grafting in 155 cases: predictive value of history and preoperative function. Otol Neurotol. 2011;32:1341-6.
26. Ferreira MC. Crossfacial nerve grafting. Clin Plast Surg. 1984;11:211-4.
27. Diels H. Facial paralysis: is there a role for a therapist? Facial Plast Surg. 2000;16(4):361-4.
28. Bianchi B, Copelli C, Ferrari S, et al. Use of the masseter motor nerve in facial animation with free muscle transfer. Br J Oral Maxillofac Surg. 2012;50:650-3.
29. Momeni A, Chang J, Khosla R. Microsurgical reconstruction of the smile-contemporary trends. Microsurg. 2013;33: 69-76.
30. Myckatyn T, Mackinnon S. The surgical management of facial nerve injury. Clin Plastic Surg. 2003;30:307-18.

31. Bianchi B, Ferri A, Ferrari S, et al. Cross-facial nerve graft and masseteric nerve cooptation for one-stage facial reanimation: principles, indications, and surgical procedure. Head Neck. 2014;36(2):235-40.
32. Harii, Ohmori K, Torii S. Free gracilis muscle transplantation, with microneurovascular anastomoses for the treatment of facial paralysis. A preliminary report. Plast Reconstr Surg. 1976;57(2):133-43.
33. Hadlock T, Cheney M, McKenna M. Facial reanimation surgery. In: Nadol JB Jr., McKenna MJ (eds), Surgery of the ear and temporal bone, 2nd edn. Philadelphia: Lippincott Williams & Wilkins; 2005:457-67, Chapter 38.
34. Hontanilla B, Marre D, Cabello A. Facial reanimation with gracilis muscle transfer neurotized to cross-facial nerve graft versus masseteric nerve: a comparative study using the facial CLIMA evaluating system. Plast Reconstr Surg. 2013;131:1241-52.
35. Harii K, Asato H, Yoshimura K, et al. One-stage transfer of the latissimus dorsi muscle for reanimation of a paralyzed face: a new alternative. Plast Reconstr Surg. 1998;102: 941-51.
36. Hadlock T. Facial reanimation: an invited review and commentary. Arch Facial Plast Surg. 2008;10(6):413-7.
37. Rofagha S. Seiff SR. Long-term results for the use of gold eyelid load weights in the management of facial paralysis. Plast Reconstr Surg. 2010;125:142-9.
38. Silver A, Lindsay R, Cheney M, et al. Thin-profile platinum eyelid weighting: a superior option in the paralyzed eye. Plast Reconstr Surg. 2009;123:1697-703.
39. Berghaus A, Neumann K, Schrom T. The platinum chain: a new upper lid implant for facial palsy. Arch Facial Plast Surg. 2003:5:166-70.
40. Tate J, Tollefson T. Advances in facial reanimation. Curr Opin Otolaryngol Head Neck Surg. 2006;14:242-8.
41. Henstrom D, Malo J, Cheney M, et al. Surgical treatment of periocular complex and improvement of quality of life in patients with facial paralysis. Arch Facial Plast Surg. 2011; 13(2):125-8.
42. Martin-Oviedo C, Garcıa I, Lowy A, et al. Hyaluronic acid gel weight: a nonsurgical option for the management of paralytic lagophthalmos. Laryngoscope. 2013;123:E91-6.
43. Mancini R, Taban M, Lowinger A, et al. Use of hyaluronic acid gel in the management of paralytic lagophthalmos: the hyaluronic acid gel "Gold Weight." Ophthal Plast Reconstr Surg. 2009;25:23-6.
44. Robey A, Snyder M. Reconstruction of the paralyzed face. Ear Nose Throat J. 2011;90(6):267-75.
45. Alford EL. Tarsorrhaphy. In: Bailey BJ, Calhoun KH, Coffey AR, Neely JG (eds), Atlas of head & neck surgery - otolaryngology. Philadelphia, PA: Lippincott - Raven; 1996:372-3.
46. Dutton JJ. Lateral Tarsorrhaphy. In: Dutton JJ (ed), Atlas of oculoplastic and orbital surgery. Philadelphia, PA: Wolters Kluwer/Lippincott Williams & Wilkins Health; 2013;106-7.
47. Coker NJ. Facial nerve grafting. In: Bailey BJ, Calhoun KH, Coffey AR (eds), Atlas of head & neck surgery—otolaryngology. Philadelphia, PA: Lippincott—Raven; 1996:364-7.
48. Suri A, Mehta VS, Sarkar C. Microneural anastomosis with fibrin glue: an experimental study. Neurol India. 2002;50 (1):23-6.
49. Knox CJ, Hohman M, Kleiss I, et al. Facial nerve repair: fibrin adhesive coaptation versus epineurial suture repair in a rodent model. Laryngoscope. 2013;123:1618-21.
50. Bacciu A, Falconi M, Pasanisi E, et al. Intracranial facial nerve grafting after removal of vestibular schwannoma. Am J Otolaryngol. 2009;30:83-8.
51. Faris C. Lindsay R. Current thoughts and developments in facial nerve reanimation. Curr Opin Otolaryngol Head Neck Surg. 2013;21:346-52.
52. Divi V, Deschler DG. Reanimation and rehabilitation of the paralyzed face in head and neck cancer patients. Clin Anatomy. 2012;25:99-107.
53. Hanasono M, Silva A, Schoracki R, et al. Skull base reconstruction: an updated approach. Plast Reconstr Surg. 2011; 128:675-86.
54. Crumley RL, Armstrong WB, Byrne PJ. Rehabilitation of facial paralysis. In: Cummings CW, et al. (eds), Cummings otolaryngology—head & neck surgery. Philadelphia, PA: Mosby; 2005:822-52.
55. Best TJ, Mackinnon SE, Evans PJ, et al. Peripheral nerve revascularization: histomorphometric study of small and large caliber grafts. J Reconstr Microsurg. 1999:15(3): 183-90.
56. Hadlock T, Cheney M. Single-incision endoscopic sural nerve harvest for cross face nerve grafting. J Reconstr Microsurg. 2008;24(7):519-23.
57. Kumar S, Jacob J. Variability in the extent of sensory deficit after sural nerve biopsy. Neurol India. 2004;52(4):436-8.
58. Ozsoy U, Hizay A, Demirel B, et al. The hypoglossal-facial nerve repair as a method to improve recovery of motor function after facial nerve injury. Annals Anat. 2011; 193:304.
59. Meltzer N, Alam D. Facial paralysis rehabilitation: state of the art. Curr Opin Otolaryngol Head Neck Surg. 2010; 18:232-7.
60. Scaramella LF. The anastomosis between the two facial nerves. [Article in Italian] Arch Ital Otol Rinol Laringol Patol Cervicofacciale. 1971;82:209-15.
61. Terzis JK, Tzaffetta K. The "babysitter" procedure: mini-hypoglossal to facial nerve transfer and cross-facial nerve grafting. Plast Reconstr Surg. 2009;123:865-76.
62. Faria JC, Scopel GP, Ferreira MC. Facial reanimation with masseteric nerve: babysitter or permanent procedure? Preliminary results. Ann Plast Surg. 2010;64:31-4.
63. Hontanilla B, Gomez-Ruiz R. Masseter nerve as "babysitter" procedure in short-term facial paralysis. Eur J Plast Surg. 2010;33:227-9.
64. Bianchi B, Copelli C, Ferrari S, et al. Facial animation with free-muscle transfer innervated by the masseter motor nerve in unilateral facial paralysis. J Oral Maxillofac Surg. 2010;68:1524-9.
65. Shipchandler T, Seth R, Alam D. Split hypoglossal-facial nerve neurorrhaphy for treatment of the paralyzed face. Am J Otolaryngol Head Neck Med & Surg. 2011;32: 511-6.
66. Manni J, Beurskens C, Van de Velde C, et al. Reanimation of the paralyzed face by indirect hypoglossal -facial nerve anastomosis. Am J Surg. 2001;182:268-73.

67. Borschel GH, Kawamura DH, Kasukurthi R, et al. The motor nerve to the masseter muscle: An anatomic and histomorphometric study to facilitate its use in facial reanimation. J Plastic Reconstr Aesthetic Surg. 2012;65:363-6.
68. Lee E, Hurvitz K, Evans G, et al. Cross-facial nerve graft: past and present. J Plast Reconstr Aesthet Surg. 2008;61:250-6.
69. Anderl H. Reconstruction of the face through cross-face nerve transplantation in facial paralysis. Chir Plast. 1973;2: 17-46.
70. Terzis JK, Kalantarian B. Microsurgical strategies in 74 patients for restoration of dynamic depressor muscle mechanism: a neglected target in facial reanimation. Plasg Reconstr Surg. 2000;105:1917-34.
71. Tomita K. Hosokawa K. Yano K. Reanimation of reversible facial paralysis by the double innervation technique using an intraneural-dissected sural nerve graft. J Plast Recostr Aesthet Surg. 2010;63:e536-9.
72. Heineke H. Die direkte einpflanzung der nerven in den muskel. Zentrabl Chir. 1914;41:465-6.
73. Terzis JK, Karypidis D. Outcomes of direct muscle neurotization in pediatric patients with facial paralysis. Plast Reconstr Surg. 2009;124:1486-98.
74. Alex J, Toriumi DM. Permanent facial paralysis. In: Gates GA (ed). Current therapy in otolaryngology-head & neck surgery, 6th edn. St. Louis, MO: Mosby; 1998:125-9.
75. Terzis J, Olivares FS. Mini-temporalis transfer as an adjunct procedure for smile restoration. Plast Reconstr Surg. 2009; 123:533-42.
76. May M. Muscle transposition techniques: temporalis, masseter and digastric. In: May M, Schaitkin BM (eds), The facial nerve, 2nd edn. New York: Thieme; 2000:635-65.
77. Cheney ML, McKenna MJ, Megerian CA, et al. Early temporalis muscle transposition for the management of facial paralysis. Laryngoscope. 1995;105:993-1000.
78. McLaughlin CR. Surgical support in permanent facial paralysis. Plast Reconstr Surg. 1953;11:302-14.
79. Labbe D, Hault M. Lengthening temporalis myoplasty and lip reanimation. Plast Reconstr Surg. 2000;105:1289-97.
80. Boahene KD. Principles and biomechanics of muscle tendon unit transfer: application in temporalis muscle tendon transposition for smile improvement in facial paralysis. Laryngoscope. 2013;123:350-5.
81. Sidle D, Simon P. State of the art in the treatment of facial paralysis with temporalis tendon transfer. Curr Opin Otolaryngol Head Neck Surg. 2013;21(4):358-64.
82. Lindsay R, Edwards C, Smitson C, et al. A systematic algorithm for the management of lower lip asymmetry. Am J Otolaryngol. 2011;32(1):1-7.
83. Hadlock T, Malo J, Cheney M, et al. Free gracilis transfer for smile in children. Arch Facial Plast Surg. 2011;13(3):190-4.
84. Zuker RM, Goldberg CS, Manktelow RT. Facial animation in children with Möbius syndrome after segmental gracilis muscle transplant. Plast Reconstr Surg. 2000;106:1-8; discussion 9.
85. Sahin S, Yaman M, Mungan SR, et al. What happens in the other eye? Blink reflex alterations in contralateral side after facial palsy. J Clin Neurophysiol. 2009;26:454-7.
86. Hadlock T, Urban L. Toward a universal automated facial measurement tool in reanimation. Arch Facial Plastic Surg. 2012;14(4):277-82.
87. Navarrete-Alvaro M, Junyent J, Torrent L. Botulinum toxin and facial palsy. Our experience. Acta Otorrinolaringol Esp. 2010;61(4):277-81.
88. Terzis JK, Karypidis D. Therapeutic strategies in post-facial paralysis synkinesis in adult patients. Plast Reconstr Surg. 2012;129:925e-39e.
89. Booth, AJ, Murray A, Tyers AG. The direct brow lift: efficacy, complications and patient satisfaction. Br J Ohthalmol. 2004;88:688-91.
90. Costantino P, Hiltzik D, Moche J. Minimally invasive brow suspension for facial paralysis. Arch Facial Plast Surg. 2003; 5:171-4.
91. Dutton JJ. Direct brow elevation. In: Atlas of oculoplastic and orbital surgery. Philadelphia, PA: Wolters Kluwer/ Lippincott Williams & Wilkins Health; 2013:72-3.
92. Dutton JJ. Eyelid shortening by lateral tarsal strip fixation. In: Atlas of oculoplastic and orbital surgery. Philadelphia, PA: Wolters Kluwer/Lippincott Williams & Wilkins Health; 2013:108-9.
93. Patel M, Shapiro M, Spinelli H. Combined hard palate spacer graft, midface suspension, and lateral canthoplasty for lower eyelid retraction: a tripartite approach. Plast Reconstr Surg. 2005;115:2105-14.
94. Yu K, Kim AJ, Tadros M, et al. Mitek Anchor augmented static facial suspension. Arch Facial Plast Surg. 2010;12(3): 159-65.
95. Alam D. Rehabilitation of long standing facial nerve paralysis with percutaneous suture based-slings. Arch Facial Plast Surg. 2007;9:205-9.
96. Mehta R, Hadlock T. Botulinum toxin and quality of life in patients with facial paralysis. Arch Facial Plast Surg. 2008;10(2):84-7.
97. Ravenni R, De Grandis D, Mazza A. Conversion ratio between Dysport and Botox in clinical practice: an overview of available evidence. Neurol Sci. 2013;34(7):1043-8.
98. Patel BCK, Anderson RL, May M. Selective myectomy. In: May M, Schaitkin BM (eds), The facial nerve, 2nd edn. New York: Thieme; 2000:467-81.
99. Henstrom D, Malo J, Cheney M, et al. Platysmectomy: an effective intervention for facial synkinesis and hypertonicity. Arch Otolaryngol Head Neck Surg. 2011;13(4): 239-43.
100. Birgfield C, Neligan P. Surgical approaches to facial nerve deficits. Skull Base. 2011;21(3):177-84.
101. Lindsay R, Robinson M, Hadlock T. Comprehensive facial rehabilitation improves function in people with facial paralysis: a 5 year experience at the Massachusetts Eye and Ear Infirmary. Phys Ther. 2010;90(3):391-7.

Index

Note: Page numbers followed by *f* and *t* indicate figures and tables, respectively.

D

E

F

G

H

I

J

K

L

O

T

W

Y

Z